MEDICAL LIBRARY ASSOCIATION GUIDES

The Medical Library Association's Master Guide to Authoritative Information Resources in the Health Sciences

Laurie L. Thompson
Editor-in-Chief

Mori Lou Higa
Esther Carrigan
Rajia Tobia
Associate Editors

Neal-Schuman Publishers
New York London

Published by Neal-Schuman Publishers, Inc.
100 William St., Suite 2004
New York, NY 10038

Printed and bound in the United States of America.

The paper used in this publication meets the minimum requirements of American National Standard for Information Sciences-Permanence of Paper for Printed Library Materials, ANSI Z39.48-1992.

Library of Congress Cataloging-in-Publication Data

The Medical Library Association's master guide to authoritative information resources in the health sciences / Laurie L. Thompson, editor-in-chief ; Mori Lou Higa, Esther Carrigan, Rajia Tobia, associate editors.
p. ; cm. — (Medical Library Association guides)
Authoritative information resources in the health sciences
Includes bibliographical references and indexes.
ISBN 978-1-55570-719-4 (alk. paper)
1. Medicine—Information services. 2. Health—Information services. 3. Reference services (Libraries). I. Thompson, Laurie L. (Laurie Lynn), 1952- II. Higa, Mori Lou. III. Carrigan, Esther. IV. Tobia, Rajia. V. Medical Library Association. VI. Title: Authoritative information resources in the health sciences. VII. Series: Medical Library Association guides.
[DNLM: 1. Medicine—Abstracts. 2. Medicine—Resource Guides. 3. Information Services—Abstracts. 4. Information Services—Resource Guides. 5. Reference Books, Medical—Abstracts. 6. Reference Books, Medical—Resource Guides. ZWB 100]

R118.2.M38 2011
610.71'1—dc22

2011009288

Contents

Contributors

Heidi Sue Adams, MS, Kalispell Regional Medical Center, Kalispell, MT. Section 9.15.

Kristine M. Alpi, MLS, MPH, North Carolina State University, Raleigh, NC. Sections 2, 9.10.4, 10.7, 10.7.2, 13.4, 17.8.2, 26.1.

Rocco Altobelli, WEMT/CCT-Paramedic, Wilderness Medical Associates, Portland, ME; ALERT, Kalispell, MT. Section 9.15

Frank Ritchel Ames, MALS, PhD, Rocky Vista University, Parker, CO. Section 8.

Richard J. Barry, MSLS, American Nurses Association, Silver Spring, MD. Section 12.

Stephen P. Bartold, MD. Section 30.2.

Debra R. Berlanstein, MLS, University of Maryland, Baltimore, MD. Sections 10.17, 10.17.1, 10.17.2, 10.17.3, 26.8.

Barbara M. Bibel, MA, MLS, Oakland Public Library, Oakland, CA. Section 33.1.

Sharon Black, MLS, Annenberg School for Communication, University of Pennsylvania, Philadelphia, PA. Section 33.2.

Paul M. Blobaum, MA, MS, Governors State University, University Park, IL. Sections 10.14, 13.1, 13.2, 13.3, 13.6, 13.7, 13.7.1, 13.8, 13.9, 13.10, 13.13, 13.14, 13.15, 13.17 13.19.

C. Trenton Boyd, MA, University of Missouri, Columbia, MO. Sections 23, 23.1, 23.2, 23.3, 23.4, 23.5, 23.6, 23.7, 23.8, 23.9, 23.10, 23.11, 23.12, 23.13, 23.14, 23.15, 26.7.

Ellen C.B. Brassil, MS, Sacred Heart University, Fairfield, CT (currently: Baystate Medical Center, Springfield, MA). Section 1.2.

Marcy L. Brown, MLS, Silverchair Science + Communications, Delmont, PA. Section 29.

Kathy Broyles, MLS, University of North Texas Health Science Center, Fort Worth, TX. Section 9.9.

Holly Ann Burt, MLIS, NN/LM Greater Midwest Region, Chicago, IL. Section 6.1.1.

Amber Burtis, MLIS, Southern Illinois University Carbondale, IL. Section 33.

Sharon Cardwell, MLS, University of Texas Southwestern Medical Center, Dallas, TX. Section 10.10.2.

Esther Carrigan, MLS, Texas A&M University, College Station, TX. Sections 11.11, 23, 23.1, 23.2, 23.3, 23.4, 23.5, 23.6, 23.7, 23.8, 23.9, 23.10, 23.11, 23.12, 23.13, 23.14, 23.15, 26.7.

Jon Crossno, MSLS, University of Texas Southwestern Medical Center, Dallas, TX. Section 10.10.8.

Peggy Cruse, MLIS, Anschutz Medical Campus, University of Colorado Denver, CO. Section 24.6.

Diana Culbertson, MALS, American Hospital Association, Chicago, IL. Sections 6, 6.1, 7, 10.8.

Heather Cunningham, MSc, MLIS, University of Toronto, Canada. Section 26.

Paul Elliott Dahl, MA, MDiv, Minnesota Department of Health. Sections 9.11, 10.15, 10.15.1, 10.15.3, 10.16, 13.18.

Christina Daley, MLS, MHA, Lancaster General Health, Lancaster, PA. Section 21.

Jackie Davis, MLIS, Sharp HealthCare, San Diego, CA. Section 30.3.

Frances Delwiche, MLIS, University of Vermont, Burlington, VT. Section 1.5.

Heather Stone Edmonds, MLIS, New England College of Optometry, Boston, MA. Section 15.

Craig S. Elam, MLS, University of North Texas Health Science Center, Fort Worth, TX. Sections 1.3, 10.7.1, 24, 24.1, 24.2, 24.3, 24.4.

Helen-Ann Brown Epstein, MLS, MS, Weill Cornell Medical College, New York, NY. Sections 10.9, 10.10, 10.10.1.

Julia M. Esparza, MLS, Louisiana State University Health Sciences Center at Shreveport, LA. Section 9.5.

Jonquil D. Feldman, MALS, University of Texas Health Science Center, San Antonio, TX. Sections 34.4, 34.5.

Jayson Felty, MSIS, Southwest Foundation for Biomedical Research, San Antonio, TX. Sections 34.1, 34.2.

Suzanne Ferimer, MSLS, MEd, University of Houston, Houston, TX. Sections 11.5, 15, 16.

Elizabeth Fine, MLIS, University of Minnesota, Minneapolis, MN. Section 13.16.

Yunting Fu, MLS, University of Maryland, Baltimore, MD. Section 17.2.

John Fullinwider, MLS, University of Texas Southwestern Medical Center, Dallas, TX. Section 9.6.

Patricia E. Gallagher, MLS, MA, New York Academy of Medicine, New York, NY. Section 32.

Margie Garner, University of Oklahoma Health Sciences Center, Oklahoma City, OK. Section 31.

Jeannine Cyr Gluck, MLS, Eastern Connecticut Health Network, Manchester, CT. Sections 10.10.4, 10.10.6.

Brenda Faye Green, MLS, University of Tennessee Health Science Center, Memphis, TN. Section 9.13.

Stephen J. Greenberg, MSLS, PhD, National Library of Medicine, Bethesda, MD. Section 32.

Gale G. Hannigan, PhD, MLS, MPH, Texas A&M University, College Station, TX. Section 6.3.

Linda M. Hartman, MLS, University of Pittsburgh, Pittsburgh, PA. Section 9.12.

Tagalie Heister, MSLS, University of Kentucky, Lexington, KY. Sections 9.10, 9.10.1, 9.10.2, 9.10.3, 9.10.4, 9.10.5.

Margaret Henderson, MLIS, Virginia Commonwealth University, Richmond, VA. Sections 9.14, 11.8.

Marcia Henry, MA, MS, California State University, Northridge, CA. Section 13.5.

Marian A. Hicks, MSLS, Cleveland Chiropractic College, Los Angeles, CA. Section 3.

Mori Lou Higa, MLS, University of Texas Southwestern Medical Center, Dallas, TX. Sections 10.15, 11.7.

Chabha Hocine, MA, MLS, Logan College of Chiropractic, Chesterfield, MO. Section 3.

Stephanie Holmgren, MLS, MBA, National Institute of Environmental Health Services, Research Triangle Park, NC. Sections 5, 17.8.1., 17.8.3.

Lisa Huang, MLS, MS, Collin College, McKinney, TX. Section 1.7.

Mary A. Hyde, MSLS, American College of Obstetricians and Gynecologists, Washington, DC. Section 11.4.

Cotina M. Jones, North Carolina Central University, NC. Sections 24.5, 24.7.

Susan K. Kendall, PhD, MS(LIS), Michigan State University, East Lansing, MI. Sections 25, 25.1, 26.2, 26.4, 26.5, 26.5.1., 26.5.2., 26.6., 27, 27.1, 27.2, 28.

John Klima, MLIS, Palmer College of Chiropractic, Davenport, IA. Section 3.

Maureen (Molly) Knapp, MA, Louisiana State University Health Sciences Center, New Orleans, LA. Sections 1.1, 1.4.

Amy Knehans, MLIS, University of Hawai'i at Hilo, HI. Section 17.6.

Sharon Leslie, MSLS, Mercer University, Atlanta, GA. Sections 17, 17.1, 17.3, 17.4, 17.5, 17.7, 22.

Jie Li, MLS, University of South Alabama, Mobile, AL. Sections 11.9, 11.10, 11.11.

Alicia A. Livinski, MPH, MA, National Institutes of Health Library, Bethesda, MD. Section 10.4.

Cynthia B. Love, MLS, Disaster Information Management Research Center, Specialized Information Services Division, National Library of Medicine, Bethesda, MD. Section 10.4.

Irene M. Lubker, MLS, MPH, RD, Virginia Commonwealth University, Richmond, VA. Sections 9.7, 9.7.1.

Tim Mason, MLS, University of North Texas Health Science Center, Fort Worth, TX. Sections 10.11, 10.19, 11.3, 11.6.

Helen G. Mayo, MLS, University of Texas Southwestern Medical Center, Dallas, TX. Section 10.5.

Tracey Minzenmayer, MIS, PhD, University of Texas Southwestern Medical Center, Dallas, TX. Sections 9.4, 20, 26.3.

Cindy Mitchell, MLS, Ivy Tech Community College Library–Lafayette, IN. Section 10.10.5.

Nicole Mitchell, MLIS, MA, University of Alabama at Birmingham, Birmingham, AL. Section 15.

David A. Nolfi, MLS, Duquesne University, Pittsburgh, PA. Section 1.9.

Elizabeth Norton, MLS, MPH, MBA, Disaster Information Management Research Center, Specialized Information Services Division, National Library of Medicine, Bethesda, MD. Section 10.4.

Brian Oliver, MLIS, American Society for Clinical Pathology, Chicago, IL. Sections 10.12, 10.12.1, 10.12.2.

Adria P. Olmi, MS, JD, U.S. Army Aviation Technical Library, Ft. Rucker, AL. Section 9.8.

Gale A. Oren, MILS, University of Michigan, Ann Arbor, MI. Sections 11.5, 16.

Annette Osenga, MLS, Life Chiropractic College West, Hayward, CA. Section 3.

Erin Palazzolo, MLIS, Rocky Vista University, Parker, CO. Section 10.3.

Emily Patridge, MLS, University of Texas Southwestern Medical Center, Dallas, TX. Sections 10.10.3, 11.1.

Holly E. Phillips, MILS, MS, University of New Mexico, Albuquerque, NM. Section 26.9.

Michael E. Piorunski, Wilmer Eye Institute, Johns Hopkins University, Baltimore, MD. Sections 11.5, 16.

Jonathan Potter, Eastern Washington University, Cheney, WA. Section 1.8.

Katherine A. Prentice, University of Texas Health Science Center at San Antonio, TX. Sections 34.3, 34.6.

Mary Fran Prottsman, MLn, University of Southern California, Los Angeles, CA. Section 10.1.

Rebecca Raszewski, MS, University of Illinois at Chicago, IL. Section 13.20.

Diane C. Rein, PhD, MLS, University at Buffalo, NY. Sections 26.10, 27.2.

Joanne Rich, University of Washington, Seattle, WA. Section 30.1.

Jean E. Riedlinger, MSLS, American College of Obstetricians and Gynecologists, Washington, DC. Section 11.2.

Elisabeth Rowan, MSLS, Shriners Hospital for Children, Lexington, KY. Sections 11.6, 13.12.

Robin Sabo, MLS, MS, RD, Central Michigan University, Mt. Pleasant, MI. Sections 9.3, 14, 14.1, 14.2.

Julie H. Schiavo, MLIS, Louisiana State University Health Sciences Center, New Orleans, LA. Sections 4, 4.4.1, 4.4.2, 4.4.3, 4.6, 4.7.1, 4.7.2, 4.7.4.

Janet G. Schnall, MS, University of Washington, Seattle, WA. Sections 12.1, 12.2.

Claire Sharifi, MLIS, Life Chiropractic College West, Hayward, CA. Section 3.

Michael Sholinbeck, MLIS, University of California, Berkeley, CA. Section 10.15.2.

Jean L. Siebert, BS Pharmacy, MLS, West Virginia University, Morgantown, WV. Section 18.

Robert Sotak, MS, MSLIS, PhD, North Carolina State University, Raleigh, NC. Sections 2, 9.10.4, 10.7, 10.7.2, 13.4, 17.8, 17.8.2, 26.1.

Lorna Springston, MIS, Ball Memorial Hospital, Muncie, IN. Sections 10.2, 10.10.9.

David C. Stewart, MSLS, Wake Forest University School of Medicine, Winston-Salem, NC. Sections 9.2, 10.10.7, 11.12.

Elizabeth A. Strother, AMLS, Louisiana State University Health Sciences Center, New Orleans, LA. Sections 4, 4.1, 4.2, 4.3, 4.5, 4.7.1, 4.7.3, 4.7.5, 4.7.6, 4.8.

David Sweet, MLS, American Health Information Management Association, Chicago, IL. Section 6.2.

Sharon Tabachnick, MSLS, PhD, Southern College of Optometry, Memphis, TN. Section 15.

Mary K. Taylor, RN, MLIS, Southern Illinois University Carbondale, IL. Section 33.

Donna F. Timm, MLS, Louisiana State University Health Sciences Center at Shreveport, LA. Section 30.4.

Rajia Tobia, AMLS, University of Texas Health Science Center, San Antonio, TX. Section 19.

Pamela Van Hine, MSLS, American College of Obstetricians and Gynecologists, Washington, DC. Section 10.18.

Mark Vrabel, MLS, Oncology Nursing Society, Pittsburgh, PA. Section 13.11.

Carol E. Vreeland, DVM, MSLS, North Carolina State University, Raleigh, NC. Section 17.8.

Carol L. Watwood, MLS, MPH, Western Kentucky University, Bowling Green, KY. Sections 1, 1.6, 9.1.

Sheree West, MLIS, Kalispell Regional Medical Center, Kalispell, MT. Section 9.15.

Laura Wilder, MLS, University of Texas Southwestern Medical Center, Dallas, TX. Sections 10.6, 30.4.

Kathy Zeblisky, MLS, MBA, Phoenix Children's Hospital, Phoenix, AZ. Sections 10.13, 10.13.1, 10.13.2.

Marcia E. Zorn, MA, MLS, National Library of Medicine, Bethesda, MD. Section 33.2.

Preface

The Medical Library Association's Master Guide to Authoritative Information Resources in the Health Sciences identified and describes 2,011 authoritative titles in the health sciences literature, including the clinical specialties, subspecialties, basic sciences, and emerging disciplines. It covers both the monographic and journal literature in print and online formats and includes online databases and other electronic resources. It is not a comprehensive bibliography; rather, selectors were limited to a maximum of ten of the most important monographs and ten of the best serials in their discipline. Titles were selected based on their quality and importance to the health care profession. Physicians, residents, students, researchers, and health care professionals of all kinds will find the titles described here to be of the highest value to their work. Whether they are caring for patients, studying for Board certifications, learning a discipline, or conducting research, these titles will help them do it better.

This work is intended to offer an updated option to the iconic publication, "Brandon/Hill Selected List of Print Books and Journals for the Small Medical Library," which ceased publication in 2003 after 38 years and 20 editions. The "Selected List" was begun in 1965 by Alfred N. Brandon, who was joined by Dorothy R. Hill in 1979 (Brandon, 1965; Brandon and Hill, 1979). After Mr. Brandon's death in 1996, Ms. Hill continued the list, which was published biennially in the *Bulletin of the Medical Library Association*, followed by the *Journal of the Medical Library Association*, for three more editions. The final edition was published only in online format (Hill, 2003). Always intended to be a list of primarily clinical titles for hospital libraries, and never including digital or online publications, the Brandon/Hill list was nonetheless used as a selection tool in small and large libraries alike (Hill, 2003). This *Master Guide* has expanded the "Selected List" by including works in the basic sciences as well as the now-common digital and online publications. Any work (of the same or preceding title) included in the *Master Guide* that also appeared in the final edition of the "Brandon/Hill" medical list, and its sister lists for nursing and allied health, have been given a "Brandon/Hill" designation (Hill and Stickell, 2002; Hill and Stickell, 2003).

Organization of the *Master Guide*

The *Master Guide* is arranged loosely by the Health Occupations (G02) and the Biological Sciences (G01) tree schedules of the National Library of Medicine's Medical Subject Headings (MeSH) (U.S. Institutes of Health, National Library of Medicine, 2009). When available, a MeSH-derived definition for each topic is included; otherwise the definition came from *Stedman's Medical Dictionary*, 28th edition, or was supplied by the topic's contributor. Each section includes general works related to the discipline as well as more specialized topics such as anatomy, physiology, diseases, pathology, diagnosis, and therapy as appropriate.

Each entry contains full bibliographic information, URLs for online versions, and an annotation describing the scope and coverage of the work. The majority of the titles will be appropriate for an academic medical library. Titles also appropriate for a hospital or consumer health collection will be indicated. Because of the scope of this work, only a few titles of primary interest to consumers have been included.

Contributors worked individually or with collaborators on assigned topics. They were permitted to assign up to five subject headings to each resource. Each resource appears under its primary subject; "see" references are made from other subjects as assigned by the contributor. In many instances, contributors working on different subjects chose the same work to review. Each review is included under its primary subject with a "see also" reference to the other subject or subjects.

Contributors

The editors selected 108 contributors for their knowledge and expertise in their various specialties. The majority are librarians (MLS, MLIS, MSLS, etc.), many with additional professional qualifications; in the list of degrees are MD, PhD, JD, DVM, MPH, MBA, MEd, MDiv, BPharm, RN, and RD. Several librarians work for professional associations and societies, such as the American Hospital Association, the American Nurses Association, the American Health Information Management Association, the American Society for Clinical Pathology, the Oncology Nursing

Society, and the American College of Obstetricians and Gynecologists. There are librarians from academic medical centers and universities; community colleges; hospitals; specialty schools such as dentistry, veterinary, optometry, chiropractic, and osteopathic; research institutes; and the National Institutes of Health and the National Library of Medicine. There is even a flight paramedic.

Selection Criteria

The editors asked each contributor: "If you could have only 10 monographs and 10 journals on your topic in your library, what would they be?" Users who wonder why a particular title may not be included will realize that not all titles they are familiar with may have made the "top 10" cut; others may have been passed over in the review of the wealth of resources currently available. The selections and annotations are the opinions of the contributors; however, the final decisions for inclusion rest solely with the editors.

The contributors chose a variety of tools to assist with selection and evaluation. Not all contributors had access to the same tools; lack of a reference to a particular tool does not indicate lack of coverage in that tool. One of the tools that was consulted frequently was *Doody's Core Titles*, and its companion, *Doody's Review Service*; titles appearing in the 2010 edition of Doody's Core Titles (http://www.doody.com/dct) are indicated. The *Journal Citation Reports* (http://go.thomsonreuters.com/jcr) published by Thomson Reuters was also used frequently; all references to impact factors and rankings are from the 2009 edition. Also used were previous Brandon/Hill lists, the *Core Collection of Medical Books and Journals* (also called *The Hague List*, an international alternative to Brandon/Hill), the "Top 100 Journals in Biology and Medicine" selected by the SLA Biomedical & Life Sciences Division, the American Association of Colleges of Pharmacy's *Basic Resources for Pharmacy Education*, and other lists.

All titles listed should be currently available. Every attempt has been made to include only the most recent editions; however, new editions and works are being published even as this manuscript goes to press.

Entries

Bibliographic information was verified by the editors using online sources; print versions were not usually consulted during review and editing. When ISBNs and ISSNs are known to be for online versions, they are also included. Publishing companies merge and change often, so consistency with their names amongst all titles published over the years was impracticable. Indexing and abstracting services' names also appear in various forms for the same reason.

URLs are listed for online versions that are available for institutional licenses or are freely available at no charge. When practical, a full URL for the work is given; otherwise, the URL is shortened to the home page of the publisher or service that makes the work available. Every attempt was made to include all URLs; however, some may have been missed or are no longer available.

Some annotations mention mobile device compatibility, but because of the rapidly transforming market, this information was not routinely included. Just during the preparation of this manuscript, the terminology changed from "PDA" to "mobile device."

Sample Monograph Entry

Walsh and Hoyt's Clinical Neuro-Ophthalmology. 6th ed.
Editors: Neil R. Miller, Nancy J. Newman, Valerie Biousse, John B. Kerrison. Lippincott Williams & Wilkins, 2005.
http://www.ovid.com/
ISBN: 9780781748148
Recommended for: Hospital, Academic Libraries
Brandon/Hill, *Doody's Core Titles* Selection

This resource has been recognized as the most comprehensive neuro-ophthalmology text since the release of the first edition in 1947. First written by a single author, the book is now a product of multiple authors. It has been condensed from a five-volume to a three-volume set without a significant change in the quality of the material. It is a clinically focused text with each chapter covering a separate disorder from history to diagnosis through treatment. All three volumes are well illustrated in black and white and also well referenced, providing an encyclopedic approach to the study of neuro-ophthalmology, with deeper coverage than that of comparable neurology and neurosurgery texts. A *Doody's Core Titles* selection for many years, it is also available electronically through Ovid. This text is a required resource for all practicing neuro-ophthalmologists and ophthalmology teaching programs. Academic and hospital medical libraries that serve neurology or neurosurgery divisions, as well as optometry libraries should have access to this resource.

The title is followed by the edition, then all authors or editors are listed. Only 13-digit ISBNs are given. Both former Brandon/Hill titles and current *Doody's Core Titles* recommendations are noted.

Many publishers make online versions of their textbooks available to individual purchasers separately from institutional subscriptions; that information may be included in the review of the work. Examples include the Evolve service and STUDENT CONSULT from Elsevier, The Point service from Lippincott/ Williams & Wilkins, and MHProfessional from McGraw Hill.

Sample Journal Entry

Archives of Ophthalmology. v. 64, American Medical Association, 1960.
http://archopht.ama-assn.org/
ISSN: 15383601 (Online)
Indexed in MEDLINE
Recommended for: Hospital, Academic Libraries

One of the major multi-specialty journals in ophthalmology, this journal superseded (in part) the *Archives of Ophthalmology and Otology* in 1869. It began under its current title in 1960. This monthly journal is one of the ten AMA consortium journals. It focuses on scholarly works in ophthalmology, including clinical trials, clinical sciences, laboratory sciences, epidemiology, and socioeconomics and health services. In addition to peer-reviewed articles, the journal offers editorials, case reports, letters, CME, news, and a surgeon's corner. The content covers the major subspecialties in ophthalmology. The main audience for this journal includes ophthalmologists, vision researchers, residents and fellows, and medical students, but is also of interest to physicians in related specialties, or anyone doing research in the field of ophthalmology. This journal ranks fourth out of 49 ophthalmology journals (2009 *Journal Citation Reports*). This international journal is indexed in dozens of abstracting and indexing sources, including MEDLINE, Embase, Scopus, and BIOSIS Previews. It is a recommended resource for hospitals, academic institutions, and ophthalmology practices. Online coverage is available back to 1929 through the publisher.

Journal information includes the title and the first volume number and year for the specific title (not for earlier titles), along with the journal's URL and ISSN. Indexing for all journal titles was verified in MEDLINE and CINAHL (core titles in the basic collection only, not CINAHL Plus). A few titles are in PubMed but are not indexed in MEDLINE; since MEDLINE is available through several vendors besides PubMed, only MEDLINE indexing is specifically noted.

Using the *Master Guide* and Recommendations

The Medical Library Association's Master Guide to Authoritative Information Resources in the Health Sciences grew out of a suggestion made during a meeting of the MLA Books Panel. The Panel members felt that there needed to be a new resource that could be used for collection development purposes, much as the Brandon/Hill lists had been used. The *Master Guide* is expected to be used by librarians for just that purpose. The reviews are written by librarians who know the needs of their clientele. The *Master Guide* will be of particular value in identifying core titles for a new program, department, service, or school. Even long-standing collections may be lacking key resources in some areas that could be identified by using this *Master Guide.*

Each title has been recommended for hospital, academic, or consumer health libraries. Recommendations are not meant to be absolute; rather, they are suggestions as to the appropriate audience for the work. Not every hospital will want or need every title recommended for a hospital library, nor will every academic or consumer health library wish to collect all the titles recommended for them. Clarifications of the recommendations are often made in the review; for example, a monograph recommended for a hospital library may only be appropriate if the hospital has a strong program in that particular subject.

The companion online version of the *Master Guide* will be updated regularly with new edition information. It is expected that a new print version of the *Master Guide* will be published on a regular basis.

References

Brandon, Alfred N. 1965. "Select List of Books and Journals for the Small Medical Library." *Bulletin of the Medical Library Association* 53 (July): 329–364.

Brandon, Alfred N. and Dorothy R. Hill. 1979. "Select List of Books and Journals for the Small Medical Library." *Bulletin of the Medical Library Association* 67, no. 2 (April): 185–211.

Hill, Dorothy R. "Brandon/Hill Selected List of Print Books and Journals for the Small Medical Library." New York: Mount Sinai Medical Center, 2003. Available: http://library.mssm.edu/brandon-hill/small_medical/index.shtml.

Hill, Dorothy R., and Henry N. Stickell. 2002. "Selected List of Print Nursing Books and Journals." *Nursing Outlook* 50, no. 3 (May/June): 100–113.

Hill, Dorothy R., and Henry N. Stickell. 2003. "Selected List of Print Books and Journals in Allied Health." *Journal of the Medical Library Association* 91, no. 1 (January): 18–33.

U.S. National Institutes of Health, National Library of Medicine. 2009. Medical Subject Headings. Bethesda, MD. Available: http://www.nlm.nih.gov/mesh/.

Acknowledgments

Little did I realize that a discussion during a Medical Library Association Books Panel meeting would result in this *Master Guide*. An idea led to a formal description and before I knew it, I was volunteering to be the editor. The *Guide* is the culmination of the work of over a hundred volunteer contributors, each of whom created the parts that make up the whole. I am thankful to each of them for their dedication to providing this new resource.

Each entry for the *Master Guide* was submitted via an online database, which was designed and programmed by Farrah Omar, and later by Joseph Tan, from the University of Texas Southwestern Medical Center Library. Farrah and Joseph were very patient with my many requests and prompt with the changes and reports I needed.

I could not have completed the *Master Guide* without the extensive assistance provided by the associate editors, Esther Carrigan, Rajia Tobia, and especially Mori Lou Higa, who assumed more than her fair share of editing responsibilities. In addition to their editorial duties, each of the associate editors also contributed sections when there were no other volunteers. I also thank two of my colleagues at the UT Southwestern Medical Center Library, Jeff Perkins and Sharon Cardwell, for their work on the bibliographic verification.

To Charles Harmon, Kathryn Suarez, and Sandy Wood at Neal-Schuman Publishers, thank you for your faith that I would be able to complete this work.

And finally, I thank Dale and Emily for listening to my complaints, tolerating my long hours on the computer, and supporting me when I needed it most.

1. Allied Health

Services in the care of patients other than a physician or registered nurse; includes a variety of therapy technicians (e.g., pulmonary), radiology technicians, and physical therapists, among many other practitioners.

—*Stedman's Medical Dictionary*, 28th ed. (2006)

Contributor: Carol L. Watwood

Monographs

Atlas of Human Anatomy. 5th ed. Author: Frank H. Netter. Saunders/Elsevier, 2010.
ISBN: 9781416059516
See Also Chapter 24. Anatomy
Recommended for: Hospital, Academic, Consumer Health Libraries
Doody's Core Titles Selection

This posthumous edition of Netter's classic atlas revises and updates the most popular anatomy book in the English language. Frank Netter, who died in 1991, was a physician-turned-medical illustrator. Netter's clear, beautiful color illustrations are instantly recognizable and suitable for study by health students in all fields. The 540 pictures include some newer plates in the Netter style. A CD-ROM included with the *Atlas* allows downloading of images for use in lectures and presentations. An accompanying STUDENT CONSULT website, which includes examination review questions and other supplementary material, is available at http://netteranatomy.com for individuals who purchase the print textbook. This work is listed in *Resources for College Libraries*, and it is considered an essential purchase by *Doody's Core Titles*. The *Atlas of Human Anatomy* is highly recommended for large consumer collections and both hospital and academic libraries.

Clinically Oriented Anatomy. 6th ed. Authors: Keith L. Moore, Arthur F. Dalley, Anne M.R. Agur. Lippincott Williams & Wilkins, 2010.
ISBN: 9780781775250
See Also Chapter 24.4. Regional Anatomy
Recommended for: Hospital, Academic Libraries
Brandon/Hill, *Doody's Core Titles* Selection

Clinically Oriented Anatomy is a *Doody's Core Titles* essential purchase selection. This textbook/reference book offers students a practical, functional approach to anatomy as it relates to primary care, emergency care, surgery, and diagnostic imaging. "Blue boxes" throughout the text relate anatomic structures to clinical conditions. Boldface type, summary tables, and icons highlight and summarize key information. Supplemental online information offered through a companion website includes searchable full text, video podcasts, case studies, and multiple-choice questions for examination review. The book is recommended for college and hospital libraries serving health sciences students; it is especially appropriate for allied health students because of its pragmatic approach.

Diseases of the Human Body. 5th ed. Authors: Carol D. Tamparo, Marcia A. Lewis. F.A. Davis, 2011.
http://www.r2library.com/ (4th ed.)
ISBN: 9780803625051
Recommended for: Hospital, Academic Libraries
Brandon/Hill Selection

This perennial best seller appears in *Resources for College Libraries* and the 2003 Brandon/Hill allied health list; it also received five stars from *Doody's Review Service*. It supplies basic information on 350 diseases and conditions. Illustrations, case studies, and patient education information are included, along with new and emerging diseases and mental disorders. The diseases are grouped by topic, in a format designed for classroom study and review rather than ready reference. Case studies and review questions aid study; an answer key, glossary, appendixes, and an index follow the text. The authors also discuss complementary and integrative medicine. The book is recommended for hospital and academic libraries serving beginning health sciences students. This review refers to the fourth edition.

Diversified Health Occupations. 7th ed. Authors: Louise Simmers, Karen Simmers-Nartker, Sharon Simmers-Kobelak. Delmar Cengage Learning, 2009.
ISBN: 9781418030216
Recommended for: Hospital, Academic Libraries
Brandon/Hill Selection

With a textbook-style layout, *Diversified Health Occupations* is designed for classroom teaching. The page design is colorful and visually appealing; key terms and concepts are highlighted. The clear color photographs and diagrams are up-to-date and of good quality. The first part of the book covers basic health care concepts and skills: history of health care, trends, health care systems (U.S. oriented), professionalism, legal and ethical responsibilities, and other topics relating to health and health promotion. The authors present basic information on searching and evaluating health information online. The second part covers special health care skills and tasks commonly performed by allied health professionals, such as patient transfer, perioperative care, and laboratory testing. A large amount of information is conveyed in this text: for example, the U.S. Health Insurance Portability and Accountability Act (HIPAA), blood pressure measure and guidelines, infection control, the food pyramid, and much more. The well-organized information contains a detailed table of contents and a glossary; its thorough index aids in quick retrieval of information. A CD-ROM with quizzes, animations, games, and supplementary activities is included with the printed textbook. A workbook, companion website, and other teaching aids are also available. This book is highly recommended for undergraduate, community college, or hospital libraries serving allied health students. It is a 2003 Brandon/Hill allied health first-purchase selection; it is also included in the 2009 *Resources for College Libraries.*

Drug Information Handbook: A Comprehensive Resource for All Clinicians and Healthcare Professionals. 18th ed. Editor: Charles F. Lacy. Lexi-Comp/American Pharmacists Association, 2009.
ISBN: 9781591952541
Recommended for: Hospital, Academic, Consumer Health Libraries

Drug information is essential for a good health reference collection, given that an estimated 12.6 prescriptions per person (excluding over the counter and herbal products) were filled in the United States in 2007 (Kaiser Family Foundation, 2008). Understanding actions and interactions among these many products is vital for all members of the health care team. The *Drug Information Handbook* contains more than 1,400 drug monographs covering over 5,000 medications. Entries give generic and proprietary names, use in pregnancy/lactation, contraindications and warnings, adverse effects ranked by frequency of occurrence, interactions, stability and storage, dosage and dosage forms, mechanism of action, pharmacokinetics/dynamics, and other patient information. Written with practitioners in mind, the *Handbook* is recommended for hospital and college libraries. It would also benefit large consumer health collections.

Encyclopedia of Careers and Vocational Guidance. 15th ed. Ferguson/Facts on File, 2011.
http://ferguson.infobasepublishing.com/
http://www.ebrary.com/
ISBN: 9780816083138
ISBN: 9781438135465 (Online)
Recommended for: Academic, Consumer Health Libraries

The wide variety of allied health careers often brings students and the public to the library to research career opportunities. In addition, some programs in the health sciences turn away applicants who may investigate other health careers. Furthermore, a common classroom assignment for entry-level students is to research a career. *Encyclopedia of Careers and Vocational Guidance*, aptly described by *Resources for College Libraries (RCL)* as "similar to an expanded version of *Occupational Outlook Handbook*," is one of the best general sources for investigating career choices. It contains health careers excluded from the *Occupational Outlook Handbook* and offers detailed information about nearly 100 industries and more than 700 careers. The history of each career is given, along with sidebars containing additional facts and information such as terminology and interesting statistics. Addresses and websites for key organizations and other sources of information about the career are supplied. Detailed articles include background information, structure of the career, and further resources. The book also provides information on job skills, job hunting, and resume writing. Black-and-white photographs, indexes, and useful appendixes are included. Ferguson is an imprint of Facts on File and publishes *Exploring Health Care Careers*, which contains different material and targets the high-school audience. The *Encyclopedia* is also available online as part of Ferguson's Career Guidance Center. This work is recommended for undergraduate, community college, and public libraries. This review refers to the fourteenth edition.

Gale Encyclopedia of Medicine. 3rd ed. Editor: Jacqueline L. Longe. Gale Cengage, 2006.
http://www.gale.cengage.com/gvrl/
ISBN: 9781414403687
ISBN: 9781414404851 (Online)
See Also Chapter 33.1. Consumer Health Information
Recommended for: Hospital, Academic, Consumer Health Libraries
Doody's Core Titles Selection

Attractively produced and illustrated, this readable, five-volume consumer health encyclopedia—with 1,750 signed, alphabetically arranged articles—is also appropriate for allied health and other undergraduate students.

Health professionals or medical writers compose articles, which are reviewed for accuracy. Disease/disorder and test/treatment articles are written in standardized sections so that readers can quickly locate information. Coverage of diseases and disorders includes causes, diagnosis, treatment, prognosis, and prevention; entries on tests and treatments cover purpose, precautions, aftercare, risks, and results. Key terms are listed and defined, and selected references are provided. Articles may be printed, e-mailed, downloaded, translated into eleven languages, or put on an MP3 player. *The Gale Encyclopedia of Medicine* is one of a number of useful health-related encyclopedias; these products are also available online through the Gale Virtual Reference Library (GVRL). Libraries can create a custom e-book collection of Gale reference books and use the GVRL to search them as a group by keyword, subject heading, or advanced search screen. The GVRL may also be cross searched with Health Reference Center Academic using Gale PowerSearch. *The Gale Encyclopedia of Medicine*, but not all the Gale health encyclopedias, is included in the Gale Health & Wellness Resource Center. This set is highly recommended for consumer health collections and hospital, undergraduate, and public libraries.

Gale Encyclopedia of Nursing & Allied Health. 2nd ed. Editor: Jacqueline L. Longe. Gale Cengage, 2006.
http://www.gale.cengage.com/gvrl/
ISBN: 9781414403748
ISBN: 9781414410449 (Online)
Recommended for: Hospital, Academic, Consumer Health Libraries

The 2002 edition of this unique, five-volume work was "highly recommended" and selected as an "outstanding title" by *Choice* in 2002, which further noted Gale's "solid reputation for publishing comprehensive encyclopedias." The second edition received five stars from *Doody's* (2007), which described it as a "worthy investment for college and hospital libraries." The 930 signed entries, many authored by allied health professionals, are written in a standardized format useful to undergraduate allied health students completing classroom assignments. Entries include diseases, tests, equipment, biology, current health issues, and nursing and allied health professions. Each entry begins with a definition, highlights key terms that may be unfamiliar to readers, and ends with a bibliography of print and online resources. According to the book's introduction, it intends to "fill a gap between health information designed for laypeople and that provided for medical professionals, which may be too complicated for the beginning student to understand." The familiar encyclopedia format serves as a helpful introduction to college-level course work. Attractively produced with good-quality color illustrations, this set is similar to Gale's other useful health encyclopedias such as those on medicine, diets, and complementary medicine. The multivolume work is available online, collectively or à la carte, as part of the Gale Virtual Reference Library. The publication's main disadvantage is its relatively high cost; libraries with limited budgets might substitute the less expensive (or free) *Merck Manuals*, *Taber's*, the *Encyclopedia of Careers and Vocational Guidance*, the various free NIH websites, and the *Occupational Outlook Handbook*. This publication is recommended for college and undergraduate libraries; it would also benefit hospital libraries serving undergraduate students.

Health Care Careers Directory 2009–2010. 37th ed. American Medical Association, 2009.
ISBN: 9781603591041
Recommended for: Hospital, Academic Libraries
Brandon/Hill Selection

This useful, annual publication provides information on 8,200 different programs preparing health sciences students for 81 different careers. A perennial favorite under several previous titles, as the *Health Professions Education Directory* it was an initial purchase selection in the 2003 Brandon/Hill allied health list. Comparison charts allow students to compare different programs within each profession. Data comparison tables allow prospective students to compare different occupations. The history, duties, job outlook, educational program descriptions, and licensure requirements are given for each field. This work is highly recommended for academic and other libraries serving students interested in allied health or other undergraduate health sciences programs.

Introduction to the Health Professions. 5th ed. Authors: Peggy S. Stanfield, Y.H. Hui, Nanna Cross. Jones & Bartlett, 2009.
ISBN: 9780763758233
Recommended for: Academic, Consumer Health Libraries
Brandon/Hill Selection

Peggy Stanfield's best-selling *Introduction to the Health Professions*, listed in the 2009 edition of *Resources for College Libraries*, provides a good overview of health occupations for beginning college students. The first part supplies an introduction to the U.S. health care system, payment for care, and health career planning. The second part discusses professions involving patient care, and part three reviews other health-related professions. Salaries, other sources of information, resumes, and job searching are also addressed. The authors cover duties, job opportunities, and training requirements for more than 75 careers. Stanfield's book, unlike the more encyclopedic works that are recommended, is suitable for a classroom text or for cover-to-cover reading. The book is recommended for undergraduate and public libraries.

Magill's Medical Guide. 4th ed. Editor: Anne Chang. Salem Health, 2008.
http://health.salempress.com/
ISBN: 9781587653841
Recommended for: Hospital, Academic, Consumer Health Libraries

This five-volume set, widely held by libraries, has more than 1,000 signed, alphabetically arranged entries in a format designed for ready reference and report writing. According to the publisher, the *Guide* covers "diseases, disorders, treatments, procedures, specialties, anatomy, biology, and issues in an A–Z format, with sidebars addressing recent developments in medicine and concise information boxes for all diseases and disorders." Articles are substantial, up-to-date, and well written. Although the set is less eye-catching and less costly than its major competitor, the *Gale Encyclopedia of Medicine*, it serves as a useful, quality reference work. *Magill's Medical Guide* is highly recommended for medical, public, and general academic libraries.

Medical Terminology: A Short Course. 5th ed. Author: Davi-Ellen Chabner. Saunders Elsevier, 2009.
ISBN: 9781416055181
Recommended for: Hospital, Academic, Consumer Health Libraries

Learning medical language is essential in all health fields. In the well-published field of medical terminology, Davi-Ellen Chabner's *Medical Terminology: A Short Course* was designed to "fill a niche in the education of allied health professionals." The book has a proven track record of successful use by students with no background in life sciences or medicine. This best seller received a four-star review from *Doody's Review Service*. Simple, clearly-labeled color photos and diagrams highlight the text; two accompanying CD-ROMs include interactive activities and animations. Chabner includes case studies and vignettes illustrating the terminology. The text/workbook format emphasizes the body as a whole. Helpful appendixes include lab tests, a glossary, word parts glossary, health careers, answer key, radiologic terms, Spanish/ English terms, and an index. Individuals can purchase this work as a combined textbook/e-book package. Although useful in many library settings, this book, like most similar titles, is better suited for individual purchase. It is recommended for undergraduate and community college libraries.

Mosby's Dictionary of Medicine, Nursing & Health Professions. 8th ed. Mosby Elsevier, 2009.
http://corp.credoreference.com/
ISBN: 9780323049375
ISBN: 9780323065665
See Also Chapter 33.1. Consumer Health Information
Recommended for: Hospital, Academic, Consumer Health Libraries
Brandon/Hill Selection

Mosby's clearly written nursing and health professions dictionary is a 2003 Brandon/Hill nursing list selection and an allied health first-purchase selection. Its easy-to-read type and thumb tabs facilitate use. This dictionary's most striking feature is its liberal use of color photographs and line drawings to add visual interest. Drugs are described in detail, and appendixes include the following useful items: units of measurement, American Sign Language medical translations, normal reference values, health promotion, nutrition, pharmacology and clinical calculations, infection control, diagnosis-related groups, and nursing data. Individuals can purchase the print textbook plus accompanying CD-ROM, which includes a medical spell-checker. Access to the supplementary Evolve website—with audible pronunciations, vocabulary and anatomy learning activities, a Spanish glossary, and other materials—is included with the print purchase for single users or educators. Individuals can also obtain as a combined print text and e-book package. The full text is available for handheld devices. Readers might also consider the competing *Stedman's Medical Dictionary of the Health Professions and Nursing*, which includes an anatomy insert and more extensive nursing appendixes. The book is recommended for hospital or academic libraries.

Structure & Function of the Body. 13th ed. Authors: Gary A. Thibodeau, Kevin T. Patton. Mosby Elsevier, 2008.
ISBN: 9780323049917
Recommended for: Hospital, Academic, Consumer Health Libraries
Brandon/Hill, *Doody's Core Titles* Selection

This best-selling textbook, selected for *Resources for College Libraries* (*RCL*) and the 2003 Brandon/Hill allied health list, provides a basic introduction to normal human anatomy and physiology. Dr. Gary Thibodeau is chancellor emeritus and professor emeritus of biology at the University of Wisconsin, River Falls; Dr. Kevin Patton is a longtime professor of life science at the two-year St. Charles Community College and an adjunct faculty member at the Saint Louis University Medical School. *RCL* describes this book as "simple and straightforward." It begins by describing introductory concepts in chemistry, cells and tissues, and organ systems; the following chapters describe the skin and membranes, skeleton, and other body systems in detail. Text boxes highlight current-interest topics, history of science, and other useful information. A semi-transparent, multi-page insert displays human anatomy in detail. The publisher also provides a separate study guide and accompanying online course. Chapter tests are included, with answer key. A companion CD-ROM contains animations and interactive activities. *Structure & Function of the Body* is recommended for undergraduate and community college libraries, for large consumer health collections, and for hospital libraries serving undergraduate health sciences students.

Taber's Cyclopedic Medical Dictionary. 21st ed. Editor: Donald Venes. F.A. Davis, 2009.
http://www.fadavis.com/
http://www.tabers.com
http://www.statref.com/
ISBN: 9780803615595
ISBN: 9780803623255 (Online)
ISBN: 9780803615601 (Online)
Recommended for: Hospital, Academic, Consumer Health Libraries
Brandon/Hill Selection

Taber's was listed in *Resources for College Libraries* (2009) and was an initial purchase in the 2003 Brandon/Hill allied health list. As the quaint title suggests (cyclopedic means "encyclopedic"), *Taber's* has a long history; the first *Taber's Medical Dictionary for Nurses* was published in 1905. Some definitions are indeed cyclopedic or quite lengthy and detailed. *Taber's* is widely used by medical students; the clear definitions make it a good choice for allied health professionals as well. Thumb tabs make it easy to use, but *Taber's* small size makes it hard to lay flat. *Taber's* contains many useful lists and tables, such as dietary guidelines and cancer statistics, and many appendixes, such as units of measurement, nutrition, integrative therapies, and nursing information. A very large amount of information is concentrated into this small, rather plain green volume. An accompanying DVD has interactive activities. The online version is available from the publisher or as part of several different online libraries; it may also be used on mobile devices. *Taber's* is appropriate for all types of hospital, academic, and medical libraries.

Journals

Journal of Allied Health. v. 1, Association of Schools of Allied Health Professions, 1972.
http://www.asahp.org/journal_ah.htm
http://www.ingentaconnect.com/content/asahp/jah
ISSN: 00907421 (Print/Online)
Indexed in: MEDLINE, CINAHL
Recommended for: Hospital, Academic Libraries
Brandon/Hill Selection

The *Journal of Allied Health* is the only major interdisciplinary allied health periodical currently being published. It is indexed in CINAHL, MEDLINE, ProQuest, and Scopus; the full text is available in ProQuest. It was an initial purchase title in the 2003 Brandon/Hill allied health list. This peer-reviewed journal is published quarterly. The target audience is "allied health leaders, educators, faculty and students." Types of articles published include "scholarly works related to research and development, feature articles, research abstracts and book reviews." The journal covers diverse allied health topics; many articles deal with allied health teaching and education. Electronic access is available through IngentaConnect; selected content is free of charge. The journal is recommended for larger collections in colleges, universities, hospitals, or other health organizations serving allied health students or professionals.

Databases and Other Electronic Resources

CINAHL Plus with Full Text. EBSCO, 1981 (some references back to 1937)
http://www.ebscohost.com/
See Also Chapter 12.1. Nursing Research, Chapter 34.2. Indexing and Database Resources
Recommended for: Hospital, Academic, Consumer Health Libraries
Brandon/Hill Selection

Originally published in print as *Cumulative Index to Nursing & Allied Health Literature*, CINAHL Plus with Full Text is the best known and the most comprehensive research database for nursing and allied health. Containing over 2 million records from more than 4,100 journals (750 of which are full-text), as well as 240 full-text monographs, it is listed in *Essential Nursing Resources* (ICIRN, 2009) as one of the three core nursing and health care databases. According to the publisher, CINAHL offers, "complete coverage of English-language nursing journals and publications from the National League for Nursing and the American Nurses' Association." The database includes "nursing, biomedicine, health sciences librarianship, alternative/complementary medicine, consumer health and 17 allied health disciplines. In addition, this database offers access to health care books, nursing dissertations, selected conference proceedings, standards of practice, educational software, audiovisuals and book chapters. Searchable cited references for more than 1,250 journals are also included." Successor to the "Red Books" used by students since the 1950s, CINAHL still has traces of its print origins and a slightly clunky feel. A more serious problem (shared by CINAHL's competitors) is the lack of full text for many important journals; EBSCOhost e-journal links to external vendors are awkward and trouble-prone. Despite these concerns, CINAHL is irreplaceable for scholarly research in nursing and allied health. A hallmark of this database is its thorough, high quality indexing with terms commonly used in the nursing and allied health fields; PubMed and Google Scholar, in particular, lack this advantage. CINAHL is essential for libraries supporting nursing and allied health programs or research by practicing nursing and allied health professionals. It is also useful for consumer health, although many consumers find this database difficult to use. Lastly, non-health sciences students needing understandable health information will benefit from this resource.

Consumer Health Complete. EBSCO, 2006.
http://www.ebscohost.com/
Recommended for: Hospital, Academic, Consumer Health Libraries

EBSCO's continuously updated Consumer Health Complete contains useful, easy-to-read health information for consumers and beginning health sciences students. It fills a niche for general health reference questions and undergraduate assignments not requiring scholarly sources. According to information supplied by EBSCO, it includes searchable full text for more than 200 reference books, Lexi-Comp's *Lexi-PALS* consumer drug information sheets, more than 800 videos, consumer health pamphlets, news, a medical image library, consumer-level evidence-based reports, magazine and journal articles, and animations. The attractive, user-friendly home page includes point-and-click options, a search box, and a medical dictionary. The advanced search screen offers more search options and a publications list. The lists of search results are similar to others offered on the standard EBSCOhost platform; however, the colorful home page of Consumer Health Complete organizes and displays the diverse sources to better advantage than its plainer, less inclusive, and less costly cousin, Health Source: Consumer Edition. Although alternative interfaces are available, the latter product uses the standard EBSCOhost platform and does not include the videos, image library, or some of the other content found in Consumer Health Complete. The less expensive Health Source: Consumer Edition or the freely available MedlinePlus may be a wiser choice for libraries with limited budgets or little demand for easy-to-read materials. Other databases should supplement both Consumer Health Complete and Health Source: Consumer Edition; they are not complete resources for scholarly research. A related EBSCOhost product, Health Source: Nursing/ Academic Edition, includes added scholarly journals; this content overlaps considerably with other EBSCOhost bibliographic databases and may be redundant if an institution subscribes to Academic Search Premier or similar products. Consumer Health Complete is recommended for undergraduate, community college, and public libraries.

Health Reference Center Academic. Gale Cengage, 199?
http://www.gale.cengage.com/
Recommended for: Hospital, Academic, Consumer Health Libraries

This multi-source online database from Gale Cengage includes the personal health information sources from Health Reference Center, plus 40 full-text nursing and allied health journals. According to the publisher, this database "integrates the full text and images of respected nursing, allied health and medical journals; consumer health magazines; newsletters; pamphlets; newspaper articles; topical overviews; and reference books." Videos and broadcast transcripts are also included. A clean, easy-to-use search screen allows users to browse subject headings or publications, enter search terms, and view search history. Many references have a high school reading level, and the attractive, colorful screen layout is familiar to users of general informational websites. This resource, with coverage from 1980 to present, conveniently includes basic, core concepts in medicine, nursing, and allied health. It does not have detailed coverage of allied health journals or specialized reference books, and it is best used in conjunction with CINAHL and other more comprehensive resources. Despite the word "academic" in the title, it is equally appropriate for general consumer health queries. This user-friendly product fills a niche for academically at-risk or preclinical health sciences students, large public libraries, and consortia. It has a high price tag; libraries with limited budgets may prefer free resources such as MedlinePlus. Potential purchasers should check the content overlap with Gale's Health & Wellness Resource Center and other health-specific and general-purpose commercial products; the material in this database may be redundant. Health Reference Center Academic is recommended for hospital, academic, or public libraries; it is not appropriate for advanced or specialized research.

Lexi-Comp ONLINE. Lexi-Comp, 1978.
http://www.lexi.com/
Recommended for: Hospital, Academic Libraries

Lexi-Comp is a leading commercial producer of point-of-care drug information. Its editorial board includes physicians, pharmacists, and other health professionals. The clean, well-designed home page links to key U.S. government drug-related websites, including NLM, and the American Society of Health-System Pharmacists (ASHP). It also has a customized web browser, drug alerts/interactions, drug ID, and a dosage calculator. The search box has a pull-down menu of searchable fields. Drug monographs include generic name with audio link for pronunciation, U.S. and international trade names, drug classes, uses (unlabeled uses are listed separately), clinically significant adverse effects, adult and pediatric patient counseling, warnings, interactions, detailed dosage information, pricing, selected readings, and other related patient care information. An optional add-in is the AHFS encyclopedic drug database sponsored by the American Society of Health-System Pharmacists. Radio buttons display additional search options, such as printable *Lexi-PALS* patient care sheets in English or Spanish. The continuously updated Lexi-Comp ONLINE encompasses a suite of products customizable for various academic and clinical settings and for use on handheld devices. For example, Lexi-Comp ONLINE for Dentistry includes dosage calculations for dental drugs, information on dental office emergencies, and access to the entire database of drug monographs so that dental professionals, including dental hygienists, may be advised of bleeding complications and other adverse effects pertinent to dental treatment. Physician assistants, dental hygienists, and other allied health professionals or students who prescribe drugs, counsel patients, or otherwise need rapid access to drug information might use Lexi-Comp ONLINE. It is recommended for hospital or academic settings where point-of-care drug information is needed; a careful needs assessment is advised before purchase.

Merck Manuals Online Medical Library (Various titles).
Merck Research Laboratories, 200?
http://www.merck.com/pubs/
Brandon/Hill Selection
Recommended for: Hospital, Academic, Consumer Health Libraries

The seven *Merck Manuals*, published under various titles since 1899, are also available in print but are more frequently updated online. The manuals are published on a not-for-profit basis as a public service. Some manuals—notably the *Home Edition*—are designed for lay readers; others, such as the *Manual of Diagnosis and Therapy*, are targeted to physicians. This authoritative, free collection of online medical reference manuals is an outstanding compilation of high-quality, comprehensive medical information. Four of the manuals are especially suited for allied health students: the *Home Edition*, *Health & Aging* (available in print or podcast formats only), *Patient Symptoms*, and *Geriatrics*. The *Manual of Diagnosis and Therapy*, a former Brandon/Hill title, is designed for physicians but might be used by allied health professionals or educated laypeople. The *Manual of Geriatrics*, published in 2000, is unfortunately becoming dated except for the revised online sections. The simple search interfaces for the online *Merck Manuals*, which vary among the different titles, permit searching by keyword, topic, or subject heading. Users of the *Home Edition* can click a link to hear the pronunciations of difficult words. Specialized functions—such as translations, podcasting, RSS feeds, iPhone applications, and e-mail newsletters—are available for some of the Merck content. Libraries should consider purchasing print copies of the frequently used *Merck Manual—Home Edition* and the *Merck Manual of Diagnosis and Therapy* due to their greater browsability and ease of use. The thorough index in the back of the print works enables readers to locate information quickly. The series is highly recommended for public, academic, and hospital libraries.

Occupational Outlook Handbook. U.S. Dept of Labor, Bureau of Labor Statistics, Published biennially.
http://www.bls.gov/OCO/
ISBN: 10767681
Recommended for: Hospital, Academic, Consumer Health Libraries

Freely available at the Bureau of Labor Statistics' website, this biennial publication is the single, best overall source of information for researching U.S. career choices. For each job category, it describes the nature of the work, training, other qualifications, advancement, employment, job outlook, projections data, national and state statistics and typical earnings, related occupations, and sources of additional information (including web addresses of national professional organizations). Additional links on this website, such as "Tomorrow's jobs," help allied health students choose and succeed in rewarding, well-paying careers. One drawback is that specialized careers are often grouped with more general ones; for example, there is no separate entry for "medical librarian" or "child life specialist." A paperback version of *Occupational Outlook Handbook* is available, but the website is so easy to use that the print edition is unnecessary where computer access is available. This work is recommended for any library where there is a need for career information.

PubMed. National Center for Biotechnology Information, 1996.
http://www.ncbi.nlm.nih.gov/pubmed/
See Also Chapter 30.4. Evidence-Based Practice, Chapter 32. History of the Health Sciences, Chapter 34.2. Indexing and Database Resources
Recommended for: Hospital, Academic, Consumer Health Libraries
Brandon/Hill Selection

PubMed is a core resource for researching the scholarly literature of allied health, though relatively few of the 5,500 journals indexed are devoted primarily to allied health. Free to the public since 1996, PubMed is a gold mine of allied health information partly due to its sheer size; 19 million records have been published from 1948 to the present. The streamlined PubMed search screen is easy to use without special training, although the use of the MeSH allied health terms and limiters ensures better results. The following search example returns 135 hits, with 11 open access articles and 17 review articles from cancer, radiology, radiologic technology, rural health, public health, and other journals: "Technology, Radiologic" [Majr:NoExpl] AND United States [MeSH Terms] AND 2004:2009 [Publication Date] with Limits: English. Google Scholar, which does not search PubMed directly, picks up many PubMed references and pushes key references to the top of the results list, as well as identifying additional sources of free full text. This renowned database is recommended for all types of libraries with a health mission.

1.1. Audiology

Hearing and hearing impairment.
—MeSH

Contributor: Maureen (Molly) Knapp

Monographs

Anatomy & Physiology for Speech, Language, and Hearing. 4th ed. Authors: Anthony J. Seikel, Douglas W. King, David G. Drumright. Delmar Cengage Learning, 2010.
ISBN: 9781428312234
Recommended for: Academic Libraries
Doody's Core Titles Selection

Designed for upper division undergraduate or graduate students in speech-language pathology and audiology, this text offers a "sequential tour" of the anatomy and physiology associated with speech, language, and hearing. Twelve chapters are organized around the four systems of speech: respiratory, phonatory, articulatory/resonatory, and nervous systems. Eight appendixes, a glossary, and an index round out the contents. A CD-ROM containing a series of software labs that offer further examination and illustration of the structures and functions of speech mechanisms is included with the text. Self-paced quizzes, flash cards, games, animations, and a medical terminology audio library are included. The CD-ROM is cross-referenced in the text to enable quick reference. It should be noted that a user review on Amazon.com noted that the CD-ROM included in the fourth edition may not work on Mac computers. The format of this textbook is quite conducive to learning anatomy and physiology. Over 100 photographs and 300 illustrations, graphs, and charts, many in full color, provide visual examples of anatomy, processes, and body systems. Margin notes identify important terminology and definitions in each chapter. Clinical notes, muscle tables, and bulleted summaries appear throughout the book to reinforce learning and relate topics directly to clinical experience. In addition, study questions and answers are included at the end of each chapter as well as references to primary and secondary sources. The appendixes at the end of the book include anatomical terms; muscles of respiration; muscles of phonation; muscles of face, soft palate and pharynx; sensors; cranial nerves; and pathologies that affect speech production. The third edition of this book was listed as a *Doody's* core title and received a three star review (85 out of 100 possible points) from *Doody's Review Service*. The most current edition has been updated to include full color throughout the text and also includes an entire chapter on swallowing physiology.

Fundamentals of Hearing: An Introduction. 5th ed. Author: William A. Yost. Elsevier/Academic, 2006.
ISBN: 9780123704733
Recommended for: Hospital, Academic Libraries
Doody's Core Titles Selection

First published in 1977 and now in its fifth edition, this classic text of audiology provides a basic understanding of normal auditory processes in order to better understand auditory diseases and disorders. The book contains

16 chapters, six appendixes, a subject index, a glossary, and references. Multimedia resources including a supplemental website and PowerPoint presentations accompany the text. The book is divided into four sections: "The Auditory Stimulus: Sound," "Peripheral Auditory Anatomy and Physiology," "Auditory Sensation," and "Auditory Perception, the Central Nervous System, and Auditory Disorders." Each chapter includes a summary and a supplement section with further readings on the topic. Appendixes include: terms, measurements, equations and conversions, anatomical and physiological measurements, a combined glossary/subject index which both defines audiological terms and refers to them in-text, references to books and journal articles, and both American National (ANSI) and International (ISO) standards useful in hearing and acoustics. While this book provides a comprehensive overview of hearing fundamentals, it does not include in-depth coverage of genetic and cellular molecular bases of auditory processing, since "such coverage would require a background in biology and chemistry that is beyond that assumed for this level," as noted in the preface.

Handbook of Clinical Audiology. 6th ed. Editor: Jack Katz. Lippincott Williams & Wilkins, 2009.
ISBN: 9780781781060
Recommended for: Hospital, Academic Libraries
Brandon/Hill, *Doody's Core Titles* Selection

First published in 1972 and now in its sixth edition, this classic text of audiology provides a broad, authoritative account of the scope of practice in audiology. Commonly referred to as "The Katz Book," it serves as both a textbook for audiology students and a reference for clinical audiologists. Its 43 chapters are divided into four broad sections. Section 1 gives an introduction to clinical audiology then covers basic audiologic tests and procedures such as the calibration of puretone, speech and noise signals, assessing bone conduction thresholds, speech audiometry, clinical masking, and case histories. Section 2 contains 15 chapters devoted to physiological principles and measures, and comprises the largest portion of the text. Chapters covering clinical topics include case studies to illustrate how physiologic tests apply to audiology. Section 3 covers special populations, including hearing loss assessment in children, educational audiology, central auditory processing disorders, noise exposure and issues in hearing conversation, individuals with multiple disabilities, and hearing loss in the elderly. Section 4 discusses the management of hearing disorders, including room acoustics and auditory rehabilitation technology; hearing aids, including troubleshooting and fitting in adults and children; cochlear implants; audiology practice management; the management of adults and children with hearing impairment; and counseling patients undergoing hearing loss. Each chapter includes tables, flowcharts, and photographs, as well as references. Author and subject indexes conclude the book. Previous editions of Katz's book have been included on the Brandon/Hill list, while the sixth edition received a three-star rating (score of 83 out of 100) from *Doody's Review Service.*

Pediatric Audiology: Diagnosis, Technology and Management. Editors: Jane R. Madell, Carol Flexer. Thieme, 2008.
ISBN: 9781604060010
Recommended for: Hospital, Academic Libraries
Doody's Core Titles Selection

As described in the editor's preface, "this is a practical, how-to book about the diagnosis and technological and educational management of infants and children with hearing disorders." Designed as both a textbook for audiology students and a reference for practicing audiologists, the book covers all aspects of diagnosis, technology, and management of pediatric audiology, and includes a DVD with demonstrations of audiometry testing techniques and cochlear implant surgery. The 32 chapters of the book are organized into five major sections: "Hearing Loss," "Diagnosing Hearing Disorders in Infants and Children," "Hearing Access Technology for Infants and Children," "Educational Management of Hearing Loss," and "Disorders Requiring Special Consideration." Each chapter is authored by an expert in the field. The chapters are designed so that each opens with a list of topics to be addressed as well as key points to remember. Pearls, pitfalls, and special considerations are also scattered throughout the chapters, emphasizing important points. Tables, diagrams, and flowcharts are also included, while discussion questions and references can be found at the end of each chapter. Three chapters in the book are authored specifically on behavioral tests, organized by age group, which coincide with the topics in the DVD. Evaluating hearing loss in children with special needs has its own chapter, as does working with multicultural and multilingual families of young children with hearing loss, and educational and access laws for children with hearing loss. An appendix includes policy statements and position papers, citations to education laws, and a directory of websites. This book received an Excellent rating from *Doody's Core Titles* and is listed as an essential purchase, receiving a five-star review (97 out of a possible 100 points).

Journals

American Journal of Audiology. v. 1, American Speech-Language-Hearing Association, 1991.
http://aja.asha.org/
ISSN: 10590889
ISSN: 15589137 (Online)
Indexed in: MEDLINE, CINAHL
Recommended for: Hospital, Academic Libraries

This peer reviewed journal of clinical practice for audiologists and hearing researchers is published by the American Speech-Language-Hearing Association (ASHA), which is the credentialing association for over 135,000 members and affiliates who are audiologists, speech-language pathologists, and speech, language, and hearing scientists. AJA's subject matter pertains to all aspects of clinical practice in audiology, including: screening, assessment, and treatment techniques; prevention; professional issues; supervision; and administration. Contents include clinical forums, clinical reviews, letters to the editor, or research reports that emphasize clinical practice. The journal is indexed by numerous indexing and abstracting sources including CINAHL, Embase, MEDLINE, PsycINFO, and Scopus. Audiologists are the journal's main audience, though speech-language pathologists and hearing scientists will find it useful as well. Beginning January 2010, all ASHA journals became online-only. Online access from volume 1, 1991 is available from the publisher.

Journal of Speech, Language, and Hearing Research: JSLHR. v. 40, American Speech-Language-Hearing Association, 1997.
See Chapter 1.4. Speech-Language Pathology

Journal of the American Academy of Audiology. v. 1, American Academy of Audiology, 1990.
http://www.audiology.org/resources/journal/Pages/default.aspx
http://www.ingentaconnect.com/content/aaa/jaaa
ISSN: 10500545
Indexed in: MEDLINE, CINAHL
Recommended for: Hospital, Academic Libraries

The *Journal of the American Academy of Audiology*, or "*J-Triple-A*" as audiology students are inclined to call it, is the American Academy of Audiology's scholarly, peer-reviewed publication, issued 10 times per year. According to its website, the American Academy of Audiology is an over-10,000 member professional organization "of, by, and for audiologists," and *JAAA* is their professional journal. *JAAA* publishes articles and clinical reports in all areas of audiology, including audiological assessment, amplification, aural habilitation and rehabilitation, auditory electrophysiology, vestibular assessment, and hearing science. Publication types include: editorials, letters to the editor, original research, and continuing education units. This journal is indexed in numerous abstracting and indexing sources including CINAHL, Embase, Linguistics and Language Behavior Abstracts (LLBA), MEDLINE, PsycINFO, Science Citation Index, Scopus and Web of Science. In 2009, *JAAA* had an impact factor of 0.879 and ranked 24 out of 36 journals in the category of otorhinolaryngology. Audiologists and audiology students are the primary audience of this journal, although ear, nose, and throat specialists may also find relevant information here. It is available in both print and online formats, with online access back to 2002 available from Ingenta.

Language, Speech, and Hearing Services in Schools: LSHSS. v. 2, American Speech-Language-Hearing Association, 1971.
See Chapter 1.4. Speech-Language Pathology

1.2. Occupational Therapy

The field concerned with utilizing craft or work activities in the rehabilitation of patients. Occupational therapy can also refer to the activities themselves.

—MeSH

Contributor: Ellen C.B. Brassil

Monographs

Conditions in Occupational Therapy: Effect on Occupational Performance. 3rd ed. Editors: Ben J. Atchison, Diane K. Dirette. Lippincott Williams & Wilkins, 2007.
ISBN: 9780781754873
Recommended for: Hospital, Academic Libraries
Brandon/Hill, *Doody's Core Titles* Selection

This is an important teaching tool that offers students a framework for learning about the common disorders and conditions seen by occupational therapists, with coverage of each condition explored in depth, from etiology to prognosis. Conditions and the effect of disease on daily activities come to life through the use of case studies that can help students apply concepts to real life situations. Every chapter in this edition was significantly revised and uses language included in the *Occupational Therapy Practice Framework*. The third edition includes the authors' interpretations of the effects of occupational performance on impairment. A new chapter discusses anxiety disorders and cardiopulmonary disease. Expanded use of drawings, graphs and other visuals, and inclusion of chapter outlines, study questions, and suggested readings help to clarify concepts. An online version is available for individual purchasers. The earlier edition of the book was included in the Brandon/Hill allied health list and this edition is included in *Doody's Core Titles*.

***Cook and Hussey's Assistive Technologies: Principles and Practice*.** 3rd ed. Authors: Albert M. Cook, Susan M. Hussey. Mosby, 2007.
ISBN: 9780323039079
Recommended for: Hospital, Academic, Consumer Health Libraries
Doody's Core Titles Selection

Occupational therapists must be familiar with both the concepts and specific devices presented in this almost encyclopedic work, which provides an updated compendium of the issues and context related to both traditional and innovative aids for every activity of daily living. The book is both a teaching tool as well as a manual for the veteran occupational therapist, who will find the latest information to be technically precise and easily understood. The authors' own Human Activity Assistive Technology model is the basis of the book's focus. The chapters are grouped according to broad categories covering background information and concepts, services, activities, regulations, and more. In addition to updated content, the book includes multimedia components such as a CD-ROM demonstrating the use of specific devices. Other features include evidence-based content, chapter outlines, learning objectives, and high quality illustrations, graphs, and photographs for concrete references. Also useful are updated bibliographic references and a comprehensive glossary.

***Documenting Occupational Therapy Practice*.** 2nd ed. Author: Karen M. Sames. Prentice Hall, 2009.
ISBN: 9780131999480
Recommended for: Hospital, Academic Libraries

Documentation is critical for occupational therapists, who can turn to the new edition of this book for the best approaches. The author covers an otherwise dry subject matter so that it becomes alive and engaging, yet filled with substance. A broad perspective assures inclusion of such wide-ranging topics as plagiarism, grant-writing, evaluation reports, and even school consent forms as they relate to occupational therapy. In addition to chapter revisions, the new edition adds to the extensive appendix. Included are sample reproducible forms, a spelling and grammar review, practice standards, and answers to exercises that reinforce the principles outlined. Readers will find the technical, ethical and legal aspects of language addressed. Examples illustrate important concepts in the context of clinical, administrative, and school documentation. Steps are aligned with the new Occupational Therapy Practice Framework principles. Different forms of documentation are covered, including SOAP notes, which are required for reimbursement under Medicare and managed care. The book models exemplary note-taking for both students and practitioners wanting to improve and perfect their documentation skills.

***Functional Performance in Older Adults*.** 3rd ed. Editors: Bette R. Bonder, Vanina Dal Bello-Has. F.A. Davis, 2009.
ISBN: 9780803616882
Recommended for: Hospital, Academic Libraries
Brandon/Hill Selection

An underlying premise of this book is that rehabilitation professionals can best support the elderly they work with by better understanding the aging process. The book is divided into five main parts, starting with a theoretical perspective that includes both biological and psychosocial theories of aging, all the way to the final chapter about special issues such as the impact of emerging technologies on functional performance for older adults. Unexpected but relevant topics include the occupational therapy implications of elder abuse and loss. An international group of distinguished contributors who hail from a variety of health related fields that deal significantly with the elderly provide an interdisciplinary perspective. Practical information on concepts such as fall prevention, dementia, self-care, and palliative care are examples of the specific topics covered. The book has many useful features such as chapter review questions, a comprehensive glossary, and lengthy chapter references. This resource balances the practical with theory related to the rehabilitation process and is essential for any health care professional working with the elderly. The book's 2001 edition was included in the National Board for Certification in Occupational Therapy book rankings.

***Occupational Therapy and Physical Dysfunction*.** 6th ed. Editors: Michael Curtin, Matthew Molineux, Jo-Anne Supyk. Churchill Livingstone, 2010.
ISBN: 9780080450841
Recommended for: Hospital, Academic Libraries

The sheer scope of this work earns it top billing for occupational therapy students as well as researchers and practitioners, who will no doubt appreciate the easy translation of theory into practice. The book offers a new approach to essential skills based not on common physical impairments alone but on theories of occupation that can be adapted to any clinical situation throughout the life span. While preserving valuable content from the well-regarded earlier editions of this book, the voluminous and overhauled sixth edition is praiseworthy for capturing global changes within the occupational therapy profession both in the United States and abroad. The 39 chapters are grouped into five general sections, written by internationally recognized professionals. Key references to the literature enrich this comprehensive book, which also provides clinical scenarios for simulated practice and discussion.

Occupational Therapy for Children. 6th ed. Editors: Jane Case-Smith, Jane Clifford O'Brien. Mosby/Elsevier, 2010.
ISBN: 9780323056588
Recommended for: Hospital, Academic Libraries
Brandon/Hill, *Doody's Core Titles* Selection

Presenting both theoretical and practical considerations involved when working with an entire age group, this resource presents a multitude of issues in pediatric occupational therapy. The earlier content is now expanded with a strong emphasis on evidence-based practice as well as a chapter devoted to working with adolescents. Coverage includes foundational knowledge, occupational assessment of children and child occupations, performance limitations, and interventions. The book's life-span perspective and also the recognition of cultural competence as it influences occupational therapy strategies are both praiseworthy. While the book is aimed at students, it is complete enough and sufficiently detailed to serve as an ongoing reference for veteran therapists. Video clips on Mosby's Evolve Resources companion website reinforce important concepts and rehabilitation techniques.

The Occupational Therapy Manager. 4th ed. Editors: Guy L. McCormack, Evelyn G. Jaffe, Marcia Goodman-Lavey. American Occupational Therapy Association, 2003.
ISBN: 9781569001783
Recommended for: Hospital, Academic Libraries

This comprehensive handbook is the perfect resource for the practicing occupational therapist, who must be familiar with an increasingly complex health care environment. Organized along the lines of AOTA's *Occupational Therapy Practice Framework: Domain and Process*, this book needs to be on the bookshelves of all occupational practitioners, whether they are managers or part-time staff members. The information provided can be adapted to the needs of many health care workers, including entry-level staff, but is especially geared to occupational therapist leaders and supervisors. Historical background gives way to an exhaustive treatment of the health care delivery system as it applies to occupational therapy. Topics covered include performance appraisal, standards, regulations, and more. Several new chapters were added to this edition, including universal health care systems and also cultural competency. There are few resources as steeped in practical managerial and regulatory information, along with tables and other primary data that make this resource an invaluable reference tool. Pages of acronyms, charts, tables, and an exhaustive index ensure both ease of use and frequent use by practicing occupational therapists for any one of a number of high stakes information needs in the workplace setting.

Quick Reference to Occupational Therapy. 2nd ed. Author: Kathlyn L. Reed. Aspen, 2001.
ISBN: 9780834216310
Recommended for: Hospital, Academic Libraries

This manual provides students, practitioners, and researchers with fast access to succinct but complete evidence-based information on dozens of diseases and disabilities commonly encountered by practicing occupational therapists. The book would also be an invaluable reference tool for many rehabilitation professionals. Among the author's many impressive credentials is a master's degree in library and information science, which explains the precise and almost aesthetic order throughout. The book uses a standard format for ease of use that covers eleven broad types of disorders or body system and divides those general units further into dozens of specific entities, including sensorimotor, cognitive, and self-care. For each entry there is a description and lengthy discussion of cause, assessment, problems, treatment/intervention, and prognosis. Each section is backed by extensive lists of references and a bibliography, all thoroughly updated since the earlier edition, and several new diagnoses have been added, including autism, sensory modulation disorders, back pain, vestibular disorders, fibromyalgia, HIV in children, lymphedema, and many more. This is an essential tool for occupational therapists in all stages of their career, regardless of their work setting, and one that should be updated on a regular basis.

The Reference Manual of the Official Documents of the American Occupational Therapy Association, Inc. 14th ed. American Occupational Therapy Association, 2009.
ISBN: 9781569002827
Recommended for: Hospital, Academic Libraries

The fourteenth edition of this important manual is an indispensible compilation of official documents of the American Occupational Therapy Association. The book is essential to occupational therapy practitioners, all of whom must adhere to sound theory and standards of practice. Main components include "Ethics Standards" and the second edition of *Occupational Therapy Practice Framework: Domain and Process*, which gives an overview of the profession and is an invaluable, patient-centered decision-making tool. The annual print publication contains a wealth of assorted documents, and includes a searchable CD-ROM of concept papers. Documents also address supervisory practices, technology skills, standards and practice guidelines, position papers, and more. New content includes such documents as AOTA's "Societal Statement on Autism Spectrum Disorders," "Occupational Therapy Scholarship," "Occupational Therapy's Commitment to Nondiscrimination and Inclusion," "Guidelines in Supervision," and much more. The book should be available for frequent reference in every rehabilitation hospital library, whether for administration or supervisory concerns, role delineation, or practice documentation, and it should be accessible to occupational therapy students and educators for quick access to AOTA documentation and principles.

The Texture of Life: Purposeful Activities in the Context of Occupation. 3rd ed. Editors: Jim Hinojosa, Marie-Louise Blount. AOTA Press, 2009.
ISBN: 9781569002841
Recommended for: Hospital, Academic Libraries

This book bridges the gap between theory and practice in occupational therapy and elucidates key principles through real life scenarios. A variety of contributors have written a series of eloquent chapters that guide students and practitioners through the best interventions for many common conditions. The book explores multiple ranges of human occupation, viewed as a means of clinical intervention and therapy. The chapters lead the reader through the process of sound clinical reasoning applicable to almost any scenario. Activities and case studies are analyzed and linked to important concepts that are illustrated by photos, exercises, charts, and figures. The book examines every facet of major occupations, such as self-care. The chapter bibliographies are augmented by a comprehensive table of major research studies.

Vision, Perception, and Cognition: A Manual for the Evaluation and Treatment of the Adult with Acquired Brain Injury. 4th ed. Author: Barbara Zoltan. Slack, 2007.
ISBN: 9781556427381
Recommended for: Hospital, Academic Libraries

This book stands out among many similar works covering physical dysfunction and rehabilitation pertaining to traumatic brain injuries. Occupational therapists frequently help individuals with acquired brain injuries to overcome the many long-term effects of such impairment, and employ intervention strategies to support affected activities of daily living. This essential book was ranked highly in the last survey of occupational therapy textbooks, prepared by the National Board for Certification in Occupational Therapy, Inc. Aside from its comprehensive treatment of a critical subject area, the book offers a holistic approach to the process of evaluation through intervention. In addition to chapter revisions, new content includes visual vestibular processing, dynamic assessment, and neural plasticity, and would be applicable to occupational therapists working in isolation or on staff with a large rehabilitation hospital as part of an inpatient organization's staff. Useful features include a lengthy glossary, detailed index, figures, tables, and updated references to the literature following each chapter. Since many of the concepts are relevant to other physical conditions and disorders, this is an essential book for occupational therapy professionals as well as any student or practitioner in a care environment.

Willard & Spackman's Occupational Therapy. 11th ed. Editors: Elizabeth B. Crepeau, Ellen S. Cohn, Barbara A.B. Schell, Helen S. Willard. Wolters Kluwer Health/ Lippincott, Williams & Wilkins, 2009.
ISBN: 9780781760041
Recommended for: Hospital, Academic Libraries
Brandon/Hill, *Doody's Core Titles* Selection

Occupational therapists regard this text as second to none for its sheer comprehensiveness and authority, with contributions from dozens of prominent educators, researchers, and practitioners. The voluminous work also draws upon the expertise of ancillary disciplines such as assistive technology and rehabilitation science. The chapter units unfold in sequence, from background concepts to concrete and complex practice issues. All subjects are delineated in the context of evidence-based practice. The book's central focus is on the individuals receiving rehabilitation services, with many powerful, first-person narratives. The eleventh edition continues to expand beyond the overhauled ninth edition, with every chapter completely revised. A new unit covers social and health policy. The book explores every aspect of treatment and evaluation, including the psychometric properties of assessment instruments. New enhancements include the latest terminology of the International Classification of Function and the draft versions of the second edition of the *Occupational Therapy Practice Framework*. The text is enriched with PowerPoint presentations, supplemental readings and exercises, a companion website, and Internet resources, available for individual purchasers. The book is a long-standing Brandon/Hill allied health recommendation and a *Doody's Core Titles* essential purchase.

Journals

American Journal of Occupational Therapy. v. 1, American Occupational Therapy Association, 1947.
http://www.aota.org/Pubs/AJOT_1.aspx
ISSN: 02729490
ISSN: 19437676 (Online)
Indexed in: MEDLINE, CINAHL
Recommended for: Hospital, Academic Libraries
Brandon/Hill Selection

The official, peer-reviewed journal of the American Occupational Therapy Association is among the Association's major publications and is a staple item for any large health care institution or long-term care facilities. The journal is published six times a year and members of the Association have online access to archived abstracts and full-text articles. Non-members may view abstracts online and purchase full-text article as of November, 2009. The journal focuses on all research, practice, and health care issues in the field of occupational therapy. The journal is cited in most indexing and abstracting sources including MEDLINE, CINAHL, OT Search, and OTDBase. The primary audience is practicing occupational therapists, educators, and researchers. Content includes feature and research articles, case reports, and educational and professional announcements.

British Journal of Occupational Therapy. v. 37, no. 6, The College of Occupational Therapists Limited, 1974.
http://www.cot.co.uk/
ISSN: 03080226
ISSN: 14776006 (Online)
Indexed in: CINAHL
Recommended for: Academic Libraries
Brandon/Hill Selection

British Journal of Occupational Therapy is the official journal of London's College of Occupational Therapists. The journal publishes papers relevant to theory, practice, research, education, and management in occupational therapy. Among the group of international peer-reviewed research journals covering occupational therapy, this is the only one that is issued monthly. It is aimed at practicing occupational therapists, faculty, and students and is also available online with free full text available to members of the British Association of Occupational Therapists and to all members of the Canadian Association of Occupational Therapists through reciprocal arrangement. The journal includes book reviews, announcements of meetings, and continuing education opportunities in the United Kingdom. The journal content may be searched using Embase, PsycINFO, OTDBase, OT Search, and CINAHL. An annual online index allows for free browsing by titles, arranged according to several broad subject categories.

Canadian Journal of Occupational Therapy: Revue Canadienne D'Ergothérapie. v. 6, no. 2, Canadian Association of Occupational Therapists, 1939.
http://www.ingentaconnect.com/content/caot/cjot
ISSN: 00084174
Indexed in: MEDLINE, CINAHL
Recommended for: Hospital, Academic Libraries

The official publication of the Canadian Association of Occupational Therapy since 1933, the aim of this peer-reviewed journal is to advance occupational therapy research and the theoretical foundations of occupational therapy. The journal is published five times per year going back to 1997. The journal actively promotes occupational therapy research and status of the profession with the hope of influencing education and practice. Included are original research articles as well as brief reports. The journal also features occasional book reviews and letters to the editors. The final issue each year includes an annual index. Articles are published in the language submitted, with an abstract in both French and English. Content may be searched using several databases, such as MEDLINE, Embase, OTDBase, OT Search, PsycINFO, and others.

Journal of Hand Therapy. v. 1, American Society of Hand Therapists, 1987.
http://www.jhandtherapy.org/
ISSN: 08941130
ISSN: 1545004X (Online)
Indexed in: MEDLINE, CINAHL
Recommended for: Hospital, Academic Libraries
Brandon/Hill Selection

Journal of Hand Therapy is the official publication of the American Society of Hand Therapists and is designed for hand specialists, including occupational therapists and others involved in rehabilitation of disabling hand problems. Contributors to the journal include primarily occupational therapists, but also physicians, physical therapists, and other hand specialists. The publication is issued quarterly, and includes peer-reviewed articles for both researchers and practitioners. The journal's main section, "Scientific/Clinical Articles," contains in-depth research studies with quizzes to earn continuing education credit. The journal also lists resources such as dozens of active hand surgery journal clubs throughout the United States. Regular features also include original case reports, clinical reviews, case studies, editorials, and book reviews.

Journal of Occupational Science. v. 5, School of Occupational Therapy, University of South Australia, 1998.
http://www.jos.edu.au/
ISSN: 14427591
Indexed in: CINAHL
Recommended for: Hospital, Academic Libraries

Previously known as the *Journal of Occupational Science: Australia*, the publication defines occupation as the purposeful activity of all humans, and includes a wide range of topics that relate to the importance of occupation in human development and aging. Since its inception in 1993 by Dr. Ann Wilcock at the University of South Australia, the journal has sought to further international support for occupational science. A guiding principle of the editorial board is the view of humans as occupational beings, drawing upon the perspectives of experts in the behavioral sciences, education, and other fields. As such, the editorial board includes recognized experts from the fields of anthropology, occupational therapy, and community health. The journal is a joint publication from the University of South Australia, the University of Southern California, and the Auckland University of Technology. Sample topics range from the biological necessity for occupation to how activity contributes to health in old age. Published three times a year, the journal includes discussion papers, world class research, editorial commentary, and book reviews.

Occupational Therapy International. v. 1, Wiley, 1994.
http://onlinelibrary.wiley.com/journal/10.1002/(ISSN)1557-0703
ISSN: 09667903
ISSN: 15570703 (Online)
Indexed in: MEDLINE, CINAHL
Recommended for: Hospital, Academic Libraries

Occupational Therapy International is published quarterly and includes peer-reviewed articles and current clinical practice and research. The journal covers subject matter as varied as education, technology, industrial health, and health care administration from an international perspective, originating from both the industrialized world as well as from developing countries. The editorial board is composed of a highly diverse body of experts from around the globe. This journal is an excellent source of practice innovation that transcends any national boundaries, and not only helps foster a vital exchange and broadening of ideas internationally but also inevitably promotes future growth and expansion within the profession. This is a superb scholarly journal in occupational therapy that includes photographs, lacks advertising or a commercial presence and is relevant to any public health care practitioner, educator, or researcher in occupational therapy or other areas related to rehabilitation.

OTJR: Occupation, Participation and Health. v. 22, Slack, 2002.
http://www.OTJRonline.com
ISSN: 15394492
ISSN: 19382383 (Online)
Indexed in: CINAHL
Recommended for: Hospital, Academic Libraries
Brandon/Hill Selection

The quarterly publication *OTJR: Occupation, Participation and Health*, was previously titled *The Occupational Therapy Journal of Research* (*OTJR*) from 1980 to 2001. The name change was intended to better reflect the role of occupation in promoting health while integrating ideas from related professions such as psychology, neuroscience, economics, anthropology, sociology, geography, rehabilitation science, nursing, and social work. It is the official journal of the American Occupational Therapy Foundation, Inc., which was chartered as a charitable, scientific, literary, and educational society to "advance the science of occupational therapy and increase the public knowledge and understanding thereof." The Foundation established an Institute for the Study of Occupation and Health, organized around professional concepts as they relate to broad societal issues and needs. The journal is an important vehicle towards advancing the Institute's goals, and attests to the significance of occupational therapy expressed by AOTF founder Wilma L. West. The journal reflects her vision that occupational therapy should address the dynamics of health and social forces as well as therapeutic interventions. The journal is cited in many online databases and indexes, and is a staple item for an academic library supporting an occupational therapy curriculum.

Scandinavian Journal of Occupational Therapy. v. 1, Informa Healthcare, 1994.
http://catalogue.informahealthcare.com/pjbp/home.htm

ISSN: 11038128
ISSN: 16512014 (Online)
Indexed in: MEDLINE, CINAHL
Recommended for: Hospital, Academic Libraries

The *Scandinavian Journal of Occupational Therapy* is international in scope, focusing on highest quality research in all areas of occupational therapy. The journal includes reviews, evaluation of instruments or interventions, clinical research, occupational therapy theory, summaries of research, case reports, and editorial commentary. The journal prides itself on fast publication of the results of quality research covering all aspects of occupational therapy and related subjects. The journal is published quarterly in English and includes special themed issues. Considered essential for researchers who want to stay apprised of major research in the field of occupational therapy, the journal covers important trends and theory affecting practitioners, educators and researchers alike.

Databases and Other Electronic Resources

OT Search: The Occupational Therapy Bibliographic System. The American Occupational Foundation and the American Occupational Therapy Association, 1999.
http://www1.aota.org/otsearch/index.asp
Recommended for: Hospital, Academic Libraries

OT Search is a subscription database based on the catalog of the Wilma L. West Library, a national clearinghouse for occupational therapy information. Formerly called OTBibSys, the database is published jointly by the American Occupational Foundation (AOTF) and the American Occupational Therapy Association (AOTA). The AOTF website has a current listing of OT Search literature. Going back to 1910, OT Search includes bibliographic information and authors' abstracts when available, and indexes thousands of records from the literature of occupational therapy and related fields such as psychology, public health, rehabilitation, and education, provided that the articles are written by occupational therapists or are of interest to occupational therapy professionals. OT Source indexes monographs, journal articles, dissertations, theses, conference proceedings, audiovisuals, and materials from the archives of AOTA. Boolean searching can combine keywords with the database's "Occupational Therapy Thesaurus" of controlled vocabulary terms. Content is available at the Wilma L. West Library and can be ordered for purchase. Plans are to add full-text database links. AOTA members may subscribe at a discount. Institutional or individual subscriptions are available for this outstanding source of best research and practice information for occupational therapy students, educators, researchers, and practitioners.

OTDBASE. OTDBASE, 1970.
http://www.otdbase.org/
Recommended for: Hospital, Academic Libraries

Begun in 1986 by University of Western Ontario Professor Emeritus Marilyn Conibear (FCAOT), this occupational therapy resource is a favorite of researchers and educators, and is one of the only Internet-based journal indexing and abstracting search services that focuses specifically on occupational therapy. It contains over 10,000 abstracts from more than 20 national and international occupational therapy journals from 1970 to the present, and is geared to researchers and professionals. OTDBASE provides subject access to the journal literature two ways: first, by one or more specific keywords appearing in titles or abstracts; and secondly, by a more general search that coordinates a main subject term with one of several associated subtopics in the menu. A third advanced search feature will retrieve journal abstracts by combinations of keywords, authors' names, years, and other elements. All abstracts are categorized under main topics and multiple subtopics, such as "Developmental Disabilities" with "Assessments/Instruments." Database results are relevancy ranked according to search specifications. Professionals consider OTDBASE to be an essential tool for efficient research of the core OT journal literature.

1.3. Physical Therapy

The auxiliary health profession which makes use of physical therapy modalities to prevent, correct, and alleviate movement dysfunction of anatomic or physiologic origin.

—MeSH

Contributor: Craig S. Elam

Monographs

Guide to Evidence-Based Physical Therapy Practice. 2nd ed. Author: Dianne V. Jewell. Jones & Bartlett, 2011.
ISBN: 9780763777654
Recommended for: Hospital, Academic Libraries
Doody's Core Titles Selection (1st ed.)

With the increasing emphasis on evidence-based physical therapy practice (EBPT) in PT education programs, this recent book has become an important resource for both students and practitioners alike. It is an excellent and easily understood introduction to evidence-based practice in the classroom and the clinic. It is divided into four sections, each logically expanding on the previous one. The first presents the principles of EBPT, which is followed by a section that reviews the components of a research article, especially those that affect the quality and validity of the research along with statistical measures. The third section provides information on how to evaluate diagnostic tests, interventions, and outcomes. The final part synthesizes the previous information in a discussion on applying evidence in practice from a patient's point of view. Each chapter contains learning objectives, definitions of terms, review questions, and examples from the published literature to illustrate key concepts specific to physical therapy. The back of the text has evidence-appraisal worksheets, sample calculations, and a comprehensive index. The review for this *Doody's Core Titles* selection is for the first edition.

Motor Control: Translating Research into Clinical Practice. 3rd ed. Authors: Anne Shumway-Cook, Marjorie H. Woollacott. Lippincott Williams & Wilkins, 2007.
ISBN: 9780781766913
Recommended for: Hospital, Academic Libraries
Brandon/Hill Selection

This is the only text to bridge the gap between current motor control research and its application to physical therapy clinical practice. It applies the latest evidence-based research findings to clinical problems related to balance, mobility, and upper extremity function. Divided into four major divisions, the first section covers the theory and fundamentals of motor learning, motor control, and recovery of function. Part two details normal and abnormal postural control, while part three addresses mobility functions associated with gait, transfers, and stair walking. Part four discusses normal and abnormal reach, grasp, and manipulation. Chapters in each section follow a standard format, presenting normal control processes, age-related issues, abnormal function, and the clinical applications of current research; chapters end with a case study highlighting specific clinical management problems. Updated color tables and illustrations are clear and easy to understand. Laboratory activities and case studies reinforce key concepts. This is an excellent text for students and clinicians seeking applications of current research. According to a Federation of State Boards of Physical Therapy survey, *Motor Control* was one of the most frequently used texts in physical therapy education programs. Earlier editions of this book were listed in the Brandon/Hill allied health list.

Muscles: Testing and Function with Posture and Pain. 5th ed. Authors: Florence Peterson Kendall, Elizabeth Kendall McCreary, Patricia Geise Provance, Mary McIntyre Rodgers, William Anthony Romani. Lippincott Williams & Wilkins, 2005.
ISBN: 9780781747806
Recommended for: Hospital, Academic Libraries
Doody's Core Titles Selection

First published over 50 years ago, this classic work continues to provide unparalleled coverage of manual muscle testing, plus evaluation and treatment of faulty and painful postural conditions. The fifth edition has been thoroughly updated with new color illustrations, drawings, charts, and photographs. The content has also been completely reorganized by body region from head to toe, expanding the treatment and exercise sections of each chapter and including a new section on post-polio syndrome. The authors describe posture and its pathologies in particular detail. The photographs clearly depict specific muscle tests, allowing students to learn these techniques easily. This is an essential text for orthopedists, physical therapists, or athletic trainers. A bonus Primal Anatomy CD-ROM contains three-dimensional interactive images that can be rotated and layers of anatomy that can be added or removed. The senior author is a recognized authority in the field. This sentinel work is a *Doody's Core Titles* selection and the second most commonly held book in a 2007 survey of practicing physical therapists.

Orthopedic Physical Assessment. 5th ed. Authors: David J. Magee. Saunders/Elsevier, 2008.
ISBN: 9780721605715
Recommended for: Hospital, Academic Libraries
Brandon/Hill, *Doody's Core Titles* Selection

This is the most comprehensive text available on the assessment of the neuromusculoskeletal system. It is well organized to provide a systematic approach to assessment, with rationales for the various aspects involved. Beginning with the principles of assessment, the chapters that follow cover every joint of the body, head and face, gait, posture, emergency sports care, and evaluation prior to participation in sports. The book offers unparalleled coverage of the extremities, with clear explanations of positions and movements. The latest edition is updated with extensive full-color illustrations and more evidence-based information on the reliability and validity of the many specific tests and techniques presented. This is an essential resource for students and practicing clinicians in an outpatient setting, including physical therapists, athletic trainers, physician assistants, primary care physicians, and orthopedists. It is a *Doody's Core*

Titles selection, with earlier editions listed in the 2003 Brandon/Hill allied health list. A 2007 study found it to be widely held in the personal libraries of practicing physical therapists, and a Federation of State Boards of Physical Therapy survey showed it to be one of the most often used texts in physical therapy education programs.

Pathology: Implications for the Physical Therapist. 3rd ed. Authors: Catherine Cavallaro Goodman, Kenda S. Fuller. Saunders/Elsevier, 2009.
ISBN: 9781416031185
Recommended for: Hospital, Academic Libraries
Brandon/Hill Selection

The only pathology textbook written specifically for physical therapists, this standard text offers guidelines, precautions, and contraindications for interventions with patients who have systemic diseases or conditions. It emphasizes health promotion and disease prevention strategies and those issues affecting patient/client management, such as injury, inflammation, the lymphatic system, and biopsychosocial and spiritual aspects of health care. "Special Implications for the Therapist" sections present the most likely practice patterns associated with each disease or disorder and address precautions, contraindications, and considerations specific to PTs. "Preferred Practice Patterns" from the second edition of the *Guide to Physical Therapist Practice* are used throughout the book. Numerous tables and text boxes summarize important information. As a practical and evidence-based text, now enhanced with full-color illustrations, this work is one of the most frequently used texts in physical therapy education programs in a Federation of State Boards of Physical Therapy survey. An earlier edition of this book was listed in the 2003 Brandon/Hill allied health list.

Physical Rehabilitation. 5th ed. Authors: Susan B. O'Sullivan, Thomas J. Schmitz. F.A. Davis, 2007.
ISBN: 9780803612471
Recommended for: Hospital, Academic Libraries

This is an essential text on the rehabilitation management of adult patients organized according to the structure and language of the second edition of the *Guide to Physical Therapist Practice*. The book clearly explains, based on a medical diagnosis, how to select the appropriate evaluation procedures and make specific evidence-based recommendations for treatment. After introductory chapters, the book is divided into five color-coded sections, the first four covering the preferred practice patterns found in the *Guide*: musculoskeletal, neuromuscular, cardiovascular/pulmonary, and integumentary. The fifth section addresses material applicable to all areas, such as gait assessment, assistive devices, orthotics, and community mobility. Chapters within each section describe the various disorders of that system following a consistent format: an outline and learning objectives; a description of the diagnosis accompanied by excellent summaries of important information presented in tables or illustrations; the proper examination, evaluation, and prognosis of a patient with this particular diagnosis; discussion of the most effective intervention strategies for that diagnosis; and, finally, case studies and extensive references. This updated fifth edition has enhanced, additional color photographs, illustrations, and tables, resulting in a more user-friendly presentation. This text is highly recommended as a quick reference source for physical therapy students and practicing clinicians. According to a Federation of State Boards of Physical Therapy survey, it is one of the most used texts in physical therapy education programs and the fourth most commonly held book in a 2007 study of practicing physical therapists.

Therapeutic Exercise: Foundations and Techniques. 5th ed. Authors: Carolyn Kisner, Lynn Allen Colby. F.A. Davis, 2007.
http://www.statref.com
http://www.ebrary.com/
http://www.r2library.com/
http://extranet.netlibrary.com/TitleSelect/
ISBN: 9780803615847 (Print)
ISBN: 9780803619265 (Online)
ISBN: 9781429495806 (Online)
Recommended for: Hospital, Academic Libraries
Brandon/Hill, *Doody's Core Titles* Selection

The latest edition of this classic text has been thoroughly revised and updated with standard terminology, use of disablement model language, more emphasis on evidence-based practice and functional outcomes, and, for the first time, a hard cover. It continues to offer basic therapeutic exercises for musculoskeletal and cardiopulmonary disorders in an easily accessible format, now with more full-color illustrations. The content has expanded to five sections, the first introducing general concepts, including the disablement model and a new chapter on prevention and wellness. The second section covers the basic principles of therapeutic exercise and functional techniques, with a new chapter on exercise for impaired balance. The third section presents an expanded discussion of the principles of intervention, with new content on surgical interventions, connective tissue and bone disorders, and peripheral nerve disorders. Exercise interventions by body region follow in the fourth section, with each of the nine chapters including a table linking preferred practice patterns to the pathologies and surgeries presented. The last section deals with special areas such as vascular, pulmonary, and obstetric topics. *Therapeutic Exercise* is included in *Doody's Core Titles* and selected as an Essential Purchase; an earlier version of this essential text appeared on the final Brandon/Hill list. It was also one of the top 10 books most commonly held by practicing physical therapists in a 2007 study, and a Federation of State Boards of Physical Therapy survey showed it to be one of the most often used texts in physical therapy education programs.

Journals

Archives of Physical Medicine and Rehabilitation. v. 34, W.B. Saunders/Elsevier, 1953.
http://www.sciencedirect.com/science/journal/00039993
ISSN: 00039993 (Print/Online)
See Also Chapter 3. Chiropractic, Chapter 10.14. Physical Medicine and Rehabilitation
Indexed in: MEDLINE, CINAHL
Recommended for: Hospital, Academic Libraries
Brandon/Hill Selection

International in scope, this is the premier multidisciplinary journal for physical therapists, presenting original, peer-reviewed research and clinical articles from the broad fields of physical medicine and rehabilitation. It also presents information on nonclinical aspects of rehabilitation professional practice. It is the official journal of the American Congress of Rehabilitation Medicine and the American Academy of Physical Medicine and Rehabilitation. Published continually for over 90 years, its authority and quality is evidenced through various rankings. It serves as one of the top three core titles in a recent citation analysis of the physical therapy literature; it appears on the Special Library Association's list of "Top 100 Journals in Biology and Medicine" over the past 100 years; and it is ranked 6 of 33 rehabilitation titles in impact factor in the 2009 *Journal Citation Reports*. Accordingly, it is widely indexed by all major biomedical abstracting and indexing services.

Journal of Orthopaedic and Sports Physical Therapy (JOSPT). v. 1, Orthopaedic and Sports Physical Therapy Sections of the American Physical Therapy Association, 1979.
http://www.jospt.org
ISSN: 01906011 (Print/Online)
See Also Chapter 9.12. Sports Medicine
Indexed in: MEDLINE, CINAHL
Recommended for: Hospital, Academic Libraries
Brandon/Hill Selection

The *JOSPT*, founded in 1979, is the official journal of the Orthopaedic Section and the Sports Physical Therapy Section of the American Physical Therapy Association (APTA). It is an essential source of peer-reviewed, evidence-based basic scientific and clinical information in musculoskeletal and sports-related rehabilitation and health. Originally released on a quarterly basis, it is now published monthly to an international audience of physical therapists, orthopedic physicians, athletic trainers, and researchers. It is recognized as an official journal of many physical therapy and sports science associations outside the United States. A measure of its influence is seen in its ranking second of 33 rehabilitation journals and ninth of 72 sports sciences journals in the 2009 *Journal Citation Reports*. The journal's quality and productivity is confirmed in a recent citation analysis of the core physical therapy literature, where it placed among the top five titles. It is indexed in major medical and nursing indexes.

Journal of Physiotherapy. v. 56, Australian Physiotherapy Association, 2010.
http://www.ovid.com
http://physiotherapy.asn.au/index.php/quality-practice/ajp/about-ajp
ISSN: 18369553
ISSN: 18369561 (Online)
Indexed in: MEDLINE, CINAHL
Recommended for: Hospital, Academic Libraries

Published for fifty-five years as the *Australian Journal of Physiotherapy*, this quarterly journal was renamed in March 2010 to reflect its growing reputation as a major international journal. It remains the official journal of the Australian Physiotherapy Association and is one of the most widely read and authoritative journals in the field. Within the past five years, the journal has increased the rigor and type of articles published, being the first physical therapy journal to require registration for all randomized controlled trials. In addition, a recent analysis showed that the quality of systematic reviews in the journal was above the average for the field. Identified as a core title in a recent citation analysis of the physical therapy literature, its increased quality and breadth is reflected by being ranked thirteenth of 33 journals in the rehabilitation category and twenty-third among 72 journals in the sports sciences category in the 2009 *Journal Citation Reports*. It is indexed in major medical and nursing indexes. Full text is available from 2001, although the Association provides access to all back volumes except the four most recent issues at its website.

Physical Therapy. v. 44, American Physical Therapy Association, 1964.
http://www.ptjournal.org
ISSN: 00319023
ISSN: 15386724 (Online)
Indexed in: MEDLINE, CINAHL
Recommended for: Hospital, Academic Libraries
Brandon/Hill Selection

As the official journal of the American Public Therapy Association (APTA), this is a leading publication for research and practice in physical therapy and related fields. Established in 1921, the journal publishes original, peer-reviewed articles providing basic and applied research and evidence to guide clinical practice for practitioners. Evidence for the quality and quantity of its publications is seen in a recent citation analysis, identifying it as the most cited journal in the core physical therapy literature. It is also ranked ninth of 33 rehabilitation titles in impact factor in the 2009 *Journal Citation Reports*. The online edition offers content back to 1980, with supplemental data files, clinical summaries, podcasts, RSS feeds, and videos from its website. It is widely indexed in medical, nursing, and allied health databases. APTA provides free, full-text online access from 1980 after a one-year embargo.

Physiotherapy. v. 34, Elsevier for the Chartered Society of Physiotherapy, 1948.
http://www.sciencedirect.com/science/journal/00319406
ISSN: 00319406 (Print/Online)
Indexed in: MEDLINE, CINAHL
Recommended for: Hospital, Academic Libraries
Brandon/Hill Selection

Serving as the official journal of the Chartered Society of Physiotherapy (CSP), this is the premier journal of the British branch of the profession. The journal publishes original, peer-reviewed research articles, critical reviews, brief reports, and case histories on a quarterly basis. It has a distinguished history, dating back to 1915. It was reinvigorated as a research journal in 2004, when Elsevier assumed publication and established the goal of becoming the leading international journal in physical therapy and rehabilitation. The success of its resurgence is evident in its listing as the sixth most cited journal by a recent citation analysis of the core physical therapy literature. It is currently indexed in the major medical, nursing, and allied health services and ranks twenty-second of 33 rehabilitation titles in impact factor in the 2009 *Journal Citation Reports*.

1.4. Speech-Language Pathology

Speech or language disorders and their diagnosis and correction.

—MeSH

Contributor: Maureen (Molly) Knapp

Monographs

Anatomy & Physiology for Speech, Language, and Hearing. 4th ed. Authors: Anthony J. Seikel, Douglas W. King, David G. Drumright. Delmar Cengage Learning, 2010.
See Chapter 1.1. Audiology

Aphasia and Related Neurogenic Language Disorders. 4th ed. Editor: Leonard L. LaPointe. Thieme, 2011.
ISBN: 9781604062618
ISBN: 9781604062625
Recommended for: Hospital, Academic Libraries
Brandon/Hill, *Doody's Core Titles* Selection

First published in 1990 and now in its third edition, this book offers in-depth coverage of aphasia and related neurogenic language disorders. Seventeen chapters offer material on: functional neuroimaging; naming and word-retrieval problems; acquired dyslexia; acquired agraphias; the pathophysiology, nature, evaluation and treatment for many types of aphasia, including Broca's, Wernicke's, conduction, transcortical, and global; dementia; right hemisphere syndrome; traumatic brain injury; and pragmatics of communication. New to the third edition are chapters on social and group models of intervention, neurobiological aspects of recovery secondary to treatment, and research on issues following prefrontal cortex damage. Each chapter is written by an expert in the field, and includes black-and-white photographs, tables, and references. Four pages of color photographs accompany the chapter on functional neuroimaging. The final chapter covers family, caregiver, and clinician resources. This chapter is presented in a directory format, offering addresses, websites, telephone numbers, and annotations of many organizations that support clinicians, families, and caregivers of persons with neurologic impairment. Recommended Internet sites, videos, books, and other literature are also included, as well as references to articles about life with neurologic impairment from the perspectives of survivors and caregivers. The second edition of this book was included in the 2003 Brandon/Hill list, while the third edition is listed in *Doody's Core Titles* essential purchase, receiving a four-star *Doody's* review (92 out of a possible 100 points). This review refers to the third edition.

Assessment in Speech-Language Pathology: A Resource Manual. 4th ed. Authors: Kenneth G. Shipley, Julie G. McAfee. Delmar Cengage Learning, 2008.
ISBN: 9781418053284
Recommended for: Hospital, Academic Libraries
Doody's Core Titles Selection

The purpose of this book is to provide students and professionals with a variety of information, materials, and procedures for use in the assessment of communication disorders. The book is organized into three sections. Part one includes preparatory considerations, incorporating foundations of assessment and multicultural considerations. Part two covers obtaining, interpreting, and reporting assessment information, such as taking case histories, conducting interviews, and reporting assessment information to clients, caregivers, and other professionals. Part three makes up the bulk of the book, providing materials and suggestions for the assessment of many communication disorders. It includes common assessment procedures such as oral-facial examination and conversation starters for eliciting a speech-language sample (including pictures and narratives with pictures) as well as tools and information for the assessment of: articulation and phonological disorders; language, fluency, voice and resonance; neurologically based communication disorders (dysarthria, apraxia, traumatic brain injury, and dementia); dysphagia; special populations (autism, augmentative/alternative communication, laryngectomies, cleft lip or palate) and hearing. This book is quite useful for the many tables, norms, and forms for diagnostics in a variety of areas. An accompanying CD-ROM includes reproducible copies of forms, stimulus materials, and illustrations in PDF, RTF, and Microsoft Word and Excel formats. The PDF version allows the clinician to input client data directly into the document, while the Word, Excel, and RTF versions can be customized. This book received a four-star *Doody's* review (94 out of a possible 100 points) and is currently a *Doody's Core Titles* essential purchase. Beginning and experienced clinicians will find this book provides time-saving, "one-stop-shopping" for assessment in communication disorders.

Clinical Decision Making in Fluency Disorders. 3rd ed. Author: Walter H. Manning. Delmar Cengage Learning, 2010.
ISBN: 9781418067304
Recommended for: Hospital, Academic Libraries

This engaging textbook presents therapeutic tools for speech-language pathologists who assist clients who stutter. Created for graduate students, this book is also useful for practicing speech language pathologists in clinical settings, and is readable enough that a layperson with an interest in stuttering could also benefit. The book is organized into 12 chapters. Chapter 1 describes the personal characteristics and clinical skills of an effective clinician and how these affect the therapeutic process. Chapter 2 addresses the nature of fluent and non-fluent speech and the characteristics of early childhood stuttering. Chapter 3 gives an historical perspective of stuttering etiologies, as well as offering evidence for and against each point of view. Recent research on anatomical and physiological abnormalities underlying the onset of stuttering, as well as neuroimaging and genetic investigations are also discussed. Chapters 4 and 5 address the assessment process in adults and children, while Chapter 6 discusses facilitating the therapeutic process. Chapter 7 describes various counseling theories. Chapters 8 and 9 discuss the management of stuttering for adolescents, adults, and children, while Chapter 10 is devoted to the assessment and management of atypical fluency disorders such as cluttered speech, malingering, and neurogenic and psychogenic stuttering. Chapters 11 and 12 discuss indicators of successful change during and following treatment. Each chapter begins by introducing learning objectives and concludes with discussion questions and recommended readings. Boxes throughout the book highlight clinical decision making and clinical insight, while many sample assessment measures, clinical checklists, and tables are also included. References and an author and subject index conclude the book, while an online companion supplements the text with video comments from the author, PowerPoint slides to accompany chapters, and video and audio examples of fluency problems and therapy sessions. As the author states in the preface, "a primary goal of this book is to convey to the reader the enthusiasm and creativity associated with assisting people who stutter." This book received a five-star *Doody's* review (100 out of 100 possible points) and was considered "an indispensible tool."

Medical Speech-Language Pathology: A Practitioner's Guide. 2nd ed, Editors: Alex F. Johnson, Barbara H. Jacobson. Thieme, 2007.
ISBN: 9781588903204
Recommended for: Hospital, Academic Libraries
Brandon/Hill Selection

Designed as both a textbook for medical speech-language pathology coursework and a reference text for those who work in health care settings, this book gives a general overview of the information needed for speech language pathologists practicing in medical settings. The book is organized into five sections: "Medical Speech Language Pathology: an Orientation," "Neurocognitive Communication Disorders," "Disorders of Swallowing and Voice," "Topics in Clinical Collaboration and Service Delivery," and "Medical Perspectives." An index is also included. Each chapter begins with an outline of topics and includes black-and-white photographs, tables, case discussions, study questions and references. The last two sections of the book are useful for the coverage of current topics in the field and multidisciplinary interaction with other health care providers. Chapters of note include evidence-based practice and outcomes-oriented approaches, clinical documentation, working in specialized settings such as the ICU, acute care, and issues in geriatric medicine. The first edition of this book was included in the 2003 Brandon/Hill list, while the current (second) edition received a four-star *Doody's* review (93 out of a possible 100 points).

Journals

American Journal of Audiology. v. 1, American Speech-Language-Hearing Association, 1991.
See Chapter 1.1. Audiology

American Journal of Speech-Language Pathology: A Journal of Clinical Practice: AJSLP. v. 1, American Speech-Language-Hearing Association, 1991.
http://ajslp.asha.org/
ISSN: 10580360
ISSN: 15589110 (Online)
Indexed in: MEDLINE, CINAHL
Recommended for: Academic Libraries

AJSLP is the quarterly, peer-reviewed publication from the American Speech-Language-Hearing Association (ASHA). ASHA is the professional, scientific, and credentialing association for speech-language pathologists, audiologists, and speech, language, and hearing scientists. *AJSLP* publishes articles on all aspects of clinical practice in speech-language pathology, including: screening, assessment, and treatment techniques; prevention; professional issues; supervision; and administration. Issue contents include: editorials, letters to the editor, original research, clinical forums, and clinical reviews ("tutorials"). It ranks 11 out of 92 titles in the linguistics category, and 9 out of 52 titles in the rehabilitation category, with an impact factor of 1.879 (2009 *Journal Citation Reports*). This journal is indexed in CINAHL, Embase, MEDLINE, PsycINFO, Scopus, and Web of Science. Beginning January 2010, all ASHA journals became online-only. Online access from volume 1, 1991 is available from the publisher.

Journal of Speech, Language, and Hearing Research: JSLHR. v. 40, American Speech-Language-Hearing Association, 1997.
http://jslhr.asha.org/
ISSN: 10924388
ISSN: 15589102 (Online)
Indexed in: MEDLINE, CINAHL
Recommended for: Academic Libraries

The *Journal of Speech, Language, and Hearing Research: JSLHR* has a long and storied history going back to 1936, when it was first published as the *Journal of Speech and Hearing Disorders*. Several journal merges and name changes later, *JSLHR* is now published bimonthly, with subject coverage spanning the processes and disorders of hearing, language, and speech as well as the diagnosis and treatment of such disorders. Publication types include: original research reports; theoretical, tutorial, or review pieces; research notes; and letters to the editor. This peer-reviewed journal ranked 4 of 92 titles in the linguistics category and 5 of 52 titles in the rehabilitation category with an impact factor of 2.347 (2009 *Journal Citation Reports*). *JSLHR* is indexed in a number of databases, including: Education Index, Embase, MEDLINE (1997–present), the Annual Bibliography of English Language and Literature, Biological Abstracts (1997-present) and Web of Science. Beginning January 1, 2010, all ASHA journals became online-only. Online access from v. 40, 1997 is available from several vendors.

Language, Speech, and Hearing Services in Schools: LSHSS. v. 2, American Speech-Language-Hearing Association, 1971.
http://lshss.asha.org/
ISSN: 01611461
ISSN: 15589129 (Online)
Indexed in: MEDLINE, CINAHL
Recommended for: Academic Libraries

Language, Speech, and Hearing Services in Schools (*LSHSS*), first published in 1970, is a quarterly peer-reviewed publication by the American Speech-Language-Hearing Association (ASHA). Topic coverage pertains to speech, language, and hearing disorders and differences in children and adolescents, as well as professional issues affecting service delivery in educational settings. Contributions appear under the following headings: articles, reports, clinical exchange, clinical forum, software perspectives, letters to the editor, and supplements. The journal ranked 24 of 92 titles in the linguistics category and 21 of 52 titles in the rehabilitation category, with an impact factor of 1.273 (2009 *Journal Citation Reports*). It is indexed in Language and Language Behavior Abstracts (LLBA), Education Index, Embase, MEDLINE, Scopus, and Web of Science. Beginning in January 2010 it became online only. Online access to issues from 1970 is available from HighWire.

1.5. Clinical Laboratory Science

Performance of techniques in clinical pathology such as those in hematology, microbiology, and other general clinical laboratory applications.

—MeSH: Technology, Medical

Contributor: Frances Delwiche

Monographs

Bailey & Scott's Diagnostic Microbiology. 12th ed. Editors: Betty A. Forbes, Daniel F. Sahm, Alice S. Weissfeld. Mosby Elsevier, 2007.
ISBN: 9780808923640
ISBN: 9780323030656
Recommended for: Hospital, Academic Libraries
Brandon/Hill, *Doody's Core Titles* Selection

Continuing a tradition that began over 60 years ago, the twelfth edition of *Bailey & Scott's Diagnostic Microbiology* remains one of the most popular microbiology textbooks for clinical laboratory science. Like its predecessors, the book is intended to serve as a reference text for both practicing technologists and instructors of diagnostic microbiology. Its 65 chapters are organized into eight major parts: "Basic Medical Microbiology," "General Principles in Clinical Microbiology," "Bacteriology," "Parasitology," "Mycology," "Virology," "Diagnosis by Organ System," and "Clinical Laboratory Management." The "Bacteriology" section, comprising nearly one-third of the book, is of particular value to both students and practitioners. It begins with an overview of bacteriological identification methods and procedures and is followed by separate chapters on the general characteristics, pathogenesis, and laboratory workup of over thirty medically important genera. The "Diagnosis by Organ System" section is very useful as well, including a review of normal flora and the most common diseases and infections found in each of the major organ systems. Many chapters incorporate a case study and questions, with answers and explanations provided in an appendix. The textbook contains a large number of content-rich, highly detailed tables and charts. Color photographs and illustrations and a pleasing layout add to the textbook's appeal. Ancillary materials, including an instructor's manual, test bank, laboratory manual, image collection, and study aids for students, are provided on an associated website. Overall, this textbook meets and exceeds its goal effectively by providing a practical, authoritative text for clinical microbiologists of all levels.

Clinical Chemistry: Theory, Analysis, Correlation. 5th ed. Editors: Lawrence A. Kaplan, Amadeo J. Pesce. Mosby/Elsevier, 2010.
ISBN: 9780323036580
Recommended for: Hospital, Academic Libraries
Brandon/Hill Selection

At nearly 1,200 pages, this comprehensive textbook of clinical chemistry is a weighty tome. Despite its size, its attractive layout and numerous learning aids render it very readable and user friendly for the undergraduate student, while serving as an excellent resource for advanced students and professionals. It represents a monumental effort by multiple primary editors, supporting editors, reviewers, and contributors to both the book and the online-only "Methods of Analysis" section. The first 26 chapters, comprising just under half the book, discuss laboratory techniques and laboratory management. Coverage includes traditional chemistry methods such as spectral techniques, chromatography, electrophoresis, and enzymology, as well as contemporary issues such as point-of-care testing, laboratory information systems, and molecular diagnostics. The second and larger section of the book is devoted to the pathophysiology of primary organ systems and its correlation to clinical chemistry analytes. In this section, the book moves well beyond the traditional boundaries of clinical chemistry by delving into topics such as neoplasia, transplantation, genetic diseases, serology testing, body fluids, and human nutrition. Chapters begin with an outline and definitions of key terms, which are subdivided into several sections with individual objectives and key concepts. Abundant black-and-white illustrations, drawings, charts, and tables break the text into manageable bites. Chapters end with a bibliography, optional references, and a list of relevant Internet sites. The "Methods of Analysis" section further expands the book's scope by providing detailed methods for 144 chemical analyses.

Clinical Hematology and Fundamentals of Hemostasis. 5th ed. Editor: Denise M. Harmening. F.A. Davis, 2009.
ISBN: 9780803617322
Recommended for: Hospital, Academic Libraries
Brandon/Hill, *Doody's Core Titles* Selection

Substantially expanded from the previous edition, this comprehensive hematology textbook is an admirable achievement. At just over 1,000 pages, it verges on being daunting—until the book is opened. From that point forward, the reader's imagination is captivated by the hundreds of color photographs, illustrations, and tables that support the authoritative text. Edited by a long-time clinical laboratory science educator and respected author, the book represents the collaborative efforts of 56 contributors and 35 reviewers. The layout of the book is somewhat unique, with 36 chapters organized into five main parts. The first part immerses the reader immediately into the heart of the subject with an overview of blood and marrow cell morphology. With this foundation, the reader is prepared for subsequent parts that cover the anemias, white blood cell disorders, and principles of hemostasis and thrombosis. The final section on laboratory methods could almost serve as a standalone procedure manual. It covers manual and automated techniques, quality control, flow cytometry, molecular diagnostics, cytochemistry, plus a special chapter on body fluids. Many chapters are very detailed, such as the chapter on automated differential analysis, which includes 23 case studies and over 30 pages of text and figures. Learning aids include objectives, chapter outlines, case studies, study questions, (often quite lengthy) chapter summaries, and references. A CD-ROM, which contains a test bank, instructor's guide, and images for use in PowerPoint lectures, is available for instructors who adopt the text.

Clinical Hematology Atlas. 3rd ed. Authors: Jacqueline H. Carr, Bernadette F. Rodak. Saunders Elsevier, 2009.
ISBN: 9781416050391
Recommended for: Hospital, Academic Libraries
Doody's Core Titles Selection

Few resources are as indispensable to the clinical hematologist as a good atlas of blood cell images, and this is one of the finest available. With spiral binding that allows it to lie flat, this atlas is designed to sit beside the microscope rather than on a shelf. Its most distinguishing feature is the hundreds of outstanding photomicrographs depicting both normal and abnormal blood cells. The book begins with a visual description of blood smear preparation and staining, followed by hematopoiesis and maturation of normal cell lines, and concludes with cellular abnormalities seen in a wide range of hematologic diseases. Additional chapters cover cytochemical staining, microorganisms, blood parasites, and artifacts. The chapter on normal newborn blood cell morphology is a unique addition, and the brief chapter on non-blood body fluids is very helpful. The book contains minimal text with the expectation that a standard hematology textbook will be consulted for background information. Utilizing fine glossy paper, the photos are clear and crisp, with accurate color representation. Arrows identify critical cellular elements, and photos of normal cells are often provided for comparison against the abnormal. Ample white space allows the image gallery to have maximum visual impact. Explanatory text, often in outline form, describes cellular features and associated disease conditions, while tables and color illustrations highlight important concepts. An accompanying website provides study materials for students and an electronic image collection for instructors. The beauty and quality of this atlas will make it a favorite among students and practitioners alike.

Hematology: Clinical Principles and Applications. 3rd ed. Editors: Bernadette F. Rodak, George A. Fritsma, Kathryn Doig. Saunders/Elsevier, 2007.
ISBN: 9781416030065
Recommended for: Hospital, Academic Libraries
Brandon/Hill, *Doody's Core Titles* Selection

Vibrant images of human blood cells on the outside cover allude to the contents of this excellent hematology textbook. Now in its third edition, this resource is very popular among clinical laboratory science faculty and students, as well as nurses, medical students, residents, and other health care professionals. The book is edited by three noted clinical laboratory science educators, with contributions from over 30 experts. Though over 800 pages, its abundant photomicrographs, tables, and color illustrations make the book highly readable and appealing. It is organized into nine major sections, including an overview of basic laboratory principles, hematopoiesis, routine hematology testing, non-blood body fluids, erythrocyte disorders, leukocyte disorders, pediatric and geriatric hematology, automation, and hemostasis and thrombosis. Veteran technologists in particular will appreciate coverage of perennially difficult topics such as hematology in pediatric and geriatric populations as well as the examination of bone marrow and body fluids. Chapters on supporting diagnostics such as cytochemistry, cytogenetics, flow cytometry, and molecular diagnostics are also very helpful. Numerous learning aids are employed throughout the book: objectives and chapter outlines, case studies, "Chapter at a Glance" boxes at the end of each chapter, and review questions that are presented in certification exam format. Hematology and hemostasis reference ranges are provided on the inside front and back covers for rapid access. New to this edition are online resources available for students and instructors, including downloadable images for use in presentations. This book serves as a source of inspiration for both students and seasoned practitioners.

Modern Blood Banking and Transfusion Practices. 5th ed. Editor: Denise M. Harmening. F.A. Davis, 2005.
http://www.r2library.com/
http://www.ebrary.com/
ISBN: 0803612486
Recommended for: Hospital, Academic Libraries
Brandon/Hill, *Doody's Core Titles* Selection

Long a favorite of clinical laboratory science faculty and students, this work should be a first choice for libraries that can only afford one book on blood banking and transfusion science. Although written expressly for clinical laboratory scientists, this book is well suited for blood bank specialists, medical students, pathology residents, nurses, and other health care professionals needing a concise yet thorough guide to immunohematology and transfusion practices. It is authored by a long-term, highly respected professor of medical technology, with the help of nearly 40 expert contributors, primarily from across the United States. Consisting of 27 chapters, the book opens with a review of basic science concepts, followed by a comprehensive coverage of routine blood bank practices. Additional chapters cover blood collection and component preparation, transfusion therapy and apheresis, quality assurance and regulatory requirements, information systems, and medicolegal and ethical considerations. At over 500 pages, the book is effectively designed and highly readable, with hundreds of two-tone illustrations, tables, and black-and-white photographs. Of particular value to the practicing technologist are the color plates depicting procedures for basic ABO typing and interpretation of antigen-antibody reactions as well as the handy charts on the inside front and back covers that summarize the major blood group systems. Additional features include learning objectives for each chapter, tables and charts summarizing key points, in-context procedural appendixes, case studies, review questions, and references. This book effectively conveys not only the science but also the passion and ethos of blood banking.

Technical Manual. 16th ed. Editor: John D. Roback. AABB, 2008.
ISBN: 9781563952609
Recommended for: Hospital, Academic Libraries
Brandon/Hill, *Doody's Core Titles* Selection

As plain in appearance as its title, the *Technical Manual* nevertheless contains the essential information for clinical blood banking and transfusion medicine. Published by the AABB (formerly the American Association of Blood Banks), this venerable resource contains nary a superfluous word in its more than 1,000 pages. The book has a pleasing, no-nonsense layout with ample tables and black-and-white illustrations. What this weighty tome lacks in colorful graphics and sophisticated formatting, it more than makes up for in the wealth of information contained within its pages. Spearheaded by a team of four editors, the bulk of the book consists of 32 chapters written by individual or multiple expert authors, with review by AABB committees and program units. The major sections of the book include "Quality Issues," "Blood Donation and Collection," "Immunologic and Genetic Principles," "Blood Groups," "Antigen and Antibody Testing," "Transfusion Practice," and "Transplantation." The writing is comprehensive yet succinct, and the chapters are abundantly referenced. The book closes with a compendium of routine and special methods representative of current practice, including basic red cell typing; antibody detection, identification, and compatibility testing; investigation of a positive DAT; testing for fetomaternal hemorrhage; blood collection and preparation of components; and transplantation of cells and tissue. With this latest edition, this time-honored resource will continue to play a pivotal role in the education and practice of clinical blood banking and transfusion medicine.

Textbook of Diagnostic Microbiology. 3rd ed. Editors: Connie R. Mahon, Donald C. Lehman, George Manuselis. Saunders Elsevier, 2007.
ISBN: 9781416025818
Recommended for: Hospital, Academic Libraries
Brandon/Hill Selection

This comprehensive and authoritative textbook provides a strong foundation in medical microbiology for clinical laboratory science students and bench technologists. Edited by three experienced clinical laboratory science educators, it boasts contributions from 48 expert authors from across the United States. Despite being a hefty 1,200 plus pages, the book's abundant illustrations, attractive design, and pedagogical aids make it particularly appealing and easy to read. Laid out in three major parts, it begins with basic principles and procedures of clinical microbiology, follows with a detailed examination of medically important organisms, and concludes with a discussion of infectious diseases by organ system. The chapter on direct examination of microbiological samples is particularly impressive, with over 100 color plates from a wide variety of clinical specimens. The hundreds of photomicrographs of colonial morphology sprinkled throughout the text are equally memorable. In addition to commonly encountered organisms, the book covers anaerobes, spirochetes, rickettsiae, Mycobacterium spp., fungi, parasites, and viruses. Also addressed are contemporary issues such as emerging pathogens, antibiotic resistance, bioterror agents, and microbial biofilms. Each chapter opens with an outline, objectives, key terms, and a case study. The chapters conclude with a brief synopsis of key points, bibliography, and study questions. Answers to the study questions, which frequently include detailed explanations, are provided in an appendix. A separate appendix describes the use, composition, incubation requirements, and color reactions of various bacteriological culture media. Online ancillaries for students and instructors include content updates, a test bank, electronic image collection, and customizable laboratory manual.

Tietz Fundamentals of Clinical Chemistry. 6th ed. Editors: Carl A. Burtis, Edward R. Ashwood, David E. Bruns, Barbara G. Sawyer. Saunders Elsevier, 2008.
ISBN: 9780721638652
Recommended for: Hospital, Academic Libraries
Brandon/Hill Selection

Now in its sixth edition, *Tietz Fundamentals of Clinical Chemistry* continues to keep pace with advances in medical technology, enabling it to retain its position as one of the most popular clinical chemistry textbooks. With the combined expertise of three editors, an educational consultant, and 77 contributors from around the world, this is a truly monumental work. At just over 950 pages, the book consists of 45 chapters organized into six main sections. The first section provides an introduction to principles of laboratory safety, specimen collection, and evidence-based laboratory medicine. The second section is a compendium of analytical techniques and instrumentation, which is followed by a discussion of statistical principles, clinical laboratory informatics, and quality management. The fourth section, which comprises nearly one-third of the volume, describes the basic biochemistry, clinical significance, and methods of analysis for a broad range of biochemical analytes. These analytes are then correlated to the pathophysiology of each of the major organ systems in the fifth section. The final section provides reference information, therapeutic and toxic levels of drugs, and critical values. Despite its comprehensive nature, the book remains highly readable through the use of plentiful black-and-white and two-tone illustrations, line drawings, and tables. The chapters open with a list of objectives and key words with definitions. Review questions are provided in the appendix, followed by a glossary and index. Online materials for instructors and students serve as ancillaries, making this resource one of the most highly respected in the field.

Urinalysis and Body Fluids. 5th ed. Authors: Susan K. Strasinger, Marjorie S. DiLorenzo. F.A. Davis, 2008.
http://www.r2library.com/
http://extranet.netlibrary.com/TitleSelect/
http://www.ebrary.com/
ISBN: 9780803616974
ISBN: 9781435694040 (Online)
Recommended for: Hospital, Academic Libraries
Brandon/Hill, *Doody's Core Titles* Selection

This lovely book provides comprehensive coverage of the theoretical and practical knowledge needed for the analysis of urine and non-blood body fluids. It opens with a discussion of clinical laboratory safety and normal renal function, followed by five chapters that cover the physical, chemical, and microscopic analysis of urine. Abundant tables highlight the procedures, interpretation, and clinical significance of the various tests that comprise a complete urinalysis. The most commonly encountered renal diseases and select metabolic disorders are discussed next in the context of urinalysis and other laboratory testing. The remaining six chapters are devoted to the analysis of other body fluids, including cerebrospinal fluid, semen, synovial fluid, serous fluids, amniotic fluid, and fecal analysis. In designing the book, the authors, both clinical laboratory science educators, have achieved the perfect balance between informative text and supporting graphics. The layout of the book is eminently appealing, with subtle but effective use of formatting, color images, tables, and drawings. The photomicrographs of urinary sediment and normal and pathologic cells of CSF and other body fluids are exemplary in terms of quality and clarity. Each chapter opens with learning objectives and key terms and then closes with a list of references, study questions, and case studies. Appendixes include a discussion of urinalysis automation and answers to study questions, and the book ends with a glossary and index. The superb quality and value of this book will no doubt earn it a prominent place on the bench of many practicing technologists.

Journals

Clinical Laboratory Science. v. 1, American Society for Clinical Laboratory Science, 1988.
http://www.ascls.org/leadership/cls/index.asp
http://ejournals.ebsco.com/direct.asp?JournalID=113968
ISSN: 0894959X
Indexed in: MEDLINE, CINAHL
Recommended for: Hospital, Academic Libraries
Brandon/Hill Selection

This is the official publication of the American Society for Clinical Laboratory Science (ASCLS), the professional organization for clinical laboratory scientists in the United States. Published quarterly, it is a peer-reviewed, scholarly/academic journal that covers all subspecialties of the discipline. The journal was started in 1988 as a continuation of the *Journal of Medical Technology*. Articles range from the very practical to the theoretical. The "Dialogue and Discussion" column provides updates on domestic legislation and regulations related to the clinical laboratory, as well as occasional editorials. The "Clinical Practice" section covers topics of practical importance, including case studies, reports, articles, and reviews of books, computer programs, and similar materials. The "Research and Reports" section offers articles describing original research, as well as literature reviews and reports about new technological developments. Finally, the "Focus" section provides a series of articles on specific topics, which offer continuing education credits. The publication has a straightforward, scholarly appearance, and articles are abundantly referenced. It contains minimal advertising, which is mostly related to Society activities. The editorial board is comprised of an editor-in-chief and three section editors, who are registered with either the National Credentialing Agency for Laboratory Personnel (NCL) or the American Society for Clinical Pathology (ASCP), plus seven contributing editors and a substantial review board. The journal is indexed in MEDLINE, CINAHL, Scopus, and other databases. Individual ASCLS members receive a subscription to the journal as a society benefit.

Laboratory Medicine. v. 1, ASCP, 1970.
http://labmed.ascpjournals.org/
ISSN: 00075027
ISSN: 19437730 (Online)
Indexed in: CINAHL
Recommended for: Hospital, Academic Libraries
Brandon/Hill Selection

Laboratory Medicine, which is also known as *LABMEDICINE*, is a monthly, peer-reviewed journal for laboratory professionals published by the American Society for Clinical Pathology (ASCP). Its general purpose is to provide "continuing education, career development, and new technologies to the laboratory community." Started in 1970, it was formed as a result of the merger of the *Bulletin of Pathology* and the *Technical Bulletin of the Registry of Medical Technologists*. Various article types, which rotate from one issue to the next, include a cover story or feature article, review articles, special reports, case studies and rounds reports, and original research articles. Articles frequently contain lengthy lists of references. Topics of monthly columns include image quizzes, quality control, standards and guidelines, laboratory management, continuing education, historical biographies, new products, and book and media reviews. The journal makes liberal use of color, both within the articles and in the plentiful advertisements. *Laboratory Medicine* is indexed by CINAHL, Academic Search Premier, Embase, Scopus, and other databases. Subscriptions are included with annual ASCP memberships and may be purchased by individual non-members and institutions.

1.6. Radiologic Technology

The application of scientific knowledge or technology to the field of radiology. The applications center mostly around x-ray or radioisotopes for diagnostic and therapeutic purposes but the technological applications of any radiation or radiologic procedure is within the scope of radiologic technology.

—MeSH: Technology, Radiologic

Contributor: Carol L. Watwood

Monographs

Comprehensive Radiographic Pathology. 4th ed. Authors: Ronald L. Eisenberg, Nancy M. Johnson. Mosby Elsevier, 2007.
ISBN: 9780323036245
Recommended for: Hospital, Academic Libraries
Doody's Core Titles Selection

Selected by *Doody's* as a core title in radiologic technology, this best seller is the product of a collaboration between a radiologist and radiologic technologist who "concentrate on the radiographic appearance of diseases and injuries that are most likely to be diagnosed with medical imaging." Material is organized by body system and is illustrated using multiple imaging modalities; treatment is also discussed. The book includes summary tables; word prefixes, suffixes, and roots; laboratory tests; and review questions. It is useful as "a student text and a quick review for practicing professionals." The book's binding could be improved as some readers have noted that the pages fall out easily. *Comprehensive Radiographic Pathology* is recommended for hospital, undergraduate, or community college libraries serving radiologic technology students.

Essentials of Dental Radiography for Dental Assistants and Hygienists. 9th ed. Authors: Evelyn M. Thomson, Orlen N. Johnson. Pearson Prentice Hall, 2012.
See Chapter 1.8. Dental Auxiliaries

Merrill's Atlas of Radiographic Positioning & Procedures. 11th ed. Authors: Eugene D. Frank, Bruce W. Long, Barbara J. Smith. Mosby Elsevier, 2007.
ISBN: 9780323033176
Recommended for: Hospital, Academic Libraries
Brandon/Hill, *Doody's Core Titles* Selection

This three-volume set was named for Vinita Merrill, who wrote the first edition in 1949. The classic encyclopedic reference includes more than 400 projections and covers the full range of commonly performed procedures and the practice of radiologic technologists. Normal and pathologic findings are shown. Projections are accompanied by photographs and color diagrams, allowing students to perfect their positioning skills. Various chapters cover bone groups, body parts, anatomy, filters, body systems, and imaging modalities, which include mobile and surgical radiography, CT, MRI, ultrasound, nuclear medicine, bone densitometry, and radiation oncology. The *Atlas* is accompanied by an instructor's website and Mosby's Radiography Online, a companion website with animations and interactive activities. It was selected as a 2003 Brandon/Hill allied health initial purchase title and a *Doody's Core Titles* suggestion. This set is recommended for academic, hospital, and departmental libraries serving radiologic technologists and radiologic technology students.

MRI in Practice. 3rd ed. Authors: Catherine Westbrook, Carolyn K. Roth. Blackwell, 2005.
ISBN: 9781405127875
Recommended for: Hospital, Academic Libraries

According to the publisher, this text and reference book for radiologists and radiologic technologists aims for a "middle ground between simple and complicated texts." It prepares readers for the advanced level MRI examination of the ARRT (American Registry of Radiologic Technologists). Analogies relate complex subjects to everyday phenomena. This book describes MRI instrumentation, principles, pulse sequences, image acquisition, and imaging parameters. This book is suitable for hospital, undergraduate, and community college libraries supporting radiography students specializing in MRI.

Nuclear Medicine and PET/CT: Technology and Techniques. 6th ed. Editors: Paul E. Christian, Kristen M. Waterstram-Rich. Mosby Elsevier, 2007.
ISBN: 9780323043953
ISBN: 9780323061322
Recommended for: Hospital, Academic Libraries
Brandon/Hill, *Doody's Core Titles* Selection

This is a textbook for nuclear medicine technologists; this specialized area of practice uses radioactive isotopes to diagnose and treat disease. It was chosen as a Brandon/Hill allied health initial-purchase selection and a *Doody's Core Titles* selection. It includes mathematics, physics, instrumentation, computer and laboratory science, chapters on various body systems and special topics, a table of radiopharmaceuticals, and a glossary. In addition to the print textbook, individuals may also purchase the publisher's combined text and e-book package. This book is recommended for hospital and academic libraries serving nuclear medicine technology students.

Patient Care in Radiography, with an Introduction to Medical Imaging. 7th ed. Authors: Ruth A. Ehrlich, Joan A. Daly. Mosby Elsevier, 2009.
ISBN: 9780323051781
ISBN: 9780323063258
Recommended for: Hospital, Academic Libraries
Doody's Core Titles Selection

This is a *Doody's* core title. As a student text following ASRT (American Society of Radiologic Technologists) curriculum guidelines, it covers professional roles, behavior, standards, organizations, patient assessment, care, transfer, safety, medications, GI tract exam care, and other topics. It includes appendixes addressing topics such as informed consent and infection control procedures. The publisher provides a print textbook and e-book package option for individual purchase. Lippincott Williams & Wilkins offers a similar publication, *Patient Care in Imaging Technology* (Torres, Dutton, and Linn-Watson, 2009, ISBN: 9780781771832), which is also well reviewed and widely used. *Patient Care in Radiography* is recommended for academic and hospital libraries serving student radiographers.

***Principles and Practice of Radiation Therapy*.** 3rd ed. Editors: Charles M. Washington, Dennis T. Leaver. Mosby Elsevier, 2010.
ISBN: 9780323053624
ISBN: 9780323066761
Recommended for: Hospital, Academic Libraries
Doody's Core Titles Selection

Radiation therapists produced this *Doody's* essential purchase title for radiation therapy students and practitioners. Other contributors represent a range of occupations. Chapters include learning objectives, summaries, review problems, and critical thinking questions. The book provides an overview of cancer and radiobiology, ethics, basic principles, physics, anatomy, instrumentation, dosage, practical applications by organ system, and a glossary. The publisher also offers this book to individuals as a combined print textbook and e-book package. It would be useful for hospital and academic libraries serving radiation therapy students and professionals.

***Principles of Radiographic Imaging: An Art and a Science*.** 4th ed. Authors: Richard R. Carlton, Arlene M. Adler. Delmar Cengage Learning, 2006.
ISBN: 9781401871949
Recommended for: Hospital, Academic Libraries
Doody's Core Titles Selection

Principles of Radiographic Imaging is the standard textbook on principles and techniques of radiographic imaging, a required part of the radiologic technology curriculum. According to the publisher, this best-selling title informs readers about "radiographic contrast, density, detail and distortion." It builds from the simple to the complex, beginning with basic principles of physics, mathematics, and radiation science. The book, which is accompanied by a CD-ROM, includes a new section on managing digital images and a glossary. A companion workbook, web tutor, electronic course manager, and instructor's manual are also available. This book is listed by *Doody's* as an essential purchase title. It is recommended for academic and hospital libraries serving radiologic technology students.

***Radiation Protection in Medical Radiography*.** 6th ed. Authors: Mary Alice Statkiewicz-Sherer, Paula J. Visconti, E. Russell Ritenour. Mosby Elsevier, 2011.
ISBN: 9780323066112
Recommended for: Hospital, Academic Libraries
Brandon/Hill, *Doody's Core Titles* Selection

Doody's selected this classic text as a core title for radiologic technology, and the 2003 Brandon/Hill allied health list also recommended it as an initial purchase title. First published in 1983, Mary Alice Statkiewicz-Sherer's text is still the standard work for students on the important topic of radiation protection and biology. Mary Anne Kuk, a 2006 reviewer for *Radiologic Technology*, said it was also an "excellent reference to anyone who works in the radiography profession." According to the publisher, "building from basic to more complex concepts, this book also presents radiation physics, cell structure, effects of radiation on humans at the cellular and systemic levels, regulatory and advisory limits for human exposure to radiation, and the implementation of patient and personnel radiation protection practices." A discussion of radiation protection from radioisotopes is included. The publisher also provides an accompanying workbook, e-text, and instructional website. The book is recommended for college, hospital, and clinical libraries serving radiologic technology students.

***Radiography PREP: Program Review and Exam Prep*.** 5th ed. Author: Dorothy A. Saia. McGraw-Hill Medical, 2009.
http://www.ebrary.com/
http://extranet.netlibrary.com/TitleSelect/
ISBN: 9780071502788
ISBN: 9780071643283
Recommended for: Hospital, Academic Libraries

This best-selling exam review, which received a four-star rating from *Doody's*, is also sold in combination with another volume by Dorothy A. Saia, Lange *Q & A: Radiography Examination*, 7th ed., 2009, ISBN: 9780071508148. The combined set's ISBN is 9780071635813. The author of this program review and examination study guide for the ARRT (American Registry of Radiologic Technologists) is an educator with 35 years experience teaching radiologic technology students. Other print and online study materials may be found on the website of the American Society of Radiologic Technologists, or students may wish to contact their advisers or program directors for additional review materials. This study guide will be a popular addition for hospital or academic libraries supporting radiologic technology students, perhaps for the reference or reserve collections. Outdated editions should be discarded since radiologic technology changes rapidly.

***Radiologic Science for Technologists: Physics, Biology and Protection*.** 9th ed. Author: Stewart C. Bushong. Mosby Elsevier, 2008.
ISBN: 9780323048378
Recommended for: Hospital, Academic Libraries
Brandon/Hill, *Doody's Core Titles* Selection

Stewart Bushong's *Radiologic Science for Technologists* is the standard textbook on the physics, mathematics, and underlying principles of radiography for radiologic technology students who are preparing for part of the ARRT (American Registry of Radiologic Technologists) examination. *Doody's* lists this book as an essential purchase title, and the seventh edition appeared on the final 2003 Brandon/Hill allied health list as an initial purchase item. The book's end sheets provide quick-reference information. Important math information and key concepts are highlighted in boxes. According to the publisher, each chapter has "objectives, key terms, outlines, introductions, and summaries," and different types of review questions follow each chapter. An accompanying workbook is available. Some users say the mathematical examples have too many mistakes and misprints, but, with little competition, this perennial best seller is still widely used and read. This book is recommended for academic and hospital libraries.

Textbook of Diagnostic Ultrasonography. 6th ed. Author: Sandra L. Hagen-Ansert. Mosby Elsevier, 2006.
ISBN: 9780323028035
Recommended for: Hospital, Academic Libraries
Brandon/Hill, *Doody's Core Titles* Selection

Included in *Doody's Core Titles*, this popular, two-volume textbook/reference book contains nearly 800 images visualizing soft-tissue structures examined by sonographers. An icon highlights sonographic findings for different procedures; attractive photographs and color diagrams further highlight and explain anatomic structures. The first volume covers general principles and protocols, the abdomen, superficial structures, and pediatrics. The second volume is devoted to cardiovascular, obstetric, and gynecologic sonography. Each chapter begins with learning objectives and includes glossaries, tables, and a selected bibliography. An accompanying workbook and web resources are also available. This set is suitable for hospital and academic libraries serving student and practicing sonographers.

Textbook of Radiographic Positioning and Related Anatomy. 7th ed. Authors: Kenneth L. Bontrager, John P. Lampignano. Mosby Elsevier, 2009.
ISBN: 9780323054102
Recommended for: Hospital, Academic Libraries
Brandon/Hill, *Doody's Core Titles* Selection

This textbook of radiographic anatomy and positioning contains essential information for all radiography students. It is one of the best-known and most widely respected radiography textbooks. Each positioning page has a title bar and is laid out clearly and attractively in a "show and tell" format that displays each procedure, gives summary information, and helps students understand why each procedure is performed. The information includes an anatomy overview and common pathologic findings. The book is organized by body areas and imaging modalities; it includes over 200 commonly used projections. It is a Brandon/Hill allied health initial purchase and *Doody's* core title. This publication is recommended for academic and hospital libraries serving radiography students.

Journals

Applied Radiology: the Journal of Practical Medical Imaging and Management. v. 5, no. 4, Anderson, 1976.
http://www.appliedradiology.com/
ISSN: 01609963
Indexed in: CINAHL
Recommended for: Hospital, Academic Libraries
Brandon/Hill Selection

Indexed in CINAHL, this practice-oriented journal targets radiologists and radiologic technologists. It has a physician editorial board. The *Applied Radiology* website includes continuing medical education, job advertisements, news, a message board, and discussion groups. Articles cover diagnostic radiology, radiation therapy, CT, ultrasound, thermography, MRI, and nuclear medicine. The journal, known as *Applied Radiology and Nuclear Medicine* from 1975–1976, is free to AMA members registered in appropriate specialties. The online content is available to professionals registering on the journal's website and through CINAHL with full text. This title is appropriate for clinically oriented collections serving students or practicing radiologists and radiologic technologists.

Journal of Diagnostic Medical Sonography. v. 1, Sage/Society of Medical Diagnostic Sonography, 1985.
http://jdm.sagepub.com/
ISSN: 87564793
ISSN: 15525430 (Online)
Indexed in: CINAHL
Recommended for: Hospital, Academic Libraries
Brandon/Hill Selection

This bimonthly title is a 2003 Brandon/Hill allied health initial purchase selection for the diagnostic medical sonography category. It is published by Sage on behalf of the Society of Medical Diagnostic Sonography and is provided as a free benefit to members. It is indexed in various sources such as CINAHL and Scopus. Continuing medical education (CME) and book reviews are included. Articles cover all aspects of the allied health field of diagnostic medical sonography, which refers to the use of sound waves to diagnose and assess health conditions in various parts of the body. Articles include topics such as case reports, image interpretation, imaging techniques, cost effectiveness, safety, equipment, contrast agents, and occupational issues. This title is suitable for libraries supporting diagnostic medical sonography educational programs and may be useful for specialized collections in large hospitals or clinics.

Journal of Medical Imaging and Radiation Sciences. v. 39, Elsevier, 2008.
http://www.jmirs.org/home
http://www.sciencedirect.com/science/journal/19398654
ISSN: 19398654
Indexed in: CINAHL
Recommended for: Hospital, Academic Libraries
Brandon/Hill Selection

This journal, which began in 1943, has had several previous titles, most recently *Canadian Journal of Medical Radiation Technology*, ISSN 19872007. The former title appeared in the 2003 Brandon/Hill allied health list. This peer-reviewed publication is the official journal of the Canadian Association of Medical Radiation Technologists. According to the publisher, articles include "recent research, new technology and techniques, professional practices, as well as relevant book reviews." Most articles are practice oriented. The journal has limited indexing, currently indexed in Embase and CINAHL and formerly indexed in MEDLINE. It is suitable for large, specialized collections.

Journal of Nuclear Medicine Technology. v. 1, Society of Nuclear Medicine, 1973.
http://tech.snmjournals.org/
ISSN: 00914916
ISSN: 15355675 (Online)
Indexed in: MEDLINE, CINAHL
Recommended for: Hospital, Academic Libraries
Brandon/Hill Selection

This quarterly, peer-reviewed journal was listed in the 2003 Brandon/Hill allied health list as an initial purchase title for the nuclear medicine technology category. It is indexed in CINAHL and MEDLINE. The journal includes practice-oriented articles for nuclear medicine technologists, who are allied health professionals trained in the technology of using radionuclides to diagnose and treat disease. Articles discuss "imaging and instrumentation, radiopharmacy, quality assurance, radiation safety, and more." Continuing education is a major focus. The technologist section of the Society of Nuclear Medicine publishes this journal, and Society members receive the journal as a benefit. It is appropriate for large hospital and clinical libraries dealing with this specialized field and for libraries supporting educational programs in nuclear medicine technology. All journal articles are freely available on HighWire, the Society's host platform, after a twelve-month embargo period.

Radiologic Technology. v. 35, American Society of Radiologic Technologists, 1963.
http://www.radiologictechnology.org/
ISSN: 00338397
ISSN: 19435657 (Online)
Indexed in: MEDLINE, CINAHL
Recommended for: Hospital, Academic Libraries
Brandon/Hill Selection

Originally titled *X-ray Technician*, this peer-reviewed, bimonthly publication is the largest and oldest journal for radiologic technologists. It is indexed by CINAHL, Scopus, and MEDLINE. It was also a 2003 Brandon/Hill allied health, initial purchase recommendation. It is published by the American Society of Radiologic Technologists, and members have free access to the online journal. *Radiologic Technology* "covers all disciplines and specialties within medical imaging, including radiography, mammography, computed tomography, magnetic resonance imaging, nuclear medicine imaging, sonography, and cardiovascular-interventional radiography." The journal includes a variety of research, teaching, and practice-oriented articles, along with CE and book and literature reviews. This publication is probably the top journal devoted specifically to radiologic technology, but research has shown that authors in this field make extensive use of the literature of radiology and other areas of clinical medicine. In a study of citation patterns in three radiologic technology journals, *Radiologic Technology* was the sixth most frequently cited title. The top five journals focused on clinical medicine: *Radiology*, *AJR*, *Journal of Nuclear Medicine*, *Journal of Computer Assisted Tomography*, and *AJNR*. (Burnham J. *Bull Med Lib Assoc* 1997; 85(3):289–292). The publication would be useful for libraries supporting radiologic technology and for large hospital and clinical libraries.

Radiology Today. v. 1, Great Valley, 2000.
http://www.radiologytoday.net
ISSN: 15390101
Recommended for: Hospital, Academic Libraries

Radiology Today is a free, current awareness magazine for radiologists and radiologic technologists. It includes practice-oriented articles, news, jobs, meetings, a vendors' guide, podcasts, and a blog. It contains newsworthy information for libraries serving students or clinicians in the imaging professions, especially those with limited resources.

1.7. Respiratory Therapy

Care of patients with deficiencies and abnormalities associated with the cardiopulmonary system. It includes the therapeutic use of medical gases and their administrative apparatus, environmental control systems, humidification, aerosols, ventilatory support, bronchopulmonary drainage and exercise, respiratory rehabilitation, assistance with cardiopulmonary resuscitation, and maintenance of natural, artificial, and mechanical airways.

—MeSH

Contributor: Lisa Huang

Monographs

Cardiopulmonary Anatomy & Physiology: Essentials for Respiratory Care. 5th ed. Author: Terry R. Des Jardins. Thomson Delmar Learning, 2008.
http://www.r2library.com/
ISBN: 9781418042783
Recommended for: Academic Libraries
Brandon/Hill, *Doody's Core Titles* Selection

This updated Brandon/Hill allied health title and *Doody's Core Titles* selection is by a well-recognized expert in the field. Des Jardins succinctly guides the student through the structure and functions of the respiratory system. The new edition is well organized and accessible to its intended audience, respiratory therapy students. It is organized into three sections: cardiopulmonary system; advanced cardiopulmonary essentials; and the cardiopulmonary system during unusual environmental conditions. Each chapter is concisely laid out with objectives, new terms, a summary with review questions at the end as well as numerous illustrations, tables, and graphs. This new edition includes over 70 new and revised illustrations; a new chapter on sleep physiology; restructured chapters on oxygen transport, carbon dioxide transport, and acid-base balance; as well as expanded clinical scenarios. Of special interest to students is the StudyWare software on the accompanying CD-ROM, which includes case studies, quizzes, and learning games to facilitate learning. This book is highly recommended for academic institutions supporting respiratory therapy students, practitioners, and educators.

Clinical Application of Mechanical Ventilation. 3rd ed. Author: David W. Chang. Thomson Delmar Learning, 2006.
ISBN: 9781401884857
Recommended for: Academic Libraries
Doody's Core Titles Selection

A *Doody's Core Titles* selection, Chang's textbook integrates the essential concepts of respiratory physiology with the clinical application of mechanical ventilation. Chang provides the latest updates on innovations, changing techniques, and clinical applications of mechanical ventilation, airways, airway management, and hemodynamic monitoring. The book covers airway management and weaning criteria as well as pharmacotherapy for mechanical ventilation. The chapters are well laid out with visual examples, key points and terms, and assessment questions in NBRC format for future exams. The last chapter contains 15 case studies for students to exercise real-world critical situations. The appendixes nicely supplement the textbook; students will find the respiratory care calculations, pressure conversions, and hemodynamic and oxygen transport ranges to be quite helpful. The book's main strength is Chang's comprehensiveness in covering all aspects of mechanical ventilation. This authoritative title is highly recommended as a required resource for academic institutions supporting respiratory therapy students, practitioners, and educators.

Clinical Assessment in Respiratory Care. 6th ed. Editors: Robert L. Wilkins, James R. Dexter, Albert J. Heuer. Mosby Elsevier, 2010.
ISBN: 9781416059233
Recommended for: Academic Libraries
Brandon/Hill, *Doody's Core Titles* Selection

Now in its sixth edition, this is "the" book for respiratory care assessment. In fact, it is the only respiratory care textbook devoted exclusively to patient assessment. This comprehensive title covers the gamut of assessment from the detailed Chapter 1, "Preparing for the Patient Encounter" to "Documentation" with a streamlined learning format and useful "Ask About" questions. The sixth edition includes a new chapter on neurological assessment and procedure checklists for common assessment procedures in the appendix. Expanded content for individual purchasers is on the Evolve website, including the new *NBRC Exam Matrix Correlation Guide* to help students pass the CRT exam and additional case studies. This book is a Brandon/Hill allied health title selection and is highly recommended for academic institutions supporting respiratory therapy students, practitioners, and educators.

Clinical Manifestations and Assessment of Respiratory Disease. 6th ed. Authors: Terry R. Des Jardins, George G. Burton. Mosby/Elsevier, 2011.
ISBN: 9780323057271
Recommended for: Hospital, Academic Libraries

In this updated edition, Des Jardins and Burton reveal the standards for correctly identifying and assessing respiratory diseases and disorders in line with implementing therapist-driven protocols (TDPs). They describe how to systematically gather clinical data, formulate an assessment, make an objective evaluation, identify the desired outcome, and design a safe and effective treatment plan, while documenting each step along the way, for common respiratory diseases and disorders. The anatomy, etiology, clinical manifestations, and treatment for each disease or disorder are concisely discussed in a systematic manner. This new edition has been vibrantly enhanced with a full color design, overviews, and 15 additional case studies with answers on the companion Evolve website. The book is student friendly with its format separated into 11 parts, allowing for easy searching. This book is highly recommended for a hospital library collection and for academic institutions supporting respiratory therapy students, practitioners, and educators.

Comprehensive Respiratory Therapist Exam Review: Entry and Advanced Level. 5th ed. Authors: James R. Sills. Mosby Elsevier, 2010.
ISBN: 9780323067010
Recommended for: Academic Libraries

Sills authored this versatile text to help respiratory therapy students prepare for their CRT and RRT exams. The text includes the 2009 National Board of Respiratory Care content outlines. It provides coverage of all subject areas such as CPAP/BiPAP titration during sleep, hemodynamic monitoring, hyperinflation therapy, laryngeal mask airway, high frequency ventilation, oxygen titration, thoracentesis, ultrasound, and ventilator-associated pneumonia protocols as well as plentiful self assessment questions and study hints. The companion CD and Evolve website offers pre- and post-testing with realistic practice for the entry-level certification exam and the advanced-level Written Registry Exam (WRE) and Clinical Simulation Exam (CSE). Other useful features are the question randomizing feature in which each practice test is different and has the same number of questions as the actual exam. The strengths of this text are its practical approach (covering both exams) and its supporting resources for respiratory therapy students preparing for the CRT and RRT exams. This should be a required resource for academic institutions supporting respiratory therapy programs.

Egan's Fundamentals of Respiratory Care. 9th ed. Editors: Robert L. Wilkins, James K. Stoller, Robert M. Kacmarek. Mosby/Elsevier, 2009.
ISBN: 9780323036573
Recommended for: Hospital, Academic Libraries
Brandon/Hill, *Doody's Core Titles* Selection

The bible of respiratory therapy textbooks for over 40 years, this best-selling, comprehensive textbook is a Brandon/Hill allied health initial-purchase selection and a *Doody's Core Titles* pick. New editor, Robert Kacmarek, co-author of *Essentials of Respiratory Care*, joins Robert Wilkins and James Stoller in discussing the art and science of being a successful respiratory therapist. The authors focus on promoting a thorough understanding of the role of respiratory therapists (RTs), a scientific basis for treatment, and clinical applications. In-depth discussions progress from the principles of respiratory care to applied anatomy and physiology, assessment, discussion of specific respiratory illnesses, basic therapy, acute and critical care, and preventive and long-term care. Clinical Practice Guidelines (CPGs) and Therapist Driven Protocols (TDPs) in appropriate chapters familiarize the novice with patient care guidelines and decision trees as they are used in practice. The book, divided into seven sections, is easily accessible with a full-color format, bulleted key point summaries, and rules of thumb highlights. Some of the new content in the ninth edition includes updates on HIPAA, expanded coverage of evidence-based care, and nutritional impacts on the respiratory system. The appendixes are helpful for students preparing for the CRT and RRT exams. This authoritative title is highly recommended for academic institutions supporting respiratory therapy students, practitioners, and educators. This text should also be a required resource for any hospital collection.

Manual of Pulmonary Function Testing. 9th ed. Author: Gregg L. Ruppel. Mosby Elsevier, 2009.
ISBN: 9780323052122
Recommended for: Hospital, Academic Libraries
Brandon/Hill Selection

Ruppel has established his text as the reference for anyone interested in the rationale and procedures for pulmonary functioning testing. The updated edition contains in-depth information on the tests used to determine the presence, extent, and progression of lung disease and abnormality in revealing conditions including asthma, chronic bronchitis, emphysema, and cystic fibrosis. Ruppel has expanded the chapters on cardiopulmonary exercise testing, specialized test regimens, and pulmonary function testing equipment, as well as case studies and self assessment questions. The latest practice guidelines and standards from the American Thoracic Society/European Respiratory Society (ATS/ERS) and the American Thoracic Society/American College of Chest Physicians (ATS/ACCP) are incorporated throughout the text. Each chapter is concisely organized and accessible to the reader. The detailed appendixes on equations, calculations, and self assessment answers will be extremely useful for the student entering the lab or the therapist needing a reference text. This well-researched text is beneficial for anyone pursuing the Certified Pulmonary Function Technologist (CFPT) exam. This book was selected as a Brandon/Hill allied health initial purchase and is highly recommended as a required resource for academic institutions supporting respiratory therapy students, practitioners, and educators and for any hospital library collection.

Mosby's Respiratory Care Equipment. 8th ed. Editors: Jimmy M. Cairo, Susan P. Pilbeam. Mosby/Elsevier, 2010.
ISBN: 9780323051767
Recommended for: Academic Libraries
Brandon/Hill, *Doody's Core Titles* Selection

An update of the previous 2002 edition, editors Cairo and Pilbeam review the latest techniques and equipment used in respiratory therapy. The new edition includes the latest on general use devices with an emphasis on transport, home-care, and alternative ventilators; the chapter on infection control issues in mass casualty situations has been updated. Each chapter has been well organized with outlines, learning objectives, and key terms; students will find the NBRC style questions useful in preparing for exams. Additional resources such as websites and review materials are supported by the Evolve Student Resource. The strength of this book is its vast clinical applications to respiratory equipment; Cairo and Pilbeam provide their in-depth clinical knowledge and expertise in utilizing the equipment in respiratory settings. Students will find this text to be a very practical aid in their clinical studies. This book, a Brandon/Hill allied health initial purchase and a *Doody's Core Titles* selection, is highly recommended for academic institutions supporting respiratory therapy students, practitioners, and educators.

Perinatal and Pediatric Respiratory Care. 3rd ed. Editors: Brian K. Walsh, Michael P. Czervinske, Robert M. DiBlasi. Saunders/Elsevier, 2010.
ISBN: 9781416024484
Recommended for: Hospital, Academic Libraries

Czervinske has added two new editors to this updated textbook, offering the latest advances and most complete respiratory care theory and clinical application for neonates, infants, and pediatric patients. This edition includes a new chapter on pediatric thoracic trauma and a companion Evolve student website for additional supplementary resources. This new text is a vast improvement from the previous 2002 edition. Its efficient chapter organization, vibrant visuals, and useful assessment NBRC-style questions, make it a user friendly reference tool for students and practitioners. Students and practitioners will find the text helpful when preparing for the NBRC neonatal/pediatric specialty exam. Each chapter includes learning objectives that break down key concepts into measurable behaviors, criteria, and conditions. As in previous editions, the text emphasizes clinical application of respiratory medicine in perinatal and pediatric medicine. This textbook is highly recommended for academic institutions supporting respiratory therapy students, practitioners, and educators and should be a required resource for a hospital library.

Rau's Respiratory Care Pharmacology. 7th ed. Authors: Douglas S. Gardenhire, Joseph L. Rau. Mosby Elsevier, 2008.
ISBN: 9780323032025
Recommended for: Hospital, Academic Libraries
Brandon/Hill, *Doody's Core Titles* Selection

After over 30 years, this classic title on respiratory care pharmacology for respiratory therapy students and practitioners needing a review has a new author. Gardenhire was handpicked by Joseph Rau. Gardenhire has thoroughly updated and revised the text with a full-color design and highlighted learning objectives, key terms, and key points, in addition to an expanded glossary and a list of helpful websites. The book is well organized and accessible to readers. This authoritative text reflects the current state of respiratory pharmacology. The book is divided into three units on basic concepts and principles in pharmacology, drugs used to treat the respiratory system, and critical care and cardiovascular drug classes. Units are further divided into thematic chapters, and each chapter concludes with a clinical scenario and multiple self-assessment questions. The appendixes contain answers to assessment questions and clinical scenarios, units and systems of measurement, recommendations on the use of aerosol generators, and pharmacological management of asthma and chronic obstructive pulmonary disease. This book is highly recommended for academic institutions supporting respiratory therapy students, practitioners, and educators and for hospital library collections. The book is also a Brandon/Hill allied health list selection and on the *Doody's Core Titles* list.

Respiratory Physiology: The Essentials. 8th ed. Author: John B. West. Lippincott Williams & Wilkins, 2008.
See Chapter 10.10.8. Pulmonary Disease, Chapter 29. Physiology

Journals

American Journal of Respiratory and Critical Care Medicine (AJRCCM). v. 149, American Thoracic Society, 1994.
http://ajrccm.atsjournals.org/
ISSN: 1073449X
ISSN: 15354970 (Online)
See Also Chapter 10.10.8. Pulmonary Disease
Indexed in: MEDLINE, CINAHL
Recommended for: Hospital, Academic Libraries

This journal was first published in March 1917 as the *American Review of Tuberculosis*. Since then the title has changed several times until 1994, when it became the *American Journal of Respiratory and Critical Care Medicine*. It is the official journal of the American Thoracic Society and is published semi-monthly. The journal focuses on human biology and disease, as well as animal and in vitro studies related to the pathophysiology and treatment of respiratory disease and critical care conditions. The intended audience is respiratory and critical care clinicians and health professionals. This peer-reviewed journal and has an international scope. In addition to original research articles, the journal publishes state-of-the-art review articles, perspectives, case reports, and commentaries between readers. The journal is indexed by numerous abstracting and indexing sources such as CAB Abstracts, CINAHL, Embase, MEDLINE, Scopus, and Web of Science. Its *Journal Citation Reports* impact factor for 2009 is 10.689. This journal is a required resource for academic institutions supporting respiratory therapy students, practitioners, and educators and for hospital libraries supporting critical care departments and researchers. Full online coverage back to 1997 is available at HighWire Press.

Chest. v. 57, American College of Chest Physicians, 1970.
http://chestjournal.chestpubs.org
ISSN: 00123692
ISSN: 19313543 (Online)
See Also Chapter 10.10.8. Pulmonary Disease
Indexed in: MEDLINE, CINAHL
Recommended for: Hospital, Academic Libraries

This peer-reviewed journal is the official publication of the American College of Chest Physicians (ACCP). Published monthly, it features original research articles that cover the many specialty areas of chest medicine. The intended audience is clinicians and non-physician specialists and researchers involved in cardiopulmonary and critical care medicine. In addition to original research articles, journal issues include contemporary review articles, recent advances, and commentaries in correspondence. The online version offers readers multimedia features such as physiology grand rounds and procedure videos. This journal's *Journal Citation Reports* 2009 impact factor was 6.36 and it ranked third among 43 respiratory journals. The journal is indexed in numerous abstracting and indexing sources including CAB Abstracts, CINAHL, Embase, MEDLINE, Scopus, and Web of Science. This journal is highly recommended for all hospital libraries and any academic institution supporting respiratory therapy programs, practitioners, and educators. Full online coverage back to 1970 is available through HighWire Press.

Respiratory Care. v. 16, Daedalus Enterprises for The American Association for Respiratory Care, 1971.
http://rcjournal.com
ISSN: 19433654 (Online)
See Also Chapter 10.10.8. Pulmonary Disease
Indexed in: MEDLINE, CINAHL
Recommended for: Hospital, Academic Libraries
Brandon/Hill Selection

Begun in 1956 (as *Inhalation Therapy*) and a Brandon/Hill allied health journal selection, *Respiratory Care* is the official science journal of the American Association for Respiratory Care (AARC). It provides current information on the care of patients with respiratory diseases/disorders, applied clinical pulmonary medicine, respiratory-related critical care, rehabilitation, and home care. It is also the only peer-reviewed scientific publication dedicated specifically and exclusively to respiratory care. In addition to original, peer-reviewed research articles, the journal publishes review articles, case reports, teaching case, reviews, and commentaries. It promotes research studies in respiratory care and attempts to keep its readers aware of the rapid technological advances in respiratory care equipment and devices. This journal is indexed in several indexing and abstracting sources including CINAHL, Embase, MEDLINE, Scopus, and Web of Science. This journal is a required resource for academic institutions supporting respiratory therapy students, practitioners, and educators and for hospital libraries. Full online coverage back to volume 1, number 1, 1956, is available through EBSCOhost EJS and back to 1990 on the journal website.

1.8. Dental Auxiliaries

Personnel whose work is prescribed and supervised by the dentist. Includes assistants, hygienists, technicians and denturists.

—MeSH

Contributor: Jonathan Potter

Monographs

Clinical Practice of the Dental Hygienist. 10th ed. Editor: Esther M. Wilkins. Wolters Kluwer/Lippincott Williams & Wilkins, 2009.
ISBN: 9780781763226
Recommended for: Academic Libraries
Doody's Core Titles Selection

A *Doody's* core title with a long and venerable publication history dating back to 1959, this text is often cited with such superlatives as "cornerstone," "gold standard," and "bible" of dental hygiene. The book is arranged in eight sections, beginning with two sections that provide an orientation and overview of dental hygiene practice, followed by five sections that correspond to the dental hygiene process of care: assess, diagnose, plan, implement, and evaluate. The concluding section covers 22 different categories of special-needs patients. Each section begins with an outline of the process of care, highlighting the step or steps covered, as well as a brief summary of the ethical applications relevant to the section. The text is rife with illustrations, usually in color, and tables or pop-outs listing key words or ethical concerns ("Everyday Ethics"). Five appendixes provide American, Canadian, and international codes of ethics; infection control guidelines; and a table of average tooth measurements. The index is thorough, with many subtopics and cross-references. A supplemental CD-ROM includes seven video clips illustrating a variety of techniques, an NCLEX test review and practice test, and audio pronunciations of select clinical terms. Single-user access to ThePoint website provides additional resources for instructors, including PowerPoint slides and lecture notes. This book should be at the very top of the list of core titles for any collection supporting a dental hygiene program or clinical practice.

Dental Assisting: A Comprehensive Approach. 3rd ed. Authors: Donna J. Phinney, Judy H. Halstead. Thomson Delmar Learning, 2008.
http://www.r2library.com/
ISBN: 9781418048730
Recommended for: Academic Libraries
Brandon/Hill Selection

At over 1,000 pages, "comprehensive" accurately describes the scope this expansive text. Designed to be used in conjunction with Delmar's practice software, workbook, exam review, videos, and instructor support materials, the book also stands on its own as a tool for both Dental Assisting National Board (DANB) certification preparation and as a ready reference suitable for the shelf of any dental assistant or library supporting a dental assisting program. Divided into sections covering the fundamentals of dental assisting as well as such related topics as professional communication, cosmetic dentistry, and HIPAA standards, the book can be followed chapter-by-chapter or consulted as needed for a wealth of clearly written, beautifully illustrated, up-to-date information. The third edition builds on the excellence of the first two editions, with a text that is well organized, easy to navigate, and thoughtfully punctuated with color illustrations and real-world clinical examples. The book also includes a CD-ROM with interactive modules that nicely supplement and complement material covered in the book.

Dental Hygiene Theory and Practice. 3rd ed. Editors: Michele Leonardi Darby, Margaret M. Walsh. Saunders Elsevier, 2010.
ISBN: 9781416053576
Recommended for: Academic Libraries
Doody's Core Titles Selection

While similar in scope to Wilkins' more established *Clinical Practice of the Dental Hygienist*, this book, as the title implies, takes a more intentional and sophisticated approach to unifying theory and practice in an evidence-based knowledge framework. As stated in the preface: "Human needs theory serves as a unifying theme" for the various strands of theoretical and practical concerns covered in the book. The book is divided into eight sections and an entire chapter in the first section on conceptual foundations is devoted to human needs theory. The second section covers more practical concerns relating specifically to the client appointment. The middle three sections correspond generally to the process of care for dental hygiene. The final three sections cover pain and anxiety control, individuals with special needs, and practice management, with a concluding chapter on legal and ethical concerns. A lengthy glossary and thorough index complete the volume. Each chapter begins with a bulleted list of competencies to be covered and concludes with an outline of key concepts and critical thinking exercises. The color photographs and other illustrations and tables are elegantly laid out and nicely complement the text. As suggested by its high *Doody's Core Titles* rating, this volume deserves a place alongside Wilkins in any academic or clinical dental hygiene collection.

Essentials of Dental Radiography for Dental Assistants and Hygienists. 9th ed. Authors: Evelyn M. Thomson, Orlen N. Johnson. Pearson Prentice Hall, 2012.
http://www.statref.com/ (8th ed.)
http://www.r2library.com/ (8th ed.)
ISBN: 9780138019396
Recommended for: Academic Libraries
Doody's Core Titles Selection

Radiography is a key area of the health sciences that has been and will continue to be affected by the universal shift to digital technology. This edition of a classic text devotes a chapter to the topic of digital radiography, which is useful but already somewhat outpaced by current technology. In the meantime, the text remains an important resource for dental assistants and hygienists. Logically divided into nine sections that progress from the history of dental radiography to advanced techniques, the book succeeds at clearly and concisely communicating key information for the student. It stresses the connection between theory and practice with case studies and lab activities that apply to both the dental assistant and the dental hygienist. This review refers to the eighth edition.

Foundations of Periodontics for the Dental Hygienist. 3rd ed. Authors: Jill S. Nield-Gehrig, Donald E. Willman. Wolters Kluwer/Lippincott Williams & Wilkins, 2011.
ISBN: 9781605475738
Recommended for: Academic Libraries
Doody's Core Titles Selection

A *Doody's* core title with a rating midway between "very good" and "excellent," the text is divided into seven modules that form a logical and relatively easy-to-follow approach to periodontics, culminating in a section on resources and case studies. Each module is prefaced by an outline of the content along with learning objectives and key terms. The book is well illustrated, although the reader must go to the supplemental CD-ROM for full-color versions of most of the images included only in black and white within the pages of the book. In addition to two full chapters devoted to patient cases, a series of "Focus on Patients" items are scattered throughout the text, providing a catalyst for applying the material to clinical situations. Each chapter also includes a list of suggested readings, highlighting research relevant to an evidence-based approach to periodontology for the dental hygienist. This is an important learning tool for dental hygiene students and a valuable reference for practitioners. This review refers to the second edition.

Oral Pharmacology for the Dental Hygienist. Authors: Mea A. Weinberg, Cheryl Westphal, James Burke Fine. Pearson Prentice Hall, 2008.
http://www.r2library.com/
ISBN: 9780130492869
Recommended for: Academic Libraries

This book is a practical and elegantly straightforward guide to pharmacology from the perspective of the dental hygienist. It is aimed at the student of dental hygiene: each chapter includes a series of review questions to use in preparing for the pharmacology section of the board exam. In light of its accessible approach to the subject, however, this book will also prove to be a handy reference for practicing hygienists and other dental health professionals. Arranged in four sections, the book moves logically, clearly, and concisely from general principles to drugs used in dentistry to drugs used by patients, concluding with a section on special topics, including chapters on oral manifestations of drug reactions and medical emergency drugs in dentistry. The text is supplemented throughout by "Rapid Dental Hints" and "Did You Know?" facts that add interest and value. Each chapter includes a "Dental Hygiene Notes" subsection, highlighting clinical considerations specific to a dental hygiene context. The index, which is of great import for any guide to drugs or pharmacology, is extensive and detailed.

Torres and Ehrlich Modern Dental Assisting. 9th ed. Authors: Doni L. Bird, Debbie S. Robinson. Saunders Elsevier, 2009.
ISBN: 9781416042457
Recommended for: Academic Libraries
Doody's Core Titles Selection

This hefty volume is divided into eleven sections, beginning with historical and scientific overviews of dentistry and continuing with comprehensive coverage of a wide range of competencies for the well-rounded dental assistant. Major sections cover oral health, infection control, occupational health and safety, patient information and assessment, clinical dentistry fundamentals, radiology, dental materials, and administrative skills. Within each section, the arrangement of individual chapters is very student and educator oriented, beginning with key terms and learning outcomes and concluding with summary boxes on patient education, law and ethics, future trends, and critical thinking. Although the volume is daunting in size and scope, it is extremely well-organized and easy to navigate. The glossary and index are functional and easy to use. A supplemental DVD provides videos and animations that further complement the well-illustrated text. An interactive CD-ROM includes case studies and review exercises. This title is included in *Doody's Core Titles* for dental auxiliaries and is additionally designated as an "essential purchase title." It should be included in any academic collection that supports a dental assistant program. The volume would also likely complement a general dentistry or dental hygiene specialized collection.

Journals

Dental Assistant. v. 63, American Dental Assistants Association, 1994.
http://www.dentalassistant.org/
ISSN: 10883886
Indexed in: MEDLINE, CINAHL
Recommended for: Academic Libraries

This official quarterly, peer-reviewed journal of the American Dental Assistants Association (ADAA) has a respected publication history dating back to 1931, albeit with several title changes along the way. The journal focuses on academic and continuing education for dental assistants. It publishes articles covering theoretical, technical and methodological advances, ADAA news, and information on trends in dental assisting education and practice. The journal is indexed by CINAHL and MEDLINE, among many others. Full-text access is available from EBSCOhost, Gale, Health Communication Network, and ProQuest. Although editorials and Association news pieces dominate its pages, the journal also publishes original and significant research. Any collection supporting a dental assisting educational program or practice should include this journal among its subscriptions.

Dimensions of Dental Hygiene. v. 1, Belmont Publications, Inc., 2003.
http://www.dimensionsofdentalhygiene.com
ISSN: 15427838
ISSN: 15427919 (Online)
Indexed in: CINAHL
Recommended for: Academic Libraries

Although this journal describes itself as a peer-reviewed publication, the scope of that label and the review process employed by the journal is not entirely clear. The primary orientation appears to be more that of a trade journal weighted towards the practical concerns of the professional dental hygienist. It is also, in both its online and print versions, somewhat cluttered with advertising and other commercial and product-oriented trappings. The benefit of that commercial element, however, is that subscriptions to the print journal are offered for free from the publisher. The journal's website also provides full-text access to articles going back to the journal's inception in 2003. Additionally, the website provides access to practitioner forums, product reviews, and continuing education modules. Although libraries supporting dental hygiene programs and practitioners might be put off by its commercial veneer, the journal does in fact publish original research, it is indexed in CINAHL, and it boasts an impressive editorial advisory board made up of academics and practitioners from across the U.S. and Canada. For these reasons, as well as being budget-friendly, it earns a place among the core journals for dental auxiliaries.

International Journal of Dental Hygiene. v. 1, Wiley-Blackwell, 2003.
http://onlinelibrary.wiley.com/journal/10.1111/(ISSN)1601-5037
ISSN: 16015029
ISSN: 16015037 (Online)
Indexed in: MEDLINE, CINAHL
Recommended for: Academic Libraries

This is the official, peer-reviewed, quarterly journal of the International Federation of Dental Hygienists (IFDH) and one of only two dental hygiene journals indexed in MEDLINE. In 2009, the journal reported an increase in overall submissions as well as a greater percentage of articles written by practicing dental hygienists, reflecting a growing awareness of the importance of research and evidence-based practice in the field and in the allied health sciences generally. The international character of the journal makes it unique and serves to complement its U.S.-focused counterparts. Articles published in 2008, for example, came from 25 different countries, making this journal a truly international forum with a vibrant array of voices and points of view. The opportunities for intellectual cross-pollination and multi-cultural insights make this an important journal for practitioners, educators, dental hygiene students, and the libraries that support them. Full-text access is available from CASPUR, EBSCOhost, Health Communication Network, Ingenta, OCLC, Ovid, Swets, and Wiley-Blackwell.

Journal of Dental Hygiene. v. 62, American Dental Hygienists' Association, 1988.
http://www.ingentaselect.com/rpsv/cw/www/adha/15530205/
http://www.adha.org/jdh/subscription.htm
ISSN: 1043254X

ISSN: 15530205 (Online)
Indexed in: MEDLINE, CINAHL
Recommended for: Academic Libraries

The *Journal of Dental Hygiene* (*JDH*) is the official, peer-reviewed quarterly publication of the American Dental Hygienists' Association. Like other allied health sciences, dental hygiene has been invigorated in recent years by the evidence-based health care movement. Since 1993, *JDH* has been a primary venue for the association's National Dental Hygiene Research Agenda. In 2009, the journal reported that submissions of original research articles related to dental hygiene education and practice increased more than 100 percent. These positive trends can only reinforce the quality of the publication and its importance for practitioners, educators, and students. The journal transitioned to online-only in 2004, but due to popular demand it reintroduced a paper format in 2008. In 2009, the journal introduced a new feature called "Critical Issues in Dental Hygiene" for in-depth consideration of hot topics in the field. *JDH* is one of only two dental hygiene journals indexed in MEDLINE. Full-text online access is available from EBSCOhost, Gale, Health Communication Network, and Ingenta.

1.9. Physician Assistants

Persons academically trained, licensed, or credentialed to provide medical care under the supervision of a physician. The concept does not include nurses, but does include orthopedic assistants, surgeon's assistants, and assistants to other specialists.

—MeSH

Contributor: David A. Nolfi

Monographs

Danforth's Obstetrics and Gynecology. 10th ed. Editors: Ronald S. Gibbs, Beth Y. Karlan, Arthur F. Haney, Ingrid E. Nygaard. Lippincott Williams & Wilkins, 2008.
http://www.ovid.com/
ISBN: 9780781769372
See Also Chapter 11.4. Obstetrics
Recommended for: Hospital, Academic Libraries
Brandon/Hill, *Doody's Core Titles* Selection

According to the Accreditation Review Commission on Education for the Physician Assistant, obstetrics and gynecology is a required practice experience for all physician assistant students. Additionally, 25 percent of physician assistants work in family practice, and slightly more than 2 percent work specifically in obstetrics and gynecology practice settings (American Association of Physician Assistants, 2009). Thus, a general obstetrics and gynecology textbook is an essential part of a collection supporting practicing physician assistants or students. If *Williams Obstetrics* is the most well-respected general textbook in obstetrics and gynecology, *Danforth's* is perhaps second on the list. It is currently listed as a *Doody's Core Titles* essential purchase and was regularly named to the Brandon/Hill list. *Danforth's* editors specifically aim to create a book for a diverse group of clinicians ranging from attending physicians to residents, medical students, and nurses, which makes it an appropriate selection for physician assistants. The book's 64 chapters are divided roughly between those that focus on obstetric issues and those that focus on other gynecologic issues. Obstetrics chapters cover all major topics such as prenatal diagnosis and care, drugs in pregnancy, fetal diagnosis, complications, labor and delivery problems, and much more. The gynecology chapters deal with age-related issues, surgical methodologies, cancer, office-based gynecology, and surgical procedures. Throughout the book, the editors have taken care to ensure that chapters are well written and approachable. Numerous figures and tables supplement the text, and references in the Books@Ovid electronic version include links to MEDLINE records.

Ethics and Professionalism: A Guide for the Physician Assistant. Editors: Barry A. Cassidy, J. Dennis Blesssing. F.A. Davis, 2008.
http://extranet.netlibrary.com/TitleSelect/
http://www.r2library.com/
http://www.ebrary.com/
ISBN: 9780803613386
ISBN: 9781441604569 (Online)
Recommended for: Academic Libraries

In order to be effective practitioners, physician assistants must have a foundation in medical ethics and an understanding of the application of ethical principles in their unique professional experiences. Although thousands of books have been written about medical and health care ethics, Barry Cassidy and J. Dennis Blessing have created one of the few ethics books written specifically for physician assistants. Given that physician assistants must practice under the supervision of physicians, ethical questions must take into account the relationships and decision-making processes that occur between the patient, physician assistant, and physician. This text supports academic coursework of physician assistant trainees, helping students to prepare for ethical questions in the practice setting. Chapter contributors include physician assistant educators, physicians, and ethicists. The first three chapters address basic issues that apply to physician assistant students as well as ethical principles and decision making in everyday practice. The later chapters cover critical topics such as ethical questions related to treatment of diverse populations, reproductive issues, end of life care, and informed consent. The five case studies provide opportunities for educators and students to discuss the physician assistant's ethical role in current, relevant issues. This book provides an excellent foundation for students or newly licensed physician assistants to begin understanding their roles and obligations when facing ethical questions in practice.

Harrison's Principles of Internal Medicine. 17th ed. Editors: Anthony S. Fauci, Eugene Braunwald, Dennis L. Kasper, Stephen L. Hauser, Dan L. Longo, J. Larry Jameson, Joseph Loscalzo. McGraw-Hill, 2008.
http://www.accessmedicine.com/
http://extranet.netlibrary.com/TitleSelect/
http://www.ebrary.com/
http://www.statref.com/
ISBN: 9780071476911
ISBN: 9780071641142 (Online)
See Also Chapter 10.10. Internal Medicine
Recommended for: Hospital, Academic Libraries
Brandon/Hill, *Doody's Core Titles* Selection

Without question *the* classic text in internal medicine, *Harrison's* is perhaps the most recognized medical text in English. Since 36 percent of physician assistants work in primary care and another 11 percent work in internal medicine subspecialties (American Association of Physician Assistants, 2009), *Harrison's* is an essential purchase for any collection supporting practicing physician assistants or students. The book is divided into 17 sections and nearly 400 chapters that provide a comprehensive approach to internal medicine and related aspects of clinical medicine. The print version includes a DVD with 39 additional chapters, extra images, charts, tables, and videos. *Harrison's Online* is a part of McGraw-Hill's AccessMedicine platform and includes the full text of the seventeenth edition. It seamlessly integrates the DVD elements as well as online-only features such as *Harrison's* lecture notes, grand rounds, podcasts, RSS feeds, photo galleries, and self-assessments. The publisher incorporates new developments by adding "Latest Updates" that summarize relevant findings from the medical literature. The clearly labeled updates display in the table of contents and provide the reader with the option to view them within the context of relevant chapters. The search feature enables a quick review of topics across multiple chapters. Additionally, AccessMedicine presents the option to narrow results using subheadings; for example, a search for "lung cancer" includes options such as complications, imaging studies, mortality, prognosis, treatment, and more. The AccessMedicine version offers additional features such as a diagnosis tool, drug monographs, images, guidelines, and patient education handouts.

Nelson Textbook of Pediatrics. 18th ed. Editors: Robert M. Kliegman, Richard E. Behrman, Hal B. Jenson, Bonita F. Stanton. Saunders/Elsevier, 2007.
http://www.mdconsult.com/
http://www.nelsonpediatrics.com/
ISBN: 9781416024507
See Also Chapter 10.13. Pediatrics
Recommended for: Hospital, Academic Libraries
Brandon/Hill, *Doody's Core Titles* Selection

This well-respected, general pediatric textbook strives to represent the current standard of practice for the medical care of infants, children, and adolescents. Given that nearly 4 percent of all physician assistants in 2009 worked in pediatric settings and another 25 percent in family medicine (American Association of Physician Assistants, 2009), an excellent pediatric textbook is a strong need for any library supporting practicing physician assistants or students. The editors' intended audience for the book includes attending physicians, residents, medical students, and others involved in the care of pediatric patients, making it a fitting resource for physician assistants. The book is broken into 33 sections and includes 714 relatively brief chapters (averaging fewer than five pages per chapter). Sections of the book address pediatric care from a variety of perspectives such as subspecialties, diseases, body systems, and more. Individuals who purchase the print version receive free access to an online version. It is also possible to purchase institutional online access to the book as part of Elsevier's MD Consult service. Like many larger textbooks, this one proves to be much easier to use and search in electronic format. This textbook is currently a *Doody's Core Titles* essential purchase. The publisher is planning to release the nineteenth edition in June 2011.

Physician Assistant: A Guide to Clinical Practice. 4th ed. Editors: Ruth Ballweg, Edward M. Sullivan, Darwin Brown, Daniel Vetrosky. Saunders/Elsevier, 2008.
http://www.sciencedirect.com/science/book/9781416044857
ISBN: 9781416044857

Recommended for: Hospital, Academic Libraries
Brandon/Hill Selection

The Duke University School of Medicine implemented the first physician assistant program in 1965, and the first class graduated in 1967. As a relatively new profession, a very small corpus of literature exists in this field. First published in 1994, the initial edition represented one of the earliest physician assistant textbooks. The second edition was named in the final Brandon/Hill list for allied health; it was also included in Grodzinski's book collection for physician assistants (*Bull Med Lib Assoc* 2001 Jul; 89(3):277–286). The first five chapters comprise an overview of the profession, addressing history, international growth, education, credentialing, certification, licensing, financing, reimbursement, and political issues. The remaining sections reflect the six professional competencies defined by the four national physician assistant accrediting/credentialing organizations: "Medical Knowledge," "Interpersonal Communication and Skills," "Patient Care," "Professionalism," "Practice-Based Learning and Improvement," and "Systems-Based Practice." The book's key contributions lie in its coverage of unique issues facing physician assistants. This relatively new profession needs literature that documents its history and culture, as well as its place in the spectrum of health care disciplines. Since physician assistants practice in virtually every medical setting, the book includes chapters about major medical specialties and types of practice settings. Although intended as a textbook, this work provides valuable information for practicing physician assistants or other health care practitioners who would like to learn more about this relatively new and fast-growing profession.

Rosen's Emergency Medicine: Concepts and Clinical Practice. 7th ed. Editors: John A. Marx, Robert S. Hockberger, Ron M. Walls, James G. Adams. Mosby/Elsevier, 2010.
http://www.mdconsult.com/
http://www.rosensemergencymedicine.com/
ISBN: 9780323054720
See Also Chapter 10.5. Emergency Medicine
Recommended for: Hospital, Academic Libraries
Brandon/Hill, *Doody's Core Titles* Selection

Approximately 10 percent of physician assistants work in emergency medicine practice settings (American Association of Physician Assistants, 2009), making a comprehensive textbook a necessity for libraries supporting students or physician assistants in hospital settings. The book divides its chapters into seven major parts dealing with fundamental clinical concepts, trauma, medicine and surgery (two parts), environment and toxicology, special populations, emergency medical services, and practice of emergency medicine. Starting with this update, the print edition is divided into two smaller volumes. Although still large at 2,604 pages, the editors reduced its length by 500 pages by moving references to an online version (available until the release of the next edition). The print version, along with its companion website, is offered to individual users through Elsevier's Expert Consult service. *Rosen's* is also available for institutional online purchase through the easy-to-use MD Consult platform. Both online versions include updates, question and answer sections, and other features. The book includes more than 1,200 color illustrations and hundreds of tables to support either emergency clinicians or students. "Cardinal Presentations" are provided throughout the book, guiding readers through differential diagnosis and further testing. *Rosen's* is one of the first emergency medicine books written by emergency medicine physicians. Physicians and librarians alike have long recognized *Rosen's* as an essential purchase (Brandon/Hill and *Doody's Core Titles*). It provides a strong foundation for practicing physician assistants working in emergency departments or for physician assistant students learning about emergency practice.

Schwartz's Principles of Surgery. 9th ed. Editors: F. Charles Brunicardi, Dana K. Andersen, Timothy R. Billiar, David L. Dunn, John G. Hunter, Jeffrey B. Matthews, Raphael E. Pollock. McGraw-Hill, 2010.
http://www.accessmedicine.com/
http://online.statref.com/
ISBN: 9780071547697
ISBN: 9781429458498 (Online)
See Also Chapter 11.9. Surgery
Recommended for: Hospital, Academic Libraries
Brandon/Hill, *Doody's Core Titles* Selection

Approximately 25 percent of physician assistants worked in surgical subspecialties or general surgery practice settings in 2009 (American Association of Physician Assistants, 2009). Thus, facilities that employ or educate physician assistants need to have good surgery information sources. Long recognized as a classic surgery textbook, this work offers a comprehensive review of surgical principles and techniques. The 48 chapters cover fundamental concepts for physician assistants in surgical practice settings, including systemic responses to surgery, fluid and electrolytes, infections, bleeding and hemostasis, and patient safety issues. Several chapters address major surgical subspecialties such as pediatric, neurosurgery, urology, gynecology, orthopedics, and plastic and reconstructive surgery. The book also covers major organ systems and other topics of interest in surgery; these include issues related to surgery in the elderly, anesthesia, palliative care, and end-of-life considerations. Starting with this edition, the chapters now include quick-reference guides, highlighted evidence-based practice references, and full color illustrations. The print book includes a companion DVD showing surgical videos. Currently listed in *Doody's Core Titles*, this book is an excellent source of information for surgical residents as well as medical students, thus making it an excellent source for physician assistants working in surgical practices.

Textbook of Family Medicine. 7th ed. Editors: Robert E. Rakel. Saunders/Elsevier, 2007.
http://www.mdconsult.com/
ISBN: 9781416024675
See Also Chapter 10.6. Family Practice
Recommended for: Hospital, Academic Libraries
Brandon/Hill, *Doody's Core Titles* Selection

As a current *Doody's Core Titles* essential purchase and regular Brandon/Hill list selection, Rakel's work is a recognized, standard textbook in family medicine. This book is intended for family physicians as well as other primary care practitioners. Since more than 36 percent of physician assistants work in primary care settings and 25 percent work in family practice, an excellent family medicine text is essential for any collection supporting practicing physician assistants or students. The book is divided into four major sections covering principles of family medicine, family medicine in the community, communication in family medicine, and practice of family medicine. The appendixes provide quick reference guides relevant to physician assistants working in family medicine, including complementary and alternative medicine information sources, energy healing modalities, and a guide for evaluating medical evidence. Throughout the book, the authors provide clearly marked Level A evidence-based medicine recommendations using the Strength of Recommendation Taxonomy (SORT) commonly employed in family medicine journals (Ebell et al., *J Am Board Fam Pract* 2004 Jan/Feb; 17(1):59–67). The book includes more than 600 illustrations and 650 tables with a focus on providing practical information for all primary care providers. Each of the 66 chapters includes color-coded key points to help the reader quickly find the most important information. Although the print edition is easy to use, the electronic version available through MD Consult takes ease of use to another level and makes the book available on any computer or mobile device connected to the Internet.

The 5-Minute Clinical Consult. Wolters Kluwer/Lippincott Williams & Wilkins, Annual.
http://www.ovid.com/
http://5minuteconsult.com/
ISBN: 9781608312597
See Also Chapter 10.10. Internal Medicine
Recommended for: Hospital, Academic Libraries
Brandon/Hill Selection

Available in various formats, this reference is well loved by physician assistant students and others on clinical rotations. It provides concise answers to hundreds of questions students and practitioners face when dealing with patients. The editors' goal is to create a reference that enables readers to find an answer in thirty seconds or less. The book begins with a quick reference guide to preventive screening and prevention recommendations from the U.S. Preventive Services Task Force (USPSTF), the U.S. Centers for Disease Control (CDC), the American Academy of Pediatrics, and the American Academy of Family Physicians. More than 900 entries organized in alphabetical order comprise the body of work and cover topics ranging from "Abnormal Pap and Cervical Dysplasia" through "Wilms Tumor." In order to provide quick, well-organized overviews, each entry includes clearly labeled sections: "Basics," "Diagnosis," "Treatment," "Ongoing Care," "Codes," and "Clinical Pearls." Entries also include references and further readings with links to MEDLINE records in the electronic versions of the book. Another section includes algorithms for diagnosis and treatment. Each entry includes a flow chart showing possible causes for clinical presentations, recommended tests, potential diagnoses, and treatments. The book ends with reproductions of *MMWR* (*Morbidity and Mortality Weekly Report*) Quick Guides showing CDC immunization recommendations for children and adults. Although the printed book is too large for point of care, individual book purchasers receive free access to a mobile version, which is ideal for students and clinicians.

Journals

American Family Physician. v. 2, American Academy of Family Physicians, 1970.
http://www.aafp.org/online/en/home/publications/journals/afp.html
http://www.mdconsult.com/
ISSN: 0002838X
ISSN: 15320650 (Online)
See Also Chapter 10.6. Family Practice
Indexed in: MEDLINE, CINAHL

Recommended for: Hospital, Academic Libraries
Brandon/Hill Selection

American Family Physician is the official journal of the American Academy of Family Physicians (AAFP), making it one of the most recognized journals in family medicine. *American Family Physician* does not publish research articles. Its primary goal is practical: to provide high quality continuing medical education for family physicians and other primary care clinicians. The editors select articles with strong foundations in evidence-based medicine and focus on clinical reviews that reflect family medicine approaches to common clinical questions. In the journal's "Close-ups" feature, patients describe their own medical cases, and their physicians add brief commentaries explaining how they treated the patients. Suggested resources for other patients or clinicians are provided. Practicing physician assistants and student will benefit from the journal's practical focus, because it enables them to learn about types of cases that they are likely to face in primary care practice. The journal is covered in numerous abstracting and indexing databases such as MEDLINE, Embase, and CINAHL, and the National Library of Medicine has long considered *American Family Physician* to be a core clinical title. Both AAFP and MD Consult offer current institutional online subscriptions. Selected archives are freely available on the AAFP website after a 13-month embargo period. Additionally, some journal aggregator services continue to offer online access to a smaller subset of the back years.

Annals of Internal Medicine. v. 1, American College of Physicians, 1927.
http://www.annals.org/
http://www.ovid.com/
ISSN: 00034819
ISSN: 15393704 (Online)
See Also Chapter 10.10. Internal Medicine
Indexed in: MEDLINE, CINAHL
Recommended for: Hospital, Academic Libraries
Brandon/Hill Selection

Generally considered to be the premier internal medicine journal, *Annals of Internal Medicine* is a key publication for any clinician working in primary care. Although focused on internal medicine, the journal seeks to make contributions to advance health care by publishing, "a wide variety of original research, review articles, practice guidelines, and commentaries relevant to clinical practice, health care delivery, public health, health care policy, medical education, ethics, and research methodology." As the most frequently cited internal medicine journal and the fifth most frequently cited general medicine journal (according to *Journal Citation Reports* 2009), the journal succeeds at influencing the science and scholarship of medicine. Subscriptions to the journal include monthly *ACP Journal Club* issues that summarize the best, new clinically-relevant evidence from more than 100 major medical journals and enable clinicians to keep abreast of important developments in medicine. *Annals of Internal Medicine* is a required subscription for any facility that employs or educates physician assistants. The journal is cited in numerous abstracting and indexing databases including MEDLINE, Embase, CINAHL, Chemical Abstracts, and BIOSIS Previews. The journal is available in online format from the journal's website, Journals@Ovid, and several journal aggregators. Full online coverage back to volume 1, number 1, 1927 is available through the American College of Physicians.

JAAPA: Journal of the American Academy of Physician Assistants. v. 7, Haymarket Media, 1994.
http://www.jaapa.com/
ISSN: 15471896
Indexed in: MEDLINE, CINAHL
Recommended for: Hospital, Academic Libraries
Brandon/Hill Selection

As the official journal of the American Academy of Physician Assistants, *JAAPA* is the primary professional journal for practicing physician assistants and students. Types of articles published include review, continuing medical education (CME), and case reports. The journal's "Departments" provide unique publishing opportunities for physician assistants including, "A Day in the Life," "Critically Appraised Topics," "When the Patient Asks," and "POEMs (Patient-oriented evidence that matters)." Other "Departments" are based on medical specialties including dermatology, surgery, and diagnostic imaging. *JAAPA* also provides a forum for the Academy through commentaries, editorials, and special articles. The journal includes original research with a focus on issues related to physician assistant practice, education, and professional issues. MEDLINE, CINAHL, Embase, Scopus, and other abstracting and indexing services cover this journal. The journal is sold only in print format, but the online version is available free of charge. Access to selected portions requires a free registration process, and archives are available starting with volume 18 (2005). Several ProQuest databases provide access starting with volume 14 (2001), and several Gale databases provide access starting with volume 12 (1999).

JAMA: Journal of the American Medical Association. v. 173, American Medical Association, 1960.
http://www.jama.ama-assn.org/
http://www.ovid.com/
ISSN: 00987484
ISSN: 15383598 (Online)
See Also Chapter 10.10. Internal Medicine, Chapter 33.1. Consumer Health Information
Indexed in: MEDLINE, CINAHL
Recommended for: Hospital, Academic Libraries
Brandon/Hill Selection

JAMA is one of the most widely circulated and cited medical journals in the world. Since its broadly stated goal is "to promote the science and art of medicine and the betterment of the public health," the journal covers a broad range of medical and health sciences topics. Published 48 times per year, *JAMA* is read regularly by physicians, other clinicians, health care administrators, policy makers, and many others. Anyone who wishes to keep abreast of news, discussion, and debate regarding current health care questions needs to read, or at least skim, *JAMA* on a regular basis. The journal includes original research articles as well as features such as Grand Rounds, commentaries, editorials, book and media reviews, and news. More than just a research journal, *JAMA* helps to shape the culture of medicine and health care in the United States. It is a required subscription for any facility that employs or educates physician assistants. The journal is cited in numerous abstracting and indexing databases, including MEDLINE, Embase, CINAHL, Chemical Abstracts, and BIOSIS Previews. The journal is available in online format from the journal's website, Journals@Ovid, and several journal aggregators. Full online coverage back to volume 1, 1883 is available at the journal's website.

Journal of Physician Assistant Education. v. 17, Physician Assistant Education Association, 2006.
http://www.paeaonline.org/
ISSN: 19419430
ISSN: 19419449 (Online)
Indexed in: MEDLINE, CINAHL
Recommended for: Academic Libraries

Although not well known outside of the community of physician assistant educators, this journal is essential for any library supporting physician assistant education. The journal's goals are to publish "scholarly manuscripts germane to PA educators" and to provide "a forum for the sharing of ideas and innovations that will enhance the education of PA students." Potential authors may submit research or special articles for peer review on any relevant topic, but authors are encouraged to consider a list of topics developed by the Physician Assistant Education Association Research Institute. The journal also includes "Features" sections that address critical issues in physician assistant education, including academic law, higher education, cultural issues, evidence-based medicine, technology, and ethics. The *Journal of Physician Assistant Education* is essential reading for any person responsible for the education of physician students. Indexing is available in CINAHL, Embase, and Scopus. This journal's former title is *Perspective on Physician Assistant Education* (volume 1–16, 1998–2005). The journal is sold only in print format, but the online version is available free of charge, with archives back to volume 10, 1999.

New England Journal of Medicine. v. 198, Massachusetts Medical Society, 1928.
http://content.nejm.org/
http://www.ovid.com/
ISSN: 00284793
ISSN: 15334406 (Online)
See Also Chapter 10.10. Internal Medicine, Chapter 33.1. Consumer Health Information
Indexed in: MEDLINE, CINAHL
Recommended for: Hospital, Academic Libraries
Brandon/Hill Selection

The *New England Journal of Medicine* (*NEJM*) is one of the most widely recognized and circulated medical journals in the world. It had the highest impact factor and total citations of all general medicine journals according to the 2009 *Journal Citation Reports*. The journal publishes original clinical research articles as well as special articles dealing with economic, legal, and ethical issues in health care. The editors solicit review articles on a variety of topics aimed at general physicians rather than specialists. The journal includes a number of additional features such as "Perspective" articles on current health care topics and "Clinical Implications of Basic Research." The online version is free with print subscriptions. Its additional features include online first articles, interactive cases, videos, podcasts, and special interest sites such as the "Health Care Reform Center." *NEJM Mobile* provides access via any mobile device with a connection to the Internet. Long known as an authoritative source of medical information, *NEJM* is regularly cited in newspaper and television stories, thus leading to patients' questions. *NEJM* is a required subscription for any facility that employs or educates physician assistants. The journal is cited in numerous abstracting and indexing databases including MEDLINE, Embase, CINAHL,

Chemical Abstracts, and BIOSIS Previews. The journal is available in online format from the journal's website, Journals @Ovid, and several journal aggregators. Online coverage back to volume 328, 1993 is available at the journal's website or through Journals@Ovid; however, Ovid does not include PDFs.

Databases and Other Electronic Resources

***The Cochrane Library*.** Wiley, 1996.
http://www.thecochranelibrary.com/
http://www.ovid.com/
http://www.ebscohost.com/
ISBN: 14651858 (ISSN)
Recommended for: Hospital, Academic Libraries

The Cochrane Library is a collection of six databases intended to inform clinical decision making by providing access to the highest levels of evidence. The best known of these databases, the Cochrane Database of Systematic Reviews (CDSR), includes more than 4,000 reviews of questions related to medical practice or health care policy. Each review attempts to gather and assess the highest quality research related to a question and then establish whether or not there is conclusive evidence to support specific interventions. Although systematic reviews are available in many sources, Cochrane is generally recognized as setting the standard for quality reviews. Access to the Cochrane Library is essential for practicing physician assistants and students. In addition to the publisher's option, Ovid Technologies provides access to the Cochrane Library through its Evidence-Based Medicine Reviews database and supplements it with the full text of *ACP Journal Club*, an EBM review service included with *Annals of Internal Medicine*. EBSCOhost offers another variation, which is known as Cochrane Collection Plus. MEDLINE, Embase, CINAHL, and other databases index the Cochrane Reviews in *CDSR*. Libraries that use link resolvers such as Ex Libris' SFX or SerialsSolutions' 360 Link can connect searchers directly from these abstracting and indexing databases to full-text reviews.

***Facts & Comparisons eAnswers*.** Wolters Kluwer Health, 2010.
http://www.factsandcomparisons.com/
Recommended for: Hospital, Academic Libraries

Since physician assistants enjoy some form of prescribing authority in all 50 states, both practitioners and students need ready access to comprehensive and reliable sources of drug information. The database, which was formerly known as Facts & Comparisons 4.0, provides access to the same content as its print counterpart, *Drug Facts and Comparisons* (ISSN 02779714), as well as additional online resources. This standard reference provides several advantages compared to other drug information compendia such as off-label or investigational uses, tables comparing drugs within therapeutic categories, summary charts to help identify comparable drugs, and incidence data for adverse effects (Snow, B. "Pharmacology and Therapeutic Reference Sources." In: *Drug Information: A Guide to Current Resources*, 3rd ed., 2008. p. 183–225). The online resources include useful information such as a drug-to-drug interaction tool, clinical calculators, FDA Black Box warnings, information on herbal remedies, and a drug identifier. Although numerous free drug information resources are available, Facts & Comparison eAnswers brings together a number of useful drug information sources and related tools that make it an invaluable resource for practicing physician assistants and students. Subscribers to the online version may also access the mobile version of the database, which is accessible using any mobile device with access to the Internet and a standard web browser. Individuals may also purchase downloadable versions of the database through Skyscape or Unbound Medicine.

2. Biomedical Engineering

Application of principles and practices of engineering science to biomedical research and health care.

—MeSH

Contributors: Kristine M. Alpi and Robert Sotak

Monographs

Basic Orthopaedic Biomechanics & Mechano-Biology. 3rd ed. Editors: Van C. Mow, Rik Huiskes. Lippincott Williams & Wilkins, 2005.
http://www.ovid.com/
ISBN: 9780781739337
Recommended for: Hospital, Academic Libraries

The editors consider the third edition a new book compared to the second edition since they have added contributors, added a co-editor who brings a European perspective, included mechano-biology in the title, updated and enlarged chapters, and added a chapter on biomechanics. The text begins with a history of orthopaedic biomechanics going back to Aristotle, although the most significant advances have happened in the past 50 years. Also covered are musculoskeletal systems and analysis, kinetics of locomotion, and structure of articular cartilage, ligaments, and tendons. Principles of tissue engineering of bone and cartilage are explained as well as imaging and lubrication of joints. Biomaterials, their classes, mechanical behavior, and wear resistance are all discussed. The final chapters cover more applied aspects of biomechanics such as fracture fixation and healing, artificial joints, and total hip arthroplasty and total knee replacement. This book can be used as an advanced undergraduate textbook in biomechanics or in an introductory graduate level course and is recommended for all libraries serving these types of students. This title would also be useful in hospital libraries serving an orthopedics residency or fellowship program.

Biomaterials: An Introduction. 3rd ed. Authors: Joon Park, Roderic S. Lakes. Springer, 2007.
http://springerlink.com/content/r81635/
ISBN: 9780387378794
Recommended for: Academic Libraries

Biomedical engineering professors from the University of Iowa and the University of Wisconsin collaborated on this introduction to the use of materials in the human body with an emphasis on materials science and biological responses. Originally developed as a senior biomedical engineering student course textbook, *Biomaterials* features worked examples and provides unanswered problems. High quality black-and-white illustrations and photographs and tables of data are primarily reprinted from other publications with permission. New topics for the third edition include tissue engineering and regenerative medicine. Each chapter ends with definitions and a bibliography with references as current as 2006. Simple appendixes offer constants, conversions, SI units, and properties of elements and selected engineering materials. A name index and a subject index that indicates figures and tables make the book useful for quick reference. For additional coverage of biomaterials consider the second edition of Ratner et al.'s *Biomaterials Science: an Introduction to Materials in Medicine* (Elsevier, 2004) or *Biological Performance of Materials: Fundamentals of Biocompatibility*, 4th ed., by Jonathan Black (CRC, 2005).

Biomedical Engineering Handbook. 3rd ed. Editor: Joseph D. Bronzino. CRC Press/Taylor & Francis, 2006.
http://www.crcnetbase.com/isbn/978-0-8493-2121-4
http://www.crcnetbase.com/isbn/978-0-8493-2122-1
http://www.crcnetbase.com/isbn/978-0-8493-2123-8
ISBN: 9780849321214 (v.1)
ISBN: 9780849321221 (v.2)
ISBN: 9780849321238 (v.3)
ISBN: 9780849321245 (Set)
Recommended for: Hospital, Academic Libraries

Part of the *Electrical Engineering Handbook* series, the third edition of this work known collectively as *Biomedical Engineering Handbook* is now in three volumes, bringing together the contributions of those working in hospitals and academia across a variety of health and science disciplines, laboratories, biomedical engineering, industry, and management. Volume 1, *Biomedical Engineering Fundamentals*, covers physiology, modeling, bioelectric systems, biomaterials, mechanics, rehabilitation and human performance engineering, and a new chapter on neuroengineering. Volume 2, *Medical Devices and Systems*, covers biomedical signal analysis, imaging, sensors, clinical engineering, medical devices and instrumentation, and medical informatics. Volume 3, *Tissue Engineering and Artificial Organs*, addresses molecular biology, transport phenomena and biomimetic systems, biotechnology, bionanotechnology, tissue engineering, artificial organs, and prostheses. The ethics section at the end of each volume is duplicate content for those who purchase all three—the volumes are also designed to stand alone as individual books. Each volume also has its own index. The handbook chapters are separately numbered and are well-organized with introductions, clear subheadings, concluding summaries, and references. They are generally well illustrated with black-and-white photos, scans, graphs and schematics; one has a color thermogram section. The second edition won the Association of American Publishers Best New Professional/Scholarly Publication—Engineering award. The *Handbook* is available online at CRCNetBase as separate volumes. The online version entitled *Biomedical Engineering Handbook* is the second edition of the handbook which has only two volumes. The fourth edition is expected to be published in March 2012.

Biomedical Engineering Principles. 1st ed. Authors: Arthur B. Ritter, Stanley Reisman, Bozena B. Michniak. Taylor & Francis, 2005.
ISBN: 9780824796167
Recommended for: Academic Libraries

This book was written as an introduction to biomedical engineering for students with some background in engineering, physics, and mathematics. The chapters are organized by the following categories: transport processes, cell physiology and the cardiovascular system, and tissue engineering. The first chapter explains the basic concepts of model building and how to validate models. Aspects of cell physiology are explained in detail, such as transport of molecules into and out of cells and muscle contraction. Principles of hemodynamics are described well and applied to specific biomedical conditions such as abnormal heart sounds. Aspects of the cardiovascular system such as blood pressure and volume regulation, mechanical events of the cardiac cycle, and the failing heart are covered. Signal acquisition and processing is explained, as are specific techniques for physiological signal processing when the standard Fourier technique may not be applicable. Principles of biomechanics involved in areas such as human movement and muscle mechanics are discussed. That is followed by a chapter on application of biomechanics, such as optimization of human power generation and mechanisms for augmenting human power. Materials used in tissue engineering and their biological interactions are explained, as well as some recent applications in this field. The final chapter provides a brief survey of future trends in devices and concepts such as cardiac care, imaging, and prostheses. All chapters except the final one have a references section and some chapters have a problems section. This text is recommended for libraries serving undergraduate biomedical engineering programs or health sciences libraries with clinicians collaborating on biomedical engineering projects.

Biomedical Instrumentation. 1st ed. Author: Raghbir S. Khandpur. McGraw-Hill Professional, 2004.
ISBN: 9780071447843
Recommended for: Academic Libraries

Biomedical Instrumentation is a dense, single-author volume covering the basics of measuring, recording, and monitoring systems; imaging systems; and therapeutic equipment. R.S. Khandpur has extensive experience in technology research, development, and training and is currently a fellow of the Institute of Electronics and Telecommunication Engineers. This book was previously published by Tata McGraw-Hill and was written with British English spellings. Geared towards an engineering and technician audience, the content is comprehensive for the time and describes the operating principles of many instruments still in use today, such as lithotriptors and lasers. Each chapter is divided into numbered sections and there are many tables and illustrations. Some of the material is awkwardly constructed and inconsistent in format, and there are no summaries at the end of the chapter to help digest what has been covered. Instrumentation is a fast moving field and the most recent reference cited is 2000; therefore, many recent devices are not addressed. However, there is no recent volume that covers the diversity of devices. For a more recent, but very basic guide to instrumentation for students and new technicians, consider Barbara L. Christe's *Introduction to Biomedical Instrumentation: The Technology of Patient Care* (Cambridge University Press, 2009).

Design of Biomedical Devices and Systems. 2nd ed. Authors: Paul H. King, Richard C. Fries. CRC Press, 2009.
ISBN: 9781420061796
Recommended for: Academic Libraries

Although this book is primarily intended for senior year design students, it also can be used by lower level undergraduates and designers who are new to the medical device field. The sequence of chapters in the book follows the design process. The first three chapters present the basics of design, design tools, such as flowcharts and objective trees, and design management. Procedures for defining, documenting, and developing products are well presented. Human factors and safety engineering which must be taken into account during the design process are carefully laid out. Methods to test reliability of devices and liability issues such as defectiveness are covered. An overview of professional societies, ethics, consulting, and intellectual property issues is provided. The final chapter discusses future design issues and the driving forces behind them. At the ends of chapters are exercises and a bibliography. Appendixes include a chi square table, percent rank tables, contradiction table, and a glossary. This book is an excellent resource and is recommended for libraries serving universities with a biomedical engineering program or health sciences libraries with clinicians collaborating on device development.

An Introduction to Biomedical Optics. 1st ed. Authors: Robert Splinter, Brett A. Hooper. Taylor & Francis, 2007.
ISBN: 9780750309387
Recommended for: Academic Libraries

The three sections of this book are "General Biomedical Optics Theory," "Therapeutic Applications of Light," and "Diagnostic Applications of Light." In the first section, the introductory chapter provides a brief history of optical discoveries, optical devices, and theory and applications. Subsequent chapters present an overview of optical principles including electromagnetic wave theory, classical optics such as Huygens' Principle, and optical interaction properties such as scattering. The remainder of the first section covers theories, mechanisms, and applications of light-tissue interaction. The second section covers photophysical, photochemical, and photobiological aspects of therapeutic applications. The final section uses the same three aspects to present diagnostic applications of light. All chapters conclude with a summary, list of further reading, and problems. The text is very clear to read but the mathematics may be beyond the understanding of many biology students. This book is recommended for upper level undergraduates, graduate students, and researchers in biomedical engineering and physics, and will benefit anyone interested in diagnostic and therapeutic optical methods.

Nanomaterials for Medical Diagnosis and Therapy. Editor: Challa Kumar. Wiley-VCH, 2007.
ISBN: 9873527313907
Recommended for: Academic Libraries

This is the capstone tenth volume in the series *Nanotechnologies for the Life Sciences*. Series and volume editor Dr. Challa Kumar is a synthetic organic chemist who has coordinated the work of an international group of contributors from basic sciences, engineering, pharmacy, and medicine. The 16 chapters represent well-organized reviews of different clinical applications of nanotechnologies with more than half of them focused on drug delivery, making this title especially relevant for pharmaceutical company libraries and libraries serving pharmacy training programs. It does not cover cancer therapy and diagnosis as these topics were covered in volumes six and seven of the series. Chapters are consistently organized, well-illustrated with clear images, and end with conclusions and references. This title is not available online from Wiley Online Library. For more on techniques, tools, and applications, see *Nanofabrication Towards Biomedical Applications* (Wiley-VCH, 2005) also co-edited by Dr. Kumar.

Nanotechnology in Biology and Medicine: Methods, Devices, and Applications. Editor: Tuan Vo-Dinh. CRC Press, 2007.
http://www.crcnetbase.com/doi/book/10.1201/9781420004441
http://extranet.netlibrary.com/TitleSelect/
ISBN: 9870849329494
ISBN: 9781420004441 (Online)
Recommended for: Academic Libraries

This book was written to serve as a reference source for a wide audience. Nearly 100 experts, ranging from chemistry, computer science, materials science, and engineering departments, have contributed to this book. It focuses on interdisciplinary interaction between nanotechnology and fields like biotechnology, genomics, and proteomics, and points out the potential of nanotechnology to improve fields of diagnosis and therapy. This book is divided into two sections: "Nanomaterials, Nanostructures, and Nanotools" and "Applications in Biology and Medicine." Section 1 covers topics such as bionanomanufacturing, structurally (e.g., peptide nucleic acids) and functionally (e.g., mussel-adhesive protein) inspired biomaterials, and quantum dots as molecular imaging agents. Applications are covered in section 2 including designing gene circuits for use in gene therapy, metallic nanoshells for gene and drug delivery, and the use of nanoparticles for diagnosis and therapy. Each chapter has its own table of contents, has an introductory section, conclusion, and references in addition to the main text. There are numerous black-and-white illustrations with color photographs on glossy paper in a separate section in the middle of the book. *Nanotechnology in Biology and Medicine* is appropriate for students and researchers in any field impacted by nanotechnology and all health sciences libraries as knowledge of this developing field is important for all clinicians.

Journals

Annals of Biomedical Engineering. v. 1, Springer, 1972.
http://www.springerlink.com/content/0090-6964
ISSN: 00906964
ISSN: 15739686 (Online)
See Also Chapter 11.8. Regenerative Medicine
Indexed in: MEDLINE
Recommended for: Academic Libraries

In addition to research articles, *Annals of Biomedical Engineering* publishes technical reports, special communications on methods and technology, rapid communications, history and teaching articles, and letters to the editor. It is interdisciplinary in approach, publishing articles in bioengineering and biomedical engineering, and tries to balance theory and modeling with experimental data. Some recent special issues were devoted to nanobioengineering; cellular biomechanics and biorheology; and systems biology, bioinformatics, and computational biology. *Annals of Biomedical Engineering* is published monthly and is an official journal of the Biomedical Engineering Society. It is indexed in BIOSIS Previews, Compendex, Inspec, MEDLINE, Science Citation Index, and Scopus among others and is available online via SpringerLink. The online version features Online First articles. *Annals of Biomedical Engineering* is recommended for graduate students and practicing biomedical engineers interested in interdisciplinary approaches.

Annual Review of Biomedical Engineering. v. 1, Annual Reviews, 1999.
http://arjournals.annualreviews.org/loi/bioeng
ISSN: 15239829
ISSN: 15454274 (Online)
See Also Chapter 11.8. Regenerative Medicine
Indexed in: MEDLINE
Recommended for: Academic Libraries

In August of each year, the print volume of *Annual Review of Biomedical Engineering* is published with 10-25 in-depth reviews of engineering technologies applied to biomedical problems and areas with the potential for industrial efforts to improve health. Recent volumes online offer tables of contents for each review, term definitions in the margins, high-quality color figures, summary points, and extensive lists of literature cited. The 2009 impact factor of 11.235 is the highest in the biomedical engineering category of *Journal Citation Reports.* Indexing coverage includes Biological Abstracts/BIOSIS Previews, Biotechnology & Bioengineering Abstracts, Chemical Abstracts, Embase, MEDLINE, Science Citation Index, and Scopus. The audience for these state-of-the art reviews includes students in engineering, physics, computer science, and the life sciences; practicing clinicians; hospital administrators; engineers; and inventors. Full online coverage back to volume 1, number 1, 1999 is available through Annual Reviews.

Biomaterials. v. 1, Elsevier, 1980.
http://sciencedirect.com/science/journal/01429612
ISSN: 01429612
ISSN: 18785905 (Online)
See Also Chapter 11.8. Regenerative Medicine
Indexed in: MEDLINE
Recommended for: Academic Libraries

Biomaterials is an international journal covering the science and application of biomaterials and associated medical devices. Their definition of biomaterials is "all those materials used in medical devices in which contact with the tissues of the patient is an important and guiding feature of their use and performance." Thirty-six issues per year cover the basic science and engineering aspects of biomaterials, including their mechanical, physical, chemical, and biological properties; design and production characteristics of devices constructed of these materials; and their clinical performance. Associate editors represent two areas: clinical outcomes and biomaterials science and engineering. Its impact factor 7.365 for 2009 *Journal Citation Reports* ranks it second in the biomedical engineering category and first in the materials science, biomaterials category, but it is a relatively expensive journal. Indexing coverage includes Biological Abstracts/BIOSIS Previews, CAB Abstracts, Ceramic Abstracts, Chemical Abstracts, Compendex, EBSCOhost, Embase, Gale Group, MEDLINE, Science Citation Index, and Scopus. Full online coverage back to volume 1, number 1, 1980 is available through Elsevier ScienceDirect.

Biomedical Microdevices. v. 1, Springer, 1988.
http://www.springerlink.com/content/1387-2176
ISSN: 13872176
ISSN: 15728781 (Online)
Indexed in: MEDLINE
Recommended for: Academic Libraries

A specialized journal in a cutting edge area, the six issues per year of *Biomedical Microdevices* cover research in the diagnostic and therapeutic applications of Micro-Electro-Mechanical Systems (MEMS), microfabrication, and nanotechnology. Design, characterization, testing, modeling, and clinical validation of microfabricated systems are addressed for areas of interest such as neural stimulation and recording; bioseparation technologies such as nanofilters and electrophoretic equipment; miniaturized analytic and DNA identification systems; biosensors; microtechnologies for cell and tissue research; tissue engineering; cell transplantation; and the controlled release of drugs and therapeutic proteins. Images are of acceptable quality and in color where appropriate. Its 2009 impact factor of 3.323 ranks it seventh in the biomedical engineering category of *Journal Citation Reports.* Indexing coverage includes AGRICOLA, Chemical Abstracts, Compendex, CSA/ProQuest, Elsevier Biobase, Embase, Gale, OCLC, MEDLINE, Science Citation Index, and Scopus. Libraries serving academic researchers and microdevice research and development should find this journal useful.

IEEE Engineering in Medicine and Biology Magazine. v. 1, IEEE, 1982.
http://ieeexplore.ieee.org/servlet/opac?punumber=51
ISSN: 07395175
ISSN: 19374186 (Online)
Indexed in: MEDLINE
Recommended for: Academic Libraries

Each issue of *IEEE Engineering in Medicine and Biology Magazine* covers a specific theme. Recent themes include wavelet-related technologies in biomedical signal processing; pattern discovery in bioinformatics; and multiscale modeling of biomedical, biological, and behavioral systems. Readers are expected to be technologically knowledgeable but not experts in each theme topic. Articles are classified in the table of contents as themes, features and departments. Other types of articles are editorials, society news, book reviews, patent descriptions, and letters to the editor and point of view. More than 20 regularly scheduled columns include "Student's Corner," which allows students to write on topics of interest. The "Retrospectroscope" column provides a historical look at biomedical topics. The magazine also publishes unsolicited features. The magazine is primarily intended for members of the IEEE Engineering in Medicine and Biology Society and others with an interest in the field. This journal is indexed in Engineering Index, Inspec, MEDLINE, and other indexes. It is published bimonthly by the IEEE Engineering in Medicine and Biology Society. Online access is available through IEEE Xplore Digital Library starting with volume 2, issue 4 1983. It is recommended for students, faculty and practicing biomedical engineers and for biomedical researchers interested in the interdisciplinary aspects of medicine and biology.

IEEE Reviews in Biomedical Engineering. v. 1, IEEE, 2008.
http://ieeexplore.ieee.org/servlet/opac?punumber=4664312
ISSN: 19373333
ISSN: 19411189 (Online)
Recommended for: Hospital, Academic Libraries

As journals are published in more narrowly specialized fields, research is also becoming more multidisciplinary. This recently launched journal attempts to integrate these two trends. The journal has three sections: "In the Spotlight," "Methodological Reviews," and "Clinical Application Reviews." "In the Spotlight" contains brief reports written by area editors about important advances in their fields of research. There are area editors for bioinstrumentation, biomedical imaging, biomedical informatics, biomedical signal processing, cardiovascular, health information systems, neural engineering, and tissue and molecular engineering. "Methodological Reviews" present state-of-the-art scientific advances. "Clinical Application Reviews" emphasize developments relevant to biomedical engineering and how they are being used in translational research. *IEEE Reviews in Biomedical Engineering* is an annual publication of the IEEE Engineering in Medicine and Biology Society and is technically co-sponsored by the IEEE Consumer Electronics Society. It is indexed by Biotechnology & Bioengineering Abstracts and Compendex and is available online through IEEE Xplore Digital Library; it is not currently indexed by MEDLINE. This journal is recommended for graduate students, biomedical and related engineers, researchers, and clinicians.

IEEE Transactions on Medical Imaging. v. 1, Institute of Electrical and Electronics Engineers (IEEE), 1982.
http://ieeexplore.ieee.org/xpl/RecentIssue.jsp?punumber=42
ISSN: 02780062
ISSN: 1558254X (Online)
Indexed in: MEDLINE
Recommended for: Academic Libraries

Imaging is an important functional area within biomedical engineering and this monthly journal is co-published by several IEEE societies, most importantly, the IEEE Engineering in Medicine and Biology Society. Studies primarily deal with imaging of body organs through modalities such as ultrasound, X-rays, computed tomography, magnetic resonance, radionuclides, and microwaves, as well as medical image processing and analysis, visualization, pattern recognition, and related methods. The focus on instrumentation systems, computer hardware and software, mathematics, and physics contribute to the practical engineering content. As expected for a journal on imaging, large numbers of high-quality color and black-and-white images are featured, but are packed tightly into dense articles and presented in PDF which limits image examination to the zoom capacities of Adobe Acrobat. Electronic access is important to being able to enlarge the images for a close look at the rich details. With an impact factor of 3.540 in the 2009 *Journal Citation Reports*, the journal ranked sixth in the biomedical engineering category and second in the imaging science and photographic technology category. Indexing coverage includes Biotechnology & Bioengineering Abstracts, CAB Abstracts, Ceramic Abstracts, Compendex, EBSCOhost, Gale Group, INSPEC, Mechanical Engineering Abstracts from CSA, MEDLINE, Science Citation Index, and Scopus. Radiologists and imaging technicians, medical physicists, as well as those developing imaging instrumentation will find this journal of interest. IEEE also publishes the *IEEE Transactions on Image Processing*.

IEEE Transactions on Neural Systems and Rehabilitation Engineering. v. 9, IEEE, 2001.
http://ieeexplore.ieee.org/servlet/opac?punumber=7333
ISSN: 15344320
ISSN: 15580210 (Online)
Indexed in: MEDLINE
Recommended for: Academic Libraries

The journal publishes full papers, brief manuscripts, and review articles which range from experimental research to clinical applications. Four broad categories of articles are reviews and special topics, neural engineering, rehabilitation engineering, and neural-rehabilitation interfaces. Specific areas include functional electrical stimulation, human performance measurement and analysis, nerve stimulation, motor control and stimulation, and hardware and software applications. Recent special sections on emerging fields have been published such as "Neuroeconomics: Modeling and Imaging the Brain Activity during Economic Transactions," "Neural and Myoelectric Control of Prostheses," "Lower Extremity Exoskeletons for Gait Rehabilitation," "Modeling the Connectivity of the Neural Systems," and "Wireless Neural Interfaces." Online access is via IEEE Xplore Digital Library from 2001. Links are provided to top accessed articles for the month. *IEEE Transactions on Neural Systems and Rehabilitation Engineering* is published bimonthly and is sponsored by the IEEE Engineering in Medicine and Biology Society. It is indexed by Compendex, Inspec, MEDLINE, Scopus and others. It is recommended for biomedical graduate students and researchers interested in neural systems, rehabilitation engineering, and assistive technology.

Physics in Medicine & Biology. v. 1, Institute of Physics, 1956.
http://www.iop.org/EJ/0031-9155
ISSN: 00319155
ISSN: 13616560 (Online)
Indexed in: MEDLINE
Recommended for: Hospital, Academic Libraries

Some of the topics covered by *Physics in Medicine & Biology* are radiotherapy physics, biomedical imaging, image analysis and computer-aided detection, and biomedical optics and radiobiology. It is published semi-monthly and contains letters to the editor, notes, topical reviews, and research papers. IOP Publishing is the publisher of *Physics in Medicine & Biology* on behalf of the Institute of Physics and Engineering in Medicine. *Physics in Medicine & Biology* is also an official journal of the following societies: the Canadian Organization of Medical Physics, the Deutsche Gesellschaft für Medizinische Physik, the Japanese Association of Radiological Physics, the European Federation of Organisations for Medical Physics, and the International Organization for Medical Physics. The online journal articles have a general scientific summary in order to improve accessibility for non-experts. An online archive from IOP Publishing is available for 1956–1998. *Physics in Medicine & Biology* is indexed in BIOSIS Previews, Compendex, Inspec, MEDLINE, Science Citation Index, and others. Its 2009 impact factor of 2.781 places it 15 out of 59 journals in the engineering, biomedical category of *Journal Citation Reports*. This journal is recommended for those interested in theoretical and applied aspects of physics in medicine and biology.

3. Chiropractic

Chiropractic is a health care discipline concerned with utilizing the relationship between structure, particularly the spine, and function coordinated by the nervous system. Chiropractic technique emphasizes manual adjustment of vertebrae and other joints in the preservation and restoration of health.

—Adapted from *Stedman's Medical Dictionary for the Health Professions and Nursing*, 6th ed. (2008)

Contributors: Annette Osenga, Marian A. Hicks, Chabha Hocine, John Klima, Claire Sharifi

Monographs

Basic and Clinical Anatomy of the Spine, Spinal Cord, and ANS. 2nd ed. Authors: Gregory D. Cramer, Susan A. Darby. Elsevier Mosby, 2005.
ISBN: 9780323026499
Recommended for: Academic Libraries

This very readable textbook and clinical resource has three sections: (a) general anatomy; muscles that influence the spine; and characteristics of the cervical, the thoracic region, and the lumbar region, with clinical considerations; (b) neuroanatomy, autonomic nervous system, and pain of spinal origin; and (c) spinal development, pediatric spine, and microscopic anatomy. This edition has a new chapter on the pediatric spine and a sizable amount of revised material on scoliosis and other conditions, based on more than 700 relevant research papers from the last decade. The author and the six contributors provide a valuable service by having mined the literature for clinically relevant and valid material. More than 170 of the 475 illustrations are new. The illustrations include drawings, dissections, brilliant photographs, and reproductions of high resolution CT and MR images, in place of the older scans in the earlier edition. Clinically relevant information is extensive and marked with a red rule. References conclude each chapter. This book is recommended as a textbook for the study of spinal disorders and the mechanisms of manipulation, and for reference at any practice focused on the spine.

Chiropractic Technique: Principles and Procedures. 3rd ed. Authors: Thomas F. Bergmann, David H. Peterson. Elsevier/Mosby, 2011.
ISBN: 9780323049696
Recommended for: Academic Libraries
Doody's Core Titles Selection

Optimal pedagogical organization, updated references, 1,340 illustrations (photographs, line drawings, and tables), and excellent writing contribute to the authors' goal to have the text be "a comprehensive service to assist in the standardization of teaching chiropractic diagnostic and adjustive methods." This well-accepted textbook for "diversified technique" courses also serves as a useful clinical reference for students and experienced practitioners seeking correlation among varied chiropractic approaches and evidence for various procedures. The second edition received a *Doody's* rating of 2.8 in 2009. For this third edition, the authors have updated discussions of the evidence for procedures and thoughtfully fine-tuned the presentation of material, particularly in the chapters on technique, adding many illustrations. Photographs are overlaid with directional graphics and paired with line drawings depicting the procedure and the involved joints or tissues. The brief first chapter, a comprehensive overview of chiropractic concepts and current developments, serves as both a highly recommended introduction and an update. The second chapter discusses the anatomy and biomechanics of joint systems of the spine, pelvis, and extremities, along with the effects of loads on connective tissue and human motion. The third chapter covers joint assessment principles and procedures, presenting traditional and current views of the subluxation complex and defensible concepts of the effect of joint function on health. Subsequent chapters cover principles of assessment and technique and provide detail for functional anatomy, biomechanics, evaluation, and adjustive procedure for each body region. The naming protocol for procedures concurs with the format used by the National Board of Chiropractic Examiners. While thrust procedures are emphasized, the final chapter provides the rationale and methods used for nonthrust adjustive procedures as well as mobilization, traction, and soft tissue techniques. The text concludes with a glossary of common terms; a list of named chiropractic techniques; a compilation and synopsis of reliability studies on several joint evaluation procedures, particularly motion palpation; and extensive references. Online access to the electronic text and ancillary content such as video clips for the evaluative and adjustive procedures are available for individual purchasers through the Evolve website at http://evolve.elsevier.com.

Chiropractic: An Illustrated History. Editors: Dennis Peterson, Glenda Wiese. Mosby, 1995.
ISBN: 9780801677359
Recommended for: Academic, Consumer Health Libraries

This commemorative book marked the centennial of the founding of the chiropractic profession. With 939 illustrations and chapters by 20 contributors, it blends historical accounts based on primary materials with contemporary interpretation of significant events and prominent figures. The opening chapters, "Antecedents to Chiropractic" and "American Medicine in the Nineteenth Century," set the stage for the discovery of chiropractic principles. Subsequent chapters cover politics, development of techniques, early instrumentation and equipment, education, legislation, professional associations, profiles of influential people, women in chiropractic, status of the profession in regions around the world, and, finally, an epilogue about the future of the profession. Several contributors continue to publish, primarily in the journal *Chiropractic History*. *Doody's* supplied this book with a 2.8 rating in 2009. The attractive design and accessible scholarly content make this "coffee table" book suitable for chiropractors' offices and collections at public and academic libraries.

Differential Diagnosis and Management for the Chiropractor: Protocols and Algorithms. 4th ed. Author: Thomas A. Souza. Jones & Bartlett, 2009.
ISBN: 9780763752828
Recommended for: Hospital, Academic Libraries
Doody's Core Titles Selection

This comprehensive textbook and reference provides a consistent approach to evaluation, decision making, and management. It avoids formulaic guidelines and instead offers evidence-based diagnostic tools as aids for individualized care. It also offers help for the practitioner's decision to accept, refer, or co-manage a patient. Typical entries include context, general strategy, relevant anatomy and physiology, evaluation, management, and algorithms (flowcharts) concerning clinical presentations that a chiropractor can expect to encounter. The author consistently explains the availability and quality of research, particularly for management. Categorical arrangement of complaints covers the following: musculoskeletal, neurological, general concerns, gastrointestinal, genitourinary, cardiopulmonary, head and face, special conditions, and special patient groups—pediatric, adolescent, geriatric, and female. It includes an appendix addressing the effect common medications may have on presentation and management outcomes. The quick index inside the front and back covers, with pages for figures in italics, is especially useful when looking for illustrations such as photographs of orthopedic tests. *Doody's* supplied a 2.7 rating in 2009. Primarily a textbook for chiropractic students, it is also recommended for libraries supporting academic programs and for primary care practices that focus on conservative care for musculoskeletal complaints.

Essentials of Skeletal Radiology. 3rd ed. Authors: Terry R. Yochum, Lindsay J. Rowe. Lippincott Williams & Wilkins, 2005.
ISBN: 9780781739467 (2 v.)
Recommended for: Hospital, Academic Libraries
Doody's Core Titles Selection

The authors of *Essentials of Skeletal Radiology* are excellent teachers and writers who have incorporated content from a wide network of colleagues. Originally created for the chiropractic profession, the osteopathic and allopathic medical fields have adopted this comprehensive, two-volume text as a teaching tool and clinical reference aid. It is a highly rated (2.9) *Doody's Core Titles* selection. Accessible writing, effective presentation suited to the content at hand, and thoughtful design of headings, tables, diagrams, and captions successfully integrate knowledge of a disease process with clinical considerations. Additional features including correlations between normal and pathological images, sections on common pitfalls and synonyms, and a list of mnemonics emphasize the book's value as both a teaching text and a reference for correct diagnosis. Capsule summaries show the evolution of knowledge and highlight essential points. The third edition includes material from eleven contributing authors and incorporates updated cases, illustrations, and references. The 4,500 carefully reproduced images include x-ray, musculoskeletal diagnostic ultrasound, bone scan, CT, and MRI. Chapters in the first volume addressing history, relevant anatomy, positioning, common conditions, imaging and interpretation precede those on various categories of disorders. A typical chapter on a condition begins with a content outline and general considerations, followed by pathology, radiologic features, treatment and prognosis, applicable imaging, and differential diagnosis. Beyond the revisions, the second volume also offers new material: the addition of exemplary critiques of case studies in the chapter on report writing and a new piece, "Masqueraders of Musculoskeletal Disease." An accompanying CD features selected images from Primal Pictures.

Functional Neurology for Practitioners of Manual Therapy. Author: Randy W. Beck. Churchill Livingstone/Elsevier, 2008.
ISBN: 9780443102202
Recommended for: Hospital, Academic Libraries
Doody's Core Titles Selection

Randy Beck states in the preface that he has gathered and integrated complex information from anatomy, clinical neurology, and manual therapies into a "guide for practitioners and/or students who wish to learn a general approach to manipulation as an afferent stimulation technique as well as a motion restoration tool." The suite of chapters begins with fundamental concepts about the nervous system and its examination, moves through a detailed discussion of each subsystem, considers the role of the nervous system in immunity and mind-body relationships, and concludes with approaches to treatment and patient management. Treatment includes manipulation as a safe, available modality and rehabilitative exercises and activities for stimulating specific parts of the central nervous system. Those who have studied the material can use the text as a reference. However, its arrangement better suits study and review. "Clinical Cases for Thought" initiate each chapter and serve as a stimulus to self-evaluation. Highlighted quick facts and clear anatomical drawings clarify the well-written discussions, and each chapter closes with extensive references and clinical case answers. Its emphasis on function in health and disease, rather than pathology, allows the practitioner to take into account the complex interchange between neurophysiology and environment in order to understand more fully the individual patient. This work benefits primary care manual therapists who have the prerequisite knowledge of anatomy, neurology, and therapy and the desire to deepen their understanding.

Introduction to Chiropractic: A Natural Method of Health Care. 12th ed. Author: Louis Sportelli. Practice Makers Products, 2009.
ISBN: 9780970383938
Recommended for: Consumer Health Libraries

This 57-page softcover book has been produced for over 20 years and marketed to chiropractors for distribution to their patients. Within this general overview of chiropractic concepts and typical care, the author mentions a variety of conditions where chiropractic manipulation may be beneficial, including some conditions common in children and seniors. However, the author attends more to low back pain and neck injury. This edition has 100 additional and updated references and a revised section on nutrition regarding chronic inflammation and the role of poor diet. Although the author tends to present background material before catching the reader's interest with practical recommendations, the discussions for self-care are nicely arranged in tables or brief paragraphs, often with a color illustration. The last chapter provides illustrated prescriptions for rehabilitation and strengthening of the low back and neck. The accompanying CD-ROM is a 49-minute lecture for chiropractors on the importance of patient education, staff training, and, especially, doctor-patient collaboration in today's environment. The text itself is appropriate for chiropractors' offices and consumer libraries. The heavy-paper cover on this edition needs reinforcement in order to survive multiple circulations. It is written at a high-school reading level, grade 11 on the Flesch-Kincaid scale. Most sections are one page in length, with simple but colorful graphic design and drawings.

Low Back Pain: Mechanism, Diagnosis, and Treatment. 6th ed. Author: James M. Cox. Williams & Wilkins, 1999.
ISBN: 9780683303582
Recommended for: Hospital, Academic Libraries
Doody's Core Titles Selection

This classic text is noted for its practicality and thoroughness. Dr. James Cox, the developer of the flexion-distraction technique, organized content from eight contributors into a comprehensive textbook and clinical reference. Although the extensive references no longer represent current research, the book still provides a broad foundation for further investigation of clinically relevant aspects of low back pain, particularly in light of recent studies. Early on, Dr. Cox identified fruitful areas of inquiry and included chapters on fibromyalgia, rehabilitation, and psychological perspectives. All of these generated much attention in research subsequent to 1999. Some chapters are devoted entirely to biomechanics, neurophysiology, and diagnosis. Other chapters incorporate these topics in more detail and in the context of conditions or regions. The chapters on spinal stenosis, intervertebral disc, and the sacroiliac joint exemplify a successful union of basic and clinical knowledge. The discussions of treatment methods describe a wide range of common interventions and their likely outcomes. Management focuses on conservative care through rehabilitative exercise, physical therapy, and distraction manipulation. Easily interpreted line drawings, photographs, tables, algorithms, and illustrative cases enhance the discussions throughout the text. The ubiquity of low back pain and the value of conservative care make this clinical reference particularly useful to both medical doctors and chiropractors. Chiropractors who employ manipulative methods other than flexion-distraction can use this text to gain a thorough understanding of low back pain in order to formulate an optimal care plan.

Principles and Practice of Chiropractic. 3rd ed. Editors: Scott Haldeman, Simon Dagenais. McGraw-Hill, 2005.
ISBN: 9780071375344
Recommended for: Academic Libraries
Doody's Core Titles Selection

Principles and Practice of Chiropractic provides an overview of the history, philosophy, and practice of chiropractic that is appropriate for students and practicing physicians seeking a textbook or reference. The editors have compiled the work of seventy-eight eminent scholars from the fields of chiropractic, neurology, geriatrics, pediatrics, biomechanics, acupuncture, and radiology. The evolution of this text since its first edition in 1980 reflects the development of chiropractic in academic and research settings. It is comprehensive in coverage and densely packed with well-researched information, making each section a challenging but effective introduction to an aspect of chiropractic. Readers will need to refer to the index to discover some aspects. For example, the author discusses chiropractic subluxation in context within several chapters on philosophy, theory, and anatomical regions. Using this text, students investigating the meaning of this term immediately discover the breadth of application of the concept, but they would need to refer to other works dedicated to theory and subluxation, such as those by Robert Leach and Meridel Gatterman, for a concentrated discussion. This book is organized effectively for study. The clear and precise illustrations and tables often present complex information. Each chapter begins with an outline, a list of objectives, and an introduction; each closes with a brief conclusion, summary, questions and answers, key references, and a complete reference list. The text is divided into five major sections that introduce the reader to different areas. The first section focuses on the history and philosophy of spinal manipulation with an emphasis on factors that influenced this field, including clinical trials in chapters 8 and 9. The second section adopts an interdisciplinary approach that highlights the influence of basic sciences—neurology, neurophysiology, and biomechanics—on chiropractic. The last three sections address practical aspects: namely, the skills and techniques required for current, evidence-based diagnosis and care. A *Doody's Core Titles* selection, this book is highly recommended as an introductory textbook and a reference for chiropractic students, practicing chiropractors, and other physicians involved in manual therapies.

Rehabilitation of the Spine: A Practitioner's Manual. 2nd ed. Editor: Craig Liebenson. Lippincott Williams &Wilkins, 2007.
http://www.ovid.com/
ISBN: 9780781729970
Recommended for: Hospital, Academic Libraries
Doody's Core Titles Selection

The second edition of Liebenson's *Rehabilitation of the Spine: A Practitioner's Manual* is an essential text for chiropractors, physical therapists, medical doctors, and other practitioners involved in back care. The text advocates an active, patient-centered model of spinal rehabilitation, as opposed to the patient's passive reception of treatment. Liebenson organizes the book into 39 chapters spread out over seven sections: overview, basic science, assessment, acute care management, recovery care management, practical application by region, and implementation of the functional paradigm. Each chapter begins with a list of learning objectives and concludes with an "audit process," a series of questions that serve as a "self-check of the chapter's learning objectives." The text features numerous images, figures, and photographs that support the reader's learning process through their clarity and design. The list of contributing authors is a veritable who's who of spinal therapy practitioners from a wide variety of disciplines. The accompanying DVD is intended to provide a clearer visual demonstration of the application of techniques discussed in the text. Sections of the text that have an accompanying presence on the DVD are denoted with a DVD icon. Among others, these include the sections on Brugger's micro-break, abdominal bracing, Vojta's basic reflex locomotion positions, and McGill's side bridge endurance test. This book builds upon the strong foundation Liebenson created with the first edition and will doubtless, among spinal therapy practitioners and health science academic institutions, be considered a must-have for a long time to come, or until the third edition is published.

Journals

Archives of Physical Medicine and Rehabilitation. v. 34, W.B. Saunders, 1953.
http://www.archives-pmr.org/home
http://www.sciencedirect.com/science/journal/00039993

ISSN: 00039993
ISSN: 1532821X (Online)
See Also Chapter 1.3. Physical Therapy, Chapter 10.14. Physical Medicine and Rehabilitation
Indexed in: MEDLINE, CINAHL
Recommended for: Hospital, Academic Libraries
Brandon/Hill Selection

In publication for over fifty years, the *Archives of Physical Medicine and Rehabilitation* (*APMR*) is a trustworthy, authoritative resource for information on the care and support of those with disabling conditions. The journal is a product of the American Congress of Rehabilitation Medicine, a multidisciplinary professional organization that has been advocating research and disseminating best practices in the field of rehabilitative medicine since its inception in 1923. Every article goes through a multistep, double-blind review process that includes pre-peer review assessment by the editorial board, peer review by at least one recognized subject expert in the field, and a final assessment for publication by one of the 35 members of the editorial board. The publication's target audience of clinicians, physical and occupational therapists, speech pathologists, chiropractors, and other rehabilitation practitioners will find the timely, authoritative articles eminently useful in the practice of evidence-based patient care, as well as administrative and nonclinical decision making. *APMR* publishes a variety of article types, including original research, reviews, case reports, commentary, and letters. This journal is essential for chiropractic and other manipulative, rehabilitative, or sports therapy practitioners and students, as well as hospitals and research institutions. *APMR* is widely indexed in sources such as CINAHL, Scopus, and MEDLINE—where it is considered a core clinical journal. It ranked sixth among 33 rehabilitation titles and thirteenth among 72 sport sciences titles on the 2009 *Journal Citation Reports*. Full online coverage back to volume 76, 1995 is available through Elsevier ScienceDirect.

Chiropractic Journal of Australia. v. 21, Chiropractors' Association of Australia, 1991.
http://www.ebscohost.com/
ISSN: 10360913
Indexed in: CINAHL
Recommended for: Academic Libraries

This quarterly, peer-reviewed publication includes case studies, educational and clinical best practices, historical articles, news briefs, and book reviews. Not surprisingly, it focuses on Australasian concerns, often covering health care laws of Australia, New Zealand, and the greater region. The material, however, is relevant to practitioners anywhere, particularly to those in educational or clinical settings. Several members of the editorial board are senior chiropractic faculty from North America, and the journal has a growing international audience. First published in 1966 as the *Journal of the Australian Chiropractors' Association*, its title changed after the merger in 1990 of the Australian Chiropractors' Association and the United Chiropractors Association of Australasia. It is indexed in specialized indexes: AMED (Allied and Complementary Medicine), ICL (Index to Chiropractic Literature), MANTIS, and CINAHL. The journal is available primarily in print. Abstracts are available at the journal's website for the former and current titles, from 1984 to the present. The journal was first offered online in 2005. EBSCOhost access is available in Rehabilitation & Sports Medicine Source from 2008 to the present, and volumes published from 2005 through 2007 are offered through ProQuest.

Clinical Chiropractic. v. 6, Elsevier/College of Chiropractors, 2003.
http://www.sciencedirect.com/science/journal/14792354
ISSN: 14792354
ISSN: 1878125X (Online)
Indexed in: CINAHL
Recommended for: Hospital, Academic Libraries

Aimed at the clinically practicing chiropractor, the journal also serves as a valuable resource at academic libraries that support preclinical programs for manual therapy and a source of authoritative information about chiropractic for other health professionals. It maintains a large contingent of expert reviewers in its double-blind, peer-review process, as well as international editorial and advisory boards. It successfully provides information for the development of clinical skills and performance to meet its goal of optimizing patient care. A typical issue opens with a case challenge and closes with an extensive discussion of that case. Original papers focus on topics that can be implemented into patient care. Reports on conferences, literature reviews, and editorials help develop the profession. Originally published as the *British Journal of Chiropractic* from 1997–2002, the journal shifted to its new title in 2003 when the British organization, the College of Chiropractors, relaunched the journal for an international audience through Elsevier. It is indexed in multiple sources, such as AMED (Allied and Complementary Medicine), CINAHL, MANTIS, ICL (Index to Chiropractic Literature), Scopus, and some aggregator services. Online access via Elsevier ScienceDirect is available from volume 6, 2003 to present.

Journal of Bodywork and Movement Therapies. v. 1, Elsevier, 1996.
http://www.bodyworkmovementtherapies.com/
http://www.sciencedirect.com/science/journal/13608592
ISSN: 13608592
ISSN: 15329283 (Online)
Indexed in: MEDLINE, CINAHL
Recommended for: Hospital Libraries

This journal is essential reading for professional and allied health practitioners who are directly involved in the assessment, diagnosis, treatment, and rehabilitation of musculoskeletal dysfunctions. The publication takes a cross-disciplinary approach in helping these providers define and clarify their roles, while discussing the broad range of issues that affect both independent and integrated care. The journal employs a double-blind review process and publishes editorials, summaries, and technique papers that explore practical approaches. While the journal has historically published articles on both the prevention and rehabilitation of injuries, it has recently devoted a section to those two areas. Well-executed illustrations are an important asset, and most articles feature a high number of photographs, drawings, and diagrams. The articles represent a wide variety of therapies, including chiropractic, cranial therapy, Feldenkrais, lymph drainage, yoga therapy, dance, tai chi, Pilates, shiatsu, and others. Founded in 1997, this is the official journal of the Association of Neuromuscular Therapists, the Australian Pilates Method Association, and the National Association of Myofascial Trigger Point Therapists (USA). Therapists and trainers of many backgrounds will apply some techniques to their own practice and will appreciate the perspective of other disciplines. The information can facilitate successful co-management, referral, and meaningful interdisciplinary communication. Indexing for MEDLINE began in 2008, and Elsevier ScienceDirect provides access from 1996 to present.

Journal of Manipulative and Physiological Therapeutics (JMPT). v. 1, Mosby Elsevier for National University of Health Sciences, 1978.
http://www.sciencedirect.com/science/journal/01614754
http://www.jmptonline.org/
ISSN: 01614754
ISSN: 15326586 (Online)
Indexed in: MEDLINE, CINAHL
Recommended for: Hospital, Academic Libraries

In addition to a large readership among chiropractors, this leading journal's audience includes radiologists, osteopaths, physical therapists, and sports medicine specialists. It is the official scientific journal of the American Chiropractic Association and the first chiropractic journal to be indexed in MEDLINE. Each issue typically includes an editorial, issue highlights, original articles, case reports, literature reviews, commentaries, and new media reviews. The *JMPT* Highlights feature—capsule summaries with small illustrations—is especially useful since readers can quickly scan the single page and turn to the referenced article. This page also appears in the online version. Occasionally, the editors issue a call for papers for a special theme issue. The March issue often incorporates award-winning papers from the previous year's annual Association of Chiropractic Colleges and Research Agenda Conference (ACC-RAC), which is a valuable service for chiropractors unable to attend. The journal's large editorial board comprises leading international low-back and spine researchers from medicine, osteopathy, chiropractic, and post-secondary education. Over 100 board members and peer reviewers participated in manuscript reviews in 2009. The National University of Health Sciences began publishing the journal in 1978 and retains the copyright today. Elsevier provides online content at ScienceDirect from 1999 to present.

Journal of the Canadian Chiropractic Association (JCCA). v. ?, Canadian Chiropractic Association, 196?
http://www.jcca-online.org
http://www.ncbi.nlm.nih.gov/pmc/journals/293/
ISSN: 00083194
ISSN: 17156181 (Online)
Indexed in: CINAHL
Recommended for: Academic Libraries

First published in 1957 as the *Canadian Chiropractic Journal*, the *Journal of the Canadian Chiropractic Association* (*JCCA*) is the official, peer-reviewed research publication of the Canadian Chiropractic Association. *JCCA* publishes peer-reviewed research papers, historical reviews, case studies, commentaries, and editorials relevant to the practice of chiropractic. The quarterly publication frequently profiles the activities and personnel of the Canadian Chiropractic Research Foundation and other members of the editorial board. Although the articles focused on the health care system may have little relevance for non-Canadian practitioners, most articles concern clinical care, legislation, education, and research initiatives of interest to chiropractors everywhere. Original articles and case reports far outnumber literature reviews. Despite the journal's close association with a well-known research community, authors reporting on clinical trials tend to publish elsewhere. Nonetheless, the journal succeeds in presenting well-vetted information on a broad array of topics relevant to the chiropractic profession. The journal is indexed in multiple sources such as PubMed (but not MEDLINE) from 1978 to the present, AMED (Allied and Complementary Medicine), and CINAHL. The Association provides open access to full-text articles from 1999 forward.

Manual Therapy: An International Journal of Musculoskeletal Therapy. v. 1, Churchill Livingstone, 1995.
http://www.sciencedirect.com/science/journal/1356689X
ISSN: 1356689X
ISSN: 15322769 (Online)
Indexed in: MEDLINE, CINAHL
Recommended for: Hospital Libraries

The diverse nature of the field of manual therapies makes the publication of a journal that caters to this audience quite a challenge, but *Manual Therapy* meets this challenge head on. The editorial board consisting of representatives from over fifteen countries, including South Africa and Australia, reinforces the diverse, international perspective of this peer-reviewed publication. The Manipulation Association of Chartered Physiotherapists (MACP) sponsors the journal. This organization consists of 900 full members, who have received approved training at the post-graduate or master's level, and 200 associate members, who are in the process of obtaining the required training and education. The publication covers a wide variety of topics associated with the human neuromusculoskeletal system, including scientific evidence for manual therapies, administrative and legal issues relating to manual therapy practice and research surrounding pathologies, biomechanics, and ergonomics and anatomy as they relate to manual therapies. This publication also features a variety of article types, including original research, case reports, review articles, "masterclass" features, technical reports, and commentary/letters. The journal is indexed in MEDLINE and other databases. Varied article types, the scientific rigor of the peer-review process, and the diverse, international perspective of the authors and editors make *Manual Therapy* a valuable resource for students, researchers, and practitioners of manual therapies. Full online coverage from volume 1 to the present is available through Elsevier ScienceDirect.

Spine. v. 1, Lippincott Williams & Wilkins, 1976.
http://www.spinejournal.com/
http://www.ovid.com/
ISSN: 03622436
ISSN: 15281159 (Online)
See Also Chapter 11.6. Orthopedics
Indexed in: MEDLINE, CINAHL
Recommended for: Hospital, Academic Libraries

Considered the leading journal in the field of spinal disorder treatment, this peer-reviewed, bi-weekly publication is at the forefront of spine research and does not publish material that other publications have discussed in detail. A typical print issue contains abstracts of case reports and other types of articles that are published exclusively online: well-researched, original articles grouped into categories such as anatomy, biomechanics, clinical case series, health services research, and surgery, as well as letters. Coverage of the outcome of surgical methods for treating spinal disorders resulting from trauma and disease is a major component. Research comparing invasive and conservative care is incorporated, though not the primary focus. Of more than 12,000 citations in MEDLINE, fewer than 200 have the keyword "chiropractic." Nevertheless, chiropractors look to the journal for relevant, up-to-date coverage of anatomy, basic science, biomechanics, case reports, and clinical trials. Among such articles are studies both supportive and critical of spinal manipulation. It is the official journal of 14 international associations, including the Cervical Spine Research Society, the Spine Society of Europe, and the Chinese Orthopaedic Association. The journal was ranked seventh out of 56 orthopedic subspecialty journal in the 2009 *Journal Citation Reports*. The publisher uses the Ovid interface for delivery of digital content from volume 1, 1976 to present.

Spine Journal. v. 1, Elsevier, 2001.
http://www.sciencedirect.com/science/journal/15299430
ISSN: 15299430
ISSN: 18781632 (Online)
Indexed in: MEDLINE, CINAHL
Recommended for: Hospital Libraries

The official journal of the North American Spine Society (NASS), an international and multidisciplinary organization, *Spine Journal* is a blend of peer-reviewed articles concerning research about the spine and treatment of disorders and other content such as major reviews of specific topics, technical notes, editorials, and special features. NASS emphasizes evidence-based, ethical spine care and furthers continuing education, research, and advocacy among its members. The Society presents an annual award for up to three outstanding papers, which are published along with the proceedings of the NASS annual meeting as a supplement to the journal. Clinical studies cover surgery and conservative care, and basic science topics discuss material likely to be of interest to clinicians. While the primary audience comprises professionals from a wide range of disciplines, its chiropractic articles are some of the most cited, as reported by Elsevier's Scopus. The journal is available online from Elsevier ScienceDirect, from its initial volume in 2001 to the present. Since 2009, the journal's case reports are published exclusively online with the corresponding abstracts appearing in the print edition.

Databases and Other Electronic Resources

Index to Chiropractic Literature (ICL). Chiropractic Library Collaboration, 2000.
http://www.chiroindex.org
Recommended for: Hospital, Academic Libraries

Begun in 2000, the Index to Chiropractic Literature (ICL) is an open access database that provides cover-to-cover indexing of peer-reviewed literature and selected trade magazines from chiropractic publishers beginning with 1985 to the present. At hospitals and academic institutions that support manual therapy programs, librarians can take advantage of its flexible search interface and its downloading capabilities in the collection development process. Searching for a specific journal will display all indexed citations, revealing the topical content and the incidence of significant publication types such as case reports and clinical trials. Similarly, searching by a publication type and sorting the retrieval after the download reveals which journals most frequently include particular types of articles. As an example, in evaluating *JACA Online* from the American Chiropractic Association, a user will likely notice the coverage of practical and timely topics, presence of peer-reviewed articles in the research and science section, and inclusion of patient education handouts in each issue. To open full text and evaluate the quality of references for the articles in *JACA Online*, a user needs a subscription. For journals published in online format, the abstract view links to the article or to the table of contents at the publisher's website and clearly identifies the items as either open access or subscription based. The editors of ICL now use a content management system to categorize links to additional resources. The Open Access Library tab lists free, peer-reviewed journals and provides convenient Google searches for chiropractic magazines and newspapers. The More Resources tab provides links to information about getting published, including instructions for authors for each journal, practice guidelines, organizations, and websites. As this content grows, researchers will be able to explore and evaluate even more resources using both the index and its accessory resources. Development of the index by volunteer editors and indexers progressed steadily from 1980 to the present. The print compilation of citations for 1980–1984 is no longer available.

4. Dentistry

The teeth, oral cavity, and associated structures, and the diagnosis and treatment of their diseases including prevention and the restoration of defective and missing tissue.

—MeSH

Contributors: Elizabeth A. Strother, Julie H. Schiavo

Monographs

ADA/PDR Guide to Dental Therapeutics. 5th ed. Editor: Sebastian G. Ciancio. American Dental Association, 2009.
ISBN: 9781563637698
Recommended for: Academic Libraries

A comprehensive source on medications encountered in dental practice, this American Dental Association publication is updated every three years. In the most recent two editions, the ADA has collaborated with the *Physician's Desk Reference*®. The book is arranged into three sections: drugs used in dentistry, drugs used in medicine, and drug issues in dental practice. Chapters are arranged by drug or product class. Each chapter begins with an overview of the pharmacologic category and dental considerations, but the majority of the information is presented in tables, allowing dentists to quickly find and read pertinent data. By arranging the information according to drug class, dentists can easily compare warnings, precautions, contraindications, and adverse effects of similar drugs. A separate table of drug interactions appears at the end of each chapter. Of particular note is "Oral Manifestations of Systemic Agents," which lists drugs according to type of oral adverse reaction. Sixteen appendixes provide additional information such as updated guidelines for prevention of infective endocarditis, drugs prescribed for tobacco cessation, and dental considerations of HIV and antiretroviral medications. This concise and authoritative guide, indispensable to clinicians as well as dental students, is a required purchase for all dental school libraries.

Contemporary Implant Dentistry. 3rd ed. Author: Carl E. Misch. Mosby Elsevier, 2008.
ISBN: 9780323043731
Recommended for: Academic Libraries
Brandon/Hill, *Doody's Core Titles* Selection

Dental implants are now accepted as a standard method of tooth replacement. In this Brandon/Hill selection, Carl Misch, an acknowledged expert in dental implants, presents a detailed overview of the science of implant dentistry, focusing on attaining predictable outcomes. This textbook is directed towards dental students, residents, postgraduates, general dentists, and specialists. The 42 chapters are arranged into six parts: "Rationale for Treatment," "Treatment Planning," "Fundamental Science," "Implant Surgery," "Soft and Hard Tissue Rehabilitation," and "Implant Maintenance." New chapters on treatment planning, bone grafting, and implant surgery have been added to the third edition. Extensive bibliographies are included at the end of each chapter and high-quality color photographs and drawings illustrate concepts in the text. This is a first purchase recommendation on the MLA Dental Section's *Booklist*. Implants are related to all aspects and specialties of dentistry and as the most widely accepted source for basic information on this significant topic, this textbook is required for all dental school library collections.

Craig's Restorative Dental Materials. 12th ed. Editors: John M. Powers, Ronald L. Sakaguchi. Mosby Elsevier, 2006.
ISBN: 9780323036061
Recommended for: Academic Libraries
Doody's Core Titles Selection

Renamed for the editor of the fourth to eleventh editions, this classic textbook provides an overview of restorative dental materials for the dental student. Chapters cover topics such as biocompatibility of dental materials, resin composite restorative materials, preventive materials, impression materials, and cements. Two new chapters on dental implants and tissue engineering have been added to the twelfth edition. A first purchase on the MLA Dental Section's *Booklist*, the book presents fundamental concepts as well as clinical and laboratory applications for restorative dental materials. Black-and-white photographs, tables, and drawings accompany the text. Each chapter includes problems and solutions to enable students to review the material presented; "Mind Maps" in appendix B also serve as a study aid by presenting a graphic outline of each chapter. Lengthy lists of references at the end of chapters are arranged by broad topic. An effective dental materials textbook and resource for data on materials, this book is a required purchase for all libraries serving dental schools.

Critical Thinking: Understanding and Evaluating Dental Research. 2nd ed. Author: Donald M. Brunette. Quintessence, 2007.
http://www.quintpub.com/
http://online.statref.com/titleinfo/fxid-235.html
ISBN: 9780867154269
Recommended for: Academic Libraries

Responding to the increased trend in the dental school curriculum to promote critical thinking and lifelong learning, this book introduces dental students, residents, and faculty to all aspects of the research process. With an emphasis on teaching dentists to critically evaluate scientific papers, the book also provides in-depth information for dentists interested in participating in research and publication. Through a realistic view of the requirements, pitfalls, and rewards of scientific research, this excellent work serves as a textbook in dental research methods. The book begins with an overview of scientific publications and describes searching the dental literature in online databases such as MEDLINE. Chapters then progress through logical analysis, the different types of research strategies and designs, and statistical analysis. In the last chapter, thirty- eight exercises allow the reader to practice critical thinking skills. This title is available electronically via STAT!Ref. A resource for all programs that encourage student understanding of, if not involvement in, dental research, this book should be in the collection of all libraries serving dental programs.

Drug Information Handbook for Dentistry. 16th ed. Authors: Richard L. Wynn, Timothy F. Meiller, Harold L. Criossley. Lexi-Comp, 2010.
http://www.lexi-comp.com
ISBN: 9781591952824
Recommended for: Academic Libraries

Over 1,600 medications are listed alphabetically by generic name in this annually updated handy reference book for dentists. Each entry includes standard drug information such as pharmacologic category, use, adverse effects, restrictions, dosage, mechanism of action, contraindications, warnings and precautions, and drug interactions. Additional information of interest to dentists includes local anesthetic and vasoconstrictor precautions, effects on dental treatment, effects on bleeding, and dental comment (as necessary). Following the alphabetical list are sections on natural products, herbal and dietary supplements, and oral medicine topics, including medically compromised patients and sample prescriptions for oral conditions. Appendixes include normal blood values and the top 200 prescribed drugs. Appearing at the end of the book are the pharmacologic category index, which serves as a brief guide to drug names for various uses, and the alphabetical index with generic and brand names. In Lexi-Comp Online, drugs can be searched by generic or brand names and information is updated daily. Supplemental material from other sections of the book is listed under Charts/Special Topics. This book includes everything a dentist needs to know about prescribing drugs and managing patients who take drugs for medical conditions. It is a required resource for dental school libraries.

Handbook of Local Anesthesia. 5th ed. Author: Stanley F. Malamed. Mosby Elsevier, 2004.
ISBN: 9780323024495
Recommended for: Academic Libraries

In *Handbook of Local Anesthesia*, Malamed presents the latest techniques and drugs used to prevent pain during dental procedures. The book is divided into four main sections covering pharmacology, armamentarium, techniques, and complications. The last section includes a new chapter on legal considerations, written by an expert oral and maxillofacial surgeon/attorney. High-quality color photographs, new to this edition, enable students to clearly see how to administer injections. The last chapter, with questions and answers on specific, practical issues in local anesthesia, serves as a review for the student. This detailed yet comprehensive volume is the preferred textbook in dental school pain control courses and also serves clinicians as an authoritative reference source. A companion DVD, sold separately or as a package with the book, follows the structure of the textbook to provide visual enhancement of written concepts. This title is a first purchase recommendation on the MLA Dental Section's *Booklist*. Because of the depth of coverage, this book is a required purchase for all collections serving dental schools.

Mosby's Dental Drug Reference. 9th ed. Editor: Arthur H. Jeske. Mosby Elsevier, 2010.
ISBN: 9780323065207
Recommended for: Academic Libraries
Doody's Core Titles Selection

This pocket-size book lists brief information for over 800 drugs of interest to dentists. Arranged alphabetically by generic name, each drug monograph includes brand names, drug class, mechanism of action, uses, pharmacokinetics, indications, dosages, side effects, precautions and contraindications, and serious reactions. Of particular significance to dentists is the inclusion of drug interactions of concern to dentistry and dental considerations for each drug. Because entries are limited to drugs likely to be encountered in dental practice, most medications used in hospitalized patients are not found in this book. A new feature of this edition is the arrangement of drug names under diseases and disorders in the generic and trade name index. "Therapeutic Management of Common Oral Lesions," and "Medically Compromised Patients," both adapted from other sources, appear at the beginning of the book. A supplemental CD-ROM includes a pill atlas, small image collection, and glossary of terms. The Evolve website also has additional material such as drugs of abuse and alternative drugs. Eleven appendixes, with information such as drugs that affect taste, drugs associated with dry mouth, and herbal medications and supplements, enhance the usefulness of the book to dentists. *Mosby's Dental Drug Reference*, an important resource for dental students, residents, and clinicians, should be in every collection supporting dental school programs.

Phillips' Science of Dental Materials. 11th ed. Author: Kenneth J. Anusavice. Saunders Elsevier, 2003.
ISBN: 9780721693873
Recommended for: Academic Libraries
Doody's Core Titles Selection

Although this edition is somewhat dated, *The Science of Dental Materials*, first published in 1937, remains the classic textbook in the field of dental materials. The comprehensive, detailed coverage of dental materials is divided into four broad parts: general classes and properties of dental materials, auxiliary dental materials, direct restorative materials, and indirect restorative and prosthetic materials. Each chapter begins with an outline and a glossary of key terms and ends with a list of selected readings. Critical thinking questions throughout the text provide topics for classroom discussion. High-quality drawings and photographs, mainly black and white, are interspersed with numerous tables and graphs. This book aims to provide students and dentists with knowledge of materials science principles so they can wisely select appropriate materials for patient treatment. This book, a first purchase recommendation on the MLA Dental Section's *Booklist*, is a required textbook for all libraries serving dental schools.

Sedation: A Guide to Patient Management. 5th ed. Author: Stanley F. Malamed. Mosby Elsevier, 2010.
ISBN: 9780323056809
Recommended for: Academic Libraries
Doody's Core Titles Selection

Written by the acknowledged expert on dental anesthesia, *Sedation: A Guide to Patient Management* provides dental students, residents, and dentists with a comprehensive overview of techniques for pain and anxiety control in outpatient settings. Chapters focus on routes of administration, inhalation and intravenous sedation, and general anesthesia. By discussing the clinical pharmacology of drugs, the author emphasizes use of drugs currently accepted as safe and effective. Safety and preparation are stressed in the section on emergencies. Separate chapters are devoted to sedation for pediatric, geriatric, disabled, and medically compromised patients. This edition includes an updated chapter on oral, rectal, and intramuscular sedation and new chapters on medicolegal considerations and the history of anesthesiology in dentistry. All photographs and drawings are in full color and numerous tables summarize important information. Each chapter ends with references for further reading. Covering both theoretical and step-by-step procedures, this book is intended to supplement classroom training in preparing dentists to safely and effectively administer drugs for the management of patient pain and anxiety. A first purchase recommendation on the MLA Dental Section's *Booklist, Sedation: A Guide to Patient Management* is required for all libraries serving dental schools.

Journals

Dental Clinics of North America. v. 1, Elsevier, 1957.
http://dental.theclinics.com/
ISSN: 00118532
ISSN: 15580512 (Online)
Indexed in: MEDLINE, CINAHL
Recommended for: Academic Libraries

Published quarterly, each issue of *Dental Clinics of North America* is devoted to a special topic. Guest editors invite authors to submit review articles covering all aspects of dentistry. Recent issues have focused on current topics such as oral health care access, the special care patient, and evidence-based dentistry. The journal is available online via ScienceDirect starting with 2002 and indexed in MEDLINE and CINAHL. The wide range of topics covered by this dental journal makes it popular among students writing research papers, dental school faculty, and dentists in private practice. Articles include high quality color and black-and-white photographs. With its in-depth coverage of the latest issues in dentistry, this journal enables clinicians to keep up with both patient care and professional developments. Of the three dental journals in *The Clinics* series, it is the only one applicable to all dentists as the other two titles are focused on oral and maxillofacial surgery. *Dental Clinics of North America* is a required subscription for all dental school libraries and a necessary title for any dental collection.

International Journal of Oral & Maxillofacial Implants. v. 1, Quintessence, 1986.
http://www.quintpub.com/
ISSN: 08822786
ISSN: 19424434 (Online)
Indexed in: MEDLINE, CINAHL
Recommended for: Academic Libraries

The official journal of the Academy of Osseointegration, this bimonthly publication contains three categories of articles: implant science, clinical applications, and technology and case reports. Additional features are editorials, thematic abstracts of articles from other journals, and a meetings calendar. This peer-reviewed journal is of interest to oral surgeons, periodontists, prosthodontists, and other dentists working in the field of oral implantology. One of the few major journals devoted to the study of dental implants, the *International Journal of Oral & Maxillofacial Implants (JOMI)* ranks 17 out of 64 dental journals in the 2009 *Journal Citation Reports*. Over twenty articles on new materials, techniques, and procedures appear in each issue. *JOMI* is indexed in MEDLINE, Science Citation Index, and CINAHL. The list of associate editors and review board members comprises international experts in oral implantology. High quality photographs and diagrams, many in color, accompany the articles. All issues of the journal are available electronically through Quintessence Publishers. This is a highly recommended journal subscription for dental school libraries.

Journal of Dental Research. v. 1, Sage for the International & American Associations for Dental Research, 1919.
http://jdr.sagepub.com/
ISSN: 00220345
ISSN: 15440591 (Online)
Indexed in: MEDLINE
Recommended for: Academic Libraries

The major research journal in the field of dentistry, this peer-reviewed monthly publication covers all aspects of basic research in the oral and craniofacial sciences. In addition to original research articles, each issue includes two or three review articles under the heading "Critical Reviews in Oral Biology and Medicine." Research articles are arranged in sections labeled clinical, biological, and biomaterials and bioengineering. Abstracts of papers and posters presented at the annual meetings of the International and American Associations for Dental Research (IADR, AADR), published in special issues of this journal, are now searchable on the IADR website. *Advances in Dental Research*, an electronic supplement to the *Journal of Dental Research*, contains review articles focused on a specific topic. Ranked second among dental journals by *Journal Citation Reports* (2009), the *Journal of Dental Research* is the most significant research journal for dentistry. It is indexed in numerous databases including MEDLINE, Biological Abstracts, and Chemical Abstracts. All volumes are available online via Sage and full-text access to articles older than one year is free. *The Journal of Dental Research* is a required subscription for all dental school libraries.

Journal of the American Dental Association. v. 26, American Dental Association, 1939.
http://jada.ada.org/
ISSN: 00028177
ISSN: 19434723 (Online)
Indexed in: MEDLINE, CINAHL
Recommended for: Hospital, Academic Libraries
Brandon/Hill Selection

As the official journal of the American Dental Association, this monthly peer-reviewed publication reaches all members of the major professional dental association and appeals to both general dentists and specialists wanting to keep up with the latest issues and trends in dentistry. Basic and clinical research articles explore advances in all areas of dentistry including implants, restorative procedures, care for medically compromised patients, dental materials, and esthetics. News, letters, and commentaries address the major contemporary issues of the profession, and columns on practice management and ethics provide dentists with information they can apply to their own work situations. This title ranks twenty-first out of 64 dental journals in the 2009 *Journal Citation Reports*. It is indexed in numerous databases such as MEDLINE, Biological Abstracts, Chemical Abstracts, and CINAHL. The journal is available online, with full text provided by HighWire Press starting in 1995. As the "best-read dental journal" in the United States, *JADA* is a major resource for dentistry and is required for all libraries supporting dental schools or hospital dental clinics.

Journal of Dental Education. v. 1, American Dental Education Association, 1936.
http://www.jdentaled.org
ISSN: 00220337
ISSN: 19307837 (Online)

Indexed in: MEDLINE
Recommended for: Academic Libraries

The *Journal of Dental Education* is the official journal of the American Dental Education Association. It has been published since 1936 and is recognized as the foremost journal in academic dentistry. This journal is one of the few that publish articles on the newest research in dental education and education research. The peer-reviewed articles deal with subjects such as testing methodologies, curriculum reform, student surveys, and systematic reviews of clinical trials. The journal supports all varieties of scientific and educational research within dental education. *Journal of Dental Education* is indexed in MEDLINE, CINAHL Plus, and ERIC. The full text of the journal is available online from 2001, and abstracts and/or tables of contents are available back to 1968. This journal is an essential purchase for a library supporting a dental education program

4.1. Operative Dentistry

That phase of clinical dentistry concerned with the restoration of parts of existing teeth that are defective through disease, trauma, or abnormal development, to the state of normal function, health, and esthetics, including preventive, diagnostic, biological, mechanical, and therapeutic techniques, as well as material and instrument science and application.

—MeSH: Dentistry, Operative

Contributor: Elizabeth A. Strother

Monographs

Fundamentals of Operative Dentistry. 3rd ed. Editors: James B. Summitt, J. William Robbins, Thomas J. Hilton, Richard S. Schwartz. Quintessence, 2006.
ISBN: 9780867154528
Recommended for: Academic Libraries
Doody's Core Titles Selection

This book presents current concepts of prevention and management of dental caries and restoration of individual teeth to an audience of both dental students and practitioners. The 20 chapters, written by international experts in the field of operative dentistry and biomaterials, present a blend of traditional methods and recent scientific developments with an emphasis on conservative dentistry. Chapters include esthetic techniques such as tooth bleaching, porcelain veneers, and esthetic inlays and onlays. The authors include the scientific basis for all concepts described and each chapter has an extensive list of references. The third edition has been updated with information derived from new scientific evidence. High-quality black-and-white and color photographs enhance the text. This book, a first-purchase recommendation on the MLA Dental Section's *Booklist*, should be considered for purchase by all dental school libraries.

Sturdevant's Art and Science of Operative Dentistry. 5th ed. Editors: Theodore M. Roberson, Harald O. Heymann, Edward J. Swift, Jr. Mosby Elsevier, 2006.
ISBN: 9780323030090
Recommended for: Academic Libraries
Doody's Core Titles Selection

In this comprehensive textbook on operative dentistry, twenty-one chapters are divided into five major sections: "Fundamentals of Operative Dentistry," "Instrumentation and Preparation," "Composite Restorations," "Amalgam Restorations," and "Metal Restorations." Chapters 1–8 present background information including dental anatomy, cariology, and biomaterials. Chapters 9–21 cover treatment planning and clinical techniques for the various types of restorations. The book discusses both traditional and new developments in operative dentistry with emphasis on treating underlying causes of the patient's problem as well as restoring the immediate damage. The fifth edition has been updated with additional coverage of dental treatment for elderly patients and new strategies and materials for bonded composite restorations. Each chapter ends with an extensive list of references. Over 2,550 black-and-white illustrations, both photographs and drawings, highlight the text. Contributors are predominantly from the University of North Carolina. Additional instructional tools are located online at the Evolve website. This detailed textbook, a *Doody's* essential purchase title and recommended first purchase title on the MLA Dental Section's *Booklist*, is a required purchase for collections serving dental schools.

Journals

Operative Dentistry. v. 1, Indiana University School of Dentistry, 1976.
http://www.jopdentonline.org/
ISSN: 03617734
ISSN: 15592863 (Online)
Indexed in: MEDLINE
Recommended for: Academic Libraries

Operative dentistry is the branch of dentistry that involves the functional and esthetic restoration of individual teeth. The refereed bimonthly publication, *Operative Dentistry*, is the official journal of the Academy of Operative Dentistry, the American Academy of Gold Foil Operators, and the RV Tucker Academy. Articles focus on dental materials and techniques for the conservation and restoration of teeth with dental caries, fractures, and wear defects. The journal also includes articles on dental education and the social, political, and economic aspects of dental practice. Clinical and laboratory research articles, literature reviews, clinical technique articles, and case reports appear in this journal. Each article begins with a brief statement of clinical relevance, followed by a lengthy abstract. Selected articles contain full-color photographs. Except for classified ads for faculty positions, the journal does not accept advertising. Full-text articles are available online beginning in 2006. *Operative Dentistry*, the major journal for research articles investigating all aspects of tooth restoration, is a required subscription for all libraries supporting dental education programs.

4.2. Forensic Dentistry

The application of dental knowledge to questions of law.

—MeSH

Contributor: Elizabeth A. Strother

Monographs

Forensic Dentistry. 2nd ed. Editors: David R. Senn, Paul G. Stimson. CRC Press, 2010.
ISBN: 9781420078367
Recommended for: Academic Libraries

In its first revision in 13 years, this authoritative text on forensic odontology has grown by over 100 pages. Covering all aspects of dental forensic identification, the book is an important resource for the dentist or any member of the forensic team preparing to participate in dental identification procedures. The editors and contributors discuss the development, current state, and future of forensic dentistry. Chapters cover various methods of forensic identification such as DNA, fingerprints, radiography, photography, and bite marks. Other topics include the role of dentists in identifying abuse, jurisprudence and legal issues, age estimation, and mass disasters. Black-and-white and color photographs illustrate the text. Extensive lists of references at the end of each chapter support the information discussed. *Forensic Dentistry*, a first purchase recommendation on the MLA Dental Section's *Booklist* for the first edition, is a highly recommended addition to all dental school libraries.

Manual of Forensic Odontology. 4th ed. American Society of Forensic Odontology, 2007.
ISBN: 9780965022361
Recommended for: Academic Libraries

This reference manual provides a basic overview of evidence-based knowledge in forensic dentistry. Chapters cover forensic dentistry as a career, techniques for human identification, accident and mass disaster management, bite mark analysis, abuse and neglect, technological aides in forensic dentistry, and dental jurisprudence. Each detailed chapter has been written by multiple forensic experts and is accompanied by an extensive list of references. Color and black-and-white photographs accompany the text. Each chapter ends with outcome assessments or learning objectives to reflect the skills demanded of a forensic dentist. Updated information in the fourth edition includes HIPAA regulations, revised guidelines from the American Board of Forensic Odontology, new technology for identification and record management, and protocols from the 9/11/2001 World Trade Center disaster, the 2004 Indian Ocean tsunami, and Hurricane Katrina. This book is recommended for all dental school library collections and for any dental professional interested in a career in forensic dentistry or participating in forensic identification procedures.

4.3. Dental General Practice

Nonspecialized dental practice which is concerned with providing primary and continuing dental care.

—MeSH

Contributor: Elizabeth A. Strother

Monographs

Dental Ethics at Chairside: Professional Principles and Practical Applications. 2nd ed. Authors: David T. Ozar, David J. Sokol. Georgetown University Press, 2002.
ISBN: 0878403760
Recommended for: Academic Libraries
Doody's Core Titles Selection

This book presents dentists with fundamental tools for ethical decision making in all aspects of dental practice. Fifteen cases illustrate ethical situations encountered by dentists. Detailed explanations of issues surrounding each case provide guidelines for dentists reflecting on ethical actions. The cases and complex analysis of each case are well-written, interesting, and easy to read. As a textbook in professional development courses, this book provides dental students with the framework for understanding their professional obligations and approaching difficult situations with ethical behavior. Among the issues discussed in the book are patients with limited financial means, poor work by previous dentists, uncooperative pediatric patients, obligations of dentists toward their employees, and HIV/AIDS in patients or dentists. A "Bibliographic Essay," at the end of the book is a compilation of annotated references arranged by chapter. This book, a guide to ethical behavior for the dental profession, should be required reading for all oral health professionals and is recommended for all dental school libraries.

Functional Occlusion: From TMJ to Smile Design. Author: Peter E. Dawson. Mosby Elsevier, 2007.
ISBN: 9780323033718
Recommended for: Academic Libraries

Peter Dawson, an acknowledged expert on the temporomandibular joint (TMJ) and dental occlusion, advocates an interdisciplinary approach to patient treatment that combines functional and esthetic principles. Based on scientific evidence, this book emphasizes the interrelationship of the TMJ and occlusion in striving for harmony in the total masticatory system. The goal of this book, providing dentists with the information required to achieve predictable clinical success, is accomplished through a combination of theory and specific clinical procedures. Chapters are divided into three main sections: "Functional Harmony," "Dysfunction," and "Treatment." Over 1,200 excellent color photographs and drawings enhance the text. This comprehensive volume, applicable to both general dentists and specialists, is the authoritative source on the treatment of TMJ and occlusal disorders. Because faculty members, residents, and students will seek out this book, it is a required acquisition for all dental school libraries.

Medical Emergencies in the Dental Office. 6th ed. Author: Stanley F. Malamed. Mosby Elsevier, 2007.
ISBN: 9780323042352
Recommended for: Hospital, Academic Libraries
Doody's Core Titles Selection

This authoritative textbook teaches dental professionals how to effectively recognize and manage medical emergencies in the dental office. The book begins with a section on prevention, preparation, and legal considerations of emergencies in the dental office. Remaining chapters are divided into signs and symptoms of physical emergencies: unconsciousness, respiratory distress, altered consciousness, seizures, drug-related emergencies, chest pain, and cardiac arrest. The accepted textbook for dental and dental hygiene students, this volume should also be reviewed periodically by members of the dental office staff. Changes in the sixth edition include a new medical history questionnaire in chapter two, rewriting of the chapter on legal considerations, and a new chapter on pediatric emergencies. Questions from the medical history questionnaire related to specific conditions are located in chapters on the conditions. The book also incorporates American Heart Association guidelines revised in 2005 for BLS, ACLS, and PALS. Numerous color photographs clearly illustrate treatment techniques and tables effectively summarize key concepts. It is a recommended first purchase title on the MLA Dental Section's *Booklist*. The depth of coverage of this book makes it a required purchase for all libraries in hospitals with dental departments and all dental school libraries.

Oral Radiology: Principles and Interpretation. 6th ed. Editors: Stuart C. White, Michael J. Pharoah. Mosby Elsevier, 2009.
ISBN: 9780323049832
Recommended for: Academic Libraries
Brandon/Hill, *Doody's Core Titles* Selection

This comprehensive textbook provides dental students with an in-depth introduction to dental radiography and imaging. The contents of this edition have been updated to include the latest techniques and standards. The text is generously illustrated with high-quality black-and-white radiographic images, photographs, and diagrams. Preliminary chapters cover radiation physics, biologic effects, and safety. The two main sections include chapters on imaging principles and techniques and radiographic interpretation of various diseases and conditions. Among the new material is a chapter on the rapidly developing technique of cone-beam computed tomography. Other new information includes bisphosphonate-related jaw osteonecrosis and an expanded chapter on dental implants. Other topics include digital imaging, MRI and CT scanning, normal radiographic anatomy, and guidelines for prescribing dental radiographs. Lengthy bibliographies at the end of each chapter are arranged by specific topic. The Evolve website offers students and instructors additional resources for instruction and review. As the most thorough and authoritative textbook currently available on dental radiology, this book is a first purchase title on the MLA Dental Section's *Booklist* and required for all libraries serving dental schools.

Treatment Planning in Dentistry. 2nd ed. Editors: Stephen J. Stefanac, Samuel P. Nesbit. Mosby Elsevier, 2007.
ISBN: 9780323036979

Recommended for: Academic Libraries
Doody's Core Titles Selection

A core textbook in the dental school curriculum, this book introduces the dental student to the fundamental knowledge required for devising patient treatment plans. Students and experienced practitioners also learn how to compromise between ideal and practical plans for their patients. The text is divided into three main sections: an overview of the treatment planning process including evidence-based treatment; five phases of the treatment plan; and planning treatment for special needs patients. Three new chapters in the third section address special care patients, oral cancer, and alcohol and substance abuse. A chapter on ethical and legal issues, including obtaining consent to treatment, provides important information. Clinical cases, scientific evidence, and the role of other members of the dental staff are highlighted in boxes throughout the text. Black-and-white photographs, radiographic images, and tables illustrate the narrative and each chapter ends with review questions, suggested projects, and suggested readings. A CD-ROM accompanying the book includes five interactive patient simulations of increasing complexity. Because it provides the dental student with tools for creating effective treatment plans for all types of adolescent and adult patients, this title is a required purchase for all libraries supporting dental schools.

4.4. Special Populations

4.4.1. Geriatric Dentistry

Dental problems of older people.

—MeSH

Contributor: Julie H. Schiavo

Monographs

Clinician's Guide to Oral Health in Geriatric Patients. 3rd ed. Editors: Joel M. Laudenbach, Jonathon A. Ship. American Academy of Oral Medicine, 2009.
http://www.atlasbooks.com
ISBN: 9781936176014
ISBN: 9781936176175 (Online)
Recommended for: Hospital, Academic Libraries

This third edition of *Oral Health in Geriatric Patients* is newly revised and updated to provide oral health practitioners the newest and best guide to treating geriatric patients. The guide offers summaries of the influences of aging, systemic diseases, and the treatment of systemic diseases on the oral health of the elderly. It also presents the etiology, clinical appearance, and treatment of common oral diseases that are prevalent in the geriatric population. The guide stresses the importance of treatment of oral conditions and the consequences of these conditions on the functionality and quality of life of the elderly. The chapters conclude with pharmacological therapies in respect to the physiological differences of the elderly. The material is presented in list and table format with color pictures of oral conditions. The appendix of this edition contains selected websites and additional readings for clinicians interested learning more. *Oral Health in Geriatric Patients* is also available in e-book format from the publisher. This is a very valuable and easy to use reference for oral health practitioners who treat the elderly.

4.4.2. Pediatric Dentistry

Dental problems of children, proper maintenance, and treatment. The dental care may include the services provided by dental specialists.

—MeSH

Contributor: Julie H. Schiavo

Monographs

Fundamentals of Pediatric Dentistry. 3rd ed. Authors: Richard J. Mathewson, Robert E. Primosch. Quintessence, 1995.
ISBN: 9780867152623
Recommended for: Academic Libraries

A staple text in the pediatric dentistry field, Mathewson's *Fundamentals of Pediatric Dentistry* is in its third edition. The text is extensively revised and reorganized from previous editions. The objective of this book is to provide the dental practitioner or student with step-by-step guidelines in the treatment of children. The chapters are divided into large sections covering diagnosis, prevention, child management, and clinical procedures. Each chapter begins with clearly defined learning goals and ends with multiple choice questions for the student to gauge his understanding of the material. Most of the illustrations included in this book are black-and-white line drawings or photographs. This title is included in the MLA Dental Section's *Booklist*.

Gorlin's Syndromes of the Head and Neck. 5th ed. Editors: Raoul C.M. Hennekam, Ian D. Krantz, Judith E. Allanson. Oxford University Press, 2010.
ISBN: 9780195307900

Recommended for: Hospital, Academic Libraries
Doody's Core Titles Selection

This text is considered the gold standard in head and neck diagnosis, covering a very large number of syndromes affecting the head and neck region. These include, but are not limited to, syndromes resulting from teratogenic agents, chromosomal syndromes, metabolic disorders, syndromes affecting the bone, short stature syndromes, overgrowth syndromes, syndromes affecting the skin and mucosa, syndromes of abnormal craniofacial contour, orofacial clefting syndromes, syndromes with gingival/periodontal components, and syndromes with unusual dental findings. *Gorlin's Syndromes of the Head and Neck* is in its fifth edition and has been revised in this printing, covering more than 700 different genetic syndromes. Each condition is described with the phenotype spectrum, epidemiology, mode of inheritance, pathogenesis, and profile. This text is a vital addition to any hospital library, especially one that serves a pediatric population. It is essential to the hospital-based pediatric dentist or any dentist serving special needs patients.

McDonald and Avery's Dentistry for the Child and Adolescent. 8th ed. Editors: Jeffrey A. Dean, David R. Avery, Ralph E. McDonald. Mosby-Year Book Inc., 2010.
ISBN: 9780323057240
Recommended for: Hospital, Academic Libraries
Doody's Core Titles Selection

This staple of the pediatric dentistry literature contains current diagnosis and treatment recommendations based on research, clinical experience, and current literature. The text covers such relevant topics as oral examination, child abuse and neglect, development and morphology of primary teeth, tumors of the oral region, trauma management, medically compromised patients, problems of children with disabilities, and community oral health. The ninth edition has been revised significantly in three main areas: color illustrations have been added, the text is connected to Elsevier's Evolve website, and several chapters have been revised and improved. The text is intended for dental students, post graduate pediatric residents, and practitioners. This title is included in *Doody's Core Titles* and the MLA Dental Section's *Booklist*.

Paediatric Dentistry. 3rd ed. Editors: Richard R. Welbury, Monty S. Duggal, Marie-Therese Hosey. Oxford University Press, 2005.
http://www.oup.com/us/
http://online.statref.com/titleinfo/fxid-124.html
ISBN: 9780198565833
Recommended for: Hospital, Academic Libraries

Paediatric Dentistry is designed for the use of dental students but is also highly recommended for postgraduates and practitioners of pediatric dentistry. In this third edition, several chapters have been rewritten by different authors. Each chapter is clearly outlined and contains boxes set apart from the text with "key points" to aid the student in focusing while studying. The chapters end with a summary of the material and a bibliography for the student seeking more information on the topics. The book contains a large number of colorful charts and full-color photographs illustrating the topics presented or steps for a procedure. This title is included in the MLA Dental Section's *Booklist* and is available electronically through STAT!Ref.

Pediatric Dentistry: Infancy through Adolescence. 4th ed. Editor: Jimmy R. Pinkham. Elsevier Saunders, 2005.
ISBN: 9780721603124
Recommended for: Academic Libraries
Brandon/Hill, *Doody's Core Titles* Selection

Currently in its 4th edition, *Pediatric Dentistry: Infancy through Adolescence* has been a vital text in the pediatric dentistry literature since its first publishing. The authors cover all aspects of dental care for the child and adolescent from basic fundamental concepts to age specific concerns. This book is uniquely designed as it is divided into five parts, with one part focused on fundamentals of pediatric dentistry and the other four parts focused on specific age groups. Each age group deals with the physical, emotional, cognitive, and social changes experienced during these years, along with the dental diseases, examination requirements, prevention, and treatment for the group. This title is included in the last Brandon/Hill list, *Doody's Core Titles*, and the MLA Dental Section's *Booklist*.

Textbook and Color Atlas of Traumatic Injuries to the Teeth. 4th ed. Editors: Jens O. Andreasen, Frances M. Andreasen, Lars Andersson. Wiley-Blackwell, 2007.
ISBN: 9781405129541
Recommended for: Hospital, Academic Libraries
Doody's Core Titles Selection

The editors of *Textbook and Color Atlas of Traumatic Injuries to the Teeth* have compiled the gold standard of reference books on dental traumatology. This edition has taken a biological approach to understanding the nature of trauma and healing and how treatment interventions can assist these events. The editors also give special consideration to the impact dental implants have made on the field of dental traumatology since the publication of the last edition of this text. This edition takes an evidence-based approach to dental traumatology; all of the treatments presented in the book are carefully screened for the effect on healing. The included chapters cover the full scope of the field from the biological basis of wound healing and tissue response to trauma, socio-psychological aspects of dental trauma, practical techniques for dealing with many types of dental trauma, prevention of injury, and the economic aspects of dental trauma. This is a large book, over 800 pages and 35 chapters, all extensively illustrated with color photographs, radiographs, graphs, and diagrams. Each chapter concludes with an "Essentials" section that summarizes the chapter and an extensive references section. This title is included in *Doody's Core Titles* and the MLA Dental Section's *Booklist*. This book is an essential tool for all dental students, pediatric dentists, oral surgeons, endodontists, or general practitioner.

Traumatic Dental Injuries: A Manual. 2nd ed. Authors: J. O. Andreasen, F. M. Andreasen, L. K. Bakland, M. T. Flores. Wiley-Blackwell Munksgaard, 2003.
ISBN: 9781405111089
Recommended for: Hospital, Academic Libraries

In this slim manual, Drs. Andreasen, Bakland, and Flores have created an extremely useful, ready reference on dental traumatology. Each chapter presents a different traumatic dental injury and gives the practitioner sound principles of diagnosis and treatment of the injury. Treatment objectives and parameters are discussed along with expectations of the results of treatment based on current long-term studies. Endodontic treatment of traumatized teeth, diagnosis of pulp and periodontal healing complications, and long term prognosis of various types of trauma are included. The text includes examination forms and follow-up protocols in order to standardize diagnostic and treatment procedures. *Traumatic Dental Injuries: A Manual* concludes with information for dental patients, discussing the importance of immediate dental care of an injury and proper first aid to a person with a traumatic dental injury. The authors see immediate care and first aid as vital in assisting the dental practitioner to achieve the best possible results in treating dental trauma. The text of this book is supplemented with a large number of photos, artist's renderings, radiographs, and charts, providing the best possible reference for a dental practitioner. This text is an essential reference for pediatric dentists, hospital dentists, and dental students.

Journals

Pediatric Dentistry. v. 1, American Academy of Pediatric Dentistry, 1979.
http://www.ingentaconnect.com/content/aapd/pd
ISSN: 01641263
ISSN: 19425473 (Online)
Indexed in: MEDLINE
Recommended for: Hospital, Academic Libraries

The journal *Pediatric Dentistry* is the official journal of the American Academy of Pediatric Dentistry, the American Board of Pediatric Dentistry, and the College of Diplomates of the American Board of Pediatric Dentistry. It was first published in 1979 and has been internationally recognized as the premier journal in the field. *Pediatric Dentistry* is peer-reviewed and presents material to promote practice, education, and research in all aspects of pediatric dental practice. The journal publishes scientific articles, case reports, and abstracts of current research. The journal is listed in several indexes such as MEDLINE, Academic Search Complete, and Biological Abstracts. It is currently available online from 2004 through Ingenta Connect. This journal is a necessary purchase for any library supporting a dental program or a specialty program in pediatric dentistry. It would also be necessary for a children's hospital library or a hospital that provides pediatric dental care.

4.4.3. Public Health Dentistry

Prevention of disease and the maintenance of oral health through promoting organized dental health programs at a community, state, or federal level.

—MeSH

Contributor: Julie H. Schiavo

Monographs

Dentistry, Dental Practice, and the Community. 6th ed. Authors: Brian A. Burt, Stephen A. Eklund. Elsevier Saunders, 2005.
ISBN: 9780721605159
Recommended for: Academic Libraries
Brandon/Hill, *Doody's Core Titles* Selection

Dentistry, Dental Practice, and the Community is in its sixth edition and is a useful text on public health dentistry. It presents dentistry not as a separate entity, but as a part of the environment that surrounds it. The authors recognize that social, economic, and national situations have a great effect on the practice of dentistry. The text begins with an overview of the profession of dentistry, professional ethics, public health dentistry, and oral health promotion. This edition details the practice of dentistry, financing dental care, patient access to care, infection control and mercury safety, reading the dental literature, and evidence-based dental practice. The third section of the book deals with oral epidemiology, research designs, and the measurement of oral disease. The distribution of oral diseases is thoroughly discussed as is the prevention of oral diseases in public health. The text contains thoughtful discussions on several topics that are relevant in today's society such as infection control, mercury safety, and water fluoridation. The authors include a large number of both print and electronic references to support the information presented to allow readers to continue investigating subjects that may interest them. This title is listed on the MLA Dental Section's *Booklist*, *Doody's Core Titles* and the Brandon/Hill list. Overall, this is a useful volume for students and dental health professionals who are interested in public health dentistry and/or public health research.

Jong's Community Dental Health. 5th ed. Editors: George M. Gluck, Warren M. Morganstein. Elsevier Mosby, 2003.
ISBN: 9780323014670
Recommended for: Academic Libraries
Brandon/Hill Selection

The fifth edition of *Jong's Community Dental Health* takes a more historical perspective than previous editions of the text. It begins with an overview of the last two hundred years of public health and follows through to the first Surgeon General's report on dentistry, "Oral Health in America," issued in 2000. The chapter authors take the basics of public health in America and expound on the delivery of dental care within the public health systems, including managed care and care for the indigent or elderly, as well as the role of Medicaid. The text describes the demographic shifts and the increasing diversity of the American people. Social and cultural health behaviors are discussed along with communication strategies for a diverse patient pool. The text covers the distribution of dental disease and public health prevention programs. Research in dental public health, including biostatistics and evidence-based research, is analyzed along with the basic tenets of research design. *Jong's Community Dental Health* concludes with a discussion of public health from an ethical and legal perspective. This title provides the dental student, general practitioner, or anyone with an interest in the dental care of the United States public with a good basis in the topics of public health dentistry and community-based dental care. This title was also included on MLA Dental Section's *Booklist* for libraries supporting a dental program.

Journals

Community Dentistry and Oral Epidemiology. v. 1, Wiley-Blackwell, 1973.
http://onlinelibrary.wiley.com/journal/10.1111/(ISSN)1600-0528
ISSN: 03015661
ISSN: 16000528 (Online)
Indexed in: MEDLINE, CINAHL
Recommended for: Academic Libraries

Community Dentistry and Oral Epidemiology is a bimonthly, peer-reviewed journal that strives to expand the scientific knowledge base of community dentistry. The journal editors present a broad scope for this journal, encompassing epidemiologic studies, behavioral science studies in relation to dentistry, and methodological reports in program planning, implementation, and evaluation. *Community Dentistry and Oral Epidemiology* has an international audience. This journal is indexed in several databases such as MEDLINE, Biological Abstracts, and Academic Search Premier. This journal is ranked highly in the 2009 ISI *Journals Citation Reports* and has an impact factor of 2.418. This is a very important journal for libraries supporting a public health program or dental education.

4.5. Oral Medicine

Diseases of the oral and paraoral structures and the oral management of systemic diseases.

—MeSH

Contributor: Elizabeth A. Strother

Monographs

Bell's Orofacial Pains: The Clinical Management of Orofacial Pain. 6th ed. Author: Jeffrey P. Okeson. Quintessence, 2005.
http://online.statref.com/titleinfo/fxid-132.html
ISBN: 9780867154399
Recommended for: Hospital, Academic Libraries

Jeffrey Okeson, a recognized expert on temporomandibular joint disorders, is author of the two most recent editions of *Bell's* respected text on orofacial pain. The book is a comprehensive discussion of the nature and mechanisms of pain, principles of pain diagnosis and treatment, and specific treatment options for each type of orofacial pain disorder. The sixth edition includes new research findings on pain. This book should be of interest not only to dental students and clinicians but also to basic scientists and physicians treating facial pain. Thirty-five cases throughout the chapters give students the opportunity to test their diagnostic skills. Black-and-white photographs, radiographs, and diagrams illustrate the text. Extensive reference lists at the end of each chapter provide scientific evidence for the information presented. This edition is available in the STAT!Ref electronic dental titles. *Bell's Orofacial Pain* is highly recommended for hospital and medical libraries and is required for libraries supporting dental schools.

Burket's Oral Medicine. 11th ed. Editors: Martin S. Greenberg, Michael Glick, Jonathan A. Ship. BC Decker, 2008.
http://online.statref.com/titleinfo/fxid-111.html
ISBN: 9781550093452
Recommended for: Hospital, Academic Libraries

With increasing focus on the connection between oral and systemic disease, dentists are becoming more knowledgeable about medical disorders of their patients. This book provides dental students and clinicians with comprehensive information on the diagnosis and management of maxillofacial diseases as well as information on dental treatment of patients with systemic diseases. Many of the 45 contributors to the eleventh edition of this title are authors of other well-regarded titles in oral medicine. A chapter on pharmacology, new in this edition, provides dentists with information on drug therapy of oral conditions via tables displaying comparative data on commonly prescribed drugs. The first half of the book covers lesions of the oral cavity, oral cancer, salivary gland diseases, temporomandibular disorders, orofacial pain, and headache. Chapters in the second half of the book discuss major medical disorders, including renal, hematologic, immunologic, and infectious diseases. The last chapter provides an overview of genetics for dental practitioners. Radiographs and color photographs aid in the identification of oral disorders. Information is highlighted in numerous tables. The book is accompanied by a CD with supplemental information and a complete bibliography. This title, a first purchase recommendation on the MLA Dental Section's *Booklist*, is also available electronically via STAT!Ref. *Burket's Oral Medicine* is a required acquisition for libraries serving dental schools.

Dental Management of the Medically Compromised Patient. 7th ed. Authors: James W. Little, Donald A. Falace, Craig S. Miller, Nelson L. Rhodus. Mosby Elsevier, 2008.
ISBN: 9780323045353
Recommended for: Hospital, Academic Libraries
Brandon/Hill, *Doody's Core Titles* Selection

Because dentists are seeing more patients with medical conditions affecting oral health care, it is critical that they understand the relationship between oral and systemic diseases and possible risks of dental treatment to medically compromised patients. This textbook focuses on dental procedures for patients with medical complications, but also provides an overview of common medical disorders such as hypertension, diabetes, HIV infection, and bleeding disorders. Oral complications and manifestations are included for each condition. A table at the beginning of the book summarizes dental concerns for the management of medical problems. The last chapter describes the effects of aging and dental treatment for older adults. Three new chapters in this edition address smoking and tobacco use cessation, tuberculosis, and sleep-related breathing disorders. Appendixes summarize medical emergencies in the dental office, infection control guidelines, management of oral lesions, drug interactions, and alternative drugs. Abundant color photographs, drawings, and tables enhance the text. The title is a Brandon/Hill selection and MLA Dental Section's *Booklist* first purchase recommendation. As the major textbook covering dental care for medically compromised patients, this book is required for all dental school libraries and highly recommended for hospital libraries with dental services and medical school libraries.

Management of Temporomandibular Disorders and Occlusion. 6th ed. Author: Jeffrey P. Okeson. Mosby Elsevier, 2008.
ISBN: 9780323046145
Recommended for: Academic Libraries
Doody's Core Titles Selection

This textbook integrates scientific investigation into the study of the intricate relationship between occlusion and mastication. As an authoritative textbook for dental students, it clearly explains the complexities of the temporomandibular joint. The sixth edition incorporates new scientific evidence discovered since the previous edition. The book is divided into four sections: functional anatomy, etiology and identification of functional disturbances in the masticatory system, treatment of functional disturbances of the masticatory system, and occlusal therapy. Chapters include case studies for each treatment option discussed. The author advocates scientifically supported treatment options that are conservative, cost effective, and in the best interest of the patient. Over 2,200 references support the concepts described in this edition. Black-and-white photographs, drawings, and tables accompany the text. An appendix contains a "Diagnostic Algorithm for Masticatory Muscle Disorders," which summarizes treatment options for 11 types of TMJ disorders. The most comprehensive textbook on the temporomandibular joint and dental occlusion, this title serves as a resource for clinicians as well as for dental students. A recommended first purchase on the MLA Dental Section's *Booklist*, this is a required purchase for all dental school libraries.

Journals

Oral Surgery, Oral Medicine, Oral Pathology, Oral Radiology and Endodontology. v. 79, Mosby Elsevier, 1995.
http://www.journals.elsevierhealth.com/periodicals/ymoe/home
ISSN: 10792104
ISSN: 1528395X (Online)
Indexed in: MEDLINE, CINAHL
Recommended for: Academic Libraries
Brandon/Hill Selection

Oral Surgery, Oral Medicine, Oral Pathology, Oral Radiology and Endodontology, published monthly, provides dentists with peer-reviewed articles covering medical and surgical techniques in five dental specialties. The journal includes research articles, literature reviews, and case reports discussing the latest techniques and procedures. Print and online only articles are arranged by specialty. Articles cover dental treatment of medically compromised patients, dental implants, diagnosis and treatment of oral and head and neck lesions, state-of-the-art radiographic techniques, and new instruments for root canal therapy. The current title continues *Oral Surgery, Oral Medicine, Oral Pathology* which began publication in 1948; all issues of both titles are available electronically via ScienceDirect. Articles are indexed in MEDLINE, CINAHL, and Scopus. As the official journal of five professional organizations, including the Organization of Teachers of Oral Diagnosis, the title is read by numerous practicing dentists and educators. It is one of three dental journals appearing on the Brandon/Hill list for the small medical library and ranks twenty-ninth in the 2009 *Journal Citation Reports*. As a single source for peer-reviewed articles in different specialties, this journal is a required subscription for every library serving dental schools.

4.6. Preventive Dentistry

Prevention of disease and the maintenance and promotion of oral health.

—MeSH

Contributor: Julie H. Schiavo

Monographs

The Prevention of Oral Disease. 4th ed. Editors: John J. Murray, June H. Nunn, James G. Steele. Oxford University Press, 2003.
ISBN: 9780192632791
Recommended for: Academic Libraries

This text provides a broad overview of the field of preventive dentistry, encompassing both traditional issues and newer topics. The editors of this edition stay true to the initial intention of the book, to assemble the scientific evidence to support the prevention of oral diseases. This edition has undergone several changes of chapter authors to expand upon the field beyond the first editions. *The Prevention of Oral Disease* begins with an overview of oral health in the twenty-first century. The book is divided into three sections. Specific diseases such as dental caries, pulpal and periapical disease, periodontal disease, and oral mucosal disease are presented in the first section. The next section describes specific environments in which prevention of oral disease is important, such as the aging dentition, physical or mental impairment, or social inequalities. The last section presents national issues dealing with oral health and disease prevention. This edition is well illustrated with pictures, charts, and graphs. It also includes conclusions and a bibliography for each chapter. *The Prevention of Oral Disease* is included in the MLA Dental Section's *Booklist*. This title is ideal for the dental student but could also be very useful for residents or practitioners with an interest in preventive and public health dentistry.

Primary Preventive Dentistry. 7th ed. Editors: Norman O. Harris, Franklin Garcia-Godoy, Christine N. Nathe. Prentice Hall/Pearson Education, 2009.
http://online.statref.com/titleinfo/fxid-104.html
ISBN: 9780132412230
Recommended for: Academic Libraries

The goal of this edition of *Primary Preventive Dentistry* remains unchanged from previous editions, to present the science and practice of assessment and treatment modalities of preventive dental care; however, in this edition, the authors strive to make the text more readable for dental and dental hygiene students. The authors accomplish this by including clear objectives and a list of key terms at the beginning of every chapter and by arranging the book in four logical units. The first unit discusses preventive dentistry from a historical perspective through current methods of assessment, diagnosis, and therapy. The second unit presents the etiology of oral disease and risk factors inherent in the development of oral disease. The next section offers strategies to prevent these diseases and to maintain health. The last section discusses target populations, public health approaches to prevention of disease, and maintaining health. This title is included in the MLA Dental Section's *Booklist* and is available electronically through STAT!Ref. This text is very useful for dental students and dental hygiene students.

4.7. Dental Specialties

4.7.1. Endodontics

Maintenance of the dental pulp in a state of health and the treatment of the pulp cavity (pulp chamber and pulp canal).
—MeSH

Contributors: Julie H. Schiavo, Elizabeth A. Strother

Monographs

Cohen's Pathways of the Pulp. 10th ed. Editors: Kenneth M. Hargreaves, Stephen Cohen, Louis H. Berman. Mosby Elsevier, 2011.
ISBN: 9780323032766
Recommended for: Academic Libraries
Brandon/Hill, *Doody's Core Titles* Selection

Pathways of the Pulp is the definitive reference book in the field of endodontics. The tenth edition includes access to a regularly updated website, *Expert Consult*, which combines the fully searchable text of the book with links to PubMed, weekly content updates, a self-study component, a monthly case presentation, video clips, a bonus chapter, and links to relevant websites. The intent of the website is to ensure the information presented is always the most authoritative, current, relevant and reliable for the reader. The full-color tenth edition of this valuable text has been redesigned and organized into three major sections: core science, advanced science, and clinical topics. The new edition contains five new chapters. A title regularly included in the Brandon/Hill list, *Doody's Core Titles*, and the MLA Dental Section's *Booklist*, this new edition combines the scientific and clinical aspects of endodontic treatment and results in a truly useful book for all types of dental practitioners.

Endodontics: Principles and Practice. 4th ed. Editors: Mahmoud Torabinejad, Richard E. Walton. Elsevier Saunders, 2009.
ISBN: 9781416038511
Recommended for: Academic Libraries
Doody's Core Titles Selection

The text of this valuable reference book stresses the dentist's primary role to prevent tooth loss. It presents both the art and science of endodontics. The art is the technical procedures performed during treatment and the science refers to the biological and pathological basis of endodontic treatment. This vital book is a good reference in the field, providing a scientific and clinical basis for treatment of pulpal and periapical diseases. The authors also present endodontic procedures in an easy to understand step-by-step format. Chapters include a large number of color pictures and radiographs to aid the student's understanding. Concepts are presented in a logical manner, beginning with healthy tooth structure, etiology of disease, diagnosis, treatment planning, anesthesia, emergency treatment, treatment preparation, procedures, and treatment outcomes. There is an appendix containing self-assessment questions developed by endodontists who were not involved in the writing of the chapters. This assures the reader of his understanding of the purpose of the chapter and assesses the reader's knowledge of the material presented in the chapter. This edition of *Endodontics: Principles and Practice* includes a companion DVD. The DVD contains videos of procedures and review questions that track student performance. This title is listed in *Doody's Core Titles* and the MLA Dental Section's *Booklist*.

Ingle's Endodontics 6. 6th ed. Editors: John I. Ingle, Lief K. Bakland, J. Craig Baumgartner. BC Decker, 2008.
http://www.bcdecker.com/
http://online.statref.com/titleinfo/fxid-93.html
ISBN: 9781550093339
Recommended for: Academic Libraries
Doody's Core Titles Selection

Long considered the bible of endodontics, *Ingle's Endodontics* has been published for over 40 years. This textbook is designed for graduate endodontics students and practicing endodontists as the authoritative reference book on the specialty. It is very text dense, containing 41 chapters written by over 75 contributing authors; illustrations are sparse, with an emphasis on narrative description of techniques and conditions. The book includes a DVD containing video presentations of endodontic techniques and procedures and illustrative plates. This excellent text is divided into six sections: "The Discipline of Endodontics," "Pathobiology," "Examination, Evaluation, Diagnosis, and Treatment Planning," "Management," "Surgical Procedures in Endodontics," and "Related Endodontic Treatment." A chapter introducing osseointegrated dental implants has been added to this edition of the book. Each chapter concludes with an extensive bibliography supporting the research presented. *Ingle's Endodontics* is included on the *Doody's Core Title* list and the MLA Dental Section's *Booklist*. This title is available in electronic format through STAT!Ref and is a necessity for any library supporting a graduate endodontic program or practicing endodontists.

Problem Solving in Endodontics: Prevention, Identification, and Management. 5th ed. Authors: James L. Gutmann, Paul E. Lovdahl. Mosby Elsevier, 2010.
ISBN: 9780323068888
Recommended for: Academic Libraries

Problem Solving in Endodontics offers students, residents, and practicing endodontists practical ways to deal with common clinical problems and issues in endodontic treatment. This new edition provides chair side guidance for common endodontic procedures, expands on previously discussed concepts, integrates new technology, and correlates optimal patient outcomes with an evidence-based approach to endodontics. Every chapter in the fifth edition of this book has been revised while retaining the succinct, user-friendly format presented in previous editions. The fourth edition of this title is included in *Doody's Core Titles* and the MLA Dental Section's *Booklist*. The authors stress the need for the practitioner to strive for the utmost quality of service to the patient and present the solutions in the book as an important tool in the delivery of a high standard of care.

Journals

Journal of Endodontics. v. 1, Elsevier, 1975.
http://www.sciencedirect.com/science/journal/00992399
http://www.jendodon.com/
ISSN: 00992399
ISSN: 18783554 (Online)
Indexed in: MEDLINE
Recommended for: Academic Libraries

The Journal of Endodontics, a peer-reviewed journal, has been published since 1975. It is the official publication of the American Association of Endodontists and is designed to keep both specialists and general dentists apprised of the state of the art of root canal treatment as well as advanced techniques and instrumentation. The editors accept scientific articles, case reports, and comparison studies on endodontic treatment, pulp conservation, materials, or methods. This journal is ranked seventh in the 2009 *Journal Citation Reports* and has an impact factor of 2.727. It is indexed in MEDLINE. *Journal of Endodontics* is available in electronic format through ScienceDirect and includes the entire backfile of issues. This journal is an essential purchase for any library supporting endodontists or a dental program.

Oral Surgery, Oral Medicine, Oral Pathology, Oral Radiology and Endodontology. v. 79, Mosby Elsevier, 1995.
See Chapter 4.5. Oral Medicine

4.7.2. Orthodontics

Prevention and correction of dental and oral anomalies (malocclusion).

—MeSH

Contributor: Julie H. Schiavo

Monographs

Contemporary Orthodontics. 4th ed. Authors: William R. Proffit, Henry W. Fields, Jr., David M. Sarver. Mosby Elsevier, 2007.
ISBN: 0323040462
Recommended for: Academic Libraries
Doody's Core Titles Selection

Contemporary Orthodontics is a very comprehensive and indispensable resource for the study of orthodontics. This edition is the first to be illustrated in full color and boasts a large number of illustrations, photographs, radiographs, charts, and graphs. The authors present the material in a gradual, building, logical style that clearly explains the concepts of orthodontics to the student and then delves into the complexities of the field for the orthodontic resident or specialist. Beginning with an overview of malocclusion and dentofacial deformity in society, it progresses to the development of orthodontic problems, then diagnosis and treatment planning. There is also a section devoted to biomechanics and orthodontic appliances. The text contains sections dealing with the treatment of preadolescent children, patients in the early stages of permanent dentition, and adults. Each chapter begins with a clearly delineated outline and ends with an extensive bibliography containing both classic works in the field and newer research. In addition to the monograph, the book is supplemented with a continually updated website that contains the searchable full text of the book, and select illustrations that can be downloaded. This title is included in *Doody's Core Titles* and the MLA Dental Section's *Booklist*. This book is an invaluable tool for dental students, residents studying the specialty, and orthodontic practitioners.

Orthodontics: Current Principles and Techniques. 4th ed. Editors: Thomas M. Graber, Robert L. Vandarsdall, Jr., Katherine W.L. Vig. Elsevier Mosby, 2005.
ISBN: 9780323026215
Recommended for: Academic Libraries
Doody's Core Titles Selection

Graber's *Orthodontics* has become one of the most widely used and well-respected textbooks in the field of orthodontics. The contributors are all respected experts in the field, and together they present a comprehensive text. The editors of this edition provide basic science, diagnostic aids, critical use, and therapeutic mechanisms in order to instruct the reader to achieve the best possible treatment outcome for the patient. The text is divided into two parts. The first part contains subjects relevant to diagnosis and treatment planning, such as special considerations, craniofacial imaging, tissue reactions, bioengineering, temporomandibular disorder, and biomaterials. Part two focuses on techniques and treatment of the patient, including functional appliances, patients with mixed dentition, bracket placement, sagittal corrections in noncompliant patients, periodontal-orthodontal connections, orthodontics' role in cleft patients, and retention and relapse. The text is highly illustrated with full color photographs and illustrations. Each chapter concludes with a comprehensive bibliography and additional readings for the student. The title is included in *Doody's Core Titles* and the MLA Dental Section's *Booklist*. It is is a vital resource for the student, resident, and practicing orthodontist or pediatric dentist.

Journals

American Journal of Orthodontics and Dentofacial Orthopedics. v. 90, Elsevier, 1986.
http://www.sciencedirect.com/science/journal/08895406
ISSN: 08895406
ISSN: 10976752 (Online)
Indexed in: MEDLINE, CINAHL
Recommended for: Academic Libraries

The American Journal of Orthodontics and Dentofacial Orthopedics has been an important resource in the field of orthodontics for over 93 years. It has undergone many name changes during that time, but its value to practitioners, researchers, and students has remained the same. This peer-reviewed publication is the official journal of the American Association of Orthodontists, the American Board of Orthodontists, and the College of Diplomates of the American Board of Orthodontists. *AJO-DO* publishes articles that cover all aspects of orthodontic treatment, diagnosis, imaging, bracket and archwires, extraction and impaction of teeth, orthognathic surgery, temporomandibular joint disorders, and adult therapy. *AJO-DO* is indexed in MEDLINE, CINAHL, and Scopus and is available with a complete backfile through ScienceDirect. This is an essential purchase for a library serving a professional dental population.

4.7.3. Oral Pathology

Pathology of the oral cavity.
—MeSH

Contributor: Elizabeth A. Strother

Monographs

Contemporary Oral and Maxillofacial Pathology. 2nd ed. Authors: J. Philip Sapp, Lewis R. Eversole, George P. Wysocki. Mosby Elsevier, 2004.
ISBN: 9780323017237
Recommended for: Academic Libraries

The distinguished authors of *Contemporary Oral and Maxillofacial Pathology* have written a concise book suitable for inclusion in the dental school curriculum. Although the book focuses on essential diseases based on their prevalence in the Western world, it also includes unique entities and information not found in other oral pathology books. Much new and updated information has been added to the second edition, including more craniofacial syndromes, additional skin lesions, and more recent knowledge about AIDS and HIV. Each chapter begins with an outline and a list of additional key terms that are also defined in boxes within the chapter. Discussion of each entity includes clinical features, radiographic features, histopathology, and treatment. High-quality color micrographs, clinical photographs, and drawings illustrate these points. A unique aspect of this book is the diagrams that accompany photomicrographs, pointing out the key features of lesions. References at the end of each chapter have been reduced to the most significant and up-to-date citations. A comprehensive glossary of terms has been included at the end of the book. This book presents an introduction for the dental student and resident to oral disorders and pathologies and is recommended for all dental school libraries.

Oral and Maxillofacial Pathology. 3rd ed. Authors: Brad W. Neville, Douglas D. Damm, Carl M. Allen, Jerry E. Bouquot. Saunders Elsevier, 2009.
ISBN: 9781416034353

Recommended for: Hospital, Academic Libraries
Doody's Core Titles Selection

This text, covering the nature, identification, and management of diseases of the oral and maxillofacial regions, is considered the gold standard for oral and maxillofacial pathology. It is intended for all dental professionals and for physicians specializing in otolaryngology, pathology, and dermatology. Written for students as well as clinicians, the comprehensive contents are arranged by source of disease process, including periodontal diseases, viral infections, epithelial pathology, soft tissue tumors, odontogenic cysts and tumors, and dermatologic diseases. Excellent color photographs show both clinical and histological aspects of pathological conditions. References in the extensive bibliographies at the end of each chapter are delineated by topic headings, making it easier to locate relevant citations. An appendix provides the differential diagnosis of oral and maxillofacial diseases. Among the new topics included in the third edition are bisphosphonate-associated osteonecrosis and oral manifestations of methamphetamine abuse. This book is highly recommended for hospital libraries and is required for all libraries serving dental and medical schools.

Oral and Maxillofacial Pathology: A Rationale for Diagnosis and Treatment. Authors: Robert E. Marx, Diane Stern. Quintessence, 2003.
http://online.statref.com/titleinfo/fxid-135.html
ISBN: 9780867153903
Recommended for: Hospital, Academic Libraries

The intended audience of this oversized volume is oral and maxillofacial surgeons as well as other surgeons treating head and neck pathologies. The authors present modern concepts and techniques in this clinical guide to the diagnosis and treatment of over 425 diseases. The information presented for each disease follows a consistent format: clinical presentation, differential diagnosis, diagnostic work-up and treatment, histopathology, and prognosis. The treatments are recommended by the authors based on their experience or research. The majority of the 2,100 photomicrographs and clinical photographs are in color, and surgical procedures are illustrated in great detail. Chapter 1 provides an overview of biopsy principles and procedures for various types of lesions. Subsequent chapters cover diseases divided into broad ccategories such as hyperplasias, hamartomas and neoplasms; salivary gland neoplasms; and odontogenic and nonodontogenic cysts. To aid in the simplification of terminology, the last chapter, "Where Have All the Great Terms Gone?" reviews and explains original and updated names for 30 diseases. All references are listed by chapter at the end of the book. This title is available electronically via STAT!Ref. Due to the comprehensive coverage and detailed clinical information, this book is recommended for libraries serving hospitals, medical schools, and dental schools.

Oral Pathology: Clinical Pathologic Correlations. 5th ed. Authors: Joseph A. Regezi, James J. Sciubba, Richard C.K. Jordan. Saunders Elsevier, 2008.
http://www.mdconsult.com/
ISBN: 9781416045700
Recommended for: Hospital, Academic Libraries

A significant resource for the dental resident and practitioner, *Oral Pathology: Clinical Pathologic Correlations* presents information for identification and diagnosis of diseases in a clear and concise manner. Pathologies are grouped by appearance and presentation. The book begins with a clinical overview, comprising photographs and tables listing clinical features, cause, and significance of each disease. Subsequent chapters discuss the etiology, clinical features, histopathology, differential diagnosis, treatment, and prognosis of each entity. Additional chapters cover metabolic and genetic diseases, tooth abnormalities, and common skin lesions of the head and neck. Numerous high-quality color photographs, photomicrographs, and radiographic images enhance the text. Key points of each disease are highlighted in boxes and tables. Bibliographies at the end of each chapter, arranged by type of condition, provide significant references for further reading. A companion CD has 30 case studies for student review or homework and a question bank of 680 multiple-choice questions and answers for self-assessment. Further supplemental material on the Evolve website is available for students and instructors. This oral pathology resource is a recommended purchase for hospital libraries and required for libraries serving dental schools with advanced education programs.

World Health Organization Classification of Tumours. Pathology and Genetics of Head and Neck Tumours. Editors: Leon Barnes, John W. Eveson, Peter Reichart, David Sidransky. IARC Press, 2005.
ISBN: 9283224175
Recommended for: Hospital, Academic Libraries

Over 100 international experts contributed to the detailed discussions of head and neck tumors included in this volume. This ninth of 10 books in the *WHO Classification of Tumours* series consolidates the contents of four previous books covering head and neck neoplasms. Each of the eight chapters, arranged by location of tumor, begins with tables listing the WHO classification and

TNM classification for malignancies followed by a narrative introduction. Descriptions of each tumor include definition, synonyms, epidemiology, etiology, clinical features, macroscopic and histopathologic descriptions, differential diagnosis, genetics, and prognosis and predictive factors. Numerous high-quality color images consisting of photomicrographs, gross specimens, and clinical photographs enhance the discussion of each tumor. A list of 2,918 references, arranged by author, follows the text. This volume is highly recommended for hospital, dental school, and medical school libraries.

Journals

Oral Surgery, Oral Medicine, Oral Pathology, Oral Radiology and Endodontology. v. 79, Mosby Elsevier, 1995.
See Chapter 4.5. Oral Medicine

4.7.4. Periodontics

Histology, physiology, and pathology of the tissues that support, attach, and surround the teeth, and of the treatment and prevention of disease affecting these tissues.

—MeSH

Contributor: Julie H. Schiavo

Monographs

Atlas of Cosmetic and Reconstructive Periodontal Surgery. 3rd ed. Author: Edward S. Cohen. BC Decker, 2007.
ISBN: 1550092677
Recommended for: Hospital, Academic Libraries

This comprehensive atlas is an indispensable tool for students and periodontal specialists alike. It focuses on the esthetic, surgical treatment of periodontal diseases. The *Atlas of Cosmetic and Reconstructive Periodontal Surgery* is highly illustrated in full color to demonstrate surgical procedures and give esthetic guidance. Special consideration is given to the facial, dentofacial, and dentogingival elements of an esthetic reconstruction. The text focuses on the treatment of periodontal diseases and the retention of teeth as long as possible rather than the quick use of dental implants. This book is divided into four parts; each deals with separate topics in periodontal surgery yet each builds upon the other. Part 1 covers the basics of periodontal surgery; part 2 covers the basics of dental esthetics. Parts 3 and 4 build upon the previous sections to present advanced procedures, both periodontal and surgical. The monograph is accompanied by a CD-ROM that contains the searchable text of the book complete with images. This title is included in the MLA Dental Section's *Booklist*. This text is a very important resource for dental students learning periodontal surgical techniques, periodontal residents who are refining their skills, and seasoned specialists seeking a reference.

Carranza's Clinical Periodontology. 11th ed. Editors: Michael G. Newman, Henry H. Takei, Perry R. Klokkevold, Fermin A. Carranza. Saunders Elsevier, 2012.
ISBN: 9781437704167
Recommended for: Academic Libraries

Carranza's Clinical Periodontology is the gold standard for periodontics texts. The editors have completely revised the tenth edition but have maintained the comprehensiveness and organization that have earned this title such respect. The fundamentals of anatomy, physiology, etiology, and pathology that have always been vital in this work are retained while new, current techniques and concepts that make up the important clinical aspects of the field were added. This edition is accompanied by the *Clinical Periodontology* e-dition, which is constantly updated to keep the reader current in state-of-the-art research. The electronic edition contains all the content, illustrations, tables, and photographs of the print edition with the addition of being fully searchable. The print edition of this text has added a primer of evidence-based periodontology, chapters devoted to ethics, jurisprudence, and finance. The "Science Transfer" box in each chapter expands the concepts presented in the chapter, sometimes linking basic science to clinical practice, sometimes introducing new techniques. This title is included in *Doody's Core Titles* and the MLA Dental Section's *Booklist*. This title is a must-have reference for all dental professionals who might treat patients with periodontal problems. Students, residents, periodontists, general practitioners, and even dental hygienists will find this book very useful. This review refers to the tenth edition.

Clinical Periodontology and Implant Dentistry. 5th ed. Editors: Jan Lindhe, Niklaus P. Lang, Thorkild Karring. Blackwell Munksgaard, 2008.
http://online.statref.com/titleinfo/fxid-323.html
http://extranet.netlibrary.com/TitleSelect
ISBN: 9781405160995
Recommended for: Academic Libraries
Doody's Core Titles Selection

With the fifth edition of *Clinical Periodontology and Implant Dentistry*, Lindhe and his fellow editors have produced an indispensable resource on all aspects of periodontology. This edition is divided into two volumes as the editors have included a large amount of new material not previously covered by the text. Each chapter is written by experts and thoroughly covers the concepts presented. The editors have also presented implant dentistry as a vital and growing part of the field of periodontology and every concept is followed by the implications on implantology. Volume one covers the basic concepts of periodontology and implantology. Subjects range from basic anatomy, epidemiology, microbiology, to pathology. The second volume presents clinical concepts such as examination protocols, periodontal and reconstructive therapy, implant installation, occlusal and prosthetic therapy, and supportive care. The text is supported by a large number of color and black-and-white pictures, radiographs, and microscopic slides. Chapters begin with an outline of presented material and conclude with an extensive references section. This title is included in *Doody's Core Titles* and the MLA Dental Section's *Booklist*. This book is an essential purchase for the support of a periodontology residency program or for a library serving the specialist.

Foundations of Periodontics for the Dental Hygienist. 3rd ed. Authors: Jill S. Nield-Gehrig, Donald E. Willman. Wolters Kluwer/Lippincott Williams & Wilkins, 2011.
See Chapter 1.8. Dental Auxiliaries

Fundamentals of Periodontics. 2nd ed. Editors: Thomas G. Wilson, Jr., Kenneth S. Kornman. Quintessence, 2003.
ISBN: 9780867154054
Recommended for: Academic Libraries

The editors of *Fundamentals of Periodontics* have assembled a valuable text to introduce the dental student to the art and science of periodontics. It functions as a guide for the student to properly diagnose and treat periodontal diseases. The editors have brought together the perspectives of several outstanding clinicians and educators to produce a solid introduction and guide for the student. The second edition of this text has been extensively updated with new developments in the field, both clinical and biological. *Fundamentals of Periodontics* is divided into four sections that follow the treatment of the patient: essential information for clinical decision making, clinical management of the periodontal patient, restorative and esthetic treatment, and dental implants. The chapters are relatively short, presenting the important information in a concise manner, and contain full color pictures, charts, and graphs to aid the student in understanding the concepts. Each chapter ends with a comprehensive reference section to support the assertions made in the text and aid the student looking for more information on the topics. This title is included in the MLA Dental Section's *Booklist* and is an excellent reference for both dental students and periodontics residents.

The Periodontic Syllabus. 5th ed. Editors: Arthur R. Vernino, Jonathan L. Gray, Elizabeth Hughes. Lippincott Williams & Wilkins, 2008.
ISBN: 9780781779722
Recommended for: Academic Libraries

With this fifth edition of *The Periodontic Syllabus* the editors continue the tradition set by the former editor, Dr. Peter Fedi, by compiling an essential companion to other periodontic texts. Developed initially as a companion to a periodontics course given by the United States Navy, *The Periodontic Syllabus* is not intended as a standalone reference, but as a companion to more detailed texts and course work. It is a quick reference for topics and techniques that are vital in the practice of periodontology. Covered topics include plaque control, scaling and root preparation, the role of the dental hygienist in periodontal therapy, wound healing, management of soft tissues, management of hard tissues, and dental implants. This is a thin volume, just over 271 pages, but it is packed with important, practical information for the dental professional. The pictures, radiographs, and drawings in the book are almost all black and white. The editors have included a reference section concluding each chapter, along with self-assessment questions for the reader to gauge his understanding of the material. Originally intended solely for an audience of dental students, *The Periodontic Syllabus* is useful to periodontists and both dental and dental hygiene students and professionals.

Journals

Journal of Periodontology. v. 41, American Academy of Periodontology, 1970.
http://www.joponline.org/loi/jop
ISSN: 00223492
ISSN: 19433670 (Online)
Indexed in: MEDLINE
Recommended for: Academic Libraries

Journal of Periodontology, the official journal of the American Academy of Periodontology, is a peer-reviewed publication. It publishes original scientific articles that promote practice, education, and research in periodontics and related areas including dental implantology. These articles include, but are not limited to, scientific research, reviews, and case reports. *Journal of Periodontology* is currently available in electronic format from 1999 to the present. It is indexed in several sources including

MEDLINE, Biological Abstracts, Chemical Abstracts, and Science Citation Index. According to the 2009 *Journal Citation Reports*, the *Journal of Periodontology* is ranked second in total number of citations per year in the dentistry and oral surgery category. This journal would be a necessity for a library supporting a dental program and/or a specialty program in periodontology.

4.7.5. Prosthodontics

Restoration and maintenance of oral function by the replacement of missing teeth and structures by artificial devices or prostheses.

—MeSH

Contributor: Elizabeth A. Strother

Monographs

Contemporary Fixed Prosthodontics. 4th ed. Authors: Stephen F. Rosenstiel, Martin F. Land, Junhei Fujimoto. Mosby Elsevier, 2006.
ISBN: 9780323028745
Recommended for: Academic Libraries
Brandon/Hill, *Doody's Core Titles* Selection

This encyclopedic work on fixed prosthodontics, defined as "the replacement and restoration of teeth by artificial substitutes that are not readily removable from the mouth," covers crowns, veneers, and partial dentures. Intended for preclinical, clinical, and postdoctoral training, this textbook is also appropriate as a reference book for practitioners. In a change from previous editions, all illustrations, including photographs and line drawings, are in color. The book is arranged into four sections following the steps for creating and delivering a restoration: planning and preparation, clinical procedures—part 1, laboratory procedures, and clinical procedures—part 2, with the last chapter focusing on postoperative care. Each chapter includes study questions, a glossary, and references. The two appendixes provide detailed lists of materials, equipment, and manufacturers. They are followed by the full "Glossary of Prosthodontic Terms," reprinted from the *Journal of Prosthetic Dentistry*. The third edition of this book was a Brandon/Hill selection for dentistry and the current edition is a first purchase recommendation on the MLA Dental Section's *Booklist*. With its comprehensive detailed coverage and numerous high-quality photographs, *Rosenstiel's Contemporary Fixed Prosthodontics* is a highly recommended textbook for dentistry and required for all dental school libraries.

McCracken's Removable Partial Prosthodontics. 12th ed. Authors: Alan B. Carr, David T. Brown. Mosby Elsevier, 2010.
ISBN: 9780323069908
Recommended for: Academic Libraries

The definitive textbook in removable partial prosthodontics for over 40 years, *McCracken's* offers comprehensive coverage of clinical and laboratory aspects of tooth replacements for patients with missing teeth. Dentists as well as dental students will find this book to be a valuable resource. Chapters are divided into three main sections: general concepts and treatment planning, clinical and laboratory procedures, and maintenance. This edition incorporates more material on dental implant considerations than earlier editions. The chapter on maxillofacial prosthetics offers an overview of prosthesis design for patients with maxillofacial defects. As a means of clearly delineating between two levels of text, paragraphs with advanced information appear in shaded boxes. Self-assessment questions at the end of each chapter enable students to thoroughly review and test their comprehension of the material. Updated high-quality color photographs and drawings vividly illustrate procedures for creating removable prosthetics. "Selected Reading Resources," compiled into one bibliography at the end of the book, includes both classic and contemporary textbooks and journal articles. With coverage of basic principles and detailed techniques and procedures, this book on removable partial prosthodontics is a required purchase for all libraries supporting dental programs.

Prosthodontic Treatment for Edentulous Patients: Complete Dentures and Implant-Supported Prostheses. 12th ed. Editors: George A. Zarb, Charles L. Bolender, Steven E. Eckert, Aaron H. Fenton, Rhonda F. Jacob, Regina Mericske-Stern. Mosby Elsevier, 2004.
ISBN: 9780323022965
Recommended for: Academic Libraries
Doody's Core Titles Selection

Prosthodontic Treatment for Edentulous Patients is the authoritative textbook on managing edentulism and fabricating complete dentures. Chapters in the first two parts are devoted to understanding functional and esthetics problems of the edentulous condition and preparing the patient for treatment. Part three covers procedures for fabricating complete dentures; chapters in part four provide an overview of implant prosthodontics, much expanded from the previous edition. Each chapter ends with a brief summary and a list of references. Over 800 line drawings and photographs, mostly black and white, illustrate concepts described in the text.

New to this edition is a chapter on temporomandibular disorders. Through numerous editions and editor changes, this has been the preferred complete denture textbook for educating dentists. It is a first purchase recommendation on the MLA Dental Section's *Booklist*. *Zarb's Prosthodontic Treatment for Edentulous Patients* is a required acquisition for all libraries supporting dental school programs.

Journals

Journal of Prosthetic Dentistry. v. 1, Elsevier, 1951.
http://www.journals.elsevierhealth.com/periodicals/ympr
ISSN: 00223913
ISSN: 10976841 (Online)
Indexed in: MEDLINE, CINAHL
Recommended for: Academic Libraries

The *Journal of Prosthetic Dentistry* is the peer-reviewed, official journal of 31 U.S. and international prosthodontic organizations. The branch of dentistry concerned with the restoration of appearance and function through the replacement of missing teeth with artificial substitutes, prosthodontics is broadly divided into removable and fixed prosthetics. This journal includes research articles, systematic reviews, and reports of innovative techniques, materials, and clinical procedures. Published monthly in two annual volumes, all articles back to 1951 are also available electronically via ScienceDirect. High-quality color photographs accompany articles. To help readers keep up with the current literature, abstracts of articles from other journals are interspersed with full-length articles. The journal is indexed in MEDLINE and Scopus. Aimed at residents and dentists specializing in prosthodontics, articles in this journal will also interest general dentists who provide advanced prosthetic procedures to their patients. The most significant journal for fixed, removable, partial, and full prosthodontics and restoration of dental implants, this publication is a required subscription for every dental library collection.

4.7.6. Oral Surgery

Diagnosis and surgical treatment of disease, injuries, and defects of the human oral and maxillofacial region.

—MeSH

Contributor: Elizabeth A. Strother

Monographs

Contemporary Oral and Maxillofacial Surgery. 5th ed. Editors: James R. Hupp, Edward Ellis III, Myron R. Tucker. Mosby Elsevier, 2008.
ISBN: 9780323049030
Recommended for: Hospital, Academic Libraries

Contemporary Oral and Maxillofacial Surgery provides a basic yet comprehensive description of oral surgery procedures for the general dentist. Procedures that general dentists would refer to oral surgeons are also discussed, but in less detail. The techniques of evaluation, diagnosis, and management covered in this book include surgical principles, instrumentation, tooth extraction, management of infections, implants, oral pathology, trauma, dentofacial deformities, temporomandibular disorders, and hospital dentistry. Full-color photographs and drawings, appearing in this edition for the first time, add clarity to the text. In the current edition, chapters on endodontic surgery, implants, and infection have been extensively revised and updated. Information has also been added about the newly recognized effect of bisphosphonates on jaw deterioration. The Evolve website includes video clips of basic procedures to help students visualize techniques. This excellent textbook, a first purchase recommendation on the MLA Dental Section's *Booklist*, provides dental students with information necessary for effectively performing simple oral surgery procedures and also with an awareness of the more complicated procedures reserved for the expertise of the oral surgeon. It is a required purchase for all libraries serving dental schools as well as libraries in hospitals with dental clinics.

Oral and Maxillofacial Surgery. 2nd ed. Editors: Raymond J. Fonseca, Robert D. Marciani, Timothy A. Turvey. Saunders Elsevier, 2009.
ISBN: 9781416066576 (v. 1)
ISBN: 9781416066552 (v. 2)
ISBN: 9781416066569 (v. 3)
Recommended for: Hospital, Academic Libraries

This three-volume encyclopedic work includes writings from a large number of oral surgeons, both private practitioners and academicians. Younger practitioners and residents as well as recognized experts contribute a variety of perspectives and knowledge to the book. The entire scope of oral and maxillofacial surgery is covered in these three volumes: volume 1 includes anesthesia, dentoalveolar surgery, practice management, and implant surgery; volume 2 covers trauma, surgical pathology, and temporomandibular disorders; volume 3 includes orthognathic surgery, esthetic surgery, and cleft and craniofacial surgery. Published eight years after the first edition of seven volumes, the latest work includes numerous updated techniques and new technology and 80 new chapters. High-quality color photographs are grouped at the end of each volume while black-and-white photographs and drawings illustrate each chapter. To ease maneuvering among the volumes, the table of contents for all three volumes appears inside the front cover of each book. These three densely packed volumes are recommended for hospital libraries and for libraries serving dental schools with oral and maxillofacial surgery programs.

Oral and Maxillofacial Trauma. 3rd ed. Editors: Raymond J. Fonseca, Robert V. Walker, Norman J. Betts, H. Dexter Barber, Michael P. Powers. Elsevier Saunders, 2005.
ISBN: 9780721601830
Recommended for: Hospital, Academic Libraries
Doody's Core Titles Selection

Eighty-nine experts contributed to this comprehensive two-volume work covering all aspects of oral and maxillofacial trauma, from basic principles of trauma management to principles of fixation. Written for members of the trauma team, the book includes information on systemic injuries that may be encountered in maxillofacial trauma patients. Chapters cover maxillofacial fractures and soft tissue injuries as well as traumatic injuries from firearms, burns, and bites. New to this edition are the introductory chapter, "The Societal Impact of Maxillofacial Trauma," and chapters on trigeminal nerve injuries, firearm injuries, and reconstruction of avulsive defects. Special considerations for treatment of the growing and geriatric patients are highlighted in separate chapters. Over 2,000 color and black-and-white photographs and drawings illustrate the surgical techniques and principles described. Extensive lists of references at the end of each chapter support the in-depth contents. This book, which provides all of the information required for residents and clinicians to successfully manage oral and maxillofacial trauma, is highly recommended for hospital and medical school libraries and libraries supporting dental schools with oral and maxillofacial residencies.

Journals

Journal of Oral and Maxillofacial Surgery. v. 40, Elsevier for the American Association of Oral and Maxillofacial Surgeons, 1982.
http://www.joms.org
ISSN: 02782391
ISSN: 15315053 (Online)
Indexed in: MEDLINE, CINAHL
Recommended for: Hospital, Academic Libraries
Brandon/Hill Selection

The official journal of the American Association of Oral and Maxillofacial Surgeons, this monthly publication continues the *Journal of Oral Surgery*, which began in 1943. Articles in this peer-reviewed journal report on innovative techniques and developments in jaw surgery and reconstruction, anesthesia and analgesia, facial injuries and deformities, TMJ disorders, dental implants, and oral cancer. Issues include basic and clinical research, literature reviews, reports of new techniques, and case reports. Two supplemental issues in the 2009 volume focus on effects of bisphosphonate therapy on the jaw and interdisciplinary advances in dental implants. An additional supplement each year presents abstracts of papers presented at the annual conference. Issues are available electronically via ScienceDirect back to 1993 and the journal is indexed in MEDLINE and Scopus. As the major comprehensive journal for oral and maxillofacial surgeons, this publication is a required subscription for all dental school and hospital libraries.

4.8. Dental Basic Sciences

Scientific fields such as anatomy, histology, microbiology, physiology, and pharmacology with applications for the practice of dentistry.

Contributor: Elizabeth A. Strother

Monographs

The Anatomical Basis of Dentistry. 3rd ed. Author: Bernard Liebgott. Mosby Elsevier, 2011.
ISBN: 9780323068079
Recommended for: Academic Libraries

Although it covers the entire human body, this unique gross anatomy textbook focuses on the areas of anatomy of most interest to dentists. Throughout the book, the author, who is a dentist, PhD, and professor of anatomy, correlates the basic science of anatomy with applications in clinical dentistry. In Chapter 11, "Applied Anatomy," he covers topics such as local anesthesia, imaging, facial fractures, and the spread of dental infections. The book introduces the dental student to the study of anatomy and presents detailed coverage of the back, thorax, and abdomen. Brief chapters on the limbs are also included. The head and neck are treated both by region and by system, with emphasis on the regions of clinical relevance to dentists. "Clinical Notes," presented in boxes throughout the text, also enable students to relate anatomy to clinical situations. Each chapter ends with review questions for self-testing. Numerous full-color illustrations accompany the text and Chapter 7, "The Head by Region," has full-color photographs. New material, including cone beam computed tomography, has been added to this edition, the first revision in 10 years. This book, specifically written for the dental student, is a required purchase for dental school libraries.

McMinn's Color Atlas of Head and Neck Anatomy. 4th ed. Authors: Bari M. Logan, Patricia A. Reynolds, Ralph T. Hutchings. Mosby Elsevier, 2010.
ISBN: 9780323056144
Recommended for: Hospital, Academic Libraries

This detailed collection of bone, dissection, and surface photographs covers the area from the neck up. Surface markings and superficial and deep dissections are supplemented by clinical photographs, drawings, notes, and narrative descriptions. A unique feature is the photographs of painted skulls depicting skull segmentation. The last chapter contains radiographs of the skull and vertebral column. New to this edition is a section on tooth anatomy included in the skull section. The vivid photographs and detailed labeling make this a definitive resource for any student of the head and neck, including dental students, oral and maxillofacial surgery residents, and ENT residents. Identification numbers overlaying photographs present opportunities for self-study and testing. Additional study material is found in the two appendixes. Appendix I illustrates various dental anesthesia blocks; appendix II includes lists of muscles, nerves, blood vessels, and lymph nodes. *McMinn's Color Atlas of Head and Neck Anatomy* is a highly recommended resource for hospital libraries and libraries serving medical and dental students and residents.

Netter's Head and Neck Anatomy for Dentistry. Author: Neil S. Norton. Saunders Elsevier, 2007.
ISBN: 9781929007882
Recommended for: Academic Libraries

A popular atlas among dental students and residents, *Netter's Head and Neck Anatomy for Dentistry* provides vivid color drawings which clearly illustrate anatomic features from the neck through the eye and orbit. Chapters on muscles of mastication, the temporomandibular joint, oral cavity, and intraoral injections are of specific interest to dentists. Numerous tables provide additional descriptions of the anatomic entities. To help students relate the anatomic information to dentistry, each chapter includes a series of dental clinical correlates. Many of Frank Netter's classic illustrations have been updated or modified and additional expert medical illustrators have contributed art to this volume. This concise atlas of clearly labeled, high-quality drawings is highly recommended for all libraries serving dental schools.

Pharmacology and Therapeutics for Dentistry. 6th ed. Editors: John A. Yagiela, Frank J. Dowd, Barton S. Johnson, Angelo J. Mariotti, Enid A. Neidle. Mosby Elsevier, 2011.
ISBN: 9780323055932
Recommended for: Academic Libraries
Doody's Core Titles Selection

Pharmacology and Therapeutics for Dentistry, a comprehensive textbook for students and practitioners, covers the foundations of pharmacology with an emphasis on applications in dentistry. The three major divisions of the book are principles of pharmacology, pharmacology of specific drug groups, and special subjects in pharmacology and therapeutics. Among the subjects covered in the third section are pain control, antibiotic prophylaxis, oral complications of cancer therapy, drugs of abuse, herbs and supplements, and prescription writing and drug regulations. Appendix 1 lists interactions of drugs commonly prescribed in dentistry; appendix 2 is a glossary of abbreviations. Diagrams illustrating drug actions, tables with lists of drugs in each category, and drug chemical formulas accompany the text. Each chapter presents basic information on medical conditions in addition to the detailed description of therapeutic agents and implications for dental care of patients taking the drugs. This book provides dentists with necessary background information on the mechanisms of action, adverse effects, and interactions of classes of drugs that they prescribe or that their patients take for systemic diseases. With the increase of patients taking generic, prescription, or over-the-counter drugs as well as herbal supplements, all dental students need to know pharmacological principles and applications. A first purchase recommendation on the MLA Dental Section's *Booklist*, this book is required for all dental school libraries.

Ten Cate's Oral Histology: Development, Structure, and Function. 7th ed. Editor: Antonio Nanci. Mosby Elsevier, 2008.
ISBN: 9780323045575
Recommended for: Academic Libraries
Doody's Core Titles Selection

The preeminent textbook on tooth histology, *Ten Cate's Oral Histology* provides dental students and residents with concise yet exhaustive information on microscopic anatomy, cell biology, physiology, embryology, and development of the oral structures. Of the 19 contributors to the book, over half are dentists. Chapter topics include embryology of the head, face, and oral cavity; bone; enamel; salivary glands; oral mucosa; and temporomandibular joint. Numerous high-quality photomicrographs, color diagrams, and tables illustrate and enhance the clearly written text. Each chapter includes a boxed "Topics for Consideration," highlighting clinical correlations of the subject under discussion. "Recommended Reading" lists at the end of each chapter are limited to essential sources. A supplemental CD with multiple-choice questions and interactive exercises accompanies the book, providing an opportunity for board exam review. As a comprehensive textbook on oral biology, *Ten Cate's Oral Histology* is required for libraries supporting dental students and residents.

Wheeler's Dental Anatomy, Physiology, and Occlusion.
9th ed. Authors: Stanley J. Nelson, Major M. Ash. Saunders Elsevier, 2010.
ISBN: 9781416062097
Recommended for: Academic Libraries
Doody's Core Titles Selection

Wheeler's Dental Anatomy, Physiology, and Occlusion may be the first dental textbook encountered by a dental student. The terminology, development, morphology, and function of teeth form the basis of dentistry and a student must master this material before progressing further. Subjects covered in this book include tooth development and eruption, the primary dentition, the orofacial complex, pulp chambers and canals, and occlusion. Separate chapters, such as "The Permanent Maxillary Premolars," cover each tooth in detail. Forensics and the temporomandibular joint are additional subjects discussed in less detail. Color illustrations, new to this edition, enhance the impact of line drawings and photographs. References provide evidence for statements in the text and bibliographies at the end of each chapter refer students to additional sources. Annotations in the text refer to 3-D animations, flash cards, exercises, and a virtual reality tooth identification quiz on the accompanying DVD. Perforated flashcards, bound into the book, enable self-testing of tooth forms. Additionally, the publisher's Evolve website provides resources for instructors and students. The numerous illustrations and study aids provide students with multiple opportunities to learn the foundation material covered by this book. A first purchase recommendation on the MLA Dental Section's *Booklist*, *Wheeler's* is a required purchase for all libraries serving dental schools.

5. Environmental Health

Controlling or modifying those conditions, influences, or forces surrounding man which relate to promoting, establishing, and maintaining health.

—MeSH

Contributor: Stephanie Holmgren

Monographs

Calculated Risks: The Toxicity and Human Health Risks of Chemicals in Our Environment. 2nd ed. Author: Joseph V. Rodricks. Cambridge University Press, 2007.
http://ebooks.cambridge.org/
http://extranet.netlibrary.com/TitleSelect
http://www.ebrary.com/
ISBN: 9780521788786
ISBN: 9780511248641
ISBN: 9780511250248
ISBN: 9780521783088
ISBN: 9780511535451
Recommended for: Academic Libraries

Written for nontoxicologists, *Calculated Risks* explains the science behind the degree to which chemicals pose a threat to human health. The book's prologue begins by supplying the broad framework of risk assessment through the case example of aflatoxin. The rest of the book is well organized, beginning with chapters on the nature of chemicals and types of exposure, how exposure leads to the body receiving a dose, and the types of harmful responses given the dose amount. Four chapters detail the broad framework of risk assessment—its evolution, principles and techniques, applications, and use in the courtroom. The final chapters investigate the challenges of managing risk and discuss the potential for better risk assessment in the future. Sources and recommended readings are provided as an appendix. This book clearly spells out the challenging and complex nature of determining whether a chemical is hazardous to human health. It also addresses the interplay between science and the regulatory process. Explained simply are fundamental risk assessment concepts such as exposure types, environmental epidemiology, kinetics, mechanisms of toxic action, dose-response relationship, and others. The challenge of extrapolating animal study results to humans, assessing low-dose exposure risk, and issues associated with susceptible populations are highlighted. This edition also incorporates more discussion of international developments in risk management and safety. The first edition of *Calculated Risks* won an 'Honourable Mentions' award from the American Medical Writers Association. This book is intended for public health, environmental protection, and public policy audiences, and it is recommended for academic, health sciences, and special libraries.

A Community Guide to Environmental Health. Authors: Jeff Conant, Pam Fadem. Hesperian Foundation, 2008.
http://hesperian.org/publications_download_EHB.php
ISBN: 9780942364569
Recommended for: Hospital, Academic, Consumer Health Libraries

This recent addition to the Hesperian collection of "how to" guides is a practical resource for health officials, development workers, or environmental activists needing to create a positive environmental health community. The book covers the broad spectrum of environmental health issues stemming from land management, water quality, food security and sustainable farming, indoor and outdoor pollution, waste management, and energy resource production. Especially useful for community groups are the two chapters on environmental justice and environmental rights law. The guide's intent is to provide communities with a tool kit for promoting local, community-based sustainable solutions to reduce their risk of environmental exposures and to create a healthy local environment. For each topic area, the authors first describe the potential environmental exposure, how it happens, and the likely health problems that result. Only then do they discuss the means for preventing or mitigating the problems. Interspersed throughout the guide are three innovative features: (a) personal stories highlight the health effect of an exposure or how a community has taken action; (b) community activities stimulate critical thinking to understand the nature of the environmental health situation; and (c) the "how-to" is a step-by-step guide to preventing or remediating the problem. This guide is a collaborative project utilizing the expertise of specialists from over 33 countries and incorporating best practices from around the world. The proposed solutions have been developed and field tested by many of these grassroots organizations and community groups. Given the intended audience, well-designed illustrations aid in understanding particular concepts. The content is extremely well organized and easy to follow. The appendix contains a resources section with a list of organizations, printed materials, and Internet resources providing further information on the topics addressed in the book. A useful vocabulary section provides definitions to new or difficult concepts used in the guide. The book is freely available online, and print copies and a CD-ROM are also available. Selected chapters in Spanish are available for download at the publisher's website. Besides the global health audience, this guide would be useful for health professionals and aid workers operating in disaster relief, rural communities, and even some urban environments. This book is recommended for academic libraries, special libraries, and some public libraries.

Current Occupational & Environmental Medicine. 4th ed. Editor: Joseph LaDou. McGraw-Hill, 2007.
http://www.r2library.com/
ISBN: 9780071443135
See Also Chapter 10.15.2. Occupational Medicine
Recommended for: Academic Libraries
Doody's Core Titles Selection

Geared toward the clinician, *Current Occupational and Environmental Medicine* serves as a practical guide to diagnosing, treating, and even preventing occupational and environmental health illnesses and injuries. As with many other books, this one is divided into easily browsable sections. The first five chapters describe the nature of occupational health in terms of its practice, history, and issues associated with workers' compensation, disability, and liability. The next 14 chapters delve into occupational illnesses, beginning with the principles of clinical toxicology and immunology. Much attention is paid to toxicity on various organ systems—cardiovascular, liver, renal, neural, and reproductive. In each of these chapters, the authors begin by describing the biomedical principles behind the adverse health effects and then describe how to diagnose, evaluate, manage, and prevent the resulting illnesses. Section four covers occupational exposures to toxic substances (metals, chemicals, solvents, gases and inhalants, and pesticides) most likely to be encountered in a work setting. These chapters serve as a quick reference guide for health professionals. Specific toxic substances are listed with details of exposure limits; nature of use and exposure; how the substance is absorbed, metabolized, and excreted; signs and symptoms of acute and chronic exposure; differential diagnosis; pathogenesis laboratory findings; and ways to prevent and treat. References are provided for each exposure. For specific exposures, authors note the occupations most at risk. The book turns to program management, which addresses issues surrounding occupational stress, employee assistance programs, occupational safety and hygiene, and biological monitoring. The last section is devoted to environmental health, encompassing air and water pollution, industrial emissions, effect of smoking on occupational exposures, establishing surveillance systems, and conducting risk assessments. An appendix reviewing key biostatistics and epidemiological methods supports the literature on these topics. Given the extensive updating of the third edition, this fourth edition does not include any new subject chapters. However, many of the individual chapters have been updated to incorporate new knowledge and recent advances. More practical tools such as diagnostic checklists have been included to help speed diagnosis and treatment. The layout is easy to scan and makes for a quick reference guide. One useful feature is the addition of PMID (PubMed Unique Identifier) numbers for every reference, as well as a brief description of how to use PubMed to find the articles or search the literature. Intended audiences include medical students, residents, physicians, and other allied health professionals. This book is a *Doody's Core Titles* recommendation. It is recommended for academic and hospital libraries.

Environmental and Occupational Medicine. 4th ed. Editors: William N. Rom, Steven B. Markowitz. Lippincott Williams & Wilkins, 2007.
http://www.ovid.com/
ISBN: 9780781762991
Recommended for: Hospital, Academic Libraries

Another long-standing textbook, the fourth edition of *Environmental and Occupational Medicine* continues to offer comprehensive coverage of occupational and environmental disease and injury. At 121 chapters, the breadth of coverage is vast. The first section addresses environmental and occupational diseases, with the beginning chapters introducing the discipline of occupational medicine, aspects of disease surveillance, principles of epidemiology and biostatistics, and practical aspects of taking an occupational history. Unlike other occupational and environmental medicine books, this one explains the biomolecular mechanisms and methods behind occupational and environmental illness. Individual chapters are dedicated to genetic susceptibility, biomarkers, and environmental mutagenesis. The remainder of the section is broken down by organ system, with the majority of the chapters devoted to understanding environmental insults to the respiratory tract. Entire chapters are devoted to other conditions which do not usually receive this much attention, such as Gulf War illness, multiple chemical sensitivity, and non-specific low back pain. The second section touches upon the environmental and occupational exposures from metals; organic chemicals; elements in the physical environment such as noise, radiation, and vibration; and general environmental areas, including air, buildings, and climate. The final section encompasses a variety of topics related to the control of occupational and environmental exposures and disease. The chapters touch on regulatory and legislative efforts, the role of specific government agencies, issues surrounding workers compensation, and industrial hygiene. Special environmental and occupational concerns at the international level and those affecting children and minority populations are given attention as well. This book reads more like a reference guide rather than a textbook; however, it does incorporate many examples and case studies to highlight concepts. Most chapters make very limited use of tables, figures, or photographs. This edition has been significantly revised and edited with 14 new chapters, and most of the remaining chapters have been completely rewritten with updated references. This version has expanded content in the area of environmental science, addressing the micro level of gene-environment interactions at one end of the spectrum and relating the health impact of global environmental change at the other end. Contributors include Nobel laureates, department chairs, practicing clinicians, and bench scientists. The work is geared towards medical students, residents and practitioners, and the public health community. It is recommended for academic and hospital libraries.

Environmental Epidemiology: Principles and Methods. Author: Ray M. Merrill. Jones & Bartlett, 2008.
ISBN: 9780763741525
Recommended for: Academic Libraries

This ambitious, well-written work by a single author seeks to present basic concepts and research methods used in environmental epidemiology, which is the study of the frequency and pattern of disease due to environmental causes. The first six chapters provide the fundamental principles underlying environmental epidemiology: elements of the research process, environmental health monitoring, epidemiological study design, statistical modeling, and causal inference. The second section describes techniques for assessing environmental health exposures at a population level using cluster analysis, geographic information systems, and time series analysis. The remaining chapters look at specific applications of environmental epidemiology within specific exposure contexts, including indoor air quality, water, radiation, climate change, and soil or food contamination. Five appendixes augment the chapters. The measures and data sources for environmental public health indicators are very useful, as are the list of selected statistical techniques and sample exposure history questionnaire. This book is designed to be used in introductory courses in environmental epidemiology for either upper-level undergraduates or graduate students in public health fields. It does not cover statistical methods or software packages in depth. Chapters begin with learning objectives and end with exercises, study questions, and references. The content is well formatted, with good use of tables and figures to summarize and clarify concepts. While numerous examples are used throughout the book, the majority are U.S.-based studies. The book could benefit from the incorporation of more international studies and discussion of regulatory policies. Key words are displayed in bold font and defined in the glossary. The statistical sections include easily understandable examples. This book is recommended for academic and health science libraries.

Environmental Epidemiology: Study Methods and Application. Editors: Dean Baker, Mark J. Nieuwenhuijsen. Oxford University Press, 2008.
ISBN: 9780198527923
Recommended for: Academic Libraries

This advanced textbook provides detailed coverage of the study methods and applications involved in environmental epidemiology. It emphasizes how to conduct a research study with elements of best practice. The beginning chapter explains the history and rationale behind environmental epidemiology. A review of epidemiological principles and terminology provides the foundation for the subsequent chapters. The core chapters focus on the issues, techniques, and tools of an environmental epidemiology study. These encompass assessment of exposure and health outcome, management of measurement error, various study designs and when to use them, and data analysis. Core chapters are followed by a chapter on special study designs unique to environmental epidemiology that are rarely described, let alone in detail, in other epidemiology books; examples include gene-environment interactions, disease clusters, panel studies, spatial epidemiology, and time series. Advantages and limitations of study designs are disclosed. A chapter devoted to health risk assessment shows how the results from the epidemiological studies are used to assess the potential impact on human health. The remaining chapters address a range of issues associated with specific situations such as studies involved with chemical or natural disasters, environmental epidemiology challenges in developing countries, and assessment of effects of global climate change. A few other chapters explore stakeholder involvement, ethics of these studies, and the role and limits that environmental epidemiological studies can play in a regulatory setting. Geared towards intermediate-level courses in public health, epidemiology, and environmental science, the book assumes basic knowledge of environmental health, epidemiology, and biostatistics. Rather than having a separate section devoted to the various types of environmental hazards, they are included as examples throughout the text to aid in understanding the techniques discussed. Many of these examples are based on air pollution, and some hazards such as noise are not mentioned. The bibliographies and further information provide good follow-up resources for readers. *Environmental Epidemiology* is recommended for academic and health science libraries.

Environmental Health Sourcebook: Basic Consumer Health Information about the Environment and Its Effects on Human Health. 3rd ed. Editor: Laura Larsen. Omnigraphics, 2010.
ISBN: 9780780810785
Recommended for: Hospital, Academic, Consumer Health Libraries

This volume is part of the classic *Health Reference Series* known for concise, current, and clear non-technical health information. Seven years after the second edition, this third edition is long overdue. This *Sourcebook* provides practical information for the layperson on the health effects of exposure to environmental agents. The book begins with a section devoted to the identification of potential health hazards and the reduction of possible exposure. Of particular importance is the emphasis given to the impact that environmental exposures have on susceptible populations such as children, the elderly, pregnant women and their fetuses, and some ethnic and minority groups. The second part explores in detail specific diseases—such as cancer, respiratory, reproductive, and others—and their associated environmental causes. The remaining chapters are organized by type of exposure: outdoor (air, water, soil); household and indoor (mold, asbestos, secondhand smoke); and foodborne hazards (genetic engineering, nanoparticles). The last chapter on consumer product and medical hazards is likely offered in response to many of the product recalls in the past few years. Content includes a discussion on nonstick pans, hand soap, fragrances, plastics, and other items. Of interest are sections relating to endocrine disruptors, specifically bisphenol A (BPA). A glossary and a useful directory of environmental health organizations and resources complete the volume. The *Sourcebook* is well organized and provides fairly comprehensive coverage of the key environmental exposures linked with human health problems, including some of the emerging issues like nanomaterials. The content is sourced primarily from documents or publications published by non-profit groups, international organizations, and the U.S. government. References to resources used are provided for each chapter. The series is geared towards the general public and would be useful for academic, consumer health, hospital, and public libraries.

Environmental Toxicants: Human Exposures and Their Health Effects. 3rd ed. Editor: Morton Lippman. John Wiley & Sons, 2009.
http://onlinelibrary.wiley.com/book/10.1002/9780470442890
http://extranet.netlibrary.com/TitleSelect
http://www.ebrary.com/
ISBN: 9780471793359
ISBN: 9780470442883 (Online)
ISBN: 9780470442890 (Online)
Recommended for: Academic Libraries

Morton Lippman has updated this second edition considerably. Experts in each of the subject areas have critically reviewed the scientific literature and summarized the current state of knowledge on the human health effects associated with 25 specific chemicals and other environmental exposures. The first chapter sets the background by discussing some of the basic principles of environmental health. The next two chapters focus on risk decision making and risk management from the perspectives of the individual, the community, and the environmental engineer. The following two chapters are quite unique. One is geared toward pulmonologists or respiratory biologists, helping them to recognize exposure-related pulmonary diseases. The other provides corporate managers with the knowledge and tools to minimize the footprint of plant operations on the environment and reduce their products' impact on public health. The subsequent chapters focus on specific chemical agents or physical factors where human exposure is most likely to occur. When appropriate, each environmental agent chapter discusses the properties associated with the agent, level and nature of exposure, biological or health effects, available biomarkers, means to mitigate effects, risk assessment, and other aspects. Of particular interest are new chapters on arsenic and endocrine active chemicals and new sections discussing nanoparticles and epigenetics. Two other chapters on noise and secondhand smoke are not typically seen in a traditional environmental health book. Each chapter is written by experts providing comprehensive, detailed reviews of the scientific literature. A balance is achieved with a discussion of results from animal models and human studies. The content is well cited with references and incorporates study or experimental examples. The book provides public health authorities, primary care physicians, industrial hygienists, and policymakers with the latest ideas needed for solid risk assessment. In addition, the breadth and depth of content would act as a useful reference for toxicologists, epidemiologists, and even clinicians. In this edition, the editor has addressed the previous edition's U.S. bias and has added more international examples. One flaw in the book is the index, which is rather shallow and nondescriptive. Despite a section being devoted to vinyl chloride and bisphenol A, neither of those two chemicals exists in the index. The descriptive table of contents does provide a useful substitute to some degree. The in-depth nature of the content makes this book more suitable for graduate students or professional environmental health practitioners. This book is recommended for academic health science and special libraries.

Essentials of Environmental Health. Author: Robert H. Friis. Jones & Bartlett, 2007.
http://www.jbpub.com/essentialpublichealth/friis/
http://www.ovid.com/
ISBN: 9780763747626
Recommended for: Academic Libraries

Robert Friis has crafted a non-technical approach to the key concepts in environmental health. The book is divided into three sections. The first section has chapters devoted to the fundamental principles of epidemiology, toxicology, and environmental policy and regulation. The second section addresses the agents of environmental disease such as infectious diseases, metals, pesticides and other organic chemicals, and radiation. Finally, specific applications are covered in the areas of water and air quality, food safety, solid and liquid wastes, occupational health, and the practice of environmental health. The content is well organized. Each chapter begins with learning objectives. The layout includes a proper mixture of text, tables/figures, and highlight boxes. Friis' epidemiology background is reflected in his strong use of epidemiological case studies to show evidence of the human impact of environmental exposures. The chapters end with study questions and exercises, along with a solid list of references. For individuals who purchase the print edition, instructor and student resources are available at the companion website. Institutional online access is also available through Ovid. The glossary is quite disappointing; for example, it does not define morbidity or mortality but defines composting toilets. Despite the book being thin, Friis is able to cover a good mix of health, environmental science, ecology, and environmental management topics in those pages. *Essentials of Environmental Health* is the first volume in the *Essential Public Health* series. The *Essentials* series content is based on the new public health core competencies identified for certification by the National Board of Public Health Examiners. The textbook is geared toward all levels of students. Health professionals and researchers needing a broad overview of environmental health will find it understandable and readable. The work is recommended for academic health science and special libraries.

Fourth National Report on Human Exposure to Environmental Chemicals. 4th ed. Centers for Disease Control and Prevention, 2009.
http://www.cdc.gov/exposurereport/
ISBN: None
Recommended for: Hospital, Academic, Consumer Health Libraries

The Centers for Disease Control's (CDC) freely available *Fourth National Report* represents the CDC's assessment of the U.S. population's exposure to environmental chemicals. This latest report incorporates population data covering 1999–2004 for 212 chemicals. Data is collected from blood and urine samples taken from participants in the National Health and Nutrition Examination Survey (NHANES). An additional 75 new chemicals—including arsenic, bisphenol A, triclosan, and perchlorate—have been included in this 2009 *Report*. Chemicals were selected because of their known high-level exposure, harmful degree of health effects, or need to assess effects due to reduced exposures. General categories of chemicals being biomonitored include tobacco smoke, metals, polycyclic aromatic hydrocarbons, pesticides, phthalates, phytoestrogens, and polychlorinated biphenyls. For each chemical or group, the *Report* provides information regarding use, sources of human exposure, disposition in the body, and major effects if known. This publication provides unique quantitative evidence of the amount of environmental exposure to Americans, which is useful for scientists, physicians, and health professionals who need to know human exposure rates. The *Fourth National Report* is recommended for academic health science, hospital, and special libraries.

Handbook of Environmental Health. 4th ed. Authors: Herman Koren, Michael S. Bisesi. Lewis/CRC, 2003.
http://extranet.netlibrary.com/TitleSelect
http://www.crcnetbase.com/isbn/978-1-56670-536-3 (v.1)
http://www.crcnetbase.com/isbn/978-1-56670-547-9 (v.2)
ISBN: 9781566705363 (v.1)
ISBN: 9781566705479 (v.2)
ISBN: 9781566705486 (set)
ISBN: 9780849377952 (v.1 online)
ISBN: 9780849378003 (v.2 online)
Recommended for: Academic Libraries

Although this latest edition is somewhat outdated, the *Handbook of Environmental Health* has been a standard reference book since the first edition was published more than twenty years ago. Given that the National Environmental Health Association co-published the book, its focus is predominantly on understanding the interrelated nature of environmental science, environmental management, and environmental health. The content is divided into two volumes. The first volume, subtitled *Biological, Chemical, and Physical Agents of Environmentally Related Disease*, addresses the indoor environment with coverage on food safety, insect and rodent control, air quality, and specific environments (hospitals, homes, work). The second volume, subtitled *Pollutant Interactions in Air, Water, and Soil*, covers the outdoor environment with attention to the usual air, sewage, water, and waste management issues. It also addresses the unusual—swimming areas, plumbing, geographic information systems, disaster emergency health needs, and ocean dumping. Except for the few beginning chapters, the majority follow the same structure, providing information on background; scientific or technical evidence; problem definition in terms of sources of exposure, nature and extent of impact, potential for disease or injury, and economic impact; potential for intervention; helpful scientific, public, or government resources; standards of practice and innovative techniques; modes of surveillance and evaluation; relevant controls, laws, and regulations; summary of chapter; and discussion of future research needs. The chapters utilize graphs, figures, and flowcharts to consolidate or clarify material in an effective manner. While much of the information is still applicable, updates are needed on issues that are of paramount importance today. The toxicology and epidemiology principles sections could be expanded. Because many of the topics are interrelated, they are often discussed in multiple sections, which help to reinforce the concepts. Graduate students involved in environmental science or environmental management will gain a clear understanding of the connection with environmental health. Professionals such as industrial hygienists, allied health professionals, resource managers, food quality managers, and others will find the book informative as well. The *Handbook* is recommended for academic health science libraries or special libraries.

Hot Zone Forensics: Chemical, Biological, and Radiological Evidence Collection. Author: Steven C. Drielak. Charles C. Thomas, 2004.
See Chapter 17.8.2. Forensic Toxicology

Occupational and Environmental Health: Recognizing and Preventing Disease and Injury. 5th ed. Editors: Barry S. Levy, David H. Wegman, Sherry L. Baron, Rosemary K. Sokas. Lippincott Williams & Wilkins, 2006.
http://www.r2library.com/
http://www.ovid.com/
ISBN: 9780781755511
Recommended for: Hospital, Academic Libraries
Doody's Core Titles Selection

This long-standing textbook has been revised recently to inform health professionals on how to recognize, treat, and prevent occupational and environmental disease and injury at both the individual and population levels. The book seeks a holistic approach by weaving together the relationship among employment, environment, and health. The range of material covered is extensive. The book is subdivided in five sections. The first section on work, environment, and health explores the social, political, legal, and ethical contexts within which occupational and environmental exposures occur. The next part is devoted to recognition, assessment, and prevention. Those seven chapters detail the practice of occupational medicine, including hygiene, safety, and ergonomics. A specific chapter is devoted to epidemiological principles. The hazardous exposures chapters include new content covering chemical; physical—noise, vibration, temperature, or other; biological; and air, water, and waste exposures. A separate chapter discusses occupational stress. A worthwhile new chapter introduces the impact of global environmental changes on work. The next section covers the cause, diagnosis, treatment, and prevention of occupationally and environmentally-generated adverse health effects. Finally, the book concludes with chapters dedicated to outlining an integrated approach to prevention. Content focuses on issues ranging from disparities; the role of labor unions, non-profits, and communities in ensuring good environmental health; and the practice of conducting workplace investigations. Some variation in writing styles and levels exists across the chapters, but, nonetheless, the explanations are clear and concise. Photographs, drawings, graphs, tables, and case studies are well utilized to highlight or exemplify points of interest. Authors from several countries offer expertise in various disciplines such as medicine, industry, labor, and government. The index is quite good for such wide-ranging coverage. This book is listed as a *Doody's* core title. Various professionals, occupational and environmental medicine physicians, allied health professionals, toxicologists, industrial hygienists, and others will find the book useful. This book is recommended for academic, hospital, and special libraries.

Pediatric Environmental Health. 2nd ed. Editors: Ruth A. Etzel, Sophie J. Balk, American Academy of Pediatrics Committee on Environmental Health. American Academy of Pediatrics, 2003.
ISBN: 9781581101119
Recommended for: Academic, Consumer Health Libraries

From the American Academy of Pediatrics Committee on Environmental Health, this handbook provides parents and practitioners with detailed information regarding environmental effects on children's health. The book begins by explaining how environmental exposures have varying effects across ages and stages of childhood development and the importance of breastfeeding. Two other chapters describe the details of taking an environmental history and conducting a home inventory of environmental hazards. The second section contains 22 chapters on chemical and physical hazards that are most likely to affect children: endocrine disruptors, secondhand smoke, herbs/dietary supplements, noise and ultraviolet light, and the other usual suspects. New content includes arsenic, gasoline and its additives, food irradiation, and metals. These chapters are similarly structured to provide a quick reference. After a description of each hazard, details are provided regarding the routes and sources of exposure, the organ systems affected, clinical symptoms, diagnostic methods, treatment, and prevention. In addition, a list of frequently asked questions and answers of interest to parents and pediatricians is included. The next part highlights environmental hazards within specific settings, such as child care, schools, workplace, and waste sites. A unique and necessary chapter has been added that describes the effects on in utero development of the child due to preconception and prenatal exposures of the parent. The section on complex threats incorporates an interesting mix of situations that pose unusual and complex exposures for children—for example, arts and crafts, non-therapeutic use of antibiotics in animal agriculture, and chemical-biological terrorism. Specific chapters also touch upon multiple chemical sensitivity, cancer, and asthma. Attention is also given to children's health in developing countries and environmental health disparities. The last section addresses how environmental health information and risks need to be communicated given the scientific uncertainties. New chapters have been added on environmental health advocacy and risk assessment and management. In keeping with its role as a practical reference guide, this book includes six appendixes that offer more resources for pediatricians and/or parents. Of particular interest are the resources for environmental health and the patient education materials. In revising this edition, the editor received substantial input from different sections and committees of the AAP. In addition to new and updated content, more tables and figures were added to clarify information, and additional references to patient education materials available on the web are listed. Although an updated edition is overdue and this one lacks some environmental concerns, such as plasticizers, phthalates, and polybrominated flame retardants, *Pediatric Environmental Health* still provides a useful guide for parents.

Risk Assessment for Environmental Health. Editors: Mark G. Robson, William A. Toscano. Jossey-Bass/Wiley, 2007.
http://extranet.netlibrary.com/TitleSelect
http://www.ebrary.com/
ISBN: 9780787983192
ISBN: 9780787988593 (Online)
Recommended for: Academic Libraries

This textbook provides a comprehensive review of the tools for and approaches to risk assessment in environmental health. The book is roughly divided into two sections. The chapters in the first section cover the major principles and techniques in the field; the second section utilizes case studies to exemplify the content presented in the preceding section. The beginning chapters cover the broad context of risk assessment, risk management, and the role risk assessment plays in regulatory decision making on risk. The next four chapters delve into the experimental and computational methods for conducting risk assessment. The remaining, first-section chapters focus on conducting risk assessment for special situations, whether in the workplace, regarding children, or due to radiological or microbial exposure. One useful chapter explores the field of biomonitoring and the challenge of monitoring exposure throughout stages of life.

Another chapter addresses various laws and regulations and the role risk played in establishing them. The book also includes a unique chapter devoted solely to the precautionary principle. The 11 case studies demonstrate many of the principles and methods discussed in the earlier chapters. Each chapter begins with summary points and ends with thought questions and further reading sources. Concepts are often discussed multiple times throughout various chapters, thereby reinforcing the material. This book is a product of the Environmental and Occupational Health Council of the Association of Schools of Public Health (ASPH). A majority of the authors are faculty from member schools of the ASPH. The resource is intended for students in public health, environmental science, environmental engineering, and other disciplines. The publication is recommended for academic and special libraries.

Silent Spring. Author: Rachel Carson. Houghton Mifflin, 1962.
ISBN: 9780618249060 (40th anniversary ed., 2002)
ISBN: 9780618253050 (40th anniversary ed., 2002)
Recommended for: Hospital, Academic, Consumer Health Libraries

A letter from a woman in Massachusetts disclosing that DDT was killing birds was the igniter for Rachel Carson, a marine biologist, to finally write *Silent Spring*. Although the book focuses on the indiscriminate use of pesticides and their effects on wildlife and human health, the book's theme more broadly seeks to raise awareness of society's relationship and responsibility vis-à-vis the natural world. Her book, which was loved by the public but reviled by industry, has been credited with launching the modern environmental movement. As a result of her book, not only did the government call for the eventual elimination of DDT and other persistent toxic pesticides, but it also established the Environmental Protection Agency in 1970. Carson set a precedent for scientists to write for the general public; notable other works include *The Closing Circle: Nature, Man & Technology* (Barry Commoner, 1971); *Only One Earth: The Care and Maintenance of a Small Planet* (Barbara Ward and René Dubos, 1972); and *Currents of Death* (Paul Brodeur, 1989). The more recent *Our Stolen Future* (Theo Colborn, Dianne Dumanoski, and John Peterson Myers, 1996) mirrors Carson's work by divulging evidence of chemicals that block hormones (endocrine disrupting chemicals), causing developmental and reproductive abnormalities in wildlife and humans. *Silent Spring* should be part of any general health collection in a library. Along with other subsequent re-releases, Houghton Mifflin offers a 2002 fortieth anniversary edition, which includes a new introduction and an epilogue providing historical context for the book.

Journals

Environmental Health Perspectives. v. 1, National Institute of Environmental Health Sciences, 1972.
http://ehp03.niehs.nih.gov/home.action
http://www.ncbi.nlm.nih.gov/pmc/journals/253/
ISSN: 00916765
ISSN: 15529924 (Online)
See Also Chapter 10.15.1. Environmental Medicine, Chapter 17.8. Toxicology
Indexed in: MEDLINE, CINAHL
Recommended for: Academic, Consumer Health Libraries

Environmental Health Perspectives (*EHP*) is one of the few peer-reviewed research journals still being published by the U.S. government. Its intent is to "serve as a forum for the discussion of the interrelationships between the environment and human health by publishing in a balanced and objective manner the best peer-reviewed research and most current and credible news of the field." Content includes both peer-reviewed research articles and sections devoted to environmental medicine and children's environmental health, summaries of selected research papers, current environmental health news, and book reviews. Unique for a publication of this type is its international outreach. Besides publishing a quarterly Chinese-language edition, *EHP* also contributes content to two Spanish journals and hosts the online journal *Mali Médical*. Complimentary copies are provided to readers in the developing world. *EHP's* Science Education program includes a student version of *EHP* tied to lesson plans. While the peer-reviewed articles are predominantly of interest to environmental health and toxicology researchers, the journal's other content would hold appeal for all health professionals, emergency responders, teachers and students, and members of the public. With an impact factor of 6.191 (*Journal Citation Reports*, 2009), *EHP* is the fourth-ranked journal in public, environmental, and occupational health, and it is the third-ranked journal in environmental sciences. Full online coverage back to volume 1 is available through the Institute's website as well as through PubMed Central. The online version is open access, but a fee is charged for the print version to recover costs.

Journal of Exposure Science and Environmental Epidemiology. v. 16, Nature Publishing Group, 2006.
http://www.nature.com/jes/archive/index.html

ISSN: 155900631
ISSN: 1559064X (Online)
See Also Chapter 10.15.1. Environmental Medicine
Indexed in: MEDLINE
Recommended for: Hospital, Academic Libraries

The *Journal of Exposure Science and Environmental Epidemiology* publishes original research, reviews, and feature articles on a range of topics related to exposure assessment. Priority is given to content that addresses the following areas: (a) advances in measurements, modeling, or instrumentation used in exposure analysis; (b) pathway mechanisms that lead to routes of exposure; (c) biomarkers of exposure and their relationship to health effects and susceptibility; and (d) population-based studies of exposure to toxic substances. Although this journal has a relatively average impact factor, its niche nature makes it an important resource for an environmental health collection, and it would be useful for academic health science and special libraries. Online content is available back to volume 9, 1999. It was originally titled *Journal of Exposure Analysis and Environmental Epidemiology* (1991–2005). Although the earlier title was not indexed by MEDLINE, the current title's indexing includes MEDLINE, Scopus, Web of Science, and other major biomedical literature sources.

Journal of Occupational and Environmental Medicine. v. 37, Lippincott Williams & Wilkins, 1995.
http://journals.lww.com/joem/
http://www.ovid.com/
ISSN: 10762752
ISSN: 15365948 (Online)
See Also Chapter 10.15.2. Occupational Medicine
Indexed in: MEDLINE, CINAHL
Recommended for: Hospital, Academic Libraries

The *Journal of Occupational and Environmental Medicine* is the official publication of the American College of Occupational and Environmental Medicine. Directed toward the interests of its membership, this journal offers a range of content related to the prevention, diagnosis, and rehabilitation of environmentally-induced conditions and work-related injuries and illnesses. Content includes peer-reviewed, clinically oriented research articles, technical reports on new developments or techniques, brief communications summarizing noteworthy epidemiological studies, an occupational medicine forum, book reviews, news highlights, and calendar of events. A unique feature is the section on articles of interest for clinicians combined with a CME credit option. This journal is recommended for academic health science libraries and hospital libraries. Although some of the content is not directly applicable to the environmental health topic, this journal is one of the few with a strong impact factor and editorial board that focuses on environmentally-related occupational conditions. The current title was preceded by the *Journal of Occupational Medicine* (1959–1994). It is indexed in all the major biomedical literature databases such as MEDLINE, Web of Science, Science Citation Index Expanded, and Scopus.

Databases and Other Electronic Resources

CHE Toxicant and Disease Database. Collaborative on Health and the Environment, 200?
http://database.healthandenvironment.org/
Recommended for: Academic, Consumer Health Libraries

The CHE Toxicant and Disease Database is a free, searchable database that summarizes links between chemical contaminants and approximately 180 human diseases or conditions. Diseases and toxicants can be viewed by clicking on the disease name; browsing by organ system, disease name, or toxicant; or searching by keyword or CAS registry number. The search results are grouped by "strength of evidence"—strong, good, and limited/conflicting. For each disease, the causes are color coded to coincide with the strength of evidence. Notes and references to the literature are provided. The CHE Toxicant and Disease Database provides readily accessible information for members of the general public as well as allied health professionals. Data is collected from major textbooks, such as *Casarett and Doull's Toxicology: The Basic Science of Poisons*, (McGraw-Hill, 2001); *Occupational and Environmental Medicine* (McGraw-Hill, 2004); and *Environmental and Occupational Medicine* (Lippincott, 1998). Given the outdated nature of the textbooks, more epidemiological studies and reviews of diseases were incorporated in the database. On the "About the Database" page, CHE explains in detail the background of the database's development, including the "significant limitations." The Collaborative is an international organization composed of individuals and organizations, including scientists, non-profit associations, health professionals, and others who are interested in promoting the scientific basis for understanding the effects of environmental factors and exposures on human health. Given the rising awareness of environmentally related health effects, this resource is worthwhile for academic health science and public libraries.

6. Health Services Administration

Organization and administration of health services dedicated to the delivery of health care.

—MeSH

Contributor: Diana Culbertson

Monographs

Slee's Health Care Terms. 5th ed. Authors: Debora A. Slee, Vergil N. Slee, H. Joachim Schmidt. Jones & Bartlett, 2008.
ISBN: 9780763746155
Recommended for: Hospital, Academic, Consumer Health Libraries

This is the leading dictionary for non-medical terms used in health care. It is useful for anyone involved with health care, especially board members or others who may be new to the field. Over 8,000 terms, phrases, and acronyms related to health care administration, health insurance, and health policy are clearly defined.

The Well-Managed Healthcare Organization. 7th ed. Authors: Kenneth R. White, John R. Griffith. Health Administration Press, 2010.
ISBN: 9781567933574
Recommended for: Hospital, Academic Libraries

This often-used textbook covers a range of administrative aspects of running a hospital or other type of health care provider organization. The book is organized into three sections: (1) governing and making organizations responsive to their environment; (2) the caring organization; and (3) learning and meeting support needs. The governing section covers the stakeholders, purpose, functions, governing board, and general management of the health care organization. The second section addresses clinical performance, physicians/medical staff, nursing staff, clinical support services, and community health. The last section focuses on information services, financial management, human resource systems, plant and guest services, planning and internal consulting, and marketing and strategy. Both authors have extensive experience in the graduate education of health administrators. The book is co-published with AUPHA Press, the publishing arm of the Association of University Programs in Health Administration. This review refers to the sixth edition.

Journals

Medical Care. v. 1, Lippincott Williams & Wilkins, 1963.
http://journals.lww.com/lww-medicalcare
ISSN: 00257079
ISSN: 15371948 (Online)
Indexed in: MEDLINE, CINAHL
Recommended for: Hospital, Academic Libraries

Medical Care is the official journal of the American Public Health Association, Medical Care Section. It is a peer-reviewed, monthly journal publishing scholarly articles on all aspects of health care delivery and administration, including the planning, organization, financing, and evaluation of health services. Individual articles may be purchased online from the publisher's website. The journal is indexed in MEDLINE.

6.1. Health Care Quality Assurance

Activities and programs intended to assure or improve the quality of care in either a defined medical setting or a program. The concept includes the assessment or evaluation of the quality of care; identification of problems or shortcomings in the delivery of care; designing activities to overcome these deficiencies; and follow-up monitoring to ensure effectiveness of corrective steps.

—MeSH: Quality Assurance, Health Care

Contributor: Diana Culbertson

Monographs

The Healthcare Quality Book: Vision, Strategy, and Tools. 2nd ed. Editors: Elizabeth R. Ransom, Maulik S. Joshi, David B. Nash, Scott B. Ransom. Health Administration Press, 2008.
ISBN: 9781567933017
Recommended for: Hospital, Academic Libraries

This guide should be useful to anyone who wants to better understand health care quality issues and improvement strategies. The book first presents chapters on the basic concepts of health care quality, laying the foundation for the chapters that follow, which are focused on the organization and microsystem. Quality measurement, provider profiling, patient safety and medical errors, leadership, organizational infrastructure, changing clinician behavior, the role of accreditation, and the purchaser perspective are topics addressed. The editors have compiled chapters written by prominent leaders in quality of health care.

Patient Safety and Quality: An Evidence-Based Handbook for Nurses. Editor: Rhonda G Hughes. Agency for Healthcare Research and Quality, 2008.
See Chapter 6.1.1. Patient Safety

Quality and Performance Improvement in Healthcare: A Tool for Programmed Learning. 4th ed. Authors: Patricia L. Shaw, Chris Elliott. American Health Information Management Association, 2010.
See Chapter 6.2. Medical Records

Safe Practices for Better Healthcare—2009 Update: A Consensus Report. National Quality Forum, 2009.
ISBN: 9781933875231
Recommended for: Hospital, Academic Libraries

First released in 2003, *Safe Practices for Better Healthcare* currently presents 34 practices that have been shown effective in reducing adverse health care events, making care safer for patients. The safe practices are based in part on a consensus development process involving other health care organizations and experts. The best practices selected are those supported by strong evidence and can be generalized across care settings and types of patients, are likely to have a significant benefit, and are easily understood by patients, providers, purchasers, and researchers. The safe practices are grouped into seven categories: culture of safety; informed consent, life-sustaining treatment, disclosure, and care of the caregiver; matching health care needs to service capability; information transfer and clear communication; medication management; prevention of health care associated infections; and condition or site specific practices. Each safe practice presented defines the problem, provides examples of implementation approaches, lists opportunities for patient and family involvement, suggests performance measures, indicates care setting considerations, and briefly discusses areas for research.

To Err Is Human: Building a Safer Health System. Editors: Linda T. Kohn, Janet M. Corrigan, Molla S. Donaldson. National Academy Press, 2000.
http://www.nap.edu/
http://extranet.netlibrary.com/TitleSelect/
http://www.ebrary.com/
ISBN: 9780309068376
ISBN: 9780585212739 (Online)
See Also Chapter 6.1.1. Patient Safety
Recommended for: Hospital, Academic Libraries
Doody's Core Titles Selection

This report stirred headlines when released in 1999, estimating that as many as 98,000 hospital patients were dying annually due to errors. Issued by the Committee on Quality of Health Care in America, Institute of Medicine, it is widely credited as the catalyst for greatly advancing the patient safety movement. The Committee report frames the problem of errors in health care—both their frequency and causes—and makes a series of recommendations for preventing them. The recommendations focus on leadership, error reporting systems, setting performance standards, and creating safety systems in health care organizations. In addition to the print version, the report or its individual chapters may be purchased in a PDF format. The full report can also be read page by page or searched online at no charge.

Understanding Patient Safety. Author: Robert M. Wachter. McGraw-Hill Lange, 2008.
http://www.r2library.com/
ISBN: 9780071482776
Recommended for: Hospital, Academic Libraries

This book is a clearly-written introduction to patient safety, organized into four key sections: an introduction to the nature and frequency of medical errors and basic principles of patient safety, types of medical errors, solutions, and appendixes with other useful information. The types of errors discussed include medication, surgical, diagnostic, human or human-machine interface, transition and hand-off, teamwork and communication, nosocomial infections, and other complications (venous thromboembolism, falls, press ulcers). Real cases of errors are used to add interest and understanding. Solutions are addressed in chapters on information technology, reporting systems, organizational culture, workforce, training, malpractice, accountability, legal issues, and patients. Key patient safety resources, a glossary, a list of milestones, patient safety indicators developed by the Agency for Healthcare Research and Quality, the Joint Commission's National Patient Safety Goals, the National Quality Forum's list of "never events," and a checklist of what patients and families can do to prevent errors are all included among the appendixes. The book is written for all levels and is appropriate for clinicians, administrators, board members, and others interested in patient safety.

Journals

Quality & Safety in Health Care. v. 11, BMJ Group, 2002.
See Chapter 6.1.1. Patient Safety

6.1.1. Patient Safety

Activities and programs intended to prevent accidents, injuries, and other adverse occurrences in patients in an institutional setting.

—MeSH

Contributor: Holly Ann Burt

Monographs

Human Error in Medicine. Editor: Marilyn Sue Bogner. Lawrence Erlbaum, 1994.
ISBN: 9780805813869
ISBN: 9780805813852
Recommended for: Hospital, Academic Libraries

This classic work examines avoidable medical error from a problem-oriented, systems perspective. For the authors of this book, this means considering human error in the context in which it is observed, identifying factors within a system that contribute to human error in medical care, and suggesting efforts to alleviate those factors and reduce the likelihood of error. The chapter authors are leaders who have hands-on experience in medical care or research into factors contributing to error in medicine and who are from diverse fields, including psychology, medicine, engineering, cognitive science, human factors, gerontology, and nursing. This interdisciplinary approach provides a comprehensive look at the diverse facets involved in human error. In the forward, James Reason reviews the Chernobyl incident, defines active and latent failures, and introduces parallels to health care. Other authors examine the inadequacies or ambiguity in the design of medical devices, responses to antagonistic environmental conditions, types of cognitive errors, medication missteps, and using statistics in clinical practice. Extensive references and a closing chapter on taxonomy are included. This book is recommended as a tool for practitioners and government agencies in addressing error and for academics and researchers in all fields of patient safety. A substantially updated second edition is planned for April 2012.

Keeping Patients Safe: Transforming the Work Environment of Nurses. Editors: Committee on the Work Environment for Nurses and Patient Safety, Board on Health Care Services, Ann Page. National Academies Press, 2004.
http://www.nap.edu/
ISBN: 9780309090674
Recommended for: Hospital, Academic Libraries

Building on the Institute of Medicine reports *To Err is Human* and *Crossing the Quality Chasm*, this book draws on the experiences of nurses to examine the key aspects of their work environment with an impact on patient safety and to identify potential improvements in health care working conditions. After introducing the critical link between nursing and patient safety, the report describes a framework for building patient safety defenses into nurses' work environments through linking needed changes in management and leadership (Chapter 4), workforce deployment and capability (Chapter 5), work processes, including workspace design, to prevent and mitigate errors (Chapter 6), and organizational culture (Chapter 7). Also discussed in this report are the characteristics of the nursing workforce and the nature of the activities nurses typically perform, evidence-based management practices, and elements needed to create and sustain a culture of safety. The book closes with encouragement for implementation of the changes recommended throughout the report and a call for additional research. Published by the National Academies Press, *Keeping Patients Safe* may be read online or purchased as a hardcover book, a single PDF, or as individual chapters in PDF format. This Institute of Medicine report is recommended for nurses, nurse leaders, healthcare organization leadership, and academic institutions training the nursing workforce and those who employ and lead them.

Patient Safety and Quality: An Evidence-Based Handbook for Nurses. Editor: Rhonda G Hughes. Agency for Healthcare Research and Quality, 2008.
http://www.ahrq.gov/QUAL/nurseshdbk/
http://www.ncbi.nlm.nih.gov/bookshelf/br.fcgi?book=nursehb
ISBN: 1587633531 (v.1)
ISBN: 158763354X (v.2)
ISBN: 1587633558 (v.3)
Recommended for: Hospital Libraries

This comprehensive handbook examines a broad range of issues and includes peer-reviewed discussions and reviews of topics and literature regarding patient safety and quality health care. Addressing the need for nurses to know what proven techniques and interventions they can use to enhance patient outcomes, this work was sponsored by the Agency for Healthcare Research and Quality (AHRQ) with additional funding from the Robert Wood

Johnson Foundation. The publication is divided into six sections: patient safety and quality, evidence-based practice, patient-centered care, working conditions and the work environment for nurses, critical opportunities for patient safety and quality improvement, and tools for quality improvement and patient safety. Chapters include a background section, an analysis of the literature and an evidence table based on the literature, a discussion of both practice and research implications, and references. *Patient Safety and Quality*, AHRQ Publication No. 08-0043, may be read online or be downloaded as single PDF or as individual chapters; it may also be ordered in a three volume printed handbook or in a CD-ROM version. The online version is available both on the AHRQ site and through the *Bookshelf* of the National Center for Biotechnology Information (NCBI) of the National Library of Medicine. This book is recommended for nurses in practice, nurse-educators, nurse-researchers, nursing students, and nursing leaders and is dedicated to nurses everywhere.

Patient Safety: Achieving a New Standard for Care. Editors: Philip Aspden, Janet M. Corrigan, Julie Wolcott, Shari M. Erickson, Committee on Data Standards for Patient Safety, Board on Health Care Services. National Academies Press, 2004.
http://www.nap.edu/
ISBN: 9780309090773
Recommended for: Hospital, Academic Libraries

This report, part of the Institute of Medicine's *Quality Chasm Series*, combines two important areas of research in patient safety: that of improving the quality of care and that of fostering the use of information technology within the health care system. *Patient Safety* describes a detailed plan to facilitate the development of data standards for the collection, coding, and classification of patient safety information. Recommendations in the report include implementation of national computerized information systems and a robust applied research agenda in patient safety. Part I of this report examines the issues surrounding building a national health information infrastructure and discusses requirements for establishing health care data standards. Part II looks at establishing comprehensive patient safety programs within health care settings, which will require a culture of safety and a commitment to analyzing adverse events and near-misses. Part III focuses on patient safety reporting systems, including methods for streamlining these systems and developing standardized reporting. With extensive references, lists of reporting systems around the country and an appendix focusing on electronic heath records, this book is an important resource for health care leaders, systems managers, patient safety researchers, and health professionals involved with reporting issues and other aspects of information technology. Available through the National Academies Press, *Patient Safety* may be read online or purchased as a hardcover book, a single PDF, or as individual chapters in PDF format.

To Err Is Human: Building a Safer Health System. Editors: Linda T. Kohn, Janet M. Corrigan, Molla S. Donaldson, Committee on Quality of Health Care in America. National Academies Press, 2000.
http://books.nap.edu/
ISBN: 9780309068376
See Also Chapter 6.1. Health Care Quality Assurance
Recommended for: Hospital, Academic, Consumer Health Libraries
Doody's Core Titles Selection

This seminal work launched the modern patient safety movement and became the first of the Institute of Medicine's *Quality Chasm Series*. Acknowledging the New York study that revealed over 98,000 Americans die every year as a result of medical error, *To Err is Human* identifies patient safety as a critical component of quality and presents a national agenda for reducing medical errors and improving patient safety. To design a safer health system, recommendations from the report involve the government at all levels, industry, health care organizations and providers, and consumers. *To Err is Human* uses detailed case studies to describe types of errors in health care and why they occur and to examine how legislation, regulation, and market activity influence the quality of care provided by health care organizations. Additional topics include the need for and importance of nationwide error reporting systems; a patient safety center to build leadership and knowledge of patient safety; protection for voluntary reporting systems and data from legal discovery; performance standards and expectations for patient safety; and strategies for creating safety systems in health care organizations. Each chapter contains a reference list for further research and focuses on the question, "How can we learn from our mistakes?" Published by the National Academies Press, *To Err is Human* may be read online or purchased as a hardcover book, a single PDF, or as individual chapters in PDF format. This landmark report is recommended for everyone interested in patient safety.

Understanding Patient Safety. Author: Robert M. Wachter. McGraw-Hill Lange, 2008.
See Chapter 6.1. Health Care Quality Assurance

Wall of Silence: The Untold Story of the Medical Mistakes That Kill and Injure Millions of Americans. Authors: Rosemary Gibson, Janardan Prasad Singh. Lifeline Press, 2003.
ISBN: 9780895261120
Recommended for: Hospital, Academic, Consumer Health Libraries

Written for and presented from the viewpoint of the patient, the authors share stories of families who have suffered devastating injuries from medical mistakes—including their own. These true stories of pain, including the loss of a loved one or a livelihood, place a human face on medical error and challenge a system that failed to care for patients and their families. The authors define types of medical mistakes through actual examples and describe a health care system that hides behind a wall of silence rather than working together to prevent medical errors. The anguish of patients and families who seek and are denied answers is revealed, along with the impact on the health professionals involved in these events. The final chapters lift up the actions of individuals, families, groups, and organizations—including health care leaders—that are working to change this system and break down the walls of silence. One chapter is devoted specifically to the steps individuals can take to help protect themselves and their families. *Wall of Silence* is recommended for everyone who uses the health care system.

Why Hospitals Should Fly: The Ultimate Flight Plan to Patient Safety and Quality Care. Author: John J. Nance. Second River Healthcare Press, 2008.
ISBN: 9780974386065
ISBN: 9780974386058
Recommended for: Hospital, Academic, Consumer Health Libraries

Evidence-based research in safety across three industries is gathered by medical safety and aviation safety expert and founding member of the National Patient Safety Foundation, John Nance, to answer the question: What would a safe hospital look like? This fictional work describes methods for supporting front-line hospital staff in providing safe, high-quality care for patients. It is introduced through the eyes of a physician turned CEO who has experienced a devastating medical error and comes to St. Michael's Memorial to learn how the hospital could have such a stellar record in patient safety and patient satisfaction. Building on experiences from the aviation and medical industries, the fictional St. Michael's represents how an ideal health care environment could look and feel. In this example of a patient-centered culture, the hospital supports, and is extremely responsive to, the needs and limitations of the people who physically care for the patients. Written for those with some knowledge of hospitals and health systems, the story incorporates and references current research on leadership, communication between health professionals, expectation of and prevention of both human and system error, checklists, and methods of changing the health care culture. It is an enjoyable and informative book with rich insights into what may be needed to provide a truly safe healthcare environment.

YOU: The Smart Patient: An Insider's Handbook for Getting the Best Treatment. Authors: Michael F. Roizen, Mehmet C. OZ. Free Press, 2006.
ISBN: 9780743293013
ISBN: 9780786287192
ISBN: 9780739467589
Recommended for: Consumer Health Libraries

This humorous and comprehensive handbook calls for everyone to become a *Smart Patient* in order to get the best possible health care. Written in conjunction with the Joint Commission, the book shows readers in clear, easy steps how to be in control of their own healthcare and address the different issues that may come up. Topics include choosing the right doctor, hospital, and insurance company; dealing with prescription drugs, specialists, treatment options, alternative medicine, and second opinions; and recommended preparations for doctor's visits and hospitals stays. Chapter 8, for example, focuses on knowing about patient rights and responsibilities and includes a discussion of living wills, do-not-resuscitate orders and the health care power of attorney. A medical jargon glossary, sample forms, extensive checklists, and additional resources are included. Filled with detailed and authoritative information, *You: The Smart Patient* is a book for every patient and every family dealing with medical issues.

Journals

Joint Commission Journal on Quality and Patient Safety. v. 31, Joint Commission Resources, 2005.
http://www.ingentaconnect.com/content/jcaho/jcjqs/
ISSN: 15537250
ISSN: 1938131X (Online)
Indexed in: MEDLINE, CINAHL
Recommended for: Hospital, Academic Libraries

This monthly, peer-reviewed journal provides a forum to focus on practical approaches to improve quality and safety in health care. Each issue identifies a specific patient safety theme and features at least one article on performance improvement. Health professionals, administrators, and specialists share their experiences and concerns, as well as their methods and successes in improving safety in their institutions. Topics in this publication cover the entire safety spectrum including human factors engineering, patient and family involvement, teamwork and communication, information technology and reporting systems, disclosure, and responses to the National Patient Safety Goals. The journal's online version is available through IngentaConnect. Indexed in MEDLINE, previous titles are: *Joint Commission Journal on Quality and Safety* [2003–2004], *Joint Commission Journal on Quality Improvement* [1993–2002], and the *Quality Review Bulletin* [1974–1993]. Although the journal addresses the mission of the Joint Commission, articles may express views that diverge from Joint Commission policies and standards. Because of the comprehensive nature of the journal, it is recommended for both hospital systems and for academic institutions focusing on training health professionals, hospital leadership, and patient safety leaders.

Journal of Patient Safety. v. 1, Lippincott Williams & Wilkins, 2005.
http://www.journalpatientsafety.com/
ISSN: 15498417
ISSN: 15498425 (Online)
Indexed in: MEDLINE
Recommended for: Hospital Libraries

This quarterly, peer-reviewed, scholarly publication is the official journal of the National Patient Safety Foundation. Started in 2005, the journal focuses on translational research (moving from research findings to patient settings), clinical applications of research, and best practices in the hospital setting. In addition to its research emphasis, the journal also publishes articles describing lessons learned from near-miss and adverse event experiences, reducing error through system modifications, and the impact of regulatory changes on healthcare delivery. Original articles cover a wide variety of patient safety topics and most issues include a section on solutions for leaders and on patient education. Additional topics in the journal include case reports, review articles and conference proceedings. A number of *Patient Guides* from the early issues of the *Journal of Patient Safety* are offered free on the journal website. Available through Wolters Kluwer Health or Lippincott Williams & Wilkins, the journal is currently indexed in MEDLINE and is recommended for health professionals and patient safety leaders.

Quality & Safety in Health Care. v. 11, BMJ Group, 2002.
http://qshc.bmj.com/
ISSN: 14753898
ISSN: 14753901 (Online)
Indexed in: MEDLINE, CINAHL
Recommended for: Hospital, Academic Libraries

Quality & Safety in Health Care is a bi-monthly international peer-reviewed forum for researchers, clinicians, nurses, clinical managers, and researchers in organizational development and behavior. It is the official journal of the International Forum on Quality & Safety in Health Care, a partnership of the Institute for Healthcare Improvement (IHI) and the BMJ Publishing Group Ltd. The journal covers the development of quality and safety initiatives, their integration into practice, practical experiences in improving health care services, the influence of management and organizational learning on the quality and safety of clinical care, involvement of patients and family members in promoting quality and safety improvements, and research relevant to health care quality and safety across all industries. In addition to original articles, each issue includes a quality improvement report and the identification of one quality and safety hero or martyr. Other regular topics include developing research and practice, education and training, and error management. Occasional supplements focus on a single issue such as safe design (2006), simulation (2004) and leadership (2001). The *Quality & Safety in Health Care* journal (formerly *Quality in Health Care* [1992–2001]) is available through the BMJ Group and is currently indexed in MEDLINE, with many articles also available through PubMed Central. The website offers a comprehensive online archive and volumes 1–16 are available with free registration. This journal is a recommended source of information on patient safety issues.

6.2. Medical Records

Recording of pertinent information concerning patient's illness or illnesses. Includes electronic health records and personal health records.

—MeSH

Contributor: David Sweet

Monographs

Documentation for Medical Records. Editors: Barbara Odom-Wesley, Diann Brown. American Health Information Management Association, 2009.

ISBN: 9781584261834
Recommended for: Hospital, Academic Libraries

This book is an overview of basic healthcare documentation principles. It covers documentation in ambulatory, home and hospice, behavioral, and long-term care settings, as well as the transition to electronic medical records. Also included are introductions to industry policies, procedures, and regulations that impact medical record documentation.

Electronic Health Records: A Practical Guide for Professionals and Organizations. 4th ed. Author: Margret K. Amatayakul. American Health Information Management Association, 2009.
ISBN: 9781584262190
Recommended for: Hospital, Academic Libraries
Doody's Core Titles Selection

This book is the industry standard on electronic health records (EHRs). It contains step-by-step guidelines for developing and implementing EHR strategies for healthcare organizations. Topics include legality of EHRs, quality measurement and reporting, financial impact analysis, consumer healthcare concerns and identity theft, and personal health records. Other key features are goal setting and strategic planning, EHR selection and contract negotiation, and system design and implementation.

Health Information Management: Concepts, Principles, and Practice. 3rd ed. Authors: Kathleen M. LaTour, Shirley E. Eichenwald. American Health Information Management Association, 2010.
ISBN: 9781584262176
Recommended for: Hospital, Academic Libraries
Doody's Core Titles Selection

This is the premier work on medical records and health information management (HIM). This new edition includes material on emerging issues such as electronic health records, information management, hybrid records, HIM standards development, personal health records, and many other topics. Instructor resource materials such as chapter outlines, lesson plans, and exercises are included. This work is written by HIM educators and industry experts. Self-quizzes are included within each chapter.

Health Information Management Technology: An Applied Approach. 2nd ed. Editor: Merida L. Johns. American Health Information Management Association, 2007.
ISBN: 9781584261414
Recommended for: Hospital, Academic Libraries

This work is the standard U.S. textbook in health information management technology (HIT). Useful for both students and practicing professionals, it contains easy-to-understand explanations of the major HIT principles and practical applications to approach real-world situations. There are case studies and quizzes included in each chapter.

ICD-9 Coding Handbook with Answers. Authors: Faye Brown, Nelly Leon-Chisen. American Hospital Association, 2009.
ISBN: 9781556483608
Recommended for: Hospital, Academic Libraries
Doody's Core Titles Selection

This guide helps coders understand the principles behind the ICD-9 classification system. It contains more than 100 exercises and review questions that allow coders to practice coding skills, plus an additional 269 case summary exercises that are based on real patient records.

The Personal Health Record. Editor: Julie Wolter. American Health Information Management Association, 2009.
ISBN: 9781584262060
Recommended for: Hospital, Academic, Consumer Health Libraries

This guide assists both practitioners and consumers in understanding current trends and processes in personal health records (PHRs). It discusses how health information management (HIM) professionals can help consumers develop their own PHRs. It provides an overview of why the PHR is needed; presents values and concerns of HIM professionals, provider organizations, physicians, consumers, and other parties; provides PHR models; and explains the benefits of PHRs to consumers.

Quality and Performance Improvement in Healthcare: A Tool for Programmed Learning. 4th ed. Authors: Patricia L. Shaw, Chris Elliott. American Health Information Management Association, 2010.
ISBN: 9781584262169
Recommended for: Hospital, Academic Libraries

This work covers the latest trends in healthcare quality control and performance. It also covers Performance Improvement (PI) foundations and fundamentals. Topics covered include national patient safety goals, pay for performance, and community-acquired and healthcare-associated infections. Learning is enhanced with key features such as figures and tables to illustrate PI concepts and quality improvement toolbox techniques.

Journals

Health Affairs. v. 1, Project HOPE, 1981.
http://www.healthaffairs.org/
ISSN: 02782715
ISSN: 15445208 (Online)
See Also Chapter 10.16. Public Health
Indexed in: MEDLINE, CINAHL
Recommended for: Hospital, Academic, Consumer Health Libraries

Health Affairs is the leading journal of health policy thought and research. The peer-reviewed journal was founded in 1981 under the aegis of Project HOPE, a nonprofit international health education organization. *Health Affairs* explores health policy issues of current concern in both domestic and international spheres. It is a multidisciplinary journal covering a wide range of health issues. Topics covered include access to care, health spending, quality, Medicare, Medicaid, prescription drug coverage and costs, physician practice, nursing trends, mental health, malpractice and health law, insurance reform, hospitals, global health, and disparities in health care. It is health policymakers' most frequently read journal and is consulted by 55 percent of staff members on U.S. congressional committees with jurisdiction in health.

Journal of AHIMA. v. 62, no. 11, AHIMA, 1991.
http://journal.ahima.org/
ISSN: 10605487
Indexed in: MEDLINE, CINAHL
Recommended for: Hospital, Academic Libraries
Brandon/Hill Selection

The *Journal of AHIMA* is the official publication of the American Health Information Management Association. It is the premier U.S. journal covering medical records and related topics. The journal serves as a professional development tool for health information managers. It keeps readers current on issues that affect practice, and it contributes to the field by publishing best practices and new knowledge. The journal, formerly known as *American Medical Record Association Journal* and *Medical Record News*, began in 1921. It was on the final Brandon/Hill list for allied health.

The Journal of Healthcare Information Management. v. 12, no. 3, Healthcare Information and Management Systems Society, 1998.
ISSN: 1099811X
Indexed in: MEDLINE
Recommended for: Hospital, Academic Libraries

JHIM is a quarterly, peer-reviewed journal specifically for health care information and management systems professionals. Each issue of *JHIM* examines a specific topic in the areas of clinical systems, information systems, management engineering, and telecommunications in health care organizations. Upcoming issues will feature articles on "Health Information Exchange: Case Studies in Interoperability and Integration," "Outcomes Improvement/Clinical Decision Support/Reporting," "Case studies in CPOE Implementation and Change Management," and "Case Studies in Meaningful Use." Online access is provided only to members of the Healthcare Information and Management Systems Society (HIMSS).

Journal of the American Medical Informatics Association: JAMIA. v. 1, American Medical Informatics Association, 1994.
http://jamia.bmj.com/
ISSN: 10675027
ISSN: 1527974X (Online)
See Also Chapter 6.3. Informatics
Indexed in: MEDLINE, CINAHL
Recommended for: Hospital, Academic Libraries
Brandon/Hill Selection

JAMIA is a journal of peer-reviewed articles that assist physicians, informaticians, scientists, nurses, and other health care professionals to develop and apply medical informatics to patient care, teaching, research, and health care administration. Issues contain reviews, discussion forums, and invited editorials presented as brief reviews or full-length papers. *JAMIA* had an impact factor of 3.974 and ranked first in both the medical informatics and computer science, interdisciplinary applications categories and third in the computer science, information system category in the 2009 *Journal Citation Reports*. It was listed on the final Brandon/Hill list for small medical libraries.

Databases and Other Electronic Resources

MyPHR.com. American Health Information Management Association, 2010
http://www.myPHR.com
Recommended for: Hospital, Academic, Consumer Health Libraries

This comprehensive website covers all aspects of personal health records (PHRs), from defining them, assisting consumers in developing PHRs for themselves or their family, discussing privacy, and providing a list of PHR vendors. Also included are news, blogs, and upcoming events as they relate to PHRs.

6.3. Informatics

The analysis and dissemination of data through the application of computers. Include medical, dental, nursing, public health informatics.

—MeSH

Contributor: Gale G. Hannigan

Monographs

Biomedical Informatics: Computer Applications in Health Care and Biomedicine. 3rd ed. Editors: Edward H. Shortliffe, James J. Cimino. Springer, 2006.
http://www.springerlink.com/content/978-0-387-28986-1
http://extranet.netlibrary.com/TitleSelect/
ISBN: 9780387289861
ISBN: 9780387217215 (Online)
Recommended for: Academic Libraries
Brandon/Hill Selection

First published in 1990 with the title *Medical Informatics: Computer Applications in Health Care*, this text continues to be a standard introduction to the field. The book has three main sections: "Recurrent Themes in Biomedical Informatics," "Biomedical Informatics Applications," and "Biomedical Informatics in the Years Ahead." The various authors, all recognized experts, review fundamental concepts such a cognitive science, probabilistic clinical reasoning, systems design, and standards. They also describe how these concepts are applied in computerized patient care systems, such as telehealth. Many of the topics covered, plus a chapter titled "Clinical Decision-Support Systems," highlight the relationship of informatics to medical decision making, which is another topic in this guide. There are also overviews of the public health infrastructure and computers in education. This book is often used for instruction in informatics education programs. As noted in the 1st edition, informatics is a rapidly developing field. While coverage of the concepts will not become outdated, the information about applications will need to be supplemented with journal articles until a new edition is published.

Clinical Bioinformatics. Editor: Ronald J.A. Trent. Springer/Humana Press, 2008.
See Chapter 26.1. Computational Biology

Clinical Decision Support: The Road Ahead. Editor: Robert A. Greenes. Elsevier Academic Press, 2007.
See Chapter 30.2. Medical Decision Making

Consumer Health Informatics: Informing Consumers and Improving Health Care. Editors: Deborah Lewis, Gunther Eysenbach, Rita Kukafka, P. Zoe Stavri, Holly Jimison. Springer, 2005.
http://www.springerlink.com/content/t622217041627p16/
http://extranet.netlibrary.com/TitleSelect/
http://www.ebrary.com/
ISBN: 9780387239910
ISBN: 9780387276526
Recommended for: Hospital, Academic, Consumer Health Libraries
Doody's Core Titles Selection

There are few books devoted to consumer health informatics, and libraries covering the topic should collect whatever they can find. This book is a comprehensive overview and part of the longstanding *Health Informatics Series*. In the first chapter, the authors present several definitions of consumer informatics and note that the "paradigm shift from physician-centered to patient-centric care and the impact of Internet access to health information has formed the basis for the development of consumer health informatics" (p. 1). Readers will learn about the design and evaluation of consumer health information websites, methods of delivery, and ethical issues; they will also find many case studies and anecdotes illustrating how consumers use information and technology to answer their health care questions.

Decision Making in Medicine: An Algorithmic Approach. 3rd ed. Editors: Stuart B. Mushlin, Harry L. Greene II. Mosby/Elsevier, 2010.
See Chapter 30.2. Medical Decision Making

Essentials of Nursing Informatics. 4th ed. Editors: Virginia K. Saba, Kathleen A. McCormick. McGraw-Hill, 2006.
http://online.statref.com/titleinfo/fxid-151.html
ISBN: 9780071441971
Recommended for: Hospital, Academic Libraries

This comprehensive review of nursing informatics is edited by leaders in the field with chapter contributions from more than 40 authors. Authors address historic perspectives, practical background information, theory, and the application of informatics in specific contexts, including nursing practice, administration, education, and research. There are two chapters about consumers' use of informatics: "Consumer and Patient Use of Computers for Health" and "Decision Support for Consumers." A unique feature is the section titled "International Perspectives" with chapters about nursing informatics in Canada, Europe, the Pacific Rim, Asia, and South America. The final section, "The Future of

Informatics," is a good overview of trends that relate to informatics, including the growing importance of genetics in health care, federal initiatives to support the development and use of electronic health records, and other topics. This book is a key source for nursing informatics. Due to the rapidly advancing nature of this field, one should look for the fifth edition before making a purchase.

Evaluation Methods in Biomedical Informatics. 2nd ed. Authors: Charles P. Friedman, Jeremy C. Wyatt. Springer, 2005.
http://www.springerlink.com/content/978-0-387-25889-8/
http://www.ebrary.com/
http://extranet.netlibrary.com/TitleSelect/
ISBN: 9780387258898
ISBN: 9780387306773
Recommended for: Academic Libraries
Doody's Core Titles Selection

Informatics initiatives are expensive, time-consuming, and complex, and they usually involve many groups of people with different needs and viewpoints such as users, vendors, technical staff, and administrators. Information systems are built, implemented, revised, and replaced often without a fair assessment that answers questions such as: "Was the system designed to do what it was intended to do?" and "Did the system in fact work as intended?" A significant and acknowledged problem with electronic health records is acceptance by users, who often are unconvinced that their personal or professional effectiveness will be improved. Evaluating information systems must be a key step in the design and use of information systems, and this book is a good place to learn appropriate methods for doing so. Why a book specifically about evaluation in informatics? In their preface, the authors point out that the evaluation of informatics resources involves three complex areas: "biomedicine as a field of human endeavor, computer-based information systems, and the general methodology of evaluation. . . ." (p. 5) The authors possess combined expertise in all of these areas and are well known in the medical informatics community. They acknowledge the value of both qualitative as well as quantitative methods, insisting on rigor in both. The index illustrates the wide variety of methods covered: ANOVA (analysis of variance), demonstration studies, nested design, sensitivity analysis, and usability studies to name a few. This is a unique book and should be on the library shelf wherever information systems are in place.

Handbook of Informatics for Nurses and Health Care Professionals. 4th ed. Authors: Toni Hebda, Patricia Czar. Pearson Prentice Hall, 2008.
See Chapter 9.13. Telemedicine

Health Care Information Systems: A Practical Approach for Health Care Management. 2nd ed. Authors: Karen A. Wager, Frances W. Lee, John P. Glaser. Jossey-Bass, 2009.
http://www.ebrary.com/
ISBN: 9780470387801
ISBN: 9780470451687
Recommended for: Hospital, Academic Libraries
Doody's Core Titles Selection

The focus of this book is on information generated or used by health care organizations. The target audience is health care administrators, information technology (IT) leaders, and informatics students needing to understand information systems in the organizational context. This management perspective distinguishes this title from others on the list. It is a suitable textbook for a formal course or self-directed study. Each chapter begins with learning objectives and ends with a summary, key terms, and learning activities. The final chapter consists of 16 case studies. Information and issues surrounding the implementation of an electronic health records system are center stage, as expected, because that is a primary goal of many health IT executives. But, the authors also address the systems development life cycle, trends in user interactions with systems, standards, the development process, evaluating IT effectiveness, strategic planning, and other topics that apply to managing information systems in general. Now in its second edition, this book belongs on the shelf of most health sciences libraries.

Health Informatics for Medical Librarians. Authors: Ana D. Cleveland, Donald B. Cleveland. Neal-Schuman, 2009.
ISBN: 9781555706272
Recommended for: Academic Libraries
Doody's Core Titles Selection

The Drs. Cleveland have written a book about health informatics that begins with the nature of health information and the emergence of the field of health informatics. They review the current state of the health care system and the incorporation of informatics into various health disciplines, such as veterinary medicine, nursing, and dentistry. Unique to this book are the discussions about the intersection of health informatics with librarianship—two fields primarily concerned with information—and various roles and opportunities for medical librarians and libraries. The second part of the book reviews the fundamental knowledge needed by any health informatics practitioner, including an understanding of health information organization and technology, the quest for an electronic health record (the "holy grail" of informatics), health information systems, medical imaging, and related ethical and legal issues. A separate chapter is devoted to bioinformatics and genomics, a field of growing research and incredible importance. A description of education, research, and careers in health informatics gives the interested reader guidance in pursuing further training in the field. Here is a book primarily for information professionals and for use in schools of library and information science; but, because it clearly lays out the fundamentals of this evolving and interdisciplinary field, this book would also be a useful resource for undergraduate courses in health informatics or biomedical sciences information management.

Information Retrieval: A Health and Biomedical Perspective. 3rd ed. Author: William Hersh. Springer, 2009.
http://www.springerlink.com/content/1386-4564/
http://www.ebrary.com/
http://extranet.netlibrary.com/TitleSelect//
ISBN: 9780387787022
ISBN: 99780387787039
Recommended for: Academic Libraries
Doody's Core Titles Selection

Given the vast amount of information in increasingly varied formats, the importance of information retrieval (IR) and the need to continuously improve IR capability cannot be overestimated. The author defines IR as consisting of "content, computer hardware to store and access that content, and computer software to process user input in order to retrieve it" (p. 6). This book provides a comprehensive review of the current state of information retrieval, from how health and biomedical information is produced, organized, indexed, retrieved, and used. The author also identifies research directions and results. The book is an essential reference for everyone associated with IR, including librarians, system developers, and informatics researchers. Sections are appropriate for graduate-level courses in informatics, information science, and computer science. The chapter on digital libraries, new to this edition, provides a good introduction to the characteristics and issues related to these evolving entities.

Medical Informatics: Knowledge Management and Data Mining in Biomedicine. Editors: Hsinchun Chen, Sherrilynne S. Fuller, Carol Friedman, William Hersh. Springer, 2005.
http://www.springerlink.com/content/978-0-387-24381-8/
ISBN: 9780387243818
ISBN: 9780387257396 (Online)
Recommended for: Academic Libraries
Doody's Core Titles Selection

The tremendous increase in the amount of data and the application of information technology has made the field of data mining not only possible but essential. Readers of this book will learn about concepts, technologies, and practices involved in text and data mining that support biomedical knowledge management. The stated audience is IT and biomedical students and professionals; the book or selected chapters could serve as a text for a course that covers the topic. The authors and editors are recognized leaders in the field. The book is divided into three units: "Foundational Topics in Medical Informatics," "Information and Knowledge Management," and "Text Mining and Data Mining." Each chapter begins with an overview and ends with questions for discussion. Of special interest to all informatics students and professionals is the chapter "Mapping Medical Informatics Research," which applies domain visualization techniques to the literature to identify important topics and researchers. Other examples and case studies illustrating concepts and techniques abound. For some informatics texts, this can limit a book's usefulness over time; that is not the case here. It will be some time before the content is outdated due to the comprehensive nature of the text and the fact that many of the projects described represent research that is in development or of proven value. This text will most likely be a key resource about this topic for some time to come.

Medical Informatics: Practical Guide for Healthcare and Information Technology Professionals. 4th ed. Editor: Robert E. Hoyt. Lulu.com, 2010.
http://www.lulu.com/
ISBN: 9780557608089
Recommended for: Hospital, Academic Libraries

This introductory text is available in paperback and also as a PDF downloadable file compatible with several e-book readers. The book is neither a technical nor theoretical treatment of the topic, but rather an attempt to explore current issues and applications. The fact that a new edition has been published each year attests to the commitment to updating the content. In this most recent edition, the chapter on electronic health records includes information about recent legislation and "hot" topics, such as meaningful use. Chapter titles range from "Online Medical Resources" to "Consumer Health Informatics" to "Picture Archiving" and "Communication Systems." Most chapters are fewer than 20 pages but each has many examples, references, and links to websites.

Unfortunately, older editions will not be that useful. This book would be a good text for a survey course in health sciences informatics or as a quick, current reference to important issues in the field.

Public Health Informatics and Information Systems. Editors: Patrick W. O'Carroll, William A. Yasnoff, M. Elizabeth Ward, Laura H. Ripp, Ernest L. Martin. Springer, 2003.
http://www.springerlink.com/content/978-0-387-95474-5/
http://www.ebrary.com/
http://extranet.netlibrary.com/TitleSelect/
ISBN: 9780387954745
ISBN: 9780387227450
Recommended for: Academic Libraries

When it was first published in 2003, this book met an important need for those teaching informatics courses to public health students and professionals. In 2010, there have been advances that should be covered in a new edition, but, lacking one, the original publication still serves as a solid overview of the field when supplemented by recent articles and websites. The editors and contributors are acknowledged experts in the various topics covered, including the core competencies for practitioners and the content, context, evaluation, and issues characteristic of public health information systems. The text has numerous examples, as well as nine case studies describing systems at the community, state, national, and international level. The book is well organized and clearly written. Chapters follow a set template of learning objectives, overview, introduction, and questions for review, which contributes to standardizing what could otherwise be a chaotic mix of writing styles.

Shared Decision Making in the Patient-Physician Relationship: Challenges Facing Patients, Physicians, and Medical Institutions. Author: Dennis J. Mazur. American College of Physician Executives, 2001.
See Chapter 30.2. Medical Decision Making

Journals

BMC Medical Informatics and Decision Making. v. 1, BioMed Central, 2001.
http://www.biomedcentral.com/bmcmedinformdecismak/
ISSN: 14726947 (Online)
Indexed in: MEDLINE
Recommended for: Hospital, Academic Libraries

This electronic-only, open access journal publishes peer-reviewed research on "the design, development, implementation, use, and evaluation of health information technologies and decision-making within the healthcare setting." Articles span the multiple topics of informatics—from models to web-based tools for consumers, to physician attitudes toward e-prescribing, and to data mining and risk. Supplements contain conference proceedings, meeting abstracts, or thematic reviews. The website is easy to navigate and has special features such as tags for highly accessed articles and article alerts for registered users. Both the scope and editorial board are international. There is also an impressive list of statistical advisers, suggesting rigor in the review process. All health sciences libraries would benefit from linking to this publication.

CIN: Computers, Informatics, Nursing. v. 20, Lippincott Williams & Wilkins, 2002.
http://www.cinjournal.com
http://www.ovid.com/site/catalog/Journal/566.jsp
ISSN: 15382931
ISSN: 15389774 (Online)
Indexed in: MEDLINE, CINAHL
Recommended for: Hospital Libraries
Brandon/Hill Selection

CIN: Computers, Informatics, Nursing, which was formerly known as Computers in Nursing, is a bimonthly publication about informatics, research, and technology from a nursing perspective. A stated goal is to provide "a forum for communication among nurses who use computers," which is now a quite inclusive audience. Each issue provides a mix of research and practical information about the use of technology. Peer-reviewed articles span topics such as electronic health records, social networks, and computerized support for patient education. Each issue also includes news, a calendar, and a continuing education activity. Since 2005, *CIN* has collaborated with the Alliance for Nursing Informatics (ANI) to publicize news, events, and other activities of the various nursing informatics organizations. Members of ANI organizations include the American Nursing Informatics Association (ANIA), the American Medical Informatics Association (AMIA), the Healthcare Information and Management Systems Society (HIMSS), and various regional and state nursing informatics organizations. *CIN* is the only specifically nursing informatics journal indexed by MEDLINE. It is also the only one that appears in the top twenty medical informatics journals according to the 2009 *Journal Citation Reports*, making it the obvious selection choice for libraries with nursing clientele.

Healthcare Informatics. v. 7, Vendome Group, 1990.
http://www.healthcare-informatics.com
ISSN: 10509135

ISSN: 19381441 (Online)
Indexed in: MEDLINE, CINAHL
Recommended for: Hospital, Academic Libraries

Healthcare Informatics is a longstanding trade magazine covering news and technology in the health care industry and is written for health care executives. The printed magazine is free to "qualified individuals involved in healthcare technology." The website is searchable and free. Issues include news, product information, advice, case studies, editorials, and articles. The publication has been indexed in MEDLINE since its first publication in 1984 under the title *Healthcare Computing and Communications*, establishing it as a key resource for administrators and other people interested in the business of the field.

Informatics for Health & Social Care. v. 33, Informa Healthcare, 2008.
http://www.informaworld.com/smpp/title~content=t713736879
ISSN: 17538157
ISSN: 17538165 (Online)
Indexed in: MEDLINE, CINAHL
Recommended for: Academic Libraries

Published since 1976 under various titles, *Informatics for Health & Social Care* "promotes evidence-based informatics as applied to the domain of health and social care." The use of personal information is its central focus. There are no restrictions on the type of health information discussed, and articles about research and practice are welcome, as are experiences related to implementation. A sample of recent article titles include: "Comprehension of Internet-based numeric cancer information by older adults" (Canada); "A web-based survey on students' conceptions of *accident*" (Brazil); and "The role of quality tools in assessing reliability of the Internet for health information" (U.K.). There are public health and social value of information aspects to this journal that are not as apparent in many other informatics titles. As such, it should find authors and readers among public health, information, and education professionals.

International Journal of Medical Informatics. v. 44, Elsevier Ireland Ltd., 1997.
http://www.elsevier.com/locate/ijmedinf
http://www.sciencedirect.com/science/journal/13865056
ISSN: 13865056
ISSN: 18728243 (Online)
See Also Chapter 9.13. Telemedicine
Indexed in: MEDLINE
Recommended for: Academic Libraries

The *International Journal of Medical Informatics* is the official journal of the European Federation of Medical Informatics (EFMI) and one of the official journals of the International Medical Informatics Association (IMIA). The journal is published monthly and continues the *International Journal of Bio-medical Computing*. A goal of the journal is to provide "an international medium for dissemination of original results and interpretative reviews concerning the field of medical informatics." The scope is broad and covers information systems, computer-aided medical decision support systems, and computer-based educational programs pertaining to medicine, with emphasis on the evaluation of systems, including "the organizational, economic, social, clinical impact, ethical and cost-benefit aspects of IT applications in health care." A review of the top cited and most downloaded articles illustrates the international and evaluative characteristics of the publication. Popular article titles include: "Health information systems—past, present, future" (Germany); "Adopting electronic medical records in primary care: Lessons learned from health information systems implementation experience in seven countries" (Canada); "Help seeking behavior and the Internet: A national survey" (United States); and "A review of content-based image retrieval systems in medical applications—Clinical benefits and future directions" (Switzerland). Those working in computing applied to the medical and life sciences will find this journal of value, and those interested in the field will get a high-quality sampling of the field's major trends.

International Journal of Technology Assessment in Health Care. v. 1, Cambridge University Press, 1985.
http://journals.cambridge.org/action/displayJournal?jid=THC
ISSN: 02664623
ISSN: 14716348 (Online)
Indexed in: MEDLINE
Recommended for: Hospital, Academic Libraries

This quarterly journal is the official journal of Health Technology Assessment International, a society for the promotion of health technology. It ranks in the top ten medical informatics journals according to the 2009 *Journal Citation Reports*. The journal differs from many of the others in this category because its goal is to report the implications of health technology and technology's impact on the organization and management of health care systems and public health. The intended audience is health policy makers and professionals. A review of current journal issues indicates a strong international presence, which some may appreciate as a way to learn from others and some may consider as information from contexts too different from the United States to be useful.

Journal of the American Medical Informatics Association: JAMIA. v. 1, AMIA and BMJ Group, 1994.
http://www.jamia.org/
http://jamia.bmj.com/
http://www.ncbi.nlm.nih.gov/pmc/
ISSN: 10675027
ISSN: 1527974X (Online)
See Also Chapter 6.2. Medical Records
Recommended for: Hospital, Academic Libraries
Indexed in: MEDLINE, CINAHL
Brandon/Hill Selection

Journal of the American Medical Informatics Association: JAMIA is a bimonthly journal that publishes peer-reviewed articles about medical informatics in patient care, teaching, research, and health care administration. The intended audience is physicians, informaticians, scientists, nurses, and other health care professionals. Individual issues include position papers, original investigations, and articles related to the practice of informatics. The journal ranks first among 23 medical informatics journals according to the 2009 *Journal Citation Reports* and is indexed in MEDLINE, Embase, CINAHL, Web of Science, and Current Contents. Subscribers to the paper version receive access to the online journal. Free full text for all but the most recent six months is available through PubMed Central. Non-AMIA members and nonsubscribers can purchase short-term access to an article or the entire journal. Anyone can subscribe to RSS feeds of current, recent, preprints, most frequently read, and most frequently cited articles. On the easy-to-navigate *JAMIA* website, one can search for specific articles or browse by sections such as "Consumer Health," "Neuroinformatics," "Simulation," and "Computerized Provider Order Entry." Starting in 2010, *JAMIA* is copublished by AMIA and the BMJ Group, which may affect some of the access characteristics mentioned above, but it will most likely not affect the purpose or quality of this publication.

Journal of Biomedical Informatics. v. 34, Academic Press/Elsevier, 2001.
http://www.sciencedirect.com/science/journal/15320464
ISSN: 15320464
ISSN: 15320480 (Online)
Indexed in: MEDLINE
Recommended for: Academic Libraries

The *Journal of Biomedical Informatics*, which continues *Computers and Biomedical Research*, is a scholarly research publication about information processing management and knowledge-based methodologies rather than applications. The editorial intent is to publish the scientific basis of the field, which is not limited to bioinformatics but includes the broad spectrum of informatics research, clinical application, and education. The focus is on methodologies that might be generalizable. Article titles will typically use terms such as "approach," "ontologies," "taxonomies," "methods," "analysis," "prediction," and "classification." The journal is published six times a year, is widely indexed, and should be included in libraries that serve informatics research clientele.

Journal of Medical Internet Research. v. 1, Gunther Eysenbach, Centre for Global eHealth Innovation, University Health Network,Toronto, 1999.
http://www.jmir.org/
http://www.ncbi.nlm.nih.gov/pmc/journals/224/
ISSN: 14394456
ISSN: 14388871 (Online)
See Also Chapter 9.13. Telemedicine, Chapter 33.2. Health Communications
Indexed in: MEDLINE
Recommended for: Hospital, Academic, Consumer Health Libraries

Considered a pioneer in open access publication, the *Journal of Medical Internet Research* (*JMIR*) is ranked second among 23 medical informatics journals, according to the 2009 *Journal Citation Reports*. The term "Internet" in the title is misleading as the journal publishes articles on "the development, evaluation, and application of... e-technologies in the health care setting." A goal of the journal is "to stimulate research and debate around e-health applications." Articles are welcomed from behavioral science, library science, social sciences, and other fields. Health care consumers, administrators, policy makers, members of the e-health business community, health professionals, and informatics researchers will find items of interest. *JMRI* is indexed in eighteen databases including MEDLINE, CINAHL Plus, Embase, and LISA. Articles are submitted online, peer-reviewed within ten days, and posted as soon as they are available. HTML versions of articles are free; one can purchase PDF versions. Individual and institutional paid memberships are available. Individual issues can include editorials, original papers, tutorials, and reviews, including systematic reviews. Theme issues focus on one of a variety of topics and have included e-health ethics and online cancer services. The journal also features an RSS feed. This high-quality, international, and interdisciplinary journal belongs on the virtual shelf of all health sciences libraries.

Methods of Information in Medicine. v. 1, Schattauer, 1962.
http://Methods-Online.com
ISSN: 00261270 (Print/Online)
Indexed in: MEDLINE
Recommended for: Academic Libraries

Published six times per year, *Methods of Information in Medicine* is an official journal of the International Medical Informatics Association (IMIA) and of the European Federation for Medical Informatics (EFMI). The journal differs from the majority of health informatics journals in its emphasis on publishing "original research on basic methodology in health care from an information-processing perspective." Topics covered include: health information systems, biomedical data, signal, and image interpretation; data analysis and statistical studies; expert systems and knowledge representation; and simulation and modeling. International leaders in informatics serve as editors and members of the editorial board; the journal also has a student editorial board. Starting in 2006, the *Yearbook of Medical Informatics* appears as a supplement of *Methods of Information in Medicine*, providing an overview of recent developments, comprehensive introductory reviews, and notable informatics articles published during the year. Its long-standing presence (since 1962) and focus on processing data, information, and knowledge in medicine and health care—rather than on technology—make *Methods of Information in Medicine* a core journal for researchers and students in information science and informatics.

7. Hospital Administration

Management of the internal organization of the hospital.
—MeSH

Contributor: Diana Culbertson

Monographs

AHA Guide to the Health Care Field. Author: American Hospital Association. Health Forum, Annual.
ISBN: 9780872588493
See Also Chapter 34.5. Directories and Biographical Sources
Recommended for: Hospital, Academic, Consumer Health Libraries
Brandon/Hill Selection

The *AHA Guide to the Health Care Field* has long been a widely used directory of hospitals in the United States. Hospitals are listed geographically by state and city. For each hospital listing, information is provided on address, phone, name of the CEO and other senior executives, county location, accreditations and approvals, health system affiliation, staffed beds, admissions, census, outpatient visits, births, total expenses, payroll expenses, total full-time equivalent personnel, website, Medicare ID number, ownership type, and primary service type. The AHA currently tracks 142 special services and facilities a hospital may offer, and each of these services/facilities reported by an individual hospital is noted. Some hospitals may not report complete data, resulting in occasional data gaps for some hospitals. Hospital information in the book is based on the American Hospital Association's (AHA) own annual survey sent to all U.S. hospitals, regardless of AHA membership. A separate section of the *Guide* alphabetically lists multi-hospital systems headquarters and affiliated hospital addresses, phones, websites, and CEO. An indication of the size, ownership, and classification level of integration of each system is provided. Separate listings of networks and of alliances also include contact information for the organizational headquarters and each affiliated hospital. Finally, the last section of the book provides addresses and phone numbers for other types of health care organizations, including state hospital associations, state licensure agencies, quality improvement organizations, regional health information organizations, state planning agencies, and more. A CD version of the book may also be purchased separately or with the book. The CD is in a PDF format with some limited search options. Data from the CD cannot be exported or resorted.

AHA Hospital Statistics. Author: American Hospital Association. Health Forum, Annual.
ISBN: 9780872588523
See Also Chapter 34.4. Statistics
Recommended for: Hospital, Academic Libraries
Brandon/Hill Selection

This annual publication from the American Hospital Association provides a statistical overview of the U.S. hospital sector, including national historical trend data since 1946 on the number of hospitals, hospital beds, utilization volume, employed personnel, and expenses. Separate tables provide similar data for the past five years for nine geographic regions, each state and the District of Columbia, and for eight hospital bed size categories. Current year data only is available at the metropolitan level. Another table indicates the number and percentage of hospitals that reported offering each of 142 services, covering services such as neonatal intensive care, robotic surgery, chiropractic care, heart transplants, trauma care, optical colonoscopy, indigent care clinic, oncology care, and many more. In additional to the statistical tables, an introduction provides commentary on general trends in hospitals and health care. Included with each book purchase is a separate 17" × 22" wall map of the United States with quick statistics on hospitals overlaid on each state. The data are based on AHA's own annual survey sent to all U.S. hospitals. The book is available for purchase with or without a CD-ROM that includes the tables from the book in an Excel format. For the national, regional, and state tables, the CD includes additional years of data not in the book, dating back 15 rather than five years. This resource is a useful overview of the hospital sector not just for those working in it, but also for those that market to hospitals.

Almanac of Hospital Financial and Operating Indicators. Ingenix, Annual.
ISBN: 9781601511898
Recommended for: Hospital, Academic Libraries

Benchmarks for 147 hospital financial and operating performance measures are published annually in this report available in either a print or CD format. About half of the benchmarks included are based on Medicare Cost Report analyses, while the other half are from audited hospital financial statements or other strategic operating data directly submitted by hospitals. Ingenix has audited financial statements available from about 3,500 hospitals, which it claims is the largest U.S. repository available. The financial benchmarks address profitability, liquidity, capital structure, asset efficiency, payer mix, price, and costs. Volume, length of stay, intensity of service, and efficiency measures are included with the operating benchmarks. A paragraph summarizing key trends and providing a very brief forecast introduces the data presented for each benchmark. Five-year trend data is presented for hospitals grouped by revenue range, bed size, urban/rural, teaching/non-teaching, system/non-system, geographic region and state, and control (government, non-profit, for-profit). The benchmarking figures are further classified for critical access, psychiatric, rehabilitation, and pediatric facilities. Additional data segmentation is presented for hospitals falling into upper and lower quartiles based on case mix index, wage index, operating margin, and quality scores. This is a handy resource for administrators and researchers concerned with strategic and financial performance of the hospital as a whole. It does not provide data at the unit/department level or for individual hospitals. The Almanac is similar in scope to *The Comparative Performance of U.S. Hospitals: Sourcebook* published by Thomson Reuters annually. Each publication has some benchmarks not available in the other. The 2009 edition of the Almanac includes data through fiscal year 2007. New editions are released in December.

Comparative Performance of U.S. Hospitals: Sourcebook.
Thomson Healthcare, Annual.
ISBN: 9781573723848
Recommended for: Hospital, Academic Libraries

This annual compilation of financial and operating benchmarks for hospitals will be of special interest to hospital administrators and researchers concerned with comparative costs and efficiencies, particularly if the hospital is not participating in an electronic benchmarking service. The performance indicators cover measures related to hospital capacity and utilization; patient and payer mix; capital structure; financial liquidity; revenues, expenses, and profitability; productivity and efficiency; and pricing strategies. In addition to national indicators for all hospitals, the data are further segmented by hospital subsets, including bed size range, urban vs. rural, teaching vs. non-teaching, system-affiliated vs. independent, high vs. low case-mix complexity, high vs. low managed care, ownership type (government, not-for-profit, and investor-owned), geographic location (by Census Division and state), and for rural referral centers, sole community providers, and disproportionate share hospitals. The benchmarks are not provided at unit or departmental levels or for individual hospitals. Five-year trends in median and quartiles for each benchmark are provided, with the 2009 edition covering benchmarks through fiscal year 2007. A brief trend overview and graph precedes each table of the roughly 70 performance indicators. The benchmarks are based primarily on analyses of Medicare cost reports that each hospital participating in the Medicare program must file with the federal government. This *Sourcebook* is similar in scope to the *Almanac of Hospital Financial and Operating Indicators*, published annually by Ingenix. While there is overlapping coverage, each report has some performance measures not provided by the other. The 2010 edition was released in December 2010. The publication is available in print, in a PDF format, on CD, or as an ASCII data file.

Health Care Administration: Managing Organized Delivery Systems. 5th ed. Editor: Lawrence F. Wolper. Jones & Bartlett, 2011.
ISBN: 9780763757915
Recommended for: Hospital, Academic Libraries
Brandon/Hill Selection

This classic health administration text addresses the broader aspects of the health delivery system and then focuses particularly on the hospital within the health system. A wide range of contributors were involved in writing this book. In looking at the health delivery system, the U.S. system is compared internationally in the initial chapter. Legal implications of business arrangements, stakeholder management, financial management, human resources, nursing services, planning and developing facilities, financing, marketing, information systems, ambulatory care, managed care, ethics, and bioterrorism preparedness are covered in separate chapters about the health system. Turning to hospitals in particular, the chapter authors look at the history of hospitals, their organization and management, patient access services, laboratories, pharmacy, material and resource management, legal and regulatory compliance programs, quality assurance and improvement, and physician practices. This review refers to the fourth edition.

Health Care Information Systems: A Practical Approach for Health Care Management. 2nd ed. Authors: Karen A. Wager, Frances W. Lee, John P. Glaser. Jossey-Bass, 2009. *See* Chapter 6.3. Informatics

Journals

HFM. v. 36, Healthcare Financial Management Association, 1982.
http://www.hfma.org/hfm/
ISSN: 07350732
Indexed in: MEDLINE, CINAHL
Recommended for: Hospital, Academic Libraries

HFM is a monthly periodical focused on a health care topics that could impact the financial bottom-line of healthcare organizations. Its key audiences are administrators and researchers. Recent articles have covered improving patient flow with a support service call center, the legal aspects of hospital-physician relationships, and improving patient safety and quality of care with information technology. *HFM* is indexed in MEDLINE and available full text in DataStar, Dialog, EBSCOhost, FirstSearch, LexisNexis, ProQuest, Westlaw, and WilsonWeb databases. Members of the Healthcare Financial Management Association have member access on the HFMA website, sometimes with supplemental web extras not included in the print issues.

Hospitals & Health Networks. v. 67, Health Forum/ American Hospital Association, 1993.
http://www.hhnmag.com
ISSN: 10688838
Indexed in: MEDLINE, CINAHL
Recommended for: Hospital, Academic Libraries
Brandon/Hill Selection

Currently published monthly by the American Hospital Association, this periodical focuses on issues of concern to hospital leaders. Recent articles have covered clinical effectiveness, patient satisfaction, construction, the green environmental movement, privacy, quality improvement, community benefit, and other administrative topics. While not peer-reviewed or refereed, it is indexed in MEDLINE as a core journal. Full-text articles are available from 1994 on the publication's website. The website also includes some online-only exclusive articles not included in the print version. *Hospitals & Health Networks* is currently available full text in a number of EBSCOhost, ProQuest, and FirstSearch databases.

Journal of Healthcare Management. v. 43, Foundation of the American College of Healthcare Executives, 1998.
http://www.ache.org/pubs/jhmsub.cfm
ISSN: 10969012
Indexed in: MEDLINE, CINAHL
Recommended for: Hospital, Academic Libraries
Brandon/Hill Selection

Published six times a year, this is the official journal of the American College of Healthcare Executives. Each issue includes an interview with a healthcare executive and other articles focused on timely topics of interest to administrators. Recent articles have addressed physician relations, reporting community benefit, financial improvement, the impact of nurse staffing ratio mandates, and information technology implementation in a rural hospital. The journal is indexed in MEDLINE and full-text is available in DataStar, Dialog, EBSCOhost, FirstSearch, Lexis/Nexis, Ovid, ProQuest, and Westlaw databases.

Modern Healthcare. v. 1, Crain Communications, 1974.
http://www.modernhealthcare.com
ISSN: 01607480
ISSN: 19447647 (Online)
Indexed in: MEDLINE, CINAHL
Recommended for: Hospital, Academic Libraries

Modern Healthcare is a weekly magazine focused on news about health care business. In addition to current news stories, it regularly publishes popular articles ranking the largest health systems, executive search firms, foundations, associations, finance companies, law firms, management consulting companies, fraud settlements, insurers, medical groups, pharmaceutical manufacturers, medical schools, and more in the health care sector. Online access is available, and many of the special surveys, rankings, and data reports can be purchased separately online in a variety of formats. *Modern Healthcare* is indexed in MEDLINE and is currently available full text in EBSCOhost, ProQuest, Dialog, and DataStar databases.

8. Medical Illustration

Illustrative clarification of biomedical concepts, as in the use of diagrams and drawings. The illustration may be produced by hand, photography, computer, or other electronic or mechanical methods.

—MeSH

Contributor: Frank Ritchel Ames

Monographs

The Guild Handbook of Scientific Illustration. 2nd ed. Editor: Elaine R.S. Hodges. Wiley, 2003.
ISBN: 9780471360117
Recommended for: Hospital, Academic Libraries

Though only one chapter of *The Guild Handbook of Scientific Illustration* is devoted to medical illustration (pp. 484–498), the breadth and relevance of the information and examples make the volume an essential resource for medical illustrators and libraries. The volume serves as a textbook that offers the novice a comprehensive introduction to the purposes, techniques, objects, processes, and business of illustration (as outlined in the table of contents) and as a reference work that quickens the understanding of the expert (who can mine the excellent index). The handbook—a massive 624 pages with over 620 illustrations—answers the question, "What are the essential elements in the production of a scientific illustration?" (p. 1), and the answer is full, nuanced, and reflects the collective wisdom of the Guild of Natural Science Illustrators, which sponsored the work. Less expensive and intimidating are Phyllis Wood's enduring textbook, *Scientific Illustration: A Guide to Biological, Zoological, and Medical Rendering Techniques, Design, Printing, and Display* (2nd ed., 1994, ISBN: 9780471285250), Mike de la Flor's *The Digital Biomedical Illustration Handbook* (2004, ISBN: 9781584503378), with its digital orientation and useful tutorials, and Frances W. Zweifel's *A Handbook of Biological Illustration* (1988, ISBN: 9780226997001), which best serves the needs of the non-professional.

Journals

Journal of Biocommunication. v. 1, The Journal of Biocommunication, Inc, 1974.
www.jbiocommunication.org/
ISSN: 00942499
ISSN: 19364563 (Online)
Indexed in: MEDLINE
Recommended for: Academic Libraries

This affordable multimedia journal offers scholarly, peer-reviewed articles that describe, evaluate, and foster effective visual communication in the fields of biology and medicine. Featured articles treat technical, historical, analytical, and professional aspects of illustration, photography, animation, and graphic design in established and emerging media of all types, and columns offer news, retrospectives, reviews, and commentary. The journal's first goal is to "serve as an exemplary showcase of biocommunication techniques," and it does this well. Publication is managed by representatives of the Association of Biomedical Communications Directors, Association of Medical Illustrators, Australian Institute of Medical and Biological Illustration, BioCommunications Association, and, until 2008, the Health Sciences Communication Association. The publication is essential reading in the profession, and a subscription is recommended for libraries that support hospital-based photography units, college-based illustration courses, and well-rounded health sciences collections. The journal supercedes *Medical Art*, formerly the *Association of Medical Illustrators Journal*, and since 2000, has incorporated the *Journal of Biological Photography*, which was published from 1932 to 1979 as the *Journal of the Biological Photographic Association*. The BioCommunications Association maintains a cumulative index for years 1932 to 1997 and offers years 1974 to 2001 on CD-ROM. Three volumes are published each year, and the journal is indexed in MEDLINE, Current Index in Journals in Education, and Hospital Literature Index.

Journal of Visual Communication in Medicine. v. 28, Informa Healthcare, 2005.
http://http://informahealthcare.com/jau
ISSN: 17453054
ISSN: 17453062 (Online)
Indexed in: MEDLINE
Recommended for: Hospital, Academic Libraries

This useful but not inexpensive quarterly publication explores the development and use of images and other audiovisuals to record and communicate medical information. Contributions are scholarly, peer-reviewed and span historical, technical, and professional topics. Issues typically include an event calendar, editorial, papers and articles, reports and announcements, book and technology reviews, and a retrospective piece from twenty-five years in the past. The publication, which serves as the official journal of the Institute of Medical Illustrators, is intentionally interdisciplinary in scope and international in perspective, though scope and perspective are largely shaped by professionals from the United Kingdom. This does not lessen the value of the work. The journal is essential reading for professionals in the field and for libraries supporting educational programs in medical illustration; and a subscription is recommended for libraries supporting illustration and photography units in hospitals and health sciences libraries seeking to develop or maintain comprehensive, robust collections. Published from 1978 to 2004 as the *Journal of Audiovisual Media in Medicine*, the journal is indexed in MEDLINE, Cambridge Scientific Abstracts, Contents Pages in Education, Educational Technology Abstracts, and Library Information Science Abstracts, with full text available online from EBSCO, informaworld, and other providers.

9. Medicine

9.1. Adolescent Medicine

Diagnosis and treatment of diseases occurring during the period beginning with puberty until the cessation of somatic growth.

—MeSH

Contributor: Carol L. Watwood

Monographs

Adolescent Health Care: A Practical Guide. 5th ed.
Editors: Lawrence S. Neinstein, Catherine M. Gordon, Debra K. Katzman, David S. Rosen, Elizabeth R. Woods. Lippincott Williams & Wilkins, 2008.
http://www.ovid.com/
http://www.r2library.com/
ISBN: 9780781792561
Recommended for: Hospital, Academic Libraries
Doody's Core Titles Selection

Now in its fifth edition, Dr. Lawrence Neinstein's *Adolescent Health Care: A Practical Guide* is a high quality, in-depth discussion and reference guide for adolescent health care, intended, according to its foreword, for "physicians, nurses, faculty members . . . and other health practitioners" in "private practice and public health settings." Dr. Neinstein and his four coeditors have assembled a distinguished panel of contributors, mostly U.S. academic physicians, many with public health credentials. Some contributors are Canadian, and some have mental health, law, or other backgrounds. Although this book is targeted to a professional audience, it is accessible to educated laypeople. This volume's academic flavor and in-depth subject coverage make it especially appropriate for libraries and examination review. This title is available electronically from R2 Library and OvidSP, but the long table of contents and detailed entries are easier to use in print. A condensed, portable version, *Handbook of Adolescent Health Care* (2009, ISBN 9780781790208), is also available. Physical growth and development during adolescence is covered extensively, as are key adolescent issues such as sleep disorders, body image, gender identity, back pain, and reproductive health. Coverage of college health and public health issues, such as teen pregnancy and youth violence, is particularly strong; effective use of U.S. government data such as "Monitoring the Future" provides a solid scientific basis for discussions of substance abuse and similar topics. Females are the principal authors of chapters dealing with pregnancy, contraception, and other topics especially pertinent to girls. An experienced attorney wrote the chapter on legal aspects of care. Coverage of psychological and mental health issues has been expanded but is not encyclopedic; for example, self-injury behaviors are not described in detail. An outstanding feature of this book is the extensive list of websites, references and additional reading following each chapter, and two appendixes listing reference materials on adolescence, resources and services for adolescents, online discussion lists, hotlines, adolescent health services, how to find counseling, health portals, and websites. Dr. Neinstein has also developed an online, adolescent curriculum with cases and review questions, which is freely available at http://www.usc.edu/student-affairs/Health_Center/adolhealth/. *Adolescent Health Care* received a four-star, general medicine rating by *Doody's Core Titles*. This one-volume, scholarly textbook on adolescent medicine is recommended for health professionals, academic libraries, college health services, and clinical libraries. Readers preferring a more concise adolescent medicine text might also consider the widely used works by Victor C. Strasburger (*Adolescent Medicine: A Handbook for Primary Care*, 2006, ISBN 97807817531 59), Gail Slap (*Adolescent Medicine*, 2008, ISBN 97803 23040730), or Donald Greydanus (*Essential Adolescent Medicine*, 2006, ISBN 9780071438438).

Adolescent Health Services: Missing Opportunities.
Editors: Robert S. Lawrence, Jennifer Appleton Gootman, Leslie J. Sim. National Academies Press, 2009.
http://extranet.netlibrary.com/TitleSelect/
ISBN: 9780309114677
ISBN: 9780309114684 (Online)
Recommended for: Hospital, Academic Libraries

In understanding adolescent medicine, a broad grasp of adolescent health and public policy is essential; *Adolescent Health Services* examines this issue with a wide lens. This title reviews the health status of 42 million U.S.

adolescents aged 10 to 19 and the health providers who treat them, both in private offices and in "safety net" settings such as hospitals, schools, community health centers, and local health departments. This study began in 2006 when the (U.S.) National Academies' Board on Children, Youth, and Families created the Committee on Adolescent Health Care Services and Models of Care for Treatment, Prevention, and Healthy Development to study adolescent health. The committee chair and principal editor of this report, Robert S. Lawrence, MD, was chosen to head a multidisciplinary panel including representatives from nursing, law, psychiatry, pediatrics (including the subspecialty of adolescent medicine), dentistry, social work, health insurers, public policy research, and government agencies. The committee found that most U.S. adolescents are thriving, but many engage in habits and behaviors that have serious consequences immediately and throughout adult life. Certain groups of adolescents are especially vulnerable, including the poor (many of whom are members of racial or ethnic minorities); recent immigrants; lesbian, bisexual, gay, and transgender (LBGT) teens; those in the juvenile justice system; and runaways. Health services for adolescents can include a variety of potentially successful models and health professionals in many disciplines who can participate in treating adolescent patients. Currently available adolescent health services and providers are fragmented, poorly coordinated, and not ideally suited to the behavioral and developmental needs of adolescents. Health care services are too often problem-oriented, focusing on specific, acute conditions, rather than broader prevention, health promotion, or behavioral issues of adolescence. An absence of insurance and health professionals' lack of knowledge and skills in dealing with adolescent patients also hamper adolescent health services. Committee recommendations include greater coordination of primary health services for adolescents among federal and state government agencies, private foundations, and private insurers; paying more attention to the needs of vulnerable populations; and making disease prevention, health promotion, and behavioral health services a major part of routine health care. Overall, *Adolescent Health Services* gives a balanced, detailed picture of the key stakeholders and issues in U.S. adolescent medicine and health. Statistical tables and charts, several appendixes, and a detailed index are included. This book is highly recommended for academic and clinical collections with an emphasis on adolescent health.

Adolescent Health Sourcebook. 2nd ed. Editor: Joyce Brennfleck Shannon. Omnigraphics, 2007.

ISBN: 9780780809437

Recommended for: Hospital, Academic, Consumer Health Libraries

Adolescent Health Sourcebook, part of Omnigraphics' popular *Health Reference Series*, is a consumer health publication on adolescent health and development, wellness, diseases, injuries, mental health, and substance abuse. The advisory board for the *Health Reference Series* is composed of librarians, with the assistance of a medical consultant. Many of Omnigraphics' books are available online; however, at this writing, the *Adolescent Health Sourcebook* is offered in print format only. The target audience includes parents, teens, and other laypeople. Information is mostly gleaned from secondary sources, including U.S. government agencies, nonprofit health organizations, and consumer health websites. The sources used, such as http://www.kidshealth.org, are widely regarded as reputable and were generally less than five years old when the *Sourcebook* was published. A third edition of the *Adolescent Health Sourcebook* (ISBN 9780780811409) is in preparation, but was not yet available for review. The reading level in this volume varies according to the source material; it is mostly suited for older teens, college students, and adults. Information is divided into ten parts organized around general themes and divided into chapters; for example, part 1, "Adolescent Growth and Development Overview," includes a chapter on parenting teens, a chapter on normal adolescent growth and development, medical care of 13- to 18-year-olds, and other topics. Statistics, references, and sources of additional information are given. A glossary, list of organizations and websites, and an index appear in the back of the volume. This volume is valuable as a guide pointing older teens and adults to reliable sources of consumer health information. Like other books in the *Health Reference Series*, this book is quite useful in getting novice researchers started in the sometimes overwhelming literature of the health sciences for high school and undergraduate term papers, speeches, and presentations. This sturdy, red-and-white volume has a rather plain appearance and scattered black-and-white charts and illustrations of average quality. Although this volume uses previously published material, it is an up-to-date, versatile compilation drawn from reliable sources. The *Adolescent Health Sourcebook* is recommended for public, community college, and undergraduate libraries, in addition to consumer health collections.

Bright Futures: Guidelines for Health Supervision of Infants, Children, and Adolescents. 3rd. ed. Editors: Joseph F. Hagan Jr., Judith S. Shaw, Paula M. Duncan.

American Academy of Pediatrics, 2008.
http://www.ebrary.com/
ISBN: 9781581102239
ISBN: 9781581105186 (Online)
Recommended for: Hospital, Academic Libraries

Developed as part of the "Bright Futures" initiative begun by the U.S. Health Resources and Services Administration's Maternal and Child Health Bureau in 1990, *Bright Futures* is a set of health promotion "principles, strategies, and tools" for all levels of society from the family to the policy level. A physician and a nurse co-chair the steering committee; this committee, along with an advisory committee, represents a variety of stakeholders. Although much of the material pertains to younger children, adolescents ages 11 to 21 are also discussed in detail. Health promotion is organized around ten themes drawn partly from *Healthy People 2010*, emphasizing strengths (rather than problems), family, and community support. Each of these ten themes is discussed in detail; information on mental and oral health, which is often segregated from other health services by separate insurance/managed care agreements, is integrated with other health services. Each age group is then discussed in detail with regard to general observations, priorities for visits to health professionals, history, observation, surveillance, physical examination, screening, and immunizations. Charts and a detailed index follow the text. A 62-page section on "Adolescence" may be downloaded free of charge at http://brightfutures.aap.org/3rd_Edition_Guidelines_and_Pocket_Guide.html. Some of the material in the "Adolescence" section has a pediatric orientation that may be unrealistic for adolescents; for example, adolescents may not go for annual check-ups, have insurance, or have suitable providers. Additionally, many parents do not accompany their teens to the examining room. Although some material in *Bright Futures* is geared toward younger children, it is nevertheless a key publication for adolescents as well, representing a paradigm shift from the problem-based approach to a strengths-based emphasis on health promotion. In 1997, the American Medical Association issued a similar document, *Guidelines for Adolescent Preventive Services* (*GAPS*), available at http://www.ama-assn.org/. This book is recommended for collections serving child and adolescent health professionals.

***Cancer in Adolescents and Young Adults*.** Editors: W. Archie Bleyer, Ronald D. Barr. Springer, 2007.
http://www.springerlink.com/content/g75uu3/
http://www.ebrary.com/
http://extranet.netlibrary.com/TitleSelect/
ISBN: 9783540408420
ISBN: 9783540681526 (Online)
Recommended for: Hospital, Academic Libraries

Cancer is the most common, non-accidental cause of death in U.S. adolescents, but few books have been written about cancer in this age group. A volume in the monographic series *Pediatric Oncology*, this book, which received a five-star review from *Doody's*, is intended to be a comprehensive treatise on cancer in adolescents and young adults (15–29 years old when diagnosed). Dr. W. Archie Bleyer and Dr. Ronald Barr, aided by an international team of coeditors and contributors, reviewed all aspects of adolescent/young adult cancer, including an overall review of occurrence, diagnosis, and general aspects/types of treatment; history of adolescent oncology; general remarks on epidemiology and etiology of cancer in this age group; access to care; participation in clinical trials; detailed discussions of specific cancer types; models of care and special needs of this age group; psychosocial aspects; aftercare; late effects of treatment; ethical issues, end-of-life care, and personal narratives; financial aspects; consumer information resources; and future and global trends. Color figures, tables, and text boxes enhance the text. This book is recommended for graduate, postgraduate, and clinical libraries supporting students and practitioners in medicine, nursing, and other health and social services fields interacting with adolescent/young adult cancer patients; it is also pertinent to public health and health services.

***A Doctor of Their Own: The History of Adolescent Medicine*.** Author: Heather Munro Prescott. Harvard University Press, 1998.
ISBN: 9780674214613
Recommended for: Academic Libraries

The study of adolescent medicine, or any other discipline, is enhanced by learning its history. Heather Prescott has written the first detailed history of adolescent medicine, using primary sources such as oral histories, patient records, popular literature, and letters from teens. Dr. Prescott, a medical writer, based this book on her 1992 dissertation, *A Doctor of Their Own: The Emergence of Adolescent Medicine as a Clinical Sub-Specialty, 1904–1980*. Beginning with G. Stanley Hall's *Adolescence* in 1904, the notion of adolescence as a field of scientific research gained momentum throughout the twentieth century. Adolescent medicine became a separate discipline in the mid-twentieth century and still struggles to define itself, as did its parent discipline, pediatrics, earlier in the century. Dr. Prescott relates the development of adolescent medicine to American social history and to the pioneering work of Dr. J. Roswell Gallagher who, in 1951, established the first successful adolescent health center in the United States, the Adolescent Unit at Boston Children's Hospital, which he ran until 1967. Dr. Gallagher was an early proponent, perhaps the father, of adolescent medicine. Dr. Prescott researched records at Boston Children's Hospital, the Society of Adolescent Health and Medicine in Cincinnati, and other sources. Adolescent medicine was recognized as a board-certified subspecialty of pediatrics in 1991, but it has struggled to attract physicians and even survive. Dr. Prescott describes some of the issues in this struggle, including the low degree of "functional autonomy." Without any technology, diseases, or procedures to set it apart from other specialties, adolescent medicine faces a number of challenges. As a group, teens are healthy by traditional measures; teen health problems often result from psychosocial issues for which treatments are low technology, time-consuming, and poorly reimbursed by insurers, leading to the perception that adolescent medicine is a low-status specialty. A second edition of this work updating Dr. Prescott's research to the present would be a welcome addition. *A Doctor of Their Own* is recommended for academic libraries supporting graduate and postgraduate adolescent health and medicine programs, and for medical history collections.

Handbook of Adolescent Behavioral Problems: Evidence-Based Approaches to Prevention and Treatment. Editors: Thomas P. Gullota, Gerald R. Adams. Springer, 2005.
http://www.springerlink.com/content/978-0-387-23845-6
ISBN: 9780387238456
ISBN: 9780387238463 (Online)
Recommended for: Hospital, Academic Libraries
Doody's Core Titles Selection

Listed in *Doody's Core Titles* for psychiatric nursing, the *Handbook of Adolescent Behavioral Problems* offers a multidisciplinary "biopsychosocial approach" to adolescent behavioral problems. The principal editor, Thomas P. Gullotta, has published extensively on adolescents and on primary prevention. Most contributors are psychologists or psychiatrists, but a few are from public health, academia, or other fields. The book opens with a general introduction to adolescent development, primary prevention, family and community influences, treatment approaches and principles, and evidence-based practices. The second section deals with obesity, anxiety, eating disorders, and other common adolescent issues. The third section discusses problem behaviors such as delinquency, substance abuse, and school failure. Each topic includes an introduction; detailed discussion; family and community factors; psychopharmacology; evidence-based treatments that work, might work, and don't work; recommendations; and references. An epilogue and index end the volume. The book is nicely printed and attractively bound, with no pictures and a few tables. It is clearly targeted to psychologists, but it is also quite relevant to other professionals who work closely with adolescents. This book is one of several, good compilations of evidence-based treatments for adolescents that target psychologists and psychiatrists with relevance to other disciplines. Readers might also consider similar works by John R. Weisz, Ric G. Steele, and Craig Winston LeCroy. This book is recommended for clinical and academic collections dealing with adolescent psychology.

Lewis's Child and Adolescent Psychiatry: A Comprehensive Textbook. 4th ed. Editors: Andrés Martin, Fred R. Volkmar. Lippincott Williams & Wilkins, 2007.
See Chapter 9.10.2. Child and Adolescent Psychiatry

Pediatric & Adolescent Gynecology. 5th ed. Editors: S. Jean Emans, Marc R. Laufer, Donald P. Goldstein. Lippincott Williams & Wilkins, 2005.
http://www.ovid.com/
ISBN: 9780781744935
See Also Chapter 11.2. Gynecology
Recommended for: Hospital, Academic Libraries
Doody's Core Titles Selection

This clinically oriented text, available in print and online formats, is listed in *Doody's Core Titles* pediatrics specialty category. Office evaluation of children and adolescents is described in detail; numerous helpful pictures and diagrams illustrate procedures. Reproductive health services are also discussed, addressing one of the most common reasons adolescent girls aged 15–19 visit health providers. Common and uncommon gynecological conditions, puberty, breast examination, and anatomic variations are described. Surgery, sexually transmitted diseases, legal issues, sexual abuse, contraception, and teenage pregnancy are also discussed. Several useful appendixes include information on sexuality, informed consent and instructions for oral contraceptives, a sexual abuse protocol, and other useful information. This book is recommended for academic and clinical collections serving students, health professionals, or researchers having an interest in pediatric and adolescent obstetrics and gynecology.

Journals

Adolescent Medicine: State of the Art Reviews. v. 18, American Academy of Pediatrics, 2007.

http://ebooks.aap.org/product/am-stars-adolescent-medicine
ISSN: 19344287
See Also Chapter 11.2. Gynecology
Indexed in: MEDLINE, CINAHL
Recommended for: Hospital, Academic Libraries

Adolescent Medicine: State of the Art Reviews (*AM: STARs*) is a monographic series published three times a year by the American Academy of Pediatrics. *AM: STARs* was previously called *Adolescent Medicine Clinics* (2004–2006) and *Adolescent Medicine* (1990–2003). It is indexed in MEDLINE and CINAHL. Each issue has a separate theme that focuses on a key area of clinical practice. Individual issues may be purchased separately in print or e-book formats; additionally, the series can be purchased as a subscription. Some reviews are quite lengthy; volume 20, number 2, for example, contains an entire work called *Handbook of Adolescent Medicine*, 2nd ed. (ISBN 781581103342). Unfortunately, this title is not widely held, although the series deals with useful topics such as adolescent diabetes and asthma. *AM: STARs* is recommended for large pediatric collections; libraries and health practitioners not subscribing to the series may wish to purchase individual volumes.

Archives of Pediatrics & Adolescent Medicine. v. 148, American Medical Association, 1994.
http://archpedi.ama-assn.org/
ISSN: 10724710
ISSN: 15383628 (Online)
See Also Chapter 10.13. Pediatrics
Indexed in: MEDLINE, CINAHL
Recommended for: Hospital, Academic Libraries
Brandon/Hill Selection

Archives of Pediatrics & Adolescent Medicine, an international, peer-reviewed journal published monthly by the American Medical Association, is the oldest, continuously published pediatrics journal in the United States. Previous titles of this publication were *American Journal of Diseases of Children* (1911–1950, 1960–1993); *A.M.A. American Journal of Diseases of Children* (1950–1955); and *A.M.A. Journal of Diseases of Children* (1956–1960). This title is indexed in MEDLINE, BIOSIS, most of the major medical and health databases, and many other sources. The latest issue is posted the first Monday of each month on the *JAMA & Archives* website, http://pubs .ama-assn.org/. This website has many special features, such as job information, topics collections, and online, evidence-based medicine resources. Like many other pediatrics journals, *Archives* includes content on adolescents as well as younger children. The *Archives*' description states that it "is a vehicle for increased attention to adolescent health." Indeed, it seems to focus more on adolescents than do many other pediatrics titles. Types of articles accepted include original studies, editorials, expert reviews, practice commentaries, case quizzes, and updates on clinical science and practice management; readers may express their views in the Pediatric Forum. The *Archives* is one of the most influential pediatrics journals with a 2009 impact factor of 4.726 (*Journal Citation Reports*), and it appeared on the last Brandon/Hill list. *Archives of Pediatrics & Adolescent Medicine* is recommended for academic medical center libraries and for libraries supporting graduate- or postgraduate-level education, research, and practice in child and adolescent health.

Journal of Adolescent Health. v. 12, Elsevier for Society for Adolescent Health and Medicine, 1991.
http://www.sciencedirect.com/science/journal/1054139X
http://www.jahonline.org/
ISSN: 1054139X (Print/Online)
See Also Chapter 13.18. School Nursing
Indexed in: MEDLINE, CINAHL
Recommended for: Academic Libraries

Journal of Adolescent Health (*JAH*), formerly called *Journal of Adolescent Health Care* (1980–1990) and *Society for Adolescent Medicine Newsletter* (1965–1979), is the leading interdisciplinary research journal entirely devoted to adolescent health and medicine. It is the official journal of the preeminent U.S. professional organization in adolescent health and medicine, Society for Adolescent Health and Medicine (SAHM), which is a U.S.-based national and international "multi-disciplinary organization of health professionals who are committed to advancing the health and well-being of adolescents." Elsevier publishes this monthly journal, which is available online on the publisher's website for SAHM members and through ScienceDirect for other individual and institutional subscribers. Its impact factor in 2009 was 3.325, and it was ranked sixth out of 94 journals in pediatrics and seventeenth out of 122 journals in public health (*Journal Citation Reports*). *JAH* was listed as an essential core title in maternal/child health, public health practice, and health education/behavioral science in Yale's Core Public Health Journals—Version 2.0 (http://publichealth.yale.edu/phlibrary/phjournals/v2/). *JAH* is indexed by MEDLINE, Gale's Academic OneFile, and many other indexing/abstracting services. *JAH*, according to its website, is a "multidisciplinary scientific journal, which seeks to publish new research findings in the field of adolescent medicine and health ranging from the basic biological and behavioral sciences to public health and policy." It encompasses "anthropology, dentistry and oral health, education, health services research, international health, law, medicine, mental health, nursing, nutrition, psychology, public health and policy, social work, sociology, youth development, and other disciplines that work with or are committed to improving the lives of adolescents and young adults." In addition to original manuscripts, *JAH* accepts review articles, letters to the editor, commentaries, and case reports. The distinguished editorial board includes leading writers, teachers, and researchers in adolescent medicine; they are primarily U.S. academics but also include international researchers and representatives of hospitals and organizations such as WHO, AHRQ, and PAHO. The subject coverage of *JAH* articles is diverse with a strong emphasis on public health, prevention, education, and psychosocial issues, as evidenced by the topics of the most frequently downloaded *JAH* articles: sleep, abstinence, bullying, pregnancy prevention, sex education, exercise, mental health, and ADHD. *JAH* is highly recommended for research-oriented collections in adolescent medicine, college health, public health, advanced nursing practice, or other adolescent health fields.

Journal of American College Health. v. 30, Taylor & Francis with American College Health Association, 1982.
http://www.tandf.co.uk/journals/titles/07448481.asp
http://www.ebscohost.com/
ISSN: 07448481
ISSN: 19403208 (Online)
See Also Chapter 33. Health Education
Indexed in: MEDLINE, CINAHL
Recommended for: Academic Libraries

Journal of American College Health (*JACH*) is a refereed, bimonthly journal published in cooperation with the American College Health Association (ACHA). Content includes "clinical and preventive medicine, health promotion, environmental health and safety, nursing assessment, interventions, management, pharmacy, and sports medicine." Online access to *JACH* is free to ACHA members; print or online subscriptions are available from Taylor & Francis. The journal was previously called *Journal of the American College Health Association* (1962 to 1982) and *Student Medicine* (1952 to 1962). Various types of articles are accepted, including original research, reviews, program descriptions, brief reports, viewpoints, book reviews, and letters to the editor. The editorial board comprises academics, mostly non-MDs, from diverse fields such as public health, social work, and nursing from various types of U.S. colleges and universities. The board reviews many or most of the journal's articles. The primary target audience of *JACH* is college health professionals such as physicians, nurses, health educators, and administrators. This journal is also quite useful for students needing scholarly articles for research papers on health-related topics. The content is readable and covers topics of wide interest to college students such as body image, underage drinking, and sexual decision making. *JACH* is indexed in MEDLINE, and both indexing and online full text are widely available through EBSCOhost, WilsonWeb, and other indexing and abstracting services. Because of its readability, wide availability, and versatility, *Journal of American College Health* is recommended for students, faculty, and staff in all types of college and university settings.

Journal of Pediatric and Adolescent Gynecology. v. 9, Elsevier for North American Society for Pediatric and Adolescent Gynecology, 1996.
http://www.jpagonline.org/
http://www.sciencedirect.com/science/journal/10833188
http://www.mdconsult.com/
ISSN: 10833188 (Print/Online)
See Also Chapter 11.2. Gynecology
Indexed in: MEDLINE
Recommended for: Academic Libraries

The *Journal of Pediatric and Adolescent Gynecology* is the official journal of the North American Society for Pediatric and Adolescent Gynecology. This peer-reviewed publication, previously published by Springer as *Adolescent and Pediatric Gynecology* (1988 to 1995), produces six issues a year. The subject scope includes clinical, basic science, and molecular biology research in pediatric and adolescent gynecology. Types of articles published include "original studies, review articles, book and literature reviews, letters to the editor, and communications in brief." Indexed in: MEDLINE, this journal recently received a "debut" ISI impact factor of 0.859 and was ranked fifty-fifth out of 70 obstetrics and gynecology journals (*Journal Citation Reports*, 2009). This journal publishes a mix of basic science, clinical, and interdisciplinary articles, such as those related to public health, behavioral sciences, and public policy. A review of the most frequently cited/downloaded articles suggests that the basic science articles may be used less often. *Journal of Pediatric and Adolescent Gynecology* is recommended for academic and research collections dealing with adolescent gynecology.

Journal of Youth and Adolescence: A Multidisciplinary Research Publication. v. 1, Springer, 1972.

http://www.springerlink.com/content/104945/
ISSN: 00472891
ISSN: 15736601 (Online)
Indexed in: MEDLINE
Recommended for: Academic Libraries

The *Journal of Youth and Adolescence* is a peer-reviewed, multidisciplinary journal for "psychologists, psychiatrists, biologists, criminologists, educators, and professionals in many other allied disciplines who address the subject of youth and adolescence." It is widely indexed in sources such as MEDLINE, PsycINFO, and various Gale, EBSCOhost, and ProQuest databases. In 2009, *Journal Citation Reports* listed this journal's impact factor as 1.383. Types of articles include original research articles, reviews, theoretical articles, and book reviews. This title emphasizes research having policy or social implications. Many articles address health-related behaviors such as dieting and tobacco and alcohol use. This journal is recommended for college and university libraries, especially those serving graduate and postgraduate programs.

Databases and Other Electronic Resources

Teen Health & Wellness: Real Life, Real Answers. Rosen Publishing Online, 2007.
http://www.teenhealthandwellness.com
Recommended for: Academic, Consumer Health Libraries

Teen Health & Wellness is a subscription-based database for teens produced by Rosen Publishing, which also publishes print materials on health and wellness. Experts review articles, some written by teens. This database has won several awards and recognitions, including *Library Journal's* Best Reference Source and *School Library Journal's* Top 10 Digital Resource. It is a unique, niche product with an attractive, colorful look and feel and clean, well-designed screens. Suitable for educational use, the content follows state and national curriculum standards. Medium length articles discuss all aspects of teen health and well-being. Medical news and social issues are connected to relevant articles. Resource lists include websites, organizations, and further reading. The database features first person narratives by teens and information about 24-hour hotlines. Interactive polls and quizzes add interest. Articles include citations in MLA format and names of authors, reviewers, and dates. New features include a mobile application, video, social bookmarking, and instant translator. Teen Health & Wellness is appropriate for high school and college libraries and for consumer health collections serving teens.

9.2. Andrology

Male reproductive biology, diseases of the male genital organs, and male infertility.

—MeSH

Contributor: David C. Stewart

Monographs

Andrology for the Clinician. 1st ed. Editors: Wolf-Bernhard Schill, F.H. Comhaire, Timothy B. Hargreave. Springer, 2006.
http://www.springerlink.com/content/978-3-540-23171-4
ISBN: 9783540231714
Recommended for: Hospital, Academic Libraries

The editors of this book state that their aim is to provide condensed, systematically organized information for clinicians to aid them when they need to manage a patient with andrological concerns. *Andrology for the Clinician* is divided into two parts. Part 1, "Diagnosing and Solving Clinical Problems" presents information by defining the disease and then, in turn, discussing its etiology, taking a physical history and examination, differential diagnosis, treatment, prognosis, complications, and other considerations. Subjects presented in part 1 include disorders of sexual differentiation, abnormal pubertal development, abnormal spermatozoa, varicocele, and sexual dysfunction. Other chapters deal with testicular trauma, penile fractures, and priapism. Testicular and penile cancers as well as male breast disorders are also discussed. Part 2, "Rationale" focuses on mechanisms of dysfunction and pathology, diagnostic tools, morphological analyses, genetics, and therapeutic approaches. This textbook would be a useful addition to an academic medical library's collection. *Andrology for the Clinician* is a recommended title from the International Society of Andrology (ISA).

Andrology: Male Reproductive Health and Dysfunction. 3rd ed. Editors: Eberhard Nieschlag, Hermann M. Behre, Susan Nieschlag. Springer, 2010.
http://www.springerlink.com/content/978-3-540-78354-1
ISBN: 9783540783541
ISBN: 9783540783558 (Online)
Recommended for: Hospital, Academic Libraries

Now in its third edition, *Andrology: Male Reproductive Health and Dysfunction* continues to be one of the leading textbooks on male reproduction. The second edition received four stars from *Doody's*; the reviewer praised the book for its lack of repetition among chapters and its consistency of style among its authors, along with its superb illustrations. The second edition is also a recommended title from the International Society of Andrology (ISA). The book is intended for andrologists, endocrinologists, urologists, gynecologists, pediatricians, and internists, as well as researchers in the basic sciences. In addition to chapters on sperm maturation and fertilization, and infertility, additional chapters discuss areas not always covered in other textbooks such as environmental influences, psychology and sexual medicine, and ethics. *Andrology: Male Reproductive Health and Dysfunction* is recommended for all medical libraries.

Infertility in the Male. 4th ed. Editors: Larry I. Lipshultz, Stuart S. Howards, Craig S. Niederberger. Cambridge University Press, 2009.
ISBN: 9780521872898
Recommended for: Hospital, Academic Libraries
Doody's Core Titles Selection

Infertility in the Male has established itself as one of the essential textbooks in the field of andrology. Forty-one chapters lay out the development of the male reproductive tract, the mechanisms involved in fertilization, causes of infertility, surgical and non-surgical treatments for infertility, psychological aspects, legal aspects, sperm banking, DNA measurement, and future directions for andrology. The textbook's chapters' authors are drawn from institutions in Europe, the Middle East, and North and South America. Students planning to enter the field of andrology will find this book useful while residents and researchers will find it a helpful reference tool. Many illustrations, including two pages of color plates, help to illuminate the text's findings.

Men's Health. 3rd ed. Editors: Roger S. Kirby, Culley C. Carson III, Michael G. Kirby, Alan White. Informa Healthcare, 2009.
http://informahealthcare.com/
ISBN: 9780415447331
ISBN: 9786611964061 (Online)
Recommended for: Hospital, Academic, Consumer Health Libraries

This title is recommended by the International Society of Andrology (ISA). While many of its authors are British, *Men's Health's* information will prove useful to American readers as well. Although written for the clinician, *Men's Health* can be read by the layperson, too. It is intended as a reference source for all health care professionals who treat men. The third edition has been reorganized into disease and problem-based sections. Infertility has its own chapter. Other chapters that provide information not found commonly in other textbooks include diet, fat and cancer of the prostate, men as risk takers, men and suicide, and osteoporosis in men. *Men's Health* is recommended for hospital and all other medical libraries.

A Practical Guide to Basic Laboratory Andrology. 1st ed. Editors: Lars Björndahl, David Mortimer, Christopher L.R. Barratt, Jose A. Castilla, Roelof Menkveld, Ulrik Kvist, Juan G. Alvarez, Trine B. Haugen. Cambridge University Press, 2010.
ISBN: 9780521735902
Recommended for: Hospital, Academic Libraries

A Practical Guide to Basic Laboratory Andrology presents step-by-step descriptions of the procedures followed in the analysis and assessment of male factor infertility and the preparation of spermatozoa in assisted conception therapy. Individually authored overviews on physiology, semen analysis, sperm function tests, sperm preparation, cryobanking, and ReProxTox testing (among other topics) are followed with detailed procedural instructions. A helpful feature is the information provided on quality control considerations for the procedures discussed in the text. Appendixes provide information on basic reference values, an equipment list for setting up an andrology laboratory, a home testing overview, and sample forms. Written particularly for researchers and technicians who perform diagnostic testing, this would be a useful but not essential purchase for a hospital library but should be considered for academic medical collections.

Office Andrology. 1st ed. Editors: Phillip E. Patton, David E. Battaglia. Humana Press, 2005.
http://www.springerlink.com/content/978-1-58829-318-3
ISBN: 9781592598762
ISBN: 9781592598765 (Online)
Recommended for: Academic Libraries

The editors of *Office Andrology* in their preface state, "The goal of *Office Andrology* is to provide a practical guide for those [practitioners] requiring concise answers . . . on male infertility." Part of the *Contemporary Andrology* series, this textbook contains articles on a variety of topics including endocrinology, immunology, specialized sperm testing, and male infertility genetic problems, authored by leading experts. In a review of this title published in *Andrologia* (2005 Oct., 37(5): 195), the reviewer recommended this book "to all doctors caring for patients with fertility disorders, as it covers a really broad spectrum of aspects of male infertility in a comprehensive manner, thus providing quick access to relevant questions in this field." This textbook is one of the titles in the International Society of Andrology's (ISA) virtual library and is recommended for academic health sciences libraries.

Textbook of Men's Health and Aging. 2nd ed. Editors: Bruno Lunenfeld, Louis J.G. Gooren, Alvaro Morales, John E. Morley. Informa Healthcare, 2007.
http://informahealthcare.com/
ISBN: 9780415425803
Recommended for: Hospital, Academic Libraries
Brandon/Hill Selection

Sponsored by the International Society for the Study of the Aging Male, this text addresses issues related to the health of older men in a comprehensive fashion. The editors' stated purpose is "to draw together relevant gender-specific knowledge of men's health." The book is organized into 10 overarching sections with chapters on specific topics under each heading. The first section discusses the biology of aging and gender differences. The second section covers the clinical diagnosis and assessment of age-related health issues common to males. Subsequent sections examine how aging affects body systems such as the genitourinary, endocrine, cardiovascular, respiratory, central nervous, and skeletal systems. These sections cover important topics, such as libido changes, depression, sleep disorders, and osteoporosis. Separate sections address sexual dysfunction, body composition, and nutritional problems in the older male. All chapters include an extensive bibliography. The review of *Textbook of Men's Health and Aging* in *JAMA* called it "a significant contribution to the literature of geriatric medicine" and said it provides "clinically relevant information in an accessible and well-referenced format." This book is highly recommended for all academic and hospital libraries.

Journals

Andrologia. v. 6, Wiley-Blackwell, 1974.
http://onlinelibrary.wiley.com/journal/10.1111/(ISSN)1439-0272
ISSN: 14390272 (Online)
ISSN: 03034569
Indexed in: MEDLINE
Recommended for: Academic Libraries

The first international journal in the field of andrology, *Andrologia* began publication in 1969. It features original papers on the current clinical, morphological, biochemical, and experimental status of organic infertility and sexual disorders in men. It also publishes articles that concentrate on anatomy, endocrinology, physiology, and veterinary medicine. *Andrologia* is indexed in MEDLINE, Science Citation Index, Chemical Abstracts, Biological Abstracts, and EMBase (among others). It remains a primary source for dermatologists, endocrinologists, gynecologists, oncologists, and urologists as well as for scientists conducting andrological research. All past issues are now available online.

Asian Journal of Andrology. v. 1, Nature Publishing Group, 1999.
http://www.asiaandro.com/
http://www.nature.com/aja/index.html
ISSN: 1008682X
ISSN: 17457262 (Online)
Indexed in: MEDLINE
Recommended for: Academic Libraries

The *Asian Journal of Andrology* (*AJA*) is the official journal of the Asian Society of Andrology and is sponsored by the Shanghai Institute of Materia Medica, Chinese Academy of Sciences. It is published in English and conforms to the NIH mandate for deposit of NIH-funded research articles into PubMed Central. The AJA's peer-reviewed articles focus on new findings in basic and clinical research in the field of andrology with special emphasis on regulation of spermatogenesis, gene expression in accessory sex organs and external genitalia, feedback regulation of gonadotropins, sperm capacitation, anatomical studies of the reproductive tract, prostate diseases, and physiology of penile erectile tissue. *AJA* is indexed in MEDLINE, Biological Abstracts, Science Citation Index, Scopus, and other databases.

International Journal of Andrology. v. 1, Scriptor, 1978.
http://onlinelibrary.wiley.com/journal/10.1111/(ISSN)1365-2605
ISSN: 01056263
ISSN: 13652605 (Online)
Indexed in: MEDLINE
Recommended for: Academic Libraries

International Journal of Andrology is the official publication of the European Academy of Andrology. Its aims are to promote and integrate basic and clinical research in the field of andrology and to publish the latest ideas. *International Journal of Andrology* is peer-reviewed and publishes papers on all aspects of andrology, including anabolic steroids, androgens, endocrinology, fertility, genital tract, hormones, infertility, reproductive medicine, sexual dysfunction, and urogenital medicine. Its targeted audience includes scientists and clinicians. The journal is indexed in a variety of databases including MEDLINE, Biological Abstracts, and Science Citation

Index. Full online coverage goes back to volume 1 and is available through Wiley Online Library. *International Journal of Andrology* is highly recommended for academic health sciences libraries.

Journal of Andrology. v. 1, J.B. Lippincott, 1980.
http://www.andrologyjournal.org/
ISSN: 01963635
ISSN: 19394640 (Online)
Indexed in: MEDLINE
Recommended for: Academic Libraries

The American Society of Andrology (ASA) began publishing the *Journal of Andrology* in 1980 for the purpose of highlighting new findings of basic and clinical researchers doing work in this field. The journal is peer-reviewed and supports the NIH open access publishing policy by depositing a copy of every article into PubMed Central. Special interest areas are hormonal regulation of spermatogenesis, gene expression in accessory sex organs and external genitalia, feedback repletion of gonadotropins, sperm capacitation, anatomical studies of the reproductive tract, noncancer prostate diseases, and physiology of penile erectile tissue. The journal's audience includes urologists, endocrinologists, physiologists, fertility specialists, and scientists, biochemists, and gynecologists. The journal is indexed in MEDLINE. Full online coverage back to volume 1, number 1, 1980 is available.

9.3. Bariatric Medicine

Weight reduction in patients with obesity.
—MeSH

Contributor: Robin Sabo

Monographs

Encyclopedia of Obesity. Editor: Kathleen Keller. Sage Publications, 2008.
http://www.sage-ereference.com/
ISBN: 9781412952385
ISBN: 9781412963862 (Online)
Recommended for: Academic, Consumer Health Libraries

This two-volume, 1040 page encyclopedia from Sage is available electronically and was recommended by *Library Journal* (May 15, 2008) for both academic and public libraries. This work has 475 entries including information on hormonal control, pharmaceutical treatments, relevant organizations, and ethnic variations and disparities. According to the introduction, this reference work is intended for scholars, educators, researchers, physicians, and the general public. The "Reader's Guide" section of this book assists in finding articles by topic. Many black and white as well as color photographs are included. The editor states that this book is intended as a general, non-technical reference. As such, this book is more accessible to the lay reader than many medical volumes and is appropriate for larger consumer health collections and community college libraries. In addition, academic libraries supporting four-year universities will find this title useful.

The End of Overeating: Taking Control of the Insatiable American Appetite. Author: David A. Kessler. Rodale, 2009.
ISBN: 9781605297859
Recommended for: Hospital, Academic, Consumer Health Libraries

This is an excellent, thought-provoking book of interest to health care and public health professionals, food policymakers, and consumers looking for help in learning to control their weight. The author, former Commissioner of the U.S. Food and Drug Administration, discusses how the food industry has contributed to the worldwide obesity epidemic. Development of hyper-palatable high fat, high sugar foods coupled with an ubiquitous food supply has led to "conditioned hyper-eating." Explanations of how changed behavioral responses can break this cycle and strategies for dealing with high risk situations are helpful. A review in *Booklist* (2009 Mar 15:34) states Kessler "offers some simple, practical tools to help control one's impulses." At the end of the book, Dr. Kessler relates his own personal struggles with battling his weight. A former *New York Times* best seller for hard cover non-fiction, this book is recommended for consumer health collections, academic libraries and hospital libraries in institutions with weight management programs.

Handbook of Obesity Prevention: A Resource for Health Professionals. Editors: Shiriki Kinika Kumanyika, Ross C. Brownson. Springer, 2007.
http://www.springerlink.com/content/978-0-387-47859-3
http://site.ebrary.com/
http://www.r2ibrary.com/
http://extranet.netlibrary.com/TitleSelect/
ISBN: 9780387478593
ISBN: 9780387478609 (Online)
Recommended for: Hospital, Academic Libraries
Doody's Core Titles Selection

Appearing in the *Doody's* core title list for health sciences—nutrition, this book is recommended for public health students and professionals. The book is divided into four sections: "Overview and Background," "Understanding the Landscape," "Crafting Solutions" on both an institutional and an individual/family level, and "Conclusion." Chapters are authored by leaders in the field including Kelly Brownell, Rena Wing, and Brian Wansink. Editors Kumanyika and Brownson introduce the book with the first chapter, "Why Obesity Prevention?" This chapter discusses the obesity epidemic and the resulting public health impact. This book is recommended in *JAMA* (2008 Jun 18:2797) as "an excellent and useful volume surveying the public health perspective on obesity." At more than 500 pages, this book is comprehensive and is described as a sourcebook, overview, reference, and teaching text. It is recommended for academic libraries. In addition, hospital libraries supporting weight management programs and medical education will find this book helpful.

Obesity Epidemiology. Editor: Frank B. Hu. Oxford University, 2008.
ISBN: 9780195312911
See Also Chapter 9.7. Epidemiology
Recommended for: Academic Libraries

From Harvard Medical School, the editor also authored many of the chapters in this book. It is the first book to focus specifically on the epidemiology of obesity. Written as a textbook for graduate students, the book is also intended for clinicians and researchers in human nutrition, exercise science, and public health. The book is divided into three sections: "Student Design and Measurements," "Epidemiologic Studies of Consequences of Obesity," and "Epidemiologic Studies of Determinants of Obesity." Medical and surgical treatments for obesity are not covered. This work contains extensive lists of references and a number of tables that summarize the literature in this field. A book review from the *American Journal of Epidemiology* (2009:1277) recommends this book, describing it as an excellent reference volume. University libraries with health sciences graduate programs and large academic medical center libraries will find this to be an important resource.

Obesity in Youth: Causes, Consequences, and Cures. Editors: Leslie J. Heinberg, J. Kevin Thompson. American Psychological Association, 2009.
ISBN: 9781433804274
Recommended for: Hospital, Academic Libraries

Published by the American Psychological Association, this book is highly recommended by *Choice Reviews* (August 2009) for graduate students, researchers, and professionals. The book is edited by a professor of medicine, Heinberg, and a professor of psychology, Thompson. In addition to the editors, 22 experts from leading medical schools and universities contributed to this book. Focusing on the psychological aspects of obesity in youth, the editors point out that the book was written specifically for mental health professionals, but that others working in pediatric obesity, should also find this book to be relevant. The book is organized into three major sections: "Obesity Risk," "Psychological Effects," and "Assessment, Intervention, and Prevention." Lengthy lists of references complete each of the 10 chapters. This book is suggested for libraries in hospitals with pediatric weight management programs and for academic libraries with nutrition, public health, medical, and psychology programs.

Obesity Prevention and Public Health. Editors: David Crawford, Robert W. Jeffery. Oxford University, 2005.
http://www.ovid.com/
ISBN: 9780198566007
Recommended for: Hospital, Academic Libraries
Doody's Core Titles Selection

Appearing as an essential title in the health sciences – public health category of *Doody's Core Titles*, this book provides public health professionals with a "state of the science overview of the epidemiology of the world-wide obesity epidemic and the case for prevention" (p. xi). The book is divided into three sections: "Context," "Strategies for Prevention at a Population Level," and "Novel Approaches for Prevention of Obesity." Edited by an Australian and an American, this book brings an international perspective to bear on this growing problem. Chapters include "Nutrition Transition in the Developing World" and "Food Regulation as a Policy Instrument for Preventing Obesity in Developing Countries." This book will be a useful purchase for academic libraries with health sciences curricula and for large hospital libraries.

Journals

Appetite. v. 1, Elsevier, 1980.
http://www.sciencedirect.com/science/journal/01956663
ISSN: 01956663
ISSN: 10958304 (Online)
Indexed in: MEDLINE
Recommended for: Hospital, Academic Libraries

The target audience for this bimonthly, peer-reviewed journal includes academics and researchers in neuroscience, physiology, and nutrition. *Journal Citation Reports* 2009 ranks this journal 24 out of 66 in the nutrition and dietetics category with an impact factor of 2.582. The article, "Mapping the Literature of Dietetics" also recommends this journal as a core title (Smith AM, *Bull Med Libr Assoc* 1999 Jul; 87(3):292–297). The scope of the subject matter in this journal is behavioral nutrition and the impact of cultural, sensory, and physiological influences on dietary intake. In addition to basic and applied research studies, the journal includes short communications, review articles, special issues, abstracts from international multidisciplinary conferences, and a calendar of events. This journal is indexed and abstracted in major databases including Biological Abstracts, MEDLINE and PsycINFO. Full-text online coverage is available through Elsevier ScienceDirect. University libraries with graduate health professions and psychology programs will find this journal helpful. This title is also recommended for large hospital libraries supporting nutrition researchers or clinicians specializing in obesity and other eating disorders.

International Journal of Eating Disorders. v. 1, Wiley, 1981.
http://onlinelibrary.wiley.com/journal/10.1002/(ISSN)1098-108X
ISSN: 02763478
ISSN: 1098108X (Online)
Indexed in: MEDLINE, CINAHL
Recommended for: Hospital, Academic Libraries

The official journal of the Academy of Eating Disorders, this peer-reviewed journal has an impact of factor of 2.797 (*Journal Citation Reports*, 2009). The journal ranks 19 out of 66 in the nutrition and dietetics category, 45 of 117 in psychiatry and 23 of 71 in psychology. *Magazines for Libraries* (2009 Jan. 12) recommends this title for healthcare and mental health professionals. "Mapping the Literature of Dietetics" (Smith AM, *Bull Med Libr Assoc* 1999 Jul; 87(3):292–297) lists this as a core title. The journal publishes basic and clinical research studies dealing with obesity and other eating disorders. Other publication types include reviews, brief reports, case studies, and forums. This journal is indexed and abstracted in Biological Abstracts, CINAHL (since 1996), MEDLINE, and PsycINFO. Academic libraries with dietetics, psychology, medicine, and related health professions programs will find this helpful. This title is also recommended for large hospital libraries and other hospital libraries with weight management and mental health programs.

International Journal of Obesity. v. 29, Nature, 2005.
http://www.nature.com/ijo/index.html
ISSN: 03070565
ISSN: 14765497
Indexed in: MEDLINE
Recommended for: Hospital, Academic Libraries

The *International Journal of Obesity* is a multidisciplinary, international journal publishing basic clinical and applied research in biochemistry, physiology, genetics, and nutrition, and molecular, metabolic, psychological, and epidemiological aspects of obesity and related disorders. One of three official journals of the International Association for the Study of Obesity, this journal has an impact fact of 4.343 (*Journal Citation Reports*, 2009), ranking fourth of 66 journals in the nutrition and dietetics category and 23 of 105 in the endocrinology and metabolism category. This journal is also listed as a core journal in "Mapping the Literature of Dietetics" (Smith AM, *Bull Med Libr Assoc* 1999 Jul; 87(3):292–297). BIOSIS, Chemical Abstracts, CINAHL Plus, and Embase are some of the major databases providing citations and abstracts to this journal. Over 68,000 people receive electronic mailings for the table of contents, and weekly online articles are published ahead of print publication. Online content may also include additional materials such as video. This journal is recommended for academic libraries with medical schools and dietetics programs and for large teaching hospitals.

Obesity. v. 14, Nature, 2006.
http://www.nature.com/oby/
ISSN: 19307381
ISSN: 1930739X
Indexed in: MEDLINE
Recommended for: Hospital, Academic Libraries

Formerly called *Obesity Research*, this is the official journal of The Obesity Society. The audience for this journal includes nutrition researchers, endocrinologists, internists, psychiatrists, pediatricians, bariatric surgeons, family practice physicians, and dietitians. This peer-reviewed journal publishes original basic and applied research articles, reviews and commentaries. Periodic supplements are also published. Areas of coverage include clinical nutrition, medicine, pharmacology, genetics, epidemiology and exercise physiology. The impact factor for this journal is 3.366 (*Journal Citation Reports*, 2009), and the journal is ranked 13 out of 66 journals in the nutrition and dietetics category and 39 of 105 in endocrinology and metabolism. The journal is indexed in major databases including Chemical Abstracts, MEDLINE and PsycINFO. University libraries with medical, dietetics, and other health professions programs and large hospital libraries will find this journal useful.

9.4. Behavioral Medicine

The development and integration of behavioral and biomedical science, knowledge, and techniques relevant to health and illness and the application of this knowledge and these techniques to prevention, diagnosis, treatment, and rehabilitation.

—MeSH

Contributor: Tracey Minzenmayer

Monographs

A Compendium of Neuropsychological Tests: Administration, Norms, and Commentary. 3rd ed. Authors: Esther Strauss, Elizabeth M.S. Sherman, Otfried Spreen. Oxford University Press, 2006.
ISBN: 9780195159578
Recommended for: Hospital, Academic Libraries
Doody's Core Titles Selection

Mental health professionals practicing in a medical setting need at least a working knowledge of neuropsychological assessment, and this encyclopedic text provides extensive coverage of current neuropsychological tests. The first five chapters address key concepts in assessment, including basic psychometric principles, practical guidance for the interview and assessment processes, and tips for writing reports. In addition to revisions and updates throughout the book, the two chapters on psychometrics and norms in neuropsychological assessment are new to this edition. Chapters 6 through 16 contain reviews of neuropsychological tests for children and adults. Each of these chapters includes enough information for practitioners to choose an appropriate test and learn how to interpret its results. The summary for each test provides its purpose and description, pricing and ordering information, appropriate demographic groups, normative data, reliability and validity, and scoring and administration guidelines. Tables within the text summarize features of similar tests to make comparisons easier. As a current *Doody's Core Titles* selection for psychology, this book is an essential purchase for hospitals and academic institutions supporting clinicians, researchers, and students in the mental health fields or neurology.

Foundations of Health Psychology. 1st ed. Editors: Howard S. Friedman, Roxane Cohen Silver. Oxford University Press, 2007.
ISBN: 9780195139594
Recommended for: Academic Libraries

Named a 2007 *Choice* Outstanding Academic Title, this book explores the concepts upon which the field of health psychology has been built from a theoretical, conceptual, and psychological perspective. The 14 chapters of the book are organized into three sections: history and research methods, core concepts of the biopsychosocial approach to health, and applications to health promotion and effective treatment. Each chapter is an expert-written review on a particular concept, such as methodological issues in health psychology research, psychoneuroimmunology, and the relationship between aging and health. The diverse array of topics discussed is representative of the multitude of approaches and areas of study within health psychology itself. This text is highly recommended for academic institutions with training programs in health psychology or behavioral medicine. It is appropriate for students of health psychology from undergraduate to graduate level, experienced practitioners of health psychology, and researchers working in other areas who want to learn more about this relatively new field.

Handbook of Adolescent Behavioral Problems: Evidence-Based Approaches to Prevention and Treatment. Editors: Thomas P. Gullota, Gerald R. Adams. Springer, 2005.
See Chapter 9.1. Adolescent Medicine

Handbook of Health Psychology and Aging. 1st ed. Editors: Carolyn M. Aldwin, Crystal L. Park, Avron Spiro III. Guilford Press, 2007.
http://www.ebrary.com
ISBN: 9781593850579
Recommended for: Hospital, Academic Libraries

The relationships among biological, psychological, and social factors and the role they play in health and illness in older adults are thoroughly examined in this book. Twenty chapters written by experts in health psychology and gerontology are divided into sections on theory and methodology, biology, psychosocial topics, and clinical issues. The coverage includes how to promote coping and resilience in older adults; why some people are less affected by age-related stressors than others; how personality, social support, religion, and culture influence adult health; and which interventions have been shown to be effective in a medical setting. One chapter is devoted specifically to the health and psychological consequences of caregivers of older adults. Both researchers and clinicians who work with older adults and their caregivers will benefit from the theoretical and empirical research compiled in this resource. This handbook is highly recommended for hospitals that treat geriatric patients and for academic institutions that train future professionals in mental health, public health, nursing, or medicine.

Learning Cognitive-Behavior Therapy: An Illustrated Guide. 1st ed. Authors: Jesse H. Wright, Monica R. Basco, Michael E. Thase. American Psychiatric Publishing, 2006.
ISBN: 9781585621538
Recommended for: Hospital, Academic Libraries
Doody's Core Titles Selection

This practical guidebook to learning cognitive-behavior therapy (CBT) is a *Doody's Core Titles* choice. It is part of the *Core Competencies in Psychotherapy* series edited by Glen O. Gabbard and created to assist practitioners with the development of the competencies set by the Accreditation Council for Graduate Medical Education. CBT is an empirically supported psychotherapeutic technique that is widely used by mental health professionals who are interested in the mind-body connection. With step-by-step instructions, worksheets, checklists, and numerous case examples, this book is a thorough introduction to CBT for beginning students through experienced practitioners. It covers full explanations of effective behavioral techniques from basic to advanced levels, help with integrating CBT with psychopharmacological intervention, a biopsychosocial model for treatment, and many more CBT topics. An accompanying DVD demonstrates key concepts from the book through video vignettes of therapeutic interactions between a therapist and patient. This book is a highly recommended addition to the libraries of both academic institutions with training programs for mental health professionals and hospitals of all types.

Journals

Annals of Behavioral Medicine. v. 7, Springer, 1985.
http://www.sbm.org/annals/
http://www.springerlink.com/content/120893
ISSN: 08836612
ISSN: 15324796 (Online)
Indexed in: MEDLINE
Recommended for: Hospital, Academic Libraries

As the official publication of the Society of Behavioral Medicine, this peer-reviewed journal presents research on all aspects of the field, especially information on the biopsychosocial model and how it relates to health promotion, disease prevention and progression, risk factor modification, adjustment to physical disorders, and rehabilitation. Both empirical articles and integrative reviews on the application of behavioral interventions in health care are included. Researchers and clinicians in the medical, mental health, and nursing fields will find this an invaluable resource due to the coverage of both basic science and evidence-based clinical applications. The journal is highly recommended for academic institutions supporting the training of mental health professionals, rehabilitation specialists, or nurses, as well as hospitals providing behavior therapy or programs in preventive care. Various abstracting and indexing sources such as CINAHL Plus, Embase, MEDLINE, and PsycINFO cite this journal. Online coverage is available through SpringerLink starting with volume 17, 1995. Early articles are found under the title *Behavioral Medicine Update* (ISSN 07425554) beginning with volume 1, 1979 and continuing to the change to the current title with volume 7, 1985.

Behaviour Research and Therapy. v. 1, Elsevier, 1963.
http://www.sciencedirect.com/science/journal/00057967
ISSN: 00057967
ISSN: 1873622X (Online)
Indexed in: MEDLINE
Recommended for: Hospital, Academic Libraries

Practitioners, researchers, and students of behavioral medicine will find this peer-reviewed journal essential for its coverage of cognitive behavior therapy (CBT), one of the most common treatments used in their field. With an impact factor of 2.995 (2009 *Journal Citation Reports*) and content specifically geared toward both behavioral medicine and clinical psychology, this journal is beneficial to other mental health professionals such as psychologists and social workers. Articles focus primarily on mechanisms of behavior change; the role psychopathology plays in prevention and treatment; and the development, evaluation, and application of evidence-based treatments in clinical practice. Due to its emphasis on empirically supported treatments, this journal is highly recommended for hospitals that provide CBT. It is also highly recommended for academic institutions that have training programs for mental health professionals that include CBT in their curriculum. The journal is cited in Embase, MEDLINE, and PsycINFO, as well as a variety of other indexing and abstracting sources. Online coverage starting with volume 1, 1963 is available through Elsevier ScienceDirect.

British Journal of Health Psychology. v. 1, British Psychological Society, 1996.
http://www.bpsjournals.co.uk/journals/bjhp/
ISSN: 1359107X
ISSN: 20448287 (Online)

Indexed in: MEDLINE
Recommended for: Hospital, Academic Libraries

The British Psychological Society publishes this peer-reviewed journal to provide a forum for high quality research on all aspects of health psychology. It covers empirical, theoretical, and methodological research on every age group and at every level from the individual to the community. Systematic review articles on previously published research are also included. The content consists of such topics as health-related behaviors, how patients respond to illness, evaluations of clinical interventions, and prevention and management of illness. With an impact factor of 1.485 (2009 *Journal Citation Reports*), this publication is a highly recommended resource for academic institutions with training programs in behavioral medicine, psychology, and even public health. Hospitals are also highly advised to acquire this journal for its emphasis on publishing research about clinical interventions. Numerous abstracting and indexing sources cite this journal, including MEDLINE, PsycINFO, and Scopus. Both print and online formats, including backfiles, are available through several vendors.

Health Psychology. v. 1, American Psychological Association, 1982.
http://www.apa.org/journals/hea/
ISSN: 02786133
ISSN: 19307810 (Online)
Indexed in: MEDLINE, CINAHL
Recommended for: Hospital, Academic Libraries

This interdisciplinary peer-reviewed journal publishes empirical research on the relationship between behavior and physical health. Coverage includes the role of biopyschosocial factors in the development or prevention of disease; behavioral methods used to diagnose, treat, or rehabilitate people with physical disorders; and psychological or behavioral techniques to reduce the risk of disease. With an impact factor of 3.462 (2009 *Journal Citation Reports*) and its status as the official journal of the American Psychological Association's Division 38 (health psychology), this journal ranks as one of the most influential in behavioral health. It is highly recommended for hospitals that provide behavior therapy or rehabilitation, as well as academic institutions that have programs in mental health care and rehabilitation. Because the journal includes behavioral interventions from the individual to the community level, it is also recommended for institutions with a public health training program. This publication is cited in a variety of indexing and abstracting sources, including CINAHL, Embase, MEDLINE, and PsycINFO. Both print and online formats are available, including backfiles.

Journal of Behavioral Medicine. v. 1, Springer, 1978.
http://www.springerlink.com/content/0160-7715
ISSN: 01607715
ISSN: 15733521 (Online)
Indexed in: MEDLINE, CINAHL
Recommended for: Hospital, Academic Libraries

With an impact factor of 3.084 (2009 *Journal Citation Reports*), this interdisciplinary title ranks tenth out of 93 journals in clinical psychology. The scope of the journal includes all aspects of the application of the principles of behavioral medicine to the prevention, treatment and rehabilitation of physical illnesses. Coverage includes peer-reviewed articles on the effects of psychological stress and behavioral factors on physical health, sociocultural influences on health, compliance with medical treatments, the use of biofeedback for somatic disorders, and the relationship between the brain and behavior. Psychologists, physicians, epidemiologists, and public health administrators will all find topics of interest in this publication. This publication is recommended for hospitals that provide psychological, psychiatric, rehabilitative, or preventive care and for academic institutions that train future mental health, rehabilitation, or public health professionals. Various abstracting and indexing sources cite this journal, including CINAHL, Embase, MEDLINE, and PsycINFO. Online content is available through SpringerLink beginning with volume 1, 1978.

Journal of Psychosomatic Research. v. 1, Elsevier, 1956.
http://www.sciencedirect.com/science/journal/00223999
ISSN: 00223999
ISSN: 18791360 (Online)
Indexed in: MEDLINE
Recommended for: Hospital, Academic Libraries

Multidisciplinary in scope, this peer-reviewed journal focuses on the relationship between psychology and medicine, covering everything from basic biological and psychological research to treatment evaluations. Studies on children, adolescents, the elderly, and other special populations are included, and most articles deal with patients rather than healthy individuals. This publication is the official journal of the European Association for Consultation-Liaison Psychiatry and Psychosomatics and is affiliated with the International College of Psychosomatic Medicine. With an impact factor of 2.908 (2009 *Journal Citation Reports*), both physicians and mental health professionals will find this journal beneficial in their work. This title is highly recommended for hospitals of all types due to its heavy focus on patient populations and to academic institutions that train physicians, psychologists, or other health care professionals. The journal is cited in CINAHL Plus, Embase, MEDLINE, and PsycINFO, among numerous other indexing and abstracting sources. Elsevier ScienceDirect provides online coverage back to volume 1, 1956.

Psychological Medicine. v. 1, Cambridge University, 1970.
See Chapter 20. Medical Psychology

Psychophysiology: The International Journal of the Society for Psychophysiological Research. v. 1, Wiley-Blackwell, 1964.
See Chapter 20. Medical Psychology

Psychosomatic Medicine. v. 1, Lippincott Williams & Wilkins, 1939.
See Chapter 20. Medical Psychology

9.5. Clinical Medicine

Study and practice of medicine by direct examination of the patient.

—MeSH

Contributor: Julia M. Esparza

Monographs

Bates' Guide to Physical Examination and History Taking. 10th ed. Editors: Lynn S. Bickley, Peter G. Szilagyi. Wolters Kluwer/Lippincott Williams & Wilkins, 2009.
ISBN: 9780781780582
See Also Chapter 30.3 Diagnosis
Recommended for: Academic Libraries
Brandon/Hill, *Doody's Core Titles* Selection

Bates' Guide to Physical Examination and History Taking is an excellent resource on physical assessment with a focus on nursing. This textbook covers basic history taking and interviewing of patients. It then breaks down the different patient examinations by body system that should be conducted by students. The detailed illustrations and color photographs provide visual references for students who are studying examination techniques. Emphasis is paid to health promotion and patient communication, which are keys for nursing practice. The "Special Populations" section features chapters on pediatrics, pregnant women, and older individuals, and provides guidance to students who will deal with these different populations. Since this tenth edition contains more references, students who wish to continue their learning can easily find more resources to consult. The companion DVD and website provide critical, actual physical examinations that students can observe.

DeGowin's Diagnostic Examination. 9th ed. Editors: Richard F. LeBlond, Richard L. DeGowin, Donald D. Brown. McGraw-Hill, 2009.
http://www.accessmedicine.com/
http://www.statref.com/
http://www.myilibrary.com/
ISBN: 9780071478984
ISBN: 9780071605748
See Also Chapter 30.3. Diagnosis
Recommended for: Hospital, Academic Libraries
Brandon/Hill, *Doody's Core Titles* Selection

DeGowin's Diagnostic Examination is used frequently in medical schools to teach clinical medicine. The textbook is also a good resource for other clinicians learning physical evaluation and for recent graduates who are beginning their clinical practice. The book covers initial history taking, the patient interview, and preoperative evaluation. Divided into two sections, the book begins with general symptoms followed by in-depth coverage of each body system, highlighting the necessary physical tests to be done for evaluation. The chapter "Vital Signs" provides the most detailed information on these important assessments and places this book in this elite listing. Included illustrations provide visual maps for those learning evaluation and, with the ninth edition, color photographs enhance the text. "Alerts" located in each chapter highlight important physical findings that warrant more urgent evaluation or treatment. While a medical school may choose a different book for teaching purposes, academic medical libraries and those hospitals with residency programs should incorporate *DeGowin's* into their collections to provide additional learning material.

Mosby's Guide to Physical Examination. 7th ed. Authors: Henry M. Seidel, Jane W. Ball, Joyce E. Dains, John A. Flynn, Barry S. Solomon, Rosalyn W. Stewart. Mosby Elsevier, 2010.
ISBN: 9780323055703
Recommended for: Hospital, Academic Libraries
Brandon/Hill Selection

Mosby's Guide to Physical Examination is one of the most comprehensive guides to physical assessment. The book begins with history taking, followed by a detailed chapter on the cultural issues that could influence a patient interview. As students interact with an increasingly diverse patient population, cultural differences are growing in their importance. The textbook then provides a detailed explanation on everything from patient positions to the differences in sputum between infants, children, pregnant women, and older adults. The age and gender distinction show the inclusiveness of the textbook and make it a critical book for all students going into the health professions. The companion DVD is an excellent resource that allows the students to observe different physical assessments and hear differences in clinical states for the lung and the heart. *Mosby's Guide to Physical Examination* and its companion *Mosby's Physical Examination Handbook* are two books that all health sciences libraries should include in their collections.

Mosby's Physical Examination Handbook. 7th ed. Authors: Henry M. Seidel, Jane W. Ball, John A. Flynn, Barry S. Solomon, Rosalyn W. Stewart. Mosby Elsevier, 2010.
ISBN: 9780323065405
Recommended for: Hospital, Academic Libraries

Mosby's Physical Examination Handbook is the companion pocket guide to *Mosby's Guide to Physical Examination.* It may appear that this would not be useful in a library collection, but this guide is organized in a way that makes it a valuable resource for students. The book covers the same information as the *Guide* in a reduced format. One of the reasons the *Handbook* is useful is that each chapter has a section called "Pediatric Variations." This allows readers to focus quickly on how to assess the pediatric patient without having to carry another book. In addition, each chapter has a "Sample Documentation" section providing both subjective and objective examples for the body system. Finally, the "Aids in Differential Diagnosis" supplies students with a starting point on possible diagnoses so as to properly test the patient in order to provide excellent care. As a pocket guide, this is a very useful tool, but availability through an institution's website or on mobile devices in clinical settings would make this a valuable resource for students. The *Mosby's Physical Examination Handbook* and its companion *Mosby's Guide to Physical Examination* are two books that all medical schools and health sciences libraries should have on top of their purchase list.

The Patient History: Evidence-Based Approach. Editors: Lawrence M. Tierney Jr., Mark C. Henderson. McGraw-Hill Medical, 2005.
http://www.statref.com/
ISBN: 9780071402606
Recommended for: Hospital, Academic Libraries

A good clinical examination starts by taking a good patient history. *The Patient History* is an excellent resource that details questions for a student or new clinician to consider while talking to the patient. In "Basic Concepts," the authors address general techniques in gathering an adequate patient history. Symptoms such as dizziness or fatigue often bring a patient into the office. The "General Symptoms" section addresses these types of complaints and offers questions for consideration in providing appropriate care. The rest of the textbook is then divided into body systems with questions leading to adequate evaluation of the patient. The "Alarm Symptoms" identified in each chapter help identify those situations that may require urgent action. Additionally, the "Diagnostic Approach" algorithms at the end of each chapter provide a quick visual aid on how to evaluate the patient. Suggested readings provide additional learning opportunities for the new student or new clinician. This is an appropriate book for both the general academic medical library and hospital libraries serving residencies as a resource for interns.

Textbook of Physical Diagnosis: History and Examination. 6th ed. Author: Mark H. Swartz. W.B. Saunders, 2010.
ISBN: 9781416062035
Recommended for: Academic Libraries
Brandon/Hill, *Doody's Core Titles* Selection

Textbook of Physical Diagnosis is an excellent physical assessment textbook. The 6th edition covers patient interviews and specific assessment tools based on body system. It includes detailed illustrations and a large number of color photographs showing students exactly what they need to examine. Additionally, the textbook addresses the cultural issues involved when assessing and interviewing patients. One unique chapter evaluates the use of alternative or complementary medicine by patients as part of the assessment process. Another chapter presents focused patient assessment that prepares students to take the USMLE Step 2 CS (Clinical Skills) and OSCE (Objective Structured Clinical Examination) exams. The "Special Populations" section has a chapter focused on the "Acutely Ill Patient," a population not addressed separately in other textbooks. The accompanying, three-hour DVD showing actual physical assessments make this a resource that any academic medical library should include in its collection. Hospital libraries might consider this title if they have not purchased another physical assessment textbook.

9.6. Community Medicine

The total health of the individual within the home environment and in the community, and with the application of comprehensive care to the prevention and treatment of illness in the entire community.

—MeSH

Contributor: John Fullinwider

Monographs

A Community Guide to Environmental Health. Authors: Jeff Conant, Pam Fadem. Hesperian Foundation, 2008. *See* Chapter 5. Environmental Health

Evaluating Public and Community Health Programs. Author: Muriel J. Harris. Jossey-Bass/Wiley, 2010.
http://www.ebrary.com/
http://extranet.netlibrary.com/TitleSelect/
ISBN: 9780470400876
ISBN: 9780470586174 (Online)
Recommended for: Academic Libraries

One could profitably begin reading Muriel Harris's manual, *Evaluating Public and Community Health Programs* (2010), at the end. Her final chapter presents a case study of a fictional project to reduce the incidence of diabetes, the "Healthy Soon Project," to illustrate major steps in program design and evaluation: community assessment, intervention, evaluation design, data collection, analysis and interpretation of data, and report of the results. Dr. Harris has written a clear, down-to-earth account of how to evaluate community-based health interventions that will be helpful to practitioners and students whether they are working on HIV/AIDS prevention or designing a school-based program to address childhood obesity. Harris advocates a "participatory model of evaluation," in which community organizations and participants not only contribute to the design of a particular initiative but also take part in the evaluation and reporting of results. The book's twelve chapters are organized in a textbook format, including learning objectives, chapter summaries, key terms, and discussion questions/activities. It must be a pleasure to study with Dr. Harris, but she has produced a work with uses far beyond the classroom. Any citizen organization contemplating action on community health will benefit from engaging the practical ideas and methods in this book.

The Handbook of Health Behavior Change. 3rd ed. Editors: Sally A. Shumaker, Judith K. Ockene, Kristin A. Riekert. Springer, 2009.
ISBN: 9780826115454
Recommended for: Academic Libraries

A hundred years ago, the three leading causes of death were pneumonia/influenza, tuberculosis, and gastritis. Today heart disease, cancer, and stroke are the top three. As explained in the book's opening chapter, "The shift from infectious to chronic diseases as major causes of premature morbidity and mortality necessitated a shift in theories of prevention." In 1979, the surgeon general concluded that half of mortality from the 10 leading causes of death was a result of "unhealthy behavior or lifestyle." If, as the editors note, there is "a strong relationship among the onset, progression, and exacerbation of diseases and alteration of lifestyles," why don't more of us quit smoking, eat healthier foods, practice safe sex, adhere to our medication prescriptions, and exercise more? The 40 essays in Shumaker's compendium on health behavior change provide the theoretical and factual basis to answer this question. Contributors report on successful lifestyle interventions; describe reliable methods of measuring health behavior; explore the ways that income, gender, education, ethnicity, age and other population variables effect health behavior; and, in the final chapter, articulate "what we know doesn't work." The editors' principal audience may be graduate students in "public or population health, health psychology, health communications, and medical sociology and anthropology," but one hopes that more than a few policy makers will wade into this rich, fact-based volume.

Handbook of Urban Health: Populations, Methods, and Practice. Editors: Sandro Galea, David Vlahov. Springer, 2005.
http://www.springerlink.com/content/978-0-387-23994-1
ISBN: 9780387239941
ISBN: 9780387258225 (Online)
Recommended for: Hospital, Academic Libraries

Practicing community medicine inevitably involves an encounter with the living conditions of diverse populations. For physicians working in American cities—"elegant, sophisticated... dense, teeming, and dangerous places"—Sandro Galeo and David Vlahov have compiled an essential handbook. For the 26 essays collected here, the editors provide an introductory statistical and conceptual overview and "integrative chapters" to bridge the book's three sections. The opening guide to specific populations includes chapters on homeless and destitute people; racial, ethnic and sexual minorities; immigrants; members of drug subcultures; children "in crisis"; and older adults. Grounded in voluminous scholarship, these essays include strategies for improving the health of each group. The section on methods illustrates the cross-disciplinary analysis of health in cities that Galeo and Vlahov view as key to success, with contributions from anthropology, epidemiology, sociology, environmental health, and urban design. The last section on practice, "the most optimistic," describes "practical examples of interventions that have been implemented," ongoing efforts to improve urban health. While the editors stress the field's complexity, that "promoting health in cities requires an appreciation of the multiple levels of determinants that shape population health," they also recognize that "urban health practitioners have to move forward." That movement can only be enhanced by wide distribution of this comprehensive work.

Health Issues in the Black Community. 3rd ed. Editors: Ronald L. Braithwaite, Sandra E. Taylor, Henrie M. Treadwell. Jossey-Bass/Wiley, 2009.
http://www.ebrary.com/
ISBN: 9780470436790
ISBN: 9780470552650 (Online)
Recommended for: Hospital, Academic Libraries
Doody's Core Titles Selection

Health Issues in the Black Community has been for nearly two decades the go-to source on the health of African Americans. Braithwaite and colleagues have revised the book to include new sections on "alternative interventions" and "the impact of incarceration" and expanded chapters on pollution and health disparities. This new edition provides a multi-dimensional vision of "the health divide between the haves and the have-nots." Divided into six parts, the book addresses health status across the life span; social, mental, and environmental challenges; chronic diseases; lifestyle behaviors; alternative interventions and human resources development; and ethical, political, and ecological issues. The contribution of Bullard, Johnson, and Torres on "environmental assault" and the editors' introductory overview of African American health conditions are standouts in a uniformly powerful collection. The editors' use of international comparisons is particularly compelling; life expectancy for U.S. black men is less than that of men in Iran, Colombia, Ecuador, Sri Lanka, and the Palestinian Territories. Against such grim statistics, Hatcher, Clay, and Burley lift up the resilience of the community in their essay on the central role of the black church in fostering health. This book addresses multiple audiences—medical students, clinicians working in predominantly African American areas, consumer health and community-based organizations, health researchers, and health policy makers.

Social Movements and the Transformation of American Health Care. 1st ed. Editors: Jane C. Banaszak-Holl, Sandra R. Levitsky, Mayer N. Zald. Oxford University Press, 2010.
ISBN: 9780195388305
Recommended for: Academic Libraries

The "community" in community medicine is more often than not a disenfranchised group (ethnic, cultural) or area (inner-city, border colonias). Change rarely comes without social and political struggle. Using the insights of social movement theory, the thirty-plus scholars represented in this collection expand the understanding of social change in key ways. First, these writers enlarge the arena of social action from "movement vs. state power" to social movements interacting with various power centers in society—governmental, of course, but also the multi-institutional system that constitutes health care in the United States (e.g., professional associations, insurance and pharmaceutical companies, and academic, non-profit, and for-profit health care facilities). Second, they broaden the field of relevant social change agents from "outside protestors vs. inside government officials" to include social change actors both inside and outside multiple health-related power centers. The California Nurses Association provides a visible example of insiders (i.e., nurses) as agents of systemic change. The essays, which originated in a 2007 conference, examine health care in four basic areas: state financing and regulation, institutional fields, professions and organizations, and cultural legitimacy and norms. Here, then, is an insightful portrait of the world's most prosperous nation, and the only Western nation lacking a system of universal care, at the moment when President Obama, after the failures of five previous presidents, set out to fulfill his promises of health reform.

Youth-Led Health Promotion in Urban Communities: A Community Capacity-Enhancement Perspective. Authors: Melvin Delgado, Huiquan Zhou. Rowman & Littlefield Publishers, 2008.
ISBN: 9780742561144
Recommended for: Academic Libraries

Every hot-button health care issue in the United States today—teen pregnancy, asthma, obesity and overweight, type 2 diabetes, teen pregnancy, STDs, HIV/AIDS, violence, and tobacco, alcohol, and illegal drug use—exists in an intensified form among urban youth of color. Health promotion initiatives addressed to "at-risk" teenagers often not only fail to acknowledge the "power relationships" that put young people at risk, but also fail to engage them on a level that will produce significant behavioral changes to improve their health and well-being. Melvin Delgado and Huiquan Zhou describe an alternative approach, "youth-led health promotion," based on identifying the assets that urban youth in a particular community can bring to bear upon an issue, in opposition to the more common view of urban families and communities as a tangle of pathologies and dysfunctions. This "assets first" perspective "embraces a view that before youth needs get examined, it is imperative that their abilities, resources, or assets first get identified and marshaled for addressing needs." After a thorough, and thoroughly readable, literature review, demographic summary, and discussion of youth health issues, Delgado and Zhou provide a detailed actual case report of their approach in action. Respect for young people and hope for the future permeate every page of the vital book, which should be required reading for educators, physicians, social workers, and community organizers alike—indeed for anyone concerned about the lives of children and youth, particularly black and Latino kids in our nation's inner cities.

Journals

American Journal of Preventive Medicine. v. 1, Elsevier Science, Inc., 1985.
http://www.ajpm-online.net/
ISSN: 07493797
ISSN: 18732607 (Online)
See Also Chapter 10.15. Preventive Medicine
Indexed in: MEDLINE
Recommended for: Hospital, Academic Libraries

Published since 1985, the official journal of the American College of Preventive Medicine and the Association for Prevention Teaching and Research focuses generally on "prevention research, teaching, practice and policy." Features include original research, official policy statements of the sponsors, review articles, media reviews, and editorials concerning a wide range of interventions for the prevention of chronic disease and promotion of community health. The editors welcome papers that examine "injury and violence, infectious disease, women's health, smoking, sedentary behaviors and physical activity, nutrition, diabetes, obesity, and alcohol and drug abuse." Recent issues have reported on unhealthy food environments near public schools in New York City; the validity and utility of family history and personal genomics as tools for disease prevention; and effectiveness of mass media messages to reduce youth smoking. The journal also publishes special theme issues, which have recently featured public health approaches to preventing injuries among U.S. military personnel; strategies for linking clinical and community scholarship in the Robert Wood Johnson Community Scholars Program; and public health impacts of climate change. The journal has a five-year impact factor of 5.006 (2009 *Journal Citation Reports*). Full coverage is available online from 1998 through Elsevier Science/Sciverse Science Direct.

Journal of Community Health. v. 1, Springer, 1975.
http://www.springerlink.com/content/0094-5145
ISSN: 00945145
ISSN: 15733610 (Online)
Indexed in: MEDLINE, CINAHL
Recommended for: Hospital, Academic Libraries

In its 1975 opening article, this journal's first editor promised to "address those issues that affect the health of groups of people.... Thus, we are concerned with those factors that make people sick, as well as those that would purport to make them well again." A secondary objective was to address "the education of health professional students, particularly with their grasp of those issues that affect community health." Today the journal publishes original articles on preventive medicine, health personnel, health care delivery, environmental impact on health, and medical education, with both a national and international focus. Recent issues have included articles about research on the neighborhoods surrounding major academic medical centers in Baltimore; mental health of youth in rural Zimbabwe; how community norms affect the enforcement of underage drinking laws; ten programs in Washington's Lower Yakima River Valley funded by the National Cancer Institute's Community Network Program; the role of community health workers in Chiapas, Mexico, in tuberculosis control; and a survey of providers and patients at the nation's free clinics. The journal's five-year impact factor is 1.491. Full coverage from 1975–1996 is available through SpringerLink Behavioral Sciences Archives; 1997–present is available through SpringerLink Journals.

Journal of Epidemiology and Community Health. v. 1, BMJ Group, 1947.
http://jech.bmj.com/
ISSN: 0143005X
ISSN: 14702738 (Online)
See Also Chapter 9.7. Epidemiology
Indexed in: MEDLINE, CINAHL
Recommended for: Hospital, Academic Libraries

Published since 1947, *Journal of Epidemiology and Community Health* describes itself as "a truly international journal that encompasses all aspects of epidemiology and public health." Affiliated with the British Society for Social Medicine, whose objectives inform the editorial policy of *JECH*—to address "the broad determinants of health—income and poverty, education, environmental factors such as housing and transport—as well as health care and genetic influences," requiring an interdisciplinary approach including "medicine, epidemiology, statistics, economics, social science and many others." Regular features include essays commissioned by the editors, reports "from the field on evidence-based public policy and practice," "Speakers' Corner" (short, guest commentaries), "Gallery" (which uses "images over words" to explore "aspects of human health"), and studies that illustrate "novel methods or conceptual frameworks" to investigate research problems in epidemiology and public health. Recent issues have contained articles on tools to effectively measure the links between housing quality and health outcomes; an examination of why educational attainment impacts mortality so markedly in the U.S. but hardly at all in Costa Rica; and socioeconomic inequalities in cirrhosis mortality in a Southern European urban population. On the short list of favorite journals of most professors of public health and community medicine, *JECH* has a five-year impact factor of 3.910. Full coverage from 1947–present is available from BMJ Group and PubMed Central (the most recent three years embargoed).

Journal of Health Care for the Poor and Underserved. v. 1, Johns Hopkins University Press, 1990.
http://muse.jhu.edu/journals/journal_of_health_care_for_the_poor_and_underserved/
ISSN: 10492089
ISSN: 15486869 (Online)
Indexed in: MEDLINE, CINAHL
Recommended for: Hospital, Academic Libraries

This official journal of the Association of Clinicians for the Underserved publishes original research papers, reports and evaluations of community initiatives in health promotion and disease prevention, literature reviews, book reviews, and analyses of health legislation and policy. The journal's self-described goal is "the dissemination of information on the health of, and health care for, low-income and other medically underserved communities to health care practitioners, policy makers, and community leaders who are in a position to effect meaningful change." Available in print and online editions, the summer 2010 issue contained original research on body image in Hispanic/Latino vs. European American adolescents, pap tests among Hmong women, screening for hepatitis B in Vietnamese Americans, and the extent of and reasons for mistrust of medical research among African Americans. Many of the issues examined in *JHCPU* could easily be the subject of polemics, but the treatment herein is scholarly in every sense. The journal's first issue was the record of a 1990 conference on serving the underserved at Meharry Medical School, whose president at the time, David M. Satcher, went on to become U.S. Surgeon General. Reading over that inaugural issue, one is struck by the staying power of the articles, which addressed U.S. health care policy and the prospects for reform; a decade later, a number of the ideas presented found their way into health care legislation under President Obama. Full coverage from 1990–present is available from Project Muse/Standard Collection.

Progress in Community Health Partnerships: Research, Education, and Action. v. 1, Johns Hopkins University Press, 2007.
http://muse.jhu.edu/journals/progress_in_community_health_partnerships/
ISSN: 15570541
ISSN: 1557055X (Online)
Indexed in: MEDLINE
Recommended for: Academic Libraries

Recognizing that communities may be grounded in geography, shared interests, or social networks, the editors seek "to facilitate dissemination of programs that use community partnerships to improve public health, to promote progress in the methods of research and education involving community health partnerships, and to stimulate action that will improve the health of people throughout the world." The journal is particularly interested in presenting "studies that seek to improve health or health care delivery in underserved communities." This quarterly journal has regular sections to encourage the reporting of preliminary results ("Works in Progress"); informal, personal essays ("Community Perspectives"); health policy analysis and advocacy ("Policy and Practice"); outcome measurement ("Theory and Methods"); curricula and strategies for training researchers and community organizations in effective research partnerships ("Education and Training"); and tools to facilitate partnerships, such as advisory boards ("Practical Tools"). Recent features have included a special issue on community-based research approaches to youth violence prevention; articles concerning the use of "one-pagers," short summaries of research findings and policy proposals, as a policy advocacy tool used by a community group in Detroit; how a women's organization created "fotonovelas" to increase health literacy among Latinas; the influence of parents on child body image among first graders in Washington, DC; and barriers to and enablers of optimal chronic care for racial and ethnic minority patients of seven Boston Community Health Centers. Full coverage from 2007 to the present is available through Project MUSE.

9.7. Epidemiology

The determination of causes, incidence, and characteristic behavior of disease outbreaks affecting human populations. It includes the interrelationships of host, agent, and environment as related to the distribution and control of disease.

—MeSH

Contributor: Irene M. Lubker

Monographs

Critical Appraisal of Epidemiological Studies and Clinical Trials. 3rd ed. Editor: Mark Elwood. Oxford University Press, 2007.
ISBN: 9780199218257
Recommended for: Hospital, Academic Libraries

This book is written so that the statistical concepts related to epidemiological studies and clinical trials are explained without the use of complex mathematics. The book is useful for those seeking to learn how to critically appraise epidemiological studies. It explains the art and science of designing and evaluating clinical trials and observational studies. Chapters 1 to 9, which are the core chapters, include self-test questions with answers near the end of the book. Chapter 8 explains systematic reviews and meta-analysis, making this book a must for those concerned with evidence-based practice. Chapters 10 to 15 are dedicated to examples of critical appraisals of different studies, showing readers the application of the material discussed in the core chapters. There is an appendix with a summary of statistical methods and some tables towards the end. The audience for this book is new epidemiologists and clinicians who seek to practice evidence-based health care, as well as graduate students.

Dictionary of Epidemiology. 5th ed. Editor: Miquel S. Porta. Oxford University Press, 2008.
ISBN: 9780195314496
Recommended for: Hospital, Academic Libraries

This classic dictionary of epidemiology, now in its fifth edition, is an indispensable quick reference tool for students of epidemiology as well as practicing epidemiologists, public health workers, biologists, and biomedical scientists. It has been completely revised and updated. It is edited for the International Epidemiological Society and is considered the definitive dictionary of epidemiology. This dictionary contains definitions for the most significant terms and specialized vocabulary used in epidemiology, reflecting the multi-disciplinary nature of the field. This is an extensive epidemiology dictionary, covering all the major branches of epidemiology including general, environmental and clinical epidemiology; biostatistics; infectious disease control; genetics; health promotion; health economics; and medical ethics. The definitions were reviewed by an international network of contributors from all the major branches of epidemiology. The writing is clear and easy to understand, but more elaborate explanations are included when needed. This resource also contains website links to further information on topics.

Environmental Epidemiology: Principles and Methods. Author: Ray M. Merrill. Jones & Bartlett, 2008.
See Chapter 5. Environmental Health

Environmental Epidemiology: Study Methods and Application. Editors: Dean Baker, Mark J. Nieuwenhuijsen. Oxford University Press, 2008.
See Chapter 5. Environmental Health

Epidemiology. 4th ed. Author: Leon Gordis. Saunders Elsevier, 2009.
http://www.mdconsult.com/
ISBN: 9781416040026
Recommended for: Academic Libraries
Doody's Core Titles Selection

This is one of the best epidemiology books for beginning health professions students to learn principles and methods in epidemiology as well as its clinical applications. The author, who is an award winning instructor, draws from his long years of teaching experience in two introductory epidemiology courses, Principles of Epidemiology and Clinical Epidemiology at Johns Hopkins University. The book is divided into three sections: section 1 covers epidemiologic approach to disease and intervention; section 2 covers the use of epidemiology to identify the causes of disease; and the third section deals with the application of epidemiology to evaluate policy.

The book begins by introducing epidemiology as a subject with objectives and its relevance to both public health and clinical practice, and how observational data can be used to institute preventative measures. In addition to the usual graphs and textbook illustrations, the author uses classroom tested line diagrams, photographs, and cartoons to illustrate points. The book is clearly written, with full color format. It contains review questions at the end of each chapter, with answers to some of the questions provided. Individual purchasers of this book also have access to http://studentconsult.com with interactive resources plus an online version of the text which can be downloaded onto a handheld device. The text is also available online through MD Consult.

Fourth National Report on Human Exposure to Environmental Chemicals. 4th ed. Centers for Disease Control and Prevention, 2009.
See Chapter 5. Environmental Health

Obesity Epidemiology. Editor: Frank B. Hu. Oxford University Press, 2008.
ISBN: 9780195312911
See Also Chapter 9.3. Bariatric Medicine
Recommended for: Academic Libraries

This book focuses on observational studies and other methods of research in obesity epidemiology. The beginning chapters discuss the history of obesity research. The book is divided into three parts: The first part, chapters 1 to 7, is devoted to "Study Designs and Measurements"; the second part, chapters 8 to 13, discusses "Epidemiological Studies of Consequences of Obesity"; and part three is devoted to "Epidemiological Studies of Determinants of Obesity." The authors discuss different studies in obesity, carefully pointing out the strengths and weaknesses of the studies. The editor and the invited contributing authors (who cite some of their own research) are very knowledgeable and experienced researchers and educators in the field of obesity epidemiology. The writing is clear and uncomplicated and includes many examples to help readers understand the studies, making it one of the best books for graduate students studying obesity epidemiology. Students in dietetics, nutrition, and exercise physiology could also benefit from this book. It has been called the first comprehensive methodological oriented book in obesity epidemiology. Experienced researchers and instructors in public health and other clinical researchers in obesity could use this book as a desk reference. This book is a required resource for all academic libraries.

Journals

American Journal of Epidemiology. v. 81, Oxford University Press, 1965.
http://aje.oxfordjournals.org/
ISSN: 00029262
ISSN: 14766256 (Online)
Indexed in: MEDLINE, CINAHL
Recommended for: Hospital, Academic Libraries

This peer-reviewed journal is one of the most important epidemiological journals, with research articles from original contributions and current methodological developments in the field of epidemiological research. Each volume has a section devoted to opinion pieces, book reviews, and other review articles. The primary audience of this journal is epidemiologists, public health professionals, clinicians, graduate students in related fields, and anyone who uses epidemiological data. The journal is issued semi-monthly and is sponsored by the Society of Epidemiologic Research. *American Journal of Epidemiology* is a member of the Committee on Publication Ethics and is listed in the *Core Collection of Medical Books and Journals* (Hague List). It has an impact factor of 5.589 (2009 *Journal Citation Reports*) and is indexed in numerous indexing and abstracting sources covering a wide range of subject fields. Online access back to 1965 is available from the publisher.

American Journal of Public Health. v. 1, American Public Health Association, 1911.
http://ajph.aphapublications.org/
ISSN: 00900036
ISSN: 15410048 (Online)
See Also Chapter 10.16. Public Health, Chapter 13.16. Public Health Nursing
Indexed in: MEDLINE, CINAHL
Recommended for: Hospital, Academic Libraries
Brandon/Hill Selection

American Journal of Public Health (*AJPH*) is the official journal of the American Public Health Association. It was voted by the Special Library Association as one of the 100 most influential journals in the field of biology and medicine in the last 100 years. It has an impact factor of 4.371 and ranks ninth out of 122 journals in public, environmental and occupational health (2009 *Journal Citation Reports*). The journal publishes in-depth original research on current issues in all the disciplines of public health, both domestic and international. Articles in the journal concentrate on research methods, program evaluation in public health, and health policy. The articles are peer-reviewed by a panel of invited reviewers in the appropriate fields of public health. It also has a letter section and uniquely, a historical section that compares past public health issues and practices with current practice. The journal also acts as a health policy forum by publishing editorials and commentaries on public health issues. This journal is a must for all academic institutions with a public health program, as well as for hospitals with clinicians and public health practitioners who want to keep current with public health issues and best practices. Published monthly, this journal is cited in many abstracting and indexing sources such as MEDLINE, Ageline, Biological Abstracts, CINAHL, Criminal Justice Abstracts, Embase, Environmental Abstracts, Hospital Literature Index, PsycINFO, Science Citation Index, and (SRI)/LexisNexis.

Clinical Infectious Diseases. v. 14, University of Chicago Press, 1992.
http://www.journals.uchicago.edu/toc/cid/current
http://www.jstor.org/
ISSN: 10584838
ISSN: 15376591 (Online)
See Also Chapter 10.10.5. Infectious Disease Medicine
Indexed in: MEDLINE
Recommended for: Academic Libraries

This peer-reviewed journal is an official publication of the Infectious Diseases Society of America. It began in 1979 under the title of *Reviews of Infectious Diseases*. This journal is one of the most cited journals in the field of infectious diseases and microbiology. It was also named as one of the "100 Most Influential Journals in Biology and Medicine" of the past 100 years by the Special Libraries Association Biomedical and Life Sciences Division. Each issue has book reviews, a news section, brief reports, articles, and commentaries. Major articles in the journal cover a wide variety of topics such as the prevalence and incidence of disease, population studies, infectious disease control in populations, disease surveillance, and practice guidelines. In each issue there are special sections that focus on key relevant topics such as infectious diseases as biological weapons, HIV/AIDS, and antimicrobial resistance. Disease outbreaks or conditions affecting populations are also highlighted, such as the 2006 Escherichia coli 0157 outbreak from uncooked spinach. Some supplemental issues devoted to single topics of infectious disease are also published. The primary audience for this publication is practicing clinicians, researchers, and epidemiologists. The journal is indexed in most of the major indexing and abstracting sources. Online access back to June 1997 is available from the publisher and the full-text backfile is available from JSTOR.

Epidemiologic Reviews. v. 1, Oxford University Press, 1979.
http://epirev.oxfordjournals.org/
ISSN: 0193936X
ISSN: 14786729 (Online)
Indexed in: MEDLINE, CINAHL
Recommended for: Academic Libraries

A subscription to *American Journal of Epidemiology* includes this annual publication that collects review articles on various aspects of epidemiology and public health. Articles are peer-reviewed; some are invited. Some of the annual volumes of this journal have distinct titles. Past volumes have focused on prostate cancer, cohort study, vaccines, genetic epidemiology, and injury prevention. Some of the more recent topics have been: "Vaccines and Public Health" (2006), "Epidemiology of Obesity" (2007), "Epidemiology of Mental Disorders" (2008) and "Health Disparities" (2009). This journal had the highest impact factor (17.500) out of all public, environmental and occupational health journals, making it one of the leading journals in public health and epidemiology (2009 *Journal Citation Reports*). The primary audience for this journal is public health practitioners, researchers, and students. Online access from 1979 to the present is available from the publisher.

Epidemiology. v. 1, Lippincott Williams & Wilkins and Epidemiology Resources Inc, 1990.
http://journals.lww.com/epidem/
ISSN: 10443983
ISSN: 15315487 (Online)
Indexed in: MEDLINE
Recommended for: Academic Libraries

This peer-reviewed journal is the official journal of the International Society of Environmental Epidemiology. It is ranked sixth out of 122 journals in public, environmental and occupational health and has an impact factor of 5.511 (2009 *Journal Citation Reports*). Article content covers a wide range of topics in epidemiology including chronic diseases, reproductive diseases, environmental diseases, psychosocial diseases, infectious diseases, and genetic epidemiology. The journal also publishes review articles, meta-analyses, and descriptions and applications of new methods. It is international in scope and encourages submissions from developing countries. The primary audience for this journal is epidemiologists, clinicians, graduate students, public health researchers, and environmental scientists. It is recommended for academic libraries. Online access to back to volume 1, 1990 is available from the publisher, Ovid, and JSTOR.

International Journal of Epidemiology. v. 1, Oxford University Press, 1972.
http://ije.oxfordjournals.org/
ISSN: 03005771
ISSN: 14643685 (Online)
Indexed in: MEDLINE
Recommended for: Academic Libraries

This peer-reviewed journal is one of the most heavily cited epidemiology journals with an impact factor of 5.262 (2009 *Journal Citation Reports*). Published six times a year, the journal solicits articles from the international epidemiology community and is international in scope. The journal publishes articles from a variety of epidemiology fields including infectious and non-infectious diseases, environmental health, preventive medicine, chronic disease, risk management, and general medical care. New methods of public health data analysis are featured. The journal also publishes reprints and reflections of articles, systematic reviews, methodology, letters to the editor, book reviews, and essay reviews. This is a very important journal for public health practitioners, especially those with an interest in global public health and health care issues. The journal is a member of the Committee on Publications Ethics (COPE). It is indexed by numerous indexing and abstracting sources including Biological Abstracts, CAB Abstracts, Embase, Global Health, MEDLINE, Science Citation Index, Scopus, and Web of Science. Online access back to 1972 is available from the publisher.

Journal of Epidemiology and Community Health. v. 33, BMJ, 1979.
http://jech.bmj.com/content/current
http://www.ncbi.nlm.nih.gov/pmc/journals/167/
ISSN: 14702738 (Online)
ISSN: 0143005X
See Also Chapter 9.6. Community Medicine
Indexed in: MEDLINE, CINAHL
Recommended for: Hospital, Academic Libraries

This is a peer-reviewed international journal that publishes original papers, review articles, book reviews, and short reports in public health. The content focus is on both the study of epidemiology in communities as well as the improvement of the health of those communities world wide. The articles are generally divided into epidemiology, health services research, methods, and public health policy and practice. It is suitable for health professionals, primary care and environmental health consultants, housing and planning officials, health and safety officials, public policy makers, occupational therapists, and researchers in all areas of epidemiology, as well as graduate students. It is one of the more heavily cited journals, ranking 23 out of 122 journals in public, occupational, and environmental health (2009 *Journal Citation Reports*). All academic health sciences libraries, government agencies, and hospitals should have this journal available. This journal is indexed in all the major indexing and abstracting sources including MEDLINE and ISI Current Contents. Online access back to 1979 is available from the publisher. The archive of this journal and its earlier titles is also available in PubMed Central, from 1947 until three years prior to current.

Journal of Exposure Science and Environmental Epidemiology. v. 16, Nature Publishing Group, 2006.
See Chapter 5. Environmental Health, Chapter 10.15.1. Environmental Medicine

9.7.1. Molecular Epidemiology

The application of molecular biology to the answering of epidemiological questions. The examination of patterns of changes in DNA to implicate particular carcinogens and the use of molecular markers to predict which individuals are at highest risk for a disease are common examples.

—MeSH

Contributor: Irene M. Lubker

Monographs

Molecular Epidemiology of Chronic Diseases. Editors: Chris Wild, Paolo Vineis, Seymour Garte. Wiley Blackwell, 2008.
http://onlinelibrary.wiley.com/book/10.1002/9780470725726
ISBN: 9780470027431
Recommended for: Academic Libraries

This very useful handbook on the molecular epidemiology of chronic disease contains a collection of research papers by several expert authors. It is clearly written and accessible. Content of its 26 chapters include: an introduction to molecular epidemiology; study design; molecular epidemiological studies; family studies, haplotypes, and gene association studies; individual susceptibility and gene-environment interaction; biomarker validation; exposure assessment; carcinogen metabolites as biomarkers; biomarkers of exposure; biomarkers of mutation and DNA repair capacity; high-throughput techniques—genotyping and genomics; proteomics and molecular epidemiology; metabolic profiling; univariate and multivariate data analysis; meta-analysis and pooled analysis; analysis of complex datasets; implications of random exposure measurement errors; bioinformatics; biomarkers, disease mechanisms, and their role in regulatory decisions; biomarkers in intervention studies; biological resource centers; molecular epidemiology and ethics; biomarkers for dietary carcinogens; hormones; aflatoxin, hepatitis B virus, and liver cancer; and complex exposures. Most of the research papers highlight the applications of laboratory research techniques that aid the understanding of the epidemiological problems of chronic diseases. The text includes numerous examples from population studies to illustrate techniques. The potential audience for this book is laboratory scientists, epidemiologists, clinical researchers, and biostatisticians, since it takes a cross-disciplinary approach to focus on practical aspects of research application.

Molecular Epidemiology of Infectious Diseases: Principles and Practices. Author: Lee W. Riley. ASM Press, 2004.
ISBN: 9781555812683
Recommended for: Hospital, Academic Libraries

This is an easy-to-understand introductory molecular biology text. The first chapter starts with definitions before delving into the substance of the subject. There are a number of illustrations that explain specific examples of investigations of bacterial infectious diseases. To illustrate stratification and refinement of data in epidemiologic investigations, data and methodologies from real case studies are provided. Authors provide a glossary of terms, index and an extensive annotated bibliography of websites of databases that are useful for molecular epidemiology investigations. The terminology in the glossary provides a connection between epidemiology and molecular biology. This book would be useful to clinicians, epidemiologists, and molecular biologists new to the field of molecular epidemiology, as well as more advanced students working on research.

Molecular Epidemiology: Applications in Cancer and Other Human Diseases. Editors: Timothy R. Rebbeck, Christine B. Ambrosone, Peter G. Shields. Informa Healthcare, 2008.
http://informahealthcare.com/
http://extranet.netlibrary.com/TitleSelect/
ISBN: 9781420052916
Recommended for: Academic Libraries

This text has over 30 contributing authors from fields of cancer epidemiology, molecular epidemiology, environmental epidemiology, genetics, biostatistics, genomics, and medicine. The three editors are very experienced, having collectively written and published 405 peer-reviewed articles in their fields. The papers in this handbook focus on the connection between biology and causes of cancer and other human diseases. The text also provides best practices in conducting molecular epidemiology research. Chapters 1 to 4 discuss appropriate study designs; chapters 5 to 8 discuss data collection methods; chapters 10 to 16 discuss different tools for data analysis; and chapters 17 and 18 discuss interpretation of results and how to make useful inferences for practice. This book includes scientific tables, equations, and illustrations to provide a foundation for conducting and interpreting molecular epidemiological studies. However, since this is not a book for beginners, it does not provide a glossary of terms. The primary audience for this text is biomedical and epidemiological researchers and graduate students.

Journals

Cancer Causes and Control. v. 1, Springer Netherlands, 1990.
http://www.springerlink.com/content/0957-5243
ISSN: 09575243
ISSN: 15737225 (Online)
Indexed in: MEDLINE
Recommended for: Academic Libraries

This journal is one of the more highly cited journals in the public, environmental, and occupational health category and has an impact factor of 3.199 (2009 *Journal Citation Reports*). It is an international epidemiology journal that publishes studies of cancer in human populations. The journal is published ten times a year and has a quick turn-around, publishing articles within 30 to 60 days after acceptance. The articles in this journal are peer-reviewed by an expert panel of authors and include original research, review articles, comments, opinions, and letters to the editor. The journal's aim is to publish articles that advance the current understanding of cancer causes, distribution in populations, methods of control, and prevention. Authors are from different countries and from diverse biological and medical disciplines. The journal also publishes a large amount of information that can be used by government agencies to aid in making policies for cancer control. Any researcher, epidemiologist, medical statistician, cancer biologist, health educator, or medical economist working in oncology, especially prevention of cancer globally, should have access to this publication. This journal is indexed in many abstracting and indexing sources such as MEDLINE, Academic OneFile, AGRICOLA, Biological Abstracts,

BIOSIS Previews, CAB Abstracts, CSA/ProQuest, Embase, Global Health, JSTOR, PsycINFO and Science Citation Index. Online access back to volume 1, 1990 is available from Springer.

Cancer Epidemiology, Biomarkers & Prevention. v. 1, American Association for Cancer Research, 1991.
http://cebp.aacrjournals.org/
http://intl-cebp.aacrjournals.org/
ISSN: 15387755 (Online)
ISSN: 10559965
Indexed in: MEDLINE
Recommended for: Academic Libraries

This peer-reviewed journal is published by the American Association for Cancer Research. It is the tenth highest cited public, environmental, and occupational health journal with an impact factor of 4.310 (2009 *Journal Citation Reports*). The articles in this journal present original research on causes of cancer, mechanisms of carcinogenesis, prevention, and survivorship. The journal also has short review articles and short communications. Content covers a broad spectrum of cancer epidemiology, including descriptive, analytical, biochemical, and molecular epidemiology; biomarkers, nutrition, and behavior in prevention; chemoprevention; screening and early detection; survivorship and supportive care; the role of behavioral factors in etiology and prevention; and statistical methods and models. Experts are invited to write commentary on published papers or to write original articles from varied perspectives. The primary audience for this journal is cancer researchers and public health practitioners interested in the prevention of cancer. This journal is highly recommended for epidemiologists and biomedical researchers. It is indexed in numerous indexing and abstracting sources, including Biological Abstracts, Embase, MEDLINE, Scopus, and Web of Science. Online access back to volume 1, 1991 is available from the publisher.

Genetic Epidemiology. v. 1, Wiley, 1984.
http://onlinelibrary.wiley.com/journal/10.1002/(ISSN)1098-2272
ISSN: 07410395
ISSN: 10982272 (Online)
Indexed in: MEDLINE
Recommended for: Academic Libraries

Genetic Epidemiology is the official journal of the International Genetic Epidemiology Society. This journal is published eight times a year with a supplemental issue in some years. The sequencing of the human genome has made genetic epidemiology an important field of molecular epidemiology that is becoming increasingly popular. This journal publishes original peer-reviewed articles on genetic and environmental causes of disease and the distribution of human traits in families and populations. The articles range from applied research and innovative statistical or computational studies to methodological studies that help in the understanding of genetic epidemiology. In addition to the original articles, there are letters to the editor, review articles, and perspectives from other fields of studies. The audience for this journal is genetic scientists, epidemiologists seeking to understand the genetic component of causes and distribution of disease in families and populations, biostatisticians, and researchers and specialists in infectious and hereditary diseases. The journal is cited in many abstracting and indexing sources such as MEDLINE, Embase, BIOSIS Previews and IBIDS. Online access back to volume 1, 1984 is available from the publisher.

Infection Control and Hospital Epidemiology. v. 9, University of Chicago Press, 1988.
http://www.journals.uchicago.edu/ICHE/
ISSN: 0899823X
ISSN: 15596834 (Online)
Indexed in: MEDLINE, CINAHL
Recommended for: Hospital, Academic Libraries

This peer-reviewed journal is the official journal of the Society of Healthcare Epidemiology of America. It began in 1982 under the title *Infection Control*. With a primary focus on the control of infectious diseases in health care facilities, the journal publishes research on the study, control and evaluation of the transmission of pathogens in hospitals and other health institutions. Authors are usually infection control practitioners and epidemiologists in infection control. Articles range from those discussing the science and methods of isolating disease-causing organisms to cost effectiveness of clinical procedures aimed at controlling infections in hospitals. In addition to scientific articles, the journal publishes World Health Organization network reports, commentaries, concise communications, research briefs, and letters to the editor. The primary audience for this journal is infection control and epidemiology practitioners in health care facilities, as well as researchers and students interested in this field. The journal is indexed in numerous abstracting and indexing sources including Biological Abstracts, CAB Abstracts, Embase, MEDLINE, Scopus, and Web of Science. Online access back to volume 9, 1988 is available from JSTOR.

Journal of Clinical Epidemiology. v. 41, Elsevier, 1988.
http://journals.elsevierhealth.com/periodicals/jce

http://www.sciencedirect.com/science/journal/08954356
ISSN: 08954356
ISSN: 18785921 (Online)
Indexed in: MEDLINE
Recommended for: Hospital, Academic Libraries

This peer-reviewed journal is the twenty-fourth out of 122 most cited journal in the category of public, environmental, and occupational health (2009 *Journal Citation Reports*). It has had a long publication history and several title changes. According to its aims and scope statement, the journal promotes quality clinical and patient-oriented health services research. Its monthly issues include original research articles, systematic reviews, meta analyses, methodology articles, and commentaries from experts in different fields of public health. The journal also publishes practice and research articles to encourage innovative ways of patient care and research that can be translated into clinical care. The primary audience for this publication is practicing clinicians, researchers, and students in epidemiology and public health. All hospitals and academic health science libraries should have access to this journal. It is indexed in numerous abstracting and indexing sources including CAB Abstracts, Embase, Global Health, MEDLINE, Science Citation Index, Scopus, and Web of Science. Online access is available from the publisher back to volume 41, 1988.

9.8. Geriatrics

The physiological and pathological aspects of the aged, including the clinical problems of senescence and senility.
—MeSH

Contributor: Adria P. Olmi

Monographs

American Psychiatric Publishing Textbook of Alzheimer Disease and Other Dementias. Editors: Myron F. Weiner, Anne M. Lipton. American Psychiatric Publishing, 2009.
http://www.r2library.com/
http://extranet.netlibrary.com/TitleSelect/
http://www.ebrary.com/
ISBN: 9781585622788
ISBN: 9781585628940 (Online)
Recommended For: Hospital, Academic Libraries
Doody's Core Titles selection

The *Textbook of Alzheimer Disease* covers important topics in treating Alzheimer disease and dementias. The resource is organized into six parts and includes: (1) introductory matter discussing the history of dementia, from Ancient Greece to contemporary standards in molecular biology and epidemiology of dementia; (2) evaluation and diagnosis of dementia; (3) Alzheimer disease and other dementias, including Lewy bodies and other synucleinopathies, frontotemporal dementia, and traumatic brain injury; (4) treatment of dementia from pharmacology to behavioral management; (5) caregiving, legal, and ethical issues; and (6) the future, which discusses prevention, the future of treatment, genetics of Alzheimer disease, and the molecular basis of the disease. The work builds on an earlier American Psychiatric publication titled *Dementias: Diagnosis, Treatment and Research*. It includes copious appendixes. This textbook has been written for students and physicians in the fields of psychiatry, neurology, and geriatrics. The textbook is listed in *Doody's Core Titles*.

American Psychiatric Publishing Textbook of Geriatric Psychiatry. 4th ed. Editors: Dan G. Blazer, David C. Steffens. American Psychiatric Publishing, 2009.
http://www.psychiatryonline.com
ISBN: 9781585622771
ISBN: 9781585623754 (Online)
See Also Chapter 9.10.5. Geriatric Psychiatry
Recommended For: Hospital, Academic Libraries

This textbook, which builds on the earlier editions by Ewald W. Busse, continues the interdisciplinary approach by including contributions from the fields of medicine, medical psychology, nursing, sociology, health policy, neurology, and social work. The work's treatment of geriatrics starts with the basic science of aging, including physiology, neuroanatomy and neuropathology, genetics, and social theories. It then delves into the diagnostic interview (part II), psychiatric disorders (part III), and treatment of disorders (part IV). The work concludes with special topics in the areas of law, ethics, policy, and an overview of geriatric psychiatry's past and future. The online edition helpfully includes a DOI (digital object identifier) for each section, links to related textbook matter, journal articles in the PsychiatryOnline subscription database, and mobile device download options. The online edition's reference sections include helpful links to citations held in PubMed. The textbook's "Suggested Readings" section deepens the bibliographic knowledge base and guides readers to a wider scope of documentation. The editors have updated the work by keeping in mind Dr. Busse's earlier editorial insights, producing a work aimed at psychiatrists, other geriatric and gerontological health providers, and candidates seeking board certification in geriatrics. This resource is highly recommended for all health, academic, and hospital libraries. Institutions will receive many benefits from the online product's approach to integration with PubMed and its reliance on an easily navigated information platform.

Brocklehurst's Textbook of Geriatric Medicine and Gerontology. 7th ed. Editors: Howard M. Fillit, Kenneth Rockwood, Kenneth Woodhouse. Saunders/Elsevier, 2010.
ISBN: 9781416062318
Recommended For: Hospital, Academic Libraries
Brandon/Hill Selection

This venerable textbook, which is now in its seventh edition, begins by covering biological, medical, neurological, and social concepts in gerontology. The second section discusses medical geriatrics, which emphasizes a systems approach to disease. It starts with a discussion on disease in old age and is followed by a section on patient evaluation—including assessment, laboratory medicine, and measurement of the outcomes of interventions. While a chapter is devoted to geriatric oncology, cancer is also covered in other chapters, such as the breast, gynecologic disorders, prostrate, and large bowel. The third section focuses on problem-based geriatric medicine and covers prevention and syndromes, such as falls, delirium, and pressure sores. *Brocklehurst's* offers approximately fifty pages of indexing, and color plates precede the first chapter. The "Key Points" inset allow readers to quickly grasp the main points of chapter contents and often follow the chapter summaries. Chapters are illustrated throughout with various figures and tables. The comprehensiveness of this text is one of its most valuable benefits. The contributors are associated with institutions in the United States and the United Kingdom, and the work provides an international perspective by covering health systems in the United States, Europe, Latin America, United Kingdom, and, more briefly, other international milieus (specifically, chapter IV). Regrettably, chapter bibliographical references are only available online to individual subscribers through Elsevier's Expert Consult option. The resource is structured for practitioners, gerontologists, geriatricians, and other health care providers. It is suitable for hospital libraries, academic libraries, and other settings with scientifically informed health collections.

Essentials of Clinical Geriatrics. 6th ed. Authors: Robert L. Kane, Joseph G. Ouslander, Itamar B. Abrass, Barbara Resnick. McGraw-Hill, 2009.
http://www.r2library.com/
ISBN: 9780071498227
Recommended For: Hospital, Academic Libraries
Doody's Core Titles selection

This resource is an excellent, single-volume guide to clinical geriatrics. The 6th edition incorporates standards of evidence-based practice and includes insights from professional nursing. The tables are veritable gold mines of knowledge, especially the "evidence summary" tables that are available in many chapters. The guide offers twenty pages of indexing, discrete lists of Internet resources for providers and patients, a specific index of organizations, and chapter bibliographic references. The work includes chapters on the aging process and clinical work, evaluating the geriatric patient, demographics of the aged, chronic disease management, differential diagnosis (such as prevention, falls, and immobility), general management strategies for cardiovascular disorders, decreased vitality, sensory organs, drug therapy, available health programs, nursing home care, and ethics. *Essentials of Clinical Geriatrics* received very positive reviews from *Doody's Core Titles*. Due to its scholarly nature and its clinician-oriented features, the intended audience includes academic professionals and health care providers. The resource deserves to be added to academic and hospital library collections. Physicians and other clinicians may want to use this as a ready-reference tool. Altogether, this is an excellent resource for geriatricians.

Geriatric Nutrition: The Health Professional's Handbook. 3rd ed. Editor: Ronni Chernoff. Jones & Bartlett, 2006.
See Chapter 14.2. Dietetics

Hazzard's Geriatric Medicine and Gerontology. 6th ed. Editors: Jeffrey B. Halter, Joseph G. Ouslander, Mary E. Tinetti, Stephanie Studenski, Kevin P. High, Sanjay Asthana. McGraw-Hill, 2009.
http://www.accessmedicine.com/
http://extranet.netlibrary.com/TitleSelect/
http://www.r2library.com/
http://www.ebrary.com/
ISBN: 9780071488723
ISBN: 9780071641241 (Online)
See Also Chapter 13.5. Geriatric Nursing
Recommended For: Hospital, Academic, Consumer Health Libraries
Brandon/Hill, *Doody's Core Titles* Selection

This outstanding medical textbook contains 130 chapters that cover the principles of gerontology, geriatrics, geriatric syndromes, organ systems, and diseases. The sixth edition contains new chapters, such as rural aging and antibiotic use, and a dedicated chapter on international gerontology. The section on "Special Management Issues" includes palliative care, pain management, spirituality, ethics, rehabilitation, and alternative medicine. The contributors include a selection of international advisors, and the editors recruited many women as chapter authors. The work is well organized, attractively designed, and illustrated with tables and figures. In the chapter "Biology of Aging and Longevity," one figure creatively shows population-based associations of short stature with various cancers such as breast, prostrate, and esophageal. Color plates are included as end matter after the index. This text is included in McGraw-Hill's AccessMedicine, which offers updating features for resources that are also published as print editions. The editors have expressed a desire for this text to become interactive with *Harrison's Internal Medicine*, which is also included in AccessMedicine. This is a standard text for medical students and doctors, making it suitable for hospital collections, but is also highly useful for academic institutions and public library consumer health collections.

Handbook of Health Psychology and Aging. 1st ed. Editors: Carolyn M. Aldwin, Crystal L. Park, Avron Spiro III. Guilford, 2007.
See Chapter 9.4. Behavioral Medicine

Physiological Basis of Aging and Geriatrics. 4th ed. Editor: Paola S. Timras. Informa Healthcare, 2007.
http://extranet.netlibrary.com/TitleSelect/
http://www.ebrary.com/
ISBN: 9780849373053
ISBN: 9781420007091 (Online)
Recommended For: Academic, Consumer Health Libraries
Doody's Core Titles Selection

This fourth edition relies upon physiology as the groundwork and integral theory of aging processes. This work is an outgrowth of another title, *Developmental Physiology and Aging* (Macmillan, 1972), which is considered a landmark work. While the fourth edition is somewhat dated, the text still serves as a very useful resource for those wanting a concise descriptive treatment of cellular, molecular, and organismic aspects of aging and age-related biological changes over time. The first part discusses methods of studying aging, human longevity, geriatric functional assessment, cellular senescence, cell death, and theories of aging and the life span. The second part offers a systematic approach, while the third part covers prevention generally and, more specifically, rehabilitation, pharmacology, diet, physical exercise, and assistive technology. Insets treat important topics such as pros and cons of rodent models for studying menopause and historical research on stress in relationship to longevity. Tables and figures provide ample illustration of important concepts. The work has been written specifically to meet the needs of aging experts who are biologically focused, the elderly themselves, and others interested in longevity and continuity of care and physiology. The brevity of the work, clear writing, accessibility of language, tables and charts, sourcing, and range of topics show that it has met its target of reaching educated readers, not simply scientists or student clinicians. This is a very useful resource for academic libraries and consumer health collections.

Reichel's Care of the Elderly: Clinical Aspects of Aging. 6th ed. Editors: Christine Arenson, Jan Busby-Whitehead, Kenneth Brummel-Smith. Cambridge University Press, 2009.
http://www.cambridge.org/
http://www.r2library.com/
http://www.ebrary.com/
http://extranet.netlibrary.com/TitleSelect/
ISBN: 9780521869294
See Also Chapter 13.5. Geriatric Nursing
Recommended For: Hospital, Academic Libraries
Brandon/Hill, *Doody's Core Titles* Selection

The sixth edition of *Reichel's Care of the Elderly* continues to focus on the clinical treatment of the elderly patient, discussing diseases, injuries, disorders, and basic care principles. Each chapter is concisely written and individually referenced; many chapters include black-and-white pictures. The work contains appropriate use of tables and figures, and color plates are included. *Reichel's* offers twenty pages of indexing. This resource also places an emphasis on the physician as a formulator of a biopsychosocial-spiritual model of health care, advocating for the patient, emphasizing optimal and healthy aging, and looking at the patient in totality; it avoids simply relying on technological means of health care delivery. It discusses community-based institutional care and related issues, such as abuse of elders, preventing errors, and caregiver burden. This resource was highly recommended by *Doody's* and was regularly listed on the former Brandon/Hill lists. *Reichel's* audience includes health care providers, from medical students to working physicians. It is appropriate for hospital and academic libraries seeking a well-respected text on clinical geriatric care.

Textbook of Men's Health and Aging. 2nd ed. Editors: Bruno Lunenfeld, Louis J.G. Gooren, Alvaro Morales, John E. Morley. Informa Healthcare, 2007.
See Chapter 9.2. Andrology

Journals

Age and Ageing, v. 1, Oxford University Press/British Geriatrics Society, February 1972.
http://ageing.oxfordjournals.org/
ISSN: 00020729
ISSN: 14682834 (Online)
See Also Chapter 13.5 Geriatric Nursing
Indexed in: MEDLINE, CINAHL
Recommended For: Hospital, Academic Libraries

This journal, a publication sponsored by the British Geriatrics Society, provides access to original, refereed research and commissioned reviews on topics within geriatrics and gerontology. The audience includes medical scientists focusing on aging from the areas of clinical research, epidemiology, and psychology. The resource offers an international perspective through worldwide contributions. According to the 2009 *Journal Citation Reports, Age and Ageing's* impact factor was 3.131, which has increased steadily over the years. It is indexed by MEDLINE, CINAHL, Current Contents/Clinical Medicine, Biological Abstracts, and Embase. The journal complies with the NIH Public Access mandate and offers access to selected articles through PubMed Central, with an embargo of twelve months for open access content. The journal articles are available at the publisher's website, offering PDF and abstracts from February 1972 to November 2005; full text (HTML), PDF, and abstracts are supplied from November 2005 to the present.

Age: The Journal of the American Aging Association, v. 1, Springer Netherlands/American Aging Association, 1978.
http://springerlink.com/content/113232/
http://www.ncbi.nlm.nih.gov/pmc/journals/518/
ISSN: 01619152
ISSN: 15744647 (Online)
Indexed in: MEDLINE
Recommended For: Academic Libraries

This peer-reviewed journal is the official organ of the American Aging Association (AGE), an organization dedicated to studying the biological mechanisms of aging; promoting public health, especially in regards to healthy living and longevity; and connecting the field of gerontology with the work of physicians and health care professionals. This quarterly journal covers biology and biomedical research, encompassing the areas of molecular medicine, biological evolution, genetics, immunology, endocrinology, physiology, pharmacology, and psychology. The journal publishes clinical articles that discuss the underlying biological mechanisms of aging as well as reports from the American Aging Association. According to the 2009 *Journal Citation Reports*, the journal's impact factor is 5.839, the third highest ranked journal in the geriatrics and gerontology category. The journal is indexed by MEDLINE, various OCLC sources, Abstracts in Social Gerontology, and Scopus. It is available online at the publisher's website, SpringerLink, and PubMed Central (with a 12-month embargo). The journal is appropriate for academic university libraries and scientific research centers. The audience of the journal is clearly scientific and biomedical researchers, cellular biologists involved with research in aging studies, and medical scientists.

American Journal of Geriatric Psychiatry. v. 1, Lippincott Williams &Wilkins/American Association for Geriatric Psychiatry, 1993.
http://www.ovid.com/
ISSN: 10647481
ISSN: 15457214
See Also Chapter 9.10.5. Geriatric Psychiatry
Indexed in: MEDLINE
Recommended For: Hospital, Academic Libraries

This resource is the official journal of the American Association for Geriatric Psychiatry. The journal publishes peer-reviewed research on psychiatric disorders, psychopharmacology, and other interventions, as well as articles covering epidemiological and biological aspects of disease. The journal presently publishes twelve issues per year. In addition to more traditional research articles and letters, the journal publishes clinical reviews articles. According to the 2009 *Journal Citation Reports*, the *American Journal of Geriatric Psychiatry's* impact factor is 3.353, the ninth highest-ranked journal in the geriatrics and gerontology category. Practitioners of mental health, geriatricians, and other clinical readers form the main audience of this journal. The journal is indexed by MEDLINE, CINAHL, and Scopus. It is available online at Wolters Kluwer's Ovid/LWW website, with both table of contents service and full-text retrieval back to volume 1, 1993. This journal is appropriate for university and hospital libraries.

Journal of the American Geriatrics Society, v. 1, Wiley/American Geriatrics Society, 1953.
http://onlinelibrary.wiley.com/journal/10.1111/(ISSN)1532-5415
ISSN: 00028614
ISSN: 15325415
See Also Chapter 13.5. Geriatric Nursing
Indexed in: MEDLINE, CINAHL

Recommended For: Hospital, Academic, Consumer Health Libraries
Brandon/Hill Selection

This peer-reviewed, clinically focused journal covers principles of aging, hospital and community health care, assessment, prevention, alternative medicine, geriatric syndromes, geriatric psychiatry, and diseases and disorders. It includes articles from various disciplines such as nursing, dentistry, pharmacology, and bioscience; it also contains discussions of ethics, education, public policy, and economics. It is indexed by many leading indexing and abstracting services, including AgeLine, CINAHL, EBSCOhost (Health Source/Nursing Academic, Elite, Premier, and Complete), MEDLINE, ProQuest Health & Medical Complete, Science Citation Index, BIOSIS, and Abstracts in Social Gerontology (SAGE). *Journal Citation Reports* 2009 supplied this journal with an impact factor of 3.656, the eighth highest-ranked journal in the geriatrics and gerontology category. While the target audience is geriatricians and care providers seeking clinically reliable information, consumers and students can also find value in this resource. Given its breadth of coverage and its purposeful scholarly endeavor, this excellent journal is worthy of being included in large academic collections, scientific libraries, hospital libraries, and consumer health libraries.

Journals of Gerontology. Series A, Biological Sciences and Medical Sciences. v. 50A, Oxford/Gerontological Society of America, 1995.
http://biomedgerontology.oxfordjournals.org/
ISSN: 10795006
ISSN: 1758535X (Online)
See Also Chapter 13.5. Geriatric Nursing
Indexed in: MEDLINE, CINAHL
Recommended For: Hospital, Academic Libraries
Brandon/Hill Selection

The *Journals of Gerontology. Series A*, the official organ of the Gerontological Society of America, combines the content of two separate publications: the *Journal of Gerontology, Biological Sciences* and the *Journal of Gerontology, Medical Sciences*. The *Journals of Gerontology. Series A* offers wide-ranging coverage of the biological studies of aging and diseases, including genetics, evolutionary biology, biochemistry, pathology, and nutrition; it also incorporates clinical and basic medical research and health services research for related health fields such as nursing and dentistry. The *Journal of Gerontology, Medical Sciences* publishes original research and review essays. The journal is well received by the health and biomedical sciences academic community. It is listed as a core clinical title by NLM. *Journal Citation Reports* assigned a 2009 impact factor of 3.083. The *Journals of Gerontology. Series A* continues in part the *Journal of Gerontology*. In addition to being indexed by MEDLINE, it is also included in CINAHL and AgeLine. The editorial boards are international in scope. The present title is archived online at the Oxford Journals website back to 1995. It is available in PDF only from 1995–2000; from 2000 to the present, full-text articles in both HTML and PDF are available. The journal is recommended for hospital collections, academic libraries, and special libraries serving research institutes and government agencies.

Journals of Gerontology. Series B, Psychological Sciences and Social Sciences. v. 50B, Oxford/Gerontological Society of America, 1995.
http://psychsocgerontology.oxfordjournals.org/
ISSN: 10795014
ISSN: 17585368 (Online)
See Also Chapter 13.5. Geriatric Nursing
Indexed in: MEDLINE, CINAHL
Recommended For: Hospital, Academic Libraries
Brandon/Hill Selection

The *Journals of Gerontology. Series B* covers both the psychological sciences and the social sciences. The National Library of Medicine lists *Journals of Gerontology. Series B* as a core clinical title; in addition, this title was one of four titles recommended in the geriatrics category for the 2003 Brandon/Hill list for journals in small medical libraries. The *Journal of Gerontology, Psychological Sciences* covers an array of aspects of aging, including applied, experimental, counseling, clinical, developmental, and social psychology. The *Journal of Gerontology, Social Sciences* embraces research in the areas of anthropology, demographics, economics, public health, social work, sociology, and epidemiology. Both journals publish articles reporting original research, brief reports, reviews, and theoretical and methodological articles. The journals are ranked well by both the science and social sciences editions of the 2009 *Journal Citations Report* in the areas of geriatrics and gerontology: 17 of 40 in *JCR:Science* and six of 25 in *JCR:Social Science*. MEDLINE, AgeLine, CINAHL, various ProQuest databases, and Abstracts in Social Gerontology index this publication. *Journals of Gerontology* is traditionally well received by clinical readers, both medical and psychological, and provides excellent coverage of the various interrelated aspects of aging. This resource is appropriate for both hospital and academic libraries.

Databases and Other Electronic Resources

National Guideline Clearinghouse. Agency for Healthcare Research and Quality (AHRQ), U.S. Department of Health and Human Services, 1998
http://www.guideline.gov/
Recommended For: Hospital, Academic Libraries

The National Guideline Clearinghouse (NGC) website is a continuously updated resource. It provides access to evidence-based practice guidelines and related documents. It updates practice guidelines from professional associations and shows FDA alerts. A June 2010 search on the keyword "geriatrics" revealed 319 guidelines; a search of the keyword "dementia" retrieved 184 guidelines. These resources are created for physicians, nurses, health care plans, delivery services, and other health care organizations. The important structural components of the NGC include: (1) abstracts about the guideline and its development; (2) links to full text or descriptions of ordering information for print copies; (3) mobile device downloads of summaries; (4) ability to compare guides either through user-generated comparisons or professional staff syntheses; (5) an online forum for discussion; (6) annotated bibliographies; and (7) expert commentaries. Users can browse by disease/condition (which includes mental disorders), treatment/intervention, organization, and measures. Altogether, this is a very useful resource for updating professional association guidelines, for finding relevant information for evidence-based practice, and for contrasting and comparing resources.

9.9. Osteopathic Medicine

Therapy and medicine based on the theory that the normal body is a vital mechanical organism whose structural and functional states are of equal importance and is capable of making its own remedies against infections and toxic conditions when there are favorable environmental circumstances and adequate nutrition.

—MeSH

Contributor: Kathy Broyles

Monographs

Cranial Osteopathy: Principles and Practice. 2nd ed. Authors: Torsten Liem, John M. McPartland, Evelyn Skinner. Churchill Livingstone, 2004.
http://www.sciencedirect.com/science/book/9780443074998
ISBN: 9780443074998
Recommended for: Hospital, Academic Libraries

Cranial Osteopathy: Principles and Practice is an in-depth clinical guide to the osteopathic cranial treatment approach for common disorders affecting the head and neck. Chapters are divided by different areas of the skull, and each bone is described by its location, development, and clinical implication of dysfunction. For each of the cranial bones, there is a description of palpation, motility, and suggested techniques. Black-and-white drawings and photographs offer a step-by-step sequencing of techniques. For all cranial structures, the osteopathic methodology and treatment techniques are described. The book includes an extensive chapter on mandible and the temporomandibular joint, describing and illustrating osteopathic techniques and treatment. A glossary of cranial osteopathic terminology is included. This text is designed for the cranial osteopathic physician, student, or therapist. It would be appropriate for the hospital or academic library.

The DOs: Osteopathic Medicine in America. 2nd ed. Author: Norman Gevitz. Johns Hopkins University Press, 2004.
http://www.ebrary.com/
ISBN: 9780801878336
ISBN: 9780801878343
ISBN: 9780801897368
Recommended for: Academic, Consumer Health Libraries

Originally the author's doctoral dissertation, *The DOs: Osteopathic Medicine in America* has been in publication for over 20 years and is now in its second edition. The author has updated the 1982 text and included two new chapters, "In a Sea of Change" and "The Challenge of Distinctiveness." The text traces the history of osteopathic medicine from its inception in the 1880s by Andrew Taylor Still to present day osteopathic medicine and today's challenges. The author is a historian and professor of the history of medicine. The book is scholarly, yet easy to read. It would be of interest to physicians, students, or individuals interested in medical history. The book would be appropriate for the public or academic library.

Evidence-Based Manual Medicine: A Problem-Oriented Approach. Authors: Michael A. Seffinger, Raymond J. Hruby. Saunders, 2007.
http://www.sciencedirect.com/science/book/9781416023845

ISBN: 9781416023845
ISBN: 1416023844
Recommended for: Hospital, Academic Libraries

Evidence-Based Manual Medicine: A Problem-Oriented Approach provides an evidence-based, step-by-step manual for the treatment of somatic dysfunction. Opening chapters discuss somatic dysfunction, including its pathophysiology, biomechanics, diagnosis, and management. Other chapters include low back pain, neck and upper back pain, cervicogenic headache, temporomandibular joint dysfunction, shoulder pain, carpal tunnel syndrome, and ankle sprain. The last chapter covers manual medical coding. This text would benefit the experienced physician as well as medical students. It is appropriate for the hospital or academic library.

Foundations for Osteopathic Medicine. 2nd ed. Editors: Robert C. Ward, Raymond J. Hruby. Lippincott Williams & Wilkins, 2003.
ISBN: 9780781734974
Recommended for: Hospital, Academic Libraries

Foundations for Osteopathic Medicine is a comprehensive textbook that covers the history, philosophy, and theory of osteopathic medicine. The text covers the basic sciences, behavioral sciences, clinical problem solving, primary care, clinical specialties, and palpatory diagnosis and technique. Black-and-white illustrations and photographs help further the understanding of the various techniques used in osteopathic manipulation. The last section discusses basic and clinical research in osteopathic theory and practice. The text includes the "Glossary of Osteopathic Terminology." This book would be useful for the student of osteopathic medicine or the practicing physician, and it is appropriate for the hospital or academic library.

An Osteopathic Approach to Children. 2nd ed. Author: Jane E. Carreiro. Churchill Livingstone, 2009.
http://www.sciencedirect.com/science/book/9780443067389
ISBN: 9780443067389
Recommended for: Hospital, Academic Libraries

An Osteopathic Approach to Children is a comprehensive overview of pediatric medicine. The book is divided into two sections. The first discusses the osteopathic perspective of the physiology and development of body systems. The second section outlines pediatric pathophysiological processes, including normal changes and adaptations in structure and function. The osteopathic approach is presented, but specific techniques are not described. The book is illustrated with drawings, along with black-and-white photographs of bone and cadaver dissections. This book would be of value to individuals interested in using the osteopathic approach to treat pediatric patients, and it would also be appropriate for hospital or academic library collections.

An Osteopathic Approach to Diagnosis and Treatment. 3rd ed. Editors: Eileen L. DiGiovanna, Stanley Schiowitz, Dennis J. Dowling. Lippincott Williams & Wilkins, 2005.
ISBN: 9780781742931
Recommended for: Hospital, Academic Libraries

An *Osteopathic Approach to Diagnosis and Treatment* begins with introductory chapters on the history and philosophy of osteopathic medicine. Other chapters include somatic dysfunction, palpation, and anatomic and physiologic considerations. There is also a chapter devoted to osteopathic structural examination and documentation. The second part of the book discusses osteopathic manipulation, its history and goals. Various techniques are reviewed and illustrated with both drawings and photographs. The remaining sections discuss different areas of the body and how to evaluate and treat various conditions. Integrated throughout the text are case histories that add significantly to the volume. The last section describes the manipulative prescription and how to develop a management plan. This text would be useful for students and experienced physicians who are interested in osteopathic manipulation. It would be appropriate for the hospital or academic library.

Osteopathic Medicine: A Reformation in Progress. Editors: R. Michael Gallagher, Frederick J. Humphrey II, Marc S. Micozzi. Churchill Livingstone, 2001.
ISBN: 9780443079917
Recommended for: Academic, Consumer Health Libraries

Osteopathic Medicine: A Reformation in Progress examines the beginning of osteopathic medicine, its present role, and the future of osteopathy. The first section traces the history of medicine in America and the origins of osteopathy by Andrew Taylor Still in the late 1800s. The legal battles and fight for recognition are also covered in this section. Section two is devoted to osteopathic medicine in the present environment. Chapters include osteopathic philosophy, primary and specialty care medicine, and osteopathic medical education. The last section discusses the future of the profession. The intended audience includes current osteopathic physicians, students, and anyone interested in understanding the osteopathic medical profession. It would be appropriate for academic or public libraries.

Somatic Dysfunction in Osteopathic Family Medicine. Editors: Kenneth E. Nelson, Thomas Glonek. Lippincott Williams & Wilkins, 2007.
ISBN: 9781405104753
Recommended for: Hospital, Academic Libraries

Somatic Dysfunction in Osteopathic Family Medicine is a clinically-oriented text that addresses somatic dysfunction and the osteopathic approach to conditions other than musculoskeletal pain. The first section discusses the diagnosis of somatic dysfunction and the manipulative prescription. The second section talks about the different kinds of patients an osteopathic physician may encounter and the care that is unique to these patient groups. Patient groups covered include the psychiatric, pediatric, female, surgical, athletic, geriatric, and end-of-life patients. The third section covers conditions such as otitis media, gastrointestinal problems, hypertension, temporomandibular joint pain, respiratory infections, and congestive heart failure, along with many others. The last section discusses practice issues such as coding and the standardized medical record. This text would be of interest to osteopathic physicians and students. It would be appropriate for the academic or hospital library.

Journals

International Journal of Osteopathic Medicine. v. 8, Elsevier, 2005.
http://www.sciencedirect.com/science/journal/17460689
ISSN: 17460689
Indexed in: CINAHL
Recommended for: Hospital, Academic Libraries

The *International Journal of Osteopathic Medicine* is a peer-reviewed journal from the Australian Osteopathic Association. The scope is research and review articles relating to the principles and practice of osteopathic medicine and neuromusculoskeletal medicine. Particular emphasis is on basic science research, epidemiology, and health social science. The journal is indexed in CINAHL, Embase, Scopus, and Web of Science.

The Journal of the American Osteopathic Association: JAOA. v. 1, American Osteopathic Association, 1901.
http://www.jaoa.org/
ISSN: 00986151
Indexed in: MEDLINE, CINAHL
Recommended for: Hospital, Academic Libraries

The Journal of the American Osteopathic Association (*JAOA*) is the official scientific publication of the American Osteopathic Association (AOA). It is the oldest, continuously published osteopathic journal, having begun publication in 1901. This peer-reviewed journal is published monthly. The content includes basic and clinical research, review articles, case reports, and commentaries on the osteopathic profession. It also includes articles on medical education and special communications. On an annual basis, *JAOA* publishes the abstracts from the American Osteopathic Association conference. It is indexed in MEDLINE and OSTMED.DR (Osteopathic Medicine Digital Repository).

Osteopathic Family Physician. v. 1, Elsevier Science, 2009.
http://www.osteopathicfamilyphysician.org/
ISSN: 1877573X
Recommended for: Hospital, Academic Libraries

Osteopathic Family Physician is the official publication of the American College of Osteopathic Family Physicians. The ACOFP has published various newsletters and journals over the past 58 years. The current publication, *Osteopathic Family Physician*, replaces *Osteopathic Family Physician News* that was published from 2001 to May/June 2009. This bimonthly, peer-reviewed scientific journal covers topics such as family medicine research, public health, osteopathic principles and practices, pain management, medical education, practice management, and organizational news.

Osteopathic Medicine and Primary Care. v. 1, BioMed Central, 2007.
http://www.om-pc.com/
http://www.ncbi.nlm.nih.gov/pmc/journals/467/
ISSN: 17504732
Recommended for: Hospital, Academic, Consumer Health Libraries

Osteopathic Medicine and Primary Care is an open access, peer-reviewed journal published online at BioMed Central. Content includes research articles, review articles, commentaries, short reports, and study protocols. The scope of the journal includes all aspects of family medicine, internal medicine, pediatrics, obstetrics and gynecology, osteopathic medicine, techniques, and treatment. It is indexed in CINAHL Plus, PubMed (but not MEDLINE), and Scopus.

Databases and Other Electronic Resources

OSTMED.DR. American Osteopathic Association and the American Association of Colleges of Osteopathic Medicine, 2007.
http://www.ostmed-dr.com
Recommended for: Hospital, Academic Libraries

OSTMED.DR (Osteopathic Medicine Digital Repository) is the only searchable index devoted totally to osteopathic literature. This freely available osteopathic medicine digital library was developed in response to the cessation in 2003 of OSTMED, a bibliographic osteopathic medicine index. OSTMED.DR is supported by the American Osteopathic Association (AOA), the American Association of Colleges of Osteopathic Medicine (AACOM), and the Virginia College of Osteopathic Medicine (VCOM). OSTMED.DR combines citations with selected full-text coverage for books, journals, video, and images.

9.10. Psychiatry

The origin, diagnosis, prevention, and treatment of mental disorders.

—MeSH

Contributor: Tagalie Heister

Monographs

Clinical Neurology for Psychiatrists. 6th ed. Author: David M. Kaufman. Saunders Elsevier, 2007.
http://www.mdconsult.com/
ISBN: 9781416030744
Recommended for: Hospital, Academic Libraries

This is the newest edition of a work that has been a definitive text for board review for psychiatrists, and it continues to provide a concise, yet complete, overview of clinical neurology with special attention to those conditions that have co-morbidity or mimic psychiatric disorders. Well organized and thorough, this text works well for both board preparation and for clinicians who regularly encounter neurologically-related issues in their psychiatric patient care. It includes office and bedside diagnosis, clinical assessment tools, detailed descriptions of all conditions covered, differential diagnosis, and treatment recommendations. Also covered are topics related to medical ethics and medico-legal concerns, especially with regard to vegetative states and capacity. The work includes 1,600 sample questions similar to those found in the neurology section of the psychiatry board exam. Online access is offered through MD Consult's psychiatry e-books collection.

Diagnostic and Statistical Manual of Mental Disorders: DSM-IV-TR. 4th ed., text revision. Editor: American Psychiatric Association. American Psychiatric Publishing, 2000.
http://www.psychiatryonline.com/
ISBN: 9780890420249
ISBN: 9780890420256
See Also Chapter 30.3. Diagnosis
Brandon/Hill, *Doody's Core Titles* Selection
Recommended for: Hospital, Academic, Consumer Health Libraries

This is the complete multiaxial classification system for mental disorders including codes and diagnostic criteria that is used as the standard by all mental health professionals in the United States. This is the fourth major revision of the official diagnostic manual of the American Psychiatric Association (APA). The fifth revision is expected in May 2012, and its preparation has been a joint endeavor of the APA and the National Institute of Mental Health. This book is essential for all hospital, academic, and mental health libraries. It would also be of interest for consumer health settings. Print and electronic formats are available from American Psychiatric Publishing.

Kaplan & Sadock's Synopsis of Psychiatry: Behavioral Sciences/Clinical Psychiatry. 10th ed. Authors: Benjamin J. Sadock, Virginia A. Sadock. Wolters Kluwer/Lippincott Williams & Wilkins, 2007.
ISBN: 9780781773270
Recommended for: Hospital, Academic Libraries
Brandon/Hill, *Doody's Core Titles* Selection

The Kaplan and Sadock series of psychiatry textbooks consists of three versions, including the complete, two-volume version, this synopsis, and a concise "pocket" version. With over 1,300 pages of text, the synopsis offers a practical, yet comprehensive, review of all aspects of psychiatric medicine. There is broad subject coverage addressing topics such as normal development, the brain and behavior, clinical examination of psychiatric patients, psychiatric rating scales, and ethics. Overviews of clinical disorders are comprehensive, including both historical and theoretical information along with epidemiological, demographic, and treatment content. The text includes sections on specific populations such as children, adolescents, and the aged. It is both *DSM* (*Diagnostic and Statistical Manual of Mental Disorders*) and *ICD* (*International Classification of Diseases*) compatible. The book is targeted to physicians, especially psychiatrists, and other mental health professionals and students in those fields. Along with the *DSM*, it is the one resource that all medical libraries and mental health practitioners should have on hand.

Learning Cognitive-Behavior Therapy: An Illustrated Guide. 1st ed. Authors: Jesse H. Wright, Monica R. Basco, Michael E. Thase. American Psychiatric Publishing, 2006.
See Chapter 9.4. Behavioral Medicine

Manic-Depressive Illness: Bipolar Disorders and Recurrent Depression. 2nd ed. Authors: Frederick K. Goodwin, Kay R. Jamison. Oxford University Press, 2007.
http://www.statref.com/
ISBN: 9780195135794
Recommended for: Academic, Consumer Health Libraries

Recognized as the definitive work on manic-depressive illness, this book has been well received by clinicians as well as mental health consumers and their families. Bringing together state-of-the-art information from scientific research on neuropathology to the latest information on effective treatments, this text has everything that is currently understood about this disorder. Covering such topics as the biology and genetics of bipolar disorder, epidemiology, differential diagnosis, evidence-based clinical management, biological and somatic therapies, therapeutic alliance, and suicidality, this is an important resource for psychiatrists and other mental health providers, primary care physicians, neuroscientists, and consumers with manic-depressive illness and their families. This edition of the book was the 2008 winner of the American Medical Writers Association's Medical Book Award.

Psychiatric Interview: A Practical Guide. 2nd ed. Author: Daniel J. Carlat. Lippincott Williams & Wilkins, 2005.
http://www.ovid.com/
http://www.statref.com/
ISBN: 9780781751865
Recommended for: Academic Libraries
Brandon/Hill, *Doody's Core Titles* Selection

This is an excellent handbook for learning how to do a basic psychiatric interview and how to handle special patient populations and special interview situations. Sections include how to obtain a good psychiatric history, how to perform a diagnostic interview, and how to interview patients in order to provide the most appropriate treatment. Other sections address the therapeutic alliance and writing up the results of the interview. Additional chapters cover such timely topics as determining malingering, assessing suicidal ideation, and evaluating patients for attention deficit disorder. This resource includes forms and handouts that can be copied for use in the patient setting. A volume in the *Practical Guides in Psychiatry* series, it is written for mental health providers, physicians and nonphysicians, as well as students in those fields.

Stahl's Essential Psychopharmacology: Neuroscientific Basis and Practical Applications. 3rd ed. Author: Stephen M. Stahl. Cambridge University Press, 2008.
http://stahlonline.cambridge.org/
http://www.cambridge.org/9780521673761
ISBN: 9780521857024
ISBN: 9780521673761
ISBN: 9780521746090
See Also Chapter 17. Pharmacology
Recommended for: Hospital, Academic, Consumer Health Libraries

Intended to be used by the prescribing mental health clinician, this popular text is both theoretical and practical. It includes text and graphical explanations of the neurobiological basis of psychiatric medications and contains extensive lists of references, making this extremely complex and dynamic scientific field meaningful to the everyday practice of psychiatry. *Stahl's* provides the current state-of-the-art information on the mechanisms of action for specific medications and classes of medications. Because the author has been able to present this material in such a clear and understandable fashion, this text is also very readable for nonphysicians seeking a clearer understanding of psychotropic medications. The product is available in many formats: digital, online, or print, or a combination of these. It should be noted that this is an authored text rather than the work of a reviewing committee of experts; however, it is a work of considerable quality, providing detailed and comprehensible explanations of neurobiology in health and disease and the psychopharmacologic action of psychotropic medications.

Textbook of Psychotherapeutic Treatments. Editor: Glen O. Gabbard. American Psychiatric Publishing, 2008.
http://www.psychiatryonline.com/
ISBN: 9781585623044
ISBN: 9781585623648
Recommended for: Academic Libraries

This is a scholarly, but practical, overview of today's state-of-the-art psychotherapy. Edited by the well-respected and much-published psychiatrist Glen Gabbard—with the input of fifty proponents of various schools of psychotherapeutics—this definitive work covers, among other topics, theory, process, and treatment efficacy. All modalities are included: individual, conjoint, and group. The scientific basis for recommendations is provided, and ethical issues in psychotherapy, including professional boundaries issues, are covered in depth. Case vignettes and examples are included to provide further instruction. This text is recommended for both those training in the fields of psychotherapy and for experienced clinicians who seek to improve their knowledge and expertise in this area.

Journals

American Journal of Psychiatry. v. 78, American Psychiatric Association, 1921.
http://ajp.psychiatryonline.org/
ISSN: 0002953X
ISSN: 15357228 (Online)
Indexed in: MEDLINE, CINAHL
Recommended for: Hospital, Academic, Consumer Health Libraries
Brandon/Hill Selection

Originally published as the *American Journal of Insanity*, the *American Journal of Psychiatry* has been in continuous publication since 1844. This official journal of the American Psychiatric Association (APA) is an essential publication for any medical library collection. The peer-reviewed *American Journal of Psychiatry* is published monthly and includes APA official reports, APA practice guidelines, and timely articles on all topics related to psychiatry. It also includes letters to the editor and book reviews. A section titled "Treatment in Psychiatry Series" provides case vignettes of common diagnoses with reviews of relevant research and treatment recommendations. Every online issue includes a downloadable, 30-minute MP3 program that contains highlights from the issue, and there is a CME option for physicians. Subscriptions include electronic access to major articles in advance of print. In 2009, ISI's *Journal Citation Reports* listed this journal as having a 12.522 impact factor and ranked it second in their listing of psychiatry journals indexed.

Archives of General Psychiatry. v. 3, American Medical Association, 1960.
http://archpsyc.ama-assn.org/
ISSN: 0003990X
ISSN: 15383636 (Online)
Indexed in: MEDLINE
Recommended for: Hospital, Academic Libraries
Brandon/Hill Selection

This journal was published as the *A.M.A. Archives of General Psychiatry* until 1959. Beginning in 1960 as the *Archives of General Psychiatry*, this journal has established an international reputation and, in 2009, had the third highest impact factor, 12.257, among psychiatric journals according to ISI's *Journal Citation Reports*. Providing articles that present original and timely research, this journal is geared toward clinical psychiatrists and research scientists. Its emphasis is on scientific inquiry, and it endeavors to provide clinicians with the latest findings in clinical and bench research. This resource is essential for hospital and academic libraries.

Evidence-Based Mental Health. v. 1, BMJ Publishing Group, 1998.
http://ebmh.bmj.com/
ISSN: 13620347
ISSN: 1468960X (Online)
Indexed in: MEDLINE, CINAHL
Recommended for: Academic Libraries

This quarterly publication, one of the British Medical Journal Group's evidence-based products, provides evaluative reviews of research that has recently appeared in a wide range of international journals covering topics relevant to mental health. Studies reviewed include all ages and diagnoses. The concise reviews of research methodology, precision, and results provide psychiatrists and other mental health providers with qualitative information that informs evidence-based practice. *EBMH* also serves as an excellent resource for keeping abreast of the latest research findings. It is an appropriate and important resource for all mental health providers and the libraries that serve them.

Psychological Medicine. v. 1, Cambridge University, 1970.
See Chapter 20. Medical Psychology

Psychosomatic Medicine. v. 1, Lippincott Williams & Wilkins, 1939.
See Chapter 20. Medical Psychology

Databases and Other Electronic Resources

PsychiatryOnline. American Psychiatric Publishing, 2005.
http://www.psychiatryonline.com
Recommended for: Hospital, Academic Libraries

PsychiatryOnline provides electronic access to a superior core collection of critical resources for the practice of psychiatry, including the *DSM-IV-TR*, all the American Psychiatric Association (APA) Practice Guidelines, the *American Psychiatric Publishing Textbook of Psychiatry*, and seven of the APA and American Psychiatric Press journals: *American Journal of Psychiatry*, *Psychiatric*

Services, *Academic Psychiatry*, *Journal of Neuropsychiatry and Clinical Neurosciences*, *Psychosomatics*, and *Psychiatric News*. This searchable and comprehensive resource is invaluable for academic libraries as well as practicing psychiatrists in settings that do not have extensive libraries. For academic libraries, the Legacy Collection version of the product is essential, as it contains all the back issues of the collection's journals. The search feature is not highly specific, but this product is valuable for its inclusiveness. Options are also available for mobile devices. It includes psychiatric medication information handouts for adults and children. PsychiatryOnline offers full online access to one of its featured new publications each month. It also provides key articles from several of its journals in advance of the print.

9.10.1. Biological Psychiatry

The biological bases of behavior—biochemical, genetic, physiological, and neurological—and applying these to the understanding and treatment of mental illness.

—MeSH

Contributor: Tagalie Heister

Monographs

Clinical Handbook of Psychiatry & the Law. 4th ed. Authors: Paul S. Applebaum, Thomas G. Gutheil. Wolters Kluwer/Lippincott Williams & Wilkins, 2007.
See Chapter 9.10.4. Forensic Psychiatry

Journals

Archives of General Psychiatry. v. 3, American Medical Association, July 1960.
See Chapter 9.10. Psychiatry

Journal of Clinical Psychiatry. v. 39, Physicians Postgraduate Press, Jan 1978.
http://www.psychiatrist.com/
ISSN: 01606689
ISSN: 15552101 (Online)
Indexed in: MEDLINE
Recommended for: Hospital, Academic Libraries

Originally published as *Diseases of the Nervous System*, this significant, monthly journal provides peer-reviewed articles selected for relevance to clinical practice and biological treatments of mental disorders in particular. Its frequent supplements provide timely, topical overviews. Geared toward psychiatrists and other medical professionals, the journal publishes articles related to all age groups and psychiatric disorders. A valuable resource for libraries providing services to psychiatrists, the *Journal of Clinical Psychiatry* also offers direct continuing medical education opportunities for physicians.

Psychosomatics: The Journal of Consultation and Liaison Psychiatry. v. 1, American Psychiatric Publishing, 1960.
http://psy.psychiatryonline.org/
ISSN: 00333182
ISSN: 15457206 (Online)
Indexed in: MEDLINE
Recommended for: Hospital, Academic Libraries

Psychosomatics, the official journal of the Academy of Psychosomatic Medicine, is one of the journals published by American Psychiatric Publishing, the American Psychiatric Association's publishing venture. It is also available through their electronic product PsychiatryOnline. The journal provides peer-reviewed articles on topics relevant to co-morbid psychiatric and medical illness. Articles include major research reviews as well as case reports, letters, articles on emergency trends, and book reviews. A regular column provides reviews of psychopharmacological issues regarding treatment for comorbid disorders. This title is particularly important to general hospitals as well as those specializing in mental disorders, all mental health practitioners, and primary care health providers who often see these disorders in their clinical settings.

9.10.2. Child and Adolescent Psychiatry

The origin, diagnosis, prevention, and treatment of mental disorders in children and in individuals 13–18 years.

—Adapted from MeSH: Child Psychiatry, Adolescent Psychiatry

Contributor: Tagalie Heister

Monographs

Diagnostic and Statistical Manual of Mental Disorders: DSM-IV-TR. 4th ed., text revision. Editor: American Psychiatric Association. American Psychiatric Association, 2000.
See Chapter 9.10. Psychiatry

Dulcan's Textbook of Child and Adolescent Psychiatry. Editor: Mina K. Dulcan. American Psychiatric Publishing, 2010.
http://www.psychiatryonline.com/
ISBN: 9781585623235

ISBN: 9781585623921 (Online)
Recommended for: Hospital, Academic Libraries

This new publication is offered as both an online, monthly-updated version and a print textbook. It replaces the 2004 *Textbook of Child and Adolescent Psychiatry* edited by Jerry M. Wiener and Mina K. Dulcan, also from American Psychiatric Publishing. Containing 65 chapters by 110 contributors, this provides a new, comprehensive resource for clinicians and trainees in psychiatry, child and adolescent psychiatry, pediatrics, and behavioral pediatrics. Although it contains a substantial amount of background and theoretical materials, the emphasis is on treatment, making it a practical choice as the one major reference work for child and adolescent clinicians.

Lewis's Child and Adolescent Psychiatry: A Comprehensive Textbook. 4th ed. Editors: Andrés Martin, Fred R. Volkmar. Lippincott Williams & Wilkins, 2007.
http://www.ovid.com/
http://www.r2library.com/
ISBN: 9780781762144
Recommended for: Hospital, Academic Libraries
Brandon/Hill, *Doody's Core Titles* Selection

Editor emeritus Melvin Lewis's standard work on child and adolescent psychiatry is now in its fourth edition, updated by editors Andrés Martin and Fred Volkmar, two of Lewis's colleagues at the Yale Child Study Center. The latest edition is listed in *Doody's Core Titles*, and the previous edition appeared in the last Brandon/Hill list. This book is available in print, accompanied by a companion website with searchable full text, or as an e-book from Ovid or R2 Library; the print version is easier to use. This book is designed for teaching, critical thinking, and detailed study of child and adolescent psychiatry; it is widely used for examination review (a set of board review questions based on this text is also published separately). The editor's compelling, heartfelt introduction, "An Approach to the Discipline," explains why he was attracted to this field and discusses different ways of thinking about child and adolescent psychiatry, the interplay between nature and nurture, the evidence basis for treatment, historical perspectives, education and training, public policy, and financial matters. The seven sections of this volume outline a "modern" approach, emphasizing scientific foundations, normal development, clinical relevance, and the interface between psychiatry, other scientific disciplines, and social institutions. Sections on scientific foundations, normal and pathological development, classification and assessment, specific disorders and syndromes, treatment, and interface areas of child and adolescent psychiatry follow the editor's introduction. A postscript reflects on the history of the discipline. Normal adolescent development and psychopathology are discussed in detail. Although this work encompasses children as well as adolescents, coverage specific to adolescents is substantial for key topics such as gender identity, eating disorders, personality disorders, suicidal behavior, and legal issues. This book is highly recommended for libraries and mental health practice settings needing a scholarly, in-depth textbook on child and adolescent psychiatry.

Principles and Practice of Child and Adolescent Forensic Mental Health. Editors: Elissa P. Benedek, Peter Ash, Charles L. Scott. American Psychiatric, 2010.
See Chapter 9.10.4. Forensic Psychiatry

Journals

Child and Adolescent Psychiatric Clinics of North America. v. 1, Saunders/Elsevier, 1992.
http://childpsych.theclinics.com/
http://www.sciencedirect.com/science/journal/10564993
http://www.mdconsult.com/
ISSN: 10564993 (Print/Online)
Indexed in: MEDLINE
Recommended for: Hospital, Academic Libraries

Each volume of this quarterly monographic series is devoted to a specific subject and produced by a guest editor. It is indexed by MEDLINE, PsycINFO, and Excerpta Medica. According to the journal's website, this series "updates you on the latest trends in patient management; keeps you up to date on the newest advances; and provides a sound basis for choosing treatment options." Although this title has a psychiatric focus, many of the articles—on issues such as anxiety, depression, and substance abuse—are useful for multidisciplinary research, practice, and teaching. This journal is recommended for clinical or academic graduate- or postgraduate-level collections with an emphasis on child and adolescent psychiatry or psychosocial issues.

Journal of Clinical Child and Adolescent Psychiatry. v. 31, Routledge, 2002.
See Chapter 10.15.3. Preventive Psychiatry

Journal of the American Academy of Child & Adolescent Psychiatry. v. 26, Elsevier, 1987.
http://www.jaacap.com
http://www.sciencedirect.com/science/journal/08908567
http://www.mdconsult.com/

ISSN: 08908567
ISSN: 15275418 (Online)
Indexed in: MEDLINE
Recommended for: Hospital, Academic Libraries

As the major journal in the field of child and adolescent mental health, the *Journal of the American Academy of Child & Adolescent Psychiatry* is published monthly and is the best single source for keeping abreast of new information in the field. Coverage is broad and includes research, clinical practice, applied brain imaging, evidence-based practice, efficacy of psychopharmacologies and psychotherapeutics, mental health service and treatment effectiveness, and health policy and advocacy. The journal also includes editorials and book reviews. The American Academy publishes its official Practice Parameters in the journal and, in recent years, there have been excellent evidence-based practice reviews. This is an essential publication for anyone in the field of child or adolescent mental health and for those in pediatric practice who strive to keep abreast of child and adolescent mental health treatment and issues.

9.10.3. Community Psychiatry

The provision and delivery of a coordinated program of mental health care to a specified population. The foci included in this concept are all social, psychological and physical factors related to etiology, prevention, and maintaining positive mental health in the community.

—MeSH

Contributor: Tagalie Heister

Journals

Psychiatric Services. v. 46, American Psychiatric Association, 1995.
http://ps.psychiatryonline.org
ISSN: 10752730
ISSN: 15579700 (Online)
Indexed in: MEDLINE, CINAHL
Recommended for: Hospital, Academic, Consumer Health Libraries

Psychiatric Services, originally published as *Hospital and Community Psychiatry* beginning in 1950, provides peer-reviewed articles on mental health and its treatments. Of special interest are issues related to systems of care, model treatment programs, and, in particular, improvements to the care of psychiatric patients and those with mental disabilities. It is geared toward all mental health professionals and is essential for facilities that provide services to those with mental illnesses or mental disabilities.

9.10.4. Forensic Psychiatry

Psychiatry in its legal aspects. This includes criminology, penology, commitment of mentally ill, the psychiatrist's role in compensation cases, the problems of releasing information to the court, and of expert testimony.

—MeSH

Contributors: Kristine M. Alpi, Tagalie Heister, and Robert Sotak

Monographs

Clinical Handbook of Psychiatry & the Law. 4th ed. Authors: Paul S. Applebaum, Thomas G. Gutheil. Wolters Kluwer/Lippincott Williams & Wilkins, 2007.
http://www.ovid.com/
ISBN: 9780781778916
Recommended for: Hospital, Academic Libraries
Doody's Core Titles Selection

Medico-legal issues in the field of mental health are challenging and complicated. Written by two of the leading forensic psychiatrists in the United States, this resource provides useful overviews of many of the areas in which the law and psychiatry come together. Coverage includes confidentiality, emergency psychiatry issues such as detaining at-risk patients, competency in legal actions or in decision making, advice for expert testimony, assessing suicidality and capacity, and many others. This is the authoritative source for both clinicians and attorneys, written so that both audiences can easily understand the terminology and the issues. It is an important work for any hospital collection and all medical and legal academic libraries.

Principles and Practice of Child and Adolescent Forensic Mental Health. Editors: Elissa P. Benedek, Peter Ash, Charles L. Scott. American Psychiatric Publishing, 2010.
ISBN: 9781585623365
Recommended for: Hospital, Academic, Consumer Health Libraries

Edited by academic psychiatrists, two of whom direct Psychiatry and Law services, this work authoritatively addresses legal and ethical issues surrounding the mental health of young patients. Authors cover forensic evaluation, child abuse, and juvenile offenders as well as litigation concerns, including depositions and courtroom testimony. Expanded from the 2002 edition of *Principles and Practice of Child and Adolescent Forensic Psychiatry* which won the 2003 Manfred S. Guttmacher Award from the American Psychiatric Association and the American Academy of Psychiatry and the Law, many of its chapters have been entirely rewritten by new authors to provide fresh insight into such topics as child custody; juvenile law; abuse, neglect, and permanent wardship cases; transcultural, transracial, and gay/lesbian parenting and adoption; and the reliability and suggestibility of children's statements. A chapter on psychological autopsy covers evaluation of the circumstances surrounding pediatric suicides, describing various types of equivocal deaths and discussing legal issues such as admissibility of the autopsy in court. This is a valuable reference not only for practitioners in all areas of mental health and forensic medicine and nursing, but also for attorneys and judges. Another useful title in forensic mental health not limited to children is *Psychological Evaluations for the Courts, Third Edition: A Handbook for Mental Health Professionals and Lawyers* by Gary B. Melton, John Petrila, Norman G. Poythress, and Christopher Slobogin (Guilford Press; 3rd ed. 2007).

9.10.5. Geriatric Psychiatry

The mental health of the aged.

—MeSH

Contributor: Tagalie Heister

Monographs

American Psychiatric Publishing Textbook of Geriatric Psychiatry. 4th ed. Editors: Dan G. Blazer, David C. Steffens. American Psychiatric Publishing, 2009.
http://www.psychiatryonline.com/
ISBN: 9781585622771
See Also Chapter 9.8 Geriatrics
Recommended for: Hospital, Academic Libraries

This comprehensive work provides an authoritative, substantive review of geriatric psychiatry. It is written for those in academic institutions as well as clinicians, psychiatrists, and nonpsychiatrists who provide care to geriatric patients. This single source covers the essentials of the field, including the scientific basis of understanding mental disorders in aging, clinical disorders of the elderly, differential diagnoses, somatic and biological therapies, as well as psychosocial factors, systems of care issues, and medico-legal problems. This fourth edition provides the latest scientific information critical to understanding and treating psychiatric disorders of geriatric patients. It is recommended for all libraries serving facilities with geriatric patients and for all clinicians who provide care to the elderly.

Journals

American Journal of Geriatric Psychiatry. v. 1, Lippincott Williams & Wilkins, 1993.
http://journals.lww.com/ajgponline/pages/default.aspx
ISSN: 10647481
ISSN: 15457214 (Online)
See Also Chapter 9.8. Geriatrics
Recommended for: Hospital, Academic Libraries

This monthly publication is the official journal of the American Association for Geriatric Psychiatry (AAGP). It publishes clinically focused articles dealing with issues related to mental disorders of the aged. It contains peer-reviewed articles related to all aspects of geriatric psychiatry, including diagnosis, classification, epidemiology, psychopharmacologic treatments, and somatic therapies. Abstracts of the AAGP annual meetings are published as a supplement to this title. It is an important title for hospital and academic libraries as well as libraries that support institutions that provide services to the elderly.

9.11. Social Medicine

The role of socio-environmental factors in the occurrence, prevention and treatment of disease.

—MeSH

Contributor: Paul Elliott Dahl

Monographs

America's Social Health: Putting Social Issues Back on the Public Agenda. 1st ed. Authors: Marque-Luisa Miringoff, Sandra Opdycke. M.E. Sharpe, 2008.
ISBN: 9780765616746
Recommended for: Academic Libraries

This thought-provoking book issues a clarion call for the development of 16 social health indicators as measures to judge America's performance in social health. The authors clearly communicate that such a report of social conditions is rooted in the past (specifically in President Lyndon Johnson's administration and in unpassed legislation proposed by Senator Walter Mondale in 1967) and their initial effort of the Index of Social Health may be only the beginning of a further refined set of measures. The book has nine chapters and several supportive appendixes. The first four chapters deal with the importance of social reporting while the final five cogently present the key indicators of social health for children, youth, adults, the elderly, and for all ages. Tables and graphs are interspersed throughout the book and are effective in aiding reader comprehension and depth of knowledge. The interrelatedness and interplay of economic and social forces undoubtedly impact the health of individuals and groups within a nation-state; only by visibly viewing the social health indicators needing improvement may policy makers see the need to address social ills. While this book may not be well known, those in the field of social medicine know that its power lies in the realization that the institutional integration of social indicators may truly live on the same plane of importance as economic indicators in the future.

Social and Behavioral Foundations of Public Health. 2nd ed. Editor: Jeannine Coreil. Sage, 2009.
ISBN: 9781412957045
Recommended for: Academic Libraries

This foundational textbook examines public health from a social and behavioral sciences perspective. The book utilizes a "social ecological framework to address multilevel influences on health and enlarge the dominant risk factor approach to health behavior." The work is organized into six broad sections. The first section provides an introductory overview to social epidemiology and historical perspectives. The second section outlines the theoretical foundations of the social environment and health and illness. The third section addresses the sociocultural context of health with some cultural comparisons. The fourth section elucidates a life span perspective in examining three particular populations at different states of the life cycle. The fifth section deals with health promotion and policy advocacy. The last section presents special topics of public health concern with a focus on problem analysis and intervention design. A significant strength of this book is that it draws from a number of disciplines such as medical sociology, health psychology, medical anthropology, demographics, gerontology, and economics to create an interdisciplinary work. The book is illustrated and has effective case studies. The second edition has been thoroughly updated and revised with new content. While this is intended as a textbook for graduate students, it will also be highly useful to public health practitioners and other health professionals wanting a comprehensive examination of social medicine.

Social Injustice and Public Health. Editors: Barry S. Levy, Victor W. Sidel. Oxford University Press, 2006.
http://www.ebrary.com/
ISBN: 9780195384062
ISBN: 9780195171853
Recommended for: Academic Libraries

This invaluable primer uncovers many aspects of the linkage between social injustice and ill health by masterfully documenting the inequities in the social and economic well-being of children and their families. The book is organized into five parts. Part 1 gives the reader an introductory summary of social injustice. Part 2 explains in specific detail how the health of specific population groups is adversely impacted by social injustice. Part 3 examines how social injustice affects relevant health states such as infectious diseases, chronic diseases, mental health, and environmental health. Part 4 provides some needed prescriptions on how social injustice can be overcome. The editors have done a marvelous job of selecting the contributing authors since the book holds together as a whole and also as the sum of individual chapters standing by themselves. The illustrations used in the book are effective and keep the reader engaged. This book is a required resource for any public health professional and student in a public health program. It is also highly recommended for academic institutions since health professionals and other disciplines will appreciate how socio-economic factors influence individual and population health.

The Social Medicine Reader. 2nd ed. Editors: Nancy M.P. King, Ronald P. Strauss, Larry R. Churchill, Sue E. Estroff, Gail E. Henderson, Jonathan Oberlander. Duke University Press, 2005.
ISBN: 9780822335689 (v.1)
ISBN: 9780822335931 (v.2)
ISBN: 9780822335696 (v.3)
Recommended for: Hospital, Academic, Consumer Health Libraries

This three-volume set successfully chronicles the interplay and interaction of medicine on society and how the economic, political, social, and cultural forces existing in societal structures also impact the medical profession itself. Volume 1 covers the terrain of illness, the physician-patient relationship, health care ethics, and end of life issues. Volume 2 deals with how health and illness are viewed in the milieus of ethnicity, race, gender, and class. Volume 3 examines the health care market with its deficiencies and disadvantages and presents some pressing health policy issues needing to be addressed. The anthology contains both fiction and nonfiction selections in the multidisciplinary framework it creates by skillfully blending poetry, scholarly essays, case studies, works of fiction, medical reports, and personal narratives in its pages. There are some black-and-white illustrations found in the anthology. The readings in this work originally were brought together to support a year-long interdisciplinary course for first-year medical students at the University of North Carolina. This three-volume work is recommended for all academic collections having programs in medicine or other health care disciplines. It will also be suitable for hospital libraries and public libraries as well. It is a must read for public health professionals.

Journals

Health & Place: An International Journal. v. 1, Elsevier, 1995.
http://www.sciencedirect.com/science/journal/13538292
ISSN: 13538292
ISSN: 18732054 (Online)
Indexed in: MEDLINE, CINAHL
Recommended for: Academic Libraries

This bi-monthly journal published by Elsevier is dedicated to "the study of all aspects of health and health care in which place or location matters." The points of contact between geography, sociology, health policy, public health, and epidemiology lead to diverse convergences that affect both individual and community health in positive and negative ways. The role of the built environment is explored and evaluated so that practices in human construction, neighborhood development, and urban renewal are changed to improve health on many levels. This journal is suitable for academic institutions in general and for public health professionals, in particular those concerned with reducing the negative environmental impact of human-designed communities. This journal had an impact factor of 2.993 in 2009 and ranked eighth out of 76 journals in the public, environmental, and occupational health category (*Journal Citation Reports*). This journal is cited in several abstracting and indexing sources such as MEDLINE, CINAHL, Current Contents, and Sociological Abstracts. Full online coverage goes back to volume 1, 1995 through Elsevier ScienceDirect.

Social Science & Medicine. v. 16, Elsevier Pergamon, 1982.
http://www.sciencedirect.com/science/journal/02779536
ISSN: 02779536
ISSN: 18735347 (Online)
See Also Chapter 21. Medical Sociology
Indexed in: MEDLINE, CINAHL
Recommended for: Academic Libraries

This journal "provides an international and interdisciplinary forum for the dissemination of social science research on health." Original, peer-reviewed empirical and theoretical articles, reviews, position papers, and commentaries are found in this journal. Social scientists, health professionals, and policy makers are the main audience for this journal, which is the most cited social science journal over the last decade. The 2009 *Journal Citation Reports* impact factor for this journal is 2.710. This journal is cited in numerous abstracting and indexing sources including MEDLINE and CINAHL. This journal is highly recommended for public health professionals and academic institutions. Full online coverage to volume 16, 1982 is available through Elsevier ScienceDirect.

9.12. Sports Medicine

Physical fitness and the diagnosis and treatment of injuries sustained in sports activities.

—MeSH

Contributor: Linda M. Hartman

Monographs

Athletic Training and Sports Medicine. 4th ed. Editors: Glen Johnson, Chad Starkey. Jones & Bartlett, 2006.
ISBN: 9780763705367
Recommended for: Hospital, Academic Libraries

The twenty-four chapters are divided into three sections: overview, regional pathologies (management of injuries for each major body part), and specific populations (pediatric, adolescent, aging athlete, industrial setting, and athletes with different abilities). The appendix provides a list of manufacturer information for products referenced in the book. The index/glossary is a conventional index with embedded definitions for some terms. The inside front cover can be used as a quick reference for finding surgical and clinical techniques. The 4th edition reflects advances in diagnostic and surgical techniques as well as increased focus on prevention. The reader is expected to understand anatomy, clinical diagnostic skills, acute injury management, and therapeutic modalities and exercise. Each chapter begins with a listing of topics and the starting page, which allows the user to zone in on needed information. Text layout—along with plenty of tables, figures, and images—makes it easier to locate and understand the information provided. References are listed at the end of each chapter. *Athletic Training and Sports Medicine* is a valuable resource for any professional interested in the physical medicine and rehabilitation of musculoskeletal injuries.

Evidence-Based Sports Medicine. 2nd ed. Editors: Domhnall MacAuley, Thomas M. Best. BMJ/Blackwell, 2007.
http://extranet.netlibrary.com/TitleSelect/
ISBN: 9781405132985
ISBN: 9780470994214 (Online)
Recommended for: Hospital, Academic Libraries

The focus of this second edition is the clinical examination using an evidence-based approach. Past practices have been based on those who came before, not evidence found through research. That has changed, and the evidence is reflected in this text. The topics were chosen to represent the field's growth and potential for further research. The 30 chapters are arranged by six headings: prevention, acute injury, chronic conditions, injuries to the upper limb, injuries to the groin and knee, and injuries to the lower leg. Each chapter has an extensive list of references as well as some or all of the following: a set of multiple choice questions with answers, a list of essay questions, case studies, recommendations for clinical practice, future research, a summary, or key messages. The descriptions of studies give detailed methodologies, including the databases that were searched and the search strategies used; the inclusion and exclusion criteria were also included. These descriptions look like those seen in systematic reviews; in fact, the first chapter is a systematic review. *Evidence-Based Sports Medicine* is written for students and those practicing in the field.

Physical Rehabilitation of the Injured Athlete. 3rd ed. Editors: James R. Andrews, Gary L. Harrelson, Kevin E. Wilk. Saunders, 2004.
ISBN: 9780721600147
Recommended for: Hospital, Academic Libraries
Doody's Core Titles Selection

While the primary audience for this book is practicing clinicians, it can also be used as a textbook. The contributors are experts in athletic rehabilitation and include both clinicians and researchers. New to this edition are updated rehabilitation protocols and chapters. The protocols are not meant to be "how to's." They are meant to be guides since each athlete is different, and each patient's therapy must be individualized. Current surgical techniques have been expanded while those in declining use have been deleted. Those chapters that are not new have been expanded. An entire chapter is dedicated to the rehabilitation of the female athlete. Each of the 21 chapters starts with a list of objectives and ends with a list of summary points. Clinical pearls are listed throughout the text as are boxes highlighting important concepts. The format of the text makes it easy to read and find subtopics. There are numerous diagrams, figures, and photos to supplement the text. References are listed at the end of each chapter.

Journals

American Journal of Sports Medicine. v. 4, Sage Publications for the American Orthopaedic Society for Sports Medicine, 1976.
http://www.ajsm.org/
http://ajs.sagepub.com
ISSN: 03635465
ISSN: 15523365 (Online)
Indexed in: MEDLINE, CINAHL
Recommended for: Hospital, Academic Libraries

The *Journal of Sports Medicine* started in 1972 and changed its name to the *American Journal of Sports Medicine* in 1976. It is the official publication of the American Orthopaedic Society for Sports Medicine. According to the 2009 *Journal Citation Reports*, the journal has the third highest impact factor ranking out of 73 journals in the sports sciences category and the second highest ranking out of 56 journals in the orthopedics category. Libraries supporting clinical and academic professionals would find this journal suitable for their patrons, who might include orthopedic surgeons and specialists, sports medicine physicians, physiatrists, athletic trainers, team physicians, and physical therapists. Family physicians, emergency physicians, and pediatricians are also part of the team working to bring valuable information to the orthopedic sports medicine community through this publication. It is indexed in many different databases including MEDLINE, CINAHL, Embase, Academic ASAP, Academic Search Premier, Education Research Complete, BIOSIS Previews, Periodical Abstracts, and Global Health. The *American Journal of Sports Medicine* covers anterior cruciate ligament (ACL) injury and reconstruction; arthroscopic techniques; degenerative joint disease; imaging studies; surgical techniques for the knee, shoulder, elbow, and ankle; rehabilitation and training; and treatment techniques. It looks at anatomy, biomechanics, and cell biology as they relate to clinical sports medicine, as well as epidemiology of sports injuries. Specific populations—such as children, adolescents, and female athletes—are covered.

British Journal of Sports Medicine. v. 4, BMJ Group, 1969.
http://bjsm.bmj.com/
ISSN: 03063674
ISSN: 14730480 (Online)
Indexed in: MEDLINE, CINAHL
Recommended for: Hospital, Academic Libraries

Begun in 1964 under the title *Bulletin—British Association of Sport and Medicine*, the journal's name was changed to its present form in 1969. The publication is the official journal of the British Association of Sport and Exercise Medicine. According to the 2009 *Journal Citation Reports*, the *British Journal of Sports Medicine* had the eighth highest impact factor out of 73 journals in the sports sciences category. The journal's primary audience is physicians (sports and primary care), physiotherapists, exercise scientists, and public policy specialists. It is also of interest to kinesiologists, occupational therapists, cardiologists, dietary specialists, rheumatologists, orthopedic and emergency medicine consultants, osteopaths, and chiropractors. Some of the numerous resources indexing this journal are MEDLINE, Embase, Scopus, Web of Science, CINAHL, Academic Search Premier, Expanded Academic ASAP, and Global Health. The *British Journal of Sports Medicine* contains clinically relevant original research, editorials, and commentaries on a broad range of topics. These include clinical practice and research, management of sports injury, exercise physiology, sports psychology, physiological evaluations of sports performance, nutrition, physiotherapy, and epidemiology of exercise and health. Starting in 2004, each issue includes selected summaries from *SportsMedUpdate*. This is an evidence-based journal watch service coordinated in South Africa. Online availability begins with the first volume.

Exercise and Sport Sciences Reviews. v. 1, Lippincott Williams & Wilkins, 1973.
http://www.acsm-essr.com
http://www.ovid.com/
ISSN: 00916331
ISSN: 15383008 (Online)
Indexed in: MEDLINE
Recommended for: Hospital, Academic Libraries

Exercise and Sports Sciences Reviews is the review publication of the American College of Sports Medicine. From its start in 1973 until 2000, it was offered as an annual, hardcover monograph series; it now appears quarterly in journal format. The journal is suitable for an academic or hospital library since the main audience is students, professors, clinicians, scientists, and professionals. *Exercise and Sports Sciences Reviews* covers information related to exercise, movement, physical activity and sports. Its mission is to provide contemporary information based on novel, integrative concepts and hypotheses, which is reflected in the journal's cutting-edge issues and interdisciplinary topics. The publication is ranked fourth out of 73 journals in the 2009 *Journal Citation Reports* sports sciences category. It is indexed in MEDLINE, BIOSIS Previews, Scopus, Embase, Physical Education Index, and Web of Science. All volumes of *Exercise and Sports Sciences Reviews* are available electronically.

Journal of Athletic Training. v. 27, National Athletic Trainers' Association, 1992.
http://www.journalofathletictraining.org
http://www.ncbi.nlm.nih.gov/pmc/journals/131/
ISSN: 10626050
ISSN: 1938162X (Online)
Indexed in: MEDLINE, CINAHL
Recommended for: Academic Libraries

The *Journal of Athletic Training* has undergone a couple of name changes since it began in 1956. Not only is it the official publication for the National Athletic Trainers' Association, but also for the Taiwan Athletic Trainers' Association and Japan Athletic Trainers' Organization. Articles pertaining to qualitative and quantitative original research, meta-analysis and systematic reviews, case reports, clinical techniques, evidence-based practice, and literature reviews can be found in the various sections of each issue. Extra features include the ability to earn continuing education credits (CEUs) by taking quizzes based on readings from the journal. This publication is suitable for an academic library where the users can find its citations in several different databases including AMED (Allied and Complementary Medicine), Biological Abstracts, BIOSIS Previews, MEDLINE, CINAHL, Academic Search Premier, Education Research Index, Embase, Physical Education Index, PsycINFO, Scopus, SPORTDiscus, and Web of Science. Online availability starts with the 1992 issues.

Journal of Orthopaedic and Sports Physical Therapy. v. 1, Orthopaedic and Sports Medicine Sections of the American Physical Therapy Association, 1979.
http://www.jospt.org/
ISSN: 01906011
ISSN: 19381344 (Online)
See Also Chapter 1.3. Physical Therapy
Indexed in: MEDLINE, CINAHL
Recommended for: Hospital, Academic Libraries
Brandon/Hill Selection

Physical therapists, athletic trainers and orthopedic surgeons will find much value in the *Journal of Orthopaedic and Sports Physical Therapy* (*JOSPT*). It is the official publication of the Orthopaedic and Sports Physical Therapy Sections of the American Physical Therapy Association, as well as several professional associations in Australia, New Zealand, Europe, South America, South Africa, and Canada. MEDLINE, CINAHL, Scopus, and Web of Science index this journal. The journal is an international source of clinical, basic, and translational science in the areas of the lower body including gait, ambulation, balance, and posture; mid-upper body including hand, wrist, and elbow; spine including pelvis; TMJ and dentistry; electrostimulation; electrotherapy; exercise physiology; muscle physiology; pharmacology and drugs; and radiology and ultrasound. *JOSPT* contains case reports, editorials, book reviews, clinical commentaries, invited commentaries, literature reviews, musculoskeletal imaging, new product information, practice guidelines, research reports, resident's case problems, and technical notes. The *Journal of Orthopaedic and Sports Physical Therapy* is ranked ninth out of 73 journals in the 2009 *Journal Citation Reports* sports sciences category.

Medicine and Science in Sports and Exercise. v. 12, Lippincott Williams & Wilkins, 1980.
http://www.ovid.com/
http://www.acsm-msse.org
ISSN: 01959131
ISSN: 15300315 (Online)
Indexed in: MEDLINE
Recommended for: Hospital, Academic Libraries

Medicine and Science in Sports and Exercise changed its name in 1980 from *Medicine and Science in Sports*, which began in 1969. The publication is the official journal of the American College of Sports Medicine whose members come from many medical specialties, allied health professions, and scientific disciplines. The journal, which is ranked second out of 73 publications in the 2009 *Journal Citation Reports* sports sciences category, is read by exercise physiologists, physiatrists, physical therapists, team physicians, and athletic trainers. *Medicine and Science in Sports and Exercise* is indexed in numerous sources: AMED, AgeLine, BIOSIS Previews, Biological Abstracts, CINAHL, Academic Search Premier, Education Abstracts, Embase, Global Health, MEDLINE, PsycINFO, and Scopus. Each issue is divided into three sections—"Clinical Sciences," "Basic Sciences," and "Applied Sciences"—which contain original investigations, clinical studies and comprehensive reviews, bibliographies, and book reviews. Academic and medical libraries will find this journal to be an essential part of their collections. Online issues are available starting with 1980.

Sports Medicine. v. 1, Adis, 1984.
http://www.ingentaconnect.com/content/adis/smd
http://adisonline.com/sportsmedicine
ISSN: 01121642
ISSN: 11792035 (Online)
Indexed in: MEDLINE, CINAHL
Recommended for: Hospital, Academic Libraries

Published by Adis Press, *Sports Medicine* has the fifth highest impact factor of 73 journals in the sports sciences category according to the 2009 *Journal Citation Reports*. The journal began in 1984 and is indexed in MEDLINE, Embase, Academic Search Premier, CINAHL, SPORTDiscus, Global Health, PsycINFO, and Physical Education Index. Topics discussed include sports medicine, sports science (including performance research), exercise physiology, medical syndromes, medical use of exercise for rehabilitation and health, and application of physiological and biomechanical principles to specific sports. Along with regular monthly issues, the editors have compiled special collections on topics and emerging areas such as exercise and fatigue, soccer training and injury prevention, and strength training adaptations and recommendations.

9.13. Telemedicine

Delivery of health services via remote telecommunications. This includes interactive consultative and diagnostic services.
—MeSH

Contributor: Brenda Faye Green

Monographs

Current Principles and Practices of Telemedicine and e-Health. Editor: Rifat Latifi. IOS Press, 2008.
http://www.ebrary.com/
ISBN: 9781586038069
Recommended for: Hospital, Academic Libraries

This book provides useful information for consideration when starting up a telemedicine program, such as a listing of what to do and not to do. Also addressed are impediments and issues to overcome during planning and implementation phases. The book discusses how to leverage current infrastructure and what is involved in moving to a paperless environment. It is recommended for purchase because it includes information on the timely uses of telemedicine during natural disasters or armed conflicts, as well as in remote locations. *Current Principles and Practices of Telemedicine and e-Health* also covers the use of telemedicine in various settings such as critical care and home health; coverage includes specialties such as rehabilitation, dermatology, oncology, pathology, and wound care. The book is part of the *Studies in Health Technology and Informatics* series and will be useful for hospital, academic, and research libraries.

Handbook of Informatics for Nurses and Health Care Professionals. 4th ed. Authors: Toni Hebda, Patricia Czar. Pearson Prentice Hall, 2008.
ISBN: 9780135043943
Recommended for: Hospital, Academic, Consumer Health Libraries

The discussion of telemedicine, or telehealth, takes place in the sixteenth chapter of the third section. In addition to telehealth, this section includes the use of computers in educating health care professionals and computer applications in nursing and health care research. The same chapter includes the evolution of telehealth from a novel idea to a generally accepted delivery platform for various health care services. Attention is given to telehealth methods such as teleconferencing and its use in different countries. This book provides a good overview of both nursing informatics and health care informatics. Nurses play a vital role in the provision of telehealth services, and this book provides a background for the broader field of informatics in which telehealth is neatly situated. Now in its fourth edition, this book attempts to keep up with evolving changes in informatics and telehealth. Chapters are devoted to topics related to telehealth, such as electronic patient records, computer hardware and software terminology, data integrity, health care information systems, and community health information networks. These related topics are important issues because telehealth does not exist in a vacuum.

History of Telemedicine: Evolution, Context, and Transformation. Authors: Rashid L. Bashshur, Gary W. Shannon. Mary Ann Liebert, 2009.
ISBN: 9781934854112
Recommended for: Academic Libraries

This authoritative book is highly regarded for it comprehensive and well-researched treatment of the development of telemedicine, from its roots in ancient Greece to its present role providing patients with equal access to health care services. According to this book, telemedicine applications date back to 1905. This book also chronicles radiology and psychiatry's use of telemedicine beginning in the 1970s. Written by Rashid L. Bashshur, former editor of *Telemedicine and e-Health*, and Gary W. Shannon, author of a 2006 book on telemedicine, the *History of Telemedicine* has received excellent reviews. In his review, Dr. Donald A.B. Lindberg, director of the National Library of Medicine, highlights the authors' focus on the role of telemedicine in improving patient outcomes and advancing public health. Described by Dr. Lindberg as "interesting and balanced," the book is favored by another reviewer for the analogies between current and ancient efforts to provide care for patients from distant locations, now called telemedicine. The book covers telemedicine's transformative process, from ancient to modern times, with dates ranging from 1870 to the present. The book is supported by the National Library of Medicine and includes maps and illustrations. The *History of Telemedicine* ends with a chapter devoted to evidence of telemedicine's impact on several issues such as quality, cost, and accessibility.

Telemedicine and Telehealth: Principles, Policies, Performance, and Pitfalls. Authors: Adam William Darkins, Margaret Ann Cary. Springer, 2000.
http://extranet.netlibrary.com/TitleSelect/
http://www.ebrary.com/
ISBN: 9780826113023
ISBN: 9780826197047
Recommended for: Hospital, Academic Libraries

Although published in 2000, this book remains a good resource for libraries that support telemedicine and telehealth efforts at their institutions. Purchased by most academic health sciences libraries on campuses with active and mature telemedicine efforts, this easy-to-use book is well organized with 12 chapters, references, a glossary, and an index. The authors provide four definitions of telehealth and supply a historical overview. A patient-centered perspective, which recognizes the role of patients in managing their health care, is a welcome addition to this book. Several sections of this book consider the consumer in telehealth. An especially useful section is "Verifying the Information Given Patients in Telehealth Programs." Also included in this book is the relationship between physicians and telehealth, telehealth services, marketing, contracting, and the business side of telehealth. The authors discuss administrative issues such as contracts, management, regulations, legislation, and political considerations. Tables provide useful information such as the top specialties that use telemedicine for consultations, with mental health comprising the largest percentage of use. Another table lists barriers to sustainability, with reimbursement topping the list of barriers. This book is recommended for academic, hospital, and nursing library collections.

Journals

International Journal of Medical Informatics. v. 44, Elsevier Ireland Ltd., 1997.
http://www.sciencedirect.com/science/journal/13865056
ISSN: 13865056
ISSN: 18728243 (Online)
See Also Chapter 6.3. Informatics
Indexed in: MEDLINE
Recommended for: Hospital, Academic Libraries

This is the official journal of the European Federation for Medical Informatics, European Regional Council of the International Medical Informatics Association. Its editorial board is international in scope with a good representation of authors from the United States. With 12 issues per year, this journal's 2009 impact factor is 3.126. It is indexed extensively by 24 multidisciplinary indexing and abstracting services, including Biotechnology and Bioengineering Abstracts, Embase, International Nursing Index, and MEDLINE. Online access is available through ScienceDirect, which includes its preceding title, the *International Journal of Bio-Medical Computing*, (1970–March 1997). The audience for *International Journal of Medical Informatics* includes medical sciences personnel and radiologists, who jointly provide telemedicine services. This journal also provides several nursing-centered articles and is recommended for libraries that serve colleges of nursing, as well as staff nurses at affiliated hospitals in addition to academic and hospital library collections. The content also provides an international focus on the provision of telemedicine services in various countries and specialties such as neurosurgery, pulmonology, oncology, and health informatics.

Journal of Medical Internet Research. v. 1, Gunther Eysenbach, Centre for Global eHealth Innovation, University Health Network,Toronto, 1999.
http://www.jmir.org/
http://www.ncbi.nlm.nih.gov/pmc/journals/224/
ISSN: 14394456
ISSN: 14388871 (Online)
See Also Chapter 6.3. Informatics, Chapter 33.2. Health Communications
Indexed in: MEDLINE
Recommended for: Hospital, Academic Libraries

Founded in 1999 and considered a pioneer in open access, this peer-reviewed journal publishes articles as they are received, reviewed, and accepted for publication. The cycle takes place within a four-week time frame. Articles are collected into four issues per year and collated into an annual volume. The HTML content is free, while PDF downloads require a fee with members paying a reduced fee. While primarily an electronic journal, content has been freely distributed in CD-ROM to scientists. Libraries are encouraged to pay for a print subscription that is fulfilled through electronic PDFs. With a 2009 impact factor of 3.924, the *Journal of Medical Internet Research* covers the interdisciplinary field of e-health. Its focus goes beyond medical sciences to include communication, informatics, and behavioral, social, and library sciences. Articles are devoted to the design, impact, and effect of Internet use and applications. Journal content includes original research, reviews, and tutorials.

Journal of Telemedicine and Telecare. v. 1, The Royal Society of Medicine Press, 1995.
http://jtt.rsmjournals.com/
http://www.ebscohost.com/
ISSN: 1357633X
ISSN: 17581109 (Online)
Indexed in: MEDLINE
Recommended for: Hospital, Academic Libraries

The research section of the *Journal of Telemedicine and Telecare* frequently includes systematic reviews and articles on timely topics, such as the use of telemedicine in an emergency situation during transatlantic airline flights. Published by the Royal Society of Medicine Press, this internationally focused, bimonthly journal includes corporate, individual, student, and nurse contributions from countries such as Australia, Belgium, Denmark, Germany, the United Kingdom, and the United States. A 2009 impact factor of 0.921 may be due in part to its unique focus and bimonthly publication schedule, which results in a smaller group of articles compared to other journals in the health care sciences and services category. The 2009 impact factor is based upon 82 articles being cited 1,639 times. This journal is recommended for purchase by hospital, academic health science, and nursing libraries. The nursing literature demonstrates a close relationship between nursing and the provision of varied telemedicine resources and services. Indexed by numerous sources such as MEDLINE and the Web of Science, the *Journal of Telemedicine and Telecare* is the official publication of eight societies, including the International Society for Telemedicine and eHealth.

Telemedicine and e-Health. v. 11, Mary Ann Liebert, 2005.
http://www.liebertpub.com/products/product.aspx?pid=54
ISSN: 15305627
ISSN: 15563669 (Online)
Indexed in: MEDLINE
Recommended for: Hospital, Academic Libraries

With special interest membership groups such as nursing, pediatric, ocular, and teledermatology, the American Telemedicine Association's official journal is *Telemedicine and e-Health*. Formerly known as *Telemedicine Journal* and *Telemedicine Journal and e-Health*, it is also the official publication of the Canadian Telehealth Forum of COACH. Ten issues are published annually. The content appears in several categories such as telemedicine news, roundtable discussion, medical connectivity, original research, brief communications, and meeting reports. Articles discuss the provision of services in a variety of locations such as assisted living, battlefield, home health care, nursing home, and rural settings. Articles also address advanced technology applications and connectivity, electronic patient records, mobile devices, and related issues of interest to health care personnel, hospitals, and medical centers. *Telemedicine and e-Health* encompasses clinical medicine, technological advances, health policy, and efficacy and safety of telemedicine. The journal covers administrative aspects of telemedicine, such as cost, quality, accessibility, and medical records. Paid subscribers can take advantage of a "track citation" feature. The publisher provides full online coverage back to volume 1, 1995.

9.14. Tropical Medicine

Diseases, mainly of parasitic origin, common in tropical and subtropical regions.

—MeSH

Contributor: Margaret Henderson

Monographs

Atlas of Tropical Medicine and Parasitology. 6th ed. Authors: Wallace Peters, Geoffrey Pasvol. Elsevier Mosby, 2007.
ISBN: 9780323043649
Recommended for: Hospital, Academic Libraries

Atlas of Tropical Medicine and Parasitology is a heavily illustrated text arranged by the mechanism of transmission of the disease. Chapters cover arthropod-borne infections, soil- and mollusk-mediated helminthiases, infections acquired through the gastrointestinal tract, airborne infections, sexually transmitted diseases, infections through the skin and mucous membranes, poisonous animals, nutritional disorders, and miscellaneous disorders. Diagnosis is aided by over 1,200 photographs throughout the book. International travel is considered when discussing disease distribution. Tables, maps, and life cycle diagrams support the text. All the images are included on the accompanying CD-ROM and can be used in presentations. This book is an excellent text to support tropical medicine courses and should be included in any library collection supporting tropical medicine programs, as well as traveler or immigrant medical programs. It is also suitable for an academic library that supports programs that send health care students to tropical areas.

Lecture Notes: Tropical Medicine. 6th ed. Editors: Geoffrey V. Gill, Nick Beeching. Wiley-Blackwell, 2009.
ISBN: 9781405180481
Recommended for: Hospital, Academic Libraries

Lecture Notes: Tropical Medicine is a comprehensive introduction to tropical medicine, rather than an encyclopedic reference. The first part covers disease/infections presentations by system. The second part covers major tropical infections, and the third part addresses other diseases and conditions, grouped by gastrointestinal, respiratory, neurological, fever, and miscellaneous presentations. Treatment, prevention, and management sections are laid out for the conditions covered. This book was developed as a text for medical students or postgraduate doctors taking tropical medicine courses, but it can also serve as a reference for health professionals involved with medicine in the tropics or imported tropical disease. Figures, tables, and color photos appear throughout the book to help with diagnosis and treatment, and an extensive index is included. The book would be most useful for hospital or academic libraries supporting programs that send health care professionals to tropical areas.

Manson's Tropical Diseases. 22nd ed. Editors: Gordon C. Cook, Alimuddin I. Zumla. Saunders, 2009.
http://www.mdconsult.com/
ISBN: 9781416044703
Recommended for: Hospital, Academic Libraries
Brandon/Hill Selection

Manson's Tropical Diseases is one of the oldest, continuously published texts on tropical medicine. It starts with background information about tropical medicine—

including genetics, traditional medicine, ethics, and immunology—and then covers signs and symptoms for diagnosis. Diseases are covered by system, and specialties such as surgery, pediatrics, and obstetrics are discussed. The sections on viral, bacterial, and parasitic infections are extensive. Nutrition, plant, and animal poisons, along with heart disease and diabetes in the tropics, are also covered. There are cross references between system and disease sections for further information. Appendixes appear only online. Extensive references and a comprehensive index are included, with figures and tables highlighting key information throughout the text. Individuals who purchase the print edition can access updates online through Elsevier's Expert Consult platform. Institutional online access is offered through Elsevier's MD Consult platform. *Manson's* was developed for specialists who treat returning travelers or immigrant populations, as well as for health professionals in the field. This is considered to be one of the best texts in the field and is a three star *Doody's* title.

Oxford Handbook of Tropical Medicine. 3rd ed. Authors: Michael Eddleston, Robert Davidson, Andrew Brent, Robert Wilkinson. Oxford University Press, 2008.
ISBN: 9780199204090
Recommended for: Academic Libraries
Doody's Core Titles Selection

This handbook has been written for easy field consultation, not as a comprehensive text. The chapters are grouped roughly by medical specialty, but the most common concerns come first: pediatrics, malaria, HIV/AIDS and tuberculosis, diarrheal diseases, and acute respiratory infections. Practical protocols developed by the World Health Organization provide treatment plans for patient care. This book was developed for students and practitioners to use in the field where limited resources are available. This updated edition has been fully revised and includes an emphasis on pediatrics and public health with new material on avian flu. At 856 pages with a pocket size format (approx. 7 by 4 inches and 1 inch thick) and reasonable weight (almost 1 pound), it is quite portable when compared with most other texts. Features include illustrations of blood films and stool smears for diagnosis; consistent sections addressing clinical features, diagnosis, and management help simplify information retrieval. This book is useful for libraries that support health care workers who travel to tropical regions.

The Travel and Tropical Medicine Manual. 4th ed. Editors: Elaine C. Jong, Christopher A. Sanford. Saunders/Elsevier, 2008.
http://www.sciencedirect.com/science/book/9781416026136
http://www.mdconsult.com/
ISBN: 9781416026136
Recommended for: Hospital, Academic, Consumer Health Libraries

The Travel and Tropical Medicine Manual is intended as a reference for medical providers in the area of travel medicine, but this excellent reference book is helpful in many ways. The sections on pre-travel advice and advice for special circumstances are useful for learning about malaria, diarrhea, and other common tropical conditions. The following diagnosis sections are arranged by presenting symptom, such as fever, diarrhea, or skin lesions. Tables throughout the work help present the most important information. Multiple cross references and a good index aid in providing access to the information. While many hospital libraries will not need an encyclopedic reference on tropical medicine, their health care professionals may deal with travelers or immigrants who have come from tropical areas. This highly recommended book (four stars from *Doody's*) is a reasonably priced addition to a general reference collection and would also be useful in a consumer health collection.

Tropical Infectious Diseases: Principles, Pathogens & Practice. 2nd ed. Editors: Richard L. Guerrant, David H. Walker, Peter F. Weller. Churchill Livingstone, 2006.
http://www.sciencedirect.com/science/book/9780443066689
http://www.mdconsult.com/
ISBN: 9780443066689
Recommended for: Hospital, Academic Libraries
Doody's Core Titles Selection

Tropical Infectious Diseases: Principles, Pathogens, and Practice is an important, multidisciplinary resource on infectious diseases such as malaria, respiratory infections, cholera, and hepatitis. The principles and pathogens sections are well organized and authoritative and include information on the latest developments in immunology, genetics, and molecular approaches. The last section deals with social and cultural factors in tropical medicine or considerations when treating migrant, immigrant, or refugee patients. Tables are used throughout to convey comparative aspects of their subjects, and life cycle diagrams assist with the understanding of disease progression. Helpful bibliographic references and an extensive index are included. An accompanying CD-ROM contains the full text of this book and an image bank for individual purchasers of the print book. Institutional online access is provided on Elsevier's ScienceDirect and MD Consult platforms. The spread of many of the covered infectious diseases outside of tropical areas is considered, making this useful to any library supporting infectious disease programs.

Journals

Acta Tropica. v. 1, Elsevier, 1944.
http://www.sciencedirect.com/science/journal/0001706X
ISSN: 0001706X
ISSN: 18736254 (Online)
Indexed in: MEDLINE
Recommended for: Hospital, Academic Libraries

Acta Tropica covers topics relevant to human and animal health in the tropics and the subtropics. The major scope is biomedical and health science aspects of parasites and vectors in the areas of taxonomy, morphology, biochemistry, physiology, and immunology. The coverage includes diagnosis, disease control, clinical and community medicine, and epidemiology. Research papers, review articles, and short communications—but not case reports—are geared towards parasitologists, microbiologists, immunologists, and epidemiologists. The international scope of the articles is mirrored by the international affiliations of the authors. Special issues are published based on conferences proceedings, special workshops, or programs. This is a useful journal for institutions with tropical medicine programs. The journal is ranked sixth in the tropical medicine journals category (2009 *Journal Citation Reports*), and it is indexed in Web of Science, MEDLINE, Scopus, and others.

American Journal of Tropical Medicine and Hygiene. v. 1, American Society of Tropical Medicine and Hygiene, 1952.
http://www.ajtmh.org
http://www.ncbi.nlm.nih.gov/pmc/journals/960/
ISSN: 00029637
ISSN: 14761645 (Online)
Indexed in: MEDLINE
Recommended for: Hospital, Academic Libraries
Brandon/Hill Selection

The *American Journal of Tropical Medicine and Hygiene* is the official journal of the American Society of Tropical Medicine and Hygiene, whose mission is to promote world health by prevention and control of tropical disease. The journal covers basic and field research in the fields of tropical medicine, parasitology, immunology, infectious diseases, epidemiology, basic and molecular biology, virology, and international medicine. Begun in 1921 as the *American Journal of Tropical Medicine*, the *Journal* publishes peer-reviewed papers, invited review articles, short reports, case studies, reports on the efficacy of new drugs and methods of treatment, prevention and control methodologies, new testing methods and equipment, book reports, and letters to the editor. This journal is essential for any hospital or academic library that supports an institution with an international health care rotation or a special tropical medicine program. The journal is ranked third in tropical medicine journals (2009 *Journal Citation Reports*), but it is the leading general journal on tropical medicine. The journal is covered by BIOSIS, Embase/Excerpta Medica, MEDLINE, and others.

Annals of Tropical Medicine & Parasitology. v. 1, Maney on behalf of Liverpool School of Tropical Medicine, 1907.
http://www.ingentaconnect.com/content/maney/atmp
ISSN: 00034983
ISSN: 13648594 (Online)
Indexed in: MEDLINE
Recommended for: Academic Libraries

This journal from the Liverpool School of Tropical Medicine covers tropical medicine, global parasitology, and medical entomology. *Annals of Tropical Medicine & Parasitology* strives to publish articles that reach between specialties; field research is linked with molecular biology, microbiology with nutrition, and entomology with epidemics. Other areas of interest include medical entomology, malaria, HIV/AIDS, microbiology, and epidemiology. Although the journal started as a house journal for the Liverpool School of Tropical Medicine, it has become a journal for the worldwide dissemination of tropical medicine research. This is a useful journal for institutions with tropical medicine programs. The journal is ranked eighth in tropical medicine journals (2009 *Journal Citation Reports*) and is indexed in BIOSIS, CAB Abstracts, Embase/Excerpta Medica, MEDLINE, Web of Science, and others.

Bulletin of the World Health Organization. v. 1, World Health Organization, 1948.
http://www.who.int/bulletin/en/
ISSN: 00429686
ISSN: 15640604 (Online)
Indexed in: MEDLINE, CINAHL
Recommended for: Hospital, Academic Libraries

Like the Centers for Disease Control and Prevention's *Emerging Infectious Diseases*, this free, online publication will be useful in libraries that cannot afford specific tropical medicine journals. The *Bulletin* covers international public health concerns, with a special focus on developing countries. Authors, reviewers, and editors are drawn from World Health Organization (WHO) experts worldwide. Many WHO programs focus on rare and emerging infectious diseases, and the *Bulletin* is often the communication tool for these programs. Ranked seventh in the public, environmental, and occupational health journals category (2009 *Journal Citation Reports*) with an impact factor of 5.302, this is a useful publication for any health library. Peer-reviewed articles are indexed in MEDLINE, Web of Science, and others.

***Emerging Infectious Diseases*.** v. 1, National Center for Infectious Diseases, Centers for Disease Control and Prevention (CDC), 1995.
http://www.cdc.gov/ncidod/eid/index.htm
ISSN: 10806040
ISSN: 10806059 (Online)
See Also Chapter 10.16. Public Health
Indexed in: MEDLINE
Recommended for: Academic Libraries

This monthly publication by the Emerging Infectious Diseases Unit of the Centers for Disease Control and Prevention (CDC) covers emerging infections from a national and global perspective. Authors and reviewers from around the world communicate their knowledge of new and evolving infectious diseases. The journal is ranked third in the infectious diseases category (2009 *Journal Citation Reports*), with an impact factor of 6.794. Those libraries unable to afford more specific tropical medicine journals—but with a need to support tropical diseases through travelers or immigrant populations—can find useful information in this free, online publication from the CDC. It is indexed in MEDLINE and other databases.

***Malaria Journal*.** v. 1, BioMed Central, 2002.
http://www.malariajournal.com
http://www.ncbi.nlm.nih.gov/pmc/journals/98/
ISSN: 14752875
Indexed in: MEDLINE
Recommended for: Hospital, Academic Libraries

Malaria Journal is a peer-reviewed, online journal with open access for research articles. The journal also includes case reports and studies, methodology articles, reviews, and opinion articles. *Malaria Journal* publishes exclusively about malaria from all specialty areas, covering basic science and clinical and field research. The journal also strives to be a communication focus for malariologists, and, as such, it tries to maintain up-to-date links as well as information about meetings, initiatives, and events. Journal articles can also include large datasets, many color illustrations and moving pictures, relevant links to databases, relevant websites, or other papers. This journal is useful in hospital and academic medical libraries that may support medical personnel and students who travel to help in clinics in tropical areas or travelers returning from such areas. *Malaria Journal* ranks second in the tropical medicine journals category (2009 *Journal Citation Reports*). All articles are listed in PubMed immediately upon acceptance after peer review and are covered by CAS, CAB Abstracts, Embase, MEDLINE, Web of Science, and others.

***PLoS Neglected Tropical Diseases*.** v.1, Public Library of Science, 2007.
http://www.plosntds.org
http://www.ncbi.nlm.nih.gov/pmc/journals/532/
ISSN: 19352735
Indexed in: MEDLINE
Recommended for: Hospital, Academic Libraries

PLoS Neglected Tropical Diseases is an online-only, open access journal devoted to neglected tropical diseases (NTDs), such as elephantiasis, river blindness, leprosy, hookworm, schistosomiasis, and African sleeping sickness. *PLoS Neglected Tropical Diseases* covers the pathology, epidemiology, treatment, control, and prevention of NTDs, as well as public policy concerning these diseases. Each issue includes peer-reviewed research papers and one or more of these sections: editorials, viewpoints, debates, policy platform, reviews, expert commentary, innovations, symposia, historical perspectives, and interviews. The journal is geared toward scientific investigators, health practitioners, control experts, and advocates. The journal encourages authors from endemic countries to submit articles and will provide them with additional support. This journal is useful in hospital and academic medical libraries that support medical personnel and students who travel to help in clinics in tropical areas or travelers returning from such areas. *PLoS Neglected Tropical Diseases* is ranked first in tropical medicine journals (2009 *Journal Citation Reports*) and is indexed in Google Scholar, MEDLINE, Scopus, and Web of Science.

***Transactions of the Royal Society of Tropical Medicine and Hygiene*.** v. 14, Royal Society of Tropical Medicine and Hygiene/Elsevier, 1920.
http://www.sciencedirect.com/science/journal/00359203
ISSN: 00359203
ISSN: 18783503 (Online)
Indexed in: MEDLINE, CINAHL
Recommended for: Academic Libraries

Transactions of the Royal Society of Tropical Medicine and Hygiene is the official journal of the Royal Society of Tropical Medicine and Hygiene. The journal publishes original, peer-reviewed articles and invited reviews across a broad range of topics relevant to the Society's goals, including clinical tropical medicine, infectious diseases, parasitology, microbiology, epidemiology, translational research, and other related topics. The goal is to make the research available to workers from a range of disciplines and apply new technologies to tropical medicine. Non-communicable diseases in developing countries are also covered. Other global programs and field trials of new vaccines and therapies are included. This is a useful journal for institutions with tropical medicine programs. The journal is ranked fourth in the tropical medicine journals category (2009 *Journal Citation Reports*) and is indexed in CSA, MEDLINE, Web of Science, and others.

Tropical Medicine & International Health. v. 1, Wiley-Blackwell, 1996.
http://onlinelibrary.wiley.com/journal/10.1111/(ISSN)1365-3156
ISSN: 13602276
ISSN: 13653156 (Online)
Indexed in: MEDLINE
Recommended for: Academic Libraries

This journal succeeds, combines, and integrates these publications: *Annales de la Société Belge de Médecine Tropicale*, *Journal of Tropical Medicine and Hygiene*, *Tropical and Geographical Medicine* (incorporating *Acta Leidensia*), and *Tropical Medicine and Parasitology*. The combined journal is published on behalf of the Netherlands Society for Tropical Medicine and International Health and the Belgian Society of Tropical Medicine and the Prince Leopold Institute of Tropical Medicine. *Tropical Medicine & International Health* is a multidisciplinary journal publishing work in areas such as infectious and non-infectious disease; parasitology; clinical diseases and medicine of the tropics; epidemiological theory and fieldwork; tropical medical microbiology; medical entomology; tropical public health and community medicine; international health policy; and health economics. The journal requests that articles on fieldwork involve local authors and that studies have a quantifiable impact on human health. This is a useful journal for institutions with tropical medicine programs. The journal is ranked fifth in tropical medicine journals (2009 *Journal Citation Reports*). It is indexed in BIOSIS, CAB Abstracts, CSA, Embase/Excerpta Medica, MEDLINE, Web of Science, and others.

9.15. Wilderness Medicine

Skills and knowledge required for assessment and treatment of traumatic, environmental, and medical emergencies in remote geographic or wilderness environments.

—MeSH

Contributor: Heidi Sue Adams, Rocco Altobelli, Sheree West

Monographs

NOLS Wilderness Medicine. 1st ed. Author: Tod Schimelpfenig. Stackpole Books, 2006.
ISBN: 9780811733069
Recommended for: Academic Libraries

This publication is designed as a field textbook for the National Outdoor Leadership School's wilderness first aid curriculum. It covers topics relating to first aid care of emergencies encountered or experienced by outdoor enthusiasts. This particular resource also includes additional information relating to expedition medicine, including information on leadership, teamwork, and communication for rescue groups.

Wilderness First Aid: Emergency Care for Remote Locations. 3rd ed. Author: American Academy of Orthopaedic Surgeons. Jones & Bartlett, 2008.
ISBN: 9780763751456
Recommended for: Hospital, Consumer Health Libraries

This small, easily transportable first aid manual contains "what to look for" and "what to do" information applicable to immediate, stabilizing care for the injured person located in a remote location. It contains information on rescue techniques, victim assessment, wounds and injuries care, and bandaging techniques. Colored instructional diagrams are included. Although small, this surprisingly robust resource covers a variety of topics related to common injuries and illnesses that can occur in remote locales.

Wilderness Medicine. 5th ed. Editor: Paul S. Auerbach. Mosby Elsevier, 2007.
http://www.mdconsult.com/
ISBN: 9780323032285
Recommended for: Hospital, Academic Libraries
Doody's Core Titles Selection

The author is one of the pioneers of the Wilderness Medical Society, and, to date, this large textbook is still considered the preeminent resource on the topic of emergencies in the natural environment. With a varied list of contributors, this resource covers a wide variety of topics relating to the management of human emergencies resulting from interactions in the mountains, jungles, deserts, or oceans. Such emergency encounters may be the result of hazardous weather or encounters with plants, animals, or insects, both on land and in the sea. In addition to supplying information about the management of medical emergencies, there are sections relating specifically to prevention. The chapter on equipment and special knowledge, for example, includes knot tying and wilderness navigation techniques. The latest edition also incorporates a new chapter on aerospace medicine.

Journals

Prehospital Emergency Care. v. 1, Informa Healthcare, 1997.
http://informahealthcare.com/
ISSN: 10903127
ISSN: 15450066 (Online)
See Also Chapter 10.5. Emergency Medicine
Indexed in: MEDLINE, CINAHL
Recommended for: Hospital Libraries

Prehospital Emergency Care was enthusiastically endorsed by an aeromedical flight paramedic as "the best peer-reviewed journal for transport medicine." Published quarterly, it is tilted towards emergency medical services, although it does cover flight physiology and critical care transport medicine on occasion. A highlight of this resource is its great operational studies on system management and other issues. Each article is peer-reviewed with the exception of policy statements for groups associated with the journal (such as Emergency Medical Service—EMS—physicians). Although this publication is useful for paramedics, it is also valuable to doctors functioning as medical directors for local ambulance services.

Wilderness & Environmental Medicine. v. 6, Elsevier, 1995.
http://www.wemjournal.org
ISSN: 10806032
ISSN: 15451534 (Online)
Indexed in: MEDLINE
Recommended for: Hospital, Academic Libraries

A continuation of the *Journal of Wilderness Medicine*, *Wilderness & Environmental Medicine* is a quarterly, peer-reviewed journal from the Wilderness Medical Society. This publication's editorial board represents an international group of renowned experts whose focus is on the science and practice of wilderness medicine. Articles are submitted from an international base of experts on topics relating to the many aspects of wilderness medicine. Formerly published by the Alliance Communications Group, Elsevier assumed publishing responsibilities beginning with volume 21, 2010.

10. Medical Specialties

10.1. Aerospace Medicine

The health and medical problems of man in aviation (aviation medicine) and space flight.

—MeSH

Contributor: Mary Fran Prottsman

Monographs

Aeromedical Transportation: A Clinical Guide. 2nd ed. Author: Terence Martin. Ashgate, 2006.
ISBN: 9780754641483
Recommended for: Hospital, Academic Libraries

From history to the organizational, operational, and medicolegal aspects of aeromedical transport, Terence Martin provides valuable information regarding the atmosphere, altitude, flight biodynamics, transmeridian flight, the medical flight crew, and aeromedical equipment. Using anecdotes, evidence-based studies, and practical case studies, he enumerates the clinical indications for aeromedical transport for spinal injured patients, burn patients, obstetric patients, neonates, and children. Ample illustrations and two new chapters on nursing care and critical care transfer round out this book. This work is strongly recommended for clinical and academic libraries with an interest in the field of aerospace medicine.

Aviation Psychology and Human Factors. Authors: Monica Martinussen, David R. Hunter. CRC Press/Taylor & Francis, 2010.
http://extranet.netlibrary.com/TitleSelect/
http://www.crcnetbase.com/isbn/978-1-4398-0843-6
ISBN: 9781439808436
ISBN: 9781439808443
Recommended for: Hospital, Academic Libraries

Aviation Psychology and Human Factors explores the application of psychological principles and techniques to the specific situations and problems of aviation. It provides a complete overview of the role of psychology in the field of aviation. The authors address the contribution of psychology to the design of aviation systems, the selection and training of pilots, the psychological characteristics of pilots that may relate to aviation safety, and to the behavior of passengers. They cover key concepts of psychological research and data analysis at a depth that fosters a greater appreciation for the use of these tools in the development of new psychological knowledge. A keener understanding of aviation psychology will better prepare pilots for the demands of aviation. While many books cover this subject for psychologists, very few, if any, customize content for pilots. With balanced coverage of the material for both audiences, this book makes pilots aware of the positive impact psychology and its application can have on improving aviation operations, providing specific information that pilots can use in their daily operations. It gives psychologists a better understanding of how their discipline is applied to aviation, while giving pilots the tools to better evaluate and implement future products in the field of aviation psychology. The book is recommended for clinical and academic libraries.

Clinical Aviation Medicine. 4th ed. Authors: Russell B. Rayman, John D. Hastings, William B. Kruyer, Richard A. Levy, Jeb S. Pickard. Professional Publishing Group, 2006.
ISBN: 9780971301771
Recommended for: Hospital, Academic Libraries

In order for Aviation Medical Examiners (AME) and military flight surgeons (FS) to determine a pilot's fitness to fly, they must understand the stresses of flight, aircraft operations, and the appropriate medical standards. *Clinical Aviation Medicine* provides these practitioners with clinical information on a wide range of diseases relevant to aeromedical disposition and waiver/exemption decisions for flight certification, emphasizing their significance in an aviation environment. In 2000, a review in *Aviation, Space, and Environmental Medicine* proclaimed that "everybody who practices this specialty needs to have a copy, and keep it close at hand in the examination room." The fourth edition contains updated information on multiple sclerosis, deep venous thrombosis, bleeding peptic ulcer disease, glaucoma, hepatitis, HIV, coronary artery and valvular disease, sleep disorders, and mild cognitive impairment. It provides new material on therapeutic medications, including a section on herbals. This text is recommended for libraries that support clinical and teaching programs in the field of aerospace medicine.

Ernsting's Aviation Medicine. 4th ed. Editors: David J. Rainford, David P. Gradwell. Oxford University Press, 2006.
ISBN: 9780340813195
Recommended for: Hospital, Academic Libraries

Another standard in the field, *Ernsting's Aviation Medicine* examines daily stresses faced by civil and military aircrew, applying physiological and behavioral sciences. Originally edited by John Ernsting, former Commandant of the Royal Air Force, the text has an international reputation and complements *Fundamentals of Aerospace Medicine*. While both texts cover physiological and clinical issues of each body system, *Ernsting's* provides additional coverage of the ageing pilot, commercial passenger fitness to fly, international standards, naval air operations, accident investigation, in-flight communication, aircraft hygiene, aeromedical aspects of air traffic control, and escape from the aircraft. Concluding with chapters on the medical aspects of aeromedical evacuation and aeromedical transfer of the critically ill patient, the text is recommended for academic and clinical libraries serving aviation medicine practitioners and those interested in the field.

Fundamentals of Aerospace Medicine. 4th ed. Editors: Jeffrey R. Davis, Robert Johnson, Jan Stepanek, Jennifer A. Fogarty. Lippincott Williams & Wilkins, 2008.
http://www.ovid.com/
ISBN: 9780781774666
Recommended for: Hospital, Academic Libraries

Known as "DeHart's" for many years, *Fundamentals of Aerospace Medicine* has been the bible of aviation medicine programs for decades. It was preceded by Louis Bauer's *Aviation Medicine*, the first volume on the topic published in the United States in 1926, and Harry Armstrong's *Principles and Practice of Aviation Medicine*. With its first edition published in 1985, *Fundamentals of Aerospace Medicine* became the introductory text for physicians, physiologists, researchers, and residents. Roy L. DeHart, former commander of the U.S. Air Force School of Aerospace Medicine, edited the first three editions. Now in its fourth edition with a new editorial team, this comprehensive text addresses the history of aviation medicine, pilot health, and recertification, as well as the medical and public health issues involved in the care of crews, passengers, and support personnel of aircraft and space vehicles. Coverage includes human physiology under flight conditions, clinical medicine in the aerospace environment, and operational issues including human factors and safety issues. The fourth edition contains new chapters on radiation, toxicology and microbiology, dentistry, women's health issues, commercial human space flight, and parachuting. Amply illustrated with tables and photographs, it is required for clinical and academic programs that support aerospace medicine residencies, flight surgeons, and aeromedical emergency transport.

Fundamentals of Space Medicine. Author: Gilles Clément. Springer, 2005.
http://www.springerlink.com/content/978-1-4020-3246-2
http://www.ebrary.com/
http://extranet.netlibrary.com/TitleSelect/
ISBN: 9781402015984
ISBN: 9781402032462
ISBN: 9781402034343 (Online)
Recommended for: Academic Libraries

What have we learned from human space flights? *Fundamentals of Space Medicine* answers this question, beginning with an introduction to space biology and the space life sciences. It includes a description of the environment, a history of space flight, and challenges facing humans in space. The text describes the effect of space on each body system, space health hazards, and psychosocial issues of space flight, including selection criteria for the mission. It concludes with a description of space life sciences missions and future challenges. The book is recommended for academic libraries with an interest in the field. Gilles Clément presents a detailed description of how to fly a space experiment based upon his work with Salyut-7, Mir, Spacelab, and the Space Shuttle. The text is eminently readable and well illustrated.

Principles and Practice of Aviation Psychology. Editors: Pamela S. Tang, Michael A. Vidulich. Lawrence Erlbaum, 2003.
http://extranet.netlibrary.com/TitleSelect/
ISBN: 9780805833904
ISBN: 9781410606242 (Online)
Recommended for: Academic Libraries

A volume in the *Human Factors in Transportation* series, *Principles and Practice of Aviation Psychology* provides a comprehensive overview and an important addition to the literature of aviation psychology. Not only does it cover the history of aviation, but it also describes the actual pilot actions and tasks pilots are involved with today. The editors have discovered and convinced leaders in this field to contribute to this work. The text presents psychological principles and research pertinent to the interface between a pilot and the cockpit. Understanding the cognitive demands and the capabilities and limitations of the pilot has important implications on selection and training of pilots and display/control designs in the cockpit. Emphasis is placed on the scientific methods of achieving this understanding and the view that theories and principles of human behavior would have much to learn from practical problems and applied studies. Reviews in journals such as *Ergonomics* and the *International Journal of Aviation Psychology* are overwhelmingly favorable, calling this text thought provoking and utterly engaging. It is recommended for academic libraries.

Principles of Clinical Medicine for Space Flight. Editors: Michael R. Barratt, Sam L. Pool. Springer, 2008.
http://extranet.netlibrary.com/TitleSelect/
http://www.springerlink.com/content/978-0-387-98842-9
http://www.ebrary.com/
ISBN: 9780387988429
ISBN: 9780387681641 (Online)
Recommended for: Hospital, Academic Libraries

A successor to Douglas Busby's *Space Clinical Medicine* published in 1968, this comprehensive text, edited by physicians of the NASA/Johnson Space Center in Houston, Texas, describes how to diagnose and treat conditions that occur during or as result of space flight. Including dental, dermatological, and gynecologic concerns, it describes the underlying physiological and psychological aspects of the field, which include topics such as the human response to space flight, medical evaluation and standards, and telemedicine. Amply illustrated with figures, tables, and photographs, the text draws heavily upon the experience of the U.S. Skylab and Space Shuttles programs, the Russian experiences aboard the Salyut and Mir space stations, and the joint work on the International Space Stations (ISS). As a standard of care for supporting humans in space, it is recommended for all academic and clinical medical libraries serving civil, military, and commercial sector medical practitioners.

Journals

Aviation, Space, and Environmental Medicine. v. 1, Aerospace Medical Association (AsMA), 1975.
http://www.ingentaconnect.com/content/asma/asem
ISSN: 00956562 (Print/Online)
Indexed in: MEDLINE, CINAHL
Recommended for: Hospital, Academic Libraries

Affectionately known as the "blue journal," *Aviation, Space, and Environmental Medicine* has provided a forum for aeromedical practitioners (physicians, life scientists, bioengineers, and medical specialists) to publish case studies, research findings, technical notes, news items, and book reviews since 1975. Sponsored by Aerospace Medical Association (AsMA), it is the most used and cited journal in its field and is distributed to more than eighty nations. It is required reading for all who need to stay abreast in the field. The monthly journal publishes occasional supplements on topics such as advances in clinical space medicine and performance enhancement techniques. It is indexed by Embase, PsycINFO, MEDLINE, SPORTDiscus, and Scopus. It is required for clinical and academic libraries that serve practitioners in the field. Former titles for this journal include the *Journal of Aviation Medicine* (1930–1959) and *Aerospace Medicine* (1959–1974).

Human Factors. v. 1, Sage on behalf of Human Factors and Ergonomics Society, 1958.
http://hfs.sagepub.com/
ISSN: 00187208
ISSN: 15478181 (Online)
Indexed in: MEDLINE
Recommended for: Hospital, Academic Libraries

Published bimonthly by Sage Publications as the official publication of the Human Factors and Ergonomics Society, *Human Factors* publishes original research on the study of ergonomic impact, the role of humans in complex systems, the design of equipment and facilities, and the development of human-compatible environments. Many of the articles published are of value to aerospace medicine, such as those related to pilot performance, pilot decision making, crew resource management, automated cockpits, and factors contributing to aircraft incidents. The journal, which is indexed by PsycINFO and MEDLINE, is recommended for academic and clinical libraries.

10.2. Allergy and Immunology

The hypersensitivity of the individual to foreign substances and protection from the resultant infection or disorder.
—MeSH

Contributor: Lorna Springston

Monographs

Allergens and Allergen Immunotherapy. 4th ed. Editors: Richard F. Lockey, Dennis K. Ledford. Informa Healthcare, 2008.

http://extranet.netlibrary.com/TitleSelect/
http://www.ebrary.com/
ISBN: 9781420061970
ISBN: 9781420061987 (Online)
Recommended for: Hospital Libraries
Doody's Core Titles Selection

Modernized and updated, the 4th edition of *Allergens and Allergen Immunotherapy* addresses all major areas of allergens and immunotherapies: pollens, animal/insect, fungi, food, the manufacture and standardization of allergen vaccines, the new method of sublingual swallow immunotherapy, the administration of vaccines, and the avoidance and treatment of adverse effects. *Allergens and Allergen Immunotherapy* is filled with quick reference charts, tables, and indexes. Allergists, immunologists, and otolaryngologists will find this text to be an essential practical reference for diagnosis, treatment, and management of allergies. The textbook focuses on the most relevant information related to allergens and immunotherapy; topics are concise for easier use as a daily reference. The textbook is listed as a *Doody's Core Titles* recommendation within the allergy/clinical immunology subcategory of clinical medicine.

Allergy in ENT Practice. 2nd ed. Authors: Hueston C. King, Richard L. Mabry, Cynthia S. Mabry, Bruce R. Gordon, Bradley F. Marple. Thieme Medical, 2005.
See Chapter 11.7. Otolaryngology

Middleton's Allergy: Principles and Practice. 7th ed. Editors: N. Franklin Adkinson Jr., William W. Busse, Bruce S. Bochner, Stephen T. Holgate, F. Estelle R. Simons, Robert F. Lemanske Jr. Mosby/Elsevier, 2009.
http://www.mdconsult.com/
ISBN: 9780323056595
ISBN: 9780323048842
Recommended for: Hospital, Academic Libraries
Brandon/Hill, *Doody's Core Titles* Selection

This best-selling, multi-format resource is the leader in its field. It is comprised of contributions from hundreds of international authorities offering expertise to address any clinical challenge. It provides comprehensive coverage of basic science as well as authoritative guidance on the practical aspects of day-to-day diagnosis and management. This edition includes 400 new illustrations, or 700 in all. The seventh edition offers a new format—The Expert Consult Edition—for busy practitioners, making information retrieval easier and quicker. The Expert Consult Edition offers online access to the complete contents of the two-volume set for individuals. It includes a glossary of allergy and immunology for easy reference, highlighted key points and clinical pearls to find important information quickly, and links to authoritative online resources for professionals and patients, including links to MEDLINE abstracts for all of the references. *Middleton's* covers hot topics such as food allergy and immunotherapy, and it includes the latest guidelines from the National Asthma Education and Prevention Program (NAEPP). In addition to the Expert Consult version, institutional online access is offered on Elsevier's MD Consult platform. The textbook is a former Brandon/Hill allergy recommendation and a *Doody's Core Titles* essential purchase recommendation within the allergy/clinical immunology subcategory of clinical medicine.

Pediatric Allergy: Principles and Practice. Editors: Donald Y.M. Leung, Hugh A. Sampson, Raif S. Geha, Stanley J. Szefler. Mosby, 2003.
ISBN: 9780323018029
Recommended for: Hospital, Academic Libraries
Doody's Core Titles Selection

The goal of the editors of *Pediatric Allergy: Principles and Practice* was to document and summarize the numerous recent changes in the field of pediatric allergy/immunology. Leung and his colleagues have fulfilled their goal. This textbook on allergic disorders in infants and children covers a wide range of topics, including food allergy in nine, well-written chapters with topics ranging from the mechanisms of mucosal immunity to the diagnosis and management of food allergy. Of particular note is the chapter on the prevention of atopy, which presents and discusses various controversies. The section on asthma is provided in twelve chapters that cover immunopathology, new directions in research, the clinical aspects of asthma, the education of patients about asthma, and the promotion of compliance to treatment and self management. Sections on pediatric immunology and immunodeficiency are included. All sections are concise and offer practical algorithms and tables. However, rhinitis and drug allergies are covered in lesser detail, and readers may have to refer to other sources for more comprehensive information. This well-written text displays solid organization. The "key concepts" boxes throughout each chapter are invaluable for highlighting important points and summarizing information. This companion to *Middleton's Allergy* is a practical guide to the diagnosis and management of all pediatric allergies. The textbook is a *Doody's Core Titles* recommendation within the allergy/clinical immunology subcategory of clinical medicine.

Journals

American Journal of Rhinology & Allergy. v. 23, Ocean-Side, 2009.
See Chapter 11.7. Otolaryngology

The Journal of Allergy and Clinical Immunology. v. 1, Mosby, 1971.
http://www.jacionline.org/
http://www.sciencedirect.com/science/journal/00916749
ISSN: 00916749
ISSN: 10976825 (Online)
Indexed in: MEDLINE
Recommended for: Hospital, Academic Libraries
Brandon/Hill Selection

An official publication of the American Academy of Allergy, Asthma, and Immunology, *The Journal of Allergy and Clinical Immunology* provides timely clinical papers, instructive case reports, and detailed examinations of the latest equipment and techniques available to clinical allergists, immunologists, dermatologists, internists, and other physicians concerned with clinical manifestations of allergies in their practice. Articles cover such topics as allergic and immunologic diseases; the latest therapies and treatment programs; occupational and industrial allergy; and studies of antigens, allergens, and the environment. According to the 2009 *Journal Citation Reports*, the journal ranks first of 21 titles in the allergy category and eighth of 128 in the immunology category. *The Journal of Allergy and Clinical Immunology* is a former Brandon/Hill selection. Full online coverage back to volume 93, 1994 is available through Elsevier.

10.3. Dermatology

The skin, its structure, functions, diseases, and treatment.
—MeSH

Contributor: Erin Palazzolo

Monographs

Clinical Dermatology: A Color Guide to Diagnosis and Therapy. 5th ed. Author: Thomas P. Habif. Mosby Elsevier, 2010.
ISBN: 9780723435419
Recommended for: Hospital, Academic, Consumer Health Libraries
Brandon/Hill, *Doody's Core Titles* Selection

This text is recommended for academic institutions, hospitals, and practitioners' offices that field dermatologic complaints. The chapters are arranged consistently, presenting photographs and descriptions for identification, information about testing, and treatment options. The latest edition of *Clinical Dermatology* includes over 1,000 color photographs, 500 of which are new and include updated information for the diagnosis and treatment of different ethnic skin types. Habif's text includes a dermatologic formulary, a chapter on dermatologic procedures, and, new to this edition, a chapter on anatomy and diagnosis that acts as a quick visual reference directing the reader to extended reading options in later chapters. For individual purchasers of the print book, Expert Consult online access is included. This access combines the contents of the text with additional images, links to PubMed, and the updated DDx Mannequin, which allows the user to find the most probable differential diagnosis by body region. Previous editions of this text have been included in *Doody's Core Titles* and have been selected for the Brandon/Hill small medical libraries list.

Color Atlas of Pediatric Dermatology. 4th ed. Authors: Samuel Weinberg, Neil S. Prose, Leonard Kristal. McGraw-Hill, 2008.
ISBN: 9780071455435
Recommended for: Hospital, Academic, Consumer Health Libraries
Doody's Core Titles Selection

This four-star 2009 *Doody's Core Titles* selection is a required text for academic institutions, hospital libraries, and those who treat pediatric dermatological complaints. The *Atlas* contains more than 900 color photographs (230 new images from the last publication), with each including a few sentences describing the condition or discussing its treatment. From the common to the very rare conditions, this book provides a good pictorial reference that will aid medical staff with diagnosis. The *Atlas* is divided into 27 sections, from "Bacterial Disorders" and "Drug Eruptions" to "Disorders of Nails and Hair." This edition includes references to new and emerging infectious diseases and biological and chemical weapons; it also contains updated clinical findings and treatment guidelines where applicable.

Differential Diagnosis for the Dermatologist. Authors: Scott M. Jackson, Lee T. Nesbitt. Springer, 2008.
http://www.springerlink.com/content/978-3-540-75886-0/
http://extranet.netlibrary.com/TitleSelect/
http://www.r2library.com/

http://www.ebrary.com/
ISBN: 9783540758860
ISBN: 9783540758877
Recommended for: Hospital, Academic Libraries

Practicing dermatologists and dermatology residents are the audience for this resource, which is intended to streamline the time spent on constructing a differential diagnosis. For ease of use, this book is ordered alphabetically and provides an appendix with syndromes and their symptoms; when appropriate, a workup is recommended to confirm the diagnosis. Entries also provide references for further reading. The print textbook is accompanied by a mobile version that offers physicians easy portability. The *Doody's* reviewer described it as "the best differential book to date."

Ethnic Dermatology: Clinical Problems and Skin Pigmentation. 2nd ed. Author: Clive B. Archer. Informa Healthcare, 2008.
http://www.ebrary.com/
http://extranet.netlibrary.com/TitleSelect/
ISBN: 9780415471190
ISBN: 9780203092149
Recommended for: Hospital, Academic, Consumer Health Libraries
Doody's Core Titles Selection

Academic institutions, hospitals, and libraries that serve residents, physicians, and other medical professionals who treat dermatologic complaints should provide access to this specialized text. Its unique focus on skin complaints in patients with Indian or African ethnic origins sets this book apart. Where so many other dermatologic texts focus on light-skinned individuals, this valuable text helps fill a void by acting as a reference to dermatological complaints and their manifestations in individuals with darker skin. This text contains an excellent collection of color images that will aid in diagnosis. This publication is included in *Doody's Core Titles*.

Fitzpatrick's Color Atlas and Synopsis of Clinical Dermatology. 6th ed. Editors: Klaus Wolff, Richard A. Johnson. McGraw-Hill Medical, 2009.
http://www.accessmedicine.com/
http://extranet.netlibrary.com/TitleSelect/
http://www.statref.com/
http://www.r2library.com/
ISBN: 9780071599757
ISBN: 9780071633420
Recommended for: Hospital, Academic, Consumer Health Libraries
Brandon/Hill, *Doody's Core Titles* Selection

This atlas should be required in all academic institutions and hospitals that serve residents, physicians, and other medical professionals who treat dermatologic complaints. Each disorder is listed with the epidemiology, pathogenesis, clinical manifestation, course, laboratory examinations, diagnosis, and differential diagnosis. Most entries contain multiple color images and include added tables and sections where appropriate. For example, the entry for allergic contact dermatitis includes a table providing the "Top Ten Contact Allergens (North American Contact Dermatitis Group) and Other Common Contact Allergens." The laboratory sections go into detail on which tests to run and the results that are sought. This text is a *Doody's* essential purchase.

Fitzpatrick's Dermatology in General Medicine. 7th ed. Editor: Klaus Wolff. McGraw-Hill, 2008.
http://www.accessmedicine.com/
http://www.r2library.com/
http://www.ebrary.com/
ISBN: 9780071466905
ISBN: 9780071544481
Recommended for: Hospital, Academic Libraries
Brandon/Hill, *Doody's Core Titles* Selection

This two-volume encyclopedic resource starts with an introduction to the science of skin as an organ and proceeds to explore dermatologic conditions in depth within its 39 sections and 257 chapters. Similar to its peers, *Fitzpatrick's* contains the usual array of photographs, diagnosis criteria, and treatment, but it excels with more comprehensive text delving into the how and why cutaneous reactions occur in the body. It provides a multitude of figures that will help medical students better understand the integument system and allow seasoned instructors to provide visual resources for complex topics. In the newest edition, the basic science chapters are grouped with appropriate clinical chapters within the different sections. For individual purchasers, the print textbook is accompanied by an online version that allows for quick searching and the ability to download images. Institutional online access is provided through AccessMedicine and other platforms. The most recent edition of this book is a *Doody's* core title, and previous editions were selected for the Brandon/Hill small medical libraries list.

Lever's Histopathology of the Skin. 10th ed. Editor: David E. Elder. Lippincott Williams & Wilkins, 2009.
http://www.ovid.com/
http://www.r2library.com/
ISBN: 9780781773638

Recommended for: Hospital, Academic Libraries
Doody's Core Titles Selection

Lever's is a classic text that has been in publication for 50 years. Currently in its tenth edition, the text is still a standard in histopathology for dermatologists, pathologists, residents, and the libraries that serve them. This resource contains over 1,400 color illustrations and an appendix of black-and-white electron micrographs. The tenth edition follows the "traditional clinicopathologic classification of cutaneous disease," the structure of all previous editions. This edition was favorably reviewed in the *Journal of the American Academy of Dermatology* (2009 Jul; 61(1):171) as it "continues the tradition of scholarship and practicality that have made the text one of the best-known names in medical publishing." The tenth edition was also named as a *Doody's Core Titles* selection.

Skin Cancer. Editor: Keyvan Nouri. McGraw-Hill, 2008.
http://extranet.netlibrary.com/TitleSelect/
http://www.ebrary.com/
http://www.r2library.com/
ISBN: 9780071472562
ISBN: 9780071593595
Recommended for: Hospital, Academic Libraries

Skin Cancer is an elegant resource that covers all aspects of cutaneous malignancies. The more than 450 illustrations take the reader through the clinical presentation of the malignancy to the pathology and diagnosis. The text delves into the genetic alterations, treatments, epidemiology, and prognosis of each type of cancer. This is an excellent resource for residents and physicians who diagnose and treat skin cancers. The text is divided into three sections: "Cancer and Tumors," "Techniques and Treatments," and "Related Issues and Frontiers." The *JAMA: Journal of the American Medical Association* reviewer concluded, "with the excellent clinical and histopathologic images and the exhaustive list of references, this textbook will become the major source of information about skin cancers."

Surgery of the Skin: Procedural Dermatology. 2nd ed. Authors: June K. Robinson, C. William Hanke, Daniel M. Siegel, Alina Fratila. Mosby Elsevier, 2010.
ISBN: 9780323065757
Recommended for: Hospital, Academic Libraries

Awarded five stars by *Doody's*, this text was described in the *Journal of the American Academy of Dermatology* as a "complete, well-written, well-thought-out and beautifully presented book." *Surgery of the Skin* is recommended for libraries that act as a resource for dermatologic surgeons and residents. This book covers the most common dermatologic procedures and extends its coverage to related topics, such as accreditation issues and surgical suite design. Included with the print text is a DVD of surgical procedures performed by the senior author of each chapter. These procedures are accompanied by running commentary and act as a useful learning tool for new surgeons. This review refers to the first edition. The second edition includes new procedures in both the written text and the accompanying DVD, online access for individual purchases of the print textbook, and bonus images showing alternative techniques or additional therapies at Elsevier's Expert Consult website.

Journals

Archives of Dermatology. v. 82, American Medical Association, July 1960.
http://archderm.ama-assn.org/
ISSN: 0003987X
ISSN: 15383652 (Online)
Indexed in: MEDLINE
Recommended for: Hospital, Academic Libraries
Brandon/Hill Selection

This journal started publication in 1920 as the *Archives of Dermatology and Syphilogy* and, after several name changes, became the *Archives of Dermatology* in July 1960. This resource was a recommended purchase from the Brandon/Hill list and is currently ranked second in dermatology journals by the 2009 *Journal Citation Reports*. With its broad coverage, this journal is appropriate for both academic and hospital libraries and will be used by medical professionals ranging from students to practicing physicians. Both generalists and specialists will find this to be a valuable resource. This journal is widely indexed and is considered a core clinical journal by the National Library of Medicine.

British Journal of Dermatology. v. 63, British Association of Dermatologists/Wiley-Blackwell, 1951.
http://onlinelibrary.wiley.com/journal/10.1111/(ISSN)1365-2133
ISSN: 00070963
ISSN: 13652133 (Online)
Indexed in: MEDLINE
Recommended for: Hospital, Academic Libraries

This resource is the official publication of the British Association of Dermatologists and has been in publication under various titles for over 120 years. The journal covers both the clinical and experimental aspects of dermatology and "serves equally the laboratory worker and the clinician." Because of its broad coverage, this journal supports medical professionals in academia, research, and hospital environments. Issues include original articles addressing the following topics: cutaneous biology, clinical and laboratory investigations, contact dermatitis and allergy, dermatological surgery and lasers, dermatopathology, epidemiology and health services research, pediatric dermatology, photobiology, and therapeutics. *Journal Citation Reports* (2009) ranks this widely indexed publication fourth, with an impact factor of 4.260, among 48 dermatology journals.

Dermatology Nursing. v. 1, A.J. Jannetti, 1989.
http://www.dermatologynursing.net/
http://www.ebscohost.com/
ISSN: 10603441
Indexed in: MEDLINE, CINAHL
Recommended for: Hospital, Academic Libraries

Dermatology nurses in training and in practice will utilize this resource. The journal provides clinical information on all aspects of skin and wound care and offers continuing nursing education (CNE) opportunities that practicing nurses will appreciate. This publication also offers practical advice for medical assistants in the successful management of a dermatology office. *Dermatology Nursing* is appropriate for libraries that support nursing students and environments that include nurses who specialize in dermatological care and research.

Experimental Dermatology. v. 1, John Wiley, 1992.
http://onlinelibrary.wiley.com/journal/10.1111/(ISSN)1600-0625
ISSN: 09066705
ISSN: 16000625 (Online)
Indexed in: MEDLINE
Recommended for: Academic Libraries

Experimental Dermatology is an important resource for institutions that support faculty and staff in dermatological research. This resource is the official publication of several organizations, including the European Immunodermatology Society, the Australasian Hair and Wool Research Society, Arbeitsgemeinschaft Dermatologische Forschung, and the Hidradenitis Suppurativa Foundation. The journal focuses on cutting-edge research and experimental design and methodology. Though a relatively new journal, it has already reached an impact factor of 3.329 and is ranked in the top ten journals in dermatology (2009 *Journal Citation Reports*). This publication is indexed and abstracted in multiple sources such as MEDLINE, Embase, and Science Citation Index.

Journal of Dermatological Science. v. 1, Elsevier, 1990.
http://www.sciencedirect.com/science/journal/09231811
ISSN: 09231811
ISSN: 1873569X (Online)
Indexed in: MEDLINE
Recommended for: Academic Libraries

The *Journal of Dermatological Science* serves as the official journal of the Japanese Society for Investigative Dermatology. A multi-national editorial board supports this English-language journal. This resource includes broad coverage of dermatological science and supports both laboratory and clinical practice. Although a relatively new publication, it has achieved an impact factor that places it sixth in dermatological journals, as determined by the 2009 *Journal Citation Reports*. This is a good choice for academic libraries and institutions that support dermatological research.

Journal of Investigative Dermatology. v. 1, Nature Publishing Group, 1938.
http://www.nature.com/jid/index.html
ISSN: 0022202X
ISSN: 15231747 (Online)
Indexed in: MEDLINE
Recommended for: Academic Libraries

The *Journal of Investigative Dermatology* was established in 1938, which is the same year as its founding organization, The Society for Investigative Dermatology. Based on the 2009 *Journal Citation Reports*, this resource ranks first among 48 journals in the dermatological field, with an impact factor of 5.543. The editors state that this resource is dedicated to "original research on all aspects of cutaneous biology and skin disease." Topics include "biochemistry, biophysics, carcinogenesis, cell regulation, development, skin structure, extracellular matrix, genetics, immunology, melanocyte biology, microbiology, molecular and cellular biology, pathology, physiology, pharmacology, photobiology, percutaneous absorption, clinical research, and epidemiology." This widely indexed journal provides original articles, communications, reviews, and letters to the editor. This is an essential acquisition for organizations that train or employ dermatologists, as well as large university libraries.

Journal of the American Academy of Dermatology. v. 1, Mosby, 1979.
http://www.sciencedirect.com/science/journal/01909622

http://www.mdconsult.com/
ISSN: 01909622
ISSN: 10976787 (Online)
Indexed in: MEDLINE
Recommended for: Hospital, Academic Libraries
Brandon/Hill Selection

Started in 1979 as the official publication of the American Academy of Dermatology, this peer-reviewed journal was created "to meet the continuing education needs of the Academy members and the international dermatologic community." Medical students and residents will appreciate its broad topic coverage, and faculty and other practicing physicians will value its continuing medical education (CME) opportunities. The journal is currently ranked fifth in impact factor among 48 in its subject (2009 *Journal Citation Reports*). It was a recommended purchase from the Brandon/Hill list for small medical libraries.

Pediatric Dermatology. v. 1, Wiley-Blackwell, 1983.
http://onlinelibrary.wiley.com/journal/10.1111/(ISSN)1525-1470
ISSN: 07368046
ISSN: 15251470 (Online)
Indexed in: MEDLINE
Recommended for: Hospital, Academic Libraries

This journal is the official publication of several organizations, including the Society for Pediatric Dermatology, the European Society for Pediatric Dermatology, the International Society of Pediatric Dermatology, the Dutch/Belgian Pediatric Dermatology Society, the Latin American Pediatric Dermatology Society, and the Spanish Society of Pediatric Dermatology. This resource covers all aspects of infant and child dermatology, from genetics and research to clinical diagnosis and treatment. The journal includes reviews, original research, and plentiful case reports. Physicians of varied levels of experience can practice their diagnostic skills using the sections "What's Your Diagnosis?" and "Techniques for Tots."

Pigment Cell & Melanoma Research. v. 21, Blackwell Munksgaard, 2008.
http://onlinelibrary.wiley.com/journal/10.1111/(ISSN)1755-148X
ISSN: 17551471
ISSN: 1755148X (Online)
Indexed in: MEDLINE
Recommended for: Hospital, Academic Libraries

This publication is the official journal for both the International Federation of Pigment Cell Societies and the Society for Melanoma Research. It started publication in 1987 under its previous title, *Pigment Cell Research*, and shifted to its current title in 2008. As the title suggests, this journal publishes on all topics relating to pigment cells and melanoma, including development, genetics, and disease processes. It is ranked third among 48 dermatology journals, with an impact factor of 4.344 (2009 *Journal Citation Reports*). This journal has a regular format that includes editorials, news and views, review articles, and original articles. Indexing is available through multiple sources such as Scopus, MEDLINE, and Chemical Abstracts. This journal is appropriate for researchers, residents, and physicians who specialize in this field.

Databases and Other Electronic Resources

VisualDx: Visual Diagnostic Decision Support. Logical Images, 2000.
http://www.visualdx.com
Recommended for: Hospital, Academic Libraries

Available by subscription, *VisualDx* is an electronic database that will aid residents, physicians, and dental professionals in diagnosis; it will also support faculty and students in the learning process. The database includes over 1,000 different conditions and contains over 17,000 images, with a wide range of ethnicity, age, immunity status, and disease severity. The resource covers conditions affecting the skin, external eye, oral mucosa, and pulmonary system. The database is similar to traditional atlases that allow users to look up specific diagnoses, but its unique differential diagnosis module also permits users to locate diagnoses by listing symptoms. Users can select the age of the patient, along with the type and location of the lesion; key findings, such as distress and duration of the problem, can then be added to the differential builder. The database also allows users to indicate other noncutaneous findings, such as fever or weight loss. Beginning students who are still unfamiliar with the appropriate terminology will be able to use this resource because the database provides images to help define the difference between types of dermatological findings, such as a scaly papule and eschar. Once an entry for a specific condition has been located, the user will be able to view multiple images and read about the diagnosis, testing, and treatment of the condition. Potentially life-threatening emergency warnings are posted in red at the top of each condition page, and a red [E] appears next to pictures to aid physicians in rapid assessment.

10.4. Disaster Medicine

Management and organization of public health response to disasters and major events including the special health and medical needs of a community in a disaster.

—MeSH

Contributors: Alicia A. Livinski, Cynthia B. Love, and Elizabeth Norton

Monographs

Advanced Disaster Medical Response Manual for Providers. Editors: Susan M. Briggs, Kathryn H. Brinsfield. Harvard Medical International Trauma & Disaster Institute, 2003.
ISBN: 9780972377201
Recommended for: Hospital, Academic Libraries

This spiral-bound handbook is about "delivering the greatest good to the greatest number" in disaster situations where destruction and mortality may be common. It begins with a discussion of mass casualty incidents when local medical and public health infrastructures are likely to be overwhelmed and resources, including communication and transportation, may be very limited or non-existent. The second of nine sections describes the Incident Command System that allows for an organized and coordinated response to emergency situations of any type and scope. Other sections include succinct and illustrated information on medical response to disasters, public health response to disasters, decontamination, medical response to terrorism, care of specific injuries in disasters, environmental considerations, psychological responses to disasters and care of the dead. This text is intended for use in both training and in medical response. Its easy-to-carry design is suitable for field use.

Disaster Medicine. 3rd ed. Editor: Gregory R. Ciottone. Elsevier/Mosby, 2006.
http://www.sciencedirect.com/science/book/9780323032537
http://www.mdconsult.com
ISBN: 9780323032537
Recommended for: Hospital, Academic Libraries
Doody's Core Titles Selection

This comprehensive reference text represents the work of over 200 contributors in the field of disaster preparedness, assessment, management and response. It is divided into two parts. Part 1 includes 70 concise chapters about the disaster medicine discipline, disaster response and training, ethical issues, animal management, triage, search and rescue, and the integrated management of disaster events. Particular attention is given to the Incident Command System that is widely used to manage emergency situations. Part 2 consists of 120 equally concise chapters on every disaster scenario imaginable at the time of publication, including meteoroid impact and exposure to LSD. The scenarios include a description of the event, the recommended medical treatment of casualties, unique characteristics, knowledge gaps, and risks and vulnerabilities. As a general text, it is an appropriate and ready reference guide for all types of medical and public health professionals, government authorities, and emergency managers and planners. *Disaster Medicine* is a *Doody's* core title in the emergency medicine category.

Disaster Medicine. 2nd ed. Editors: David E. Hogan, Jonathan L. Burstein. Lippincott Williams & Wilkins, 2007.
http://www.ovid.com/
ISBN: 9780781762625
Recommended for: Hospital, Academic Libraries
Doody's Core Titles Selection

Hogan and Burstein's text provides comprehensive coverage of the emerging field of disaster medicine. Directed at medical and public health practitioners who are involved in disaster preparedness and response, the book contains information ranging from basic disaster concepts to how to handle the medical consequences of intentional use of warfare agents to inflict mass casualties. The 39 chapters in this book are divided into six sections for ease of use. A particularly valuable feature of this text is the extensive coverage in the first two sections on topics related to disaster planning and incident management. Medical responders to disaster events and first recipients of victims need to understand and plan for working within the collaborative incident response framework presented in these chapters. Of note is the in-depth coverage of the role of the hospital in disaster preparedness and planning. Three sections of the book cover specific types of disasters, divided into natural disasters; industrial, technological, and transportation disasters and conflict-related disasters. The sixth section covers education, core competencies, training, and research in disaster medicine, which are important topics for this evolving, multidisciplinary field. Extensive references and resource lists follow each chapter. This text is a *Doody's* core title within the related emergency medicine subject area.

Hidden Impact: What You Need to Know for the Next Disaster—A Practical Mental Health Guide for Clinicians. Editors: Frederick J. Stoddard, Craig L. Katz,

Joseph P. Merlino. Jones & Bartlett, 2010.
ISBN: 9780763768751
Recommended for: Hospital, Academic Libraries

The main title and small paperback format should not deter consideration of this book on mental health for a collection on disaster medicine. Written primarily for clinicians in the primary care setting, it is a comprehensive and useful guide for preparing for the unexpected. Twenty-four contributed chapters are organized in four sections: preparedness, assessment, intervention and special issues. The first section focuses on how to become involved in disaster response and how to participate within the existing national disaster response framework. This section is applicable for a general audience, not solely behavioral health or clinical professionals. The second section describes screening tools, abnormal and normal disaster behaviors, and unique considerations among children and within special needs populations. The third section offers psychiatric first aid, psychological and pharmaceutical options, and the role of collaboration. Section four covers ethical and legal dimensions of working in a disaster setting and the use of telepsychiatry. The easy-to-read format of this book makes it also useful for non-clinicians who are interested in understanding the psychological and behavioral aspects of disasters.

Koenig and Schultz's Disaster Medicine: Comprehensive Principles and Practices. Editors: Kristi L. Koenig, Carl H. Schultz. Cambridge University Press, 2010.
http://www.cambridge.org/
ISBN: 9780521873673
ISBN: 9780511795602 (Online)
Recommended for: Hospital, Academic Libraries

This text is a very recent addition to the limited, but growing list of disaster medicine resources, and as such is very current in its coverage of disaster topics and the management of mass casualty situations. The book is organized into three parts with 39 chapters contributed by disaster and emergency medicine specialists from around the world. The intended audience of emergency physicians and nurses is provided a rich reference guide that describes the conceptual framework of disasters, operational issues related to disaster planning, response and management, and clinical management of specific natural and man-made disaster types. Over one-half of the text explores special topics in disaster planning and preparedness, including ethical considerations, mental and behavioral health, special needs populations, surge capacity, public health issues, mass fatality management, and crisis communications. Potential disaster situations are described in separate chapters with detailed guidance on the diagnosis and treatment of victims.

Public Health Consequences of Disasters. Editor: Eric K. Noji. Oxford University Press, 1997.
ISBN: 9780195095708
Recommended for: Hospital, Academic Libraries

This text is considered a classic reference on defining and exploring the public health impact of disasters. It is divided into four parts: general issues, geophysical events, weather-related problems, and human-generated problems. Although it was published before some of the recent significant disasters, including Hurricane Katrina and the World Trade Center attack of 9-11-2001, it provides a thorough description of basic concepts such as the practical application of epidemiologic methods in disasters, disease surveillance and control, environmental impacts, mental health issues, and media relations. This book covers specific disasters from a different perspective than texts geared toward medical professionals. The focus in this book is on the natural and man-made factors that contribute to and result from the disaster, minimizing the impact on public health through prevention and control strategies, identification of critical knowledge gaps, methodological problems, and research recommendations. Among its features is a chapter on complex emergencies, defined as wars, violent civil conflicts, and other situations that result in large-scale displacement of civilian populations and may include human rights abuses. This book adds a public health perspective to the study of disaster medicine. In-depth coverage of clinical treatment of victims, disaster response and incident management is left to other texts.

Public Health Management of Disasters: The Practice Guide. 2nd ed. Author: Linda Young Landesman. American Public Health Association, 2005.
ISBN: 9780875530451
Recommended for: Hospital, Academic Libraries

This book is a practical resource that provides guidelines, resources, and information about planning for and responding to the public health implications of disasters. Its 13 chapters are well organized and easy for health professionals to glean knowledge from experiences in previous disaster situations. Among the many updates of this second edition is information on new types of disasters, changes in federal response and organization, new communication systems, surge capacity, organizing mental health services, ensuring food safety and feeding large numbers of displaced persons, death notification, assisting people with disabilities, and handling human remains. In addition to an extensive bibliography, there are over 100 pages of appendixes that include definitions of terms and acronyms used in disaster preparedness and response, lists of websites, and content suggestions for first aid and survival kits. Public health professionals, policy makers, government officials, health professionals involved in disaster preparedness, and emergency managers will find this a comprehensive compilation of relevant resources about the implications and management of disasters affecting the community.

Textbook of Disaster Psychiatry. Editors: Richard J. Ursano, Carol S. Fullerton, Lars Weisaeth, Beverley Raphael. Cambridge University Press, 2007.
http://www.cambridge.org/
ISBN: 9780521852357
ISBN: 9780511372407 (Online)
Recommended for: Hospital, Academic Libraries

Psychological, biological and social consequences of disasters are addressed in this text dedicated to disaster psychiatry. Intended for practitioners and health planners dealing with mental health treatment and recovery, the book describes evidenced-based clinical interventions by a highly experienced range of clinicians and researchers. The contents, organized into five parts, include foundations of disaster psychology, clinical care and interventions, special topics, and public health issues. The special topics cover areas such as dealing with the behavioral, social, and emotional consequences of exposures to or fear of weapons of mass destruction, pandemics, workplace disasters, and terrorism. Chapters also address the epidemiology of disaster response, the neurobiology of disaster exposure, role of non-governmental organizations, and workplace policies. This book provides scientific and practical information that ensures the often overlooked stress-related aspects of disasters are considered in the preparedness, mitigation, and recovery activities of traumatic events. It addresses both the needs of the individual and those of the community, which makes this also a very useful reference for public health planners and professionals.

Toxico-terrorism: Emergency Response and Clinical Approach to Chemical, Biological, and Radiological Agents. Editors: Robin B. McFee, Jerrold B. Leikin. McGraw-Hill, 2008.
ISBN: 9780071471862
ISBN: 9780071593557 (Online)
Recommended for: Hospital, Academic Libraries

Given the proliferation of biological, chemical, and radiological agents as deliberate threats to social and individual safety, a text on this subject is a must-have for any disaster medicine collection. This text is directed primarily at physicians and other pre-hospital and hospital emergency personnel who need to be prepared to identify, treat, and manage victims of exposure to these agents. There are seven parts to the book, each divided into chapters contributed by professionals in the field. The first three parts of the book cover general principles of what, how, and where of toxic contaminants; emergency services issues; and preparation within the emergency department, including triage, security, and pharmacy readiness. The next three parts address in detail the specific types of agents, chemical, biological, and ionizing radiation, that victims may be exposed to. These sections include information on properties, manifestations, diagnosis, and clinical management of exposure. The last section expands the discussion to the public health considerations of deliberate releases of these agents on the population. The book also contains 11 appendixes on practical information, including laboratory guidelines and specific instructions for shipping samples. An e-book version is available for individual purchasers.

Journals

American Journal of Disaster Medicine. v. 1, Weston Medical, 2006.
http://ejournal.disastermedicinejournal.com/
ISSN: 1932149X
Indexed in: MEDLINE
Recommended for: Hospital, Academic Libraries

This peer-reviewed publication covers all aspects of disaster medicine. Geared towards physicians and medical professionals, the journal provides interdisciplinary guidance in a wide range of subjects including triage protocols, toxicological disasters, treating mass casualties, psychological trauma, biological weapons exposure, public health preparedness, humanitarian relief, and other current topics in disaster and emergency medicine. Aspects of emergency management are reported together with clinical and trauma care for an integrated perspective on the disaster medicine field. Coverage is both national and international. The bi-monthly publication includes original research articles, clinical reports, brief communications, articles related to new ideas or innovations, letters to the editor, editorials, invited book reviews, and meeting announcements. It is available in print with an online version published in a flash format. The journal is indexed in MEDLINE.

Annals of Emergency Medicine. v. 9, Mosby, Inc, 1980.
http://www.annemergmed.com/

http://www.sciencedirect.com/science/journal/01960644
ISSN: 01960644
ISSN: 10976760 (Online)
See Also Chapter 10.5. Emergency Medicine, Chapter 13.2. Emergency Nursing
Indexed in: MEDLINE, CINAHL
Recommended for: Hospital, Academic Libraries

Begun in 1972 under another title, *Annals of Emergency Medicine* is the official journal of the American College of Emergency Physicians (ACEP). This international, peer-reviewed journal includes articles on teaching and research in emergency medicine as well as general emergency medicine topics, opinion pieces, and clinical reports. This is the top emergency medicine journal, ranking number one in ISI's 2009 *Journal Citation Reports* for the emergency medicine category. In 2009, the Special Libraries Association ranked the *Annals of Emergency Medicine* as one of the 100 most influential journals of biology and medicine over the last 100 years. The intended audience is all those interested in emergency medicine and research. This journal is a required resource for hospitals with an active emergency room or trauma referral center as well as any academic medical center. It is cited in numerous abstracting and indexing sources such as MEDLINE, Embase, CINAHL, Science Citation Index (Web of Science), and Scopus. While not disaster-specific in its focus, its subject matter is closely related to disaster medicine, and it frequently publishes articles about disaster preparedness, response, and management. Other related subjects include health policy and ethics, toxicology, and out-of-hospital emergency medical services. Full online coverage is available through Elsevier ScienceDirect.

Biosecurity and Bioterrorism: Biodefense Strategy, Practice and Science. v. 1, Mary Ann Liebert, Inc, 2003.
http://www.liebertpub.com/BSP
ISSN: 15387135
ISSN: 1557850X (Online)
Indexed in: MEDLINE
Recommended for: Hospital, Academic Libraries

This journal is an authoritative source for in-depth coverage of issues related to biological weapons and bioterrorism. Published quarterly, the journal includes articles on medicine, public health law, national security, bioscientific research, agriculture and food safety, and drug and vaccine development. This is an excellent resource for anyone who works, conducts research, develops policy or has an interest in biosecurity strategy, management, science or operations. Its international and multidisciplinary focus reflects the complexity of assessing and mitigating biological vulnerabilities within any geographic or governmental arena. The journal is peer-reviewed and indexed in MEDLINE, Social Sciences Citation Index, Current Contents/Social & Behavioral Sciences, Social SciSearch, EMBiology, Scopus, and CAB Abstracts. Online access is available to volume 1, 2003 from the publisher.

Disaster Medicine and Public Health Preparedness. v. 1, American Medical Association, 2007.
http://www.dmphp.org/
ISSN: 19357893
ISSN: 1938744X (Online)
Indexed in: MEDLINE
Recommended for: Hospital, Academic Libraries

Published by the American Medical Association, this relatively new quarterly peer-reviewed journal contains original research, reviews, special studies, letters, and editorials related to disaster medicine and public health preparedness. National and global perspectives are included on subjects such as public health law, ethics, policy, mass critical care management, surge capacity, and emergency response strategy. The content of this journal is geared toward medical and public health practitioners, emergency managers, and policy makers who are involved in preparedness and response issues. The focus is on both the practical and the exchange of ideas for further research on the practice of disaster medicine and its integration with public health. In addition to the quarterly publication schedule, special topic supplements are occasionally produced. Online access is available to volume 1, 2007.

Disasters: The Journal of Disaster Studies, Policy and Management. v. 1, Wiley-Blackwell, 1977.
http://onlinelibrary.wiley.com/journal/10.1111/(ISSN)1467-7717
ISSN: 03613666
ISSN: 14677717 (Online)
Indexed in: MEDLINE
Recommended for: Hospital, Academic Libraries

As one of the oldest continuously published disaster-related journals, *Disasters* focuses on all aspects of disaster studies, policy, and management. The journal's coverage appeals to the academic sector and policymakers with its heavy emphasis on humanitarian and international relief efforts and studies. It is peer-reviewed and published quarterly on behalf of the Overseas Development Institute, an independent, international development think tank in Britain. The journal contains field studies, case studies, academic papers, book reviews, conference reports, letters, and discussions. It is considered a premier journal in international disaster studies and is indexed in several dozen sources, including MEDLINE, Current Contents, Embase, Social Sciences Citation Index, CAB Abstracts, Social SciSearch and CSA Biological Sciences Database. Online access to volume 1, 1977 is available from the publisher.

Journal of Traumatic Stress. v. 1, John Wiley & Sons, 1988.
http://onlinelibrary.wiley.com/journal/10.1002/(ISSN)1573-6598
ISSN: 08949867
ISSN: 15736598 (Online)
Indexed in: MEDLINE
Recommended for: Hospital, Academic Libraries

Disaster events trigger significant emotional, social, and psychological stress in victims and in persons assisting victims. A disaster medicine collection would not be complete without a publication dedicated to the study and research of bio-psychosocial aspects of traumatic events. This bi-monthly journal, published for the International Society for Traumatic Stress, provides peer-reviewed works related to the treatment, prevention education/training, and legal and policy issues related to stress caused by events such as disasters, war, violence, and other life-threatening situations. The contents include original articles, brief reports, review papers, commentaries, and occasional special issues devoted to a single topic. Its research and scholarly focus would appeal to researchers, clinicians, and therapists who are involved in the study and treatment of persons who have been involved in or been affected by a traumatic or disaster event. It is indexed in MEDLINE and numerous other indexing and abstracting databases, among them: Cambridge Scientific Abstracts, CSA Biological Sciences Database, Current Abstracts, Current Contents/Social & Behavioral Sciences, Embase, Psychological Abstracts, Social Sciences Citation Index, and Social SciSearch. Online access to volume 1, 1988 is available from the publisher.

Prehospital and Disaster Medicine: The Official Journal of the National Association of EMS Physicians and the World Association for Disaster and Emergency Medicine in Association with the Acute Care Foundation. v. 4, World Association for Disaster and Emergency Medicine, 1989.
http://pdm.medicine.wisc.edu/
ISSN: 1049023X
ISSN: 19451938 (Online)
Indexed in: MEDLINE, CINAHL
Recommended for: Hospital, Academic Libraries

This peer-reviewed international journal is a key resource for disaster medicine professionals. Its focus is on the practice of out-of-hospital and in-hospital emergency medical care, disaster health, and public health and safety. Coverage includes articles related to the delivery of care to victims of mass casualty events, studies of public health implications of catastrophes, and the prevention and mitigation of the negative health effects of disasters on the population and environment. As one of the few journals of its type, the journal's content appeals to a wide audience including emergency personnel, hospital administrators, disaster planners, physicians, nurses, researchers, psychologists, and others involved in the practice or study of crisis care delivery and response. Published bimonthly, the journal contains research studies, special reports, theoretical discussions, case reports, and comprehensive reviews with both a national and international focus. Articles are indexed and abstracted in dozens of indexing tools, including MEDLINE. Volumes 17, 2002 to the present are available online.

Databases and Other Electronic Resources

REMM: Radiation Event Medical Management. U.S. Department of Health and Human Services, Office of the Assistant Secretary for Preparedness and Response and National Library of Medicine, 2005?
http://www.remm.nlm.gov/
Recommended for: Hospital, Academic Libraries

Radiation Event Medical Management or REMM, is a web-based database that provides guidance for health care providers about clinical diagnosis and treatment during mass casualty radiological/nuclear events. It provides evidence-based, usable information with background and context to make complex issues understandable to those without formal radiation medicine expertise. While the audience for REMM is primarily physicians, there are content pages also for first responders, mental health professionals, hospitals, public information officers, radiation safety and protection, response planning, practices and drills, and even pet owners. The web-based content is downloadable in advance, so that it would be available during an event if the Internet is not accessible. REMM was produced by the Department of Health and Human Services, Office of the Assistant Secretary for Preparedness and Response, Office of Planning and Emergency Operations, in cooperation with the National

Library of Medicine, Division of Specialized Information Services, with subject matter experts from the National Cancer Institute, the Centers for Disease Control and Prevention, and many U.S. and international consultants. There is no charge for use of REMM.

WISER: Wireless Information System for Emergency Responders. U.S. National Library of Medicine, 2005?
http://webwiser.nlm.nih.gov/getHomeData.do
Recommended for: Hospital, Academic Libraries

The Wireless Information System for Emergency Responders or WISER is a decision support system designed to assist first responders, hazmat specialists, and emergency and other clinical personnel in hazardous material incidents. Developed by the National Library of Medicine, WISER provides a wide range of information on hazardous substances, including substance identification support, physical characteristics, human health information, and containment and suppression guidance. A key feature of WISER is the support for identifying an unknown substance based on signs/symptoms of victims of exposure, physical properties of the substance gathered by observation or sensors, hazard values from NFPA 704 placards, the ability to categorize a substance, and transportation identification such as DOT placards. It also covers radiological and biological agent support and includes an electronic searchable copy of the widely-used Department of Transportation's *Emergency Response Guidebook*. WISER is free and can be downloaded as a standalone application or used on the web.

10.5. Emergency Medicine

Resuscitation, transportation and care from the point of injury or beginning of illness through the hospital or other emergency treatment facility.

—MeSH

Contributor: Helen G. Mayo

Monographs

Atlas of Emergency Medicine. 3rd ed. Editors: Kevin J. Knoop, Lawrence B. Stack, Alan B. Storrow, R. Jason Thurman. McGraw-Hill, 2010.
http://www.accessmedicine.com
ISBN: 9780071496186
Recommended for: Hospital, Academic Libraries
Doody's Core Titles Selection

The *Atlas of Emergency Medicine* is in *Doody's Core Titles* list for emergency medicine and is included in the American College of Emergency Medicine bookstore list of the best educational products in emergency medicine. The intended audience is all health care professionals involved in emergency medicine, including prehospital care providers as well as ER nurses, physicians, residents, and medical students. Divided into 25 chapters over two parts, regional anatomy and specialty areas, The *Atlas of Emergency Medicine* is an excellent quick reference tool. New chapters have been added on tropical medicine, airway procedures, and electrocardiography; toxicological conditions now constitute a separate chapter. With 1,500 full color and radiologic images, each chapter is divided into three sections: clinical summary with differential diagnosis, emergency department treatment and disposition images, and a concise list of clinical pearls. Chapters have also been added on airway management, with equipment, technique, and images sections, and on electrocardiogram (ECG) abnormalities, with ECG findings, images, and pearls. The online version makes chapters available in HTML for handheld devices. This text is very useful in identifying key visual cues for the diagnosis and treatment of emergency conditions. The *Atlas of Emergency Medicine* is a recommended resource for hospitals with an active emergency room and for academic medical centers affiliated with such hospitals or with an emergency medicine department, division, or residency program.

Clinical Procedures in Emergency Medicine. 5th ed. Editors: James R. Roberts, Jerris R. Hedges. Saunders Elsevier, 2010.
http://www.mdconsult.com
ISBN: 9781416036234
Recommended for: Hospital, Academic Libraries
Doody's Core Titles Selection

Clinical Procedures in Emergency Medicine is included in the American College of Emergency Medicine bookstore list of the best educational products in emergency medicine and in *Doody's Core Titles* for emergency medicine. This is the standard "how to" procedural book, and is highly recommended. The intended audience is emergency residents and physicians. Divided into 71 chapters over 12 sections with an appendix of commonly used formulas and calculations, this text includes both commonly used procedures and those that are less frequently encountered in the emergency setting. This new edition is enhanced with 1,700 illustrations, 1,350 in color, with additional algorithms and tables for quicker reference. A companion website at http://expertconsult.com is available for individuals, which includes the bibliographic citations with links to their MEDLINE abstracts. A new chapter on physical and chemical restraint has been added, plus there is additional emphasis on ultrasound guided procedures. Information includes general background, indications and contraindications, equipment and anatomy, the procedure/technique, complications, and conclusions. *Clinical Procedures in Emergency Medicine* is a required resource for hospitals with an active emergency room or trauma referral center as well as any academic medical center affiliated with such hospitals or those with an emergency medicine department, division, or residency program.

Current Diagnosis & Treatment Emergency Medicine. 6th ed. Editors: C. Keith Stone, Roger L. Humphries. McGraw-Hill Lange, 2008.
http://www.accessmedicine.com/
http://online.statref.com/
http://www.r2library.com/
ISBN: 9780071443197
Recommended for: Hospital, Academic Libraries
Doody's Core Titles Selection

Current Diagnosis & Treatment Emergency Medicine is included in the American College of Emergency Medicine bookstore list of the best educational products in emergency medicine and is a *Doody's* core title for emergency medicine. The intended audience is all health care professionals involved in emergency medicine, including prehospital care providers as well as ER nurses, physicians, residents, and medical students. There is limited discussion of the basic science of emergency medicine and the text focuses on situations routinely dealt with in the ER. This concise, practical guide is divided into 48 chapters over four sections: special aspects of emergency medicine, including disasters and weapons of mass destruction, plus a step-by-step chapter on emergency procedures with equipment requirements, personnel needed, and indications and contradictions for each procedure; problem based management of common emergency problems; traumatic emergencies; and nontraumatic emergencies. Of particular usefulness are the essentials-of-diagnosis bullet points and graphic algorithms. Chapters on syncope, gastrointestinal emergencies, seizures, and neurologic emergencies have been added. The AccessMedicine online version makes chapters available in HTML for handheld devices. *Current Diagnosis & Treatment Emergency Medicine* is an appropriate resource for hospitals with an active emergency room and is recommended for academic medical center affiliated with such hospitals or with an emergency medicine department, division or residency program.

Emergency Medical Services: Clinical Practice and Systems Oversight. Editor: National Association of EMS Physicians. Kendall Hunt, 2009.
ISBN: 9780757561399
Recommended for: Hospital, Academic Libraries

Published under the auspices of the National Association of EMS Physicians (NAEMSP), this comprehensive four-volume textbook covers all aspects of prehospital emergency medical services (EMS). The intended audience is students, teachers, and practitioners of EMS. Volume 1, "Clinical Aspects of Prehospital Medicine," includes four sections: time/life critical events, such as cardiac arrest and shock; trauma, including sexual assault and child abuse, and environmental related issues; 16 chapters of individual chief complaint protocols; and special clinical considerations, such as airway management, special patient populations, and end of life issues. Instructive clinical vignettes are included in each chapter. Volume 2, "Medical Oversight of EMS," addresses the medical aspects of designing, implementing, and operating EMS systems. Although U.S. focused, information is included on international models. Chapters include topics ranging from legal and legislative issues to personnel and finance. Volume 3, "Evaluating and Improving Quality in EMS," recognizes that quality improvement and assessment is of increasing importance in healthcare, with an overview of prehospital research, including basic principles and types and areas of EMS research. Volume 4, "Special Operations Medical Support," includes sections on incident planning and response, U.S. federal response to health disasters, medical support for emergency responders, and special operations such as search and rescue and dealing with hazardous materials. The volumes may also be purchased separately. This set is a required resource for academic medical centers or hospitals with EMS/prehospital care training programs and is recommended for academic medical centers with an active emergency medicine department or division.

Forensic Emergency Medicine. 2nd ed. Editors: Jonathan S. Olshaker, M. Christine Jackson, William S. Smock. Lippincott Williams & Wilkins, 2007.
See Chapter 10.7. Forensic Medicine

Handbook of Common Poisonings in Children. 4th ed. Editor: American Academy of Pediatrics. American Academy of Pediatrics, 2010.
See Chapter 17.8.2. Forensic Toxicology

Harwood-Nuss' Clinical Practice of Emergency Medicine. 5th ed. Editor: Allan B. Wolfson. Lippincott Williams & Wilkins, 2010.

ISBN: 9780781789431
Recommended for: Hospital, Academic Libraries
Doody's Core Titles Selection

Harwood-Nuss' Clinical Practice of Emergency Medicine is in *Doody's Core Titles* list for emergency medicine and is included in the American College of Emergency Medicine bookstore list of the best educational products in emergency medicine. *JAMA* has called this one of the three most authoritative books in emergency medicine, along with *Rosen* and Tintinalli. The intended audiences are emergency physicians, physicians in training, and those preparing for board examination in emergency medicine. Chapters follow a standard format of introduction, clinical presentation, differential diagnosis, emergency department evaluation, management and critical interventions, disposition, and common pitfalls. The critical interventions and common pitfalls features are especially useful for quickly highlighting key elements. Sections on pain and pain management, resuscitation, high-risk chief complaints, and trauma are followed by sections on medical and surgical emergencies, divided by organ system. Specific sections on pediatric, toxicological and environmental emergencies are also included, with a final section on administrative and special clinical considerations. The hardcover comes with a CD-ROM of board review questions from each section and a companion website is available with fully searchable text, more than 400 self-assessment questions with answers, and additional images and tables. This is a recommended resource for hospitals with an emergency room with a residency program and is required for any academic medical center affiliated with such hospitals or with an emergency medicine department, division, or residency program.

Hot Zone Forensics: Chemical, Biological, and Radiological Evidence Collection. Author: Steven C. Drielak. Charles C. Thomas, 2004.
See Chapter 17.8.2. Forensic Toxicology

Manual of Forensic Emergency Medicine: A Guide for Clinicians. Author: Ralph J. Riviello. Jones & Bartlett, 2010.
See Chapter 10.7. Forensic Medicine

NOLS Wilderness Medicine. 1st ed. Author: Tod Schimelpfenig. Stackpole Books, 2006.
ISBN: 9780811733069
See Chapter 9.15. Wilderness Medicine

Rosen's Emergency Medicine: Concepts and Clinical Practice. 7th ed. Editors: John A. Marx, Robert S. Hockberger, Ron M. Walls. Mosby Elsevier, 2009.
http://www.mdconsult.com
ISBN: 9780323054720
See Also Chapter 1.9. Physician Assistants
Recommended for: Hospital, Academic Libraries
Brandon/Hill, *Doody's Core Titles* Selection

Rosen's Emergency Medicine is included in the American College of Emergency Medicine bookstore list of the best educational products in emergency medicine and *Doody's Core Titles* for emergency medicine, receiving four stars in the latest *Doody's* review, and was recommended in the last Brandon/Hill list. In its review of a previous edition, *JAMA* called this one of the three most authoritative books in emergency medicine. The book is based on the published literature and includes varying practice options where no consensus has been reached. The intended audiences are those interested in emergency medicine as well as full-time ER physicians. The book is divided into seven parts, including trauma and non-trauma medicine and surgery sections. Fundamental clinical concepts, such as shock, resuscitation, and common presentations; environment/toxicology; emergency medical services, including disaster preparedness; and special populations are also covered in detail. An editorial decision was made to omit specific procedures. Of interest to academic emergency physicians is the section on the practice and administration of emergency medicine. A companion website at http://expertconsult.com is available for individuals and includes the book's full bibliography, regular updates with material from new journal articles selected, and abstracted by the senior editors, a library of all book images, and certification review questions. *Rosen's Emergency Medicine* is a required resource for hospitals with an active emergency room or trauma referral center as well as any academic medical center.

Tintinalli's Emergency Medicine: A Comprehensive Study Guide. 7th ed. Editors: Judith E. Tintinalli, J. Stephan Stapczynski, David M. Cline, O. John Ma, Rita K. Cydulka, Garth D. Meckler. McGraw-Hill, 2011.
http://www.accessmedicine.com/
ISBN: 9780071484800 (set)
ISBN: 9780071744676
ISBN: 9780071744669 (CD)
Recommended for: Hospital, Academic Libraries
Doody's Core Titles Selection

Tintinalli's Emergency Medicine: A Comprehensive Study Guide is a *Doody's* core title for emergency medicine, receiving three stars in the latest review, and is included in the American College of Emergency Medicine bookstore list of the best educational products in emergency medicine. The sixth edition has 312 chapters over 28 sections contributed by more than 400 authors, including a section on disaster planning with chapters on bioterrorism and chemical agents of mass destruction. New sections include non-traumatic musculoskeletal disorders and special emergency patient populations, such as the homeless, elderly patients, and IV drug abusers. The section on vitamins and herbal preparations was revised and the online version includes links to both freely available and subscription based web sources of this information. An effort has been made to include evidence-based medicine when possible. The AccessMedicine online version includes regular updates with abstracts of relevant new studies as well as videos of various procedures. The online version also makes chapters available in HTML for handheld devices. *JAMA* has called this one of the three most authoritative books in emergency medicine and it continues to be a prime source for anyone preparing for board or recertification exams. The intended audience is emergency residents and physicians. This is a required resource for hospitals with an emergency room with a residency program as well as any academic medical center affiliated with such hospitals or with an emergency medicine department, division or residency program. This review refers to the sixth edition.

Trauma. 6th ed. Editors: David V. Feliciano, Kenneth L. Mattox, Ernest E. Moore. McGraw-Hill, 2008.
ISBN: 9780071469128
Recommended for: Hospital, Academic Libraries
Doody's Core Titles Selection

Trauma is included in the American College of Emergency Medicine bookstore list of the best educational products in emergency medicine and in *Doody's Core Titles* list for emergency medicine, receiving four stars in the latest review. *Doody's Review Service* named this text the standard in the field of trauma. The intended audience is all health care professionals involved in emergency medicine. The book is divided into 68 chapters over five sections: an overview of trauma, including trauma systems, injury scoring, and outcomes; generalized approaches to the traumatized patient, ranging from initial assessment to anesthesia and infection; detailed management of specific injures, divided by organ system, with helpful graphical algorithms; special problems, such as specific patient populations; and the management of complications after trauma, including system and multiple organ failure. Each chapter is enhanced with commentaries by an expert in that particular aspect of trauma medicine. The book has been updated to include chapters on weapons of mass destruction, acute care surgery, disaster management, and gastrointestinal failure. The new chapter on modern combat casualty care reflects experiences of the wars in Iraq and Afghanistan. *Trauma* is a required resource for hospitals with an active emergency room or trauma referral center as well as any academic medical center.

Wilderness First Aid: Emergency Care for Remote Locations. 3rd ed. Author: American Academy of Orthopaedic Surgeons. Jones & Bartlett, 2008.
See Chapter 9.15. Wilderness Medicine

Wilderness Medicine. 5th ed. Editor: Paul S. Auerbach. Mosby Elsevier, 2007.
See Chapter 9.15. Wilderness Medicine

Journals

Academic Emergency Medicine. v. 1, Wiley-Blackwell, 1994.
http://onlinelibrary.wiley.com/journal/10.1111/(ISSN)1553-2712
ISSN: 10696563
ISSN: 15532712 (Online)
Indexed in: MEDLINE, CINAHL
Recommended for: Hospital, Academic Libraries

Begun in 1989, this journal is the official journal of the Society for Academic Emergency Medicine (SAEM). The mission of the journal is to promote the advancement of emergency medicine research, education, and clinical practice. This journal is the second largest peer-reviewed publication dedicated specifically to emergency medicine, after the *Annals of Emergency Medicine*. The intended audience is emergency residents and physicians and the academic emergency medicine community. Topics include preclinical and clinical practice research as well as health policy and advances in emergency medicine education. This journal is a required resource for hospitals with an active emergency room or trauma referral center as well as any academic medical center affiliated with such hospitals or with an emergency medicine department, division, or residency program. The journal ranks third in the emergency medicine category (2009 *Journal Citation Reports*). *Academic Emergency Medicine* is cited in numerous abstracting and indexing sources such as MEDLINE, Embase, CINAHL, Science Citation Index (Web of Science), and Scopus. Full online coverage back to volume 1, 1994 is available through Wiley-Blackwell.

American Journal of Emergency Medicine. v. 1, Saunders, 1983.
http://www.sciencedirect.com/science/journal/07356757
http://www.mdconsult.com/

ISSN: 07356757
ISSN: 15328171 (Online)
Indexed in: MEDLINE, CINAHL
Recommended for: Hospital, Academic Libraries
Brandon/Hill Selection

Begun in 1983, this peer-reviewed journal "invites original research, reports, correspondence, and opinion relating to acute adult and pediatric medicine and surgery and the related fields of trauma, toxicology, critical care, resuscitation, emergency medical services, behavioral emergencies, and environmental medicine." The authorship is international in origin. The journal's online version includes interesting and unique emergency medicine case reports of up to 800 words while the print version includes abstracts of these submissions. The intended audience is emergency residents and physicians. This journal is an appropriate resource for hospitals with an active emergency room and is recommended for academic medical center affiliated with such hospitals or with an emergency medicine department, division, or residency program. The journal ranks fifth in the emergency medicine category (2009 *Journal Citation Reports*) and was one of only three emergency medicine journals listed in the last Brandon/Hill list for the small medical library. *American Journal of Emergency Medicine* is cited in numerous abstracting and indexing sources such as MEDLINE, Embase, CINAHL, Science Citation Index (Web of Science), and Scopus. Full online coverage, back to volume 1, 1983 is available through Elsevier ScienceDirect with Electronic-Extra Pages case reports available back to volume 25, number 4, 2007.

Annals of Emergency Medicine. v. 9, Mosby-Elsevier, 1980.
http://www.sciencedirect.com/science/journal/01960644
http://www.mdconsult.com/
http://www.annemergmed.com/
ISSN: 01960644
ISSN: 10976760 (Online)
See Also Chapter 10.4. Disaster Medicine, Chapter 13.2. Emergency Nursing
Indexed in: MEDLINE, CINAHL
Recommended for: Hospital, Academic Libraries

Begun in 1972 under another title, this journal is the official journal of the American College of Emergency Physicians (ACEP). This international, peer-reviewed journal includes articles on teaching and research in emergency medicine as well as general emergency medicine topics, opinion pieces, and clinical reports. It also covers disaster medicine, including disaster preparedness, response, and management. Other related subjects include health policy and ethics, toxicology, and out-of-hospital emergency medical services. This is the top emergency medicine journal, ranking number one in the emergency medicine category (2009 *Journal Citation Reports*) and was recommended in the last Brandon/Hill list. In 2009, the Special Libraries Association ranked the journal as one of the 100 most influential journals of biology and medicine over the last 100 years. The intended audience is all those interested in emergency medicine and research. This journal is a required resource for hospitals with an active emergency room or trauma referral center as well as any academic medical center. It is cited in numerous abstracting and indexing sources such as MEDLINE, Embase, CINAHL, Science Citation Index (Web of Science), and Scopus. Full online coverage back to volume 1, 1972 (earlier title) is available from Elsevier ScienceDirect.

Emergency Medicine Clinics of North America. v. 1, Saunders Elsevier, 1983.
http://www.sciencedirect.com/science/journal/07338627
http://www.mdconsult.com/
ISSN: 07338627
ISSN: 15580539 (Online)
Indexed in: MEDLINE, CINAHL
Recommended for: Hospital, Academic Libraries
Brandon/Hill Selection

Begun in 1983, the "goal of *Emergency Medicine Clinics of North America* is to keep practicing physicians up to date with current clinical practice in emergency medicine by providing timely articles reviewing the state of the art in patient care." With a separate personal subscription, individual physicians can acquire AMA PRA Category 1 Credits™ by taking an exam based on each individual volume. Each issue of this monographic serial reviews a single topic in emergency medicine under the direction of an expert guest editor. Authors are encouraged to submit multi-media files, including movies and audio, which are made available via the online subscription. Topics can vary from conditions found in the emergency room to wilderness medicine and global emergency medicine. The intended audience is all those interested in emergency medicine, especially ER physicians and residents. This journal is an appropriate resource for hospitals with an active emergency room and is recommended for academic medical centers affiliated with such hospitals or with an emergency medicine department, division, or residency program. The journal ranks ninth in the emergency medicine category (2009 *Journal Citation Reports*) and was one of only three emergency medicine journals listed in the last Brandon/Hill list.

Emergency Medicine Clinics of North America is cited in abstracting and indexing sources such as MEDLINE, Embase, CINAHL, Science Citation Index (Web of Science), and Scopus. Online coverage, back to volume 14, 1996 is available through Elsevier ScienceDirect.

Emergency Medicine Journal. v. 18, BMJ Publishing Group, 2001.
http://emj.bmj.com/
http://www.ncbi.nlm.nih.gov/pmc/journals/155/
ISSN: 14720205
ISSN: 14720213 (Online)
Indexed in: MEDLINE, CINAHL
Recommended for: Hospital, Academic Libraries

Begun in 1984 under another title, *Emergency Medicine Journal* is the official journal of the British Association for Immediate Care and the Faculty of Prehospital Care of the Royal College of Surgeons of Edinburgh and is the journal of the College of Emergency Medicine. This international peer-reviewed journal covers all aspects of prehospital and hospital emergency care and includes original articles, reviews, and research. Of particular interest are the Best Evidence Topic reports from the Manchester Royal Infirmary, which outline short evidence-based answers concerning specific clinical conditions. The online version also contains supplementary data, such as extensive tables or media files. The intended audience is emergency residents and physicians as well as nurses, paramedics, and ambulance staff. This journal is an appropriate resource for hospitals with an active emergency room involved in research as is recommended for any academic medical center affiliated with such hospitals or with an emergency care department, division or training program. The journal ranks sixth in the emergency medicine category (2009 *Journal Citation Reports*). *Emergency Medicine Journal* is cited in numerous abstracting and indexing sources such as MEDLINE, Embase, CINAHL, Science Citation Index (Web of Science), and Scopus. Full online coverage back to volume 1, 1984 is available through the BMJ Publishing Group Ltd under their *Emergency Medicine Journal* website. The online archive beginning with volume 1, 1984 is also available on PubMed Central up to issues three years before the current issue.

Injury. v. 1, Elsevier, 1969.
http://www.sciencedirect.com/science/journal/00201383
ISSN: 00201383
ISSN: 18790267 (Online)
Indexed in: MEDLINE
Recommended for: Hospital, Academic Libraries

Begun in 1969, *Injury* is the official journal of the British Trauma Society, the Australasian Trauma Society, and the Saudi Orthopaedic Association (Trauma Group), and is affiliated with the Hellenic Association of Orthopaedic Surgery and Traumatology, the Italian Society of Orthopaedics and Traumatology, and the Gerhard Kuentscher Society. This peer-reviewed journal is truly international in scope, with over 80 percent of the articles originating outside the United States. According to its scope statement, *Injury* covers all aspects of trauma care and emergency surgery, including trauma systems and management, surgical procedures, epidemiological studies, surgery (of all tissues), resuscitation, biomechanics, rehabilitation, anesthesia, radiology, basic science of local and systemic response to trauma and tissue healing. The intended audience is all members of the trauma team. This journal is a recommended resource for hospitals with an active emergency room or trauma referral center involved in research as well as any academic medical center affiliated with such hospitals or with an emergency medicine department, division, or residency program. The journal ranks fourth in the emergency medicine category (2009 *Journal Citation Reports*). Injury is cited in numerous abstracting and indexing sources such as MEDLINE, Embase, CINAHL, Science Citation Index (Web of Science), and Scopus. Full online coverage back to volume 1, 1969 is available through Elsevier ScienceDirect.

Journal of Emergency Medicine. v. 1, Elsevier, 1983.
http://www.sciencedirect.com/science/journal/07364679
ISSN: 07364679
Indexed in: MEDLINE
Recommended for: Hospital, Academic Libraries

Begun in 1983, this peer-reviewed journal publishes clinical and research articles of interest to practicing and academic emergency physicians. Selected topics include "toxicology, prehospital care, the difficult airway, aeromedical emergencies, disaster medicine, cardiology commentary, emergency radiology, critical care, sports medicine, and wound care." *Journal of Emergency Medicine* ranks eighth in the emergency medicine category (2009 *Journal Citation Reports*). This journal is cited in numerous abstracting and indexing sources such as MEDLINE, Embase, CINAHL, Web of Science, and Scopus. The journal is available with full online coverage back to volume 1, 1983 through Elsevier ScienceDirect.

Journal of Medical Toxicology. v. 1, Springer, 2005.
See Chapter 17.8.2. Forensic Toxicology

Prehospital Emergency Care. v. 1, Informa Healthcare, 1997.

http://informahealthcare.com/pec
ISSN: 10903127
ISSN: 15450066 (Online)
See Also Chapter 9.15. Wilderness Medicine
Indexed in: MEDLINE, CINAHL
Recommended for: Hospital, Academic Libraries

Begun in 1997, *Prehospital Emergency Care* is the official journal of the National Association of EMS (Emergency Medical Services) Physicians, the National Association of State EMS Directors, the National Association of EMS Educators, and the National Association of Emergency Medical Technicians. According to its scope statement, this peer-reviewed journal covers topics relevant to the practice, educational advancement, and investigation of prehospital emergency care. The intended audience is students, teachers, and practitioners of emergency medical services, especially prehospital emergency care. Articles include original contributions and research reports. Of particular interest are the articles on the education and practice of prehospital emergency care and the regular sections on specific aspects of prehospital care, such as airway management, cardiac arrest, and military medicine. This journal is a required resource for academic medical centers or hospitals with EMS or prehospital care departments, divisions or training programs and is recommended for academic medical centers affiliated with an active emergency medicine department or division. The journal ranks seventh in the emergency medicine category (2009 *Journal Citation Reports*) and is the only journal in the top ten devoted to prehospital emergency care. *Prehospital Emergency Care* is cited in numerous abstracting and indexing sources such as MEDLINE, Embase, CINAHL, Science Citation Index (Web of Science), and Scopus. The journal is available with full online coverage back to volume 1, 1997 through Informa Healthcare.

Resuscitation. v. 1, Elsevier, 1972.
http://www.sciencedirect.com/science/journal/03009572
ISSN: 03009572
ISSN: 18731570 (Online)
Indexed in: MEDLINE
Recommended for: Hospital, Academic Libraries

Begun in 1972, *Resuscitation* is the official journal of the European Resuscitation Council, an interdisciplinary council for resuscitation medicine and emergency medical care founded in 1989. This international, peer-reviewed journal covers the "etiology, pathophysiology, diagnosis and treatment of acute diseases. Clinical and experimental research, reviews and case histories and description of methods used in clinical resuscitation or experimental resuscitation research are encouraged." Basic science as well as clinical articles are welcomed. The journal encompasses a wide range of specialties: critical care and emergency medicine (both in and out of hospital), intensive care, cardiology, cardiopulmonary resuscitation, neurology, anesthesiology, and nursing. The intended audience is all emergency practitioners; *Resuscitation* also includes information of interest to critical care practitioners, anesthesiologists, neurologists, cardiologists, perinatologists and laboratory investigators. *Resuscitation* is a required resource for hospitals with an active emergency room or trauma referral center as well as any academic medical center affiliated with such hospitals or with an emergency medicine department, division, or residency program. The journal ranks second in the emergency medicine category and is in the top ten of the critical care medicine category (2009 *Journal Citation Reports*). *Resuscitation* is cited in numerous abstracting and indexing sources such as Chemical Abstracts, MEDLINE, Embase, CINAHL, Web of Science, and Scopus. The journal is available with full online coverage back to volume 1, 1972 through Elsevier ScienceDirect.

Wilderness & Environmental Medicine. v. 6, Elsevier, 1995.
See Chapter 9.15. Wilderness Medicine

10.6. Family Practice

The provision of continuing, comprehensive primary health care for the entire family.

—MeSH

Contributor: Laura Wilder

Monographs

The Color Atlas of Family Medicine. Editors: Richard P. Usatine, Mindy Ann Smith, E.J. Mayeaux, Jr., Heidi Chumley, James Tysinger. McGraw-Hill, 2008.
ISBN: 9780071474641
Recommended for: Hospital, Academic Libraries
Doody's Core Titles Selection

The Color Atlas of Family Medicine, a visual guide to daily patient care, is a valuable resource for all health professionals in family medicine. Concise, yet comprehensive in coverage, it contains almost 1,500 large, full-color clinical photographs of disease symptoms. Divided into eighteen parts, the main section of the text covers 12 different body systems or areas of medicine, such as ophthalmology, oral health, women's health, dermatology, and infectious diseases. Each topic is organized by presentation or appearance, beginning with a patient story and followed by bullet points on epidemiology, etiology and pathophysiology, diagnosis, differential diagnosis, management, and patient education. Most diagnostic and treatment recommendations are referenced and/or evidence-graded. *The Color Atlas of Family Medicine* is an extremely useful visual learning experience for medical students and residents and an outstanding visual reference for family physicians and other primary care practitioners. At present, *The Color Atlas of Family Medicine* is only available in print. Online access would make this unique textbook even more useful. A five-star *Doody's* review stated, "It is a must for the library of every primary care physician." It is also highly recommended for all hospital or academic libraries that support a family medicine residency program.

Current Diagnosis and Treatment in Family Medicine. 2nd ed. Editors: Jeannette E. South-Paul, Samuel C. Matheny, Evelyn L. Lewis. Lange/McGraw-Hill, 2008.
http://www.accessmedicine.com/
http://www.r2library.com/
http://extranet.netlibrary.com/TitleSelect/
http://www.ebrary.com/
ISBN: 9780071461535
ISBN: 9780071510042 (Online)
Recommended for: Hospital, Academic Libraries
Doody's Core Titles Selection

This updated and expanded edition of *Current Diagnosis and Treatment in Family Medicine* provides practical, up-to-date information on common conditions affecting patients of all ages that are seen in family medicine practices. As a comprehensive reference for practicing family physicians, residents, primary care trainees, and physician assistants, the work's emphasis is on disease progression, diagnostic workup tools, differential diagnosis, clinical findings, and treatment decisions. Attention is given to the importance of psychosocial factors and the culture of illness on the entire family. The body of the text is organized according to the human life cycle, while the last three chapters cover "Genetics for the Family Physician," "Pharmacogenetics," and "Complementary and Alternative Medicine." Problem-oriented and largely evidence-based, the book's 63 chapters are highlighted with tables, charts, and algorithms, making *Current Diagnosis and Treatment in Family Medicine* an ideal quick reference in the ambulatory setting. In addition to the print text, it is accessible online from AccessMedicine where individual chapters can be downloaded to a computer or handheld device. The entire book can also be purchased in a simplified version for major handhelds. Considered an essential purchase title from *Doody's Core Titles*, *Current Diagnosis and Treatment in Family Medicine* is highly recommended for hospital libraries that have residency programs and for academic medical libraries.

The 5-Minute Clinical Consult. Wolters Kluwer/Lippincott Williams & Wilkins, Annual.
See Chapter 1.9. Physician Assistants, Chapter 10.10. Internal Medicine

Pfenninger and Fowler's Procedures for Primary Care. 2nd ed. Editors: John L. Pfenninger, Grant C. Fowler. Mosby/Elsevier, 2003.
ISBN: 9780323005067
Recommended for: Hospital, Academic Libraries
Doody's Core Titles Selection

The second edition of *Pfenninger and Fowler's Procedures for Primary Care* is an updated version of its acclaimed predecessor, *Procedures for Primary Care Physicians*, which was a runaway best seller and ranked as one of the 37 best medical texts ever produced. A 1995 *JAMA* review of the first edition states, "This book is the most comprehensive source of information on primary care procedures available anywhere." Organized by specialty or anatomic system—such as anesthesia, dermatology, obstetrics, or gastrointestinal—*Procedures for Primary Care* is a comprehensive guide containing practical, step-by-step instructions to 216 medical and surgical procedures. Illustrated by line drawings and black-and-white photographs, each procedure's section outlines clinical indications, contraindications, equipment needed, patient procedural information, techniques, complications, and CPT/billing codes. Appendixes include patient handouts and consent forms. Intended for primary care physicians, family practice residents, and medical students, *Procedures for Primary Care* would also be useful to a wider audience. *Procedures for Primary Care* is only available in print. However, a related resource, *Multimedia Primary Care Procedures*, offers two DVDs, a website, and a pocket manual. The online resource offers interactive videos of 65 procedures, with a promise of more to come. *Doody's Review Service* gives *Pfenninger and Fowler's Procedures for Primary Care* four stars and calls it "an excellent publication," which is "highly recommended." This outstanding text is definitely recommended for both hospital collections and academic medical libraries.

Primary Care Medicine: Office Evaluation and Management of the Adult Patient. 6th ed. Editors: Allan H. Goroll, Albert G. Mulley Jr. Lippincott Williams & Wilkins, 2009.
http:///www.ovid.com/
http://www.r2library.com/
ISBN: 9780781775137
Recommended for: Hospital, Academic Libraries
Brandon/Hill, *Doody's Core Titles* Selection

The sixth edition of this comprehensive textbook provides family medicine physicians and other primary care practitioners with relevant, succinct clinical information on diagnosis, therapy, and health maintenance indispensable to decision making in the outpatient primary care setting. *Primary Care Medicine* is divided into 16 parts and is subdivided into 239 chapters. The first two parts cover the topics "Principles of Primary Care" and "Systemic Problems." Forming the heart of the book, the next thirteen parts are arranged by organ system and cover screening, evaluation, and management of common diseases within the organ system. Every chapter has been updated to include more images, tables, and bulleted lists; many contain lists of websites for added resource material. Some of the areas that have been revised in this edition include substance abuse, hypertension, hyperlipidemia, outpatient cancer, and HIV management. The last section, "Allied Fields," discusses herbal supplements, caring for the adolescent patient, and an approach to frailty in the elderly. An online version of *Primary Care Medicine* is contained in various Lippincott Williams & Wilkins packages, including Books@Ovid, and from Rittenhouse's R2 Digital Library. *Primary Care Medicine: Office Evaluation and Management of the Adult Patient*, a former Brandon/Hill recommended book and a current title in *Doody's Core Titles*, is a required resource both for hospital collections and academic medical libraries.

Textbook of Family Medicine. 7th ed. Editor: Robert E. Rakel. Saunders/Elsevier, 2007.
http://www.mdconsult.com/
ISBN: 9781416024675
See Also Chapter 1.9. Physician Assistants
Recommended for: Hospital, Academic Libraries
Brandon/Hill, *Doody's Core Titles* Selection

The seventh edition of this renowned textbook focuses on clinically relevant information for family physicians and other primary care practitioners. Well-organized and thorough, it covers the basics of primary care in the first three sections: principles of family medicine, family medicine in the community, and communication in family medicine. The fourth section includes all the common disorders seen by general practitioners. This latest edition contains 10 new chapters on current topics such as electronic health records, evidence-based medicine, complementary and alternative medicine, diabetes mellitus, and obesity. All the chapters contain new material, having been written by new authors, updated, or thoroughly revised. Visually appealing, the *Textbook of Family Medicine* contains 650 tables and 600 illustrations. Key points on diagnosis, therapy, and high-level (level "A") evidence-based recommendations are highlighted and easy to find in each chapter. Available in print and digital formats, the online version of *Textbook of Family Medicine* is included in MD Consult. Listed as an initial purchase suggestion in the final Brandon/Hill list and considered by *Doody's Core Titles* as an essential purchase, this is a required book for any hospital or academic medical library.

Journals

American Family Physician. v. 2, American Academy of Family Physicians, 1970.
http://www.aafp.org/afp
http://www.mdconsult.com/
ISSN: 0002838X
ISSN: 15320650 (Online)
See Also Chapter 1.9. Physician Assistants
Indexed in: MEDLINE, CINAHL
Recommended for: Hospital, Academic Libraries
Brandon/Hill Selection

As the official journal of the American Academy of Family Physicians, *American Family Physician* publishes "evidence-based, authoritative clinical review articles about conditions frequently seen by family physicians." A peer-reviewed journal emphasizing diagnosis and management of common, important diseases, *AFP* does not publish original research. Instead, it includes summaries of selected articles from other medical journals, clinical reviews, practice guidelines, and patient information. Published semimonthly, *American Family Physician* is indexed in a wide variety of databases including MEDLINE, CINAHL, Scopus, Current Contents, and SciFinder. Extending from 1998 to the present, most of the online archive for *American Family Physician* is freely available to all after one year, but online access to the latest issues is restricted to AAFP members and paid subscribers. Current online access is also available from MD Consult. Long considered an important family medicine journal, *AFP* was first introduced as the *American Family Physician/GP*. It is included in the last Brandon/

Hill list as an initial purchase suggestion for a small medical library. It is also considered to be a core clinical title by the National Library of Medicine. *AFP* has an impact factor of 1.702 (2009 *Journal Citation Reports*). *American Family Physician* is highly recommended for hospital collections and academic medical libraries.

Annals of Family Medicine. v. 1, Annals of Family Medicine, 2003.
http:// http://www.annfammed.org/
http://www.ncbi.nlm.nih.gov/pmc/journals/330/
ISSN: 15441709
ISSN: 15441717 (Online)
Indexed in: MEDLINE, CINAHL
Recommended for: Hospital, Academic Libraries

The *Annals of Family Medicine* is a peer-reviewed research journal, sponsored by the American Academy of Family Physicians (AAFP) in collaboration with six other family medicine organizations that work together to support a research forum for scientists, practitioners, and policy makers. Part of its mission, "advancing knowledge essential to understanding and improving health and primary care," is accomplished through the publication of clinical, biomedical, social, and health services research. *Annals* also includes articles on methodology and theory; selected, forward-thinking systematic reviews; and personal reflections from clinicians, patients, families, communities, and policy makers. To fulfill the second part of its mission, supporting "a learning community of those who generate and use information about health and generalist health care," *Annals* provides an open forum called TRACK (Topical Response to the Annals Community of Knowledge), which allows for online, interactive discussion of each published article and other important topics. A regular editorial feature, "On TRACK," later synthesizes these discussions. Indexed in: many databases including MEDLINE, PsycINFO, Embase, CINAHL, Scopus, and Web of Science, *Annals* is published six times a year in print, online, and mobile formats. Free, full-text access is available through HighWire Press and PubMed Central, starting with volume 1, May/June 2003. With an impact factor of 4.130 (2009 *Journal Citation Reports*), *Annals of Family Medicine* is required for hospital collections that support clinical research, well-rounded academic medical collections, and specialized collections for health insurance companies and other policy makers.

Family Medicine. v. 13, Society of Teachers of Family Medicine, 1981.
http://www.stfm.org/fmhub/
ISSN: 07423225
ISSN: 19383800 (Online)
Indexed in: MEDLINE
Recommended for: Hospital, Academic Libraries

For the past 40 years, *Family Medicine*, the official journal of the Society of Teachers of Family Medicine (STFM), has published clinical and educational research articles as well as commentary on medical education. A scholarly, peer-reviewed journal, *Family Medicine* is intended primarily for family physicians, family medicine educators, researchers, and residents. However, it also covers research of interest to psychologists, sociologists, and public health specialists. Intended for educators from various backgrounds in family medicine education, *Family Medicine* publishes a regular column, "For the Office-based Teacher of Family Medicine," that gives such instructors usable knowledge about issues of concern to family physician preceptors. Published ten times a year, *Family Medicine* is indexed in Scopus, Current Contents, MEDLINE, and Embase. *Family Medicine*, which was first released as *Family Medicine Teacher*, is published in both print and online formats. Full-text articles are available online at the STFM website starting in February, 1998 with volume 30, number 2. *Family Medicine* has an impact factor of 1.331 (2009 *Journal Citation Reports*) and is recommended for hospital libraries serving family medicine educators who oversee residency programs and academic medical libraries.

Family Practice Management. v. 1, American Academy of Family Physicians, 1994.
http://www.aafp.org/fpm
http://www.mdconsult.com/
ISSN: 10695648
ISSN: 15311929 (Online)
Indexed in: MEDLINE, CINAHL
Recommended for: Hospital, Academic Libraries

Family Practice Management (*FPM*) is a peer-reviewed journal published six times a year by the American Academy of Family Physicians. Its stated mission is "to give family physicians the tools and information they need to build better practices and improve patient care." Accordingly, it focuses on practice issues such as the fundamentals of office management, documentation and coding, ethical practice, legislation, employment issues, and computerization as a way to help family physicians adapt to the current health care environment and to future governmental reforms. Serving as a rich source of best practice tips, *FPM* is indexed in many major databases such as MEDLINE, Scopus, CINAHL, and ProQuest Central. Extending from 1998 to the present, most of the online archive for *Family Practice Management* is freely available to all after a one-year embargo, but online access to the latest issues is restricted to AAFP members and paid subscribers. Current online access is also available from MD Consult. The *FPM* website provides other resources such as the *FPM* Toolbox that offers more than 150 practice management tools and *FPM's* CME Quiz. *Family Practice Management* is unique in its coverage of practice management and the socioeconomic aspects of family medicine, and, as a result, it is recommended for family physicians in private or group practice, hospital collections, and well-rounded academic medical libraries.

Journal of Family Practice. v. 1, Quadrant HealthCom, 1974.
http://www.jfponline.com/
http://www.ebscohost.com/
http://www.gale.cengage.com/
ISSN: 00943509
ISSN: 15337294 (Online)
Recommended for: Hospital, Academic Libraries
Indexed in: MEDLINE
Brandon/Hill Selection

The *Journal of Family Practice* is a peer-reviewed, scientific journal that delivers high-quality, clinically relevant articles each month to practicing family physicians, family medicine researchers, and other primary care clinicians. *JFP* gives highest priority to studies that address clinical questions or health care delivery topics in primary care. Committed to translating evidence-based information to family physicians and family medicine researchers in useful and relevant formats, *JFP* publishes review articles known as POEMs (Patient-Oriented Evidence that Matters) and FPIN Clinical Inquiries, which are evidence-based answers from the Family Physicians Inquiries Network. *The Journal of Family Practice* is indexed by major databases, including MEDLINE, Scopus, Current Contents, Web of Science, and PsycINFO. *JFP* is available in print and online formats. Formerly listed in the prestigious Brandon/Hill list and currently included in the *Core Collection of Medical Books and Journals* (Hague List), *JFP* has an impact factor of 1.426 (2009 *Journal Citation Reports*). Considered by the National Library of Medicine to be a core clinical title, the *Journal of Family Practice* is highly recommended for hospital collections and academic medical libraries.

Journal of the American Board of Family Medicine. v. 19, American Board of Family Medicine, 2006.
http://www.jabfm.org
ISSN: 15572625
ISSN: 15587118 (Online)
Indexed in: MEDLINE
Recommended for: Hospital, Academic Libraries

The *Journal of the American Board of Family Medicine* (*JABFM*) is the official, peer-reviewed journal of the American Board of Family Medicine (ABFM). The journal's self-proclaimed emphasis is on "original material from authors with new knowledge to contribute to the understanding and advancement of family medicine research and practice." As a result, it publishes original, evidence-based primary care or health services research, as well as in-depth clinical reviews, evidence-based clinical medicine papers, clinical guidelines, health policy issues, and ethics commentaries. The journal presents original articles, brief reports, and short communications that cover clinical issues for family medicine physicians; it also provides a forum for the family medicine specialty and serves as a news source for the American Board of Family Medicine. Formerly known as the *Journal of the American Board of Family Practice* until 2006, the *JABFM* is issued six times a year in both online and print formats. Indexed in: several databases such as MEDLINE, Scopus, Embase, Current Contents, and CINAHL Plus with Full Text, it provides its articles free of charge without registration through HighWire Press from 2001 to the present. With a high impact factor of 2.106 (2009 *Journal Citation Reports*), the *Journal of the American Board of Family Medicine* is recommended for large hospital collections and all academic medical libraries.

10.7. Forensic Medicine

The application of medical knowledge to questions of law.
—MeSH

Contributor: Kristine M. Alpi and Robert Sotak

Monographs

Child Fatality Review: An Interdisciplinary Guide and Photographic Reference. Authors: Randell Alexander, Mary E. Case. GW Medical, 2008.
See Chapter 10.7.2. Forensic Pathology

Clarke's Analytical Forensic Toxicology. 1st ed. Editors: Sue Jickells, Adam Negrusz. Pharmaceutical Press, 2008.
See Chapter 17.8.2. Forensic Toxicology

Color Atlas of Forensic Medicine and Pathology. 1st ed. Editor: Charles A. Catanese. CRC Press, 2010.

http://www.crcpress.com/
http://extranet.netlibrary.com/TitleSelect/
ISBN: 9781420043204
ISBN: 9781420043228 (DVD)
ISBN: 9781420043211 (Online)
Recommended for: Hospital, Academic Libraries
Doody's Core Titles Selection

The ten chapters of *Color Atlas of Forensic Medicine and Pathology* are organized by cause of death. Each chapter begins with several pages of text providing background information on the topic followed by numerous photographs illustrating specific conditions. Brief but useful text accompanies each photograph or group of photographs. This book begins by discussing sudden natural death such as heart disease, vascular disease, and other causes. Deaths related to therapeutic interventions and the difficulties they present to the forensic pathologist are explained well. Ways to identify substance abuse and poisoning due to drugs such as alcohol, cocaine, heroin, methamphetamine and poisons such as arsenic, cyanide and ethylene glycol are covered. Early postmortem changes, decomposition, and skeletonization are presented. Blunt force injuries such as abrasions, contusions, lacerations and sharp force injuries are described and illustrated. Photographs of gunshot wounds illustrate entrance and exit wounds. Range of fire estimation and trajectory determination and evidence recovery are also covered. Text and photographs of victims of burns and asphyxia comprise the final chapter. There are excellent photographs of patterns produced in death of various causes. *Color Atlas of Forensic Medicine and Pathology* is essential for forensic pathologists and medical examiners but was written to be useful for medical and non-medical personnel.

Death Investigation: Systems and Procedures. Author: Randy Hanzlick. CRC Press, 2007.
http://extranet.netlibrary.com/TitleSelect/
http://www.crcnetbase.com/isbn/9781420044751
ISBN: 9781420044751
ISBN: 9781420044768 (Online)
Recommended for: Hospital, Academic, Consumer Health Libraries

Dr. Randy Hanzlick, board-certified forensic pathologist, has created a concise and comprehensible introduction to death investigation. Students of forensic science, pathology, epidemiology, law, and interested laypersons will better understand the workings of coroners and medical examiners with clear explanations of jurisdiction, practices in each state, principles of evidence collection, terminology, processes, and public health import of autopsies and death certificates. Samples of typical institutional, private, and medicolegal death investigation, as well as a day in the life of the medical examiner's office make everything clear. Black-and-white photos and tables from other references illustrate key points. For specifics, the author refers to guidelines such as the National Institute of Justice's *Death Investigation: A Guide for the Scene Investigator* (1999, http://www.ncjrs.gov/pdffiles/167568.pdf). Forensic pathologists may find the explanation of their work too basic, but the book provides information on the system in which they practice. A list of websites and an index round out this brief work. It is especially recommended for hospital and public libraries as it explains hospital-based death investigations and how to request death investigation as next of kin.

Effective Expert Witnessing: Practices for the 21st Century. 4th ed. Authors: Jack V. Matson, Suha F. Daou, Jeffrey G. Soper. CRC Press, 2004.
http://www.crcnetbase.com/isbn/978-0-8493-1301-1
ISBN: 9780849313011
ISBN: 9786610109050 (Online)
Recommended for: Hospital, Academic Libraries

The significance of the U.S. Supreme Court ruling in *Daubert vs. Merrill Dow Pharmaceuticals* (1993) is emphasized in this book since this case set a high standard for admissibility of expert opinion. The importance of depositions and how to prepare for them are also emphasized since many cases do not go to trial. The requirements for being an expert witness are described, as are ways to interact with lawyers, and how to market oneself as an expert. Actual cases are described to illustrate some of the difficulties encountered by expert witnesses. Lawyers are given advice on traits to look for in an expert witness. The future of expert witnessing is outlined. The text includes an *Effective Expert Testimony* CD-ROM. This book is recommended for libraries of all types as it would be useful for anyone who is considering becoming an expert witness or who needs to become more adept as an expert witness.

Forensic Emergency Medicine. 2nd Editors: Jonathan S. Olshaker, M. Christine Jackson, William S. Smock. Lippincott Williams & Wilkins, 2007.
http://www.ovid.com/
ISBN: 9780781792745
Recommended for: Hospital Libraries
Brandon/Hill Selection

Edited by experienced emergency physicians, two of whom are fellows of the American Academy of Emergency

Medicine or the American College of Emergency Physicians, this text provides emergency clinicians information about the medicolegal aspects of treating victims of violence, motor vehicle accidents, sexual assault, child abuse, elder abuse, and intimate partner abuse. It offers detailed guidelines on interviewing and examining the victim and collecting, preserving, and documenting evidence for legal proceedings. The book includes a chapter by an attorney on expert testimony and a chapter on forensic photography in the emergency department. A full-color photo insert illustrates injury patterns and key evidence. This edition provides increased coverage of motor vehicle accidents, DNA evidence, and new drugs of abuse. The first edition of this text was chosen for the Brandon/Hill list. This new edition is available in paper and is also available online via Ovid. The American emergency department setting may not resonate with European audiences—international audiences may consider *Simpson's Forensic Medicine* (Hodder Arnold, 12th ed., 2003) or the U.K.-focused *Clinical Forensic Medicine* (Cambridge, 3rd ed., 2009) and for forensics pediatrics the Edinburgh-based Keeling and Busuttil's *Paediatric Forensic Medicine and Pathology* (Hodder Arnold, 2008).

Forensic Entomology: The Utility of Arthropods in Legal Investigations. 2nd ed. Editors: Jason H. Byrd, James L. Castner. CRC Press, 2010.
http://www.crcpress.com/
http://www.myilibrary.com/
http://extranet.netlibrary.com/TitleSelect/
ISBN: 9780849392153
ISBN: 9781420008869 (Online)
Recommended for: Hospital, Academic Libraries

Authors, with affiliations ranging from universities to crime scene units, contributed to this interesting book. The introduction explains that "forensic entomology is the broad field where arthropod science and the judicial system interact." This book focuses on medicocriminal entomology, emphasizing the extended postmortem interval, which may be days or even decades, and the use of insects and other arthropods to determine that time period. Beginning with basic background information on arthropod biology and the insects that are important in forensics, mainly flies and beetles, the text continues with chapters on collection procedures and laboratory rearing. Factors that affect colonization and succession of arthropods on human remains are described. Various methods for estimating the postmortem interval are explained as are computer models of insect growth. Black-and-white photographs within the chapters and a separate section of color photographs on glossy paper illustrate the common insects of forensic importance. Each chapter has a table of contents, which will be useful for those who prefer to browse. Chapters also have reference sections and several chapters describing forensics procedures have appendixes, such as identification keys and a list of collecting materials, log sheets, and data forms. This book will serve as an excellent introduction for anyone interested in the field of forensic entomology and would be useful for libraries serving academic programs in forensics or entomology, as well as health sciences collections serving medical examiners and their teams.

Handbook of Common Poisonings in Children. 4th ed. Editors: American Academy of Pediatrics. American Academy of Pediatrics, 2010.
See Chapter 17.8.2. Forensic Toxicology

Handbook of Forensic Toxicology for Medical Examiners. Author: D.K. Molina. CRC Press, 2010.
See Chapter 17.8.2. Forensic Toxicology

Introduction to Environmental Forensics. 2nd ed. Editors: Brian L. Murphy, Robert D. Morrison. Elsevier, 2007.
ISBN: 9780123695222
Recommended for: Academic Libraries

The editors have taken a multidisciplinary approach to environmental forensics. Thirty-two experts with a wide range of backgrounds such as geochemistry, environmental science, and physics have contributed to this volume. Since environmental forensics has matured since the first edition in 2002, several new chapters have been added to this edition. This text has methods of general applicability for the forensics investigator and has a companion website. Several chapters are dedicated to properly collecting data and statistical analysis. The authors describe how to use multiple lines of evidence in an investigation. Hypothetical situations are presented in order to learn how to do site histories. The text explains how to use isotopes for determining the source of environmental contaminants. Chemical fingerprinting techniques are explained in detail as are methods for studying movement of contaminants in the subsurface and air. The final chapter covers emerging forensic techniques such as dendroecology and DNA fingerprinting. *Introduction to Environmental Forensics* is recommended for academic libraries and health sciences libraries with a strong environmental health focus as this book will be very useful to those currently working in environmental forensics as well as those new to the field. Methods for specific contaminants can be found in *Environmental Forensics: A Contaminant Specific Guide* (Elsevier, 2005; not reviewed).

A Litigator's Guide to DNA: From the Laboratory to the Courtroom. Authors: Ron C. Michaelis, Robert G. Flanders, Paula H. Wulff. Elsevier Academic Press, 2008.
See Chapter 10.7.1. Forensic Genetics

Manual of Forensic Emergency Medicine: A Guide for Clinicians. Author: Ralph J. Riviello. Jones & Bartlett, 2010.
ISBN: 9780763744625
Recommended for: Hospital, Academic Libraries

Manual of Forensic Emergency Medicine is a thorough guide to the clinical approach to criminal illness and injury. This resource offers emergency care professionals the knowledge needed to make an accurate diagnosis of abuse, neglect, sexual assault, or other conditions in which forensic investigation is needed, as well as information on victim services, patient resources, and relevant aspects of the legal system. It contains color photos, a glossary, and forensic forms that can be used in a clinical practice.

Principles and Practice of Child and Adolescent Forensic Mental Health. Editors: Elissa P. Benedek, Peter Ash, Charles L. Scott. American Psychiatric, 2010.
See Chapter 9.10.4. Forensic Psychiatry

Sexual Assault: Victimization across the Life Span, a Clinical Guide and a Color Atlas. Editors: Angelo P. Giardino, Elizabeth M. Datner, Janice B. Asher, Barbara Girardin, Diana K. Faugno, Mary J. Spencer. GW Medical Publishing, 2003.
See Chapter 13.4. Forensic Nursing

Spitz and Fisher's Medicolegal Investigation of Death: Guidelines for the Application of Pathology to Crime Investigation. 4th ed. Editors: Werner U. Spitz, Daniel J. Spitz, Russell S. Fisher, Ramsey Clark. Charles C. Thomas, 2006.
ISBN: 9780398075446
Recommended for: Hospital, Academic Libraries

Spitz and Fisher's is recommended as a core resource for the examination of the American Board of Medicolegal Death Investigators and as a reference by many other forensic texts. Totally rewritten and updated in 2006, the text is oriented to forensic pathologists, criminal investigators, and attorneys. It embraces all aspects of the pathology of trauma as it is witnessed daily by law enforcement officers, interpreted by pathologists of varying experience and expertise in forensic pathology, and used by lawyers involved in the prosecution and defense in criminal cases as well as those engaged in civil litigation. This authoritative text uses a simple and practical approach, limiting technical terminology, to reach all parties with an interest in the study of injury patterns and the practice of pathology as it relates to the law. New illustrations, diagrams and sketches showing patterns and mechanisms of injury as well as an inclusive index add value.

Journals

American Journal of Forensic Medicine & Pathology. v. 1, Lippincott, Williams & Wilkins, 1980.
http://journals.lww.com/amjforensicmedicine
http://www.ovid.com/
ISSN: 01957910
ISSN: 1533404X (Online)
Indexed in: MEDLINE
Recommended for: Academic Libraries

Editor-in-chief Dr. Vincent J.M. DiMaio, author of several well-regarded forensic pathology texts, coordinates the expertise of a large editorial board and international board of editors of leading forensic pathologists, lawyers, and criminologists. Published quarterly as the official journal of the National Association of Medical Examiners, the *American Journal of Forensic Medicine and Pathology* features coverage of forensic medical practices worldwide. Articles represent new examination and documentation procedures, retrospective epidemiologic studies, prospective studies, reviews, and of course, case reports. Eleventh in the legal medicine category of the 2009 *Journal Citation Reports* with an impact factor of 0.713, it also ranks 65 of 71 in the pathology category. It is widely indexed by many databases including Biological Abstracts/BIOSIS, CINAHL Plus, Criminal Justice Abstracts, Embase, MEDLINE, Scopus, and Web of Science.

Analytical Chemistry. v. 19, American Chemical Society, 1947.
http://pubs.acs.org/journal/ancham
ISSN: 00032700
ISSN: 15206882 (Online)
Indexed in: MEDLINE
Recommended for: Hospital, Academic Libraries

Forensics is not a major subject of *Analytical Chemistry* but the techniques and applications covered, such as bioanalysis, spectroscopy, and environmental analysis, will be of interest to forensic scientists and toxicologists. The journal is published semi-monthly and primarily covers theoretical and applied aspects of analytical chemistry. It aims to find "ways to increase accuracy, selectivity, sensitivity, and reproducibility" of analytical measurements. *Analytical Chemistry* has an applications review on forensic science on a biannual basis and also includes a Review Issue and Lab Guide. *Analytical Chemistry* includes editorials, research profiles, government and society, features, research articles, and technical notes. Features and news stories cover recent advances published in a broad range of journals. The journal website has podcasts discussing select articles. Links are provided to most-read and most-cited articles. With an impact factor of 5.214 for 2009 *Analytical Chemistry* is ranked third out of 70 journals in the chemistry, analytical category of *Journal Citation Reports*. It is indexed by CABI, Chemical Abstracts, Compendex, MEDLINE, Science Citation Index (Online), Scopus, and many others. *BioTechniques* (ISSN 07366205) is free to qualified personnel and could be used as an alternative to this journal. It features techniques with a molecular biological emphasis and publishes occasional articles related to forensics.

Forensic Science International. v. 11, Elsevier, 1978.
http://www.sciencedirect.com/science/journal/03790738
ISSN: 03790738
ISSN: 18726283 (Online)
See Also Chapter 10.7.1. Forensic Genetics
Indexed in: MEDLINE
Recommended for: Hospital, Academic Libraries

In addition to peer-reviewed research articles, *Forensic Science International* publishes reviews, preliminary communications, book reviews, case reports and forensic anthropology population data. Thirty issues are published each year. The journal is associated with the *Forensic Science International Supplement Series*. Wide-ranging subject coverage includes pathology, chemistry, serology, odontology, toxicology, psychiatry. Within these subjects some areas of interest are bitemarks, ballistics, analytical techniques, breath analyzers, and document examination. Its 2009 *Journal Citation Reports* impact factor of 2.104 ranks it third out of ten journals in the medicine, legal category. It is indexed by BIOSIS Previews, CAB Abstracts, MEDLINE, Science Citation Index, Scopus, and others. This journal is recommended for graduate students, practitioners, and researchers and would be useful in academic, law, and health sciences libraries, particularly those serving trauma centers. *Forensic Science International* is available online from ScienceDirect. Online articles have previews which present abstract, article outline, figures and tables, and references. Links are provided to related articles within ScienceDirect.

Forensic Science, Medicine, and Pathology. v. 1, Humana, 2005.
http://springerlink.com/content/1547-769x/
ISSN: 1547769X
ISSN: 15562891 (Online)
Indexed in: MEDLINE
Recommended for: Academic Libraries

Crime knows no boundaries and so an international editorial board joins with editor-in-chief Roger W. Byard to present advances in forensics through peer-reviewed papers, short communications, meeting proceedings, and case reports. In its five years of publication this quarterly journal has covered forensic science, medicine, nursing, and pathology; toxicology; human identification; mass casualties; sexual assault; veterinary pathology; and forensic applications of anthropology, archeology, entomology, botany, and other disciplines. It is indexed by Academic Search, Chemical Abstracts, MEDLINE, Scopus, TOC Premier, and Web of Science, but in several cases only since volume 4, 2008. All issues are available online via SpringerLink.

International Journal of Legal Medicine. v. 104, Springer, 1990.
http://www.springerlink.com/content/0937-9827
ISSN: 09379827
ISSN: 14371596 (Online)
See Also Chapter 10.7.1. Forensic Genetics
Indexed in: MEDLINE
Recommended for: Academic Libraries

From the International Academy of Legal Medicine and formerly known as *Zeitschrift für Rechtsmedizin*, this journal has a distinguished history from 1922 and a primarily European editorial and advisory board. The six issues per year cover topics such as forensic pathology of death and non-accidental injury and rape, forensic biology and DNA testing, forensic toxicology and traffic medicine, through original articles, case reports, review articles, and technical notes/short communications. With an impact factor of 2.793 in the 2009 *Journal Citation Reports*, it ranks first in the legal medicine category. Indexed in: Abstracts in Anthropology, Biological Abstracts/BIOSIS Previews, Embase, Gale, IBIDS, Index Copernicus, INPHARMA, OCLC, MEDLINE, Web of Science, Scopus, and others, *International Journal of Legal Medicine* also provides Online First articles on the website.

Journal of Forensic Sciences. v. 1, Wiley-Blackwell, 1972.
http://onlinelibrary.wiley.com/journal/10.1111/(ISSN)1556-4029

ISSN: 00221198
ISSN: 15564029 (Online)
Indexed in: MEDLINE
Recommended for: Academic Libraries

Journal of Forensic Sciences provides comprehensive coverage of forensic sciences including toxicology, psychiatry and behavioral sciences, physical anthropology, jurisprudence, engineering sciences, and criminalistics. It is the official journal of the American Academy of Forensic Sciences. *Journal of Forensic Sciences* is published bimonthly and is available online via Wiley Online Library. In addition to full-length research reports, it publishes review articles, technical notes, case reports, book reviews, letters, editorials, and letters to the editor. Articles are organized by subject area. The Digital and Media Sciences section is a recent addition to the journal. A *Journal Citation Reports* impact factor of 1.524 for 2009 places it fifth out of 11 journals in the medicine, legal category. *Journal of Forensic Sciences* is indexed by BIOSIS Previews, CAB Abstracts, MEDLINE, Scopus, Science Citation Index, and others. This journal is recommended for students and practitioners of all disciplines within forensic science and would be useful for academic, science, and legal libraries.

Medicine, Science & the Law. v. 1, Royal Society of Medicine Press, 1960.
http://www.rsmjournals.com/misc/msl.dtl
ISSN: 00258024
ISSN: 20421818 (Online)
Indexed in: MEDLINE
Recommended for: Academic Libraries

Each quarterly issue from the British Academy of Forensic Sciences contains original papers of interest to clinicians, lawyers, and forensic scientists. Additionally there are book reviews, letters to the editor, abstracts of recent relevant reports, and other material of interest to members of the Academy. Formerly published by Barnsbury Publishing, from v. 50, 2010 forward it is published in print and online by Royal Society of Medicine Press. While the impact factor of 0.523 puts it next to last in the legal medicine list in the science *Journal Citation Reports* 2009, it has the longest cited half-life (more than 10 years) in this category, meaning its content continues to be cited. Indexed by many databases including AgeLine, Chemical Abstracts, CINAHL Plus, Criminal Justice Abstracts, Embase, MEDLINE, Scopus, and Web of Science, the new online availability may also influence its citation by future authors.

10.7.1. Forensic Genetics

The application of genetic analyses and molecular diagnostic techniques to legal matters and crime analysis.

—MeSH

Contributor: Craig S. Elam

Monographs

A Litigator's Guide to DNA: From the Laboratory to the Courtroom. Authors: Ron C. Michaelis, Robert G. Flanders, Paula H. Wulff. Elsevier Academic Press, 2008.
http://www.ebrary.com/
http://extranet.netlibrary.com/TitleSelect/
ISBN: 9780123740366
ISBN: 9780080560403
Recommended for: Academic Libraries

This book is essential reading for those needing current information on all aspects of the use of DNA evidence in criminal and civil trials. The target audience includes judges, trial attorneys, forensic science students, and criminalists. It is authoritative, with a biology professor, a former judge, and a former prosecutor serving as authors. The first six chapters provide background information on the structure of DNA, the molecular biological basis for DNA identification tests, essential laboratory quality control and assurance practices, interpretation of evidence using population genetics and probability theory, and specialized mitochondrial DNA and Y chromosome analyses. These chapters are written specifically for those with little or no science background. The remaining four chapters are devoted to the admissibility of DNA evidence in court, examination of the legal strategies and issues involved from the prosecutor and defense counsel perspectives, and post-conviction testing. Scattered throughout are "Recapping the Main Point" boxes providing concise summaries. Appendixes offer relevant, practical statistical calculations; a sample consent form; list of references; glossary; and index. The book has been cited numerous times in a recent opinion by U.S. Supreme Court Justice Samuel Alito, demonstrating its value as a resource for all involved in the legal applications of DNA analysis.

An Introduction to Forensic Genetics. Authors: William Goodwin, Adrian Linacre, Sibte Hadi. John Wiley & Sons, 2007.
http://www.ebrary.com/
http://extranet.netlibrary.com/TitleSelect/
ISBN: 9780470010259

ISBN: 9780470010266
ISBN: 9780470010273 (Online)
Recommended for: Hospital, Academic, Consumer Health Libraries
Doody's Core Titles Selection

This British work is an accessible introduction to forensic genetics for undergraduate students. Basic information is presented in a logical sequence to guide the reader through the process used to generate a DNA profile, from the collection of evidence to its evaluation and presentation in a courtroom. The initial chapters briefly present DNA structure, the collection of samples, and the extraction of DNA from those samples. Technological methodology is limited to those most commonly used in the field, with chapters on the PCR chain reaction and analysis and assessment of short term repeat (STR) profiles. These are followed by discussions of population genetics and the statistical interpretation of STR profiles. A short chapter covers the evaluation and the presentation of DNA evidence in a legal setting. The book concludes with chapters devoted to DNA databases—primarily the UK National DNA Database (NDNAD), kinship testing, lineage markers, and single nucleotide polymorphisms (SNPs). This is a valuable guide for those seeking a brief introduction to the scientific aspects of forensic genetics, with liberal illustrations, references to case studies, web resources, additional readings, a glossary, and index. It is also available as an e-book.

DNA: Forensic and Legal Applications. Authors: Lawrence Kobilinsky, Thomas F. Liotti, Jamel Oeser-Sweat. Wiley, 2005.
http://onlinelibrary.wiley.com/book/10.1002/0471681911
http://www.ebrary.com/
ISBN: 9780471414780
ISBN: 9780471681915 (Online)
ISBN: 9780471681908 (Online)
Recommended for: Academic Libraries

This comprehensive work covers the science of DNA analysis and the use of DNA evidence in the legal system. Its primary goal is to provide those in the legal community with the scientific background to understand the benefits and limitations of this technology as applied to the criminal justice system; it also provides forensic scientists with the legal applications of these techniques. The authors assume that the reader has no knowledge of DNA biochemistry, providing that in an introductory chapter. The following chapters cover evidence gathering techniques and the various DNA identification tests, providing their strengths, weaknesses, and significance to better interpret the validity of the results. Of particular interest to legal practitioners are the discussions of statistics and population genetics in DNA analysis, the legal challenges and defenses involved in presenting admissible DNA evidence at trial, and post-conviction appeals and testing to prove innocence. This is a concise text for forensic scientists, students, analytical chemists, lawyers, judges, and law enforcement personnel. The scientific chapters include bibliographies and references; appendixes provide additional references, state and federal court cases involving the admissibility of DNA evidence, contact information for innocence projects, legislative information for post-conviction DNA testing, and a glossary. *DNA: Forensic and Legal Applications* is recommended for medical collections supporting forensic programs and law libraries, but it may be too technical for general libraries.

Forensic DNA Typing: Biology, Technology, and Genetics of STR Markers. 2nd ed. Author: John M. Butler. Elsevier Academic Press, 2005.
http://extranet.netlibrary.com/TitleSelect/
http://www.ebrary.com/
ISBN: 9780121479527
ISBN: 9780080470610
Recommended for: Academic Libraries

Although partially updated by a new edition, this remains the standard resource on the science and technology of DNA analysis. The book is divided into biology and technology sections, each progressing from basic introductory material to more advanced topics. The basic information has been collected and updated separately in a new volume, *Fundamentals of Forensic DNA Typing*, with the more complex topics to be published later. Until then, this book still offers the most comprehensive and detailed information in the exponentially growing field of forensic genetics and DNA technology. The biology chapters cover sample collection, DNA amplification, the biology of short tandem repeat (STR) markers, and more specialized topics in DNA testing. The technology section discusses DNA databases and a variety of testing methods, including electrophoresis, staining, automated systems, and instrumentation. Also addressed are population genetics, statistics, and victim identification. Valuable appendixes list STR alleles, suppliers of DNA analysis equipment and products, and DNA Advisory Board Quality Assurance Standards. High-profile cases and other interesting information are presented in Data, Notes & Applications (D.N.A.) boxes throughout the book. A digital version is available from NetLibrary and ebrary.

Fundamentals of Forensic DNA Typing. Author: John M. Butler. Academic Press/Elsevier, 2010.
ISBN: 9780123749994
Recommended for: Academic Libraries

This is an important, new text by one of the most prominent researchers in the field. Due to the rapid expansion of forensic genetics, he has split the new edition of his 2005 classic text, *Forensic DNA Typing: Biology, Technology, and Genetics of STR Markers*, 2nd edition, into two volumes—the present one supplying introductory information and a later one discussing advanced topics. The author's goal, however, remains the same: to present the current science of DNA analysis by examining the biology, technology, and genetics of STR markers, which is the most common method used today. This book contains all the fundamental information essential for students, logically progressing through the DNA testing process. It begins with a historical overview and the basic biology of DNA typing. Subsequent chapters cover crime scene sample collection, DNA extraction, PCR techniques, short tandem repeat (STR) markers, and the statistical interpretation of results. New information is found in the chapters on DNA databases, quality assurance, and lineage markers. Briefly discussed are expanded applications of DNA testing in tracing kinship, wildlife identification, and disaster victim identification. Each chapter concludes with Points for Discussion, followed by a list of references and websites, although these are not directly cited in the text. "Data, Notes & Applications" (D.N.A.) boxes highlight high-profile cases and practical topics of interest throughout the book. This is an exceptional work in terms of currency, clarity, and coverage of the field of DNA analysis. It is an excellent text for undergraduate students in forensic genetics, with an extensive glossary, list of useful websites, and appendixes addressing background information on probability and statistics. Ancillary information is available at an instructor website.

Genetic Witness: Science, Law, and Controversy in the Making of DNA Profiling. Author: Jay D. Aronson. Rutgers University Press, 2007.
http://extranet.netlibrary.com/TitleSelect/
http://www.ebrary.com/
ISBN: 9780813541877
ISBN: 9780813541884
ISBN: 9780813543833 (Online)
Recommended for: Academic, Consumer Health Libraries

This is the definitive history of the early rise of DNA typing since its 1987 introduction in the American legal system. It describes the "DNA Wars"—the intense legal challenges and controversies that eventually led to the standardization of rigorous scientific, procedural, and quality assurance protocols for producing reliable DNA profiling evidence. Several chapters review those significant courtroom and legislative actions, including one devoted to the O.J. Simpson trial, which led to today's general acceptance of DNA markers as an essential investigative tool in the criminal justice system. It concludes with a chapter on the revolutionary legacy wrought by DNA profiling, including a warning on the nature of human fallibility in producing such highly technological legal evidence. Since the book is based on the author's doctoral dissertation written several years ago, the discussion of DNA scientific techniques is somewhat outdated. The author provides the reader with extensive notes, references, and a detailed index. Written in an easily accessible style, this work will interest a wide variety of audiences, from the layman to academicians interested in the history and sociology of forensic genetics. This book is recommended for all libraries.

Journals

American Journal of Forensic Medicine & Pathology. v. 1, Lippincott, Williams & Wilkins, 1980.
See Chapter 10.7. Forensic Medicine

Forensic Science International. v. 12, Elsevier, 1978.
http://www.fsijournal.org/
http://www.sciencedirect.com/science/journal/03790738
ISSN: 03790738
See Also Chapter 10.7. Forensic Medicine
Indexed in: MEDLINE
Recommended for: Hospital, Academic Libraries

Published for over 30 years, this remains one of the most important sources of original research in forensic genetics, especially for literature published prior to the creation of the more specialized *Forensic Science International: Genetics* in 2007. This journal is especially valuable for providing a broader context for genetics within the forensic sciences and other relevant fields, including law, medicine, and public health. *FSI* publishes original, peer-reviewed research papers, review articles, preliminary communications, letters to the editor, book reviews, and case reports. It is indexed widely in major abstracting and indexing services, including MEDLINE, Biological Abstracts, Chemical Abstracts, Science Citation Index, and Scopus. Its impact factor is ranked third out of ten legal medicine titles. Full-text articles are available back to volume 1, which includes access under its preceding title *Forensic Science.*

Forensic Science International: Genetics. v. 1, Elsevier Science, 2007.
http://www.fsigenetics.com/
http://www.sciencedirect.com/science/journal/18724973
ISSN: 18724973
Indexed in: MEDLINE
Recommended for: Academic Libraries

Also known as *FSI Genetics*, this journal was created in March 2007 as an offshoot of its parent journal, *Forensic Science International* (*FSI*) in response to the rapid increase in DNA analysis and forensic genetics research. This type of research now constitutes the highest percentage of articles in major forensic science journals today. Although relatively recent, this journal reflects the maturity of the field and presents original, peer-reviewed research, short communications, case reports, and announcements of population data. Published quarterly, this journal is essential reading for all medical and legal professionals and scientists wishing to stay current with the technological advances in DNA analysis and forensic genetics. It is the official journal of the International Society for Forensic Genetics and is indexed in MEDLINE, Embase/Excerpta Medica, Scopus, and Science Citation Index. The journal's first impact factor was calculated in 2009; it is currently ranked fifth out of ten legal medicine titles.

Forensic Science International: Genetics Supplement Series. v. 1, Elsevier Science, 2008.
http://www.fsigeneticssup.com/
http://www.sciencedirect.com/science/journal/18751768
ISSN: 18751768
Recommended for: Academic Libraries

This supplement series to *Forensic Science International: Genetics* currently consists of the proceedings of the annual conference of the International Society for Forensic Genetics. The first volume, titled *Progress in Forensic Genetics 12*, presents the proceedings of the twenty-second International ISFG Congress held in 2007, which is the first completely electronic version. The supplement is indexed in Embase/Excerpta Medica and Scopus, thus making these detailed papers more accessible to those actively working in the field. The proceedings consist mainly of short manuscripts of the over 250 oral and poster presentations, with minor editing to speed publication. As a result, the second volume was published only three months after the Congress was held.

Forensic Science, Medicine, and Pathology. v. 1, Humana, 2005.
See Chapter 10.7. Forensic Medicine

International Journal of Legal Medicine. v. 104, Springer, 1990.
http://www.springerlink.com/content/1437-1596/
ISSN: 09379827
ISSN: 14371596 (Online)
See Also Chapter 10.7. Forensic Medicine
Indexed in: MEDLINE
Recommended for: Academic Libraries

This journal is one of the major journals in forensic medicine and, despite its broad scope, is a valuable source of information on forensic genetics and DNA analysis, particularly from beyond the United States. Originally published in German, it has been published in English since 1990 and is the official publication of the International Academy of Legal Medicine. It provides review articles, peer-reviewed original research papers, case reports, and letters. Of particular interest is the "Technical Notes" section, originally created for rapid publication of data in the dynamic field of DNA analysis. This section presents innovative protocols and methodologies, including DNA validation studies, population data, quality control studies, and more. It has the highest ranked journal impact factor out of ten legal medicine journals and is widely indexed. It is available in full text beginning with its first volume in 1922.

Medicine, Science & the Law. v. 1, Royal Society of Medicine Press, 1960.
See Chapter 10.7. Forensic Medicine

10.7.2. Forensic Pathology

The application of pathology to questions of law.
—MeSH

Contributors: Kristine M. Alpi and Robert Sotak

Monographs

Child Fatality Review: An Interdisciplinary Guide and Photographic Reference. Authors: Randell Alexander, Mary E. Case. GW Medical, 2008.
ISBN: 9781878060754
Recommended for: Hospital Libraries

With growing awareness of suspicious infant deaths, the child fatality review process has become mainstream. *Child Fatality Review* details common types of child fatalities for health, social services, and legal professionals to use as a reference, including sections devoted to review procedures, the roles of each team member, and full-color photographs of various causes and manners of death. Case studies illustrate abusive and accidental forms of death, including neglect, SIDS, suicide, burning, drowning, genetic diseases, natural causes, and shaken baby syndrome. Self-study and educational efforts will be enhanced by the *Child Fatality Review* CD-ROM, which allows readers to test their abilities in reviewing difficult cases from the text. Also available for a quarter of the price is the spiral-bound *Child Fatality Review Quick Reference: For Healthcare, Social Service, and Law Enforcement Professionals* (GW Medical Publishing, Inc., 2009).

Color Atlas of the Autopsy. Author: Scott A. Wagner. CRC Press, 2003.
http://extranet.netlibrary.com/TitleSelect/
ISBN: 9780849315206
ISBN: 9780203494387 (Online)
Recommended for: Hospital, Academic Libraries

The autopsy is the central component of forensic pathology and it must be understood by professionals interacting with the pathologist. Dr. Wagner is a forensic pathologist, and the creator of the video *The Autopsy, Chapter One: Unraveling Life's Mysteries. Color Atlas of the Autopsy* introduces the before, during, and after process and principles of the procedure with over 500 full-color photographs. This is recommended as a core resource for the examination of the American Board of Medicolegal Death Investigators. Dr. Wagner also authored *Death Scene Investigation: A Field Guide* (CRC 2009) to assist death scene investigators in using standard terminology and descriptions of pathological findings. The price and portability of this slim, photo-packed volume make it accessible when forensic pathology atlases are not practical.

DNA: Forensic and Legal Applications. Authors: Lawrence Kobilinsky, Thomas F. Liotti, Jamel Oeser-Sweat. Wiley, 2005.
See Chapter 10.7.1. Forensic Genetics

Essential Forensic Neuropathology. Editors: Juan C. Troncoso, Ana Rubio, David R. Fowler. Wolters Kluwer/Lippincott Williams & Wilkins, 2010.
http://www.ovid.com/
ISBN: 9780781778695
Recommended for: Hospital, Academic Libraries

Neuropathology is a complex area of forensic pathology and this guide provides the knowledge to conduct a thorough postmortem examination of the nervous system, describe and document the relevant pathological changes, and interpret these findings in a way that will be helpful in determining the cause and manner of death. A typical forensic pathology text devotes only about 50 pages to neuropathology, so there is a place for this concise but thorough 330+ page publication. High quality color photos, black-and-white scans, clear tables and interesting cases described in boxes bring essential content quickly to the reader. Most chapters are short, generally fewer than ten pages due to the small print, tight margins, and plethora of images, making this an excellent resource for residents and trainees. The text is well organized and each chapter ends with references. The index indicates figures and tables with good cross-referencing for terms and acronyms, but does not include slang terms for certain types of injuries such as hangman's fractures or Jefferson's fractures. The companion website for individual purchasers provides the complete, fully searchable text, an image bank and additional figures. For deeper coverage on all these topics, see the recent second edition of Jan E. Leestma's *Forensic Neuropathology* (CRC Press, 2009).

Forensic Pathology: Principles and Practice. Editors: David Dolinak, Evan W. Matshes, Emma O. Lew. Academic Press Elsevier, 2005.
ISBN: 9780122199516
Recommended for: Academic Libraries

Forensic Pathology: Principles and Practice is an extensively illustrated work containing more than 1,800 color photographs. The images are high quality and discussed in the text and identified with figure numbers, but they are not captioned or specifically noted in the index, making the book slightly less useful as a quick reference. Given the price and almost 10 lb. weight, this is not a portable personal book but the binding is not designed to hold up to heavy use. The text is very readable with frequent subheadings, bulleted points, take-home messages and summaries of what and what not to do at the ends of most of the chapters. References for further reading include journal articles and books covering a wide time span. This volume uses a case-oriented format to address a variety of topics from death investigation, forensic autopsy, types of injuries, postmortem changes, identification, and photography, as well as covering the life span from pregnancy to infant and child death to elder abuse. Richard Souviron, who provides a brief introduction to forensic ondontology, covers the topic in depth with co-author William Silver in *Dental Autopsy*

(CRC Press, 2009). Another topic that is better covered in other works is forensic osteology; readers interested in this topic would benefit from *The Human Bone Manual* by Tim D. White and Pieter A. Folkens (Elsevier Academic, c2005).

Handbook of Autopsy Practice. 4th ed. Editor: Brenda L. Waters. Humana Springer, 2009.
http://www.springerlink.com/content/978-1-58829-841-6
ISBN: 9781588298416
ISBN: 9781597451277 (Online)
Recommended for: Hospital, Academic Libraries
Doody's Core Titles Selection

Most autopsy and pathology reference tools are about the images. That is not the case for Brenda L. Waters' *Handbook of Autopsy Practice*, which is a core reference illustrated with black-and-white photos and diagrams. While primarily focused on general hospital autopsy procedures and clinical pathology, the discussion of the pros and cons of dissection techniques will be of great use to general and forensic pathology trainees. Part 1 includes six new chapters and sections on generally underdiscussed topics such as quality assurance, chemistry, cytogenetics, imaging, medicolegal matters, microbiology, radiation safety, and autopsy reporting, with sample letters and worksheets. According to Sperhake's review in *Forensic Science, Medicine, and Pathology* (2010; 6(1):77–78) and Hoda and Basenceney's review in *JAMA* (2009; 302(20):2260–2261), the bulk of the text is the alphabetical list of common and rare conditions with corresponding pathologic findings and the strategies used to uncover them. Part 3 provides a series of tables providing organ weights and body measurements for fetuses, children, and adults.

Handbook of Forensic Pathology. 2nd ed. Authors: Vincent J.M. DiMaio, Suzanna E. Dana. CRC Press, 2007.
ISBN: 9780849392870
Recommended for: Hospital, Academic Libraries

In its second edition, *Handbook of Forensic Pathology* is a concise, authoritative manual that illustrates the core aspects of forensic pathology, collecting evidence, determining time of death and identifying remains. It covers the natural causes of death in children and adults as well as causes such as homicide, suicide, accident, and those that remain undetermined. Written in outline format with easily understandable language, this precise resource contains detailed entries. New content in the second edition includes nursing home death, tasers, and pepper spray. With numerous instructional charts and diagrams and full-color photographs, this handbook is recommended by the American Board of Medicolegal Death Investigators as a core resource for their board examination. This is not to be confused with the 2001 second edition of DeMaio's work *Forensic Pathology*. While causes of sudden natural death in children are covered in *Handbook of Forensic Pathology*, for more detailed pediatric forensic pathology and autopsy consider *Handbook of Pediatric Autopsy Pathology* (Humana Press, 2005) by Enid Gilbert-Barness and Diane Debich-Spicer.

Karch's Pathology of Drug Abuse. 4th ed. Author: Steven B. Karch. CRC Press, 2009.
See Chapter 17.8.2. Forensic Toxicology

Sexual Assault: Victimization across the Life Span, a Clinical Guide and a Color Atlas. Editors: Angelo P. Giardino, Elizabeth M. Datner, Janice B. Asher, Barbara Girardin, Diana K. Faugno, Mary J. Spencer. GW Medical Publishing, 2003.
See Chapter 13.4. Forensic Nursing

Spitz and Fisher's Medicolegal Investigation of Death: Guidelines for the Application of Pathology to Crime Investigation. 4th ed. Editors: Werner U. Spitz, Daniel J. Spitz, Russell S. Fisher, Ramsey Clark. Charles C Thomas, 2006.
See Chapter 10.7. Forensic Medicine

Journals

American Journal of Forensic Medicine & Pathology. v. 1, Lippincott, Williams & Wilkins, 1980.
See Chapter 10.7. Forensic Medicine

Forensic Science International. v. 11, Elsevier, 1978.
See Chapter 10.7. Forensic Medicine, Chapter 10.7.1. Forensic Genetics

Forensic Science, Medicine, and Pathology. v. 1, Humana, 2005.
See Chapter 10.7. Forensic Medicine

International Journal of Legal Medicine. v. 104, Springer, 1990.
See Chapter 10.7. Forensic Medicine, Chapter 10.7.1 Forensic Genetics

Medicine, Science & the Law. v. 1, Royal Society of Medicine Press, 1960.
See Chapter 10.7. Forensic Medicine

10.8. Hospitalists

Physicians who are employed to work exclusively in hospital settings, primarily for managed care organizations. They are the attending or primary responsible physician for the patient during hospitalization.

—MeSH

Contributor: Diana Culbertson

Monographs

Comprehensive Pediatric Hospital Medicine. Editors: Lisa B. Zaoutis, Vincent W. Chiang. Mosby Elsevier, 2007.
http://www.mdconsult.com/
ISBN: 9780323030045
Recommended for: Hospital, Academic Libraries

The editors, each a hospitalist at different pediatric hospitals, have compiled a broad resource for those who focus on inpatient care of children. As such, it differs from standard pediatrics texts that put more emphasis on child development and ambulatory care. The book covers the numerous conditions a pediatric hospitalist could encounter when caring for a hospitalized child. It also covers other professional issues for the hospitalist, including quality, patient advocacy, finances, medical consultation and co-management, ethics, and legal issues.

Hospital Medicine. 2nd ed. Editors: Robert M. Wachter, Lee Goldman, Harry Hollander. Lippincott Williams & Wilkins, 2005.
http://www.ovid.com/
ISBN: 9780781747271
Recommended for: Hospital, Academic Libraries
Brandon/Hill Selection

The term hospitalist was coined by two of the three editors—Wachter and Goldman—in 1996 (Wachter, *N Engl J Med* 1996; 335(7):514–517). Since then, the field of hospital medicine has developed substantially and continues to grow. Now in its second edition, this book pulls together evidence-based clinical information geared toward caring for the hospitalized patient. In addition to the sections generally organized by organ system, the book also touches on practice management issues, such as economics, ethics, quality and safety, hospital information systems, decision analysis, and more.

Hospitalists: A Guide to Building and Sustaining a Successful Program. Authors: Joseph A. Miller, John Nelson, Winthrop F. Whitcomb. Health Administration Press, 2008.
ISBN: 9781567932836
Recommended for: Hospital, Academic Libraries

This book is written for those who want to start or improve a hospitalist program. The book is divided into two sections. The first provides a strategic perspective, covering organizational models, how hospitalists add value, return on investment, program essentials, and legal and contract issues. The second section focuses on the practice management perspective, addressing hospitalist retention and career satisfaction, communication, staffing, scheduling, night coverage, use of non-physician clinical staff, compensation, the medical director role, performance measurement, billing and revenue, and pediatric hospitalist programs. The appendixes include practical tips and sample documents: a job description for a hospitalist program medical director, sample performance dashboards, recruitment recommendations, and a sample hospitalist practice brochure.

Journals

Journal of Hospital Medicine. v. 1, Wiley, 2006.
http://onlinelibrary.wiley.com/journal/10.1002/(ISSN)1553-5606
ISSN: 15535592
ISSN: 15535606 (Online)
Indexed in: MEDLINE
Recommended for: Hospital, Academic Libraries

This is the official journal of the Society of Hospital Medicine, the professional organization representing hospitalists who focus on the general medical care of the hospitalized patient. It is particularly recommended for libraries in health facilities with hospitalist programs. The journal is indexed in MEDLINE, Embase/Excerpta Medica, PsycINFO/Psychological Abstracts, Scopus, and Science Citation Index Expanded.

10.9. Integrative Medicine

The discipline concerned with using the combination of conventional (allopathic) medicine and alternative medicine to address the biological, psychological, social, and spiritual aspects of health and illness.

—MeSH

Contributor: Helen-Ann Brown Epstein

Monographs

The ACP Evidence-Based Guide to Complementary & Alternative Medicine. Editors: Bradly P. Jacobs, Katherine Gundling. American College of Physicians, 2009.
ISBN: 9781934465042
Recommended for: Hospital, Academic, Consumer Health Libraries

This guide offers insight and guidance on alternative medical systems, such as mind-body interventions, biologically based therapies, manipulative and body-based therapies, and energy therapy. It illustrates how physicians can use these complementary and alternative (CAM) methods for common ailments and diseases. In-depth reviews of the research are thoroughly digested into concise summary tables. The book provides bottom-line recommendations for each therapy using a five-level system. The clinical evidence for the CAM therapies is evaluated by using the GRADE system. This title is also available as an e-book for individual purchasers.

Fundamentals of Complementary and Integrative Medicine. 4th ed. Editor: Marc S. Micozzi. Saunders/Elsevier, 2011.
ISBN: 9781437705775
Recommended for: Hospital, Academic, Consumer Health Libraries

The aim of this work is to provide clear and rational guides for health care professionals and students to complementary approaches to specific medical conditions and the integration of complementary therapy into mainstream medical practice. It is a survey of the basics of complementary medical systems currently available in North America and Europe. Chapters on homeopathy, chiropractic, herbal medicine, aromatherapy, nutrition, Chinese medicine, and yoga are included. Boxes, tables, and illustrations enhance the text. Suggested readings close each chapter.

Integrative Health: A Holistic Approach for Health Professionals. Authors: Cyndie Koopsen, Caroline Young. Jones & Bartlett, 2009.
ISBN: 9780763757618
Recommended for: Hospital, Academic Libraries

Written by a nurse and a public health professional, this book combines treatments from conventional medicine and clinically proven complementary and alternative medicine to address the body, mind, and spirit, as well as the environment and relationships with others. There are chapters devoted to holistic stress management, health and the human spirit, meditation, healing environments, traditional Chinese and Ayervedic medicine, humor and healing, music therapy, integrative nutrition, therapeutic massage, and physical activity. Every chapter begins with learning objectives and ends with a list of references.

Integrative Medicine. 2nd ed. Editor: David Rakel. Saunders/Elsevier, 2007.
http://www.mdconsult.com/
ISBN: 9781416029540
Recommended for: Hospital, Academic Libraries

According to the editor, "This text is focused on empowering the clinician to practice an integrative approach using therapies that address all aspects of health to facilitate healing." The authors offer an evidence-based focus on primary care with integrative therapeutic interventions. The text is divided into three sections: an overview of the field of integrative medicine, an integrative approach to disease, and practical tools for everyday practice. There are applications involving nutrition, exercise, mind-body, biochemical, biomechanical, and bioenergetic inluences on diseases, such as anxiety, migraine, Alzheimer's, HIV disease, hepatitis, hypertension, congestive heart failure, obesity, low back pain, and many others. This book is included in the MD Consult collection.

Integrative Women's Health. 1st ed. Authors: Victoria Maizes, Tieraona Low Dog. Oxford University Press, 2010.
ISBN: 9780195378818
Recommended for: Hospital, Academic, Consumer Health Libraries

This is a selection in the *Weil Integrative Medicine Library*. It is the first comprehensive guide on integrative women's care written for both health professionals and general audiences by an all-female, internationally known team of authors. The work covers a range of topics such as massage, fibromyalgia, sexuality, spirituality, and the future of women's health. *Integrative Women's Health* weaves together the best of conventional treatments with mind-body interventions, nutritional strategies, herbal therapies, dietary supplements, acupuncture, and manual medicine, providing clinicians with a roadmap for practicing comprehensive integrative care. Each chapter is highlighted with bulleted key points and breakout text boxes of essential clinical information.

Mosby's Complementary & Alternative Medicine: A Research-Based Approach. 3rd ed. Editor: Lyn W. Freeman. Mosby, 2009.
ISBN: 9780323053464

Recommended for: Hospital, Academic, Consumer Health Libraries
Brandon/Hill, *Doody's Core Titles* Selection

By consulting this book, readers will gain an understanding of the most commonly used alternative therapies, as well as those most likely to be integrated with conventional medical treatment. It provides a practical, comprehensive overview of recent medical advances, and the history and philosophy of each discipline. There are indications, contraindications, case studies, and clinical trials for each topic. Commentary is provided by well-known experts, and research is critically reviewed, with examples of exceptional and flawed studies. Part one covers mind-body integration, part two covers mind-body interventions, part three covers alternative professionals, part four reviews complementary self-help strategies, and part five covers energetics and spirituality. In this third edition are new chapters on "Measurement of the Human Biofield" and "The Future of Ethnomedicine." An appendix contains Internet resources. This work comes with a free Evolve companion website for individual purchasers, which includes regular updates of content, student activities, and full-color images.

Scientific Basis of Integrative Medicine. 2nd ed. Editors: Leonard A. Wisneski, Lucy Anderson. CRC Press, 2009.
ISBN: 9781420082906
Recommended for: Academic Libraries

The second edition of the *Scientific Basis of Integrative Medicine* continues to provide doctors and other health practitioners with information on complementary and alternative approaches to health that is authoritative, scientifically based, and epidemiologically substantiated. It offers a scientific basis for the mind-body connection. This work also investigates how hope, faith, and love aid healing.

Textbook of Complementary and Alternative Medicine. 2nd ed. Editors: Chun-Su Yuan, Eric J. Bieber, Brent Bauer. Parthenon, 2006.
ISBN: 9781842142974
Recommended for: Hospital, Academic Libraries

This book provides contemporary, evidence-based information on complementary and alternative medicine (CAM) therapies, including herbal medicine, meditation, acupuncture, and osteopathy. It presents a sound academic understanding of the approaches and systems of CAM. A highlight of the text is a section on common medical disorders, with details of which CAM therapies may be most appropriate in their treatment. Based on a successful course at the Pritzker School of Medicine of the University of Chicago and thoroughly referenced, *Textbook of Complementary and Alternative Medicine* is a science-based guide to understanding CAM applications to human health and interactions with conventional medicine.

Journals

Acupuncture in Medicine. v. 1, BMJ Publishing Group, 1983.
http://aim.bmj.com/
ISSN: 09645284
ISSN: 17599873 (Online)
Indexed in: MEDLINE, CINAHL
Recommended for: Academic Libraries

Acupuncture in Medicine, the official publication of the British Medical Acupuncture Society, is a quarterly scientific and clinical journal aimed at Western-trained physicians and other health professionals. It uses the prevailing understanding of neurophysiology and anatomy to interpret the effects of acupuncture. It contains articles on clinical, experimental, technical, and basic science aspects of medical acupuncture and related techniques. It welcomes scientific reports, systematic and general reviews, audits, and case reports.

Alternative Medicine Review. v. 1, Thorne Research, Inc, 1996.
http://altmedrev.com/
ISSN: 10895159
Indexed in: MEDLINE, CINAHL
Recommended for: Academic, Consumer Health Libraries

This is a peer-reviewed journal dedicated to providing accurate, timely, and clinically relevant original research articles and literature reviews four times yearly to the practicing health care practitioner. It has an impact factor of 3.515 and ranks first of 17 journals in the integrative and complementary medicine category in the 2009 *Journal Citation Reports*. A free online version back to volume 1, 1996 is available from the publisher.

Alternative Therapies in Health and Medicine. v. 1, InnoVision Health Media, 1995.
http://www.alternative-therapies.com/
ISSN: 10786791
Indexed in: MEDLINE, CINAHL
Recommended for: Hospital, Academic Libraries

Alternative Therapies in Health and Medicine has a mission "to promote the art and science of integrative medicine and a responsibility to improve public health." It addresses all systems of integrative medicine, with an emphasis on evaluation and appropriate use. It is peer-reviewed and includes papers about all age groups. It also includes interviews with leaders in alternative medicine. There are six issues per year. This journal is indexed in MEDLINE. Online access back to volume 1, 1995 is available.

BMC Complementary and Alternative Medicine. v. 1, BioMed Central, 2001.
http://www.biomedcentral.com/bmccomplementalternmed/
http://www.ncbi.nlm.nih.gov/pmc/journals/10/
ISSN: 14726882 (Online)
Indexed in: MEDLINE
Recommended for: Hospital, Academic, Consumer Health Libraries

This is an open access journal, electronic only, in the BioMed Central family. It publishes original peer-reviewed research articles in interventions and resources that complement or replace conventional therapies. There is a specific emphasis on research that explores the biological mechanisms of action, as well as their efficacy, safety, costs, patterns of use, and implementation. *BMC Complementary and Alternative Medicine* is indexed in MEDLINE, CAS, Embase, Scopus, CINAHL, FSTA, Web of Science, and Google Scholar. All articles are deposited in PubMed Central immediately after publication.

Complementary Therapies in Medicine. v. 1, Elsevier, 1993.
http://www.sciencedirect.com/science/journal/09652299
ISSN: 09652299
ISSN: 18736963 (Online)
Indexed in: MEDLINE, CINAHL
Recommended for: Hospital, Academic, Consumer Health Libraries

Complementary Therapies in Medicine is an international, peer-reviewed journal. Its audience is family practitioners, complementary therapists, nurses, and physiotherapists; academics, including social scientists and CAM researchers; health care managers; and patients. The journal aim is "to publish valid, relevant and rigorous research and serious discussion articles with the main purpose of improving healthcare." Each issue features research articles, abstracts of recently published research, reviews, and opinion pieces, as well as information and experiences on integrating complementary medicine into mainstream care. It ranks fourth of 17 journals in integrative and complementary medicine in the 2009 *Journal Citation Reports*. RSS feeds are available. It is indexed in MEDLINE and other major databases. Online access back to volume 1, 1993 is available through ScienceDirect.

Evidence-Based Complementary and Alternative Medicine. v. 1, Oxford University Press, 2004.
http://ecam.oxfordjournals.org/current.dtl
ISSN: 1741427X
ISSN: 17414288 (Online)
Recommended for: Hospital, Academic Libraries

Evidence-based Complementary and Alternative Medicine (*eCAM*) is an international, peer-reviewed journal that focuses on the study of "CAM modalities, particularly traditional Asian healing systems. *eCAM* emphasizes health outcomes, while documenting biological mechanisms of action." Original articles are available as open access; other articles, including reviews, editorials, and commentaries are only available through a subscription. The journal is indexed in many services including PubMed (but not MEDLINE), Embase, and Global Health.

Journal of Alternative and Complementary Medicine. v. 1, Mary Ann Liebert, 1995.
http://www.liebertonline.com/toc/acm/14/10
ISSN: 10755535
ISSN: 15577708 (Online)
Indexed in: MEDLINE, CINAHL
Recommended for: Hospital, Academic Libraries
Brandon/Hill Selection

This is the official journal of the International Society for Complementary Medicine Research and the Society for Acupuncture Research. It includes both observational and analytical articles on complementary and alternative treatments to assess their therapeutic value. Articles include discussions of clinical care and case reports to evaluate and integrate CAM therapies into patient care protocols and research strategies. The journal is indexed in a variety of sources including MEDLINE and MANTIS. RSS feeds, table of contents alerts, and an open access publishing option are available.

Databases and Other Electronic Resources

National Center for Complementary and Alternative Medicine. National Institutes of Health, 1998.
http://nccam.nih.gov
Recommended for: Hospital, Academic, Consumer Health Libraries

This is a valuable free website for health professionals and consumers from the National Institutes of Health. It links to health information topics, clinical trials, and research resources. Two of the research resources are the complementary and alternative medicine (CAM) subset in PubMed and the CAM subset in the Cochrane Library. The website also features grants and other funding opportunities. One can chat with an expert and subscribe to a RSS feed. It is also available in Spanish.

Natural Standard. Natural Standard Research Collaboration, 2003?
http://www.naturalstandard.com/
See Also Chapter 17. Pharmacology
Recommended for: Hospital, Academic, Consumer Health Libraries

Natural Standard is an international tool for health professionals and consumers that aggregates and synthesizes data on complementary and alternative therapies. It provides objective, reliable information on foods, herbs and supplements, health and wellness, medical conditions, sports medicine, nutrition, genomics and proteomics, and environmental and global health. There are interactions and symptom checkers, as well as calculators. This information aids clinicians, patients, and health care institutions to make more informed and safer therapeutic decisions. The information is evidence based, consensus based, and peer reviewed. Print versions of the tools, a handheld version, webinars, blog, podcasts, a monthly newsletter, and RSS feeds are available.

10.10. Internal Medicine

The diagnosis and treatment of diseases of the internal organ systems of adults.

—MeSH

Contributor: Helen-Ann Brown Epstein

Monographs

Cecil Medicine. 23rd ed. Editors: Lee Goldman, Dennis A. Ausiello, William Arend, James O. Armitage. Saunders/Elsevier, 2008.
http://www.us.elsevierhealth.com/product.jsp?isbn=9781416044789
ISBN: 9781416044789
Recommended for: Hospital, Academic, Consumer Health Libraries
Brandon/Hill Selection

Cecil Medicine is a required text for all types of libraries. It contains unbiased, evidence-based guidance on the evaluation and management of every medical condition. Algorithms simplify decision making. There are pertinent bibliographical references, with annotations explaining their clinical significance. Management recommendations are supported by Grade A clinical evidence. The electronic version is included in Expert Consult for individual purchasers. A new edition is expected in May 2011.

Current Medical Diagnosis & Treatment 2010. 49th ed. Editors: Stephen J. McPhee, Maxine A. Papadakis. Appleton & Lange, 2010.
http://www.accessmedicine.com/cmdt
ISBN: 9780071624442
Recommended for: Hospital, Academic, Consumer Health Libraries
Brandon/Hill, *Doody's Core Titles* Selection

Current Medical Diagnosis & Treatment is an annual classic. It covers symptoms, signs, epidemiology, and treatment for more than 1,000 diseases and disorders. For each topic there are concise, evidence-based answers to questions regarding both hospital and ambulatory medicine. New topics in this edition include H1N1, acute knee pain, caccine safety, neuromyelitis optica, and Chikungunya fever. The chapter on cancer has been rewritten and the information about antithrombotic therapy has been revised. It is available online through AccessMedicine (with four additional chapters), as well as on the Amazon Kindle platform.

Davidson's Principles & Practice of Medicine. 21st ed. Editors: Nicki R. Colledge, Brian R. Walker, Stuart H. Ralston. Churchill Livingstone/Elsevier, 2010.
ISBN: 9780702030857
Recommended for: Hospital, Academic Libraries

The previous edition of *Davidson's* was an award-winning title, for New Edition of an Edited Textbook, presented at the Royal Society of Medicine and Society of Authors 2007 Medical Book Awards. Its system-based chapters follow a standard format, beginning with an overview of relevant clinical examination, followed by an account of functional anatomy, physiology and investigations, then describing the common presentations of disease, and finishing with details of the individual diseases of that system. Throughout the book, tables and boxes carry symbols of causes, clinical features and complications, investigations, treatments and adverse effects, evidence-based medicine, approaches in old age, and other information. The book is well illustrated. There are not many references at the close of the chapters; however, suggestions are given for related websites. An online STUDENT CONSULT version is available for individual purchasers.

The 5-Minute Clinical Consult. Wolters Kluwer/Lippincott Williams & Wilkins, Annual.
http://www.5minuteconsult.com/
ISBN: 9781605470139
See Also Chapter 1.9. Physician Assistants
Recommended for: Hospital, Academic, Consumer Health Libraries
Brandon/Hill Selection

This text is offered in print, mobile, and online format, presenting information on the diagnosis, treatment, and follow-up of over 1,000 medical conditions. The online and mobile versions are updated quarterly. The 18th print edition features behavioral medicine (cognitive behavior therapy, meditation, relaxation techniques, yoga, and other therapies), more evidence-based medicine ratings, and additional complementary and alternative medicine material. Updated ICD-9 codes are highlighted within the text. The website offers over 1,000 English and Spanish patient handouts from the American Academy of Family Practice, full-color images, videos of medical procedures and physical therapy, and *Facts & Comparisons A to Z Drug Facts* monographs.

Harrison's Principles of Internal Medicine. 17th ed. Editors: Anthony S. Fauci, Eugene Braunwald, Dennis Kasper, Stephen Hauser. McGraw-Hill Medical, 2008.
http://www.mhprofessional.com/Medical/harrisons/
http://www.accessmedicine.com
ISBN: 9780071466332 (Single Volume)
ISBN: 9780071476911 (Two Volumes)
See Also Chapter 1.9. Physician Assistants
Recommended for: Hospital, Academic, Consumer Health Libraries
Brandon/Hill, *Doody's Core Titles* Selection

Harrison's Principles of Internal Medicine is considered the bible of internal medicine. The seventeenth edition includes more than 40 new chapters, including new information on global health issues. There are over 800 new illustrations and a full-color format. Harrison's is appropriate for all types of libraries as a basic reference text for internal medicine. It was a long-standing title on the Brandon/Hill list for small medical libraries. It is available in electronic format that is updated monthly and is also available through AccessMedicine. A DVD with additional content accompanies the print volume.

Oxford Textbook of Medicine. 5th ed. Editors: David A. Warrell, Timothy M. Cox, John D. Firth. Oxford University Press, 2010.
http://www.r2library.com/
ISBN: 9780199204854
Recommended for: Academic Libraries

This is a three-volume textbook of internal medicine focusing on clinical management and prevention of disease. There is an emphasis on infectious diseases with coverage of global health, molecular biology, and nutrition. Other sections of note include: pain, bioterrorism, forensic medicine, medical disorders in pregnancy, travel and expedition medicine, nutrition, the use of stem cells, regenerative medicine, psychiatry, and drug-related problems in general medical practice. Each chapter has accompanying illustrations and photographs in full color, tables, and graphs. Further readings are listed at the end of each chapter. The online edition includes links to sources of related and further reading via PubMed, ISI, and CrossRef. All the figures are downloadable to PowerPoint. Purchasers of the print edition may also purchase access to the online edition for a reduced rate by following the instructions given in the book. The *Oxford Textbook of Medicine* is a recommended title in *Doody's Core Titles.*

The Washington Manual of Medical Therapeutics. 32nd ed. Editors: Daniel H. Cooper, Andrew J. Krainik, Sam J. Lubner, Hilary Reno, Scott Micek. Lippincott Williams & Wilkins, 2007.
http://www.r2library.com/
ISBN: 9780781781251
Recommended for: Hospital, Academic, Consumer Health Libraries

The Washington Manual of Medical Therapeutics from the Department of Medicine of Washington University in St. Louis is carried in every housestaff member's pocket in its familiar spiral-bound format or in the handheld version. It is available online in the R2 Rittenhouse Digital Library. The quick-reference style covers organ system diseases as well as medical emergencies, arthritis, anemia, diabetes mellitus, antimicrobials, critical care, cardiac arrhythmias, hypertension, fluid management, and nutrition support. It is a Brandon/Hill title and a *Doody's Core Titles* essential purchase.

Journals

ACP Journal Club (within ***Annals of Internal Medicine***). v. 114, suppl. 1, American College of Physicians, 1991.
http://www.acpjc.org/
ISSN: 10568751
ISSN: 15398560 (Online)
Indexed in: MEDLINE, CINAHL
Recommended for: Hospital, Academic Libraries
Brandon/Hill Selection

ACP Journal Club selects articles from over 100 journals that report original studies and systematic reviews of important advances in internal medicine. These articles are summarized in value-added abstracts and commented on by clinical experts. The articles chosen are about therapy, diagnosis, etiology and harm, prognosis, and economics of health care. *ACP Journal Club PLUS* (*ACPJCP*), available to ACP members, provides online access to all articles that pass the *ACP Journal Club* criteria. It offers e-mail alerts that users can easily customize according to their own clinical interests. Online access to *ACP Journal Club* is available back to 2001.

American Journal of Medicine. v. 1, Elsevier, 1946.
http://amjmed.com/
http://www.sciencedirect.com/science/journal/00029343
ISSN: 00029343
ISSN: 15557162 (Online)
Indexed in: MEDLINE
Recommended for: Hospital, Academic Libraries
Brandon/Hill Selection

This is the "Green Journal." It is the official publication of the Association of Professors of Medicine. Original clinical research of interest to physicians in internal medicine, both in academia and community-based practice, are featured. Each issue has original scientific studies that have direct clinical significance, and position papers on health care issues, medical education, and public policy. This is a core title in internal medicine and is indexed in MEDLINE. It has an impact factor of 4.466 and is ranked fourteenth of 133 journals in the medicine, general and internal category of the 2009 *Journal Citation Reports*. Full online access back to volume 1, 1946 is available through ScienceDirect.

Annals of Internal Medicine. v. 1, American College of Physicians–American Society of internal Medicine, 1927.
http://www.annals.org/
ISSN: 00034819
ISSN: 15393704 (Online)
See Also Chapter 1.9. Physician Assistants
Indexed in: MEDLINE, CINAHL
Recommended for: Hospital, Academic, Consumer Health Libraries
Brandon/Hill Selection

The *Annals of Internal Medicine* is one of the core titles in internal medicine. Each issue has at least one review paper and may contain a summary for patients. RSS feeds, e-mail alerts, and a mobile format are available. It is the fourth highest-ranked general and internal medicine journal in the 2009 *Journal Citation Reports*, with an impact factor of 16.225. The journal is published twice a month and indexed in MEDLINE, ProQuest, Academic Search Premier, and other sources.

Archives of Internal Medicine. v. 1, American Medical Association, 1908.
http://archinte.ama-assn.org/
ISSN: 00039926
ISSN: 15383679 (Online)
Indexed in: MEDLINE, CINAHL
Recommended for: Hospital, Academic, Consumer Health Libraries
Brandon/Hill Selection

This is one of the family of journals from the American Medical Association. It is an international peer-reviewed journal published 22 times each year. The majority of the readership is office- and hospital-based general internists and significant numbers of internal medicine subspecialists in the United States. The Archives' mission is to promote the art and science of medicine and the betterment of human health. With an impact factor of 9.813, it ranks eighth in the general and internal medicine category of the 2009 *Journal Citation Reports*. *Archives of Internal Medicine* is indexed in all the major services, including MEDLINE, CINAHL, and Scopus. Online access back to volume 1, 1908 is available.

BMC Medicine. v. 1, BioMed Central, 2003.
www.biomedcentral.com/bmcmed
http://www.ncbi.nlm.nih.gov/pmc/journals/216/
ISSN: 17417015 (Online)
Indexed in: MEDLINE
Recommended for: Hospital, Academic Libraries

This open access, peer-reviewed journal is in the BioMed Central family. Issues may include mini-reviews, original research, technical advances, editorials and correspondence. With an impact factor of 3.985, it ranks eighteenth out of 133 journals in the general and internal medicine category of the 2009 *Journal Citation Reports*. It is available in online format only and is indexed in MEDLINE, CINAHL, Scopus, Web of Science, and many others. All articles are also deposited in PubMed Central immediately after publication.

BMJ (British Medical Journal). v. 297, BMJ Group, 1988.
http://www.bmj.com/
ISSN: 09598138
ISSN: 14685833 (Online)
Indexed in: MEDLINE, CINAHL
Recommended for: Hospital, Academic, Consumer Health Libraries
Brandon/Hill Selection

BMJ is one of the core medical journals for every library. There is a student edition. The mission of *BMJ* is "to lead the debate on health, and to engage, inform, and stimulate doctors, researchers and other health professionals in ways that will improve outcomes for patients." There are four editorially identical editions of the *BMJ* every week (*General Practice, Clinical Research, International*, and *Compact*) and the journal is received by over 100,000 doctors each week in print. *BMJ* is published in 13 territories in six non-English languages—Chinese, Greek, Portuguese, Romanian, Spanish, and Turkish. It ranks fifth in the general and internal medicine category of the 2009 *Journal Citation Reports* with an impact factor of 13.660. It is indexed by all the major abstracting and indexing services.

JAMA: Journal of the American Medical Association. v. 173, no. 9, American Medical Association, 1960.
http://jama.ama-assn.org/
ISSN: 00987484
ISSN: 15383598 (Online)
See Also Chapter 1.9. Physician Assistants, Chapter 33.1. Consumer Health Information
Indexed in: MEDLINE, CINAHL
Recommended for: Hospital, Academic, Consumer Health Libraries
Brandon/Hill Selection

JAMA is a must for any health sciences collection, including consumer health collections. Each issue includes original contributions, editorials, and letters. Other features include a work of art on the cover, a section titled "A Piece of My Mind," poetry and medicine, and "JAMA 100 Years Ago." There are book and media reviews. Some issues will feature the "Rational Clinical Examination" or the "User Guide to Health Sciences Literature." A student edition is available, as is a patient page. *JAMA* continues the *Journal of the American Medical Association* (1883–1960). E-mail alerts are available. Full online access is available back to volume 279, 1998, and tables of contents and selected content are available back to volume 1, 1883. Also available online are topic collections that are searchable for articles from 1998 forward.

The Lancet. v. 1, Lancet Publishing Group, 1823.
www.thelancet.com
http://www.sciencedirect.com/science/journal/01406736
ISSN: 01406736
ISSN: 1474547X (Online)
Indexed in: MEDLINE, CINAHL
Recommended for: Hospital, Academic, Consumer Health Libraries
Brandon/Hill Selection

The Lancet is one of the core titles in internal medicine for every health sciences library. Thomas Wakley, *Lancet's* founder, and his successors "aimed to combine publication of the best medical science in the world with a zeal to counter the forces that undermine the values of medicine, be they political, social, or commercial." It is international in scope, covering medical science and practice with medical news, high-quality clinical trials, original research, commentary, letters, and reviews on all aspects of clinical medicine and public health. *The Lancet* publishes specialty journals in infectious diseases, neurology, and oncology. *The Lancet* continually has a very high impact factor. In the 2009 *Journal Citation Reports* it ranked second of 122 titles in the medicine, general, and internal category with an impact factor of 30.758.Online access back to volume 1, 1823 is available on ScienceDirect. Podcasts and RSS feeds are available.

Medical Clinics of North America. v. 1, Saunders/Elsevier, 1917.
http://www.medical.theclinics.com/
http://www.sciencedirect.com/science/journal/00257125
ISSN: 00257125
ISSN: 15579859 (Online)
Indexed in: MEDLINE, CINAHL
Recommended for: Hospital, Academic Libraries
Brandon/Hill Selection

This Brandon/Hill selection is published bimonthly and offers comprehensive, state-of-the-art reviews to provide current, practical information on the diagnosis and treatment of conditions in internal medicine. Each issue is dedicated to a specific topic. Recent issues have included "Otolaryngology for the Internist," "Drug Hypersensitivity," "Sleep Medicine," "Chest Pain," and "Challenges in Inflammatory Bowel Disease." In the 2009 *Journal Citation Reports* it ranked thirty-fourth of 133 titles in the general and internal medicine category with an impact factor of 2.182. CME credits and RSS feeds are available.

Medicine. v. 1, Lippincott Williams & Wilkins, 1922.
http://journals.lww.com/md-journal/
ISSN: 00257974
ISSN: 15365964 (Online)
Indexed in: MEDLINE, CINAHL
Recommended for: Hospital, Academic Libraries
Brandon/Hill Selection

Medicine is a journal of in-depth review articles covering current therapeutic approaches, preventive techniques, and research in internal medicine, dermatology, neurology, pediatrics, and psychiatry. The journal also offers follow-up studies and practice-oriented reports of clinical observations. A former Brandon/Hill title, in the 2009 *Journal Citation Reports* it ranked twelfth of 133 titles in the medicine, general and internal category with an impact factor of 5.054. Online access is available back to volume 1, 1922.

New England Journal of Medicine. v. 198, Massachusetts Medical Society, 1928.
http://content.nejm.org/
ISSN: 00284793
ISSN: 15334406 (Online)
See Also Chapter 1.9. Physician Assistants, Chapter 33.1. Consumer Health Information.
Indexed in: MEDLINE, CINAHL
Recommended for: Hospital, Academic, Consumer Health Libraries
Brandon/Hill Selection

New England Journal of Medicine is one of the core titles every collection should have. A weekly publication of general medicine indexed in MEDLINE and all the other leading health sciences databases, it is available in print and electronic format with electronic table of contents service, RSS feeds, and audio summaries. An issue can be downloaded to a handheld device. There are accompanying videos and opportunities to gain CME credit. A case from the Massachusetts General Hospital is presented each week. There are reports of original research, medical perspectives, book reviews, editorials, and correspondence. In the 2009 *Journal Citation Reports* it ranked first of 133 titles in the medicine, general and internal category with an impact factor of 47.050. Full online access is available back to volume 1, 1812. "Topic Collections" of clinical interest are available since 1996.

Databases and Other Electronic Resources

eMedicine. WebMD Medscape, 1994.
http://emedicine.medscape.com/
Recommended for: Hospital, Academic, Consumer Health Libraries

This is Medscape's online, continually-updated, clinical reference. It contains more than 6,500 articles contributed by about 10,000 physicians. Search options include subject or particular disease. Articles include an overview containing the history and physical exam, differential diagnosis and workup, treatment, and medication and follow-up. There are summary tables and illustrations throughout with references at the end of each article. Articles can be sent to e-mail addresses.

MedlinePlus. National Library of Medicine, 1998.
http://medlineplus.gov
See Also Chapter 33.1. Consumer Health Information
Recommended for: Hospital, Academic, Consumer Health Libraries

MedlinePlus is produced by the National Library of Medicine and brings together authoritative information in over 40 languages from NLM, the National Institutes of Health (NIH), other government agencies, and health-related organizations. It is not only the premiere website for consumer health information but also valuable for introducing a health care practitioner to a new medical concept. It includes a dictionary; encyclopedia of more than 800 health topics, covering conditions, diseases and wellness; interactive tutorials; videos; and drug information. MedlinePlus also features the latest health news with e-mail updates and RSS feeds. *MedlinePlus* magazine is freely available online. Preformulated MEDLINE searches are included in MedlinePlus and give easy access to medical journal articles.

10.10.1. Cardiology

The heart, its physiology, and its functions.
—MeSH

Contributor: Helen-Ann Brown Epstein

Monographs

Acute Coronary Syndromes. 3rd ed. Editor: Eric J. Topol. Informa Healthcare, 2004.
ISBN: 9780824757953
Recommended for: Hospital, Academic Libraries
Doody's Core Titles Selection

This book is for clinician-cardiologists, internists, nurses, and paraprofessional staff. The third edition is written by worldwide contributors and contains chapters dedicated to the genomics of acute myocardial infarction, cardiac biomarkers, new arterial inflammatory markers, percutaneous coronary intervention, improving microcirculation perfusion in the coronary bed, the metabolic syndrome, and stem cell therapy for acute myocardial infarction. There are accompanying charts, tables, figures, pathology slides, drawings with extensive bibliographies, and index.

Braunwald's Heart Disease: A Textbook of Cardiovascular Medicine. 9th ed. Editors: Robert O. Bonow, Douglas

L. Mann, Douglas P. Zipes, Peter Libby. Saunders/Elsevier, 2012.
http://www.mdconsult.com/
ISBN: 9781437703986 (1 v.)
ISBN: 9781437727081 (set)
Recommended for: Hospital, Academic Libraries
Brandon/Hill Selection

This classic cardiovascular text is available in single volume, two volumes, and electronic format with MD Consult. There are chapters on the fundamentals of cardiovascular disease, molecular biology and genetics, physical examination and testing by EKG, stress testing, echocardiography, and nuclear testing. A reviewer of the seventh edition of *Braunwald's* in *JAMA* (2005; 294(3):376) commented "The editors have accomplished an impressive feat: improving on an already classic text... A worthy addition to the medical library of any practicing cardiologist, cardiology fellow, or health care practitioner with a special interest in heart disease." It was listed on the final Brandon/Hill list for small medical libraries. This review refers to the eighth edition.

Clinical Nuclear Cardiology: State of the Art and Future Directions. 4th ed. Editors: Barry L. Zaret, George A. Beller. Elsevier Mosby, 2010.
ISBN: 9780323057967
Recommended for: Hospital, Academic Libraries

This edition, now in full color, presents the most recent developments in technology, instrumentation, and radiopharmaceuticals in clinical nuclear cardiology. The text is presented in nine sections: "Radiopharmaceuticals/Tracer Kinetics," "Instrumentation," "Ventricular Function," "Perfusion Imaging," "Disease/Gender-Specific Issues," "Acute Coronary Syndromes," "Viability," "Tracer-Specific Imaging Techniques," and "New Molecular Approaches." The revision also includes 20 new chapters, including "Cellular Mechanisms of Tracer Uptake and Clearance," "Attenuation/Scatter Corrections: Clinical Aspects," "Hybrid Imaging; Digital/Fast SPECT," and "Imaging in Revascularized Patients." Individual purchasers have online access through http://expertconsult.com.

Current Diagnosis & Treatment: Cardiology. 3rd ed. Editor: Michael H. Crawford. McGraw-Hill Medical, 2009.
http://www.accessmedicine.com/
ISBN: 9780071442114
Recommended for: Hospital, Academic, Consumer Health Libraries

Current Diagnosis & Treatment: Cardiology is a concise discussion of the essential knowledge needed to diagnose and manage cardiovascular diseases. It is good for consumer health reference, practicing physicians, and for Board review as a quick reference tool. "Essentials of Diagnosis" bullets introduce each topic and tables summarize the text. Suggested readings close each chapter. It is available online through AccessMedicine and on the Kindle platform from Amazon.

Drugs for the Heart. 7th ed. Editors: Lionel H. Opie, Bernard J. Gersh. Saunders Elsevier, 2009.
ISBN: 9781416061588
Recommended for: Hospital, Academic, Consumer Health Libraries
Doody's Core Titles Selection

The focus of this title is cardiovascular pharmacology. Throughout the text there are dynamic full-color drawings that illustrate key pharmacological and physiological actions. All cardiovascular drugs are covered, including new drug classes and drug use for single and multiple problem management. There is a useful chapter titled "Which Drug for Which Disease." At the end of each chapter there is a summary for each drug class for quick reference. There is an accompanying website for individual purchasers at http://expertconsult.com.

Evidence-Based Cardiology. 3rd ed. Editors: Salim Yusuf, John Cairns, John Camm, Ernest L. Fallen, Bernard J. Gersh. John Wiley & Sons, 2010.
http://onlinelibrary.wiley.com/book/10.1002/9781444309768
ISBN: 9781405159258
ISBN: 9781444309768 (Online)
Recommended for: Hospital, Academic Libraries

Evidence-Based Cardiology includes chapters on evidence-based medicine principles, prevention of cardiovascular diseases, coronary artery disease, arrhythmias, acute coronary syndromes, diseases of left heart dysfunction, valvular heart disease, stroke, and cardiac disease and pregnancy. References close each chapter. A review in *JAMA* (2010; 304(6):692–693) states, "the third edition will be a welcome addition to the shelves of cardiologists or primary care physicians with an interest in the dynamic field of cardiology." It is available online from Wiley Online Library.

Feigenbaum's Echocardiography. 7th ed. Editors: William F. Armstrong, Thomas Ryan. Lippincott Williams & Wilkins, 2010.
ISBN: 9780781795579
Recommended for: Hospital, Academic Libraries
Doody's Core Titles Selection

The seventh edition of this text has been thoroughly revised. It includes over 1,600 illustrations, bibliographies, references, and index. Current American Heart Association and American College of Cardiology guidelines are included for each chapter. An accompanying DVD contains tutorials on echocardiographic interpretation with voiceover and animations. There are chapters on the history of echocardiography, specialized techniques and methods, the echocardiographic exam and the diseases that can be revealed by this test. This is a *Doody's* five-star rated book.

Hurst's The Heart. 13th ed. Editors: Valentin Fuster, Richard A. Walsh, Robert A. Harrington. McGraw-Hill Medical, 2011.
http://www.accessmedicine.com/ (12th ed.)
ISBN: 9780071636476 (DVD)
ISBN: 9780071636469 (set)
ISBN: 9780071636490 (v.1)
ISBN: 9780071747985 (v.2)
Recommended for: Hospital, Academic, Consumer Health Libraries
Brandon/Hill, *Doody's Core Titles* Selection

This is a classic work in print and also available online in AccessMedicine. The twelfth edition has a global authorship. Coverage of hypertension, including pulmonary hypertension has been expanded. Chapters concerned with the human genome, cardiovascular practice guidelines, and evolving imaging technology for assessing coronary and non-coronary atherosclerotic disease and plaque characterization have been extensively revised. Additional revised chapters focus on diseases of the aorta, cardiovascular drug interactions, and surgical and non-surgical approaches to carotid arterial disease and peripheral vascular disease. The American College of Cardiology/American Heart Association Clinical Practice Guidelines are clearly featured in this edition. Each chapter closes with references. This review refers to the twelfth edition.

Kaplan's Clinical Hypertension. 10th ed. Authors: Norman M. Kaplan, Ronald G. Victor. Wolters Kluwer/Lippincott Williams & Wilkins, 2010.
ISBN: 9781605475035
Recommended for: Hospital, Academic Libraries
Brandon/Hill, *Doody's Core Titles* Selection

This work is an up-to-date, practical, evidence-based text on treatment and prevention of all forms of hypertension. Abundant algorithms and flow charts are included to aid clinicians in decision-making. The tenth edition is highlighted with "new developments in the pathogenesis of hypertension; discussions on the significance of nighttime blood pressure; new information on the relationship of sleep apnea to blood pressure; updates on diagnosing primary aldosteronism; and detailed information on the latest antihypertensive drugs, including combination drugs." Every chapter is followed by an extensive list of references. It was a Brandon/Hill title and received a four-star review from *Doody's Review Service.*

Marriott's Practical Electrocardiography. 11th ed. Editors: Galen S. Wagner, Henry Joseph L. Marriott. Wolters Kluwer/Lippincott Williams & Wilkins, 2008.
ISBN: 9780781797382
Recommended for: Hospital, Academic Libraries
Brandon/Hill, *Doody's Core Titles* Selection

Marriott's Practical Electrocardiography is a classic text on the interpretation of ECGs. This revised edition is filled with ECG recordings, especially arrhythmias, tables, anatomical drawings, and illustrations. Glossaries at the end of each chapter reinforce new terms. An accompanying CD-ROM includes animations correlated with ECGs. It is a *Doody's Core Titles* selection.

Physiology of the Heart. 4th ed. Author: Arnold M. Katz. Lippincott Williams & Wilkins, 2006.
See Chapter 29. Physiology

Textbook of Interventional Cardiology. 5th ed. Editor: Eric J. Topol. Saunders/Elsevier, 2008.
ISBN: 9781416048350
Recommended for: Academic Libraries
Brandon/Hill, *Doody's Core Titles* Selection

The fifth edition of this text has been completely reorganized. It presents practical, evidence-based guidance on treating a full range of coronary lesions with chapters on balloons and stents, pharmacologic intervention with thrombolytics and lipid lowering drugs, "big artery" vascular interventions, intracardiac interventions, and intravascular ultrasound. Each chapter discusses the very latest techniques, devices, and adjunctive therapies and provides critical appraisals of emerging therapeutic approaches. The text is enhanced with figures, tables, graphs, full color images, and references. A DVD accompanies the text.

Journals

American Heart Journal. v. 1, Elsevier Health, 1925.
http://www.ahjonline.com/
http://www.sciencedirect.com/science/journal/00028703
ISSN: 00028703

ISSN: 10976744 (Online)
Indexed in: MEDLINE
Recommended for: Hospital, Academic Libraries
Brandon/Hill Selection

The audience for this journal is cardiologists and general practice physicians. It features articles on topics pertaining to the broad discipline of cardiovascular disease. Included are primary investigations, scholarly reviews, and opinions. The editors especially encourage "submission of three types of reports that are not frequently seen in cardiovascular journals: negative clinical studies, reports on study designs, and studies involving the organization of medical care." The journal does not accept individual case reports. It has an impact factor of 4.357 and ranks fourteenth of 95 journals in the cardiac and cardiovascular systems category of the 2009 *Journal Citation Reports*. RSS feeds are available. Full online access back to volume 1, 1925 is available through ScienceDirect.

American Journal of Cardiology. v. 1, Elsevier, 1958.
http://www.ajconline.org/home
http://www.sciencedirect.com/science/journal/00029149
ISSN: 00029149
ISSN: 18791913 (Online)
Indexed in: MEDLINE, CINAHL
Recommended for: Hospital, Academic Libraries
Brandon/Hill Selection

This is one of the core titles in cardiology. It absorbed the *Bulletin of the American College of Cardiology* and supersedes the *Transactions of the American College of Cardiology*. Coverage includes systemic hypertension, methodology, drugs, pacing, arrhythmia, preventive cardiology, congestive heart failure, valvular heart disease, congenital heart disease, and cardiomyopathy. Also included are editorials, readers' comments, and symposia. With an impact factor of 3.575, it ranks twenty-first of 95 journals in the cardiac and cardiovascular systems category in the 2009 *Journal Citation Reports*. Full online access back to volume 1, 1958 is available through Elsevier ScienceDirect. This journal is indexed in MEDLINE, CINAHL, and Scopus, among other sources.

Circulation. v. 1, Lippincott Williams & Wilkins, 1950.
http://circ.ahajournals.org/
http://www.ovid.com/
ISSN: 00097322
ISSN: 15244539 (Online)
Indexed in: MEDLINE, CINAHL
Recommended for: Hospital, Academic Libraries
Brandon/Hill Selection

Circulation is a weekly publication of the American Heart Association. Each issue may contain clinical summaries, editorials, original articles, "Basic Science for Clinicians," "AHA Scientific Statements," images in cardiovascular medicine, letters, and the European perspective. It ranks first in the 2009 *Journal Citation Reports* in all three categories to which it belongs, cardiac and cardiovascular systems, hematology, and peripheral vascular disease, with an impact factor of 14.816 and a cited half-life of over seven years. *Circulation* offers an electronic table of contents alert to stay current with its weekly contributions. The journal is indexed in MEDLINE and other leading databases. Online access to all content back to volume 1, 1950 is available at the publisher's website, and all content older than one year is offered for free. Institutional online subscriptions are available through Ovid.

Circulation Research. v. 1, Lippincott Williams & Wilkins, 1953.
http://circres.ahajournals.org/
ISSN: 00097330
ISSN: 15244571 (Online)
Indexed in: MEDLINE
Recommended for: Academic Libraries

Circulation Research is a semi-monthly publication of the American Heart Association. Each issue features news and views, editorials, review papers, and papers in molecular medicine, cellular biology, and integrative physiology. An article may contain online supplementary information, including online video files. *Circulation Research* ranks in the top five journals in three categories, cardiac and cardiovascular systems, hematology, and peripheral vascular disease, in the 2009 *Journal Citation Reports*. The journal offers an electronic table of contents alert and is indexed in all major databases. All issues back to volume 1, 1953 are available online at the journal's website and all content older than 12 months may be access at no cost.

Harvard Heart Letter. v. 1, Harvard Health Publications, 1990.
http://www.health.harvard.edu/newsletters/Harvard_Heart_Letter.htm
ISSN: 10515313
ISSN: 1943510X (Online)
Indexed in: MEDLINE, CINAHL
Recommended for: Consumer Health Libraries

This monthly newsletter is written for the consumer audience interested in cardiovascular health. Recent articles include "Beating High Blood Pressure with Food,"

"Standing Guard over Blood Vessel Health," "Choosing the Right Replacement Heart Valve," and "New Heart Rate Estimate for Women." A regular feature is "Ask the Doctor." It is indexed in MEDLINE. Articles vary in length from brief to long and suggest further readings. Issues back to 2007 are available online.

Heart. v. 75, BMJ Publishing Group, 1996.
http://heart.bmj.com/
http://www.ncbi.nlm.nih.gov/pmc/journals/159/
ISSN: 13556037
ISSN: 1468201X (Online)
Indexed in: MEDLINE, CINAHL
Recommended for: Academic Libraries
Brandon/Hill Selection

Heart is the continuation of the *British Heart Journal*. It is the official journal of the British Cardiovascular Society, covering advances in the diagnosis and treatment of cardiovascular disease. Topics covered include coronary disease, electrophysiology, valve disease, imaging techniques, congenital heart disease (fetal, pediatric, and adult), heart failure, surgery, and basic science. Each issue contains an extensive continuing professional education section ("Education in Heart") and "Journal Scan" highlighting important papers from outside the cardiology literature. It is available online back to volume 1, 1939 from the publisher and in PubMed Central until three years before the present. Beginning in 2008, only selected content is available through PubMed Central.

Heart & Lung: The Journal of Critical Care. v. 1, Mosby, 1972.
http://www.heartandlung.org/
http://www.sciencedirect.com/science/journal/01479563
ISSN: 01479563
ISSN: 15273288 (Online)
Indexed in: MEDLINE, CINAHL
Recommended for: Hospital, Academic, Consumer Health Libraries

Heart & Lung is the official publication of The American Association of Heart Failure Nurses. It presents original peer-reviewed articles on techniques, advances, investigations, and observations in acute and critical care, respiratory and heart failure nursing. The journal's acute care articles focus on critical care provided for a short time, often outside the intensive care unit. The journal's heart failure articles focus on improving heart failure patient outcomes. Other sections focus on infection control, neonatal nursing, advanced practice nursing, pharmacotherapy, ethical issues, and patient education. It is indexed in MEDLINE, CINAHL, Scopus, and other major databases. Online access is available back to volume 24, 1995.

Hypertension. v. 1, Lippincott Williams & Wilkins, 1979.
http://hyper.ahajournals.org/
ISSN: 0194911X
ISSN: 15244563 (Online)
Indexed in: MEDLINE
Recommended for: Hospital, Academic Libraries

Hypertension is one of the peer-reviewed journals of the American Heart Association. With an impact factor of 6.614, it ranks fourth in journals in the peripheral vascular disease category and the highest among other journals devoted to the study of hypertension (2009 *Journal Citation Reports*). This monthly journal contains clinical and research articles and CME credit is given with some papers. Each issue may contain brief reviews, original research, editorials, and letters. It is indexed in MEDLINE and other databases. Online access back to volume 1, 1979, is available from the AHA.

Journal of the American College of Cardiology. v. 1, Elsevier Biomedical, 1983.
http://content.onlinejacc.org/
http://www.sciencedirect.com/science/journal/07351097
ISSN: 07351097
ISSN: 15583597 (Online)
Indexed in: MEDLINE, CINAHL
Recommended for: Hospital, Academic Libraries
Brandon/Hill Selection

Each weekly issue contains original peer-reviewed clinical and experimental research. Topics covered include coronary artery and valve disease, congenital heart defects, vascular surgery, cardiomyopathy, drug treatment, new diagnostic techniques, findings from the laboratory, and large multicenter studies of new therapies. *Journal of the American College of Cardiology* also publishes abstracts of papers presented at the annual scientific sessions of the American College of Cardiology and the reports and recommendations of the Bethesda Conferences on current topics in cardiovascular disease. In the 2009 *Journal Citation Reports* it ranked second of 95 titles in the cardiac and cardiovascular systems category with an impact factor of 12.640. It is available electronically in the ScienceDirect collection. RSS feeds are also available.

Stroke. v. 1, Lippincott Williams & Wilkins, 1970.
http://stroke.ahajournals.org/
ISSN: 00392499
ISSN: 15244628 (Online)

Indexed in: MEDLINE, CINAHL
Recommended for: Hospital, Academic Libraries

Stroke is the official journal of the American Stroke Association, a division of the American Heart Association. The journal is dedicated to clinical research in cerebrovascular disease and "provides reports of clinical and basic investigation of all aspects of the cerebral circulation and its diseases from many disciplines including neurology, internal medicine, radiology, nuclear medicine, neuropathology, neurosurgery, epidemiology, vascular surgery, rehabilitation, anesthesiology, critical care medicine, vascular physiology, neuropsychology, speech pathology, and neuro-ophthalmology." In the 2009 *Journal Citation Reports* it ranked fourth of 61 titles in the peripheral vascular disease category and fifth of 167 titles in clinical neurology with an impact factor of 7.041. Each issue may contain editorials, original contributions, letters, and comments. Some issues contain progress reviews, topical reviews, a Cochrane Corner, and AHA Scientific Statements. Readers can register for electronic delivery of tables of contents, and CME is available. Full online access is available back to volume 1, 1970.

10.10.2. Endocrinology

The metabolism, physiology, and disorders of the endocrine system.

—MeSH

Contributor: Sharon Cardwell

Monographs

Atlas of Thyroid Surgery: Principles, Practice, and Clinical Cases. 1st ed. Author: Ernst Gemsenjaeger. Thieme Medical, 2009.
ISBN: 9783131450319
Recommended for: Hospital, Academic Libraries
Doody's Core Titles Selection

As a renowned endocrine surgeon and professor, Ernst Gemsenjaeger provides valuable information in a concise and well-written book for those caring for patients with surgical disorders of the thyroid. Utilizing his extensive surgical experience, Gemsenjaeger illustrates proper clinical management with detailed descriptions of surgical anatomy and surgical techniques, such as proper positioning of the surgical incision and the technique of capsular dissection to avoid injury to the laryngeal nerves or the parathyroid glands during thyroid operations. Numerous clinical cases are included with step-by-step demonstrations, illustrations, and comments relating to surgical procedures that prepare the reader for a broad range of everyday practice scenarios. An accompanying DVD provides detailed surgical techniques in five clinical cases with cross references to the text. An intended audience of general surgeons, endocrinologists, pathologists, residents, and medical students will benefit from this *Doody's Core Titles* essential purchase title available in print only with accompanying DVD.

Clinical Gynecologic Endocrinology and Infertility. 8th ed. Authors: Marc A. Fritz, Leon Speroff. Lippincott Williams & Wilkins, 2011.
http://www.ovid.com/
http://www.r2library.com/ (7th ed.)
ISBN: 9780781779685
See Also Chapter 10.18. Reproductive Medicine
Recommended for: Hospital, Academic Libraries
Doody's Core Titles Selection

Utilizing a concise and user-friendly style enhanced by numerous illustrations, this world-renowned gynecology textbook provides a complete explanation of the female endocrine system and its disorders and offers practical guidance on evaluation and treatment of female endocrine problems and infertility. This review refers to the seventh edition. Coverage includes the latest information on contraception and infertility and new guidelines on hormone replacement therapy during menopause. Several revised chapters place greater emphasis on progestins and hormone administration. Marc Fritz, prominent reproductive endocrinologist, and Leon Speroff, leader in the field of reproductive endocrinology, combine their expertise for this latest edition. Comprehensive, relevant, and highly informative, this textbook clearly outlines the improvements to patient care within clinical reproductive endocrinology. Divided into four main parts, reproductive physiology, clinical endocrinology, contraception, and infertility, the latest in clinical research developments is provided throughout. Written with an intended audience of medical students, residents, interns, and practicing endocrinologists, this *Doody's Core Titles* recommendation is available in print or online through Ovid and R2 Library.

Endocrine and Metabolic Disorders Sourcebook. 2nd ed. Editor: Joyce B. Shannon. Omnigraphics, 2007.
ISBN: 9780780809529
Recommended for: Hospital, Academic, Consumer Health Libraries

One of numerous books in the *Health Reference Series*, this reliable, comprehensive, and reader-friendly sourcebook provides basic consumer health information about diagnosis and treatment of the endocrine system and metabolic function disorders. Each book in the series is fully indexed and includes charts, tables, illustrations, and glossaries of terms. Collected within each book are publications issued by National Institutes of Health, Centers for Disease Control and Prevention, other government agencies, professional associations, research centers, and similar organizations, as well as current information from reliable journals. Topics covered in this sourcebook include: hormonal and metabolic disorders that affect the body's growth, development, and functioning, including disorders of the pancreas, ovaries and testes, pituitary, thyroid, parathyroid, and adrenal glands; growth disorders; diabetic disorders; errors of metabolism; endocrine functioning; and diagnostic and screening tests. The intended audience includes academic and public libraries, medical facilities, doctors' offices, and other health information centers serving the general public.

Greenspan's Basic and Clinical Endocrinology. 8th ed. Editors: David G. Gardner, Dolores Shoback. McGraw-Hill, 2007.
http://www.statref.com/
http://extranet.netlibrary.com/TitleSelect/
http://www.ebrary.com/
http://www.ovid.com/
ISBN: 9780071440110
Recommended for: Hospital, Academic Libraries
Brandon/Hill, *Doody's Core Titles* Selection

The updated 8th edition of *Basic and Clinical Endocrinology* remains a high-quality reference book with the latest diagnostic testing and newest approaches to medical management for the field of clinical endocrinology and the underlying basic science. Written primarily by clinicians and researchers from highly-acclaimed endocrine divisions at the University of California, San Francisco, this comprehensive and richly illustrated guide is recognized as one of the nation's most respected endocrine reference books. The contents encompass everything from the molecular biology of thyroid hormone signal transduction to the clinical approach to the patient with Cushing's syndrome. New chapters include "Evidence-Based Endocrinology" (chapter 4) and "Neurohypophysis" (chapter 6). In addition, new reference lists include web-based educational resources for physicians as well as their patients. Written for an intended audience of medical students, residents, interns, research fellows, and practicing endocrinologists, this *Doody's Core Titles* essential purchase title is available in print or online through STAT!Ref, NetLibrary, Ebrary, and Ovid.

Werner and Ingbar's The Thyroid: A Fundamental and Clinical Text. 9th ed. Editors: Lewis E. Braverman, Robert D. Utiger. Lippincott Williams & Wilkins, 2005.
http://www.r2library.com/
http://www.ovid.com/
ISBN: 9780781750479
Recommended for: Hospital, Academic Libraries
Brandon/Hill, *Doody's Core Titles* Selection

Encompassing the basic and clinical aspects of the healthy and diseased thyroid, this well-organized textbook documents the rapid pace of changes in the endocrinology subfield of thyroidology. Originated in 1955 by Drs. Werner and Ingbar, this classic textbook provides comprehensive coverage of every aspect of normal thyroid anatomy, development, biochemistry, physiology, pathophysiology, cellular mechanisms, bone/mineral interactions, clinical manifestations, thyroid function testing, treatment of thyroid disorders, management of thyroid cancer, and specific thyroid disease. The ninth edition is edited by well-respected thyroidologists, Drs. Braverman and Utiger, and includes an increase in international contributors detailing new developments on such topics as mortality in thyroid disease, oncogenes, biological effect of radioiodine treatment for carcinoma, trophoblastic tumors, and subacute and acute infectious thyroiditis. New chapters deliver clinical controversies relating to subclinical hypothyroidism and hyperthyroidism. In addition, the "function tests look-up" is improved with a reorganization of the section on laboratory assessment of thyroid function. With 1,100 pages and 350 illustrations, this *Doody's Core Titles* textbook is available in print or online through Ovid and R2Library. The intended audience includes medical students, clinical residents, interns, research fellows, and specialized clinicians.

Williams Textbook of Endocrinology. 11th ed. Editors: Henry M. Kronenberg, Shlomo Melmed, Kenneth S. Polonsky, P. Reed Larsen. Elsevier, 2008.
http://www.mdconsult.com/
ISBN: 9781416029113
Recommended for: Hospital, Academic Libraries
Brandon/Hill, *Doody's Core Titles* Selection

Originated 50 years ago by Robert Williams with his goal of "a condensed and authoritative discussion of the management of clinical endocrinopathies based upon the application of fundamental information obtained from chemical and physiological investigation," this classic work stands the test of time and is recognized as one of the essential textbooks on endocrinology. Subsequent editions include increased genetic and epidemiologic investigation and improved clinical trial data to guide practicing endocrinologists in the care of their patients. The eleventh edition includes 12 new, distinguished authors contributing new chapters that focus on such topics as "Hormones and Athletic Performance," "Neuroendocrine Control of Appetite and Body Weight," and "The Endocrinology of HIV/AIDS." In addition, prior chapters have been revised to form a new section titled, "Body Fat and Lipid Metabolism." With increased goals of affordability, easier navigation, and more concise presentations, the editors facilitate a seamless blend of scientific and clinical information into everyday patient care. Understanding of essential concepts is further enabled with new full-color illustrations. Written with an intended audience of medical students, residents, interns, and practicing endocrinologists, this *Doody's Core Titles* essential purchase title is available in print or online thru MD Consult.

Journals

Endocrine Practice. v. 1, American Association of Clinical Endocrinologists (AACE), 1995.
http://www.aace.com/
ISSN: 1530891X
ISSN: 19342403 (Online)
Indexed in: MEDLINE
Recommended for: Hospital, Academic Libraries

This peer-reviewed journal, *Endocrine Practice*, is the official journal for the American Association of Clinical Endocrinologists (AACE) and the American College of Endocrinology (ACE). Both organizations are committed to preserving relationships among hospitals, academic institutions, industry, and individuals who contribute to their basic mission "to enhance physicians' ability to provide the highest quality medical care to patients with endocrine disorders," (Garber JR, *Endocr Pract* 2009 Dec; 15(7):669). Continuing education of practicing endocrinologists enhances the health care of patients with endocrine diseases, and clinicians will benefit from reliable clinical materials and timely reviews. Published initially in 1995, the journal is indexed in Embase, MEDLINE, Scopus, Reactions Weekly, and Web of Science.

Endocrine Reviews. v. 1, The Endocrine Society, 1980.
http://edrv.endojournals.org/
ISSN: 0163769X
ISSN: 19457189 (Online)
Indexed in: MEDLINE
Recommended for: Hospital, Academic Libraries

Published bimonthly in print or online by The Endocrine Society, *Endocrine Reviews* provides peer-reviewed knowledge, perspective, and coverage of both clinical and experimental endocrinology topics. Authors relay significant clinical experience and current research in the areas of endocrinology and metabolism as well as related areas of cell biology, immunology, pharmacology, genetics, molecular biology, neuroscience, reproductive medicine, and pediatric endocrinology. This well-respected journal is currently ranked one of 105 in *Journal Citation Reports* (2009) with the highest impact factor ranking in the category of endocrinology and metabolism. Online subscriptions are hosted at Stanford University's HighWire Press and include abstracts, full-text and PDFs, table of content alerts, research alerts, RSS feeds, access to Rapid Electronic Publications (publish ahead of print), and access to back copies through 1997. Limited open access is available thru HighWire Press Free and PubMed Central after 12 months, back to January 1997. Reliable indexing sources include Embase, BIOSIS, MEDLINE, Ovid, Scopus, and Reactions Weekly. The intended audience is medical students, residents, interns, research fellows, and practicing endocrinologists. This title incorporates *Recent Progress in Hormone Research* (1947–2005, ISSN 00799963).

Endocrinology. v. 1, The Endocrine Society, 1917.
http://endo.endojournals.org/
ISSN: 00137227
ISSN: 19457170 (Online)
Indexed in: MEDLINE
Recommended for: Hospital, Academic Libraries
Brandon/Hill Selection

As the oldest journal (originally published in 1917) by the Endocrine Society, this monthly journal continually defines the science of endocrinology with a broad range of high quality basic research related to the endocrine glands and their hormones. As one of the most authoritative biomedical research journals in the world, more than 6,000 pages are published annually from such subjects as sub-cellular mechanisms to whole animal physiology. More specific topics include bone and mineral, cover receptors, growth factors, intracellular signal systems, neuroendocrinology, reproductive steroids, signal transduction, thyroid, and physiology. This journal repeatedly receives an annual high impact factor rating and is committed to the highest scientific standards with a low manuscript acceptance rate of 30 percent. Also useful for readers are employment opportunities and conference announcements. As a core journal in the field of endocrinology, this journal is appropriate for both medical and biology collections with an intended audience of practicing clinicians, faculty, residents, fellows, and students.

Online content is available via Stanford's HighWire Press with limited open access available via HighWire Press Free from 1997 with 12 months embargo and PubMed Central from 2008 with 12 months embargo.

Journal of Clinical Endocrinology & Metabolism. v. 12, The Endocrine Society, 1952.
http://jcem.endojournals.org/
ISSN: 0021972X
ISSN: 19457197 (Online)
Indexed in: MEDLINE
Recommended for: Hospital, Academic Libraries
Brandon/Hill Selection

Published by The Endocrine Society, *Journal of Clinical Endocrinology & Metabolism* (*JCEM*) is considered to be the world's foremost peer-reviewed journal for endocrine clinical research and cutting-edge clinical practice reviews. Provided in each monthly issue is the latest in-depth coverage of new developments for the diagnosis and treatment of endocrine and metabolic disorders. Regular features include clinical trials, clinical reviews, clinical practice guidelines, case seminars, and controversies in clinical endocrinology, as well as original reports of important advances in patient-oriented endocrine and metabolic research under such topics as diabetes, reproductive endocrinology, growth hormone therapy, and thyroid disease. *Journal Citation Reports* (2009) lists this journal as 10 out of 105 with an impact factor of 6.202 in the subject category of endocrinology and metabolism. Originally published in 1941 thru 1952 as the *Journal of Clinical Endocrinology*, this monthly journal is indexed in such sources as BIOBASE, BIOSIS Reviews, Embase, MEDLINE, Reactions Weekly, and Scopus with an intended audience of clinical endocrinologists and clinical scientists. This journal is currently available in print or online with additional limited access through PubMed Central.

Molecular Endocrinology. v. 1, The Endocrine Society, 1987.
http://mend.endojournals.org/
ISSN: 08888809
ISSN: 19449917 (Online)
Indexed in: MEDLINE
Recommended for: Academic Libraries

Published since 1987, this journal provides a forum for molecular and cellular biologists to publish original mechanistic studies that investigate and describe the molecular mechanisms by which hormones and related compounds regulate function. These cellular regulatory processes include such topics as: how receptors and hormones signal to regulate gene expression, development, physiological function, and disease. As a highly visible journal with up-to-date communication of cutting edge science, the average turnaround time from manuscript receipt to first decision is 28 days. Upon acceptance, manuscripts are published online within a week. *Journal Citation Reports* (*JCR*) repeatedly ranks this journal within the top 20 titles in the category of endocrinology and metabolism. This journal is intended for an audience of researchers, fellows, and students. Online content is available via Stanford's HighWire Press with limited open access available via HighWire Press Free from 1997 with 12 months embargo and PubMed Central from 2008 with 12 months embargo.

Translational Research in Endocrinology & Metabolism. v. 1, The Endocrine Society, 2010.
http://www.endojournals.org/trem/
ISSN: 21505810 (Online)
Recommended for: Hospital, Academic Libraries

Published by The Endocrine Society, this online-only collection features the latest translational research among basic science, clinical investigation, and patient care. Articles featuring patient-care application of cutting-edge research are conveniently compiled from three well-established, high impact factor journals: *The Journal of Clinical Endocrinology & Metabolism*, *Molecular Endocrinology*, and *Endocrinology*. The collection includes up-to-date scientific advances that offer new approaches to prevention and management of disease; extended online access through HighWire Press with searching, extensive linking to related resources, and personal alerts; and a reading list for the intended audience of faculty, residents, fellows and students about recent developments in endocrinology and metabolism and related applications to clinical care.

10.10.3. Gastroenterology

The physiology and diseases of the digestive system and related structures (esophagus, liver, gallbladder, and pancreas).

—MeSH

Contributor: Emily Patridge

Monographs

Atlas of Gastroenterology. 4th ed. Editor: Tadataka Yamada. Wiley-Blackwell, 2009.
http://onlinelibrary.wiley.com/book/10.1002/9781444303414
http://www.ebrary.com/

http://www.r2library.com/
http://extranet.netlibrary.com/TitleSelect/
ISBN: 9781405169097
ISBN: 9781444303414 (Online)
ISBN: 9781444303421 (Online)
Recommended for: Hospital, Academic Libraries
Doody's Core Titles Selection

This gold standard text aids both practicing gastroenterologists and trainees. There are over 1,700 full-color images, endoscopic ultrasonographs, computed tomography scans, magnetic resonance images, radionuclide images, and angiograms portrayed in this atlas. The book's contributors examine every gastroenterology condition. The atlas contains three parts: "Principles of Clinical Gastroenterology," "Gastrointestinal Diseases," and "Diagnostic and Therapeutic Modalities in Gastroenterology." *Atlas of Gastroenterology* is listed as a *Doody's Core Titles* selection.

Clinical Gastrointestinal Endoscopy. Authors: Gregory G. Ginsberg, Michael L. Kochman, Ian Norton, Christopher J. Gostout. Elsevier/Saunders, 2005.
ISBN: 9780721602820
Recommended for: Hospital, Academic Libraries
Doody's Core Titles Selection

This resource focuses on endoscopic procedures that diagnose and treat a range of gastrointestinal disorders. The authors are internationally renowned experts in endoscopy. This book would be ideal for an academic or hospital library that supports gastroenterologists, gastroenterology fellows, and other trainees. The print purchase includes a DVD that provides clinical photographs and videos covering endoscopic procedures. *Clinical Gastrointestinal Endoscopy* is included in *Doody's Core Titles.*

Essential Pediatric Gastroenterology, Hepatology, & Nutrition. Editor: Stefano Guandalini. McGraw-Hill, 2005.
ISBN: 9780071416306
Recommended for: Hospital, Academic Libraries

This guide is designed for nonspecialists in gastroenterology, but it is also useful for residents beginning gastroenterology rotations or for those with an interest in pediatric gastroenterology. This book focuses on evaluation, diagnosis, and management of the full spectrum of gastrointestinal complaints. This book also includes a drug formulary for common prescriptions. The editor of this book, Dr. Stefano Guandalini, is the immediate past president of the European Society of Pediatric Gastroenterology.

Evidence-Based Gastroenterology and Hepatology. 3rd ed. Editors: John W.D. McDonald, Andrew K. Burroughs, Brian G. Feagan, M. Brian Fennerty. Wiley-Blackwell, 2010.
http://onlinelibrary.wiley.com/book/10.1002/9781444314403
http://extranet.netlibrary.com/TitleSelect/
ISBN: 9781405181938
ISBN: 9781444314410 (Online)
Recommended for: Hospital, Academic Libraries

This is the only evidence-based resource combining gastroenterology and hepatology. It appraises the evidence for diagnosis, screening, and treatment. One of the features of this book is the inclusion of an evidence-based grade of the trials and treatment recommendations, supplying the practicing gastroenterologist with guidance on patient diagnosis and care. This third edition includes additional subjects that were not covered in the second edition, such as the management of hepatitis B and drug-induced liver disease. The book comprises two parts: "Gastrointestinal Disorders" and "Liver Disease." This book would be a useful addition for hospital and academic libraries.

Harrison's Gastroenterology and Hepatology. Editors: Dan L. Longo, Anthony S. Fauci. McGraw-Hill, 2010.
ISBN: 9780071663335
Recommended for: Hospital, Academic Libraries

Any clinician or student with an interest in gastroenterology and hepatology will find that the authority behind *Harrison's Principles of Internal Medicine* (*HPIM*) is present in this book. *Harrison's Gastroenterology and Hepatology* features the gastroenterology and hepatology chapters that first appeared in the authoritative, seventeenth edition of *HPIM*. The paperback format of *Harrison's Gastroenterology and Hepatology* makes it compact in size and very portable. The book includes updated references since the publication of the seventeenth edition of *HPIM*, "diagnosis-speeding guidelines," and an appendix of laboratory values.

Netter's Gastroenterology. 2nd ed. Editors: Martin H. Floch, Kris Kowdley, C.S. Pitchumoni, Neil R. Floch, James Scolapio, Raul Rosenthal. Saunders/Elsevier, 2010.
ISBN: 9781437701210
Recommended for: Hospital, Academic Libraries

This book encompasses the entire scope of digestive diseases, containing references to over 300 of the most commonly encountered clinical conditions. The illustrations cover key anatomic structures and highlight the important concepts of this book. The guide uses a template format for quick access to key highlights of information. The sections covered include the esophagus; stomach and duodenum; abdominal wall; small intestine; colon, rectum, and anus; infectious and parasitic diseases of the alimentary tract; pancreas; gallbladder and bile ducts; liver; and nutrition of gastrointestinal disease. This book targets any clinician seeking information on major gastrointestinal diseases and conditions.

Practical Gastroenterology and Hepatology: Liver and Biliary Disease. Editors: Nicholas J. Talley, Keith D. Lindor, Hugo E. Vargas. Wiley-Blackwell, 2010.
ISBN: 9781405182751
Recommended for: Hospital, Academic Libraries

Practical Gastroenterology and Hepatology: Liver and Biliary Disease is an invaluable resource for any academic or hospital library. The book contains seven parts: "Pathobiology of the Liver and Biliary Tract," "Diagnostic Approaches in Liver Disease," "Problem-Based Approach to Liver Disease," "Problems Related to Chronic Liver Disease," "Diseases of the Liver," "Liver Transplantation," and "Problem-Based Approach to Biliary Tract Disease and Gallbladder." In each chapter, highlighted text set aside in visible boxes emphasizes the important facts. This work's target audience includes fellows, trainees, and candidates for recertification in gastroenterology.

Practical Gastrointestinal Endoscopy: The Fundamentals. 6th ed. Authors: Peter B. Cotton, Christopher B. Williams, Robert H. Hawes, Brian P. Saunders. Wiley-Blackwell, 2008.
http://onlinelibrary.wiley.com/book/10.1002/9781444300819
Http://extranet.netlibrary.com/TitleSelect/
http://www.statref.com/
http://www.ebrary.com/
ISBN: 9781405159029
ISBN: 9781444300819 (Online)
ISBN: 9781444300826 (Online)
Recommended for: Hospital, Academic Libraries
Doody's Core Titles Selection

Some of the leading endoscopy experts in the United Kingdom authored this book. In discussing the procedures, the authors begin with the top of the gut and end at the bottom. They also discuss the bile and pancreatic ducts. In addition to procedural information, the book covers the endoscopy unit and staff; endoscopic equipment; patient care, risks, and safety; and other resources and websites. The book is illustrated with color line drawings and diagrams. *Practical Gastrointestinal Endoscopy* targets new practitioners or experienced practitioners who want to update their knowledge or improve their technique. This work is a "must have" for any hospital or academic library.

Principles of Clinical Gastroenterology. Editors: Tadataka Yamada, David H. Alpers, Anthony K. Kalloo, Neil Kaplowitz, Chung Owyang, Don W. Powell. Wiley-Blackwell, 2008.
http://onlinelibrary.wiley.com/book/10.1002/9781444300758
http://www.ebrary.com/
http://www.r2library.com/
Http://extranet.netlibrary.com/TitleSelect/
ISBN: 9781405169103
ISBN: 9781444300765 (Online)
ISBN: 9781444300758 (Online)
Recommended for: Hospital, Academic Libraries
Doody's Core Titles Selection

Over the past 20 years, thousands of physicians have come to depend on Tadataka Yamada's *Textbook of Gastroenterology*. His new textbook, *Principles of Clinical Gastroenterology* presents the major disorders in gastroenterology and hepatology from the clinical observation of signs and symptoms. There are over 31 chapters in this text, including an initial chapter on clinical decision making. This book is a "must have" for both hospital and academic libraries.

Sleisenger and Fordtran's Gastrointestinal and Liver Disease: Pathophysiology/Diagnosis/Management. 9th ed. Authors: Mark Feldman, Lawrence S. Friedman, Lawrence J. Brandt. Saunders/Elsevier, 2010.
ISBN: 9781416061892
Recommended for: Hospital, Academic Libraries
Brandon/Hill, *Doody's Core Titles* Selection

This resource is required for any academic, clinical, or hospital library. As an Elsevier Expert Consult title, the print purchase includes online full-text access for individual users, including regular updates and downloadable illustrations. Content includes the newest technologies, techniques, and treatments, with updated information on bariatric surgery, Barrett's esophagus, and many other evolving areas. A separate study guide, *Sleisenger and Fordtran's Gastrointestinal and Liver Disease: Review and Assessment*, 9th ed., 2010 (ISBN 9781437707304) includes over 1,000 review questions for the American Board of Internal Medicine's subspecialty examination in gastroenterology.

Journals

American Journal of Gastroenterology. v. 21, Nature Publishing Group for the American College of Gastroenterology, 1954.
http://www.nature.com/ajg/

ISSN: 00029270
ISSN: 15720241 (Online)
Indexed in: MEDLINE
Recommended for: Hospital, Academic Libraries

The *American Journal of Gastroenterology* is published on behalf of the American College of Gastroenterology (ACG) and provides support for practicing clinicians. Some of the topics in this journal include endoscopy, pathology, and the stomach. This journal is famous for its Red Section, "which starts each issue by summarizing What's Hot in the Red Journal and publishing articles, debates and editorials covering techniques, methodologies, ethics, practice management and other important matters of concern to the international clinical community." According to the 2009 *Journal Citation Reports*, it has an impact factor of 6.012 and ranks sixth of 65 journals in the gastroenterology and hepatology category.

American Journal of Physiology. Gastrointestinal and Liver Physiology. v. 238, American Physiological Society, 1980.
http://ajpgi.physiology.org/
ISSN: 01931857
ISSN: 15221547 (Online)
Indexed in: MEDLINE
Recommended for: Academic Libraries

The American Journal of Physiology – Gastrointestinal and Liver Physiology addresses normal and abnormal functioning of the gastrointestinal tract, hepatobiliary system, and pancreas. Original research articles may pertain to studies that focus on the molecular or cellular level, and research can involve either animal or human subjects. The journal is indexed in numerous sources such as MEDLINE, Scopus, and Web of Science. Previously titled *American Journal of Physiology – Endocrinology, Metabolism and Gastrointestinal Physiology*, this publication would be a useful addition for any academic library that supports gastroenterology researchers.

Clinical Gastroenterology and Hepatology. v. 1, Elsevier/Saunders for AGA (American Gastroenterological Association) Institute, 2003.
http://www.sciencedirect.com/science/journal/15423565
ISSN: 15423565
Indexed in: MEDLINE
Recommended for: Hospital, Academic Libraries

Clinical Gastroenterology and Hepatology is the official clinical practice journal of the AGA Institute. The 2009 *Journal Citation Reports* ranks *CGH* seventh of 65 journals in the gastroenterology and hepatology category with an impact factor of 5.6. *CGH* provides "a broad spectrum of themes in clinical gastroenterology and hepatology, including the diagnostic, endoscopic, interventional, and therapeutic advances in cancer, inflammatory diseases, functional gastrointestinal disorders, nutrition, absorption, and secretion." This would be an important addition to any hospital library.

Digestion. v. 109, Karger, 1968.
http://content.karger.com/
ISSN: 00122823
ISSN: 14219867 (Online)
Indexed in: MEDLINE
Recommended for: Hospital Libraries

This journal began publication in 1895 as *Archiv für Verdauungskrankheiten*, was renamed *Gastroenterologia* in 1939, and assumed its current title in 1968. Since its start in 1895, this journal has been a premiere resource for gastroenterologists in hospital settings. Its 2009 *Journal Citation Reports* impact factor is 1.770. The primary focus of this journal is on clinical research reports that cover a variety of topics from neuro-gastroenterology to gastrointestinal oncology. It is indexed in Current Contents/Life Sciences, MEDLINE, and Biological Abstracts.

Endoscopy. v. 1, Thieme, 1969.
https://www.thieme-connect.de/ejournals/toc/endoscopy
ISSN: 0013726X
ISSN: 14388812 (Online)
Indexed in: MEDLINE
Recommended for: Hospital, Academic Libraries

This journal is internationally known for its top quality review articles and original contributions in the field of gastrointestinal endoscopy. Some of the unique features of this journal include Annual Congress reports from Digestive Disease Week (DDW), endoscopic abstracts from the United European Gastroenterology Week, and photographic and schematic material. In the 2009 *Journal Citation Reports*, it ranks third in surgery titles and eighth in gastroenterology and hepatology titles. *Endoscopy* also serves as the official journal of the European Society of Gastrointestinal Endoscopy and is indexed in MEDLINE, Current Contents (Clinical Medicine and Life Sciences), Science Citation Index, and Embase/Excerpta Medica.

Gastroenterology. v. 1, Elsevier/Saunders for AGA (American Gastroenterological Association) Institute, 1943.
http://www.sciencedirect.com/science/journal/00165085
http://www.gastrojournal.org
ISSN: 00165085

Indexed in: MEDLINE
Recommended for: Hospital, Academic Libraries
Brandon/Hill Selection

Gastroenterology is the official journal of the American Gastroenterological Association (AGA) Institute. Sections of subject coverage include "Clinical Alimentary Tract," "Clinical Liver, Pancreas and Biliary," "Clinical Advances in Liver, Pancreas, and Biliary," "Basic Alimentary Tract," and "Basic Liver, Pancreas and Biliary." The 2009 *Journal Citation Reports* ranks *Gastroenterology* first of 65 journals in the gastroenterology and hepatology category, with an impact factor of 12.899. This is an essential part of any hospital or academic library collection that supports clinicians with an interest in gastroenterology. The AGA's journal website provides additional content—podcasts and videos—for individual subscribers.

Gastrointestinal Endoscopy. v. 12, Elsevier for American Society for Gastrointestinal Endoscopy, 1965.
http://www.sciencedirect.com/science/journal/00165107
http://www.giejournal.org
ISSN: 00165107
ISSN: 10976779 (Online)
Indexed in: MEDLINE, CINAHL
Recommended for: Hospital, Academic Libraries

This journal contains original, peer-reviewed articles on endoscopic procedures used to study, diagnose, and treat digestive disorders and diseases. With long-standing, international prestige since the journal's inception in the 1940s, it would be an important addition to any hospital or academic library collection. In the 2009 *Journal Citation Reports*, it is ranked fifth in the gastroenterology and hepatology category. Health care professionals accessing the journal at the Society's website have access to additional online features, such as the video and audio clips. Individual subscribing clinicians can also earn category one CME credit by reviewing the online material and completing the CME examination.

Gut. v. 1, British Society of Gastroenterology (BSG) and BMJ, 1960.
http://gut.bmj.com/
ISSN: 00175749
ISSN: 14683288 (Online)
Indexed in: MEDLINE
Recommended for: Hospital, Academic Libraries
Brandon/Hill Selection

Gut encompasses research articles on the alimentary tract, liver, biliary tree, and pancreas. Other content includes *Gut* podcasts and tutorials to help clinicians keep their skills updated. This is an official journal of the British Society of Gastroenterology. According to the 2009 *Journal Citation Reports*, *Gut* has an impact factor of 9.357 and ranks third of 65 journals in the gastroenterology and hepatology subject category. Online access back to volume 1, 1960 is available at the journal's website.

Hepatology. v. 1, Wiley for American Association for the Study of Liver Diseases, 1981.
http://onlinelibrary.wiley.com/journal/10.1002/(ISSN)1527-3350
ISSN: 02709139
ISSN: 15273350 (Online)
Indexed in: MEDLINE
Recommended for: Hospital, Academic Libraries

Published monthly, *Hepatology* includes peer-reviewed articles on immunology, chronic hepatitis, viral hepatitis, cirrhosis, genetic and metabolic liver diseases and their complications, liver cancer, and drug metabolism. According to the 2009 *Journal Citation Reports*, *Hepatology* has an impact factor of 10.84 and ranks second of 65 journals in the gastroenterology and hepatology subject category. *Hepatology* is published on behalf of the American Association for the Study of Liver Diseases. This is an essential journal for a basic gastroenterology collection in any academic or hospital library.

Journal of Pediatric Gastroenterology and Nutrition. v. 1, Lippincott Williams & Wilkins, 1982.
See Chapter 14.1. Child Nutrition Sciences

Nature Reviews. Gastroenterology & Hepatology. v. 6, Nature Publishing Group, 2009.
ISSN: 17595045
ISSN: 17595053 (Online)
Indexed in: MEDLINE
Recommended for: Hospital, Academic Libraries

This journal was released initially in 2004 as *Nature Clinical Practice. Gastroenterology & Hepatology*. Written by an international group of clinical academics and researchers, the journal targets practicing physicians, researchers, and academics. The journal's content includes perspectives, news & views, case studies, and research highlights. Some of the many topics addressed are cancer, the gallbladder and biliary tract, and the stomach. *Journal Citation Reports*, 2009, supplied an impact factor of 4.520 for the former title. ISI treats the *Nature Reviews* series of journals as new titles; they will be assigned their first impact factor in June 2011.

10.10.4. Hematology

Morphology, physiology, and pathology of the blood and blood-forming tissues.

—MeSH

Contributor: Jeannine Cyr Gluck

Monographs

Nathan and Oski's Hematology of Infancy and Childhood. 7th ed. Editors: Stuart H. Orkin, David G. Nathan, David Ginsburg, A.T. Look, David E. Fisher, Samuel E. Lux IV. Saunders Elsevier, 2009.
ISBN: 9781416034308
Recommended for: Hospital, Academic Libraries
Brandon/Hill, *Doody's Core Titles* Selection

Nathan and Oski's has been called "the bible of pediatric oncology" (*N Engl J Med* 1998; 338:1164, 5th edition). It is unusual that the scope of a major textbook contracts, but this is what has happened as a companion title, *Oncology of Infancy and Childhood*, split off into a separate volume. The 300-page section on oncology has been removed, as well as 40 pages devoted to psychology and infectious complications. The 7th edition, however, is less than 100 pages shorter than the previous edition. The extra space has been allocated fairly evenly to the remaining chapters and a bit more to the hemolytic anemias. The authors aim to integrate basic science and clinical medicine, and they give greater emphasis to diagnosis and treatment than in past editions. The book's 1,795 pages are divided into 37 chapters and 12 major sections: "History," "Bone Marrow Failure," "Disorders of Erythrocyte Production," "Hemolytic Anemias," "Disorders of Hemoglobin," "Phagocyte System," "Immune System," "Storage Diseases," "Hemostasis," "Supportive Therapy," and "Hematologic Manifestations of Systemic Diseases." The format is very user friendly. Chapters begin with an outline of the content, black-and-white and full-color illustrations are used effectively throughout the work, and references are provided in sufficiently-sized type for readers above the age of 50. Purchase of the book comes with a password to the online version for individual subscribers.

Wintrobe's Clinical Hematology. 12th ed. Editors: John P. Greer, John P. Foerster, George M. Rodgers, Frixos Paraskevas, Bertil Glader, Daniel A. Arber, Robert T. Means Jr. Wolters Kluwer/Lippincott Williams & Wilkins, 2009.
http://wintrobes.com
http://www.ovid.com/
ISBN: 9780781765077
See Also Chapter 10.12.1. Clinical Pathology
Recommended for: Hospital, Academic Libraries
Brandon/Hill, *Doody's Core Titles* Selection

Now in its 12th edition, *Wintrobe's Clinical Hematology* is considered "comprehensive, encyclopedic, accurate, and authoritative" (*JAMA* 2009; 302(22):2491). Editors aim to correlate basic science with clinical hematology, thus making the two volumes very useful for practicing hematologists, internists, and trainees alike. More than 2,600 pages are organized into seven major sections: "Laboratory Hematology," "Normal Hematologic System," "Therapeutic Modalities," "Disorders of Red Cells," "Disorder of Hemostasis and Coagulation," "Nonmalignant Disorders of Leukocytes, the Spleen, and/or Immunoglubulins," and "Hematologic Malignancies." New chapters cover anemia of the newborn, pathology of histiocytic disorders, tumors of the spleen, and myeloproliferative disorders and mast cell disease. Coverage of new medications has been expanded. The international panel of editors and contributors represent a wide range of relevant specialties. Black-and-white and full-color images are interspersed throughout the pages. A password to an online searchable version of *Wintrobe's* is supplied with purchase of the print book.

Journals

Blood. v. 1, American Society of Hematology, 1946.
http://bloodjournal.hematologylibrary.org/
ISSN: 00064971
ISSN: 15280020 (Online)
See Also Chapter 10.12. Pathology
Indexed in: MEDLINE
Recommended for: Hospital, Academic Libraries
Brandon/Hill Selection

Blood is the weekly, official journal of the American Society of Hematology (ASH). The editor-in-chief and associate editors are primarily from North America, while roughly one quarter of the editorial board resides in other parts of the world. The journal covers all aspects of hematology, including hematologic oncology. All research articles, which comprise the majority of the journal, are prepublished online. Many have supplemental tables and appendixes, which appear only online. With an impact factor of 10.555, *Blood* is the second ranking journal in hematology category in the 2009 *Journal Citation Reports*. The publishers are supportive of open access, with every issue offering free access to commentaries, the "How I Treat" review, and five research articles. Additionally, all issues older than 12 months are free to everyone in their entirety. An annual November supplement includes abstracts of the ASH conference.

10.10.5. Infectious Disease Medicine

Diagnosis and treatment of infectious diseases.
—MeSH

Contributor: Cindy Mitchell

Monographs

Emerging Infections 8. 8th ed. Editors: W. Michael Scheld, Scott M. Hammer, James M. Hughes. American Society for Microbiology, 2008.
http://www.ebrary.com/
ISBN: 9781555814441
ISBN: 9781555815592
Recommended for: Hospital, Academic Libraries

First published in 1998, this eighth volume in the series coincides with the joint 2008 Interscience Conference on Antimicrobial Agents and Chemotherapy (ICAAC) and the Infectious Diseases Society of America (IDSA) meeting. The authors continue the work and information provided by the earlier editions, with the increasing awareness that disease outbreaks have a global effect on the vulnerability of public health and security. This eighth edition comprises 20 chapters and provides updates on prevention and strategies for the control of emerging and reemerging infectious diseases. Each chapter, such as the one on Methicillin-Resistant Staphylococcus Aureus (MRSA), may include illustrations, photographs, tables, or charts. Also included are descriptions of the incidence, risk factors, transmission, diagnosis and treatment, prevention, and conclusions for each disease. The references at the end of each chapter and the comprehensive index add to the value of this important title. This work is a required resource for hospital collections, medical schools, and for academic institutions supporting studies in public health, nursing, and veterinary medicine.

Infections of Leisure. 4th ed. Editor: David Schlossberg. American Society of Microbiology, 2009.
ISBN: 9781555814847
Recommended for: Hospital, Academic, Consumer Health Libraries

This fourth edition continues to be a highly readable, accessible, and informative source. Suitable for academic institutions, hospital collections, and medium to large public libraries, this source identifies infectious risks surrounding leisure activities. Three new chapters have been added: "Infectious Risks of Air Travel," "Perils of the Petting Zoo," and "Infections on Cruise Ships." Each chapter includes features such as photographs, tables, charts, and references. New to this edition is a list of "practical tips" at the end of each chapter, covering the management and prevention of the infections addressed in the chapter. The extensive index adds to the book's functionality; the reader does not have to guess where to locate entries ranging from malaria to tattooing.

Mandell, Douglas, and Bennett's Principles and Practice of Infectious Diseases. 7th ed. Editors: Gerald L. Mandell, John E. Bennett, Raphael Dolin. Churchill Livingstone/Elsevier, 2010.
http://www.mdconsult.com/
ISBN: 9780443068393
Recommended for: Hospital, Academic Libraries
Brandon/Hill, *Doody's Core Titles* Selection

First published in 1979 and now in its seventh edition, this text is required for collections on infectious diseases. With 330 chapters, this two-volume set is meant for a broad audience of physicians (with a specialty in infectious diseases), pharmacologists, microbiologists, public health experts, and veterinarians, to name a few. The 7th edition includes updated coverage on H1N1, MRSA, travel medicine, and the importation of exotic pets. It is intended to assist readers in quickly finding clinical information for the diagnosis and treatment of patients. The effective use of charts, illustrations, photographs, and references allows each chapter to stand on its own. The chapter on "Hospital Preparedness for Emerging and Highly Contagious Infectious Diseases: Getting Ready for the Next Epidemic or Pandemic" is an example of such strength. The aforementioned chapter provides coverage on patient and community support, isolation techniques, examples of instructions that can be placed on patient charts, transportation of patients, and management of visitors. This work is available online for individuals with the purchase of the Expert Consult Premium edition; a scratch-off access activation code is located inside the front cover of the first volume. Institutional access is offered through Elsevier's MD Consult platform.

Rubin's Pathology: Clinicopathologic Foundations of Medicine. 5th ed. Editors: Raphael Rubin, David S. Strayer. Wolters Kluwer Health/Lippincott Williams & Wilkins, 2008.

ISBN: 9780781795166
Recommended for: Hospital, Academic Libraries
Doody's Core Titles Selection

Now in its fifth edition, *Rubin's Pathology* is the classic textbook on pathology and provides medical students with a basis to discuss the disease process and its effects. Chapters from the earlier editions are revised, and new sections are included on emerging infections, biowarfare, and stem cells. Chapters such as the one on "Infectious and Parasitic Diseases" include an overview, giving the reader some history and context as a starting point to the subsections. As in earlier editions, each topic within a chapter, such as the one on Rocky Mountain spotted fever, gives an overview, a brief description with scientific name, epidemiology, pathology, and clinical features. The use of color icons, photographs, and illustrations contributes to the highly useful nature of this title. The comprehensive index makes use of "see" and "cross" references, making the topics easy to locate in this large volume. New with this print edition for individuals is a companion website, thePoint, including interactive case studies, images, and fully searchable text. A scratch-off sticker with the logon information is located on the inside cover pages.

Journals

Clinical Infectious Diseases. v. 14, University of Chicago Press, 1992.
http://www.journals.uchicago.edu/CID/
ISSN: 10584838
ISSN: 15376591 (Online)
See Also Chapter 9.7. Epidemiology
Indexed in: MEDLINE
Recommended for: Hospital, Academic Libraries

Clinical Infectious Diseases continues *Reviews of Infectious Diseases*, 1979–1991. This scholarly, academic journal is published semimonthly. The journal publishes clinical articles on diagnosis, medical microbiology, and the treatment of diseases caused by infectious agents. Special sections may include articles on bioterrorism, food safety, and emerging infections; it features brief reports, review articles, editorials, and commentaries. A recent issue covered topics such as influenza testing, H1N1, and antituberculosis drugs. This journal is extensively indexed in various sources including Web of Science, MEDLINE, and CAB Abstracts. The 2009 *Journal Citation Reports* supplies an impact factor of 8.195, which is the second highest in the infectious diseases category. This journal is an important addition to the field of infectious diseases and will be used by medical schools, academic intuitions, and hospital libraries.

10.10.6. Medical Oncology

The study of neoplasms.
—MeSH

Contributor: Jeannine Cyr Gluck

Monographs

AJCC Cancer Staging Manual. 7th ed. Editors: Stephen B. Edge, David R. Byrd, Carolyn C. Compton, April G. Fritz, Frederick L. Greene, Andrew Trotti. Springer, 2010.
http://ajcce-staging.com
ISBN: 9780387884400
Recommended for: Hospital, Academic Libraries

The *AJCC Cancer Staging Manual* is the authoritative reference for tumor node metastasis (TNM) staging in the United States. This seventh edition contains 50 percent more pages than the previous sixth edition, which was published in 2002. There are 57 chapters that each begin with a summary of changes, reflective of new knowledge. Of these, nine chapters are new, devoted to neoplasms previously included in other sections. Chapters include discussions of cancer staging by anatomical site, references, diagrams, and staging forms. A CD-ROM packaged with the manual contains electronic staging forms. Each form now asks physicians to indicate whether treatment planning took into consideration staging and National Comprehensive Cancer Network (NCCN) or other national guidelines. The AJCC e-Staging Tool provides online access to all the forms from the *Staging Manual* as well as a comprehensive, interactive guide to the general rules of cancer staging and specific classifications for T, N, and M. The *Staging Manual* is a required reference for all cancer collections in hospital or academic libraries.

Cancer in Adolescents and Young Adults. Editors: W. Archie Bleyer, Ronald D. Barr. Springer, 2007.
See Chapter 9.1. Adolescent Medicine

Clinical Gynecologic Oncology. 7th ed. Editors: Philip J. DiSaia, William T. Creasman. Mosby Elsevier, 2007.
http://www.mdconsult.com/
ISBN: 9780323039789
Recommended for: Academic Libraries
Brandon/Hill, *Doody's Core Titles* Selection

Clinical Gynecologic Oncology is considered by many to be an essential resource for clinicians and students in the field of women's health care. Its stated audience is "the community physician, resident, and other students involved with these patients." Emphasis is on the practical aspects of patient management. Each chapter begins with a brief outline of the content that follows, and red text highlights key points throughout the work. Most pages contain at least one table or illustration, and full-color images abound. The 26 contributors discuss not only the female reproductive tract, but breast diseases, colorectal and bladder neoplasms, and cancer in pregnancy. Also presented are complications of disease and therapy; basic principles of chemotherapy; tumor immunology, host defense mechanisms, and biologic therapy; genes and cancer; palliative care and quality of life; the role of laparoscopic surgery in gynecologic malignancies; epidemiology of commonly used statistical terms; and analysis of clinical studies. References are adequate in number, grouped by subsection of the chapter, and written in a readable font size.

DeVita, Hellman, and Rosenberg's Cancer: Principles & Practice of Oncology. 8th ed. Editors: Vincent T. DeVita Jr., Theodore S. Lawrence, Steven A. Rosenberg. Wolters Kluwer/ Lippincott Williams & Wilkins, 2008.
http://www.cancerppo8.com/
http://www.ovid.com/
http://www.r2library.com/
ISBN: 9780781772075
Recommended for: Hospital, Academic Libraries
Brandon/Hill, *Doody's Core Titles* Selection

If one could afford only a single book in this field, it should be *DeVita's Cancer*. Randall Hughes, reviewing the previous edition in *JAMA* (2005; 294(6):747–748), called it "a staple reference text in the medical oncologist's library." Among the eighth edition's 221 chapters and sections, 40 are new and 70 others have been rewritten completely by new contributors. The 3,200 pages, provided in a two-volume set, are divided into four major divisions: "Molecular Biology of Cancer," "Principles of Oncology," "Practice of Oncology," and "Newer Approaches in Cancer Treatment." Surgeons, along with medical and radiation oncologists, have collaborated on the treatment chapters and discussed therapy of each cancer type by stage. The molecular biology of each cancer is presented, with a discussion of its impact on clinical management. Many high-quality, full color and black-and-white images appear throughout the work, as do references that are supportive of the 2008 publication date. The editors state that "no more than 3 years will lapse between editions to keep the book fresh." Between editions, content is updated on a bimonthly basis in *The Cancer Journal: The Journal of Principles & Practice of Oncology* (ISSN 15289117). A companion website offers searchable full text and images of the textbook.

Diseases of the Breast. 4th ed. Editors: Jay R. Harris, Marc E. Lippman, Monica Morrow, C. Kent Osborne. Wolters Kluwer/Lippincott Williams & Wilkins, 2009.
http://www.diseasesofthebreast.com/
http://www.ovid.com/
ISBN: 9780781791175
Recommended for: Hospital, Academic Libraries
Doody's Core Titles Selection

Diseases of the Breast, fourth edition, focuses on breast cancer but also covers benign disease in a 60-page section. The editors have arranged and structured the 98 chapters to maximize their accessibility to practicing clinicians. Fifteen sections address the following topics: breast anatomy and development; diagnosis and management of benign disease; imaging and image-guided biopsy techniques; epidemiology and risk; in situ carcinoma; pathology and biological markers of invasive cancer; management of primary invasive disease; preoperative systemic therapy; special therapeutic problems; evaluation after primary therapy and management of recurrent cancer; new therapeutic approaches; site-specific therapy of metastatic disease; special populations; issues in survivorship; and medicolegal and cost issues. The 186 contributors—30 of them new to this edition—represent a very wide range of disciplines. Fourteen chapters are new or completely rewritten, and each management-oriented chapter concludes with a summary. Illustrations—many in full color—and tables are sprinkled liberally throughout the work.

Oncology of Infancy and Childhood. Editors: Stuart H. Orkin, David E. Fisher, A. Thomas Look, Samuel E. Lux, David Ginsburg, David G. Nathan. Saunders Elsevier, 2009.
ISBN: 9781416034315
Recommended for: Hospital, Academic Libraries
Doody's Core Titles Selection

Oncology of Infancy and Childhood was born in the pages of *Nathan and Oski's Hematology of Infancy and Childhood*. The latter title included material on hematologic malignancies, but readers needed to look elsewhere for information on solid tumors. The section on leukemias and lymphomas had grown to over 300 pages in the sixth edition, but the editors felt they could not keep up with advances in the field. Finally, the decision was made to divide hematology and oncology into two separate titles. The 34 chapters are split into five sections: "Biology of Cancer," "Pediatric Cancer Therapeutics," "Hematologic Malignancy," "Solid Tumors," and "Supportive Care." The 92 contributors (two-thirds from the Dana-Farber Cancer Institute and other Boston medical centers) represent a broad cross section of relevant subspecialties. Therapy chapters, which together comprise more than one-half of the book, correlate basic science with clinical practice. The intended audience includes trainees, pediatric oncologists, and clinicians in other fields who see the delayed effects of treatment in their patients. Each chapter begins with an outline page for ease of use. Black-and-white and full-color illustrations appear throughout the work. References are in a legible font size and are relatively current. Purchase of the book enables individual access to a companion website, which is searchable and linked to PubMed. *Oncology of Infancy and Childhood* represents a valuable new contribution to this field.

Perez and Brady's Principles and Practice of Radiation Oncology. 5th ed. Editors: Edward C. Halperin, Carlos A. Perez, Luther W. Brady. Wolters Kluwer/Lippincott Williams & Wilkins, 2008.
http://www.perezandbradys.com
http://www.ovid.com/
http://www.r2library.com
ISBN: 9780781763691
See Also Chapter 10.17.2. Radiation Oncology
Recommended for: Hospital, Academic Libraries
Brandon/Hill, *Doody's Core Titles* Selection

When the first edition of this work was published, it was called "a superb reference for radiation oncologists" in the journal *Radiology*. Referring to the fifth edition, a reviewer in *JAMA* stated that "Since then, this text has been one of the most reliable references in the field of radiation oncology" (*JAMA* 2009; 301(19):2047–2048). Ninety-eight chapters are arranged into five sections: "Overview and Basic Science of Radiation Oncology," "Techniques, Modalities, and Modifiers of Radiation Oncology," "Clinical Radiation Oncology," "Palliative and Supportive Care," and "Economics, Ethics, and Technology Assessment." New chapters discuss stereotactic body irradiation, oncologic imaging/oncologic anatomy, photodynamic therapy, radiation and gene therapy, and radiation oncology in the developing world. The prostate cancer chapter has been divided into two sections—one on low-risk disease and another covering intermediate- and high-risk disease. Material on recent advances, such as targeted therapy, has been expanded. Even with these additions, the page count has been reduced by roughly 6 percent over the fourth edition. Color has increased the usability of this edition. Most noticeably, illustrations are now interspersed throughout the text so that the reader does not need to flip back to two sections of plates. Color is used effectively in tables and tabs as well. *Perez and Brady's* serves the needs of a wide audience, from radiation oncology students to experienced specialists.

Principles and Practice of Gynecologic Oncology. 5th ed. Editors: Richard R. Barakat, Maurie Markman, Marcus E. Randall. Wolters Kluwer/Lippincott Williams & Wilkins, 2009.
http://www.barakatoncology.com
http://www.ovid.com/
ISBN: 9780781778459
See Also Chapter 11.2. Gynecology
Recommended for: Hospital Libraries
Brandon/Hill, *Doody's Core Titles* Selection

As is the case with other oncology books from this publisher, *Principles and Practice of Gynecologic Oncology* focuses on multidisciplinary treatment. Drs. Barakat, Markman, and Randall were chosen as successors by editors of the first three editions, and they bring expertise in surgery, medical oncology, and radiation oncology to the table. Their selection of 114 chapter authors reflects this mix, which includes pathologists and other specialists as appropriate. Thirty percent of the authors are new, and they have rewritten or extensively updated all content. The book is written at a subspecialist level and is divided into the major sections of basic science, therapeutic modalities, disease sites, and special management topics (infections, complications, pain, nutrition, quality of life, and end of life). Black-and-white illustrations appear throughout the work, with 16 pages of color plates at the front of the text. Purchase of the print book includes password protected access to a searchable online companion website for individuals. This book is well suited to a hospital collection serving practicing oncologists.

Principles and Practice of Pediatric Oncology. 6th ed. Editors: Philip A. Pizzo, David G. Poplack. Wolters Kluwer/Lippincott Williams & Wilkins, 2011.
http://www.r2library.com/ (5th ed.)
http://www.ovid.com/
ISBN: 9781605476827
Recommended for: Hospital, Academic Libraries
Brandon/Hill, *Doody's Core Titles* Selection

JAMA called Pizzo's textbook "a comprehensive source of information that should prove invaluable to members of the medical professions involved with the treatment of childhood cancer" (*JAMA* 2006; 296(4):452–453). The book aims to interpret the field for pediatric oncologists at all levels of experience and training. This review refers to the fifth edition. Sections include the following:

"Biological Basis of Childhood Cancer," "Diagnosis and Evaluation of the Child with Cancer," "Principles of Multimodal Therapy," "Management of Common Cancers of Childhood," "Supportive Care of Children with Cancer," and "Other Issues Arising at Diagnosis, During Treatment and after Cessation of Therapy." The 164 contributors represent a cross section of disciplines and prominent institutions throughout the United States, with a small percentage of international experts.

Journals

Cancer. v. 1, Wiley, 1948.
http://onlinelibrary.wiley.com/journal/10.1002/(ISSN)1097-0142/
ISSN: 0008543X
ISSN: 10970142 (Online)
Indexed in: MEDLINE
Recommended for: Hospital, Academic Libraries
Brandon/Hill Selection

Cancer, the interdisciplinary International Journal of the American Cancer Society, is published on behalf of the ACS by Wiley-Blackwell. According to the stated scope, "*Cancer* is pleased to receive original articles related to human cancer including, but not limited to: biologic response modifiers (such as growth factors, interferons, interleukins, lymphotoxins), clinical observations, chemotherapy, clinical trials, detection, epidemiology, ethical issues, etiology, genetics and cytogenetics, imaging, immunology and immunotherapy, oncogenes, pathology and clinicopathologic correlations, prevention, psychosocial studies, radiation therapy, screening, staging, and surgical therapy." An annual, semimonthly subscription to *Cancer* includes the bimonthly publication *Cancer Cytopathology*. Both print and print plus online subscriptions are available. On average, issues contain one review and 20 to 25 original articles. All articles are published online in advance of print, and content older than 12 months is freely available to non-subscribers. All editorial board members except one are based in the United States. The intended audience includes medical, surgical, and pediatric oncologists; radiologists; gynecologists; urologists; basic scientists in oncology; epidemiologists; pathologists; cytopathologists; and cytologic technicians.

Journal of Clinical Oncology. v. 1, American Society of Clinical Oncology, 1983.
http://jco.ascopubs.org/
ISSN: 0732183X
ISSN: 15277755 (Online)
Indexed in: MEDLINE, CINAHL
Recommended for: Hospital, Academic Libraries

JCO, the official journal of the American Society of Clinical Oncology (ASCO), is published three times monthly. Its fifteen international editions and the composition of the editorial board reflect its worldwide span. According to the scope of coverage statement, "*JCO* publishes original research, reviews and other material related to breast cancer, gastrointestinal cancer, hematologic malignancies, molecular oncology, lung cancer, genitourinary cancer, head and neck cancer, pediatric oncology, neuro-oncology, supportive care and quality of life issues, prevention, and phase I and clinical pharmacology." Each issue offers over 20 original articles. Regular sections also include "Translational and Radiation Oncology," "Diagnosis in Oncology," and "The Biology of Neoplasia." *JCO's* 2009 impact factor is 17.793, placing it number two in the oncology category (*Journal Citation Reports*). The intended audience comprises practicing clinical oncologists, researchers, students, and allied health professionals. Beginning in 2010, institutional subscribers may choose online-only access at a lower cost than the previous print plus online option. All articles are posted online in advance of print. Roughly three-quarters of the original articles have supplementary material online. Abstracts from the annual meetings and specialty symposia are published on the journal website and in somewhat searchable databases at www.asco.org/ascov2/meetings/abstracts. The website provides non-subscribers free access to all ASCO Special Articles (evidence-based guidelines, policy statements, etc.), editorials, correspondence, and other miscellaneous articles. After one year, original research articles become freely available as well. *JCO* is a must for oncology collections in hospital or academic medical libraries.

Journal of the National Cancer Institute. v. 1, Oxford University Press, 1940.
http://jnci.oxfordjournals.org/
ISSN: 00278874
ISSN: 14602105 (Online)
Indexed in: MEDLINE
Recommended for: Hospital, Academic Libraries
Brandon/Hill Selection

Interestingly, the *Journal of the National Cancer Institute* has no affiliation with the U.S. National Cancer Institute. It is published by Oxford University Press and aims to appeal to a broad, multidisciplinary audience. Each issue of the bimonthly publication provides four or five peer-reviewed, original research articles as well as editorials, news items, memos to the media, brief communications, and correspondence. Contributors of research articles include American, British, and international authors with a focus on cancer biology, epidemiology, prevention, and treatment. Randomized controlled trials of therapy are included. Articles older than twelve months are freely available to non-subscribers, as are one or more open access articles in some issues. Pay-per-view is also available. Content prior to 1996 is not included with a current subscription, but online access can be purchased separately. Articles are published online ahead of print, and a few have supplementary material online. Patients can receive copies of individual articles by e-mailing the publishers.

Databases and Other Electronic Resources

NCCN Clinical Practice Guidelines in Oncology. National Comprehensive Cancer Network, 2003.
http://www.nccn.org
Recommended for: Hospital Libraries

The *NCCN Clinical Practice Guidelines in Oncology*, which is updated at least annually, provides recommendations for managing 97 percent of tumors seen in oncology practices. Each is developed by a panel of experts from the more than 40 member institutions that includes proponents of different cancer approaches and other, occasional stakeholders. A consensus process is used, incorporating formal elements such as stepwise review and consensus-building exercises to minimize bias. At the outset, existing algorithms are circulated by panel members to institutional colleagues for comments and suggestions for revisions, based on new knowledge. If substantial changes have been made, external validation is sought. This process affords a broader representation of views and further ensures the recognition and resolution of any inadvertent biases. Each clinical practice guideline considers a specific tumor site or type and offers an algorithm outlining care management, a discussion of the algorithm, and references. Diagnosis, workup and staging, multidisciplinary treatment (primary, adjuvant and salvage/recurrence therapy), and follow-up care are presented. The website also offers *Guidelines for Detection, Prevention, & Risk Reduction* and *Guidelines for Supportive Care*. A patient version can be found at the website. The *Guidelines* are available online free of charge with a brief registration. They also appear in the *Journal of the National Comprehensive Cancer Network* (*JNCCN*), available through Cold Spring Publishing (ISSN 15401413). Other articles and reviews in that journal discuss practical application of the guidelines and analyze relevant cancer outcomes data. *NCCN Guidelines* have become the de facto standards in oncology.

PDQ (Physician Data Query). U.S. National Cancer Institute, 198?
http://www.cancer.gov/cancertopics/pdq/cancerdatabase
Recommended for: Hospital, Academic, Consumer Health Libraries

PDQ is the National Cancer Institute's comprehensive cancer database. It contains peer-reviewed, evidence-based treatment summaries for a wide variety of adult and pediatric cancer types, written at both the professional and consumer levels. The treatment guidelines are less detailed than those published by the National Comprehensive Cancer Network (NCCN). Summaries on supportive and palliative care, screening, prevention, genetics, and complementary and alternative medicine can also be found here. A registry of more than 8,000 open and over 19,000 closed cancer clinical trials is offered, along with a directory of professionals providing genetics services. Last, two dictionaries, the first with more than 600 cancer and medical terms and the second with over 1,200 cancer medications, are contained in *PDQ*. These resources are available to all without charge.

10.10.7. Nephrology

The anatomy, physiology, and pathology of the kidney.
—MeSH

Contributor: David C. Stewart

Monographs

Brenner and Rector's The Kidney. 8th ed. Editors: Barry M. Brenner, Floyd C. Rector. Saunders Elsevier, 2008.
http://www.mdconsult.com/
ISBN: 9781416031055
ISBN: 9781416031109 (Online)
Recommended for: Hospital, Academic Libraries
Brandon/Hill, *Doody's Core Titles* Selection

Brenner and Rector's The Kidney is one of the leading textbooks in its field. A Brandon/Hill selection, *The Kidney* is now in its eighth edition, which is divided into 12 sections and printed in two volumes. The sections cover normal renal function, renal disease, and the consequences of renal failure to the treatment of kidney disease. Along the way, the genetics of kidney disease, hypertension and the kidney, and renal transplantation all receive separate sections. Companion volumes that address the latest advances in contemporary nephrology are also available. The electronic edition of *Brenner and Rector's The Kidney* is updated on a monthly basis. Dozens of relevant journals are scanned and abstracts of significant articles containing new information are added to the pertinent sections within the e-text version. It is recommended for all medical libraries.

Comprehensive Clinical Nephrology. 4th ed. Editors: Jürgen Floege, Richard J. Johnson, John Feehally. Mosby/Elsevier, 2010.
ISBN: 9780323058766
Recommended for: Hospital, Academic Libraries
Brandon/Hill, *Doody's Core Titles* Selection

This textbook has become a standard in the field of nephrology and was a Brandon/Hill recommended title. With contributions from physicians and researchers from around the world, the textbook has been written specifically for "fellows, practicing nephrologists, and internists." All aspects of clinical nephrology are covered: anatomy and physiology, fluid and electrolyte disorders, glomerular disease, diabetic nephropathy, hypertension, dialysis, and transplantation. Of special note are sections devoted to pregnancy and renal disease, hereditary and congenital diseases of the kidney, urinary tract infections, tubulointerstitial and vascular diseases, geriatric nephrology, and chronic kidney disease and the uremic syndrome. A CD containing all of the images from the book is included. These can be utilized for PowerPoint presentations. This review refers to the third edition. *Comprehensive Clinical Nephrology* is recommended for all medical libraries.

Current Diagnosis and Treatment: Nephrology and Hypertension. Editors: Edgar V. Lerma, Jeffrey S. Berns, Allen R. Nissenson. McGraw-Hill, 2009.
http://www.accessmedicine.com/
ISBN: 9780071447874
ISBN: 9786612092107 (Online)
Recommended for: Hospital, Academic Libraries
Doody's Core Titles Selection

Current Diagnosis and Treatment: Nephrology and Hypertension presents reference information on the care and treatment of patients with renal disease. Fluid and electrolyte disorders, glomerular disorders, tubulointerstitial diseases, hypertension, genetics, diabetes, and geriatrics are covered in 59 chapters. With its emphasis on the practical features of clinical diagnosis and patient management, medical students, residents, family practitioners, physician assistants, and other allied health professionals will find this a useful book. It is highly recommended for all medical libraries, but especially for small hospital libraries looking for a basic nephrology text.

Essential Atlas of Nephrology and Hypertension. 2nd ed. Editor: Robert W. Schrier. Current Medicine, 2006.
ISBN: 9781573402231
Recommended for: Academic Libraries
Brandon/Hill Selection

The contributing editors of the 2nd edition of the *Essential Atlas of Nephrology and Hypertension* have assembled over 1,000 images and illustrations covering areas pertaining to nephrology and hypertension. The areas covered include electrolyte, acid-base, and water disorders and glomerular, vascular, and tubulointerstitial disorders. Transplantation and dialysis have their own chapters, while the last chapter (chapter 8) discusses the relationship between the kidney and various systemic diseases such as diabetes, vasculitis, sickle cell, HIV, and sarcoidosis. Unfortunately, despite numerous images, only a few are in color and they are grouped together at the very back of the book, which makes it difficult to relate these images to their corresponding texts. A Brandon/Hill selection for the first edition with the title *Essential Atlas of Nephrology*, this would not be an essential purchase for hospital or small medical libraries but would make an excellent addition to larger collections.

Primer on Kidney Diseases. 5th ed. Editor: Arthur Greenberg. Saunders/Elsevier, 2009.
ISBN: 9781416051855
Recommended for: Hospital, Academic Libraries
Doody's Core Titles Selection

Primer on Kidney Diseases is designed to be a comprehensive yet succinct summary of kidney and electrolyte disorders "suitable for students, residents, fellows, and practitioners." In his preface, Dr. Greenberg outlines the great changes that have taken place in nephrology since the book's first edition in 1993. *Primer of Kidney Diseases* in its 5th edition has incorporated all changes in the terminology related to reduced kidney function and chronic kidney disease (CKD). Greater emphasis on the genetic basis of structural kidney disease can be found in chapters dealing with individual disorders. Each chapter in the textbook is subdivided into separate sections dealing with a specific aspect of clinical care. Illustrations are in color and incorporated into the text. A short bibliography at the end of each chapter references important articles from the medical literature. This text is highly recommended for all medical libraries.

Principles and Practice of Dialysis. 4th ed. Editor: William L. Henrich. Lippincott Williams & Wilkins, 2009.
ISBN: 9780781781633
Recommended for: Hospital, Academic Libraries
Brandon/Hill, *Doody's Core Titles* Selection

The fourth edition of *Principles and Practice of Dialysis* continues to be a leading textbook in the field of nephrology. It received three stars from *Doody's Rating Service* and the second edition was a Brandon/Hill title. It is intended to be a practical guide to questions that arise in the care of dialysis patients. Divided into two sections, the textbook discusses technical aspects of dialysis therapy, such as hemodialysis, vascular access, and choosing the best dialysis options. The second section discusses the clinical problems involved in dialysis including how hypertension, infections, and age complicate end-stage renal disease. With its clinically oriented focus, *Principles and Practice of Dialysis* remains a useful textbook for students, nurses, and physicians working in dialysis and is recommended for all medical libraries.

Renal and Electrolyte Disorders. 7th ed. Editor: Robert W. Schrier. Lippincott Williams & Wilkins, 2010.
ISBN: 9781608310722
Recommended for: Hospital, Academic Libraries
Brandon/Hill Selection

A Brandon/Hill selection, *Renal and Electrolyte Disorders* has been a leading textbook for students and residents for over 30 years. Its focus is to introduce its readers "to the intricacies of renal physiology and pathophysiology." Its 13 chapters, written by experts from the United States, Russia, Switzerland, Israel, and Canada, present basic renal physiologic information with emphases on the most recent developments in the fields of nephrology and urology. The renin-angiotensin-aldosterone system, metabolic acidosis, hormone activities, pathogenesis of hyperactive states, mechanisms of renal injuries, and chronic renal disease are some of the topics discussed. An extensive index provides further access to specific sections. This review refers to the sixth edition. This text is recommended for all medical libraries.

Journals

American Journal of Kidney Diseases. v. 1, W.B. Saunders, 1981.
http://www.sciencedirect.com/science/journal/02726386
http://www.ajkd.org
ISSN: 02726386
ISSN: 15236838 (Online)
Indexed in: MEDLINE, CINAHL
Recommended for: Hospital, Academic, Consumer Health Libraries

As the official journal of the National Kidney Foundation, the *American Journal of Kidney Diseases* is regarded as the leading journal in the field of clinical nephrology. It reports the latest results from the field of research in the study of kidney diseases, hypertension, dialysis therapies, and kidney transplantation. *AJKD* publishes case reports that provide clinicians with new therapeutic strategies. Teaching cases and quizzes provide an educational component to the journal's offerings. It is published in print and online. *AJKD* is indexed by MEDLINE, CINAHL, Scopus, Embase, Science Citation Index, and Current Contents, and is recommended for all medical libraries.

American Journal of Nephrology. v. 1, Karger, 1981.
http://www.karger.com
ISSN: 14219670 (Online)
ISSN: 02508095
Indexed in: MEDLINE
Recommended for: Academic Libraries

The *American Journal of Nephrology* is a peer-reviewed journal published by Karger. Recently, it changed its focus from clinical papers to basic science papers. Articles are published under three main sections: "Original Reports" consists of completed experiments that answer a given question; "In-depth Topic Reviews" covers timely topics written by experts in the field; the section entitled "Kidney and Beyond" publishes selected review articles on recently discovered molecules or molecular pathways. *AJN* has inaugurated a faster publication schedule by publishing all articles electronically shortly after the author has approved all final changes. *AJN* deposits all NIH-funded articles into PubMed Central. *AJN* would be an essential purchase for research institutions but possibly not for hospitals that do not conduct research in this field.

American Journal of Physiology. Renal Physiology. v. 41, American Physiological Society, 1997.
http://ajprenal.physiology.org/
ISSN: 03636127
ISSN: 15221466 (Online)
Indexed in: MEDLINE
Recommended for: Hospital, Academic, Consumer Health Libraries

A publication of the American Physiological Society, the *American Journal of Physiology-Renal Physiology* publishes original research on topics relating to the kidney, urinary tract, and their respective cellular and vascular systems as well as body fluid volume and composition. As with the other *American Journal of Physiology* titles, articles are written utilizing a variety of approaches to the topic at hand; for example, urinary tract research information may be written from the perspective of its biochemistry or immunology or genetics, mathematical modeling, molecular biology or physiological methodologies. Of benefit to the wider community, *AJP-Renal Physiology* makes its articles available to patients if they send a request to the journal's office. All articles are made available after an embargo period of one year. This title is recommended for all medical libraries.

Clinical Journal of the American Society of Nephrology. v. 1, American Society of Nephrology, 2006.
http://cjasn.asnjournals.org/
ISSN: 15559041
ISSN: 1555905X (Online)
Indexed in: MEDLINE
Recommended for: Academic Libraries

The *Clinical Journal of the American Society of Nephrology* (*CJASN*) publishes peer-reviewed research articles related to clinical nephrology, hypertension, organ transplantation, and critical care relevant to the clinical care of patients. The editorial board particularly encourages submittal of articles on epidemiological studies and evidence-based medicine topics. Other topics regularly covered include acid-base disturbances, fluid and electrolyte disorders, hereditary and genetic diseases, and pediatric nephrology. The journal publishes an online version as well as a print version. NIH-funded articles are deposited by the publisher into PubMed Central. *CJASN* is recommended for academic libraries only.

Current Opinion in Nephrology and Hypertension. v. 1, Lippincott Williams & Wilkins, 1992.
http://journals.lww.com/co-nephrolhypertens/
ISSN: 1062482
ISSN: 10808221 (Online)
Indexed in: MEDLINE, CINAHL
Recommended for: Academic Libraries

Each issue of *Current Opinion in Nephrology and Hypertension*, published every other month, focuses on one or two topics such as circulation, hemodynamics, the pathophysiology of hypertension, the epidemiology and prevention of hypertension, mineral metabolism, and pharmacology and therapeutics. The stated aim of the journal is to provide specialists in the field of nephrology and hypertension current information written in a clear and readable format, along with experts' annotated selections of the most interesting papers published in other journals. Along with these selections, a comprehensive bibliography of citations from the major journals in the field of nephrology and hypertension is published to give the reader a comprehensive picture of current research. This title is recommended for academic medical libraries and special collections.

Journal of the American Society of Nephrology. v. 1, Williams & Wilkins, 1990.
http://jasn.asnjournals.org/
ISSN: 10466673
ISSN: 15333450 (Online)
Indexed in: MEDLINE
Recommended for: Hospital, Academic Libraries

The *Journal of the American Society of Nephrology* (*JASN*) is the leading journal in the field. With a targeted audience of clinicians and researchers, it publishes the latest in basic research, clinical research, and clinical epidemiology. Subjects covered include cell biology, developmental biology, genetics, cell and transport physiology, hemodynamics and vascular regeneration, immunology and pathology, pathophysiology of renal disease, dialysis, and transplantation. A special feature is "Brief Communications," which expedites transmission of the latest research by publishing it in a letter format. There are two educational sections: "Science in Renal Medicine" explains a "unique concept" and "Pathophysiology of the Renal Biopsy" is devoted to "interesting renal lesions" captured by light, fluorescence, and electron microscopy. *JASN* is recommended for all medical libraries.

Kidney International. v. 1, Nature, 1972.
http://www.nature.com/ki/
ISSN: 00852538
ISSN: 15231755 (Online)
Indexed in: MEDLINE, CINAHL
Recommended for: Hospital, Academic Libraries

Kidney International (*KI*) is the official journal of the International Society of Nephrology. Ranked third out of 63 urology and nephrology journals in *Journal Citation Reports* (2009), *KI* is a leading source of current research for clinicians and basic scientists. The editorial board is composed of physicians and researchers from North and South America, Europe, Asia, and Australia. *KI* is indexed by MEDLINE, BIOSIS, Chemical Abstracts, and Science Citation Index, among others. One of *KI's* special features adds commentaries to selected articles, putting published studies in a context that then creates a research tool for clinical and basic investigators. "Nephrology sans Frontieres" discusses matters of local interest to nephrologists around the world. The "Journal Club" section synthesizes the latest research found in other journals in the field of nephrology. Teaching materials, including images, are published on a regular basis. *KI* is recommended for all medical libraries that support research.

Nature Reviews. Nephrology. v. 5, no. 4, Nature Publishing Group, 2009.
http://www.nature.com/nrneph/
ISSN: 17595061
ISSN: 1759507X (Online)
Indexed in: MEDLINE
Recommended for: Academic Libraries

Nature Reviews Nephrology (formerly known as *Nature Clinical Practice Nephrology*) publishes peer-reviewed up-to-date information geared to practicing physicians and researchers within the field of nephrology. Subjects covered include acid-base, fluid and electrolyte disorders; glomerular diseases; interstitial nephritis; and tropical nephrology. In-depth reviews present current information while discussions and opinions are presented in the "Perspectives" and "News and Views" sections. "Research Highlights" present primary research information culled from other medical journals and the "Case Studies" section provides a forum for the presentation of new and unusual clinical cases. This title is recommended for academic libraries only.

Nephron. v. 1, Karger, 1964.
http://content.karger.com/
ISSN: 00282766
ISSN: 14230186 (Online)
ISSN: 16602110 (Clinical Practice)
ISSN: 16602137 (Physiology)
ISSN: 16602129 (Experimental Nephrology)
Indexed in: MEDLINE
Recommended for: Academic Libraries

Nephron is the collective title for three separate journals: *Nephron Clinical Practice*, *Nephron Experimental Nephrology*, and *Nephron Physiology*. Each of the three journals has its own editor and editorial board. The subdivision provides the opportunity for more focused coverage in the individual titles. The three journals can be purchased individually or bundled together. *Nephron Clinical Practice* reports on research that directly relates to patient treatment. Topics that are regularly covered include clinical nephrology, dialysis, and transplantation. *Nephron Experimental Nephrology* has a special emphasis on the study of pediatric nephrology and its topics are drawn from the areas of histopathology, genetics, urology, transplantation, and fetal medicine. *Nephron Physiology's* scope encompasses the cellular and integrative function of the kidney and urinary tract in health and disease. *Nephron* is recommended for academic medical libraries.

10.10.8. Pulmonary Disease

The study of the respiratory system. It is especially concerned with diagnosis and treatment of diseases and defects of the lungs and bronchial tree.

—MeSH

Contributor: Jon Crossno

Monographs

Interpretation of Pulmonary Function Tests: A Practical Guide. 3rd ed. Authors: Robert E. Hyatt, Paul D. Scanlon, Masao Nakamura. Lippincott Williams & Wilkins, 2009.
http://www.ovid.com/
ISBN: 9780781778824
Recommended for: Hospital, Academic Libraries
Brandon/Hill, *Doody's Core Titles* Selection

The latest edition of this practical guide reviews currently available pulmonary function tests (PFTs) and offers practical examples of their interpretations in various disease states. The editors provide new information on the forced oscillation technique for measuring respiratory system resistance, the usefulness of exhaled nitric oxide in studying asthma, and the current guidelines on pulmonary function testing and interpretation from the American Thoracic Society and the European Respiratory Society. One chapter includes numerous case studies with questions and answers and indexing by disease state; each case provides clear examples of how a given pathologic condition affects PFTs and how that might present to a patient. The target audience of this book includes physicians, nurses, respiratory therapists, and other health professionals in training who will be doing primary care of pulmonary specialty disease. This title is available (for purchase or subscription) from Books@Ovid. It was a long-standing Brandon/Hill small medical library recommendation and is currently a *Doody's Core Titles* recommendation within the pulmonology and respiratory therapy specialty categories.

Kendig's Disorders of the Respiratory Tract in Children. 7th ed. Editors: Victor Chernick, Thomas F. Boat, Robert W. Wilmott, Andrew Bush. Elsevier Saunders, 2006.
http://www.sciencedirect.com/science/book/9780721636955
http://www.mdconsult.com/

ISBN: 9780721636955
Recommended for: Hospital, Academic Libraries
Brandon/Hill, *Doody's Core Titles* Selection

This completely revised textbook on respiratory disease in children provides the most authoritative and comprehensive coverage available of basic science and clinical problems related to pediatric lung disease. It is an essential resource for specialist pediatric pulmonologists, trainees, and pediatricians with an interest in respiratory medicine. The text presents information on general considerations—such as development, physiology, and investigations—followed by sections on respiratory problems in the newborn, infections of the respiratory tract, and noninfectious diseases. The organization of the book, which includes expanded chapters on asthma and cystic fibrosis as well as chapters that consolidate information about rare disorders, now reflects the relative distribution of time that most pediatric pulmonologists devote to various disorders. Information is also presented on pulmonary-function testing in infants and preschool children, diagnostic imaging, and an overview of congenital lung diseases. The title is available in electronic format on multiple Elsevier platforms. The previous edition of this book was a Brandon/Hill small medical library initial purchase recommendation, and this edition currently ranks as one of the highest scoring items within the pulmonology specialty category according to *Doody's Core Titles*.

Murray & Nadel's Textbook of Respiratory Medicine. 5th ed. Editors: Robert J. Mason, V. Courtney Broaddus, Talmadge E. King Jr., Dean E. Schraufnagel, John F. Murray, Jay A. Nadel. Elsevier Saunders, 2010.
http://www.mdconsult.com/
ISBN: 9781416047100 (2 v. set)
Recommended for: Hospital, Academic Libraries

This comprehensive textbook is now considered to be a standard reference work in the field of pulmonary medicine and is essential to the identification, treatment, and management of respiratory disorders. The work is divided into 20 sections within three distinct parts. The first part focuses on the scientific principles of respiratory medicine and their foundations in basic anatomy, physiology, pharmacology, pathology, and immunology. The second part covers the diagnosis and evaluation of respiratory disease. Part three discusses the clinical applications of respiratory medicine, including pharmacological control of asthma, drug therapies for cancer, interstitial lung disease, and thoracoscopic surgery. The book incorporates more than 1,250 illustrations, photographs, charts, tables, and diagrams. For individual purchasers, a companion website is available that provides the fully-searchable contents of the book, patient information handouts, links to PubMed, weekly content updates, and more. The title is also available in an electronic format on the MD Consult platform (by subscription). The primary audience for this book includes specialists, internists, and primary care physicians with an interest in pulmonary/respiratory medicine; however, the text does not offer comprehensive coverage of critical care medicine, which many pulmonary specialists also practice. This title should be considered for inclusion in the collections of medical school libraries and medical training programs. This review refers to the fourth edition.

Respiratory Disorders Sourcebook. 2nd ed. Editor: Sandra J. Judd. Omnigraphics, 2008.
ISBN: 9780780810075
Recommended for: Hospital, Academic, Consumer Health Libraries

This consumer health textbook provides basic, current, and comprehensive information for the general public about the symptoms, diagnosis, and treatment of diseases and disorders of the respiratory system. Topics include influenza, tuberculosis, pneumonia, asthma, chronic obstructive pulmonary disease, cystic fibrosis, and lung cancer. The book also offers tips on how to quit smoking and explains the various causes of lung disease, including genetic, environmental, and lifestyle factors. A section on disorders that may be caused by bioterrorism or chemical agents is also included. Part of the *Health Reference Series*, the book contains material collected from publications by government agencies, non-profit organizations, and periodicals, including the Centers for Disease Control and Prevention, the Environmental Protection Agency, and the American Lung Association. The book is fully indexed and includes charts, graphs, tables, illustrations, and a glossary of related terms.

Respiratory Physiology: A Clinical Approach. 1st ed. Authors: Richard M. Schwartzstein, Michael J. Parker. Lippincott Williams & Wilkins, 2006.
See Chapter 29. Physiology

Respiratory Physiology: The Essentials. 8th ed. Author: John B. West. Lippincott Williams & Wilkins, 2008.
ISBN: 9780781772068
See Also Chapter 29. Physiology
Recommended for: Hospital, Academic Libraries
Brandon/Hill, *Doody's Core Titles* Selection

This compact, concise monograph explains the key concepts and equations in respiratory physiology in an easy-to-read format. Intended to supplement a first-year physiology course, the textbook describes the structure of the lung, how gases move across the blood-gas barrier by diffusion, the carriage of the respiratory gases by the blood, the mechanics of breathing, and the regulation of gas exchange. Other features include "Key Points" boxes with USMLE-style questions and answers at the end of each chapter to reinforce learning and help students review for courses or boards. The book includes ample illustrations to clarify important equations and concepts, and updated topics include the physiology of pulmonary capillaries, hypoxic pulmonary vasoconstriction, pulmonary edema, surface tension, elastic properties of the lung and chest wall, metabolic functions of the lung, and perinatal respiration. For individual purchasers, a companion website offers fully searchable text and animations to illustrate difficult physiologic concepts. This title was a long-standing Brandon/Hill allied health recommendation and is currently a *Doody's Core Titles* essential purchase recommendation within the pulmonology and respiratory therapy specialty categories.

Journals

American Journal of Respiratory and Critical Care Medicine. v. 149, American Thoracic Society, 1994.
http://ajrccm.atsjournals.org
ISSN: 1073449X
ISSN: 15354970 (Online)
See Also Chapter 1.7. Respiratory Therapy
Indexed in: MEDLINE, CINAHL
Recommended for: Hospital, Academic Libraries
Brandon/Hill Selection

Considered a standard in the field of pulmonology and respiratory medicine, this journal publishes articles, reviews, and case reports on topics that relate to the understanding of pathophysiology and the treatment of diseases affecting the respiratory system and critically ill patients. The primary focus is on human biology and disease, but a related focus concerns animal or in vitro studies that contribute to the general knowledge in the field. First published in 1917 as the *American Review of Tuberculosis*, this journal is of one of three peer-reviewed publications from the American Thoracic Society, and it currently ranks first out of 40 respiratory medicine journals according to the 2009 *Journal Citation Reports*. The journal has been recommended as an initial, required purchase for a small medical library and continues to be listed as a core journal title by the National Library of Medicine. The journal is also cited in many abstracting and indexing sources, including Biological Abstracts, Chemical Abstracts, CINAHL, Current Contents, MEDLINE, and Scopus. Full-text articles are available online on the HighWire Press platform from July 1997 to the present; prior to that, only abstracts are provided.

American Journal of Respiratory Cell and Molecular Biology. v. 1, American Thoracic Society, 1989.
http://ajrcmb.atsjournals.org
ISSN: 10441549
ISSN: 15354989 (Online)
Indexed in: MEDLINE
Recommended for: Hospital, Academic Libraries

Begun in 1989, this journal reports significant and original observations in the area of pulmonary biology, with focuses on—but not limited to—cellular, biochemical, molecular, developmental, genetic, and immunologic studies of lung cells and molecules. Originally published to address a shift in modern pulmonary science to lung cell and molecular biology, this journal now ranks sixth out of 40 respiratory medicine journals according to the 2009 *Journal Citation Reports*. Also known as the "Red Journal," it is currently cited in several abstracting and indexing sources, including Biological Abstracts, Chemical Abstracts, Current Contents, MEDLINE, and Scopus. Full-text articles are available online on the HighWire Press platform from July 1997 to the present; prior to that, article abstracts only are offered.

Chest. v. 57, American College of Chest Physicians, 1970.
http://chestjournal.chestpubs.org/
ISSN: 00123692
ISSN: 19313543 (Online)
See Also Chapter 1.7. Respiratory Therapy
Indexed in: MEDLINE, CINAHL
Recommended for: Hospital, Academic Libraries
Brandon/Hill Selection

Started in 1935 as *Diseases of the Chest*, the journal now known simply as *Chest* features original research in the various multidisciplinary specialties of chest medicine, including pulmonology, critical care, sleep medicine, cardiorespiratory interactions, thoracic surgery, transplantation, and more. The official publication of the American College of Chest Physicians, this journal offers peer-reviewed research articles, medical writing tips, recent advances and reviews, and information about practice management to specialists and other health care professionals in the field of chest medicine. The online version also offers interactive physiology grand rounds and procedure videos. The journal is ranked third out of 40 respiratory medicine journals according to the 2009 *Journal Citation Reports*, and the National Library of

Medicine considers it to be one of the core clinical titles in this field. It is also cited in many abstracting and indexing sources, including Biological Abstracts, Chemical Abstracts, CINAHL, Current Contents, MEDLINE, and Scopus. Full online coverage back to volume 1, 1935 is available.

European Respiratory Journal. v. 1, European Respiratory Society, 1988.
http://erj.ersjournals.com/
ISSN: 09031936
ISSN: 13993003 (Online)
Indexed in: MEDLINE
Recommended for: Hospital, Academic Libraries

Featuring cutting-edge clinical and experimental work in the field of respiratory medicine, this journal is the foremost respiratory journal in Europe and, as such, publishes original peer-reviewed papers, clinical cases, topical reviews, letters, and editorials. Begun in 1988, it is the official journal of the European Respiratory Society, which promotes lung health through research, knowledge sharing, and medical and public education. The journal currently ranks fourth out of 40 respiratory medicine journals according to the 2009 *Journal Citation Reports.* The *European Respiratory Journal* is cited by many abstracting and indexing sources, including Biological Abstracts, Chemical Abstracts, Current Contents, and MEDLINE. Full online coverage back to volume 7, 1994 is available. Prior to that, only abstracts are provided.

Respiratory Care. v. 16, American Association for Respiratory Care, 1971.
http://www.rcjournal.com
ISSN: 00201324
ISSN: 19433654 (Online)
See Also Chapter 1.7. Respiratory Therapy
Indexed in: MEDLINE, CINAHL
Recommended for: Hospital, Academic Libraries
Brandon/Hill Selection

The official science journal of the American Association for Respiratory Care (AARC), this journal publishes articles pertaining to the cardiorespiratory system, including their pathogenesis, pathophysiology, manifestations, diagnostic assessment, monitoring, prevention, and management. The journal focuses on both the practice of respiratory care (including the development, evaluation, and use of equipment and devices) and the patient (emphasizing the improvement of all aspects of care for individuals affected by respiratory disease). First published in 1956, the journal is cited in many abstracting and indexing sources, including CINAHL, Current Contents, MEDLINE, and Scopus. Full-text online coverage is available back to volume 35, 1990; however, either a current, personal AARC membership or subscription is required to view the most recent content.

Thorax. v. 1, BMJ Publishing Group & British Thoracic Society, 1946.
http://thorax.bmj.com
http://www.ncbi.nlm.nih.gov/pmc/journals/179/
ISSN: 00406376
ISSN: 14683296 (Online)
Indexed in: MEDLINE
Recommended for: Hospital, Academic Libraries

First published in 1946, this journal provides clinical and experimental research articles on respiratory medicine, pediatrics, immunology, pharmacology, pathology, and surgery. Each issue covers topics such as chronic obstructive pulmonary disease (COPD), asthma, smoking, respiratory infection, and lung cancer. In addition to research articles, the journal publishes editorials, short papers, review series, case reports, thorax images, and letters. The journal currently ranks second out of 40 respiratory medicine journals (2009 *Journal Citation Reports*) and is the official journal of the British Thoracic Society. It is also cited in many abstracting and indexing sources, including Biological Abstracts, Chemical Abstracts, Current Contents, MEDLINE, and Scopus. The journal is available in both print and electronic formats. Full online coverage back to volume 1, 1946 is available.

10.10.9. Rheumatology

Inflammatory or degenerative processes and metabolic derangement of connective tissue structures which pertain to a variety of musculoskeletal disorders, such as arthritis.

—MeSH

Contributor: Lorna Springston

Monographs

Arthritis and Allied Conditions: A Textbook of Rheumatology. 15th ed. Editors: William J. Koopman, Larry W. Moreland. Lippincott Willams & Wilkins, 2005.
http:///www.ovid.com/
ISBN: 9780781746717
Recommended for: Hospital, Academic Libraries
Brandon/Hill Selection

Established as the bible of rheumatology, this two-volume reference is now in its updated fifteenth edition. More than 200 of the world's experts provide encyclopedic coverage of the entire field of rheumatology, including basic science; diagnostic and therapeutic modalities; and pathophysiology, diagnosis, and medical and surgical management of all rheumatic diseases and syndromes. Chapters include extensive references, and more than 1,200 illustrations complement the text. A new coeditor, Dr. Larry Moreland, joins Dr. Koopman for this edition. Coverage includes numerous new treatment modalities, a new chapter on anti-TNF drugs, and up-to-date molecular and genetic research. The textbook is a former Brandon/Hill rheumatology recommendation.

Kelley's Textbook of Rheumatology. 8th ed. Editors: Gary S. Firestein, Ralph C. Budd, Edward D. Harris, Iain B. McInnes, Shaun Ruddy, John S. Sergent. Saunders/ Elsevier, 2008.
http://www.mdconsult.com/
ISBN: 9781416048428
Recommended for: Hospital, Academic Libraries
Brandon/Hill Selection

Kelley's is the standard American textbook of rheumatology. It is offered on Elsevier's MD Consult platform and as a combined print/online Expert Consult Premium edition for individuals. This review focuses on the Expert Consult version, which includes a companion website that allows online access to the regularly updated content at the point of need. The textbook's online content contains both images and streaming videos that demonstrate complete musculoskeletal exams, including abnormal findings and the arthroscopic presentation of diseased joints. Links are available in the online content to PubMed, evidence-based guidelines, and self-assessment questions. The Expert Consult Premium edition also includes detailed coverage of the newest clinical algorithms to understand rheumatic disease management. More multimedia is offered so that diagnosis, monitoring, and management of rheumatic disease are more effective. The textbook is a former Brandon/Hill rheumatology recommendation.

Textbook of Pediatric Rheumatology. 5th ed. Editors: James T. Cassidy, Ross E. Petty. Elsevier Saunders, 2005.
http://www.mdconsult.com/
http://www.sciencedirect.com/science/book/9781416002468
ISBN: 9781416002468
Recommended for: Hospital, Academic Libraries
Brandon/Hill Selection

Pediatric rheumatology conditions are not that uncommon, and most clinicians will have seen children afflicted by them. Cassidy and Petty's book provides a venue to explore pediatric rheumatology in a comprehensive way, with content contributed by several experts. The textbook starts with a basic introduction to the subject and then works its way around the underlying anatomical and immunological concepts required to understand the disease processes. Individual and population genetics are reviewed and explained, as is the pharmacotherapy used for children and adolescents with inflammatory conditions. The book concentrates on the assessment and management of all the musculo-skeletal inflammatory and non-inflammatory disorders of childhood. Each group of diseases is placed into context and then described and discussed. Tables and figures are available to aid understanding and consolidate learning. The text establishes an internationally accepted nosography of classification criteria based on the ACR (American College of Rheumatology), EULAR (European League against Rheumatism), and ILAR (International League of Associations for Rheumatology) criteria. Overall, the *Textbook of Pediatric Rheumatology* will retain its place as the standard for the subject. The textbook is a former Brandon/Hill rheumatology recommendation.

Journals

Arthritis and Rheumatism. v. 1, John Wiley & Sons, 1958.
http://onlinelibrary.wiley.com/journal/10.1002/(ISSN)1529-0131
ISSN: 00043591
ISSN: 15290131 (Online)
Indexed in: MEDLINE, CINAHL
Recommended for: Hospital, Academic Libraries
Brandon/Hill Selection

Arthritis & Rheumatism is the official journal of the American College of Rheumatology. It covers all aspects of inflammatory disease. The journal contains peer-reviewed articles on diagnosis, treatment, laboratory research, and socioeconomic issues related to all forms of rheumatic disease. It ranks second of 26 journals in the rheumatology category in the 2009 *Journal Citation Reports*. Full online coverage back to volume 1, 1958 is available through Wiley Online Library.

Rheumatology. v. 38, Oxford University Press, 1999.
http://rheumatology.oxfordjournals.org/
ISSN: 14620324
ISSN: 14620332 (Online)
Indexed in: MEDLINE
Recommended for: Hospital, Academic Libraries
Brandon/Hill Selection

Rheumatology, the official journal of the British Society for Rheumatology, is an international peer-reviewed journal publishing quality scientific and clinical papers. The scope of *Rheumatology* includes a range of rheumatological conditions, musculoskeletal medicine, and surgery and translational research. *Rheumatology* publishes original articles, concise reports, reviews, editorials, guidelines, case reports, clinical vignettes, letters, and matters arising from published material. It ranks seventh of 26 journals in the 2009 *Journal Citation Reports*. Full online coverage back to volume 38, 1999 is available through Oxford University Press. *Rheumatology* was previously known as the *British Journal of Rheumatology*, along with various other titles, beginning with volume 1, 1952.

10.11. Neurology

The structures, functions, and diseases of the nervous system.

—MeSH

Contributor: Tim Mason

Monographs

Adams and Victor's Principles of Neurology. 9th ed. Authors: Allan H. Ropper, Martin A. Samuels. McGraw-Hill Medical, 2009.
http://www.accessmedicine.com/
ISBN: 9780071499927
Recommended for: Hospital, Academic Libraries
Doody's Core Titles Selection

Originally part of *Harrison's Principles of Internal Medicine, Adams and Victor's* broke away with the extensive growth of the specialty field of neurology. This text provides a comprehensive review of neurology, as well as chapters on all the neurological disorders. It is written for the practicing neurologist, but contains information for the medical student, resident, and academic physician. It comprehensively discusses the subspecialties of neurology: stroke, epilepsy, movement disorders, sleep, neuromuscular disease, multiple sclerosis, pain and headache, otoneurology, neuro-ophthalmology, cognitive and behavioral neurology, critical care neurology, spinal disorders, neuro-infectious diseases, cancer neurology, and pediatric neurology. This title is a required resource for any hospital providing neurological services, as well as academic institutions involved in the education of physicians. This is a *Doody's Core Titles* (2009) essential purchase.

Basic and Clinical Anatomy of the Spine, Spinal Cord, and ANS. 2nd ed. Authors: Gregory D. Cramer, Susan A. Darby. Elsevier Mosby, 2005.
See Chapter 3. Chiropractic

Child Neurology. 7th ed. Editors: John H. Menkes, Harvey B. Sarnat, Maria L. Bernard. Lippincott Williams & Wilkins, 2006.
http://www.r2library.com/
http://www.ovid.com/
ISBN: 9780781751049
Recommended for: Hospital, Academic Libraries
Brandon/Hill, *Doody's Core Titles* Selection

This classic text on clinical child neurology discusses complex topics such as molecular biology, genetics, neurochemistry, neurophysiology, neuropathology, neuroimaging, inherited metabolic diseases, trauma, infections, autoimmune disorders, and toxic and nutritional disorders. This edition is co-edited by Harvey B. Sarnat, MD, a leading expert in neuroembryology, muscle diseases, and neonatal neurology. The chapters are clearly written with black-and-white illustrations, ideal for medical students and residents. The editors' goal is to bring both neuroscience and neurology together. This book is recommended for hospital libraries and academic libraries. Older editions were on the Brandon/Hill list for an initial first purchase. It has a *Doody's Core Titles* recommendation.

Clinical Neurology. 7th ed. Editors: Roger P. Simon, Michael J. Aminoff, David A. Greenberg. McGraw-Hill, 2009.
http://www.ebrary.com/
Http://extranet.netlibrary.com/TitleSelect/
http://www.accessmedicine.com/
ISBN: 9780071546447
ISBN: 9780071664332 (Online)
Recommended for: Hospital, Academic Libraries
Brandon/Hill Selection

As with most other textbooks on neurology, the audience for this title is the neuroscience student, neurology residents, and neurologists. Unlike many other neurology textbooks, this one is very affordably priced. This book is concise, yet comprehensive and ideal for quick reference. It presents a clinically oriented approach by presenting a patient's symptoms first, then the diagnosis and management. Some features of this edition are: chapter outlines provide a quick reference of each topic, new advances in treatment protocols are listed, advances in neurogenetics and molecular biology are incorporated throughout, and a simplified guide to the neurological exam and the laboratory investigation. This title is recommended for any hospital providing neurological care as well as academic institutions involved in medical education. A previous edition was included on the Brandon/Hill list.

Clinical Neurology for Psychiatrists. 6th ed. Author: David M. Kaufman. Saunders Elsevier, 2007.
See Chapter 9.10. Psychiatry

A Compendium of Neuropsychological Tests: Administration, Norms, and Commentary. 3rd ed. Authors: Esther Strauss, Elizabeth M.S. Sherman, Otfried Spreen. Oxford University Press, 2006.
See Chapter 9.4. Behavioral Medicine

DeJong's The Neurologic Examination. 6th ed. Authors: William W. Campbell, Russell N. DeJong, Armin F. Haerer. Lippincott Williams & Wilkins, 2005.
http://www.ovid.com/
ISBN: 9780781727679
Recommended for: Hospital, Academic Libraries
Doody's Core Titles Selection

This classic book is intended for medical students, residents and practicing neurologists. It outlines in detail the neurologic examination. For example, the neuroanatomy and physiology of the disorders are discussed before dealing with the examination techniques, laboratory testing, and differential diagnosis. Advances in the field of neuroimaging technology are incorporated throughout the text. The book is heavily illustrated with tables and figures as well as color photos. The tables, presented as sidebars, outline procedures, tests, and syndromes that are discussed in the text. Discussions of the neurological diseases are limited, focusing on the examination of the patient. This work is a required resource for any hospital collection and is highly recommended for academic institutions supporting medical students. This title received a five-star rating from *Doody's Review Service.*

Functional Neurology for Practitioners of Manual Therapy. Author: Randy W. Beck. Chruchill Livingstone/Elsevier, 2008.
See Chapter 3. Chiropractic

Merritt's Neurology. 12th ed. Editors: Lewis P. Rowland, Timothy A. Pedley. Lippincott Williams & Wilkins, 2010.
http://www.r2library.com/
http://www.ovid.com/
ISBN: 9780781791861
Recommended for: Hospital, Academic Libraries
Brandon/Hill, *Doody's Core Titles* Selection

Merritt's Neurology is intended for medical students, house officers, practicing neurologists, non-neurologists, nurses, and other health care workers. This classic neurology textbook provides a comprehensive review of neurological disorders of all etiologies. It can be used as a quick reference textbook since most disease sections contain fewer than ten pages. The sections include disease progression, differential diagnosis, images, laboratory findings, and treatment. The twelfth edition covers endovascular neuroradiology, parkinsonian syndromes, Lewy body dementias, frontotemporal dementia, vanishing white matter, vasculitis, normal pressure hydrocephalus, neuromyelitis optica, Kennedy disease, spinal muscular atrophy, complex regional pain syndrome, and Hashimoto encephalopathy. Research in the field of molecular genetics is incorporated in all the chapters. The book contains mostly black-and-white illustrations with many radiological images. Individual purchasers of the print edition can access a companion website with full text and an image bank. This title was selected for *Doody's Core Titles.*

Neurology in Clinical Practice. 5th ed. Editors: Walter G. Bradley, Robert B. Daroff, Gerald Fenichel, Joseph Jankovic. Butterworth-Heinemann, 2008.
http:///www.mdconsult.com/
ISBN: 9780750675253
Recommended for: Hospital, Academic Libraries
Brandon/Hill, *Doody's Core Titles* Selection

This comprehensive and practical textbook on neurology covers not only the clinical neurosciences, but also provides descriptions of neurological diseases with their diagnosis, therapy, and pathophysiology. It is aimed at students beginning their neuroscience training and practicing neurologists. Beginning with the fourth edition, this two-volume set includes a website with the entire fully searchable text, video clips, full color illustrations, links to other websites, and current updates. Videos of seizure and movement disorders are extremely helpful in the diagnosis and management of neurological disorders. This new edition incorporates the advances in the rapidly changing fields of neurogenetics and neurological therapeutics. This title is a required resource for any hospital providing neurological services as well as academic institutions involved in physician education. This title is a *Doody's Core Titles* recommendation and was listed on the Brandon/Hill list.

Neurology of the Newborn. 5th ed. Author: Joseph J. Volpe. Elsevier, 2008.
http://www.mdconsult.com/
ISBN: 9781416039952

Recommended for: Hospital, Academic Libraries
Brandon/Hill, *Doody's Core Titles* Selection

This textbook is the authority on neonatal neurology. It includes an 80-page introduction to neurologic examination of the neonate, covering innovative techniques such as magnetic resonance imaging and magnetic resonance spectroscopy. The rest of the 20 chapters cover the clinical aspects of specific neurological disorders. The author discusses the latest advances in genetics and the diagnosis and management of neonatal neurological disorders. He successfully blends basic research, clinical trial results, and his own experiences to produce this definitive book on neonatal neurology. He has included hundreds of tables, photos, images, and figures to support his text throughout the book. The primary audience for this textbook is not only neonatal physicians, but pediatricians and other healthcare workers who care for the infant in the neonatal stage. Lawyers will also find this book useful in neonatal brain injury cases. This title is a required text for both hospital and health science libraries. It is a *Doody's Core Titles* purchase recommendation and appeared on the Brandon/Hill list.

Wolff's Headache and Other Head Pain. 8th ed. Editors: Stephen D. Silberstein, Richard B. Lipton, David W. Dodick. Oxford University Press, 2007.
http://www.ovid.com/
ISBN: 9780195326567
Recommended for: Hospital, Academic Libraries
Brandon/Hill, *Doody's Core Titles* Selection

This resource is a classic in the field of neurology and head pain. It comprehensively covers the diagnosis, therapy, and management of headaches. It discusses migraine, cluster, primary, and secondary headache disorders as well as headaches in children and adolescents. This edition incorporates the new international headache classification, headache pathophysiology, new therapies for primary and secondary headaches and new advances in genetics. This title is a required resource for hospitals and health science libraries. Older editions were listed on the Brandon/Hill list.

Journals

Annals of Neurology. v. 1, Wiley, 1977.
http://onlinelibrary.wiley.com/journal/10.1002/(ISSN)1531-8249
ISSN: 03645134
ISSN: 15318249 (Online)
Indexed in: MEDLINE, CINAHL
Recommended for: Hospital, Academic Libraries

This title is the official journal of the American Neurological Association and the Child Neurology Society. Its focus is on understanding the diagnosis and treatment of nervous system diseases. All research articles are peer-reviewed. Studies included cover the basic and clinical sciences, as well as cellular and molecular neurobiology, population sciences, behavior, addiction, and psychiatric disorders. Topics covered are: Alzheimer disease, ataxia, atrophy, behavior, degenerative diseases, dementia, demyelinating diseases, dystrophy, epilepsy, movement disorders, myelin myopathy, sclerosis, seizures, stroke and more. It is included in the major abstracting and indexing resources. In addition to the original articles each issue has these sections: "Historical Perspective," "Discoveries in Neuroscience," and "Neurological Perspective." This journal ranks third out 167 titles in the clinical neurology category and eleventh out of 231 titles in the neurosciences category (*Journal Citation Reports*, 2009). Full online coverage from volume 1, 1977 to the present is available from Wiley.

Archives of Neurology. v. 3, American Medical Association, 1960.
http://archneur.ama-assn.org/
ISSN: 00039942
ISSN: 15383687 (Online)
Indexed in: MEDLINE, CINAHL
Recommended for: Hospital, Academic Libraries

This journal is the official publication of the American Neurological Association and the Canadian Neurological Society. The focus is to publish timely scientific information important for those physicians and healthcare professionals caring for people with neurologic dysfunction, but also for those interested in the structure and function of the normal and diseased nervous system. Articles are peer reviewed. The journal publishes theme issues on various topics such as cerebrovascular diseases, epilepsy, neuromuscular diseases, neoplasms, multiple sclerosis, movement disorders, Alzheimer disease, neurotherapeutics, genetics, sleep disorders and more. This journal encourages authors to submit video supplements to accompany their articles that are viewable in the online edition. It is indexed in all the major abstracting and indexing services. It ranks eighth out of 167 journals in clinical neurology (*Journal Citation Reports*, 2009). This title is a required journal for both hospital and health science libraries. Full online access back to 1960 is available from the AMA.

Neurology. v. 1, Lippincott Williams &Wilkins, 1951.
http://www.neurology.org

ISSN: 00283878
ISSN: 1526632X (Online)
Indexed in: MEDLINE, CINAHL
Recommended for: Hospital, Academic Libraries
Brandon/Hill Selection

Neurology is the official publication of the American Academy of Neurology. Its audience is the practicing physician concerned with diseases and disorders of the nervous system. Some of the sections that appear in the journal include: peer-reviewed articles, "Clinical/Scientific Notes," "Views & Reviews" (including "Medical Hypothesis" papers), "Issues of Neurological Practice," "Historical Neurology," "NeuroImages," "Humanities," correspondence, book reviews, software reviews, calendar listings, and position papers from the American Academy of Neurology. Some content is solely available in the online version such as the resident and fellow page, selected neuroimages, patient page, CME quizzes, podcasts, supplementary data, and video for specific articles. This journal is included the major indexing and abstracting resources. It ranks fourth out of 167 journals in the clinical neurology category (*Journal Citation Reports*, 2009). The Special Libraries Association's Biomedical & Life Sciences Division named it one of the most influential journals of the past 100 years. This journal is a required resource for both hospital and academic medical libraries and was listed as an initial first purchase on the Brandon/Hill list. Full online access is available from 1951 to the present.

Psychophysiology: The International Journal of the Society for Psychophysiological Research. v. 1, Wiley-Blackwell, 1964.
See Chapter 20. Medical Psychology

10.12. Pathology

The nature and cause of disease as expressed by changes in cellular or tissue structure and function caused by the disease process.

—MeSH

Contributor: Brian Oliver

Monographs

Color Atlas of the Autopsy. Author: Scott A. Wagner. CRC Press, 2003.
See Chapter 10.7.2. Forensic Pathology

Comprehensive Cytopathology. 3rd ed. Editors: Marluce Bibbo, David C. Wilbur. Saunders Elsevier, 2008.
ISBN: 9780721657523
Recommended for: Hospital, Academic Libraries

In this update of the 1997 and 1991 editions, cytopathologists Bibbo and Wilbur introduce 36 well-illustrated chapters that incorporate advances in the practice of gynecologic and non-gynecologic cytology. The chapters include topics in general cytology including basic cell structure and function, cytogenetics in cancer, diagnostic quality assurance, diagnostic cytology of the female genital tract, the cytology of other body sites, and fine needle aspiration. It also includes new technologies in cell preparation of samples for diagnostic tests, for example, virtual microscopy, automation in cervical cytology, and molecular techniques. An auxiliary online Expert Consult feature is available for individual purchasers. This comprehensive work is a required resource for any academic or hospital library.

Essential Forensic Neuropathology. Editors: Juan C. Troncoso, Ana Rubio, David R. Fowler. Wolters Kluwer/Lippincott Williams & Wilkins, 2010.
See Chapter 10.7.2. Forensic Pathology

Handbook of Autopsy Practice. 4th ed. Editor: Brenda L. Waters. Humana Springer, 2009.
See Chapter 10.7.2. Forensic Pathology

Pathology: Implications for the Physical Therapist. 3rd ed. Authors: Catherine Cavallaro Goodman, Kenda S. Fuller. Saunders/Elsevier, 2009.
See Chapter 1.3. Physical Therapy

Journals

American Journal of Pathology. v. 1, American Society for Investigative Pathology, 1925.
http://ajp.amjpathol.org/
http://www.ncbi.nlm.nih.gov/pmc/journals/338/
ISSN: 00029440
ISSN: 15252191 (Online)
Indexed in: MEDLINE
Recommended for: Hospital, Academic Libraries

This peer-reviewed journal is the official journal of the American Society for Investigative Pathology. It seeks to publish "high-quality, original papers on the cellular and molecular biology of disease." The editors publish manuscripts that "advance basic and translational knowledge of the pathogenesis, classification, diagnosis, and mechanisms of disease, without preference for a specific analytic method." The journal contains original research articles that are categorized according to the following research topics: cardiovascular, pulmonary and renal pathology; immunopathology and infectious diseases; matrix pathobiology; metabolic, endocrine and genitourinary pathobiology; molecular pathogenesis of genetic and inherited diseases; musculoskeletal pathology; neurobiology; pharmacogenomics, gene therapy and radiation biology; stem cells, tissue engineering and hematopoietic elements; tumorigenesis and neoplastic progression; vascular biology, atherosclerosis, and endothelium biology. In the 2009 *Journal Citation Reports* it ranked fifth of 71 titles in the pathology category with an impact factor of 5.673. This journal is a required resource for any academic, hospital, or special library that has students, clinicians, doctors, or researchers interested in the cellular and molecular biology of disease as it relates to the field of pathology. Online access is available from volume 1, 1925 from PubMed Central.

Archives of Pathology & Laboratory Medicine. v. 100, College of American Pathologists, 1976.
See Chapter 10.12.1. Clinical Pathology

Blood. v. 1, American Society of Hematology, 1946.
http://bloodjournal.hematologylibrary.org/
ISSN: 00064971
ISSN: 15280020 (Online)
See Also Chapter 10.10.4. Hematology
Indexed in: MEDLINE
Recommended for: Hospital, Academic Libraries

This peer-reviewed weekly medical journal is the official journal of the American Society of Hematology. With an impact factor of 10.555, it is the second most cited peer-reviewed publication in the category of hematology (2009 *Journal Citation Reports*). It provides "an international forum for the publication of original articles describing basic laboratory, translational, and clinical investigations in hematology. The journal covers all aspects of hematology, including disorders of leukocytes, both benign and malignant, erythrocytes, platelets, hemostatic mechanisms, vascular biology, immunology, and hematologic oncology." It is indexed and abstracted by most of the major indexing and abstracting sources. This journal is a required resource for any academic, hospital, or special library that has students, clinicians, or researchers interested in the field of hematology. Access to online issues to volume 1 is available free from the American Society of Hematology. The online version of this journal provides access to First Edition Papers, pre-published papers that have been accepted by the journal, but are still in the editorial process. These papers are fully integrated with the regular online issues and are fully searchable.

Histopathology. v. 1, Wiley-Blackwell, 1977.
http://onlinelibrary.wiley.com/journal/10.1111/(ISSN)1365-2559
ISSN: 03090167
ISSN: 13652559 (Online)
Indexed in: MEDLINE
Recommended for: Hospital, Academic Libraries

This peer-reviewed, international journal publishes articles "reporting the results of original histopathological research and clinicopathological studies, translational studies with direct relevance to the interpretation of tissue and cellular alterations in human disease, reports of relevant technical innovations, reviews, commentaries, and an expert opinion "Lesson of the Month, a case report of practical value to surgical and diagnostic histopathologists." In the 2009 *Journal Citation Reports* it ranked twelfth of 71 pathology titles with an impact factor of 3.855. It is indexed and abstracted in all of the major indexing and abstracting sources. Online access to volume 1, 1977 is available from the publisher.

Journal of Thrombosis and Haemostasis. v. 1, Wiley-Blackwell, 2003.
http://onlinelibrary.wiley.com/journal/10.1111/(ISSN)1538-7836
ISSN: 15387933
ISSN: 15387836 (Online)
Indexed in: MEDLINE
Recommended for: Hospital, Academic Libraries

This peer-reviewed journal with a focus on thrombosis, bleeding disorders, and vascular biology is the official journal of the International Society on Thrombosis and Haemostasis. The journal publishes original research reports, state-of-the art reviews, invited commentary and debate, letters, and announcements. It is abstracted and indexed in most of the main abstracting and indexing sources. It had an impact factor of 6.069 and was ranked ninth out of 61 titles in hematology and seventh out of 60 titles in the peripheral vascular disease category (2009 *Journal Citation Reports*). Online access is available from volume 1, 2003 from the publisher.

Modern Pathology. v. 1, Nature Publishing Group, 1988.
http://www.nature.com/modpathol/
ISSN: 08933952
ISSN: 15300285 (Online)
Indexed in: MEDLINE
Recommended for: Hospital, Academic Libraries

This peer-reviewed journal is the official journal of the United States and Canadian Academy of Pathology (USCAP). It "concentrates on all aspects of diagnostic human pathology, contemporary issues pertinent to diagnostic accuracy, reviews, illustrative cases, Academy news, and clinical medicine directly related to pathology practice." It is indexed in most of the major indexing and abstracting resources. The journal has an impact factor of 4.406 and is ranked ninth of 71 journals in the field of pathology (2009 *Journal Citation Reports*). Access to online issues beginning with 2000 is available from several sources and is free from the publisher after a 12-month embargo.

10.12.1. Clinical Pathology

The use of laboratory methods in clinical diagnosis.
—MeSH: Pathology, Clinical

Contributor: Brian Oliver

Monographs

Diagnostic Surgical Pathology of the Head and Neck. 2nd ed. Editor: Douglas R. Gnepp. Saunders Elsevier, 2009.
http://www.sciencedirect.com/science/book/9781416025894
ISBN: 9781416025894
Recommended for: Hospital, Academic Libraries

This comprehensive textbook addresses the most complex part of the body, the head and neck, by taking an anatomic and pathologic perspective through the area's various organ systems and tissue types. The second edition includes discussion of numerous advances, especially in the molecular characterization of many of the lesions arising in the region. The work contains 15 chapters, each containing an introduction, general comments, specific features, and a very detailed bibliography. The book is heavily illustrated with useful photographs, charts, tables, and diagrams; it contains over 1,700 full-color illustrations from rare neoplastic and non-neoplastic lesions. Full text is available online for individual purchase or through ScienceDirect. Links to PubMed are provided within each chapter bibliography. This massive work is a required resource for any academic, hospital, or pathology library.

Manual of Clinical Microbiology. 9th ed. Editors: Patrick R. Murray, Ellen J. Baron, James H. Jorgensen, Marie L. Landry, Michael A. Pfaller. ASM Press, 2007.
See Also Chapter 26.5. Microbiology
ISBN: 9781555813710
Recommended for: Hospital, Academic Libraries
Doody's Core Titles Selection

In a two-volume set, this definitive reference guides the clinical microbiologist in the laboratory diagnosis and therapeutic testing of clinically significant bacteria, viruses, fungi, and parasites. In addition, the taxonomy, biology, habitats, and clinical significance of virtually all organisms that colonize or cause disease in humans are discussed. It presents a direct approach to organizing information with thorough but concise treatments of all the major areas of microbiology, including new microbial discoveries, changing diagnostic methods, and emerging therapeutic challenges facing clinicians. Volume 1 of this text has 78 chapters in five sections: "General Issues in Clinical Microbiology," "Clinical Microbiology Laboratory in Infection Detection, Prevention, and Control," "Diagnostic Technologies in Clinical Microbiology," and "Bacteriology." Volume 2 contains 74 chapters in six sections: "Virology," "Antiviral Agents and Susceptibility Test Methods," "Mycology," "Antifungal Agents and Susceptibility Test Methods," "Parasitology," "Antiparasitic Agents and Susceptibility Test Methods." The ninth edition has a companion CD-ROM available through ASM Press that contains nearly 500 illustrations from the book. This comprehensive work is a required resource for academic, hospital, or pathology libraries. The tenth edition of this classic is scheduled to be released in May 2011.

Quick Compendium of Clinical Pathology. 2nd ed. Editors: Daniel D. Mais, Emily E. Volk. American Society for Clinical Pathology Press, 2008.
ISBN: 9780891895671
Recommended for: Hospital, Academic Libraries
Doody's Core Titles Selection

This second edition serves as a concise yet comprehensive source for the review of clinical pathology. It is best suited for those who are familiar with the basics and desire a guidebook for board preparation. The topics are organized according to the traditional clinical pathology sections. All the sections have been updated according to the literature published since the first edition. The text explores the topics of clinical chemistry, blood banking and transfusion, microbiology, hematopathology, coagulation and thrombosis, immunology and autoimmunity, molecular methods, and laboratory statistics and quality control. This work is recommended for academic, hospital, or pathology libraries.

Robbins and Cotran Pathologic Basis of Disease. 8th ed. Editor: Vinay Kumar. Elsevier Health Sciences, 2010.
ISBN: 9781416031215
Recommended for: Hospital, Academic Libraries
Doody's Core Titles Selection

Twenty-nine American academics contribute 29 chapters to the latest edition of *Robbins and Cotran*, which was first issued in 1957. Functioning as a textbook for medical students and a reference for health care professionals, the text has been extensively revised to reflect advances since publication of the 2004 edition. Major changes include reorganization and revisions to materials on cellular responses to stress and toxic insults, tissue repair and wound healing, genetic disorders and DNA sequencing technology, environmental and nutritional diseases, the gastrointestinal tract, and the female genital tract. The new edition features 1,600 full-color illustrations, including new photographs and schematics, and digitally enhanced images from the previous edition. Individual purchasers of the print version also now have access to the full text online, enabling readers to search across the entire text, bookmark passages, add personal notes, and use PubMed to view references. Case studies, previously sold separately as the *Interactive Case Study Companion*, are also available online. This comprehensive work is recommended for academic, hospital, or pathology libraries.

Wintrobe's Clinical Hematology. 12th ed. Editor: John P. Greer. Lippcott Williams & Wilkins, 2009.
http://www.ovid.com/
ISBN: 9780781765077
See Also Chapter 10.10.4. Hematology
Recommended for: Hospital, Academic Libraries
Doody's Core Titles Selection

This is the twelfth edition of *Wintrobe's Clinical Hematology*, which first appeared in 1942. In the preface to the first edition, Wintrobe stated that his objective was to be comprehensive, complete, and authoritative. He emphasized the importance of accurate diagnosis before therapy and the value of illustration in hematology. Volume one of this edition comprises four parts: laboratory hematology, normal hematologic system, therapeutic modalities, and disorders of red cells. Volume two comprises three parts: disorders of hemostasis and coagulation; nonmalignant disorders of leukocytes, the spleen, and/or immunoglobins; and hematologic malignancies. This a classic work that is a required resource for academic, hospital, or pathology libraries.

Journals

Acta Neuropathologica. v. 1, Springer, 1961.
http://www.springerlink.com/content/0001-6322
ISSN: 00016322
ISSN: 14320533 (Online)
Indexed in: MEDLINE
Recommended for: Hospital, Academic Libraries

This peer-reviewed, international journal publishes original papers, review articles, case reports and scientific correspondence dealing with disease mechanisms, and general, experimental, comparative, and molecular pathology of the nervous tissue. The journal's scope includes the topics of morphology, biochemistry, immunology, and molecular genetics. The journal has been abstracted and indexed in most of the major indexing and abstracting sources. Although some of the articles are in German, English language summaries are usually provided. In the 2009 *Journal Citation Reports* it ranked third of 71 titles in the pathology category with an impact factor of 6.397. This journal is a required resource for any academic, hospital, or special library that has students, clinicians, or researchers interested in neuropathology. Online access is available from the publisher back to volume 1, 1961.

American Journal of Clinical Pathology. v. 1, American Society for Clinical Pathology Press, 1931.
http://www.ascpjournals.org/
ISSN: 00029173
ISSN: 19437722 (Online)
Indexed in: MEDLINE, CINAHL
Recommended for: Hospital, Academic Libraries

This peer-reviewed journal is the official journal of the American Society for Clinical Pathology and the Academy of Clinical Laboratory Physicians and Scientists. The goal of the journal is to provide current information regarding novel laboratory observations on human disease and current concepts and techniques, with a focus on the application of evolving technologies to pathologic diagnosis and patient care. Some of the fields of clinical pathology that are covered in this journal are clinical chemistry, hematopathology, microbiology and infectious disease, and anatomic pathology. In the 2009 *Journal Citation Reports* it ranked twenty-fifth of 71 titles with an impact factor of 2.473. This journal also provides physicians with the ability to continue their medical education through the Accreditation Council for Continuing Medical Education. It is a required resource for any academic, hospital, or special library that has students, clinicians, or researchers interested in the field of pathology and laboratory medicine. Online access is available beginning with issues from 2000.

Archives of Pathology & Laboratory Medicine. v. 100, College of American Pathologists, 1976.
http://www.archivesofpathology.org/
ISSN: 00039985
ISSN: 15432165 (Online)

Indexed in: MEDLINE, CINAHL
Recommended for: Hospital, Academic Libraries

This monthly, international, peer-reviewed journal is the official journal of the College of American Pathologists. Published since 1926, *Archives of Pathology & Laboratory Medicine* was voted in 2009 the only pathology journal among the top 100 most influential journals of the past 100 years by the BioMedical and Life Sciences Division of the Special Libraries Association. In the 2009 *Journal Citation Reports* it ranked twenty-third of 71 titles in the pathology category and fourth of 29 in the medical laboratory technology category with an impact factor of 2.558. This journal is a required resource for any academic, hospital, or special library that has students, clinicians, or researchers interested in the field of pathology and laboratory medicine. Access to the full text is free and begins with issues from 1999.

Journal of Thrombosis and Haemostasis. v. 1, Wiley-Blackwell, 2003.
See Chapter 10.12. Pathology

Modern Pathology. v. 1, Nature Publishing Group, 1988.
See Chapter 10.12. Pathology

10.12.2. Surgical Pathology

Living tissue is surgically removed for the purpose of diagnosis and treatment.

—MeSH: Pathology, Surgical

Contributor: Brian Oliver

Monographs

Diagnostic Surgical Pathology of the Head and Neck. 2nd ed. Editor: Douglas R. Gnepp. Saunders Elsevier, 2009.
See Chapter 10.12.1. Clinical Pathology

Wintrobe's Clinical Hematology. 12th ed. Editor: John P. Greer. Lippcott Williams & Wilkins, 2009.
See Chapter 10.10.4. Hematology, Chapter 10.12.1. Clinical Pathology

Journals

American Journal of Surgical Pathology. v. 1, Lippincott Williams & Wilkins, 1977.
http://journals.lww.com/ajsp/
ISSN: 01475185
ISSN: 15320979 (Online)
Indexed in: MEDLINE
Recommended for: Hospital, Academic Libraries

This peer-reviewed journal covers the ever-expanding field of human surgical pathology. Each month, the journal's experts present original articles, review articles, detailed case reports, and special features. It contains detailed illustrations that encompass "technical methods, diagnostic aids and frozen-section diagnosis as well as detailed pathologic studies of a wide range of disease entities" from the field of surgical pathology. It is the official journal of The Arthur Purdy Stout Society of Surgical Pathologists and the Gastrointestinal Pathology Society. In the 2009 *Journal Citation Reports* it ranked eleventh of 71 titles in the pathology category and eighth of 167 in the surgery category with an impact factor of 4.062. This journal is a required resource for any academic, hospital, or special library that has students, clinicians, or researchers interested in the field of surgical pathology. Online access to volume 1 is available at the publisher's website.

Histopathology. v. 1, Wiley-Blackwell, 1977.
See Chapter 10.12. Pathology

Journal of Hematopathology. v. 1, Springer, 2008.
http://springerlink.com/content/1868-9256
ISSN: 18655785 (Online)
Recommended for: Hospital, Academic Libraries

This is a relatively new, peer-reviewed journal in the field of pathology and is issued only online. According to the journal website, it intends to provide pathologists interested in hematopathology with the information needed to evaluate lymphoid tissues and bone marrow. "The journal publishes reviews, editorials, comments, original papers, guidelines and protocols, papers on ancillary techniques, and case reports in the fields of the pathology, molecular biology, and clinical features of diseases of the hematopoietic system." The journal intends to be international in scope to help "address the huge geographical variations in incidence of disease." Molecular biologists involved in the expanding field of molecular diagnostics and research on lymphomas and leukemia would be interested in this journal. It is currently indexed by MEDLINE and Scopus.

10.13. Pediatrics

Maintaining health and providing medical care to children from birth to adolescence.

—MeSH

Contributor: Kathy Zeblisky

Monographs

Ashcraft's Pediatric Surgery. 5th ed. Editors: George W. Holcomb III, J. Patrick Murphy. Saunders, 2010.
See Chapter 11.9. Surgery

Atlas of Pediatric Physical Diagnosis. 5th ed. Editors: Basil J. Zitelli, Holly W. Davis. Mosby/Elsevier, 2007.
http://www.mdconsult.com/
ISBN: 9780323048781
Recommended for: Hospital, Academic Libraries
Doody's Core Titles Selection

The *Atlas of Pediatric Physical Diagnosis* is a unique, visual encyclopedia of pediatrics, relied upon by medical students, residents, nurses, and practicing physicians. Twenty-three chapters contain 3,000 full-color illustrations covering the major pediatric subspecialties. Figures, tables, and photos are accompanied by text that emphasizes examination techniques, visual findings, and diagnostic methods. Laboratory and radiologic findings are also included. The heavily revised fifth edition identifies more conditions and has new coverage of malnutrition, obesity, trauma, and genetic disorders. It also tackles the topic of child abuse and neglect. Purchase of the print text includes online access for individual use. This online access is fully searchable using the table of contents or a subject index. Online access also includes an easily accessible full image library and downloadable images that can be included in users' presentations. The MD Consult platform offers institutional online access. The title is recommended by *Doody's Review Service*.

Bright Futures: Guidelines for Health Supervision of Infants, Children, and Adolescents. 3rd. ed. Editors: Joseph F. Hagan Jr., Judith S. Shaw, Paula M. Duncan. American Academy of Pediatrics, 2008.
See Chapter 9.1. Adolescent Medicine

Caffey's Pediatric Diagnostic Imaging. 11th ed. Editor: Thomas L. Slovis. Elsevier (Mosby), 2008.
See Chapter 10.17. Radiology

Child Fatality Review: An Interdisciplinary Guide and Photographic Reference. Authors: Randell Alexander, Mary E. Case. GW Medical, 2008.
See Chapter 10.7.2. Forensic Pathology

Child Neurology. 7th ed. Editors: John H. Menkes, Harvey B. Sarnat, Maria L. Bernard. Lippincott Williams & Wilkins, 2006.
See Chapter 10.11. Neurology

Comprehensive Pediatric Hospital Medicine. Editors: Lisa B. Zaoutis, Vincent W. Chiang. Mosby Elsevier, 2007.
See Chapter 10.8. Hospitalists

Current Diagnosis and Treatment: Pediatrics. 19th ed. Editors: Willam W. Hay, Jr., Myron J. Levin, Judith M. Sondheimer, Robin R. Deterding. McGraw-Hill, 2009.
http://www.accessmedicine.com/
Http://extranet.netlibrary.com/TitleSelect/
http://www.ebrary.com/
http://www.r2library.com/
ISBN: 9780071544337
ISBN: 9780071641364 (Online)
Recommended for: Hospital, Academic Libraries
Brandon/Hill, *Doody's Core Titles* Selection

Current Diagnosis & Treatment: Pediatrics (*CDTP*) is part of the Lange *Current* series of medical books. *CDTP* provides extensive coverage on the care of children from birth through infancy and adolescence. It serves medical students, residents, nurses, nurse practitioners, pediatricians, and family practitioners. It also provides coverage of the Council on Medical Student Education in Pediatrics (COMSEP) curriculum used in pediatric clerkships. The book is arranged in an easy-to-use outline format for its 44 chapters. There are numerous charts, tables, figures, and treatment algorithms. Each section contains a boxed "Essentials of Diagnosis and Typical Features" area to highlight important points. Bibliographic references contain PubMed PMID numbers. The revised nineteenth edition includes new references and websites. There are four new chapters: "Child & Adolescent Psychiatric Disorders," "Sports Medicine," "Rehabilitation Medicine," and "Pain Management and Palliative Care." Eight chapters had major revisions: "The Newborn Infant," "Immunization," "Poisoning," "Oral Medicine and Dentistry," "Cardiovascular Diseases," "Gastrointestinal Tract," "Infections: Bacterial & Spirochetal," and "Infections: Parasitic & Mycotic." *CDTP* is a *Doody's Core Titles* essential purchase recommendation and a Brandon/Hill selection.

Drennan's The Child's Foot and Ankle. 2nd ed. Editors: James J. McCarthy, James C. Drennan. Lippincott, Williams & Wilkins, 2010.
See Chapter 19. Podiatry

Handbook of Common Poisonings in Children. 4th ed. American Academy of Pediatrics, 2010.
See Chapter 17.8.2. Forensic Toxicology

The Harriet Lane Handbook: A Manual for Pediatric House Officers. 18th ed. Editors: Jason W. Custer, Rachel

E. Rau. Mosby/Elsevier, 2009.
http://www.mdconsult.com/
ISBN: 9780323053037
Recommended for: Hospital, Academic Libraries
Brandon/Hill, *Doody's Core Titles* Selection

The Harriet Lane Handbook had its start in 1953 when Chief Resident Harrison Spencer suggested that residents compile a pocket-sized "pearl book." Residents met around a table in the Harriet Lane Home, and the result was an easy-to-use manual that has helped pediatricians for over 50 years. This comprehensive book is designed for pediatric house staff, and it continues to be updated and revised by house officers. It serves as a handy reference for bedside consultation. Well-worn copies of *Harriet Lane* continue to poke out of many lab coat pockets. The book is divided into four sections: "Pediatric Acute Care," "Diagnostic and Therapeutic Information," "Reference," and "Formulary." The formulary is regularly updated online for drugs and dosages. Chapters are organized in a modified outline format, with 120 illustrations and over 50 color plates. Charts, tables, figures, and boxed areas highlight information for the reader throughout the book. The eighteenth edition offers a new chapter on palliative care. The most current recommendations and treatments are reflected in updated chapters for "Nutrition and Growth," "Poisonings," "Pediatric Life Support," "Pulmonology," and "Microbiology and Infectious Disease." A chart for Reach Out and Read milestones has been added to the "Behavior and Development" chapter. In addition to the print version, individuals can access the complete contents of the book online, fully searchable with downloadable images, through Elsevier's Expert Consult and PDA. Institutional online access is offered through MD Consult. *Doody's Review Service* assigned this title a five-star rating; it was also a Brandon/Hill selection.

Kendig's Disorders of the Respiratory Tract in Children. 7th ed. Editors: Victor Chernick, Thomas F. Boat, Robert W. Wilmott, Andrew Bush. Elsevier Saunders, 2006.
See Chapter 10.10.8. Pulmonary Disease

Nathan and Oski's Hematology of Infancy and Childhood. 7th ed. Editors: Stuart H. Orkin, David G. Nathan, David Ginsburg, A.T. Look, David E. Fisher, Samuel E. Lux IV. Saunders Elsevier, 2009.
See Chapter 10.10.4. Hematology

Nelson Textbook of Pediatrics. 18th ed. Editors: Robert M. Kliegman, Richard E. Behrman, Hal B. Jenson, Bonita F. Stanton. Saunders/Elsevier, 2007.
http://www.nelsonpediatrics.com/
http://www.mdconsult.com/
ISBN: 9781416024507
See Also Chapter 1.9. Physician Assistants
Recommended for: Hospital, Academic Libraries
Brandon/Hill, *Doody's Core Titles* Selection

The *Nelson Textbook of Pediatrics* has been a gold standard resource for medical students, residents, and physicians for almost 75 years. This comprehensive text represents state-of-the-art care for neonates, children, and adolescents. It incorporates evidence-based medicine and expert commentary from leading, international authors. The eighteenth edition offers a wealth of information in its more than 3,000 pages, 33 parts, and numerous chapters. The book now offers full-color design, figures, and tables to enhance the learning experience and allow content to be located easily. It is greatly reorganized and revised from the earlier edition, and the reader will find new chapters and diseases, more tables, figures, photographs and imaging studies, and updated references for each chapter. A new editor, Bonita F. Stanton, offers an enhanced focus on general pediatrics. Individuals can purchase *Nelson's* as a combined print and online multimedia package. In addition to the fully searchable content of the print edition, the online version offers many other features, such as updates, commentaries, case studies, review and self-assessment questions, and a new "H1N1 Resource Section." There is also an image library that can be used in PowerPoint and other presentations. "Instructions for Patients" are also available online. Institutional online access is offered by MD Consult. The title was selected by both *Doody's Review Service* and Brandon/Hill. A new edition is expected in June 2011.

Oncology of Infancy and Childhood. Editors: Stuart H. Orkin, David E. Fisher, A. Thomas Look, Samuel E. Lux, David Ginsburg, David G. Nathan. Saunders Elsevier, 2009.
See Chapter 10.10.6. Medical Oncology

Oski's Pediatrics: Principles and Practice. 4th ed. Editors: Julia A. McMillan, Ralph D. Feigin, Catherine D. DeAngelis, M. Douglas Jones Jr. Lippincott Williams & Wilkins, 2006.
http://www.ovid.com/
http://www.oskisolution.com/
http://www.r2library.com/
ISBN: 9780781738941
Recommended for: Hospital, Academic Libraries
Brandon/Hill, *Doody's Core Titles* Selection

Oski's Pediatrics: Principles and Practice is a comprehensive guide to the current practice of pediatric care. The book is designed to meet the needs of medical students, residents, and academic and practicing physicians. The book is divided into two parts: "Practice of Pediatrics" and "Diseases of Childhood." The first part consists of six sections and 131 chapters, and the second part is divided into 14 sections and 329 chapters. The appendixes are titled "Pediatrician's Companion: Things You Forget to Remember," which include "Laboratory Values," "Dysmorphology Genetic Syndromes and Associations," "Pediatric Procedures," and "Presenting Signs and Symptoms." Chapters offer numerous tables, figures, and boxes, which are displayed in color and boldface. Suggested readings are included at the end of each chapter, and color plates are provided in the center of the book. The fourth edition includes new chapters on "Genetics and Pediatric Primary Care," "Complementary and Alternative Medicine," "Type 2 Diabetes Mellitus," and "Normal Infant and Childhood Development." The entire section on mental health in children was updated. Both Ovid's LWW Book Collections and R2 Digital Library offer institutional online access to the print edition. Individuals may purchase as a combined print and multimedia package. The multimedia online access is delivered through Oski's Solution integrated website, consisting of the searchable, full-color textbook, image bank, a question bank for board exams preparation and recertification examinations, and access to select articles from LWW's pediatric journals. The title was a Brandon/Hill selection.

Pediatric & Adolescent Gynecology. 5th ed. Editors: S. Jean Herriot Emans, Marc R. Laufer, Donald P. Goldstein. Lippincott Williams & Wilkins, 2005.
See Chapter 9.1. Adolescent Medicine, Chapter 11.2. Gynecology

Pediatric Clinical Practice Guidelines & Policies: A Compendium of Evidence-Based Research for Pediatric Practice. 9th ed. American Academy of Pediatrics, 2009.
http://online.statref.com/titleinfo/fxid-310.html
ISBN: 9781581103427
Recommended for: Hospital, Academic Libraries
Brandon/Hill Selection

The book's title, *Pediatric Clinical Practice Guidelines & Policies: A Compendium of Evidence-Based Research for Pediatric Practice*, provides an accurate description of its contents. This complete collection of practice guidelines and policies issued and endorsed by the American Academy of Pediatrics (AAP) is a useful resource for medical students, residents, physicians, nurses, and allied health professionals. The book is divided into five sections: "Clinical Practice Guidelines from the AAP," "Endorsed Clinical Practice Guidelines," "2008 Policies from the AAP," "Current Policies from the AAP," and "Endorsed Policies." Policy statements include clinical and technical reports. Appendixes include policies listed by committee and AAP acronyms. The book contains more than 30 clinical practice guidelines and over 380 policy statements, clinical reports, and technical reports. "Quick Reference Tools" include patient education handouts and *ICD-9-CM* coding tips displayed in a boxed format. The ninth edition contains more than 40 new or revised AAP policy statements and a new clinical practice guideline on seizures. This edition also includes a fully searchable CD-ROM and an activation code for mobile device download. Mobile device access includes the complete clinical practice guidelines, point-and-click algorithms, and a bilirubin risk-assessment tool. Instructions and technical support contact information is included. *Doody's Review Service* assigned this work a four-star rating; it was also a Brandon/Hill selection.

Pediatric Critical Care. 3rd ed. Editors: Bradley P. Fuhrman, Jerry J. Zimmerman. Mosby/Elsevier, 2006.
http://www.mdconsult.com/
http://www.sciencedirect.com/science/book/9780323018081
ISBN: 9780323018081
Recommended for: Hospital, Academic Libraries
Brandon/Hill, *Doody's Core Titles* Selection

Pediatric Critical Care is a standard text for pediatric intensive care units and serves as a great resource for medical students, residents, fellows, and practicing physicians. Contributors include physicians, nurses, and pharmacists, resulting in a comprehensive overview of care for the critically ill child. The book is divided into 119 chapters contained within seven parts: "Discipline," "Organ System Function and Failure," "Environmental Hazards," "Trauma," "Pharmacology," "Anesthesia and Analgesia," and "Cardiopulmonary Resuscitation." The bulk of the text covers organ systems and a full range of diseases. Numerous tables and figures are included, and each chapter begins with clinical pearls. Color plates follow the table of contents. The completely revised third edition includes a new section on "Failure of Organ Systems." New chapters were added that cover congenital malformations of the brain and spinal cord, gastrointestinal pharmacology, and diagnostic and therapeutic cardiac catheterization. *Doody's Review Service* assigned this title a four-star rating; it was also a Brandon/Hill selection.

Pediatric Environmental Health. 2nd ed. Editors: Ruth A. Etzel, Sophie J. Balk, American Academy of Pediatrics

Committee on Environmental Health. American Academy of Pediatrics, 2003.
See Chapter 5. Environmental Health

Pediatric Ophthalmology and Strabismus. 2nd ed. Editors: Kenneth W. Wright, Peter H. Spiegel. Springer, 2003.
See Chapter 11.5. Ophthalmology

Principles and Practice of Pediatric Neurosurgery. 2nd ed. Editors: A.L. Albright, Ian F. Pollack, P.D. Adelson. Thieme Medical, 2008.
See Chapter 11.3. Neurosurgery

Principles and Practice of Pediatric Oncology. 6th ed. Editors: Philip A. Pizzo, David G. Poplack. Wolters Kluwer/Lippincott Williams & Wilkins, 2011.
See Chapter 10.10.6. Medical Oncology

Red Book: 2009 Report of the Committee on Infectious Diseases. 28th ed. Editors: Committee on Infectious Diseases, American Academy of Pediatrics, Larry K. Pickering, Carol J. Baker, David W. Kimberlin, Sarah S. Long. American Academy of Pediatrics, 2009.
http://aapredbook.aappublications.org/
http://online.statref.com/titleinfo/fxid-76.html
http://www.r2library.com/
ISBN: 9781581103069
See Also Chapter 10.16. Public Health
Recommended for: Hospital, Academic Libraries
Doody's Core Titles Selection

Red Book: Report of the Committee on Infectious Diseases is developed by the American Academy of Pediatrics Committee on Infectious Diseases in conjunction with the Centers for Disease Control and Prevention, the Food and Drug Administration, the National Institutes of Health, the Canadian Paediatric Society, the World Health Organization, and many other organizations. These guidelines for the control of infectious diseases in children are developed and revised approximately every three years. The *Red Book* is a unique source of information on immunizations and infectious diseases for medical students, residents, physicians, and other health professionals who treat infants, children, and adolescents. The book is divided into five sections: "Active and Passive Immunization," "Recommendations for Care of Children in Special Circumstances," "Summaries of Infectious Diseases," "Antimicrobial Agents and Related Therapy," and "Antimicrobial Prophylaxis." There are twelve appendixes with additional information. The book also includes a "Summary of Major Changes," which offers providers practical guidance. The 2009 edition updates all chapters and sections. It contains a new chapter on Fusobacterium infections, the 2009 "AAP Standards for Child and Adolescent Immunization Practices," the latest on the HPV vaccines, updated information on hepatitis A and hepatitis B, and much more. In addition to online access through STAT!Ref and R2 Digital Library, the AAP offers a more comprehensive online version and a mobile version for smartphones. AAP site licenses are available. The online version from the AAP is continually updated with new information that becomes available during the three years between editions of the hard copy, including new immunization schedules and H1N1 flu resources. The online Visual Library allows access to more than 2,000 images. Archival access to past editions of the *Red Book* is also provided. The title carries an essential purchase rating from *Doody's Review Service.*

Rudolph's Pediatrics. 22nd ed. Editors: Colin D. Rudolph, Abraham M. Rudolph, George Lister, Lewis First, Anne Gershon. McGraw-Hill, 2011.
ISBN: 9780071497237
Recommended for: Hospital, Academic Libraries
Brandon/Hill Selection

Rudolph's Pediatrics was originally published in 1897 as *Diseases of Infancy and Childhood.* The work, now in full color, has continually evolved and adapted over the years, becoming an indispensable resource for medical students, residents, and practicing and/or teaching physicians. This review refers to the twenty-first edition. The book is divided into 27 chapters, and most chapters contain sections on evaluating symptom presentations. Tables and figures are used extensively in each chapter. Twenty-six color plates follow the chapters, and the appendixes include "Growth Charts," "Changes in Growth over Time," and "Blood Pressure Nomograms." Three new coeditors helped to greatly revise the twenty-first edition. New associate editors reorganized the 27 chapters. A new chapter on contemporary diagnostic techniques was added, and the chapter on emergency medicine and critical care replaced the chapter on toxicology and accidents. The chapter on ethical issues now includes discussions on palliative care and coping with the dying child. The chapter on genetic disorders expanded into two new chapters covering metabolic disorders, genetics, and dysmorphology. The new look of the book, and the new coverage, ensures that *Rudolph's* will continue to be a valued resource for years to come. *Doody's Review Service* assigned the title a four-star rating; it was also a Brandon/Hill selection.

Smith's Recognizable Patterns of Human Malformation. 6th ed. Author: Kenneth L. Jones. Elsevier/Saunders, 2006.
ISBN: 9780721606156
Recommended for: Hospital, Academic Libraries
Doody's Core Titles Selection

Smith's Recognizable Patterns of Human Malformation is a valuable resource in the area of genetics for neonatologists, perinatologists, pediatricians, obstetricians, geneticists, and genetic counselors. The text is devoted to patterns of malformations, not deformations caused by mechanical factors. The book is divided into six chapters, with the first chapter ("Recognizable Patterns of Malformation") comprising the bulk of the resource. This chapter is further subdivided into different classes of syndromes, disorders, and defects, which are then arranged alphabetically for easy reference. Other chapters include "Genetics," "Genetic Counseling," and "Normal Standards." There are two appendixes: "Pattern of Malformation Differential Diagnosis by Anomalies" and "Nomenclature for Chromosomal Syndromes." An embryonic development chart is found on the inside front cover, and a fetal development chart is on the inside back cover. Each chapter includes a description of the specific abnormality, occasional abnormalities, natural history, etiology, and references. There are over 1,400 photographs and figures. The sixth edition was the first to include full color photographs and illustrations. The book provides new information on the molecular basis of malformations and includes 16 additional common disorders. *Doody's Review Service* assigned the title a four-star rating.

Journals

Archives of Disease in Childhood. v. 1, BMJ, 1926.
http://adc.bmj.com
http://www.ncbi.nlm.nih.gov/pmc/journals/150/
ISSN: 00036888
ISSN: 14682044 (Online)
Indexed in: MEDLINE, CINAHL
Recommended for: Hospital, Academic Libraries

In publication since 1926, *Archives of Disease in Childhood* is the official journal of the Royal College of Paediatrics and Child Health. The journal is oriented toward pediatricians, researchers, and allied health professionals. It focuses on all aspects of child health and disease through adolescence. It is published 12 times per year, plus supplements. There is also a "Fetal and Neonatal" edition. *Archives of Disease in Childhood* ranks twelfth of the 94 pediatrics journals included in the 2009 *Journal Citation Reports*, with an impact factor of 2.657. It is indexed in MEDLINE, Web of Science, and Embase. Coverage includes pediatrics, community health, epidemiology, advocacy, and ethics. In addition to original research reports, the journal offers short reports, evidence reports, commentaries, images in pediatrics, and commissioned editorials, viewpoints, and reviews. The journal includes a "Paediatric and Perinatal Drug Therapy (PPDT)" section four times a year. Online coverage is available through BMJ Journals back to 1926. The online version also offers e-mail alerts and news feeds. Online submission is available for authors.

Archives of Pediatrics & Adolescent Medicine. v. 148, American Medical Association, 1994.
http://archpedi.ama-assn.org/
ISSN: 10724710
ISSN: 15383628 (Online)
See Also Chapter 9.1. Adolescent Medicine
Indexed in: MEDLINE, CINAHL
Recommended for: Hospital, Academic Libraries
Brandon/Hill Selection

Archives of Pediatrics & Adolescent Medicine, formerly known as the *American Journal of Diseases of Children* and various other titles, dates back to 1911 and is the oldest, continuously published pediatric journal in the United States. It is published 12 times per year. This international, peer-reviewed journal is oriented toward physicians and health care professionals who care for children and adolescents. The journal focuses on adolescent health, the education of pediatric health care professionals, disease prevention, and health promotion. *Archives* has the second highest impact factor (4.726) of the 94 pediatrics journals indexed in the 2009 *Journal Citation Reports*. In addition to original, peer-reviewed research, the journal offers editorials, reviews by experts, practice commentaries, case quizzes, and updates on clinical science and practice management. Full online coverage is available back to volume 1, 1911.

Journal of Pediatric and Adolescent Gynecology. v. 9, Elsevier, 1996.
See Chapter 9.1. Adolescent Medicine, Chapter 11.2. Gynecology

Journal of Pediatric Gastroenterology and Nutrition. v. 1, Lippincott Williams & Wilkins, 1982.
See Chapter 14.1. Child Nutrition Sciences

Journal of Pediatrics. v. 1, Elsevier/Mosby, 1932.
http://www.sciencedirect.com/science/journal/00223476
http://www.mdconsult.com/

ISSN: 00223476
ISSN: 10976833 (Online)
Indexed in: MEDLINE, CINAHL
Recommended for: Hospital, Academic Libraries
Brandon/Hill Selection

The *Journal of Pediatrics*, which began in 1932, remains a premier journal for pediatricians. While oriented toward practicing physicians treating infants, children, and adolescents, it is also a valuable resource for medical students, interns, and residents. The monthly journal ranks fourth of the 94 pediatric journals included in the 2009 *Journal Citation Reports*, with an impact factor of 4.092. The *Journal of Pediatrics* is indexed in MEDLINE and CINAHL, in addition to other major abstracting and indexing services. In addition to original, peer-reviewed research, the journal offers editorials, invited and other commentaries, reviews of medical progress, clinical and laboratory observations, grand rounds and clinicopathologic conferences, current best evidence, notes from the Association of Medical School Pediatric Department Chairs (AMSPDC), and special articles and supplements. Full online coverage is available through ScienceDirect back to volume 1, 1932. The online version also offers saved search alerts, citation alerts, and electronic table of contents alerts, which deliver the table of contents directly to the reader's e-mail.

Pediatric Clinics of North America. v. 1, Elsevier/Saunders, 1954.
http://www.mdconsult.com/
http://www.sciencedirect.com/science/journal/00313955
ISSN: 00313955
ISSN: 15578240 (Online)
Indexed in: MEDLINE, CINAHL
Recommended for: Hospital, Academic Libraries
Brandon/Hill Selection

Under the guidance of a guest editor, each issue of *Pediatric Clinics* focuses on a single topic relevant to the diagnosis and management of diseases of children. Authors are invited to participate in specific issues. This quarterly journal is a valuable resource for pediatricians and family practice physicians. With an impact factor of 1.587, *Pediatric Clinics* is ranked forty-second among 94 pediatrics journals included in the 2009 *Journal Citation Reports*. It is indexed in MEDLINE, CINAHL, BIOSIS, and other major abstracting and indexing services. Institutional online coverage is available through MD Consult Core Clinics and ScienceDirect back to 1996. Online access for individuals is provided through Elsevier's The Clinics at http://www.pediatric.theclinics.com, which offers pediatric CME and saved search and e-mail alerts.

Pediatric Dermatology. v. 1, Wiley-Blackwell, 1983.
See Chapter 10.3. Dermatology

Pediatrics. v. 1, American Academy of Pediatrics, 1948.
http://pediatrics.aappublications.org
ISSN: 00314005
ISSN: 10984275 (Online)
See Also Chapter 13.18. School Nursing
Indexed in: MEDLINE, CINAHL
Recommended for: Hospital, Academic Libraries
Brandon/Hill Selection

Begun in 1948, *Pediatrics* is the official, peer-reviewed journal of the American Academy of Pediatrics (AAP). *Pediatrics* is oriented toward pediatricians and family practice physicians. Contributions relevant to pediatrics are also included from disciplines such as nutrition, surgery, dentistry, public health, genetics, psychology, sociology, and nursing. This monthly publication has the third highest impact factor (4.687) of the 94 pediatrics journals indexed in the 2009 *Journal Citation Reports* (*JCR*). The journal is one of the top 100 most-cited publications in science and medicine. According to *JCR*, *Pediatrics* received 46,408 citations in 2008, more than any other pediatrics journal. It is indexed in MEDLINE, and other major abstracting and indexing services. In addition to original, peer-reviewed research, the journal offers review articles, special articles, commentaries, case reports, state-of-the-art reviews, editorials, and updates from the AAP. The Academy and HighWire Press provide full online coverage back to volume 1, 1948. The online version offers free e-mail alerts with a table of contents, keywords, and article citations. Other e-mail alerts, RSS feeds, and a Facebook page are offered.

10.13.1. Neonatology

The newborn infant.
—MeSH

Contributor: Kathy Zeblisky

Monographs

Avery's Neonatology: Pathophysiology & Management of the Newborn. 6th ed. Editors: Mhairi G. MacDonald, Martha D. Mullett, Mary M.K. Seshia. Lippincott Williams & Wilkins, 2005.
http://www.ovid.com/
ISBN: 9780781746434
Recommended for: Hospital, Academic Libraries
Brandon/Hill Selection

Gordon B. Avery, the original editor of *Avery's Neonatology: Pathophysiology & Management of the Newborn*, began planning the book in 1972. It is now in its sixth edition with new editors, but it remains an authoritative text on clinical care of the newborn for medical students, residents, and practicing physicians. The editors' goal is to assist those in training with the six general medical competencies defined by the Accreditation Council for Graduate Medical Education (ACGME). These competencies are patient care, clinical science, practice-based learning and improvement, interpersonal skills and communication, professionalism, and systems-based medicine. Organized around clinical problems, the text is divided into seven parts: "General Considerations," "The Fetal Patient," "Transition and Stabilization," "The Low-Birth-Weight Infant," "The Newborn Infant," "Pharmacology," and "Beyond the Nursery." There are numerous appendixes. Tables and figures enhance learning, and there is a small section of color plates in the front of the book. The sixth edition contains 60 chapters, all extensively revised. Eight chapters have new authors, and there are three new chapters: "Breast Feeding," "Infection Control in the NICU," and "Telehealth in Neonatology." An online version of the print edition is available via various Ovid/Lippincott Williams & Wilkins' book collections. The title was a Brandon/Hill selection.

Fanaroff and Martin's Neonatal-Perinatal Medicine: Diseases of the Fetus and Infant. 9th ed. Editors: Richard J. Martin, Avroy A. Fanaroff, Michele C. Walsh. Mosby/Elsevier, 2011.
See Chapter 10.13.2. Perinatology

Guidelines for Perinatal Care. 6th ed. American Academy of Pediatrics [and] American College of Obstetricians and Gynecologists, 2007.
See Chapter 10.13.2. Perinatology, Chapter 11.4. Obstetrics

Manual of Neonatal Care. 6th ed. Editors: John P. Cloherty, Eric C. Eichenwald, Ann R. Stark. Lippincott Williams & Wilkins, 2008.
http://www.ovid.com/
http://www.r2library.com/
ISBN: 9780781769846
Recommended for: Hospital, Academic Libraries
Brandon/Hill Selection

The *Manual of Neonatal Care* is part of the *Spiral Manual* series, providing a comprehensive but quick reference for the evaluation and management of fetal and neonatal conditions. The book contains 37 chapters focusing on maternal, fetal, and neonatal topics ranging from fetal assessment to common neonatal procedures. The sixth edition includes updated information on fetal assessment, new guidelines for managing neonatal jaundice, and new data on perinatal asphyxia. Well-used appendixes include "Common NICU Medication Guidelines," "Effect of Maternal Drugs on the Fetus," and "Maternal Medications and Breastfeeding." Neonatal resuscitation guidelines are found on the inside covers. Intubation/sedation guidelines are also included. The outline format makes it easy to find information, and the many figures and tables enhance learning. *Doody's Review Service* supplied this work with a three-star rating; it was also a former Brandon/Hill selection.

Merenstein & Gardner's Handbook of Neonatal Intensive Care. 7th ed. Editors: Sandra L. Gardner, Brian S. Carter, Mary I. Enzman-Hines, Jacinto A. Hernandez. Mosby/Elsevier, 2011.
ISBN: 9780323067157
Recommended for: Hospital, Academic Libraries
Brandon/Hill Selection

The *Handbook of Neonatal Intensive Care* is a standard reference for neonatal nurses. The book is coedited by a nurse and a physician who emphasize the importance of collaborative care in the neonatal intensive care unit. This multidisciplinary focus also applies to the contributors, making the text appropriate for nurses, nursing students, medical students, pediatricians, and family practitioners. The book is divided into six units covering 32 chapters: "Evidence-Based Practice," "Support of the Neonate," "Metabolic and Nutritional Care of the Neonate," "Infection and Hematologic Diseases of the Neonate," "Common Systemic Diseases of the Neonate," and "Psychosocial Aspects of Neonatal Care." Tables and figures are displayed in color for easy reference. Boxed information displays crucial clinical information and critical findings in boldface, colored type. Sections addressing parent teaching are included in relevant chapters, which highlight post-discharge care. Parent resources are also included in the references section of appropriate chapters, and website references are provided when applicable. The book is a Brandon/Hill nursing list selection. This review refers to the sixth edition.

Neonatology: Management, Procedures, On-Call Problems, Diseases, and Drugs. 6th ed. Editors: Tricia Lacy Gomella, M. Douglas Cunningham, Fabien G. Eyal. McGraw-Hill, 2009.
http://online.statref.com/titleinfo/fxid-113.html
http://www.r2library.com/ (Forthcoming)
ISBN: 9780071544313

Recommended for: Hospital, Academic Libraries
Brandon/Hill, *Doody's Core Titles* Selection

Neonatology: Management, Procedures, On-Call Problems, Diseases, and Drugs has been a comprehensive, pocket-sized guide for neonatologists and pediatricians for over 20 years. The book has five sections: "Basic Management," "Procedures," "On-Call Problems," "Diseases and Disorders," and "Neonatal Pharmacology." The chapters in all sections but "Basic Management" are now arranged alphabetically so that topics can be found quickly. An outline approach highlights essential information, as do numerous tables and figures. The appendixes include popular information such as abbreviations, Apgar scoring, blood pressure determinations, chartwork, growth charts, isolation guidelines, temperature conversion tables, and a weight conversion table. The sixth edition has been updated and revised, with new chapters on "Newborn Screening," "Blood Component Therapy," "Management of the Late Preterm Infant," and "Complementary and Alternative Medical Therapies in Neonatology." The very popular "On-Call Problems" section presents 33 common and serious patient problems, including a new chapter on "Rash and Dermatologic Problems." The pharmacology section has also been extensively revised and includes a large selection of commonly used medications. *Doody's Review Service* supplied a three-star rating; *Neonatology* was also a Brandon/Hill selection.

Neurology of the Newborn. 5th ed. Author: Joseph J. Volpe. Elsevier, 2008.
See Chapter 10.11. Neurology

Smith's Recognizable Patterns of Human Malformation. 6th ed. Author: Kenneth L. Jones. Elsevier/Saunders, 2006.
See Chapter 10.13. Pediatrics

Journals

Archives of Disease in Childhood: Fetal & Neonatal Edition. v. 70, BMJ, 1994.
See Chapter 10.13.2. Perinatology

Clinics in Perinatology. v. 1, Saunders Elsevier, 1974.
See Chapter 11.4. Obstetrics

Journal of Pediatrics. v. 1, Elsevier/Mosby, 1932.
See Chapter 10.13. Pediatrics

Pediatrics. v. 1, American Academy of Pediatrics, 1948.
See Chapter 10.13. Pediatrics, Chapter 13.18. School Nursing

10.13.2. Perinatology

The fetus and infant during the perinatal period. The perinatal period begins with the twenty-eighth week of gestation and ends twenty-eight days after birth.

—MeSH

Contributor: Kathy Zeblisky

Monographs

Fanaroff and Martin's Neonatal-Perinatal Medicine: Diseases of the Fetus and Infant. 9th ed. Editors: Richard J. Martin, Avroy A. Fanaroff, Michele C. Walsh. Mosby/Elsevier, 2011.
http://www.mdconsult.com/
ISBN: 9780323065450
Recommended for: Hospital, Academic Libraries
Brandon/Hill, *Doody's Core Titles* Selection

Fanaroff and Martin's Neonatal-Perinatal Medicine is a two-volume textbook that strives to cover developments in both neonatal and perinatal medicine. The editors rely on a large group of international contributors to make this valuable resource a success. The first volume focuses on "The Field of Neonatal-Perinatal Medicine," "Fetus," "Pregnancy Disorders," "Delivery Room," and "Provisions for Neonatal Care." The second volume addresses "Development and Disorders of Organ Systems"; it also includes the appendixes that contain sections on "Therapeutic Agents," "Tables of Normal Values," and "Schedule for Immunization of Preterm Infants." Tables, figures, and boxes are used throughout the volumes to highlight information. Over 800 illustrations are included. The eighth edition focuses on evidence-based medicine and attempts to consolidate results of the Cochrane Database, meta-analyses, and multicenter, randomized trials. Guidelines and committee standards have been included or referenced. Chapters were extensively rewritten, and new chapters were included: "Legal Issues in Neonatal-Perinatal Medicine," "Neonatology in Developing Countries," "Role of Positive Pressure Ventilation in Neonatal Resuscitation," "Chest Compressions," "Environmental Influences," and "Hypoxic-Ischemic Encephalopathy." The print book includes a CD-ROM for access to the illustrations, which may be downloaded to the user's presentations. The title is a *Doody's* and a Brandon/Hill selection. This review refers to the eighth edition.

Guidelines for Perinatal Care. 6th ed. American Academy of Pediatrics/American College of Obstetricians and Gynecologists, 2007.

http://www.r2library.com/
ISBN: 9781581102703
See Also Chapter 11.4. Obstetrics
Recommended for: Hospital, Academic Libraries
Doody's Core Titles Selection

Guidelines for Perinatal Care is a joint project by the American Academy of Pediatrics (AAP) and the American College of Obstetricians and Gynecologists (ACOG). It contains the latest recommendations, policies, and best practices from the AAP and ACOG. The audience is "all personnel who are involved in the care of pregnant women, their fetuses, and their neonates in community programs, hospitals, and medical centers." The guidelines are used by physicians and other providers, administrators, facilities personnel, and even architects. The book includes ten chapters: "Organization of Perinatal Health Care," "Inpatient Perinatal Care Services," "Interhospital Care of the Perinatal Patient," "Antepartum Care," "Intrapartum and Postpartum Care of the Mother," "Obstetric and Medical Complications," "Care of the Neonate," "Neonatal Complications," "Perinatal Infections," and "Infection Control." Numerous appendixes provide additional information. The chapter on "Inpatient Perinatal Care Services" is especially popular as it defines Level I, Level II, and Level III care and their required components. The revised sixth edition contains new information and addresses evidence-based data to optimize regionalized care. The book provides updated recommendations for conducting perinatal care in a hospital setting and discusses quality improvement and patient-safety initiatives, with an emphasis on communication, team training, and hospital redesign strategies. *Doody's Review Service* supplied this work with a four-star rating.

Smith's Recognizable Patterns of Human Malformation. 6th ed. Author: Kenneth L. Jones. Elsevier/Saunders, 2006.
See Chapter 10.13. Pediatrics

Journals

Archives of Disease in Childhood: Fetal & Neonatal Edition. v. 70, BMJ, 1994.
http://adc.bmj.com
http://www.ncbi.nlm.nih.gov/pmc/journals/151/
ISSN: 13592998
ISSN: 14682052 (Online)
Indexed in: MEDLINE, CINAHL
Recommended for: Hospital, Academic Libraries

Archives of Disease in Childhood began in 1926 as the official journal of the Royal College of Paediatrics and Child Health. The *Fetal & Neonatal Edition* began in 1994. The journal is published six times per year, along with supplements. *Fetal & Neonatal* ranks sixteenth among 94 pediatrics journals included in the 2009 *Journal Citation Reports*, with an impact factor of 2.493. It is indexed in MEDLINE, Web of Science, and Embase. Journal contents include fetal and neonatal physiology and clinical practice, genetics, perinatal epidemiology, and neurodevelopmental outcomes. In addition to original research reports, the journal offers short reports, evidence reports, commentaries, images in pediatrics, and commissioned editorials, viewpoints, and reviews. Online coverage is available through BMJ Journals back to 1994. The online version also offers e-mail alerts and news feeds.

Birth: Issues in Perinatal Care. v. 9, Wiley-Blackwell, 1982.
See Chapter 11.4. Obstetrics

Clinics in Perinatology. v. 1, Elsevier/Saunders, 1974.
http://www.sciencedirect.com/science/journal/00955108
http://www.mdconsult.com/
ISSN: 00955108
ISSN: 15579840 (Online)
See Also Chapter 11.4. Obstetrics
Indexed in: MEDLINE, CINAHL
Recommended for: Hospital, Academic Libraries

Clinics in Perinatology is published quarterly, with each issue focusing on a single topic in perinatology under the guidance of a guest editor. Authors are invited to participate in specific issues. This journal is a valuable resource for perinatologists, pediatricians, and family practice physicians. *Clinics in Perinatology* has an impact factor of 1.543, ranking forty-fifth among 94 pediatrics journals indexed in the 2009 *Journal Citation Reports*. It is indexed in MEDLINE, CINAHL, BIOSIS, and other major abstracting and indexing services. Institutional online access is available through MD Consult Core Clinics and ScienceDirect back to 2000. Individual online access is available through Elsevier's The Clinics at http://www.perinatology.theclinics.com, which offers saved search and e-mail alerts, RSS feeds, and pediatric CME.

Journal of Perinatology. v. 4, Nature Publishing Group, 1984.
http://www.nature.com/jp
ISSN: 07438346

ISSN: 14765543 (Online)
Indexed in: MEDLINE, CINAHL
Recommended for: Hospital, Academic Libraries

The *Journal of Perinatology* began in 1981 as the *Journal of the California Perinatal Association*. It is the official journal of the American Academy of Pediatrics Section of Perinatal Pediatrics and the official publication of the National Perinatal Association. The monthly journal is oriented toward participants in perinatal/neonatal care, including neonatologists, perinatologists, pediatricians, obstetricians/gynecologists, neonatal and perinatal nurses, respiratory therapists, pharmacists, social workers, and nutritionists. With an impact factor of 1.593, the *Journal of Perinatology* ranks fortieth among 94 pediatrics journals indexed in the 2009 *Journal Citation Reports*. It is indexed in MEDLINE, CINAHL, and Embase, in addition to other major abstracting and indexing services. Coverage includes maternal and fetal medicine, neonatal medicine, and follow up of the infant and child. In addition to peer-reviewed, clinical research articles, the journal offers state-of-the-art reviews, commentaries, letters to the editor, and communications such as case reports and educational vignettes. Online coverage is available through the publisher back to 1999. The online version also offers table of contents alerts and RSS feeds. Online submission is available for authors.

Pediatrics. v. 1, American Academy of Pediatrics, 1948. *See* Chapter 10.13. Pediatrics, Chapter 13.18. School Nursing

Seminars in Perinatology. v. 1, Elsevier/Saunders, 1977.
http://www.sciencedirect.com/science/journal/01460005
http://www.seminperinat.com
ISSN: 01460005
ISSN: 1558075X (Online)
Indexed in: MEDLINE, CINAHL
Recommended for: Hospital, Academic Libraries

Seminars in Perinatology is published six times per year, with each issue focused on a single topic of interest. The journal is a valuable resource for "professionals who care for the mother, the fetus, and the newborn," who include perinatologists, obstetricians, pediatricians, and students. With an impact factor of 2.333, *Seminars in Perinatology* ranks nineteenth of the 94 pediatrics journals indexed in the 2009 *Journal Citation Reports*. It is indexed in MEDLINE, and other major abstracting and indexing services. ScienceDirect provides online coverage back to volume 19, 1995. The fully searchable online version includes volume and issue alerts. Online submission is available for authors.

10.14. Physical Medicine and Rehabilitation

The use of physical agents, mechanical apparatus, and manipulation in rehabilitating physically diseased or injured patients.

—MeSH

Contributor: Paul M. Blobaum

Monographs

Alternative Medicine and Rehabilitation: A Guide for Practitioners. Authors: Stanley F. Wainapel, Avital Fast. Demos, 2003.
ISBN: 9781888799668
Recommended for: Hospital, Academic, Consumer Health Libraries

Wainapel and Fast have assembled a team of expert physicians and other professionals to describe unconventional therapies under prevalent use for physical conditions seen in the rehabilitation setting, and examine the research evidence to support or disprove their efficacy. It is not a "how to" book, or a comprehensive survey of alternative therapies. It is meant to be a handbook for those practitioners who are interested in adding one or more complementary methods to their care methods, based on a critical study of the evidence. With this disclaimer, the book succeeds in looking at therapies considered "unconventional" to the allopathic medical establishment, including osteopathic manipulative interventions, chiropractic, Tai Chi Chuan, accupuncture, yoga, biofeedback, and others. Helpful chapters discuss the alternative medicine research programs of the NIH, approaches to reading the complementary and alternative medicine literature, integrating modalities into practice, and reimbursement issues. This text is recommended for specialized, hospital, academic, and consumer health libraries.

Essentials of Physical Medicine and Rehabilitation: Musculoskeletal Disorders, Pain, and Rehabilitation. 2nd ed. Editors: Walter R. Frontera, Julie K. Silver, Thomas D. Rizzo. Saunders Elsevier, 2008.
http://www.mdconsult.com/
ISBN: 9781416040071
Recommended for: Hospital, Academic, Consumer Health Libraries
Brandon/Hill, *Doody's Core Titles* Selection

In the introduction, Dr. Frontera writes that this book is intended for "the average internist/family practitioner, physiatrist, orthopedist, rheumatologist, and neurologist, addressing conditions that present in practice," but this book has a larger audience of sports medicine physicians, residents, students, nurse practitioners, and other allied health professionals, and patients. Contributions to the second edition come from over 175 experts, nearly all of whom are allopathic and osteopathic physicians, and focus on ambulatory care settings, with the recognition that hospitalization is sometimes indicated. The multidisciplinary focus of the book is revealed by the credentials of the authors. Six of the contributors have physical therapy degrees, and half of these authors also have DO or MD degrees; but the other half are co-authors with MDs or DOs. Five podiatrists contributed to the section on foot and ankle problems. The text is divided into three main sections. Part I, "Musculoskeletal Disorders," treats each topic succinctly and comprehensively with definitions, symptoms including physical examination and diagnostic studies, and treatment. Part II, "Pain" is new to this edition, and distinguishes this book from comparable textbooks. It contains a discussion of the criteria necessary for patients to qualify for social security disability based on debilitating chronic pain. Part III covers rehabilitation. This book is available online through Elsevier's MD Consult, and is the only physical medicine and rehabilitation title included in that venue. Brandon/Hill identified this book as a core medical title. It is recommended for specialized, hospital, consumer health, and academic libraries.

Exercise in Rehabilitation Medicine. 2nd ed. Editor: Walter R. Frontera. Human Kinetics, 2006.
ISBN: 9780736055413
Recommended for: Hospital, Academic Libraries
Doody's Core Titles Selection

Dr. Frontera, states that the objective of the first edition of this text was to present the basic science and clinical correlates of exercise as a therapeutic and rehabilitative intervention strategy. The second edition updates these presentations with recent research findings and by including more clinical applications. Evidence from research shows that exercise is critical to health and well-being. It is the most important part of therapeutic intervention in disease states and rehabilitation for restoration to community life. This book connects research and basic science principles to clinical practice in a way that is accessible for the non-expert. It is organized in four sections: Part I, "Biological Considerations," discusses the basics of endurance, strength, and flexibility training. Part II, "Special Clinical Considerations," discusses behavioral aspects including protocols for testing, prescription guidelines, and theories and models for exercise promotion. Part III, "Exercise in the Rehabilitation of Specific Diseases and Conditions," comprises the majority of the book. This section is organized by specific disease and impairment states such as spinal cord injury, heart disease, stroke, HIV, obesity, and cancer. Each chapter begins with a case study and discussion, and a comprehensive presentation of clinical issues, therapeutic interventions, recommendations and guidelines, and application of research findings. Part IV, "Specific Patient Populations," discusses the importance of exercise in the aging process and population groups, and assisting the rehabilitation patient who moves on to become an athlete or the disabled athlete who resumes athletic activities following rehabilitative interventions. This book will prove useful for specialists and primary care physicians practicing rehabilitation, exercise physiologists, physical therapists, occupational therapists, nurses, and recreational therapists. At 450 pages, the book is portable and easy to use. It is recommended for academic, specialized, and hospital libraries.

Medical Aspects of Disability: A Handbook for the Rehabilitation Professional. 3rd ed. Editors: Herbert H. Zaretsky, Edwin F. Richter, Myron G. Eisenberg. Springer, 2005.
http://extranet.netlibrary.com/TitleSelect/
ISBN: 9780826179739
Recommended for: Academic Libraries

Medical Aspects of Disability is a recent volume in the *Springer Series on Rehabilitation*. The third edition has been significantly updated from previous editions. Published in black and white with few illustrations and photographs, this book is well indexed and contains extensive bibliographies for each chapter. Part I, "An Introduction to Key Topics and Issues," discusses comprehensive rehabilitation services, and an overview of body systems. Part II, "Disabling Conditions and Disorders," contains chapters about clinical issues which require rehabilitative intervention, including substance abuse, communicative and swallowing disorders, orthopedic problems, and visual impairments. Part III, "Special Topics," is helpful for quick overviews of rehabilitative issues in relationship to alternative therapies, technological devices, legislation and accreditation, and outcomes measurement and quality improvements. Short discussions of social work and rehabilitation are presented. This book is intended for students of physical therapy, speech therapy, social work, psychology, nursing, vocational counseling, therapeutic recreation, and hospital administration, as well as practitioners concerned about the most current information on the etiology, diagnosis, and management of a

physical therapists, speech and language therapists, clinical and rehabilitation psychologists, and physicians. It is recommended for hospitals, academic, and specialized libraries. The journal publishes 24 issues each year, and two supplements, and is indexed in MEDLINE and CINAHL, among others.

Manual Therapy: An International Journal of Musculoskeletal Therapy. v. 1, Churchill Livingstone, 1995.
See Chapter 3. Chiropractic

Journal of Bodywork and Movement Therapies. v. 1, Elsevier, 1996.
See Chapter 3. Chiropractic

Journal of Manipulative and Physiological Therapeutics (JMPT). v. 1, Mosby Elsevier for National University of Health Sciences, 1978.
See Chapter 3. Chiropractic

Journal of Orthopaedic and Sports Physical Therapy (JOSPT). v. 1, Orthopaedic and Sports Physical Therapy Sections of the American Physical Therapy Association, 1979.
See Chapter 1.3. Physical Therapy, Chapter 9.12. Sports Medicine

Journal of Rehabilitation Medicine. v. 33, Foundation for Rehabilitation, 2001.
http://medicaljournals.se/jrm/
ISSN: 16501977
ISSN: 16512081 (Online)
Indexed in: MEDLINE, CINAHL
Recommended for: Hospital, Academic Libraries

Founded in 1969 as a forum for Scandinavian research in rehabilitation, *Journal of Rehabilitation Medicine* has become one of the two top scholarly peer-reviewed rehabilitation journals in all of Europe, according to a 2008 article by Frontera, "Publishing in Physical Medicine and Rehabilitation" (*J Rehabil Med* 2008; 40:161–165). It is the official journal of several societies: the Union of European Medical Specialists (UEMS), European Board of Physical Medicine and Rehabilitation Medicine (EBPMR), the International Society of Physical and Rehabilitation Medicine, and the European Academy of Rehabilitation Medicine. However, the journal has achieved a truly international scope, as over half of the articles originate outside of Europe. The journal is owned and published by a Swedish non-profit organization, the Foundation for Rehabilitation Information. The aim and scope of the journal is to be a broad forum for research in physical medicine, including methodology, clinical research on patient groups, epidemiological studies, and reports on socio-medical aspects of rehabilitation. The journal claims its readership to include a "wide group of healthcare professionals including specialists in rehabilitation medicine, neurology, clinical neurophysiology, general medicine, psychologists, physiotherapists, occupational therapists and social workers." The journal is published monthly with occasional supplements with a not-for-profit motive. Print subscriptions are managed through the publisher; a limited amount of current articles are published for open-access. After 12 months, all articles are available online back to 2001. The journal is indexed in MEDLINE, Embase, and CINAHL. It is recommended for academic, specialized, and hospital libraries, especially those in research settings.

PM & R. v. 1, Elsevier, 2009.
http://www.pmrjournal.org/
ISSN: 19341482
ISSN: 19341563 (Online)
Indexed in: MEDLINE
Recommended for: Hospital, Academic Libraries

PM & R is the official peer-reviewed scientific journal of the American Academy of Physical Medicine and Rehabilitation (AAPM&R). *PM & R* is published monthly, and is already indexed in MEDLINE, a significant accomplishment for a start-up journal. This scholarly journal focuses on injury, function, and rehabilitation. Topics covered include acute and chronic musculoskeletal disorders and pain, neurologic conditions involving the central and peripheral nervous systems, rehabilitation of impairments associated with disabilities in adults and children, and neurophysiology and electrodiagnosis. The journal's website states, "The various sections of the journal will highlight original research including clinical trials and outcomes studies, clinically relevant translational science, comprehensive and focused review articles, case presentations, point/counterpoint discussions and commentary, literature reviews (including structured abstracts and book reviews), ethical legal topics, practice management updates, topical study guides, editorial and opinion pieces, images, clinical pearls and emerging issues."

Spine. v. 1, Lippincott Williams & Wilkins, 1976.
See Chapter 3. Chiropractic

Databases and Other Electronic Resources

Database of International Rehabilitation Research. Center for International Rehabilitation Research Information and Exchange (CIRRIE), 1990.

http://cirrie.buffalo.edu/research.php
Recommended for: Hospital, Academic Libraries

The CIRRIE *Database of International Rehabilitation Research* currently contains almost 90,000 citations of international rehabilitation research published between 1990 and the present. The database includes citations from REHABDATA plus international journals. Searches can be conducted by keyword, author, or by browsing popular research subject headings. Results can be limited by language and country of research origin. The database is open access (free).

International Encyclopedia of Rehabilitation. Center for International Rehabilitation Research Information and Exchange (CIRRIE), Various.
http://cirrie.buffalo.edu/encyclopedia
Recommended for: Hospital, Academic Libraries

The International Encyclopedia of Rehabilitation is a collaborative effort of the Center for International Rehabilitation Research Information and Exchange (CIRRIE), at the University at Buffalo, SUNY, and the Laboratoire d'informatique et de terminologie de la réadaptation et de l'intégation sociale (LITRIS), from the Institut de réadaptation en déficience physique de Québec (IRDPQ). It is a "work in progress," pioneering in reach and scope. The co-editors of the Encyclopedia are Maurice Blouin, the Director of LITRIS, and John Stone, the Director of CIRRIE. They are assisted by their respective staff of rehabilitation terminologists, librarians, and rehabilitation specialists. Currently under development with only 80 articles completed, the encyclopedia is planned to contain four hundred articles on rehabilitation and disability topics identified through terms found in the CIRRIE and REHABDATA Thesauri, the World Health Organization's *International Classification of Functioning, Disability and Health* (*ICF*) and the *International Index and Dictionary of Rehabilitation and Social Integration* (*IIDRIS*). Links among articles and between these information resources will result in a rehabilitation encyclopedia and comprehensive knowledge database publishing in a digital open access format in English, French, and Spanish. Articles are written by subject experts and are intended to be a synthesis of the state of disabilities science, rehabilitative evaluations, and restorative interventions related to social, environmental, and physical aspects of rehabilitation. Articles are peer-reviewed, but the review is non-blinded, consultative, and collaborative. The encyclopedia is limited in that there are no illustrations, charts, or photographs; but articles are accompanied by bibliographies of source material.

REHABDATA. National Rehabilitation Information Center (NARIC), 1956.
http://www.naric.com/research/rehab/
Recommended for: Hospital, Academic, Consumer Health Libraries

According to the NARIC website, "The core mission of the Center is to collect and disseminate the results of research funded by the National Institute on Disability and Rehabilitation Research (NIDRR). Over a quarter of a century, that mission has expanded to providing information services and document delivery to the disability and rehabilitation communities across the United States." REHABDATA is an open-access index database with some full text, containing approximately 69,000 abstracts and 1,300 full-text documents of books, reports, journal articles, and audiovisual materials relating to disability and rehabilitation research. Each item includes bibliographic information, a 250-word abstract, and, when appropriate, information regarding the project that produced the document. This important index spans research from 1956 to the present. The database can be searched through a search form, or by browsing the 2005 Thesaurus. An online tutorial provides instruction on its use. Documents may be obtained through the NARIC document delivery service, or through local academic, public, and hospital libraries. REHABDATA is recommended for hospital, consumer, research, and academic libraries.

The Rehabilitation Provider's Guide to Cultures of the Foreign-Born (CIRRIE Monograph Series). Center for International Rehabilitation Research Information and Exchange (CIRRIE), 2001–2008.
http://cirrie.buffalo.edu/monographs/index.php
Recommended for: Hospital, Academic, Consumer Health Libraries

This important monograph series presents specific information on the cultural beliefs and values for the top 10 countries of origin for major immigrant populations in the United States, according to the U.S. Census Bureau, with additional monographs for Haiti and the Muslim perspective. The 13-volume series is introduced by *Culture Brokering: Providing Culturally Competent Rehabilitation Services to Foreign-Born Persons*. Each monograph presents valuable information on how the culture may view disability and rehabilitation, and how professionals may approach a therapeutic relationship with their clients. Invaluable information includes the history of a particular group's immigration to America and pertinent information about their experiences, the culture's conception of individuality vs. interdependence, role of family members in health and illness, religious beliefs and practices, dietary practices, and health and self-care practices. Bibliographies for further reading are provided by the authors. The titles of the monographs are: *China* (2001), *Cuba* (2002), *Culture Brokering* (2001), *Dominican Republic* (2002), *El Salvador* (2001), *Haiti* (2003), *India* (2001), *Jamaica* (2002), *Korea* (2001), *Mexico* (2001), *Disability and the Muslim Perspective* (2008), *Philippines* (2002), *Vietnam* (2002). The monographs can be accessed online in HTML and PDF formats for free, or print copies can be ordered for $5 per copy from the publisher, with discounts for multiple copies over 25. This series is recommended for consumers, hospital, academic, and specialized library collections.

10.15. Preventive Medicine

Prevention of disease and the promotion and preservation of health in the individual.

—MeSH

Contributors: Paul Elliott Dahl, Mori Lou Higa

Monographs

Epidemiology, Biostatistics, and Preventive Medicine. 3rd ed. Authors: James F. Jekel, David L. Katz, Dorothea Wild, Joann G. Elmore. Elsevier/Saunders, 2007.
http://www.mdconsult.com/
ISBN: 9781416034964
Recommended for: Hospital, Academic Libraries
Brandon/Hill Selection

This textbook addresses the American Board of Preventive Medicine's (ABPM) core competency areas of biostatistics, epidemiology, and clinical preventive medicine. The initial section of this clinically focused work covers basic epidemiologic concepts and principles, sources for epidemiologic data, common research designs, and approaches for understanding errors and improving decisions in clinical medicine. The biostatistics section discusses topics such as statistical interference and hypothesis testing; bivariate and multivariable analysis; and sample size, randomization, and probability theory. The authors supply an introduction to preventive medicine and public health in the last section, including methods of disease prevention and health care policy. The work contains many illustrations, tables summarizing key concepts, and USMLE-style questions and answers. MD Consult offers an institutional online version in its Medical Education Premium Collection or as an a la carte option. Individual purchasers of the textbook receive free access to an online version through Elsevier's STUDENT CONSULT website. The work would benefit academic libraries supporting instructors, undergraduate students, and graduate level students in the areas of preventive medicine and public health; it would also be useful for clinical preventive medicine providers. *Epidemiology, Biostatistics, and Preventive Medicine* is especially useful for students preparing for the USMLE, and the ABPM recommends this text as one of the core preventive medicine review sources for those preparing for the ABPM exams.

Vaccines. 5th ed. Editors: Stanley A. Plotkin, Walter A. Orenstein, Paul A. Offit. Saunders-Elsevier, 2008.
http://www.mdconsult.com/
ISBN: 9781416036111
Recommended for: Hospital, Academic Libraries
Brandon/Hill, *Doody's Core Titles* Selection

This highly respected work is completely revised and updated with the publication of the fifth edition. This comprehensive work covers all aspects of vaccination from development to use in reducing disease. This masterful work is arranged in five sections. Section one provides general information on vaccination. Section two provides detailed information on licensed vaccines; this includes disease background, epidemiology, vaccination results, and public health considerations. Section three chronicles vaccines in development and new vaccine strategies. Section four examines vaccination issues with special population groups. Section five documents public health and regulatory issues across the globe. The book is tastefully illustrated with many useful charts, tables, diagrams, and photographs. The fifth edition also includes access to a companion website that has the full content online. This authoritative work is essential for any hospital collection or academic institutions supporting students in medicine and public health. It is a required resource for public health practitioners. This book was a Brandon/Hill infectious diseases recommendation and received a perfect score of 100 in *Doody's Review Service.*

Wallace/Maxcy-Rosenau-Last Public Health & Preventive Medicine. 15th ed. Editors: Robert B. Wallace, Neal Kohatsu, John M. Last, Ross Brownson. McGraw-Hill Medical, 2008.
See Chapter 10.16. Public Health

Journals

American Journal of Preventive Medicine. v. 1, Elsevier, 1985.

http://sciencedirect.com/science/journal/07493797
ISSN: 07493797
ISSN: 18732607 (Online)
See Also Chapter 9.6. Community Medicine
Indexed in: MEDLINE
Recommended for: Hospital, Academic Libraries

Begun in 1985, this official journal of the American College of Preventive Medicine and the Association for Prevention Teaching and Research is published monthly by Elsevier. The journal succeeds quite well in meeting its aim of providing interventions for the primary and secondary prevention of chronic and acute disease and in promoting health at both the individual and community level across all age groups. Included in the journal are original peer-reviewed research articles, brief reports, review and special articles, current issues, editorials and commentary, policy statements by the two sponsoring organizations, and special supplements or thematic issues. The main audience for this journal is public health professionals. Health professionals in academic institutions and hospitals focused on prevention would find this informative as well. This journal has a 2009 *Journal Citation Reports* impact factor of 4.235 and ranks eighth out of 122 journals in public, environmental, and occupational. This journal is cited in several abstracting and indexing sources such as MEDLINE, Chemical Abstracts, Current Contents, and Embase. Full online coverage back to volume 14, 1998 is available through Elsevier ScienceDirect.

Preventing Chronic Disease. v. 1, National Center for Chronic Disease Prevention and Health Promotion, 2004. *See* Chapter 10.16. Public Health, Chapter 13.16. Public Health Nursing

Prevention Science. v. 1, Springer, 2000.
http://www.springerlink.com/content/104965/
ISSN: 13894986
ISSN: 15736695 (Online)
Indexed in: MEDLINE
Recommended for: Academic Libraries

This journal "serves as an interdisciplinary forum designed to disseminate new developments in the theory, research and practice of prevention." The journal began publishing in 2000 and is the official publication of the Society of Prevention Research. Peer-reviewed original articles on a variety of health and social problems can be found in this journal, along with literature reviews, papers with new methodological developments, and theory-based articles. Public health practitioners, academic researchers, and health policy makers are the main users of this journal, which currently ranks thirty-third out of 156 public, environmental, and occupational health journals. The *Journal Citation Reports* impact factor for this journal in 2009 was 3.018. Academic institutions would be a logical purchaser of this insightful journal. The journal is cited in numerous abstracting and indexing sources such as MEDLINE, CINAHL, Current Contents, and PsycINFO. Full online coverage back to volume 1, 2000 is available through SpringerLink.

Databases and Other Electronic Resources

The Guide to Clinical Preventive Services, 2010–2011: Recommendations of the U.S. Preventive Services Task Force. AHRQ: Agency for Healthcare Research and Quality, 2010.
http://www.ahrq.gov/clinic/pocketgd.htm
Recommended for: Hospital, Academic Libraries

The U.S. Department of Health and Human Services' Agency for Healthcare Research and Quality (AHRQ) convened the U.S. Preventive Services Task Force (USPSTF) in 1984. In support of AHRQ's overall mission to improve health care for all Americans, the USPSTF was established as an independent panel comprised of private-sector, primary care providers with a mandate to "conduct rigorous reviews of research evidence to create evidence-based recommendations for preventive services" that could be used by primary care clinicians and health systems. The 2010–2011 edition of the *Guide*, which is also known as the *Pocket Guide to Clinical Preventive Services*, includes both new and updated USPSTF recommendations on screening, counseling, and preventive medication topics released from 2002 to 2010. Authoritative disease and condition recommendations for adults, children, and adolescents range from cancer to mental health to obesity. The Task Force provides letter grades with each recommendation, which "reflect the magnitude of net benefit and the strength and certainty of the evidence supporting the provision of a specific preventive service." Given the increased national pressure to control health care costs, this evidence-based *Guide* is a critical resource that supports the expansion of preventive care and reduction of preventable disease. All hospital and academic libraries supporting health care providers who make decisions about preventive services (general practitioners, internists, family practitioners, pediatricians, nurses, and nurse practitioners) should include this free, Web-based publication in their collections. This source is also recommended by the American Board of Preventive Medicine as a study aid for those preparing for the ABPM exams.

Healthy People 2020. U.S. Department of Health and Human Services, 2010.
http://www.healthypeople.gov/2020/
Recommended for: Hospital, Academic, Consumer Health Libraries

Released in December 2010, *Healthy People 2020* continues to identify national health priorities, setting new ten-year, science-based objectives for health promotion and disease prevention. This landmark public health initiative was established to create a national prevention strategy, which would guide primary prevention activities in the United States. *Healthy People* remains committed to improving the quality of the nation's health through a broad collaboration of public health and prevention experts; various government entities; health agencies and organizations; and the public itself. This fourth effort provides more than 40 topic areas with brief introductions discussing each topic's importance to the nation's health, the topic's objectives along with baselines and target measures, and an interventions and resources section containing clinical recommendations, evidence-based intervention strategies, and links to consumer health information. *Healthy People* is not a perfect initiative. Throughout its multiyear existence, critics have expressed concerns with the measurability of indicators, data quality for inputs, and achievability of the results. *Healthy People's* open and extensive feedback process works to acknowledge and address these concerns through ongoing dialog with the public and expert stakeholders from government, academic, and the private sector. With its broad focus and target audience, *Healthy People* should be considered as an essential preventive medicine resource for academic, hospital, and consumer health libraries.

10.15.1. Environmental Medicine

Environmental factors that may impinge upon human disease, and development of methods for the detection, prevention, and control of environmentally related disease.
—MeSH

Contributor: Paul Elliott Dahl

Monographs

Environmental Engineering, 3-title set. 6th ed. Editors: Nelson L. Nemerow, Franklin J. Agardy, Patrick Sullivan, Joseph A. Salvato. John Wiley & Sons, 2009.
ISBN: 9780470083031 (***Water, Wastewater, Soil and Groundwater Treatment and Remediation***)
ISBN: 9780470083048 (***Prevention and Response to Water-, Food-, Soil-, and Air-borne Disease and Illness***)
ISBN: 9780470083055 (***Environmental Health and Safety for Municipal Infrastructure, Land Use***)
ISBN: 9780470083024 (3 v. set)
Recommended for: Academic Libraries

First published in 1958, Salvato's *Environmental Engineering* has long been the indispensable reference source for sanitarians and environmental engineers/health specialists. The sixth edition has been reworked and is now organized into three separate volumes rather than the large tome it had been with the fifth edition. The *Water, Wastewater, Soil and Groundwater Treatment and Remediation* volume focuses on the effective treatment of water and wastewater. The *Prevention and Response to Water-, Food-, Soil-, and Airborne Disease and Illness* volume explains how to deal and prevent waterborne, foodborne, soilborne, and airborne environmental disease and illness. The *Environmental Health and Safety for Municipal Infrastructure, Land Use and Planning, and Industry* volume describes how to reduce and curtail municipal waste pollution, industrial waste pollution, air pollution, and noise pollution, as well as addressing land use planning, surveying, and mapping. This set is recommended for academic libraries with a focus on public or environmental health.

Journals

Environmental Health Perspectives. v. 1, National Institute of Environmental Health Services, 1972.
http://ehp.niehs.nih.gov/
http://www.ncbi.nlm.nih.gov/pmc/journals/253/
ISSN: 00916765
ISSN: 15529924 (Online)
See Also Chapter 5. Environmental Health, Chapter 17.8. Toxicology
Indexed in: MEDLINE, CINAHL
Recommended for: Hospital, Academic Libraries

This monthly open access journal should be considered required reading for health professionals interested in a "discussion of the interrelationships between the environment and human health by publishing in a balanced and objective manner the best peer-reviewed research and most current and credible news of the field." The National Institute of Environmental Health Sciences (part of the National Institutes of Health in the U.S. Department of Health and Human Services) is able to achieve its lofty mission. One of the strengths of this environmental health science journal is that it combines both human epidemiological studies and environmental policy topics with in vitro and in vivo animal research applicable to human health. It also has a research section specifically dealing with children's environmental health in every issue. Editorials, commentaries, and book reviews are also provided in most issues. This journal is suitable for any hospital but is most useful to academic institutions and public health professionals. It has a journal impact factor of 6.19 in 2009 and is the top monthly journal in the public, environmental, and occupational health category. This journal is cited in several abstracting and indexing sources such as MEDLINE and CINAHL. Print issues are only available with a paid subscription. Full online coverage back to volume 1, 1972 is available via PubMed Central.

Environmental Science & Technology. v. 1, American Chemical Society, 1967.
http://pubs.acs.org/journal/esthag
ISSN: 0013936X
ISSN: 15205851 (Online)
Indexed in: MEDLINE
Recommended for: Academic Libraries

This bi-weekly journal from the American Chemical Society is an authoritative source of information on a wide range of environmental disciplines. It has both magazine and peer-reviewed research sections so the professional audience can keep abreast of the "major advances, trends, and challenges in environmental science, technology, and policy." It is likely to find its utilization niche among environmental health professionals in both academic institutions and in public health settings. Some of the articles contained in *Environmental Science & Technology* are highly technical in nature. This journal has an impact factor of 4.63 for 2009. It is cited in several abstracting and indexing sources such as MEDLINE and Chemical Abstracts. Full online coverage back to volume 1, 1967 is available through the American Chemical Society.

Journal of Exposure Science and Environmental Epidemiology. v. 16, Nature, 2006.
http://www.nature.com/jes/
ISSN: 15590631
ISSN: 1559064X (Online)
See Also Chapter 5. Environmental Health
Indexed in: MEDLINE
Recommended for: Academic Libraries

This bi-monthly journal is required reading for those needing current research on the health effects of exposure to environmental toxins, as well as sound environmental epidemiologic means and measures to detect unsafe exposure levels. This journal was formerly called *Journal of Exposure Analysis and Environment Epidemiology* from 1991–2005. The International Society of Exposure Analysis is the sponsoring organization. The journal includes original, peer-reviewed research articles, editorials, digest news articles, and review articles. This journal would appeal to epidemiologists, researchers in exposure analysis, chemists, and toxicologists. This journal had a *Journal Citation Reports* impact factor of 2.718 in 2009 and ranks thirtieth out of 122 journals in public, environmental, and occupational health. This journal is a "must" purchase for academic institutions and would be an essential resource for environmental health epidemiologists in public health settings. This journal is cited in numerous abstracting and indexing sources such as MEDLINE, Embase, and Current Contents. Full online coverage back to volume 9, 1999 is available through Nature Publishing Group.

Toxicological Sciences. v. 41, Oxford University Press, 1998.
http://toxsci.oxfordjournals.org/
ISSN: 10966080
ISSN: 10960929 (Online)
See Also Chapter 17.8. Toxicology
Indexed in: MEDLINE
Recommended for: Academic Libraries

The mission of this peer-reviewed journal is to "publish premier peer-reviewed, hypothesis-driven, original research articles in all areas of toxicology." This journal does practice what it proclaims by covering many distinct types of toxicology in each issue as well as providing articles on biomarkers, risk assessment, and in vitro and alternatives to animals. Chemists, biologists, and environmental health researchers would be interested in reading this journal. The *Journal Citation Reports* impact factor for this journal in 2009 was 4.814 and it ranks fourth out of 77 toxicology journals. This journal is a must read for public health professionals and is a required resource at academic institutions. This journal is cited in numerous abstracting and indexing sources such as MEDLINE, CAB Abstracts, Current Contents, Embase, and Environment Index. Full online coverage back to volume 1, 1981 is available through Oxford University Press.

10.15.2. Occupational Medicine

The promotion and maintenance of the physical and mental health of employees in occupational settings.
—MeSH

Contributor: Michael Sholinbeck

Monographs

Current Occupational & Environmental Medicine. 4th ed. Editor: Joseph LaDou. McGraw-Hill, 2007.
http://www.r2library.com/
ISBN: 9780071443135
See Also Chapter 5. Environmental Health
Recommended for: Hospital, Academic Libraries
Doody's Core Titles Selection

This relatively compact and concise text provides a good overview of clinical and other occupational medicine topics. The first section, "Occupational Health," consists of chapters on occupational medical history, workers' compensation, disability prevention and management, and liability issues. The next two sections, "Occupational Injuries" and "Occupational Illnesses," cover common occupational injuries and illnesses. Comprising the largest section of the book, these sections include diagnosis, prevention, treatment, prognosis, and clinical toxicology. The last three sections address "Occupational Exposures," "Program Management," and "Environmental Health." The book is well illustrated, and tables are arranged effectively to facilitate ease of use. The book concludes with a detailed yet concise introduction to epidemiology and biostatistics, which is useful for those studying the research literature and conducting research studies. The fourth edition includes more authors from outside North America and expanded coverage of environmental medicine. Each cited reference includes a PMID number, if appropriate, to facilitate article retrieval in PubMed. *Current Occupational & Environmental Medicine* is a valuable resource for clinicians as well as industrial hygienists.

Documentation of the Threshold Limit Values and Biological Exposure Indices. 7th ed. American Conference of Governmental Industrial Hygienists, 2001.
http://www.acgih.org/store/
ISBN: 1882417437
ISBN: 9781882417438
Recommended for: Academic Libraries

Threshold limit values (TLVs) and biological exposure indices (BEIs) represent scientific consensus that exposure at or below the level of the TLV or BEI would not result in unreasonable risk of disease or injury. The American Conference of Governmental Industrial Hygienists (ACGIH)—a private, not-for-profit, nongovernmental corporation whose members are occupational health and safety professionals—publishes the TLV and BEI guidelines. The values are health based, meaning neither economic factors nor technical feasibility of implementation was considered in their development. Scientific committees review the literature in order to establish the TLVs and BEIs. Details on TLV and BEI development may be read at the ACGIH website, http://www.acgih.org/TLV/. The *Documentation* volumes are indispensable guidelines for use in making decisions about safe exposure to substances found in the workplace. The current edition is available in a five-volume loose leaf format, with annual supplements. The loose-leaf format facilitates replacement of outdated sections with new supplements. The first three volumes (TLVs) are arranged in chemical name order, and each section includes a summary, physical and chemical properties, sources of occupational exposure, summaries of both animal and human studies (carcinogenicity, toxicity, etc.), TLV recommendations, and historical TLV information. The fourth volume (BEIs), which is also in chemical name order, starts each section with a basis for the BEI and includes uses and properties of the chemical, exposure information, analytical methods, recommendations, and historical BEIs. The final volume discusses physical agents: acoustic, electromagnetic, ergonomic, mechanical, and thermal hazards. The sections include a TLV, with information on exposure, epidemiological studies, and more. All sections include an extensive reference list. Libraries serving patrons who make decisions on workplace exposure, who research such exposures, or who treat those exposed should include this work. The *Documentation* volumes are also available on CD-ROM, and both single user and networked versions are offered. A spiral-bound pocket version including only the TLVs and BEIs is also available. *Documentation of the Threshold Limit Values and Biological Exposure Indices*, 7th ed.—2010 Supplement is now available (ISBN 9781607260288).

Encyclopaedia of Occupational Health and Safety. 4th ed. Editor: Jeanne Mager Stellman. International Labour Office, 1998.
http://www.ilo.org/
ISBN: 9789221092032 (set)
ISBN: 9789221098140 (v.1)
ISBN: 9789221098157 (v.2)
ISBN: 9789221098164 (v.3)
ISBN: 9789221098171 (v.4)
ISBN: 9789221098140 (v.5: CD ROM))
Recommended for: Academic Libraries

Since 1930 when the first edition was published, the International Labour Organization's *Encyclopaedia of Occupational Health and Safety* has provided an indispensable review of "work, workers, and the working environment." Experts from over 60 countries contributed to the *Encyclopaedia*. Union staff, researchers, managers, lawyers, regulators, and others will find useful material in this work, making it important for any library collection that serves any of these audiences. The organization of the *Encyclopaedia* demonstrates its utility and comprehensiveness. Rather than comprising a strictly A to Z list of topics, the volumes are organized by broad topic areas. The first volume focuses on systemic occupational conditions, occupational health care services, management, and policy, along with the tools used in occupational medicine, such as biological monitoring. The second volume discusses the nature and management of safety and hazards: physical, environmental, and psychological. The third volume conveys information on specific industries and occupations: processes, hazards, and safety management. The fourth and final volume consists of three guides—occupations, chemicals, and units and abbreviations—as well as a directory of experts and three indexes—subject, authors cited, and chemicals. The nearly 250 pages of indexing allow for easy access to the contents of the *Encyclopaedia*. Volume 5, which may be purchased separately, consists of a CD-ROM of the entire *Encyclopedia*. While the 4th edition is over ten years old, it remains an invaluable part of any occupational medicine collection. It is also available online by subscription from the publisher.

NIOSH Pocket Guide to Chemical Hazards. U.S. Dept. of Health and Human Services, Centers for Disease Control and Prevention, National Institute for Occupational Safety and Health, 2005.
http://www.cdc.gov/niosh/npg/
ISBN: None
Recommended for: Hospital, Academic Libraries

The *NIOSH Pocket Guide to Chemical Hazards* is intended as a source of general industrial hygiene information for workers, employers, and occupational health professionals. Key information on hundreds of chemicals and substance groupings is presented in an easy-to-find and easy-to-read format in both the print and online versions. The chemicals or substances contained in this revision include all substances for which the National Institute for Occupational Safety and Health (NIOSH) has recommended exposure limits (RELs) and those with permissible exposure limits (PELs) as found in the Occupational Safety and Health Administration (OSHA) General Industry Air Contaminants Standard (29 CFR 1910.1000). The *Pocket Guide* is described by NIOSH as designed to provide chemical-specific data to supplement general industrial hygiene knowledge. To maximize the amount of data provided in this limited space, abbreviations and codes have been used extensively. These abbreviations and codes have been designed to permit rapid comprehension. Contents include chemical name, structure/formula, identification numbers (CAS, etc.), synonyms, conversion factors, exposure limits, properties, personal protection and sanitation, first aid, respirator selection information, exposure information, symptoms, and more. The online version is organized as a series of indexes: chemical names, CAS numbers, and RTECS numbers. The indexes are followed by several appendixes. The print version is in chemical name order, with an extensive index of synonyms and trade names, CAS number, and DOT ID number indexes. The online version is searchable, downloadable as a PDF document, or downloadable as a condensed HTML file for offline viewing. The guide is in the public domain and may be freely copied or reprinted (NIOSH Publication Number 2005-149; Sudoc No. HE 20.7129:C 42/2005/CD).

Occupational Medicine. 3rd ed. Editors: Carl Zenz, O. Bruce Dickerson, Edward P. Horvath. Mosby, 1994.
ISBN: 9780801666766
Recommended for: Hospital, Academic Libraries

The most recent edition of this classic work includes 78 chapters and nine appendixes by over 100 international authors. This work is not simply a compendium of diseases or chemicals. Its organization around occupational environments, such as the following, separates this work from many other texts: the physical environment (vibration, sound, driving, etc.); the chemical environment (carbon monoxide, pesticides, metals, etc., which is the largest section at around 400 pages); work categories (women in the workplace, agricultural workers, etc.); and sections on behavioral factors and prevention and control. Significant space is also devoted to various topics such as the needs of small businesses, international travel, and occupational health in developing countries. These "special" topics were fresh at the time this book was published and remain relevant today. For example, governmental entities are currently re-evaluating the types of services and regulations appropriate for small employers, including workplace health promotion. As expected, many chapters look at clinical factors, with a very large section on pulmonary diseases. Appendixes include an Occupational Stress Questionnaire and an Occupational Health Audit, as well as conversions, TLVs (threshold limit values) and BEIs (biological exposure indices), and more. The book concludes with a 75-page index. At this time, there is no evidence that a new edition is planned. Despite the book's age, the third edition remains as a useful work.

Patty's Industrial Hygiene. 6th ed. Editors: Vernon E. Rose, Barbara Cohrssen. Wiley, 2011.
http://onlinelibrary.wiley.com/book/10.1002/0471435139 (5th ed.)
ISBN: 9780470074886 (set)
Recommended for: Hospital, Academic Libraries

Patty's Industrial Hygiene has been a standard reference in occupational health and safety for decades, and the fifth edition offers a thorough introduction to the most relevant topical areas. Besides chapters on traditional occupational health topics such as chemical and physical agents, there are also chapters on exposure analysis, occupational disease diagnostic techniques, quality control, statistical design and data analysis, engineering control of hazards, and more. In addition, such legal/regulatory aspects of occupational medicine as hygienist's liability, litigation, and health promotion warrant separate chapters. The four volumes are organized into parts representing broad topics: volume one contains part I, "Introduction to Industrial Hygiene" and part II, "Recognition and Evaluation of Chemical Agents"; volume two contains part III, "Physical Agents," part IV, "Biohazards," and part V, "Engineering Control and Personal Protection"; volume three comprises part VI. "Law, Regulation, and Management"; and volume four contains part VII, "Specialty Areas and Allied Professions." The book includes a comprehensive, 50-page index. Because of the broad scope of the four volumes, this work would be important to any library that supports occupational medicine programs or other aspects of occupational health: academic and hospital libraries, law libraries, and specialized collections. The online version features downloadable text for offline viewing. This review refers to the fifth edition.

Journals

AAOHN Journal. v. 34, SLACK for the American Association of Occupational Health Nurses, 1986.
http://www.aaohnjournal.com/
ISSN: 08910162
Indexed in: MEDLINE, CINAHL
Recommended for: Hospital, Academic Libraries
Brandon/Hill Selection

AAOHN Journal, the official journal of the American Association of Occupational Health Nurses (AAOHN), offers original articles of professional interest to occupational and environmental health nurses; it is the only occupational health nursing journal. *AAOHN Journal* includes research studies, review articles, clinical articles and case reports, Association news, and more. Each issue also offers CNE credit. Of particular interest are the "Successful Programs" articles, where the planning, implementation, and evaluation of successful workplace programs are reported, and the "Business and Leadership" articles covering business or leadership theory, issues, or process of interest to occupational health nurses. The journal is peer-reviewed by AAOHN members who have strong publishing and research backgrounds along with professional practice expertise. The journal is of particular value in clinical settings, but it would also be of use in research libraries. *AAOHN Journal* is indexed in multiple sources such as CINAHL, MEDLINE, and Health and Safety Science Abstracts.

American Journal of Industrial Medicine. v. 1, Wiley-Liss, 1980.
http://onlinelibrary.wiley.com/journal/10.1002/(ISSN)1097-0274
ISSN: 02713586
ISSN: 10970274 (Online)
Indexed in: MEDLINE
Recommended for: Academic Libraries

The *American Journal of Industrial Medicine* (*AJIM*) publishes reports of original research, review articles, and case reports in the fields of occupational and environmental health and safety. The journal also accepts commentaries, book reviews, and letters of comment and criticism. Articles consisting of analyses of policy are also included, as are those examining historical aspects of occupational medicine. Specific topics of interest include occupational disease, environmental disease, pesticides, cancer, occupational epidemiology, environmental epidemiology, disease surveillance systems, ergonomics, dust diseases, lead poisoning, neurotoxicology, and endocrine disruptors. The audience for *AJIM* includes physicians and other clinicians, epidemiologists, toxicologists, and other researchers. *AJIM* is indexed in numerous sources such as MEDLINE and Biological Abstracts (BIOSIS). Although it has been published for only a relatively short span, *AJIM* is highly regarded by both clinicians and researchers.

Journal of Occupational and Environmental Medicine. v. 37, Lippincott Williams & Wilkins, 1995.
http://www.ovid.com/
http://www.mdconsult.com/
ISSN: 10762752
ISSN: 15365948 (Online)

See Also Chapter 5. Enviornmental Health
Indexed in: MEDLINE, CINAHL
Recommended for: Academic Libraries

The *Journal of Occupational and Environmental Medicine* (*JOEM*) is the official journal of the American College of Occupational and Environmental Medicine (ACOEM), "the nation's largest medical society dedicated to promoting the health of workers through preventive medicine, clinical care, research, and education." Although ACOEM, a large and influential association, and its journal have been criticized in the past for an alleged industry bias, no library collecting occupational health material should be without this journal. Each issue begins with a section called "Articles of Interest to Clinicians" that lists these articles with a very brief—perhaps two sentences—description of the study and its relevance to the "real world" of clinical occupational medicine. This is a handy feature for busy clinicians who want to keep up on the literature in their field of practice. Besides original, peer-reviewed studies, *JOEM* includes book reviews, literature reviews, Association news, ACOEM Guidance Statements, and the "Occupational Medicine Forum," a kind of practice guide. *JOEM* also provides Continuing Medical Education-designated articles, which, together with an online CME test, can earn clinicians CME credit. *JOEM* is indexed in various sources such as MEDLINE and Excerpta Medica.

Occupational and Environmental Medicine. v. 51, BMJ Publishing, 1994.
http://oem.bmj.com/
http://www.ncbi.nlm.nih.gov/pmc/journals/172/
ISSN: 13510711
ISSN: 14707926 (Online)
Indexed in: MEDLINE, CINAHL
Recommended for: Academic Libraries

Occupational and Environmental Medicine (*OEM*) is a peer-reviewed journal concerned with areas of current importance in occupational medicine and environmental health issues throughout the world. Original contributions include epidemiological, physiological, and psychological studies of occupational and environmental health hazards, and toxicological studies of materials posing human health risks. A CPD/CME series aims to help visitors in continuing their professional development. An occasional "World at Work" series describes workplace hazards and protective measures in different workplaces worldwide. *OEM* is the adopted, official journal of the Faculty of Occupational Medicine of the Royal College of Physicians of London. Each issue includes original studies, editorials, short reports, and commentaries. *OEM* is valuable for both clinicians and those "on the ground," as well as researchers in epidemiology and environmental health topics. The journal is indexed in MEDLINE and Biological Abstracts (BIOSIS). *OEM* continues the *British Journal of Industrial Medicine*, which first was published in 1944.

Scandinavian Journal of Work, Environment & Health. v. 1, Finnish Institute of Occupational Health (Finland); National Research Centre for the Working Environment (Denmark); National Institute of Occupational Health (Norway), 1975.
http://www.sjweh.fi/
ISSN: 03553140
ISSN: 795990X (Online)
Indexed in: MEDLINE
Recommended for: Hospital, Academic Libraries

The *Scandinavian Journal of Work, Environment & Health* is published (in English) by the Finnish Institute of Occupational Health (Finland), the National Research Centre for the Working Environment (Denmark), and the National Institute of Occupational Health (Norway). The editorial board includes scientists from these three countries as well as the United States, Japan, Brazil, New Zealand, and several European Union nations, giving the journal a nice international representation. According to the journal's website, this journal's emphasis is on the intersection of work and health, including occupational epidemiology, occupational medicine, occupational health services, work safety, work organization, and more. The scope is broad and includes economic factors as well as relevant psychosocial and lifestyle issues. Peer-reviewed articles and review articles are supplemented by case reports, short communications, meeting reports, book reviews, news, editorials, and more. The issues are relatively short—around 80 pages. The journal's online archive goes back to volume 1 (1975), and free full text is available for much of the back content at this time. An online subscription is required for full online access to the past two years, although selected articles in the newer online issues are also freely available. In addition to six regular issues per year, *SJWEH Supplements* are published on an as-needed basis. Although described as a separate publication, *SJWEH Supplements* are distributed to all subscribers of *SJWEH*, and the full text of all is freely available online. *SJWEH Supplements* primarily contain conference material. *SJWEH* is indexed in MEDLINE, CINAHL, Biological Abstracts, and numerous other resources.

10.15.3. Preventive Psychiatry

The prevention of mental illness and the promotion of mental health.

—MeSH

Contributor: Paul Elliott Dahl

Monographs

Clinical Manual of Prevention in Mental Health. 1st ed. Editor: Michael T. Compton. American Psychiatric Publishing, 2010.
ISBN: 9781585623471
Recommended for: Hospital, Academic Libraries

As is pointed out by the publisher, this book is "one of the few resources of its kind available to mental health professionals today, and serves as a comprehensive guide to applying proven prevention tools in psychiatric units, outpatient clinics, consultation-liaison services, and private office settings." This book is required reading for every mental health professional since it makes the case that mental health professionals must work to make prevention part and parcel of their practice. More than 30 contributors from the United States provide prevention interventions for mood disorders, anxiety disorders, psychotic disorders, adolescent behavioral disorders, elder behavioral impairments, and somatic illnesses. Prevention and health promotion tools are also presented for alcohol and drug abuse, cigarette smoking, suicide, and family violence in this timely resource. The book contains 13 chapters and a quality index. This book would be worthy reading for any health professional in general working to prevent mental illness in communities of any size.

Preventing Mental, Emotional, and Behavioral Disorders among Young People: Progress and Possibilities. Authors: Mary E. O'Connell, Thomas Boat, Kenneth E. Warner. National Academies Press, 2009.
Http://extranet.netlibrary.com/TitleSelect/
http://www.ebrary.com/
ISBN: 9780309126748
Recommended for: Academic Libraries

This report from the National Research Council and the Institute of Medicine builds upon a 1994 report, *Reducing Risks for Mental Disorders: Frontiers for Preventive Intervention Research.* The 2009 report reaffirms the need to focus on prevention rather than treatment (and not just give prevention lip service) since many of the mental, emotional, and behavioral (MEB) disorders found in adults have their roots in childhood and adolescence. These disorders with their enormous personal, family, and societal costs are therefore preventable. This report also points out the detrimental influence of poverty in negatively impacting cognitive, emotional, and behavioral development; the future of the mental health of the nation is tied to how we reduce the pernicious effects of poverty on the young. The report is organized into three parts. Part I provides an overview and background of the problem in four detailed chapters. Part II covers the state of preventive intervention research by examining the interventions, screening tools, methodological issues, and the benefits and costs of such research. Part III deals with the new frontiers of developing a prevention infrastructure and other needed improvements in prevention enhancement. A rather extensive list of nearly 100 pages of references will be useful to those seeking more in-depth reading. The report also contains a glossary, six useful appendixes (the print copy only contains Appendix A while the online report contains all the appendixes), an index, and also acronyms used in the report. The few illustrations found in the report are effective in conveying information. A summary of the report with the basic recommendations is also provided but it is imperative to read the recommendations in complete detail to gain a full understanding. The recommendations found in the report need to be implemented by policy makers, practitioners, researchers, and educators across a spectrum of disciplines in order to create a more hopeful future for our nation's youth. This book is highly recommended for academic institutions.

Journals

Annual Review of Clinical Psychology. v. 1, Annual Reviews, 2005.
http://arjournals.annualreviews.org/loi/clinpsy
ISSN: 15485943
ISSN: 15485951 (Online)
Indexed in: MEDLINE
Recommended for: Hospital, Academic Libraries

This journal provides authoritative, comprehensive review articles of selected clinical psychology topics so it is of great benefit to and would be highly read by psychologists and psychiatrists. Public health and human service professionals are also likely to highly value this journal. A perusal of this annual review from 2005 to 2010 reveals that from 15–25 articles are provided each year. Authors are invited to submit articles by Annual Reviews and are considered authorities on the subject of the article. This journal has a high impact factor rating since such review articles are highly cited by journal authors. Its impact factor rating in 2009 was 9.613 and it ranked within the top three journals for both clinical psychology (social science) and psychology (science). This journal should also be considered a critical purchase for a hospital or an academic institution due to the comprehensive reviews provided. Full online coverage back to volume 1, 2005 is available through Annual Reviews.

Journal of Clinical Child and Adolescent Psychiatry. v. 31, Routledge, 2002.
http://www.informaworld.com/smpp/title~content=1537-4416
ISSN: 15374416
ISSN: 15374424 (Online)
Indexed in: MEDLINE
Recommended for: Academic Libraries

Renamed in 2002 (known previously as *Journal of Clinical Child Psychology* for volumes 1–30, 1971–2001), this journal is the official publication of the Society of Clinical Child and Adolescent Psychology, American Psychological Association. Peer-reviewed original research articles, case studies, and brief reports are typically found in this journal. The journal aims to provide articles that critically analyze the development and evaluation of assessment and intervention techniques for children and adolescents, as well as outlining mental health developmental issues found in youth. Clinical child psychologists, family therapists, and professionals interested in the psychological health of youth would be the natural audience for this journal. School psychologists and counselors would also likely find the journal very useful. This journal would be a required resource for academic institutions. The *Journal Citation Reports* impact factor in 2009 was 2.910. This journal ranked fourteenth out of 59 in developmental psychology journals and sixteenth out of 93 in clinical psychology journals. Full online coverage back to volume 1, 1971 is available through Taylor & Francis Group's InformaWorld.

Journal of Primary Prevention. v. 2, Springer, 1981.
http://www.springerlink.com/content/105378/
ISSN: 0278095X
ISSN: 15736547 (Online)
Recommended for: Academic Libraries
Indexed in: MEDLINE

This journal is "dedicated to a better understanding of primary prevention theory, practice, and research." To that end, the journal publishes articles on a wide spectrum of prevention research topics including intervention development and evaluation, health determinants, and meta-analyses. Some of the content areas covered are substance abuse, sexual behaviors, physical activity, and mental health. Both qualitative and quantitative research is welcomed. Publication types found in this journal include original, peer-reviewed research, practice-oriented reports from the field, literature reviews, and book reviews. The editors attach a unique summary called Strategic Implications (SI) to articles and these summaries highlight the practice or policy implications. The main audience for this journal would be public health professionals, social service professionals, health policy makers, and academic researchers. Academic institutions would find this a worthy purchase. This journal is found in numerous abstracting and indexing sources such as MEDLINE, Embase, PsycINFO, and ERIC. No impact factor or journal ranking information could be found for this publication. Full online coverage back to volume 1, 1980 is available through SpringerLink.

Psychiatric Clinics of North America. v. 1, Saunders-Elsevier, 1978.
http://www.psych.theclinics.com/
http://www.sciencedirect.com/science/journal/0193953X
ISSN: 0193953X
ISSN: 15583147 (Online)
Indexed in: MEDLINE, CINAHL
Recommended for: Hospital, Academic Libraries

"Comprehensive, state-of-the-art reviews by experts in the field provide current, practical information on the diagnosis and treatment of psychiatric disorders" is the explicit aim of this journal first published in 1978. A single topic review is found in every issue of this quarterly publication. Clinical psychiatrists and others in related disciplines would be the main audience for this journal. Some public health and social service practitioners would also be likely to find this journal applicable to their positional practice. Both hospitals and academic institutions would find this a vitally important purchase. The journal is cited in several abstracting and indexing sources such as MEDLINE, CINAHL, and PsycINFO. Full online coverage back to volume 19, 1996 is available through Elsevier ScienceDirect.

10.16. Public Health

The prevention and control of disease and disability, and the promotion of physical and mental health of the population on the international, national, state, or municipal level.

—MeSH

Contributor: Paul Elliott Dahl

Monographs

A Community Guide to Environmental Health. Authors: Jeff Conant, Pam Fadem. Hesperian Foundation, 2008.
See Chapter 5. Environmental Health

Essentials of Environmental Health. Author: Robert H. Friis. Jones & Bartlett, 2007.
See Chapter 5. Environmental Health

Handbook of Epidemiology. 1st ed. Editors: Wolfgang Ahrens, Iris Pigeot. Springer, 2005.
http://extranet.netlibrary.com/TitleSelect/
http://www.myilibrary.com/
http://www.ebrary.com/corp/
ISBN: 9783540005667
ISBN: 9783540265771 (Online)
Recommended for: Academic Libraries

The objective of this handbook as stated in the preface is to "provide a comprehensive overview of the field of epidemiology, bridging the gap between standard textbooks of epidemiology and publications for specialists with a narrow focus on specific areas." This comprehensive handbook achieves that worthy objective by effectively presenting epidemiological and statistical concepts, issues, and methods in such a way that it is useful as a quick reference and as a more detailed overview. The authors, who are primarily from North America and Europe, are reputable authorities in the realm of epidemiology and statistics. The book is organized broadly with 39 chapters contained in four major parts. Part I presents the concepts and methodological approaches in epidemiology. Part II details the statistical methods in epidemiology. Part III is devoted to the applications of epidemiology. Lastly, Part IV focuses on research areas in epidemiology. Illustrations are prudently utilized to promote understanding. A list of the contributors is provided at the end of the book. The lack of an index could be problematic but it is likely that the table of contents will be able to direct readers to the proper chapter. The handbook will be of interest to public health practitioners, especially epidemiologists. Physicians, biostatisticians, health services executives, and students in various health professions will find this a useful resource as well. This is a required resource for academic institutions supporting health profession programs. A new edition is expected in September 2011.

Human-Animal Medicine: Clinical Approaches to Zoonoses, Toxicants, and Other Shared Health Risks. Authors: Peter M. Rabinowitz, Lisa A. Conti. Saunders Elsevier, 2010.
See Chapter 23.13. Veterinary Public Health

Principles and Practice of Toxicology in Public Health. Author: Ira S. Richards. Jones & Bartlett, 2008.
See Chapter 17.8. Toxicology

Public Health Communication: Evidence for Behavior Change. Editor: Robert C. Hornik. Lawrence Erlbaum Associates, 2002.
See Chapter 33.2. Health Communications

Red Book: 2009 Report of the Committee on Infectious Diseases. 28th ed. Editors: Larry K. Pickering, Carol J. Baker, David W. Kimberlin, Sarah S. Long. American Academy of Pediatrics, 2009.
http://aapredbook.aappublications.org/
ISBN: 9781581103069
See Also Chapter 10.13. Pediatrics
Recommended for: Hospital, Academic Libraries
Doody's Core Titles Selection

The *Red Book* is considered the bible of pediatric infectious diseases since it provides authoritative information on immunization and infectious diseases for health care professionals. The twenty-eighth edition of the *Red Book* was rigorously updated and all the revisions are explained on pages xxix–xxxvi. This resource is arranged in six sections. Section one provides information on active and passive immunization. Section two chronicles the recommendations made for the care of children in special circumstances. Section three contains the summaries of infectious diseases written for adults. Section four lists antimicrobial agents and related therapy utilized in combating infectious disease. Section five details the proper antimicrobial prophylaxis measures to use. The book also contains 12 useful appendixes. This is a required resource for hospitals and academic institutions to have in their collections. The audience for this resource is physicians, nurses, public health practitioners, health care administrators, and health policy makers. This is a *Doody's Core Titles* essential purchase recommendation within both the pediatrics and infectious disease specialty categories.

Silent Spring. Author: Rachel Carson. Houghton Mifflin, 1962.
See Chapter 5. Environmental Health

Sustaining Life: How Human Health Depends on Biodiversity. 1st ed. Editors: Eric Chivian, Aaron Bernstein. Oxford University Press, 2008.
See Chapter 26.3. Ecology

Wallace/Maxcy-Rosenau-Last Public Health & Preventive Medicine. 15th ed. Editors: Robert B. Wallace, Neal Kohatsu, John M. Last, Ross Brownson. McGraw-Hill Medical, 2008.
http://online.statref.com/
http://www.r2library.com/
ISBN: 9780071441988
Recommended for: Hospital, Academic Libraries
Brandon/Hill Selection

This noteworthy one-stop resource for public health and preventive medicine information is sponsored by the Association for Prevention Teaching and Research. First published in 1913, the fifteenth edition has been updated with new diseases, additional public health practice and policy issues, and revisions in chronic conditions. Over 200 well-respected authorities are contributors to the resource. The book is organized in seven sections with a total of 81 chapters covering 1,334 pages (not including the index). Section I examines the core principles in public health and preventive medicine. Section II covers communicable diseases. Section III discusses environmental health issues. Section IV recounts behavioral factors affecting health. Section V outlines noncommunicable and chronic disabling conditions. Section VI elucidates critical health-care planning, organizational, and evaluation issues. Section VII covers injury and violence issues. This guide to public health and preventive medicine is highly recommended for public health practitioners and other health professionals. The additional resources provided for further reading are excellent sources to study for the board exam in public health and preventive medicine. This reference work is essential for hospital collections and academic institutions possessing health professional programs like medicine, public health, and nursing. This resource was a recommendation on the Brandon/Hill medical library list for public health and preventive medicine.

Journals

American Journal of Public Health. v. 61, American Public Health Association, 1971.
http://ajph.aphapublications.org/
http://www.ncbi.nlm.nih.gov/pmc/journals/258/
ISSN: 00900036
ISSN: 15410048 (Online)
See Also Chapter 9.7. Epidemiology, Chapter 13.16. Public Health Nursing
Indexed in: MEDLINE, CINAHL
Recommended for: Hospital, Academic Libraries
Brandon/Hill Selection

This journal is indispensable to those wanting current, authoritative information across all disciplines in the field of public health. First published in 1911, this journal is the official journal of the American Public Health Association (APHA). The journal is able to successfully fulfill its mission "to advance public health research, policy, practice, and education." The journal contains original, peer-reviewed research articles, editorials, commentaries, and department submissions. Special supplement issues are also published each year. Public health professionals at all levels are the main audience for this journal but other health professionals concerned about population health will also find it worthwhile reading. The impact factor of this journal was 4.371 in 2009. It ranks within the top ten of all journals in the public, environmental, and occupational health category for both the science and the social science *Journal Citation Reports*. This journal is cited in numerous abstracting and indexing sources such as MEDLINE, Chemical Abstracts, CINAHL, Embase, and PsycINFO. The National Library of Medicine considers this to be a core clinical title. Full online coverage back to volume 1, 1911 is available through the American Public Health Association.

Annual Review of Public Health. v. 1, Annual Reviews, 1980.
http://arjournals.annualreviews.org/loi/publhealth
ISSN: 01637525
ISSN: 15452093 (Online)
Indexed in: MEDLINE
Recommended for: Hospital, Academic Libraries

This journal provides authoritative, comprehensive review articles of selected public health topics annually so it is accordingly of great benefit to and highly read by public health professionals. Between 2006 and 2010, 21–30 articles were published per year. The categories of epidemiology and biostatistics, environmental and occupational health, health services, public health practice, and social environment and behavior often have articles each year, although special topics may appear. Those who author articles in this journal are invited by Annual Reviews to review a subject and are considered authorities in the field. This journal has a high impact factor rating since such review articles are highly cited by journal authors. Its impact factor rating in 2009 was 7.915 and it ranked within the top three journals in the public, environmental, and occupational health category for both the science and social science *Journal Citation Reports*. This journal should be considered a critical purchase for a hospital or an academic institution due to the comprehensive reviews provided. Full online coverage back to volume 1, 1980 is available through Annual Reviews.

Emerging Infectious Diseases. v. 1, National Center for Infectious Diseases, 1995.
http://www.cdc.gov/ncidod/eid/index.html
http://http://www.ncbi.nlm.nih.gov/pmc/journals/782/
ISSN: 10806040
ISSN: 10806059 (Online)
See Also Chapter 9.14. Tropical Medicine
Indexed in: MEDLINE
Recommended for: Hospital, Academic Libraries

This monthly journal published by the Centers for Disease Control and Prevention has a twofold publication purpose: to provide "recognition of new and reemerging infections and understanding of factors involved in disease emergence, prevention, and elimination" and to ensure "fast and broad dissemination of reliable information on emerging infectious diseases." This worthy publication successfully disseminates needed information on emerging infectious diseases from around the globe. Peer-reviewed research articles as well as perspective, synopsis, and dispatch articles are found in every issue. General practitioners as well as infectious disease specialists and epidemiologists read this journal to keep abreast of infectious disease changes or the development of new infectious agents. This journal had an impact factor of 6.794 in 2009 and it ranked third out of 57 infectious disease journals in the *Journal Citation Reports*. This journal would be suitable for a hospital and is a must for academic institutions. Public health professionals would also consider this a crucial resource. The journal is cited in several abstracting and indexing sources such as MEDLINE and Current Contents. Print subscriptions are available to public health professionals where online facility is limited. Full online coverage back to volume 1, 1995 is available through the Centers for Disease Control and Prevention (CDC).

Environmental Health Perspectives. v. 1, National Institute of Environmental Health Sciences, 1972.

See Chapter 5. Environmental Health, Chapter 10.15.1. Environmental Medicine, Chapter 17.8. Toxicology

Health Affairs. v. 1, Project Hope, 1981.
http://www.healthaffairs.org/
ISSN: 02782715
ISSN: 15445208 (Online)
See Also Chapter 6.2. Medical Records
Indexed in: MEDLINE, CINAHL
Recommended for: Hospital, Academic Libraries

Founded in 1981 under the sponsorship of Project HOPE, this monthly peer-reviewed journal is the leading journal "dedicated to the serious exploration of domestic and international health policy issues." Multidisciplinary in scope, this journal publishes both thematic and "variety" issues each year attracting health policymakers, academic researchers, and health care leaders with its substantive content. Besides original feature articles, this journal also contains field reports, viewpoints, interviews, personal narratives, timely legislative updates, summaries of technology, grant, and data trends, and timely book reviews. Web exclusive articles are also published first on the web before being incorporated into a later print issue. This journal is a must read for any hospital and academic institution dedicated to authoritative analysis. This journal had an impact factor of 3.582 for 2009 and is ranked number four in the category of health care sciences and services and number two in the category of health policy and services (*Journal Citation Reports*). This journal is cited in several abstracting and indexing sources such as MEDLINE, Current Contents, and Lexis-Nexis. Full online coverage goes back to volume 1, 1981 through Project HOPE.

Journal of Public Health Management and Practice. v. 1, Lippincott Williams & Wilkins, 1995.
http://journals.lww.com/jphmp/
http://www.ovid.com/
ISSN: 10784659
ISSN: 15505022 (Online)
See Also Chapter 13.16. Public Health Nursing
Indexed in: MEDLINE, CINAHL
Recommended for: Academic Libraries

Begun in 1995, this journal is recognized as the leading practice-based public health journal. It is required reading for those in public health wanting to keep informed on pressing population health practice issues. All types of practice issues are covered including emergency preparedness, community health assessment, academic-practice linkages, and chronic disease prevention and promotion. The bi-monthly journal provides peer-reviewed, evidence-based original articles, departmental columns, editorials, and commentaries. Academic institutions, especially those with public health programs, will find this a vitally important purchase. Its 2009 *Journal Citation Reports* impact factor is 1.413 and the journal was ranked forty-second out of 95 journals in public, environmental, and occupational health. Full online coverage back to volume 1, 1995 is available through Ovid.

MMWR. Morbidity and Mortality Weekly Report. v. 25, Centers for Disease Control and Prevention, 1976.

http://www.cdc.gov/mmwr/weekcvol.html
ISSN: 01492195
ISSN: 1545861X (Online)
See Also Chapter 13.16. Public Health Nursing
Indexed in: MEDLINE, CINAHL
Recommended for: Hospital, Academic Libraries

The *MMWR* (*Morbidity and Mortality Weekly Report*) series, often called "the voice of CDC (Centers for Disease Control and Prevention)," is CDC's principal route to issue timely, authoritative public health information and recommendations to both health professionals and the general public. *MMWR* is published on a weekly basis; *MMWR Surveillance Summaries* and *MMWR Recommendations and Reports* are published on irregular schedules. Public health professionals undoubtedly will consider *MMWR* as a vital resource. Both hospitals and academic institutions will consider this an essential resource as well. The online format is available at no cost since it is a U.S. governmental publication. Full online coverage back to volume 31, number 5, 1983 is available through the Centers for Disease Control and Prevention.

Preventing Chronic Disease. v. 1, National Center for Chronic Disease Prevention and Health Promotion, 2004.
http://www.cdc.gov/pcd/
http://www.ncbi.nlm.nih.gov/pmc/journals/245/
ISSN: 15451151 (Online)
See Also Chapter 13.16. Public Health Nursing
Indexed in: MEDLINE
Recommended for: Academic Libraries

The mission of this open access peer-reviewed journal is to "address the interface between applied prevention research and public health practice in chronic disease prevention." The first issue of this bi-monthly journal was published in 2004. It strives to prevent and lower the incidence of such chronic diseases as cancer, diabetes, heart disease, and stroke. The audience for this journal is public health practitioners and researchers in the areas of chronic disease prevention and health promotion. The content includes peer-reviewed original research, community case studies, and special topic articles. Editorials, roundtable articles, tools and techniques, and essays may make an appearance. Academic institutions will find this journal a well-used resource. This journal is only available in an online format. Full online coverage back to volume 1, 2004 is available through the National Center for Chronic Disease Prevention and Health Promotion.

Public Health Reports. v. 89, Association of Schools of Public Health, 1974.
http://www.publichealthreports.org/index.cfm
ISSN: 00333549
ISSN: 14682877 (Online)
See Also Chapter 13.16. Public Health Nursing
Indexed in: MEDLINE, CINAHL
Recommended for: Hospital, Academic Libraries

Begun in 1878, this venerable public health journal is the official journal of the U.S. Public Health Service. This bimonthly journal strives to provide sound research and ground-breaking work on the issues facing the public health community. At least two supplement issues are also published each year. Original, peer-reviewed feature, practice, and research articles are the foundation of this journal. This journal also has eight special columns of interest: "Surgeon General's Perspectives," "Environmental Health," "Global Health Matters," "Law and the Public's Health," "Local Acts," "Public Health Chronicles," "NCHS Dateline," and "From the Schools of Public Health." The primary audience for this journal would be practitioners, professors, researchers, and students of public health. Professionals in related disciplines would also find it worth reading. Both hospitals and academic institutions would find the purchase of this journal highly worthwhile. This journal is cited in several abstracting and indexing sources such as MEDLINE, CINAHL, Current Contents, and Embase. The National Library of Medicine has always considered this to be a core clinical title.

Databases and Other Electronic Resources

Healthy People 2020. U.S. Department of Health and Human Services, 2010.
http://www.healthypeople.gov/2020/
See Chapter 10.15. Preventive Medicine

10.17. Radiology

The use of x-ray and other forms of radiant energy in the diagnosis and treatment of disease.

—MeSH

Contributor: Debra R. Berlanstein

Monographs

Atlas of Normal Roentgen Variants That May Simulate Disease. 8th ed. Authors: Theodore Keats, Mark W. Anderson. Mosby, 2006.
ISBN: 9780323043007

Recommended for: Hospital, Academic Libraries
Doody's Core Titles Selection

This atlas is an invaluable resource for comparing normal images and disease entities. It includes over 6,000 excellent quality images that cover common and rare entities. The update of this classic has a new format and includes the latest imaging techniques and computed tomography and magnetic resonance images. This is one of the only resources that assists practicing radiologists, residents, and students to avoid false positives by focusing on the comparison of normal and abnormal images, with head-to-toe coverage. This atlas is a must-have for every radiology department and library.

***Bone and Joint Imaging*.** 3rd ed. Editors: Donald Resnick, Mark J. Kransdorf. Saunders Elsevier, 2004.
ISBN: 9780721602707
Recommended for: Hospital, Academic Libraries
Doody's Core Titles Selection

Drs. Resnick and Kransdorf, along with 38 other specialists present a comprehensive overview of musculoskeletal imaging. The beginning chapters address basic science and diagnostic techniques, followed by chapters covering all major metabolic, degenerative, and infectious bone and joint disorders. This recent edition recognizes the advances in musculoskeletal (MSK) imaging and focuses on more current techniques including arthrography, tenography, ultrasonography, magnetic resonance imaging, and needle biopsy of bone and soft tissue. Several of these sections also include computed tomography images, with 3,800 images included in total. This comprehensive work is excellent for students and residents learning MSK radiology as well as practitioners who are reviewing the subject.

***Breast Imaging*.** 3rd ed. Author: Daniel B. Kopans. Lippincott Williams & Wilkins, 2006.
ISBN: 9780781747684
Recommended for: Hospital, Academic Libraries
Brandon/Hill, *Doody's Core Titles* Selection

The third edition of this best-selling reference combines an atlas and text that covers all aspects of breast imaging. Included are anatomy, histology, physiology, pathology, and cancer staging. All modalities are included: mammography, digital mammography, ultrasound, digital breast tomosynthesis, and percutaneous breast biopsy. Over 2,100 images are included. All but two chapters are written by Kopans and he expertly addresses the timely controversies concerning screening, radiation risk, and medicolegal issues. The many outstanding references make this work an excellent starting point for further research.

***Caffey's Pediatric Diagnostic Imaging*.** 11th ed. Editor: Thomas L. Slovis. Mosby Elsevier, 2008.
ISBN: 9780323045209
Recommended for: Hospital, Academic Libraries
Doody's Core Titles Selection

The completely revised eleventh edition of the seminal text on pediatric radiology has complete coverage of anatomy, embryology, and physiology as well as all imaging modalities from x-ray to cutting-edge multislice cardiac computed tomography, magnetic resonance imaging, and CT-PET. Included are new sections on cardiac, pericardial, and abdominal imaging as well as interventional radiology. The concise writing style also offers highlighted bullet lists and differential diagnosis charts that make it easy to review. This edition has high-quality images and presentation, and also offers access to the Expert Consult website, with images, self-assessment and video for individual purchasers. Caffey's is the clear choice for comprehensive coverage of pediatric radiology.

***CT and MRI of the Whole Body*.** 5th ed. Author: John Haaga. Mosby Elsevier, 2008.
ISBN: 9780323053754
Recommended for: Hospital, Academic Libraries

A complete and thorough review of all organ systems with correlation between computed tomography and magnetic resonance imaging, this is an indispensable work for any radiologist. Presented in two volumes, all systems are covered: brain, head and neck, spine, chest, gastrointestinal, genitourinary, and musculoskeletal. In addition, the book includes a chapter on image-guided intervention. This edition contains new generation multi-slice computed tomography images and is presented in full color.

***Diagnostic Ultrasound*.** 4th ed. Editors: Carol M. Rumack, Stephanie R. Wilson, J. William Charboneau, Deborah Levine. Mosby Elsevier, 2011.
ISBN: 9780323053976 (2 v.)
Recommended for: Hospital, Academic Libraries
Doody's Core Titles Selection

This review refers to the third edition of what is considered the standard textbook of diagnostic ultrasound. It has been expanded to include all the developments in the field over the seven years since the previous edition, including color and power Doppler, hysterosonography, laparoscopic sonography, and ultrasound guided interventional procedures. The four editors and 100 contributors offer comprehensive coverage of the field. Over 5,000 images are included in the two-volume set. Volume one covers physics, the thorax, abdomen, pelvis, small parts, vascular and intraoperative ultrasound. The second volume includes obstetrics, fetal and pediatric sonography. Particularly useful are the excellent color Doppler images and the color boxes highlighting critical diagnostic criteria. This work is equally useful for sonographers, radiologists-in-training, and practicing radiologists.

Essentials of Skeletal Radiology. 3rd ed. Authors: Terry R. Yochum, Lindsay J. Rowe. Lippincott Williams & Wilkins, 2005.
See Chapter 3. Chiropractic

Felson's Principles of Chest Roentgenology. 3rd ed. Author: Lawrence R. Goodman. Elsevier (Saunders), 2007.
ISBN: 9781416029236
Recommended for: Hospital, Academic Libraries
Doody's Core Titles Selection

In the preface to the earlier second edition, Goodman writes that *Felson's Principles of Chest Roentgenology* has been one of the best-selling books in the history of radiology "because the book is simple, relevant, interactive, repetitive, manageable, and fun." The third edition continues the popular format that presents digital quality images on the left with text and questions appearing on the right. This classic work on chest radiology incorporates all modalities (CT, MR, PET, radiographs). Goodman includes the anatomy seen on the radiograph rather than assuming the reader already has the anatomical information. He builds on this in a programmed approach highlighting specific signs to look for in radiographs and the interpretation of more complex findings. The book concludes with Felson's "Ten Axioms for a Lifetime of Medical Learning." This is a must-have text that expertly explains the art and science of chest radiology—a critical element in the education of any radiologist.

Fundamentals of Diagnostic Radiology. 3rd ed. Editors: William E. Brant, Clyde A. Helms. Lippincott Williams & Wilkins, 2006.
http://www.ovid.com/
ISBN: 9780781761352
Recommended for: Hospital, Academic Libraries
Doody's Core Titles Selection

Brant and Helms provide a complete print and multimedia package that is an introduction to radiologic imaging and a comprehensive review of the fundamental practice of diagnostic radiology. Included are the newly revised text plus instant access to online resources to benefit daily practice, residency, board review, and teaching. An accompanying website offers an interactive resource for individual purchasers to complement the hardbound or softbound versions. Viewed as a must-have overview of the ten subspecialities of radiology, this work is key for medical students in radiology rotations, first year residents, and on through to preparation for board examinations. Included are more than 2,700 illustrations, interactive test bank, and continuously updated cases. This edition includes continuous updates and newer multi-slice computed tomography and musculoskeletal imaging modalities.

Head and Neck Imaging. 4th ed. Editors: Peter M. Som, Hugh D. Curtin. Elsevier, 2004.
ISBN: 9780323009423
Recommended for: Hospital, Academic Libraries
Brandon/Hill, *Doody's Core Titles* Selection

When this edition was first published the publisher's description called this work "the field's definitive reference on the interpretation of images of the head and neck. An international cast of 'who's who' in the field discuss all modalities with an emphasis on CT scans and MRIs as well as plain film, providing encyclopedic and detailed coverage." This is still regarded as the gold standard of texts covering this field of radiology. Including 777 more pages than the prior edition, the editors have added more pathology, new techniques, new images, and an overall deeper look at head and neck imaging. The book is divided into six major anatomical areas, including midface and sinonasal cavities, mandible and temporomandibular joints, upper aerodigestive tract, neck, orbit and visual pathways, and skull base and temporal bone. This is a necessary purchase for both neuroradiologists and head and neck specialists. A new edition is planned for April 2011.

Squire's Fundamentals of Radiology. 6th ed. Author: Robert A. Novelline. Harvard University Press, 2004.
ISBN: 9780674012790
Recommended for: Hospital, Academic Libraries
Doody's Core Titles Selection

The classic text for teaching radiology to medical students pioneered by Lucy Frank Squire in 1964 is now in its 6th edition. Her style is maintained by Novelline, her former colleague. He includes an array of new techniques for diagnosing disease and injury, such as vertebroplasty, uterine artery embolization, and radiofrequency ablation. Hundreds of computed tomography, ultrasound, magnetic resonance imaging, 3-D digital, functional MRI and PET-CT images are combined with anatomical cross sections and plain films to illustrate the radiological presentation of common diseases. This remains the definitive introductory radiology text for medical students in their clinical years. It should be added to all academic collections.

Journals

Abdominal Imaging. v. 18, Springer, 1983.
http://www.springerlink.com/content/0942-8925
ISSN: 09428925
ISSN: 14320509 (Online)
Indexed in: MEDLINE
Recommended for: Hospital, Academic Libraries

Formed in 1993 by the merger of *Gastrointestinal Radiology* and *Urologic Radiology*, *Abdominal Imaging* has the mission of bringing together disparate information valuable to radiologists, internists, and surgeons involved in diagnosis of diseases of the alimentary tract and the genitourinary system. Published bimonthly, it offers peer-reviewed original research articles, case reports, technological updates, and invited review articles. Also included is a section highlighting abstracts from the current literature, book reviews and conference updates. It includes articles on abdominal imaging from all modalities—computed tomography, ultrasound, magnetic resonance, nuclear medicine, and interventional radiology. This is a highly regarded journal that should be in all radiology collections. Online access back to volume 1, 1976 of *Gastrointestinal Radiology* is available through SpringerLink.

American Journal of Neuroradiology. v. 1, American Society of Neuroradiology, 1980.
http://www.ajnr.org
ISSN: 01956108
ISSN: 1936959X (Online)
Recommended for: Hospital, Academic Libraries

Published 10 times a year by the American Society of Neuroradiology, the journal contains original clinical articles on imaging diagnosis of the central nervous system, including the spine, for an audience of radiologists, neuroradiologists, neurosurgeons, and neurologists. Each issue contains approximately 200 pages and covers the entire gamut of topics in the field beginning with the spectrum of diagnostic and functional imaging of the brain, head, neck, and spine, and continuing on with more specialized areas such as imaging and interventional techniques, pediatric neuroradiology, and cerebrovascular diseases to name just a few. Over 350 peer-reviewed articles are published in the journal each year, and it is considered the major journal in neuroradiology. It has an impact factor of 3.296 and ranks fourth of 13 neuroimaging journals and sixteenth of 104 radiology, nuclear medicine, and medical imaging journals in the 2009 *Journal Citation Reports*. Full text is available online from volume 16, 1995.

American Journal of Roentgenology (AJR). v. 1, American Roentgen Ray Society, 1906.
http://www.ajronline.org
ISSN: 0361803X
ISSN: 15463141 (Online)
Indexed in: MEDLINE
Recommended for: Hospital, Academic Libraries
Brandon/Hill Selection

American Journal of Roentgenology (*AJR*) was started by the American Roentgen Ray Society (ARRS), the oldest radiology society in the United States. Published monthly for over 100 years, the "yellow journal" offers high quality peer-reviewed original articles. Articles are grouped by system subspeciality (musculoskeletal imaging, gastrointestinal imaging, etc.). Also included are a resident's section, editorials, and medico-legal discussion. With an impact factor of 2.951, it ranks twenty-first out of 104 radiology, nuclear medicine, and medical imaging journals in the 2009 *Journal Citation Reports*. Full text is available online from volume 95, 1965.

IEEE Transactions on Medical Imaging. v. 1, Institute of Electrical and Electronics Engineers (IEEE), 1982.
See Chapter 2. Biomedical Engineering

Investigative Radiology. v. 1, Lippincott Williams & Wilkins, 1966.
http://www.ovid.com/
ISSN: 00209996
ISSN: 15360210 (Online)
Indexed in: MEDLINE
Recommended for: Hospital, Academic Libraries

Investigative Radiology is a monthly journal devoted to the early publication of research findings in diagnostic radiology, including CT, PET, MRI, ultrasound, and angiography. The emphasis is on timely publication of cutting edge research in radiology. The 2009 *Journal Citation Reports* list it as second of 104 radiology, nuclear medicine, and medical imaging journals with an impact factor of 4.850. This is an important title for any collection needing to support basic and clinical research in this field. It is available online through a variety of collections at Ovid.

Journal of Clinical Ultrasound. v. 1, John Wiley & Sons, 1973.

http://onlinelibrary.wiley.com/journal/10.1002/(ISSN)1097-0096
ISSN: 00912751
ISSN: 10970096 (Online)
Indexed in: MEDLINE
Recommended for: Hospital, Academic Libraries

An international journal published nine times a year, the *Journal of Clinical Ultrasound* includes radiologists, sonographers, obstetricians, gynecologists, pediatricians, urologists, and gastroenterologists among its subscribers. Coverage focuses on sonography of the gastrointestinal tract, genitourinary tract, vascular system, nervous system, head and neck, chest, breast, musculoskeletal system, obstetrics, and pediatrics. Doppler and interventional sonography are also covered. Original articles often compare ultrasound with other modalities; also included are discussions of new techniques, contrast agents, and equipment in the field. It has an impact factor of 0.910 and ranks thirteenth out of 28 acoustics journals and eighty-fifth out of 104 radiology, nuclear medicine, and medical imaging journals (2009 *Journal Citation Reports*). Online access is available back to volume 2, 1974.

Journal of Computer Assisted Tomography. v. 1, Lippincott Williams & Wilkins, 1977.
http://www.ovid.com/
ISSN: 03638715
ISSN: 15323145 (Online)
Indexed in: MEDLINE
Recommended for: Hospital, Academic Libraries

Each bi-monthly issue contains approximately 20 original peer-reviewed articles on a wide range of topics that focus on the use of computed tomography as a modality. Also included are case reports from leading radiologists on noteworthy and educational cases. These cases are presented with high quality images that highlight unique findings and diagnostic dilemmas, and also present their resolution. The journal also includes the abstracts of major CT meetings as well as book reviews and editorials. Since this field is such an important part of the day-to-day function of any modern radiology department, this journal is an important addition to all academic and hospital collections. It is available online through a variety of Ovid collections.

Radiographics. v. 1, Radiologic Society of North America, 1981.
http://radiographics.rsnajnls.org/
ISSN: 02715333
ISSN: 15271323 (Online)
Indexed in: MEDLINE
Recommended for: Hospital, Academic Libraries

This bi-monthly publication of the Radiological Society of North America (RSNA) states that its mission "is to publish the best in peer-reviewed educational material, emphasizing that presented at the annual meeting of the RSNA, for radiologists, trainees, physicists, and other radiologic professionals." Dedicated to CME and lifelong learning, *Radiographics* is an invaluable tool for the practicing radiologist and trainee. Covering all radiological subspecialties, the journal offers outstanding images and educational content allowing the reader to stay abreast of new research and techniques across the wide spectrum of radiology topics. It ranks twenty-eighth out of 104 radiology, nuclear medicine, and medical imaging journals with an impact factor of 2.747 (2009 *Journal Citation Reports*). Online full text is available back to volume 1, 1981.

Radiologic Clinics of North America. v. 1, W.B. Saunders, 1963.
http://radiologic.theclinics.com/
ISSN: 00338389
Indexed in: MEDLINE, CINAHL
Recommended for: Hospital, Academic Libraries
Brandon/Hill Selection

Each bi-monthly issue focuses on one clinical radiology topic under the direction of a guest editor who is a prominent leader in that field. The articles are lengthy and detailed with excellent quality images and written by experts. This is an outstanding resource for thorough coverage of major topics in radiology, and a personal subscription earns the reader CME credits. Finding an issue of *Radiologic Clinics* that focuses on one's topic of interest is a like discovering a gold mine of information. Examples of recent topics include foot and ankle imaging, breast imaging, magnetic resonance imaging of the knee, and imaging of the geriatric patient. This is an excellent review source for residents and students. It ranked forty-fourth out of 104 radiology, nuclear medicine, and medical imaging journals with an impact factor of 2.025 (2009 *Journal Citation Reports*). Online full text is available back to volume 36, 1998.

Radiology. v. 1, Radiologic Society of North America, 1923.
http://radiology.rsnajnls.org
ISSN: 00338419
ISSN: 15271315 (Online)
Indexed in: MEDLINE
Recommended for: Hospital, Academic Libraries
Brandon/Hill Selection

Published monthly by the Radiologic Society of North America (RSNA), this is the first journal title that comes to mind when looking for current, high-quality research related to all aspects of radiology. Each issue contains over 300 pages of peer-reviewed research articles, commentary and reviews, as well as coverage of new technologies and techniques. *Radiology* has the largest circulation in the field of radiology. In the 2009 *Journal Citation Reports*, it ranked second out of 104 radiology, nuclear medicine, and medical imaging journals with an impact factor of 6.341. Full text online access is available back to volume 1, 1926.

Skeletal Radiology. v. 1, Springer, 1976.
http://www.springerlink.com/content/100487/
ISSN: 03642348
ISSN: 14322161 (Online)
Indexed in: MEDLINE
Recommended for: Hospital, Academic Libraries

Skeletal Radiology is the official journal of the International Skeletal Society and this is reflected in its interdisciplinary approach. While radiology is the main focus, there is also substantial coverage of the anatomical, pathological, physiological, clinical, metabolic and epidemiological aspects of skeletal disease. The monthly issues contain original articles, case reports, review articles and meeting overviews. Since musculoskeletal radiology is such an important and growing subspecialty, this journal is an important title to include in a radiology collection. In the 2009 *Journal Citation Reports*, it ranked fifty-eighth out of 104 radiology, nuclear medicine, and medical imaging journals with an impact factor of 1.568. SpringerLink offers full text online access back to volume 1, 1976.

10.17.1. Nuclear Medicine

Diagnostic, therapeutic, and investigative use of radioactive compounds in a pharmaceutical form.

—MeSH

Contributor: Debra R. Berlanstein

Monographs

Breast Cancer Imaging: A Multidisciplinary, Multimodality Approach. 1st ed. Authors: Marie Tartar, Christopher E. Comstock, Michael S. Kipper. Mosby/Elsevier, 2008.
See Chapter 10.17.2. Radiation Oncology

Breast Cancer: Nuclear Medicine in Diagnosis and Therapeutic Options. 1st ed. Editors: Emilio Bombardieri, Gianni Bonadonna, Luca Giani. Springer, 2008.
http://www.springerlink.com/content/vp7576/
ISBN: 9783540367802
Recommended for: Hospital, Academic Libraries

This work offers a complete look at the diagnostic and therapeutic aspects of nuclear medicine as it relates to the critical area of breast cancer management. The audience includes radiologists, oncologists, and surgeons. The authors focus on nuclear medicine techniques and compare them with other approaches to breast cancer diagnosis and treatment. It is the combination of diagnostic and therapeutic coverage that makes this work especially valuable, and the authors' style make complex subjects clear and easy to understand.

Essentials of Nuclear Medicine Imaging. 5th ed. Authors: Fred A. Mettler, Milton J. Guiberteau. Elsevier (Saunders), 2006.
ISBN: 9780721602011
Recommended for: Hospital, Academic Libraries
Brandon/Hill Selection

Now in its fifth edition, this work is often considered the best introduction to nuclear medicine, and contains over 600 images. The first chapters offer introductions to the physics and science of nuclear medicine, followed by chapters covering all the body systems. This edition also covers PET/CT, cardiac-gated SPECT, and tumor-specific radionuclides. Each chapter includes basic physics, instrumentation, artifacts, and quality control. Added value includes clinical pearls and case scenarios. Overall, this is a concise, complete book useful in the daily work of nuclear medicine.

Fundamentals of Nuclear Medicine Dosimetry. 1st ed. Author: Michael G. Stabin. Springer, 2008.
http://www.springerlink.com/content/978-0-387-74578-7
ISBN: 9780387745787
Recommended for: Hospital, Academic Libraries

This work falls into the "everything you wanted to know about nuclear medicine dosimetry" category. The description indicates that this book includes "fundamental concepts, including standardized models, methods of calculation, and software applications. It also covers biological effects of radiation on living systems and regulatory aspects related to radiation dosimetry and radiation protection." This convenient pocket-sized manual includes all the tips and tricks needed to assist the nuclear medicine physician and physicist in dose calculations. Especially useful are the case studies and the coverage of the regulatory aspects of the topic.

Nuclear Medicine. 2nd ed. Editors: Gary L. Dillehay, Robert E. Henkin, Robert H. Wagner, Stephen M. Karesh, James R. Halama. Elsevier, 2006.
ISBN: 9780323028981 (2 v.)
Recommended for: Hospital, Academic Libraries
Doody's Core Titles Selection

Ten years after the original work, this second edition reflects all of the advances that nuclear medicine has seen during this period. This complete and authoritative set includes everything from basic physics to complex imaging of all body systems. Despite its encyclopedic coverage, it is easy to use and is useful for all members of the nuclear medicine team. Included are 3,000 images (1,300 in color) which make this an extremely attractive set. If a library were to only purchase one nuclear medicine title, this should be it.

Practical Nuclear Medicine. 3rd ed. Editors: Peter F. Sharp, Howard G. Gemmel, Alison D. Murray. Springer, 2005.
http://www.springerlink.com/content/k55286/
ISBN: 9781852338756
Recommended for: Hospital, Academic Libraries
Doody's Core Titles Selection

Despite recent advances in magnetic resonance imaging and computed tomography technology, nuclear medicine continues to have a unique role because of its ability to represent physiological function. This practical work begins with a review of the science of nuclear medicine, followed by different clinical applications. It includes newer technologies of PET, SPECT and tumor imaging and contains excellent images. The authors state that this edition "continues the text's tradition of guiding readers through not only the most commonly performed clinical nuclear medicine tests but the scientific bases on which they were built." They specifically address diagnostic dilemmas and try to highlight the upcoming advances in radiopharmaceuticals, instrumentation, and molecular imaging. This is an invaluable resource for radiologists, physicists, and technologists.

Journals

BMC Medical Physics. v. 1, BioMed Central, 2001.
See Chapter 26.8. Radiobiology

Clinical Nuclear Medicine. v. 1, Lippincott Williams & Wilkins, 1976.
http://journals.lww.com/nuclearmed/
ISSN: 03639762
ISSN: 15360229 (Online)
Recommended for: Hospital, Academic Libraries

This excellent journal, published monthly, provides practical clinical information in nuclear medicine with articles that address all aspects of scanning and imaging. This is the most practice-oriented journal in the field and includes numerous illustrations of all applications of nuclear medicine. Contents include both original articles and interesting image/case presentations. The *Journal Citation Reports* (2009) ranks it eleventh out of 104 journals in the radiology, nuclear medicine, and medical imaging category. Online full text access is available from volume 1, 1976.

Journal of Nuclear Cardiology. v. 1, Springer, 1994.
http://springerlink.com/content/1071-3581
ISSN: 10713581
ISSN: 15326551 (Online)
Indexed in: MEDLINE
Recommended for: Hospital, Academic Libraries

A publication of the American Society of Nuclear Cardiology, the *Journal of Nuclear Cardiology* is the only journal that focuses on this growing field that bridges nuclear medicine and cardiology. Published bi-monthly, the original articles focus on the interpretation and diagnosis of studies as well as updates on radiopharmaceuticals and equipment in this evolving field. Several review articles also appear in each issue along with the society's position papers, news, and technology updates. It is ranked twenty-sixth of 104 journals in the radiology, nuclear medicine, and medical imaging category in the 2009 *Journal Citation Reports*. Full-text online access is available from volume 1, 1976.

Journal of Nuclear Medicine. v. 1, Society of Nuclear Medicine, 1960.
http://jnm.snmjournals.org
ISSN: 01615505
ISSN: 15355667 (Online)
Indexed in: MEDLINE
Recommended for: Hospital, Academic Libraries
Brandon/Hill Selection

The flagship publication of the Society of Nuclear Medicine, the *Journal of Nuclear Medicine* holds the top impact factor ranking from *Journal Citation Reports* (2009) for all imaging journals. The journal includes original peer-reviewed research articles on basic science and clinical topics, news from the Society of Nuclear Medicine, book reviews and sections that focus on molecular imaging and continuing education. The full content of the journal is online from volume 1, 1960. This journal should be the mainstay of the nuclear medicine collection in any hospital or academic library.

Nuclear Medicine and Biology. v. 1, Elsevier, 1973.
See Chapter 26.8. Radiobiology

Seminars in Nuclear Medicine. v. 1, W.B. Saunders, 1971.
http://www.journals.elsevierhealth.com/periodicals/ysnuc
ISSN: 00012998
ISSN: 15584623 (Online)
Indexed in: MEDLINE
Recommended for: Hospital, Academic Libraries

This is a clinically oriented journal that focuses on new developments and techniques in nuclear medicine. Articles provide excellent overviews of topics relevant to the practice of nuclear medicine. Contributing authors are highly regarded experts in their field. The journal is published four times a year and each issue has a specific clinical focus. Several recent examples of topics covered include bone update, infection, and pharmacologic interventions. This is a very valuable resource for review of current practice in nuclear medicine. Ranked tenth of 104 journals in its category in the 2009 *Journal Citation Reports*, it has an impact factor of 3.962. Online access is available back to volume 1, 1971.

10.17.2. Radiation Oncology

Radiotherapy of cancer.
—MeSH

Contributor: Debra R. Berlanstein

Monographs

AJCC Cancer Staging Atlas. 1st ed. Editor: Frederick L. Greene. Springer, 2006.
http://www.springerlink.com/content/w0ruh1/
ISBN: 9780387331263
Recommended for: Hospital, Academic Libraries
Doody's Core Titles Selection

The American Joint Commission on Cancer developed this atlas as a companion to their staging manual, now in its 6th edition. This title is recommended for oncologic surgery, as well as for radiation oncology collections. There are over 400 illustrations that cover anatomic extent for tumor (T), regional lymph nodes (N), and metastasis (M) for multiple sites including head and neck, digestive system, thorax, musculoskeletal, soft tissue, breast, genitourinary, and gynecologic tumor sites. This is a concise manual that fits into a coat pocket and serves a much-needed purpose as a visual representation of cancer staging for the practicing physician.

Breast Cancer Imaging: A Multidisciplinary, Multimodality Approach. 1st ed. Authors: Marie Tartar, Christopher E. Comstock, Michael S. Kipper. Mosby/Elsevier, 2008.
ISBN: 9780323046770
Recommended for: Hospital, Academic Libraries

This multimodality book bridges the gap between the diagnosing of breast cancer and the therapeutic approaches to breast cancer. Chapters include screening of general and high-risk populations, diagnosing symptomatic patients, strategies for biopsy, staging of metastatic disease, and surveillance for recurrence. The authors use real-world examples to demonstrate their points and discuss current guidelines. They also include examples of neurologic, nuclear, and body-imaging correlations. This head-to-toe approach makes this a unique and especially helpful text, since much of the information would otherwise be available in a disparate group of texts. Over 1,000 excellent images are included in this unique work that attempts to address this specialization of radiologists.

Clinical Radiation Oncology. 2nd ed. Editors: Leonard L. Gunderson, Joel E. Tepper. Churchill Livingstone, 2007.
ISBN: 9780443068409
Recommended for: Hospital, Academic Libraries
Doody's Core Titles Selection

This is a comprehensive textbook that is considered by many to be the definitive source for radiation oncology. It is divided into three sections that cover scientific foundations, techniques and modalities, and disease sites. Included are full-color graphs, figures and diagrams, and the writing is concise and readable. There is a focus on evidence-based techniques and discussions of future areas of growth in radiation oncology as well. There is excellent coverage of the therapeutic management of specific disease sites, with discussion of single-modality and combined-modality approaches. New topics in this edition include biologics, related imaging modalities such as computed tomograpy, magnetic resonance imaging, and nuclear medicine. New disease site sections address brain tumors, management of the neck, melanoma, uncommon thoracic malignancies, and penile cancer, to name a few. This is a go-to resource written by experts in the field.

Handbook of Evidence-Based Radiation Oncology. 1st ed. Editors: Eric K. Hansen, Mack Roach. Springer, 2007.
ISBN: 9780387306476
Recommended for: Hospital, Academic Libraries
Doody's Core Titles Selection

This is an outstanding pocket guide geared to residents and fellows that offers a framework for each organ system that is easy to reference, organized, and very readable. Many of the chapters are written in part by a resident, so it is extremely practical and focused on the information that trainees need to know: treatment guidelines, staging, and the related literature that supports current evidence-based practice. Of special value are the clinical pearls on epidemiology, anatomy, pathology, and clinical presentation. Also included are practical instructions about patient set-up for simulation, dose/fractionation schema, acute/chronic toxicities, and dose-limiting structures. The appendixes are also useful and include performance status scales, radionucleotides used in brachytherapy, radiation safety, tumor markers, immunophenotyping and cytogenetics, and commonly prescribed drugs. This is a critical purchase for any institution with a residency in radiation oncology.

Perez and Brady's Principles and Practice of Radiation Oncology. 5th ed. Editors: Edward C. Halperin, Carlos A. Perez, Luther W. Brady, David E. Wazer, Carolyn Freeman, Leonard R. Prosnitz. Lippincott Williams & Wilkins, 2008.
http://www.perezandbradys.com/
ISBN: 9780781763691
See Also Chapter 10.10.6. Medical Oncology
Recommended for: Hospital, Academic Libraries
Brandon/Hill, *Doody's Core Titles* Selection

This is the leading textbook in radiation oncology, now in its fifth edition. It is arranged in five color-coded sections for easy reference. This edition is comprehensive in scope and includes background, history, biology, physics, clinical topics, and controversies. Each section is written by recognized experts and is geared toward therapists, dosimetrists, physicists, medical students, residents, and also experienced physicians. The book is full color and emphasizes the use of radiation oncology in palliative and supportive care as well as therapy. Six new chapters cover stereotactic irradiation outside the central nervous system, photodynamic therapy, radiation and gene therapy, prostate treatment, oncologic imaging, and economics. There is also coverage of molecular biology, radiosurgery, and other innovations. The companion website is fully searchable. This should be regarded as an essential purchase for libraries serving this specialty.

Radiation Therapy: A Guide to Patient Care. 1st ed. Editors: Marilyn L. Haas, William P. Hogle, Giselle J. Moore-Higgs, Tracy A. Gosselin-Acomb. Elsevier, 2007.
ISBN: 9780323040303
Recommended for: Hospital, Consumer Health Libraries
Doody's Core Titles Selection

Aimed at patient management and nursing, this work includes 13 chapters that focus on combined modality chemotherapy/radiation, evidence-based guidelines, special patient populations, and patient teaching. Also included are special sections on geriatrics and complementary medicine, and clinical trials. The book is organized into seven sections, including treatment and planning, integrative systems and clinical sites, adjuvant therapies, dimensions of clinical practice, and supportive nursing care, to name a few. This work will complement the larger and more detailed textbooks in radiation therapy with its focus on nursing issues and patient management.

Treatment Planning in Radiation Oncology. 2nd ed. Editor: Faiza M. Khan. Lippincott Williams & Wilkins, 2007.
ISBN: 9780781785419
Recommended for: Hospital, Academic Libraries
Doody's Core Titles Selection

The subtitle of this useful work is "Comprehensive guide to state-of-the-art treatment planning techniques in radiation oncology," and the second edition serves as an important update in a field exploding with new techniques and technology. Written for the entire treatment planning team—radiation oncologists, medical physicists, and medical dosimetrists—this text offers over 600 illustrations that detail specific methodologies with excellent examples. This edition includes new chapters on image-guided radiation therapy, high-dose rate brachytherapy, and brachytherapy treatment-planning algorithms, along with updates to the other chapters. By omitting obsolete modalities and concentrating on newer, relevant treatments, this work is a very useful and important addition to the radiation oncology library.

Journals

BMC Medical Physics. v. 1, BioMed Central, 2001.
See Chapter 26.8. Radiobiology

International Journal of Radiation: Oncology-Biology-Physics. v. 1, Elsevier, 1976.
http://www.redjournal.org/
http://www.sciencedirect.com/science/journal/03603016
ISSN: 03603016
ISSN: 1879355X (Online)
Indexed in: MEDLINE
Recommended for: Hospital, Academic Libraries

Often referred to in the field as the *Red Journal*, this is the official journal of the American Society for Radiation Oncology and contains original articles that connect new research and technologies to clinical applications. These include experimental studies of combined modality treatment, tumor sensitization and normal tissue protection, molecular radiation biology, particle irradiation, brachytherapy, treatment planning, tumor biology, and clinical investigations of cancer treatment that include radiation therapy. Technical advances related to dosimetry and conformal radiation treatment planning are also included. The journal is published 15 times during the year and ranks sixth out of 104 journals in its category in the 2009 *Journal Citation Reports*.

Radiation Oncology. v. 1, BioMed Central, 2006.
http://www.ro-journal.com/
ISSN: 1748717X
Indexed in: MEDLINE
Recommended for: Hospital, Academic Libraries

Radiation Oncology is an open access, peer-reviewed online journal that covers all aspects of research aimed at the treatment of cancer with radiation. It includes articles in the subject areas of molecular and cellular radiation biology, radiation physics, radiation technology, and clinical oncology. Original research, review articles, case reports, and study protocols are all included. Ranking thirty-second out of 104 titles in radiology, nuclear medicine, and medical imaging, it has an impact factor of 2.529 (2009 *Journal Citation Reports*).

Seminars in Radiation Oncology. v. 1, W.B. Saunders, 1991.
http://www.semradonc.com/
ISSN: 10534296
ISSN: 15329461 (Online)
Indexed in: MEDLINE, CINAHL
Recommended for: Hospital, Academic Libraries

Following the format of other seminar titles, this quarterly journal invites a guest editor for each issue and focuses on a key topic in radiation oncology. Many of the articles report new scientific information and topics fall in the categories of tumor biology, diagnosis, medical and surgical management of the patient, and new technologies. Recent issues have focused on head and neck cancer, stem cells in radiation oncology, and locally advanced breast cancer. It ranks ninth in its category of radiology, nuclear medicine, and medical imaging (*Journal Citation Reports*, 2009). This review journal is extremely useful to the practicing radiation oncologist. All volumes back to volume 1, 1991 are available online.

10.17.3. Interventional Radiology

Radiology that combines organ system radiography, catheter techniques and sectional imaging.

—MeSH

Contributor: Debra R. Berlanstein

Monographs

Abrams' Angiography: Interventional Radiology. 2nd ed. Editors: Stanley Baum, Michael J. Pentecost. Lippincott, Williams & Wilkins, 2006.
ISBN: 9780781740890
Recommended for: Hospital, Academic Libraries
Doody's Core Titles Selection

This update of the fourth edition of *Abrams' Angiography* is a complete reference for interventional radiology. The more than 60 contributors are leaders in the field and the organization is excellent. The book begins with an overview of the techniques and tools used in interventional radiology, followed by chapters covering different organ systems, including vascular, gastrointestinal, genitourinary, central nervous system, thoracic, trauma related, and pediatric interventions. The last two sections address drainage, foreign body retrieval, and ecanalization of dialysis fistulas. This revision also includes 15 new chapters that cover cutting-edge innovations, such as stent-grafts, radiofrequency ablation, computed tomography angiography, magnetic resonance angiography, uterine fibroid embolization, and vertebroplasty. This would be the go-to interventional text for any medical library.

Grossman's Cardiac Catheterization, Angiography, and Intervention. 7th ed. Editor: Donald S. Baim. Lippincott Williams & Wilkins, 2006.
ISBN: 9780781755672
Recommended for: Hospital, Academic Libraries
Brandon/Hill, *Doody's Core Titles* Selection

Written for interventional radiologists and cardiologists, this seventh edition of a classic work has been revised with a focus on therapy since the field has evolved in that direction. In addition, a DVD with useful cases is provided to complement the text. Organized into eight sections, the chapters cover general principles; basic techniques; hemodynamic principles; basic and special angiographic, catheter, and interventional techniques; the evaluation of cardiac function; and profiles of specific disorders. The book excels at explaining the basics as well as the more complex issues in interventional cardiology and radiology and includes evidence-based clinical studies as well as technique. This work has been described as a benchmark for cardiac catheterization and its applications and should be an essential addition to any interventional radiology collection.

Image-Guided Intervention. 1st ed. Editors: Matthew A. Mauro, Kieran P.J. Murphy, Kenneth R. Thomson, Anthony C. Venbrux, Christoph L. Zollikofer. Elsevier Saunders, 2008.
ISBN: 978141629649
Recommended for: Hospital, Academic Libraries

This two-volume set is a comprehensive, state-of-the-art textbook that includes all interventional procedures done by radiologists. It is organized with introductory chapters covering the history of the field followed by sections on vascular and non-vascular procedures. It is organized by a concise, practical approach, and includes over 1,600 large, digital-quality images that include magnetic resonance, multislice computed tomography, ultrasonography, and CT angiography. Also included are anatomical drawings. Good coverage is included on protocols, algorithms and guidelines from a variety of international experts. Step-by-step instructions on techniques, discussion of contrast agents and best practices makes this an especially important work. One reviewer wrote, "this book should be available in every interventional department and in every institution confronted with patients prior to or after interventional treatments" (Loewe C. *Eur J Radiol* 2009; 72: 188–189).

Interventional Neuroradiology. 1st ed. Editors: Robert W. Hurst, Robert H. Rosenwasser. Informa Healthcare, 2008.
ISBN: 9780849395628
Recommended for: Hospital, Academic Libraries
Doody's Core Titles Selection

Written like a surgical manual for interventional neuroradiologists by leading experts in the field, this work covers anatomy and techniques and includes coverage of embolization of aneurysms, treatment of acute strokes, and disorders of the vertebral bodies. Chapters are also devoted to computer tomography, magnetic resonance, and ultrasonographic evaluation of cerebrovascular disease. This serves as a quick reference in a rapidly growing field that treats patients who are not candidates for traditional surgery and bridges the fields of neurosurgery, neuroradiology, and neurology. This is highly recommended as a manageable but inclusive reference.

Journals

American Journal of Neuroradiology. v. 1, American Society of Neuroradiology, 1980.
See Chapter 10.17. Radiology

Cardiovascular and Interventional Radiology. v. 3, Springer, 1980.
http://www.springerlink.com/content/100121/
ISSN: 01741551
ISSN: 1432086X (Online)
Indexed in: MEDLINE
Recommended for: Hospital, Academic Libraries

This is the official journal of the Cardiovascular and Interventional Radiological Society of Europe, the Japanese Society of Interventional Radiology, and the British Society of Interventional Radiology, which makes it an excellent European/Asian companion to the *Journal of Vascular and Interventional Radiology* from the United States. Each bi-monthly issue includes peer-reviewed, original research from both laboratory and clinical studies, as well as technical notes, case reports, review articles, and editorials. The journal ranks forty-seventh out of 104 titles in radiology, nuclear medicine, and medical imaging with an impact factor of 1.949 (*Journal Citation Reports*, 2009). It is available online back to volume 1, 1978 (under its previous title, *Cardiovascular Radiology*).

Journal of Vascular and Interventional Radiology. v. 1, Elsevier, 1990.
http://www.jvir.org/
ISSN: 10510443
ISSN: 15357732 (Online)
Indexed in: MEDLINE
Recommended for: Hospital, Academic Libraries

This is the official journal of the Society of Interventional Radiology and it covers both clinical and laboratory studies in interventional radiology. The audience includes radiologists, cardiologists, vascular surgeons, and neurosurgeons. All approaches are included: medical, minimally invasive, radiological, pathological, and socioeconomic, all of which are important to vascular and interventional radiologists. This is a key purchase to insure coverage in this large subspecialty of radiology. The journal ranks fifty-second out of 104 titles in radiology, nuclear medicine, and medical imaging with an impact factor of 1.805 (*Journal Citation Reports*, 2009). It is available online back to volume 1, 1990.

Seminars in Interventional Radiology. v. 1, Thieme, 1984.
https://www.thieme-connect.de/ejournals/toc/sir

ISSN: 07399529
ISSN: 10988963
Recommended for: Hospital, Academic Libraries
Seminars in Interventional Radiology is a quarterly review journal. Each issue focuses on a particular topic of importance in interventional radiology. Articles are geared toward practicing radiologists and residents in training, and cover a multitude of important topics including cardiovascular imaging, oncologic interventional radiology, abdominal interventional radiology, metallic stents, renal intervention, angiography, neurointerventions, and CT fluoroscopy. No impact factor is available. The journal is online from volume 1, 1984.

Techniques in Vascular and Interventional Radiology. v. 1, W.B. Saunders, 1998.
http://www.techvir.com/
http://www.sciencedirect.com/science/journal/10892516
ISSN: 10892516
ISSN: 15579808 (Online)
Indexed in: MEDLINE
Recommended for: Hospital, Academic Libraries

Because the field of cardiovascular and interventional radiology is so technique driven, this journal, published quarterly, is heavily dependent on visuals making it almost atlas-like in its format. Each issue has an esteemed guest editor and focuses on a particular technique or problem. The journal describes its mission as follows: "To improve patient care by educating interventionalists on the latest techniques in catheter-based therapies from experts in the field." No impact factor is available. This is an extremely useful title for the practicing interventionalist, unique from the other journals in the field. Online access is available back to volume 1, 1998.

10.18. Reproductive Medicine

The morphology, physiology, biochemistry, and pathology of reproduction in man and other animals, and on the biological, [and] medical... problems of fertility and lactation. It includes ovulation induction, diagnosis of infertility and recurrent pregnancy loss, and assisted reproductive technologies such as embryo transfer, in vitro fertilization, and intrafallopian transfer of zygotes.

—MeSH

Contributor: Pamela Van Hine

Monographs

Breastfeeding and Human Lactation. 4th ed. Editors: Jan Riordan, Karen Wambach. Jones & Bartlett, 2010.
http://extranet.netlibrary.com/TitleSelect/
http://www.ebrary.com/ (3rd ed.)
ISBN: 9780763754327
ISBN: 9780763758820
See Also Chapter 13.7. Maternal-Child Nursing
Recommended for: Hospital, Academic Libraries

This review refers to the third edition. According to the editor, "this text brings together in a single volume the latest clinical techniques and research findings that direct evidence-based clinical practice." It has a clear, practical, clinical focus aimed primarily at nurses, lactation consultants, and other health care providers. The editor and 21 chapter authors are all breastfeeding experts. Half of the authors are lactation consultants; the rest are a mix of physicians, scientists, and nurses. The text is divided into five sections: historical and work perspectives; anatomical and biological imperatives; prenatal, perinatal, and postnatal periods; beyond postpartum; and sociocultural and research issues. Each chapter includes a summary and key concepts, extensive references, Internet resources, extensive black-and-white illustrations, and many tables and charts. All aspects of breastfeeding are covered. Unusual chapters include several on research methodology, the culture of breastfeeding, lactation consultant training and work experience, education of health care providers and patients, and extensive sections on infant growth patterns. The book also includes a glossary and eight appendixes, including the International Board of Lactation Consultant Examiners' code of ethics, clinical competencies, certification, and a sample of the useful Wellstart International patient history. This book offers practical, nurse-oriented information on breastfeeding. There is less focus on complications that need to be addressed by physicians and less detailed information on the underlying biology of lactation than is included in Lawrence and Lawrence's *Breastfeeding: A Guide for the Medical Profession*. This text is an excellent addition to any type of medical collection, including the hospital library, academic library, and special collection.

Breastfeeding Handbook for Physicians. Editors: Richard J. Schanler, Sharon Dooley. American Academy of Pediatrics [and] American College of Obstetricians and Gynecologists, 2006.
ISBN: 9781581100907
ISBN: 9781932328172
See Also Chapter 14.1. Child Nutrition Sciences

Recommended for: Hospital, Academic, Consumer Health Libraries

Breastfeeding Handbook for Physicians was written "to provide health care professionals in all specialties with a concise and inexpensive teaching and reference aid on breastfeeding and human lactation. The overall goal of the handbook is to enhance physicians' knowledge of breastfeeding physiology and clinical practice so that they become comfortable encouraging and supporting breastfeeding." Written by multiple contributors, consultants, committees, and staff, it includes 15 chapters covering three broad areas. The first topical area, breastfeeding basics, includes definitions, rates in the United States, recommended practices, importance of breastfeeding, who can and cannot breastfeed, and the basic anatomy and physiology of lactation. The second broad area is the management and encouragement of breastfeeding for normal women and infants. Coverage includes preconception and prenatal counseling, the peripartum transition to lactation, hospital-based postpartum care, and support of the continuing maintenance of breastfeeding from the perspectives of the infant and the mother. How to implement a breastfeeding-friendly medical office is the final chapter. The third area covers breastfeeding complications, including separation of the maternal-infant dyad, breastfeeding technology, drug interactions, contraception, and infants with special needs. Important topics include breastfeeding Down syndrome infants, tandem nursing, nursing multiples, and ethics. Each chapter, written in an outline form, has a brief list of selected key references, extensive tables, and simple black-and-white illustrations. Appendixes include breastfeeding resources and reprints of selected AAP and ACOG guidelines. This is an important handbook for any type of medical library collection, including a consumer health collection.

Breastfeeding: A Guide for the Medical Profession. 6th ed. Authors: Ruth A. Lawrence, Robert M. Lawrence. Elsevier/Mosby, 2005.
ISBN: 9780323028233
Recommended for: Academic Libraries

According to the first edition, "this book was written in an effort to provide the medical profession with an easily accessible reference for the clinical management of the mother-infant nursing couple." The 23 chapters, written by the two authors, cover all aspects of breastfeeding. Each chapter includes dozens of references, extensive black-and-white illustrations, and many tables, charts, and boxes that summarize key data and points. Historical perspectives are included when relevant. The chapters on anatomy, physiology, biochemistry, and immunology are much more detailed and comprehensive than in most other breastfeeding textbooks. This book has 17 appendixes, including human milk composition, dietary guidelines, normal serum values of breastfed infants, drug interactions, maternal infections, storage, Academy of Breastfeeding Medicine protocols, and American Academy of Pediatrics (AAP) hyperbilirubinemia guidelines. The drug interactions appendix is unusual, including more than just AAP information. The appendixes with guidelines could be improved with a warning to check the society website for more recent guidelines. The appendix on resources for education and training, although useful, should also include websites. This guide is an excellent addition for an academic or special collection.

The Breastfeeding Answer Book. 3rd ed. Authors: Nancy Mohrbacher, Julie Stock. La Leche League International, 2003.
ISBN: 9780912500928
Recommended for: Hospital, Academic, Consumer Health Libraries

This book, designed to help answer a mother's breastfeeding questions, uses non-medical language to help communicate with the mother and to be accessible to the wide range of medical and non-medical breastfeeding counselors who use this work. The two authors, both lactation consultants, have written 22 chapters. Initial chapters cover how to address breastfeeding questions and basic information on the breast and breastfeeding. The majority of the book focuses on specific breastfeeding questions arranged in 19 chapters, covering positioning and latching on, weight gain and nutrition, working mothers, maternal and newborn health issues, breastfeeding multiples, relactation and induced lactation, and tandem nursing. Sections on contraception and health problems are not as detailed as in more clinically-focused books. The text is presented in one column on each page, with lines separating each topic. A blank column next to the text is used to highlight key points and questions. Black-and-white illustrations are included when needed. Each chapter starts with a list of the broad topics covered in that chapter and ends with resources for parents, publications for parents, and dozens of references. This book includes two supplements: American Academy of Pediatrics' (AAP) transfer of drugs and other chemicals into human milk, and use of breast pumps and other products. This book provides practical information for breastfeeding women, lactation consultants, and others who are counseling them. It is useful in any type of medical collection, including consumer health, hospital, academic, and selected special collections.

Clinical Gynecologic Endocrinology and Infertility. 8th ed. Authors: Marc A. Fritz, Leon Speroff. Lippincott Williams & Wilkins, 2011.
http://www.r2library.com/ (7th ed.)
ISBN: 9780781779685
See Also Chapter 10.10.2. Endocrinology
Recommended for: Hospital, Academic Libraries
Brandon/Hill, *Doody's Core Titles* Selection

This review refers to the seventh edition. This book is divided into four parts: reproductive physiology, clinical endocrinology, contraception, and infertility. The 33 chapters, which do not have separate authors, are relatively brief overviews of each topic. Each chapter includes simple, but appropriate, red, black and white illustrations and a brief set of references. The appendixes include a useful listing of laboratory values in reproductive medicine and SI unit conversions. The authors' intent was to provide a "formulation of clinical diagnoses and management founded on physiologic principles," not a comprehensive encyclopedia of gynecologic endocrinology and infertility. Although this book is designed for the clinician, it has greater emphasis on reproductive physiology than Falcone and Hurd's *Clinical Reproductive Medicine and Surgery*, and it does not include chapters on reproductive imaging or surgery. This book is a classic textbook in reproductive medicine that is valuable in any type of medical library, whether in the hospital, the academic center, or a specialized collection. *Doody's* considers this Brandon/Hill book a core title in obstetrics and gynecology. The seventh edition is the first edition with a new author, Mark Fritz, and the first step in a "planned transition to a completely new authorship."

Clinical Reproductive Medicine and Surgery. Editors: Tommaso Falcone, William W. Hurd. Mosby/Elsevier, 2007.
ISBN: 9780323033091 (includes DVD)
Recommended for: Hospital, Academic Libraries

Designed as a textbook for physicians in training and those in their early years of practice, this book "provides a broad understanding of basic science of reproductive medicine and a comprehensive approach to the reproductive patient." This book is divided into seven sections: basic science, pediatric and adolescent disorders, adult reproductive endocrinology, contraception, reproductive imaging, infertility and recurrent pregnancy loss, and reproductive surgery. The 53 individual chapters are written by 95 authors who are experts in the field. Each chapter has beautiful illustrations, with colored flow charts and color photographs. Each chapter includes Pearls, which summarize the key points for each chapter, and dozens of references. Three chapters on imaging—hysterosalpingography, pelvic ultrasound/sonohysterography, and MRI—are an unusual feature for a book on reproductive medicine. The section on reproductive surgery is also strong for a general reproductive medicine book. Although the book includes pediatric and adolescent disorders and contraception, these sections are brief. This book is a practical, clinically oriented book, with basic sciences included as necessary. It is a valuable addition for any library collection that includes reproductive medicine. If the editors and authors are able to produce future editions of continuing high quality, all medical libraries will have a new, must-have classic in reproductive medicine.

Contraceptive Technology. 19th rev. ed. Editors: Robert A. Hatcher, James Trussell, Anita L. Nelson, Willard Cates Jr., Felicia H. Stewart, Deborah Kowal. Ardent Media, 2007.
ISBN: 9781597080026 (Includes CD-ROM)
Recommended for: Hospital, Academic, Consumer Health Libraries
Doody's Core Titles Selection

This ready-reference family planning handbook has 27 chapters, most of which cover all the types of contraception currently available in the United States. Additional chapters cover contraceptive efficacy, abortion, abstinence and non-coital sexual activity, sexually transmitted infections, female genital tract cancer screening, pregnancy testing and management of early pregnancy, infertility, and perimenopause. The six author-editors, 26 chapter authors, and 27 reviewers are all experts in family planning. Chapters on specific methods start with bulleted key points and include management of problems and follow-up, patient instructions, relevant line drawings, and dozens of key citations. Many chapters also include a brief history. The text is data driven, with dozens of tables covering contraceptive failure rates, risks, precautions, laboratory studies, and normal values. Efficacy, safety, noncontraceptive benefits, and personalized decision making for each method are addressed. Four appendixes provide selected websites, professional organizations, pharmaceutical company phone numbers and websites, and hotlines/websites. The pharmaceutical listing, which includes the relevant family planning products, and the hotlines/websites appendixes are especially helpful resources. Also useful is an insert that includes color photographs of combined and progestin-only oral contraceptives and a section on pills as emergency contraceptives. This handbook is aimed at the clinician who provides family planning services, but it provides valuable, easily accessible information for anyone with questions about contraception and family planning. It is an essential resource for any library, including a consumer health collection and hospital libraries.

Knobil and Neill's Physiology of Reproduction. 3rd ed.
Editor: Jimmy D. Neill. Elsevier, 2006.
http://extranet.netlibrary.com/TitleSelect/
ISBN: 9780125154000
ISBN: 9780080535272
Recommended for: Academic Libraries

This massive, two-volume work is divided into eight broad topics: gametes, fertilization, embryogenesis; female reproductive system; male reproductive system; pituitary and hypothalamus; reproductive behavior and its control; reproductive processes and their control; pregnancy; and lactation. Each section has an individual editor, and the sections are divided into 59 chapters, written by 122 authors. Each chapter has a miniature table of contents, a summary, and hundreds of references. Only black-and-while illustrations are included, but they are clear and appropriate. This book is designed for the basic scientist in reproductive medicine rather than the clinician. It does not cover therapy or surgery. Rather, it addresses the underlying physiology of reproduction, including genetics, microanatomy, and biochemistry. It compares reproductive physiology in humans to other mammals, primarily laboratory animals commonly used in reproductive biology—i.e., rats, mice, pigs, guinea pigs, and sheep. *Doody's* gives this book a score of 95, and the review states that it is "the leading comprehensive work on the physiology of reproduction." It is an essential resource for any academic or special collection that supports reproductive research.

Journals

Breastfeeding Medicine. v. 1, Mary Ann Liebert, 2006.
http://www.liebertonline.com/
ISSN: 15568253
ISSN: 15568342 (Online)
Indexed in: MEDLINE
Recommended for: Hospital, Academic Libraries

Breastfeeding Medicine, the official journal of the Academy of Breastfeeding Medicine (ABM), is published quarterly, with occasional supplements such as the recently published "First Annual Summit on Breastfeeding." The journal also includes new and revised ABM protocols. Created by physicians dedicated to the advancement of breastfeeding worldwide, this academic, peer-reviewed journal provides a scientific forum on breastfeeding and human lactation. The journal focuses on all medical aspects pertaining to breastfeeding and addresses the wide spectrum of research and clinical applications that impact the optimal care of mother and infant. *Breastfeeding Medicine* publishes original scientific articles, reviews, and case studies on a variety of topics in lactation medicine, including clinical, cultural, epidemiologic, physiologic, and psychological issues. Also covered are consequences of artificial feeding and the impact of "baby-friendly" hospitals. A review of websites relevant to breastfeeding and lactation is a regular feature. *Breastfeeding Medicine* is indexed in MEDLINE, Embase, PsycINFO, and CAB Abstracts. The journal is recommended for academic and special collections and hospital libraries with strong perinatal centers.

Contraception. v. 1, Elsevier, 1970.
http://www.sciencedirect.com/science/journal/00107824
ISSN: 00107824
Indexed in: MEDLINE
Recommended for: Hospital, Academic Libraries

Contraception, the official journal of the Association of Reproductive Health Professionals and the Society of Family Planning, is published 12 times per year, with occasional supplements. *Contraception* provides a venue for the rapid communication of advances and new knowledge in all areas of contraceptive research, including chemistry, biochemistry, physiology, endocrinology, biology, medical science, and demography. Editorials are often on family planning policy issues, but the focus of most of the articles is basic research in family planning and contraception. Results of international randomized trials on new contraceptives are frequently included. The target audience is clinicians and researchers in family planning and reproductive science. *Contraception* is indexed in MEDLINE, BIOSIS, POPLINE, Human Reproduction Update, Embase, and several other databases. This journal is recommended for academic and special collections and hospital libraries with a strong women's health program.

Fertility and Sterility. v. 1, Elsevier, 1950.
http://www.sciencedirect.com/science/journal/00150282
ISSN: 00150282
ISSN: 15565653 (Online)
Indexed in: MEDLINE
Recommended for: Hospital, Academic Libraries
Brandon/Hill Selection

Fertility and Sterility is the monthly, official journal of the American Society for Reproductive Medicine (ASRM) and its four affiliated societies, the Pacific Coast Reproductive Society, and the Canadian Fertility and Andrology Society. ASRM publishes new ASRM guidelines in the journal and includes a biennial compendium of Practice Committee Reports and ASRM meeting abstracts as supplements. According to the ASRM website, "now in its sixth decade, *Fertility and Sterility* publishes juried original articles of scientific excellence in clinical and laboratory research relevant to reproductive endocrinology, physiology, immunology, genetics and menopause.... The journal is an indispensable resource to reproductive endocrinologists, obstetricians, gynecologists, urologists, and basic scientists who treat and investigate the problems of fertility, sterility and the physiology of reproduction." Publication aims of the journal include: (a) peer-reviewed, original, innovative basic and clinical research articles in reproductive medicine and in systems-based practice that serve as an authoritative resource for knowledge and skills in reproductive medicine and that will support evidence-based opinions in reproductive science and clinical practice; (b) peer-reviewed review articles that promote continuous and practice-based learning; and (c) editorial and committee opinions that encourage professionalism and set high ethical standards for reproductive medicine. *Fertility and Sterility*, a Brandon/Hill journal indexed in MEDLINE, BIOSIS, Embase, and other databases, is highly recommended for all medical library collections.

Human Reproduction. v. 1, Oxford University Press, 1986.
http://humrep.oxfordjournals.org/
ISSN: 02681161
ISSN: 14602350 (Online)
Indexed in: MEDLINE
Recommended for: Academic Libraries

Human Reproduction, published monthly with occasional supplements, is the official journal of the European Society of Human Reproduction and Embryology (ESHRE). New ESHRE guidelines and reports are published frequently in the journal. According to the journal's website, *Human Reproduction* features full-length, peer-reviewed papers reporting original research and clinical case histories, as well as opinions and debates on topical issues. Papers published cover the scientific and medical aspects of reproductive physiology and pathology, endocrinology, andrology, gonad function, gametogenesis, fertilization, embryo development, implantation, pregnancy, genetics, genetic diagnosis, oncology, infectious disease, surgery, contraception, infertility treatment, psychology, ethics, and social issues. The highest scientific and editorial standard is maintained throughout the journal along with a rapid rate of publication. *Human Reproduction* is somewhat more basic science oriented and European oriented than *Fertility and Sterility*. It is indexed in MEDLINE, BIOSIS, Embase, Index Veterinarius, and many other databases. It is highly recommended for academic and special collections. Hospital librarians will occasionally need to request current, newsworthy articles through interlibrary loan.

Journal of Family Planning and Reproductive Health Care. v. 27, Pavilion, 2001.
http://www.ingentaconnect.com/content/ffp/jfp
ISSN: 14711893
Indexed in: MEDLINE, CINAHL
Recommended for: Academic Libraries

The Faculty of Sexual and Reproductive Healthcare of the Royal College of Obstetricians and Gynaecologists publish the quarterly *Journal of Family Planning and Reproductive Health Care*, formerly known as the *British Journal of Family Planning*. The *Journal* is a peer-reviewed, international publication that provides articles on all aspects of contraception and reproductive health, including papers reporting original quantitative or qualitative research, reviews, meta-analyses, consensus statements, case reports, short communications, and commentaries or personal views. Also included are papers relating to service delivery, education and training, public health, or clinical governance, including audits. Typical issues offer a short article on the history of contraception and a review on specific types of contraception, contraceptive complications, and sexually transmitted diseases. Additional articles cover commentaries on current topics in family planning, practical articles on the management of family planning services, and the provision of care in the ambulatory setting. This journal has UK-oriented advice and emphasis, although it is international in scope. It is indexed in MEDLINE, POPLINE, Embase, and other key databases. It is recommended for academic and special collections.

Journal of Human Lactation. v. 1, Sage, 1985.
http://jhl.sagepub.com/
ISSN: 08903344
ISSN: 15525732 (Online)
Indexed in: MEDLINE, CINAHL
Recommended for: Hospital, Academic Libraries

The *Journal of Human Lactation*, the official journal of the International Lactation Consultant Association (ILCA), is published quarterly. Written for lactation professionals by lactation professionals, the *Journal of Human Lactation* deals with the practical, routine topics that nurses, lactation consultants, midwives, nutritionists and dieticians, public health and social workers, therapists, and physicians face every day. Topics include patient counseling, sociological and ethnic issues in dealing with breastfeeding, practical discussions of breast diseases and conditions, care plans developed to help mothers and babies that require special care, economics of breastfeeding, education of physicians, hospital administration and other departments, and practical training for lactation consultants. The *Journal of Human Lactation* offers more practical articles on breastfeeding and fewer articles on basic science and medical complications than *Breastfeeding Medicine*. Its galactopharmacopedia feature, which provides a comprehensive review of the effects of a particular drug, is especially valuable. Because of its practical emphasis, this journal is recommended for hospital as well as academic library collections.

Perspectives on Sexual and Reproductive Health. v. 34, Guttmacher Institute and Wiley-Blackwell, 2002.
http://onlinelibrary.wiley.com/journal/10.1111/(ISSN)1931-2393/issues
ISSN: 15386341
ISSN: 19312393 (Online)
Indexed in: MEDLINE, CINAHL
Recommended for: Hospital, Academic Libraries

The Guttmacher Institute in partnership with Wiley-Blackwell publishes *Perspectives on Sexual and Reproductive Health* (formerly *Family Planning Perspectives*) four times a year. According to the journal's website, *Perspectives on Sexual and Reproductive Health* provides the latest peer-reviewed, policy-relevant research and analysis on sexual and reproductive health and rights in the United States and other developed countries. For more than four decades, *Perspectives* has offered unique insights into how reproductive health issues relate to one another; how they are affected by policies and programs; and how they impact individuals and societies. *Perspectives on Sexual and Reproductive Health* includes original research, special reports, and commentaries on the latest developments in the field of sexual and reproductive health, as well as staff-written summaries of recent findings in the field. Compared to other journals in family planning, *Perspectives on Sexual and Reproductive Health* has more of a family-planning policy focus than a strictly clinical or basic science focus. The journal also has a more American focus than the *Journal of Family Planning and Reproductive Health Care*. This journal is indexed in MEDLINE, CINAHL, Biological Abstracts, POPLINE, and many other medical and non-medical databases. It is an excellent addition for all medical library collections, including hospital, academic, and special collections.

Reproductive Toxicology. v. 1, Elsevier, 1987.
http://www.sciencedirect.com/science/journal/08906238
ISSN: 08906238
ISSN: 18731708
Indexed in: MEDLINE
Recommended for: Academic Libraries

Eight times a year, *Reproductive Toxicology* publishes timely, original research on the influence of chemical and physical agents on reproduction. This official journal of the European Teratology Society is a forum for communication among researchers and practitioners in diverse fields. Articles focus on the application of in vitro, animal, and clinical research to the practice of clinical medicine. All aspects of reproduction are within the scope of *Reproductive Toxicology*, including the formation and maturation of male and female gametes, sexual function, the events surrounding the fusion of gametes and the development of the fertilized ovum, nourishment and transport of the conceptus within the genital tract, implantation, embryogenesis, intrauterine growth, placentation and placental function, parturition, and lactation and neonatal survival. In addition to original research articles, *Reproductive Toxicology* also publishes interpretative review articles, editorials, letters, book reviews, and conference announcements. The first section of each journal issue is devoted to an in-depth, timely review of research on the effect of particular chemical or physical agents on reproduction. *Reproductive Toxicology* is indexed in MEDLINE, Embase, BIOSIS, and other biomedical databases. This journal is recommended for academic and special collections.

10.19. Venereology

Sexually transmitted disease.
—MeSH

Contributor: Tim Mason

Monographs

AIDS Therapy. 3rd ed. Editors: Raphael Dolin, Henry Masur, Michael S. Saag. Elsevier, 2008.
http://www.mdconsult.com/
ISBN: 9780443067525
Recommended for: Hospital, Academic Libraries
Doody's Core Titles Selection

This edition gives comprehensive guidance on the latest therapy for AIDS/HIV and the full range of related disorders and syndromes. Also, it connects the individual purchaser to a companion website with the most current advances in therapy and new drugs. Chapters cover a range of issues: antiretroviral therapy, management of patients in acute infection and pregnancy, and opportunistic processes. Unfortunately, this online access is only available for one user and of no benefit to libraries. This reference text is for the clinician who manages AIDS/HIV patients. It is a required resource for any hospital providing care for AIDS/HIV patients as well as academic health science libraries. This is a *Doody's Core Titles* recommendation.

Current Diagnosis & Treatment of Sexually Transmitted Diseases. Editors: Jeffrey D. Klausner, Edward W. Hook. McGraw-Hill, 2007.
http://www.accessmedicine.com/
http://www.ebrary.com/
http://www.r2library.com/
ISBN: 9780071456067
Recommended for: Hospital, Academic Libraries

This title is a byproduct of the classic book, *Current Diagnosis and Treatment* and a volume in the respected Lange *Current* series. It is an authoritative quick reference guide to STDs, featuring point-of-care guidelines, prevention and control, and counseling. It has treatment tables that list specific drugs, doses, and schedules. It is an essential guide for residents, family physicians, and other healthcare professionals who see patients with STDs. Each disease is fully discussed, covering biology, epidemiology, clinical manifestations, diagnosis, treatment, prevention, and social issues. The appendixes include diagnostic protocols, treatment tables, and websites. One appendix contains the 2006 "Treatment Guidelines for Sexually Transmitted Diseases" by the CDC. This title is a required resource for any hospital or clinic providing care for sexually transmitted diseases, as well as academic institutions involved in the training of physicians. It is available in e-book format from several providers.

Sexually Transmitted Diseases. 4th ed. Editors: King K. Holmes, Frederick P. Sparling, Walter E. Stamm, Lawrence Corey, Judith N. Wasserheit, Peter Piot. McGraw-Hill, 2008.
http://www.statref.com/
http://www.r2library.com/
http://www.ovid.com/
www.ebrary.com/
ISBN: 9780071417488
See Also Chapter 11.2. Gynecology
Recommended for: Hospital, Academic Libraries
Brandon/Hill, *Doody's Core Titles* Selection

This textbook addresses all aspects of sexually transmitted diseases (STDs), including etiology, transmission, epidemiology, biology, and clinical management. This is the bible on STDs. This edition covers the latest issues in this field: long-term management of HIV patients, drug use and STDs, new research and clinical data on prevention and control, and emerging and re-emerging diseases. Complete coverage of essential medical, legal, and social issues is also provided to provide broad-based coverage and understanding that goes beyond diagnosis and treatment. The full-color format enhances this edition. It is required for any hospital or clinic providing care for sexually transmitted diseases as well as academic health science libraries. This title is a *Doody's Core Titles* recommended purchase and a Brandon/Hill selection. It is available in e-book format on several platforms.

Journals

AIDS Patient Care and STDs. v. 10, Mary Ann Liebert, Inc., 1996.
http://www.liebertpub.com/products/product.aspx?pid=1
ISSN: 10872914
ISSN: 15577449 (Online)
Indexed in: MEDLINE, CINAHL
Recommended for: Hospital, Academic Libraries
Brandon/Hill Selection

This journal focuses on the latest research and advances in the diagnosis and therapy of sexually transmitted diseases and in the care of AIDS/HIV patients. It includes: AIDS medication; therapies and antiretroviral agents; HIV/AIDS-related diseases, infections, and complications; current prevention techniques for HIV; and the latest news and developments on other STDs. Articles on epidemiology, education, prevention, policy issues, and psychosocial concerns are covered. Articles are peer-reviewed and indexed in all the major abstracting and indexing resources. This journal is a required resource for any hospital providing care of AIDS patients as well as health science libraries. It ranks twenty-second out of 57 titles in the infectious disease category (*Journal Citation Reports*, 2009). This title was listed on the last Brandon/Hill list. Full online coverage from its beginning in 1987 to the present is available from the publisher.

AIDS: Official Journal of the International AIDS Society. v. 1, Lippincott Williams & Wilkins, 1987.
http://journals.lww.com/aidsonline/

ISSN: 02699370
ISSN: 14735571 (Online)
Indexed in: MEDLINE
Recommended for: Hospital, Academic Libraries
Brandon/Hill Selection

This popular journal on AIDS is for clinicians, researchers, and policy makers. It features the latest ground-breaking research and data on HIV and AIDS. Each issue includes feature articles in the basic and clinical sciences, epidemiology, editorial reviews, social issues, and updated CDC statistics. Articles are peer-reviewed and indexed in the major indexing and abstract resources. It ranks fifth out of 57 journals on infectious diseases (2009 *Journal Citation Reports*). This title was listed on the last Brandon/Hill list. It is recommended for all hospital and academic libraries. Articles older than 12 months, back to 1997, are freely accessible on their website. Full online coverage from volume 1, 1987 is available through Ovid and other vendors.

***Journal of Acquired Immune Deficiency Syndromes*.** v. 21, Lippincott Williams & Wilkins, 1999.
http://journals.lww.com/jaids/
ISSN: 15254135
ISSN: 19447884 (Online)
Indexed in: MEDLINE, CINAHL
Recommended for: Hospital, Academic Libraries

This interdisciplinary title covers clinical virology, molecular biology, epidemiology and social science. It blends the clinical and basic sciences on HIV and AIDS research. Edited by the leaders in this field, it provides peer-reviewed articles, critical reviews of current research, case reports, discussion of national policy issues, and clinical trials information. Supplements accompany many of the issues, covering specific topics and summaries of conferences. This title is a required resource for any hospital providing care to AIDS/HIV patients as well as academic libraries involved in research and education of physicians and researchers. It ranks ninth out of 57 journals in the infectious diseases category (*Journal Citation Reports*, 2009). Full online coverage is available from 1999 to the present through the publisher.

***Sexually Transmitted Diseases*.** v. 4, Lippincott Williams & Wilkins, 1977.
http://journals.lww.com/stdjournal/
ISSN: 01485717
ISSN: 15374521 (Online)
Indexed in: MEDLINE, CINAHL
Recommended for: Hospital, Academic Libraries
Brandon/Hill Selection

The journal has gone through multiple title changes, as well as association name changes in the twentieth century. Currently, this journal is the official journal for the American Sexually Transmitted Diseases Association. It publishes original, peer-reviewed articles on clinical, laboratory, immunologic, epidemiologic, sociologic, and historical subjects concerning sexually transmitted conditions and related fields. It keeps up to date on the latest developments from the CDC and NIH. Each issue contains studies and developments from around the world. It is indexed in the major indexing and abstracting resources. This title ranks twenty-sixth out of 57 infectious disease journals (2009 *Journal Citation Reports*). This title was listed on the last Brandon/Hill list and is a required title for any hospital or clinic providing care for sexually transmitted diseases as well as health science libraries. Full online coverage from 1996 to the present is available from the publisher. Online content from 1977 to the present is available from Ovid.

***Sexually Transmitted Infections*.** v. 1, BMJ Publishing Group, 1925.
http://sti.bmj.com/
ISSN: 13684973
ISSN: 14723263 (Online)
Indexed in: MEDLINE
Recommended for: Hospital, Academic Libraries

As one of the oldest international journals on sexual health, having gone through several title changes since its inception in 1925, *Sexually Transmitted Infections* publishes articles on the clinical, epidemiological, social, and laboratory aspects of this specialty. Each issue includes editorials, review articles, research methodology, social and global issues, and correspondence. Video reports are also included. Though edited in Britain, associate editors are located in the United States and around the world. This title is indexed in the major indexing and abstracting resources. Articles are peer reviewed. The journal ranks thirty-fifth out of 57 titles in the infectious diseases category (2009 *Journal Citation Reports*). This is a required resource for any hospital or clinical laboratory providing care for sexually transmitted diseases as well as health science libraries. This title is available in both print and online formats. Full online coverage to volume 1, 1925, is available under its current title through BMJ Publishing.

11. Surgical Specialties

11.1. Colorectal Surgery

The diagnosis and treatment of disorders and abnormalities of the colon, rectum, and anal canal.

—MeSH

Contributor: Emily Patridge

Monographs

ASCRS Manual of Colon and Rectal Surgery. Editors: David E. Beck, Patricia L. Roberts, John L. Rombeau, Michael J. Stamos, Steven D. Wexner. Springer, 2009.
http://www.springerlink.com/content/978-0-387-73438-5
http://extranet.netlibrary.com/TitleSelect/
http://www.ebrary.com/
ISBN: 9780387734385
ISBN: 9780387734408 (Online)
Recommended for: Hospital, Academic Libraries

This manual was designed to be a pocket reference for residents, fellows, private clinicians, and allied health professionals who care for patients with colorectal surgical disease. It is the only colorectal surgery manual that includes the ASCRS (American Society of Colon and Rectal Surgeons) Practice Guidelines. The manual includes surgery and disease chapters, anatomical and technique drawings, operative photos, and algorithms.

Atlas of Colonoscopy: Techniques, Diagnosis, Interventional Procedures. Editor: Helmutt Messman. Thieme, 2006.
http://extranet.netlibrary.com/TitleSelect/
http://www.ebrary.com/
ISBN: 9781588904317
ISBN: 9781588906786 (Online)
Recommended for: Hospital, Academic Libraries
Doody's Core Titles Selection

The editor of this book, Dr. Helmut Messman, and his team of specialists perform over 13,000 endoscopies annually. With their expertise in the field of colonoscopy, the contributors provide an atlas that encompasses necessary instruments and examination techniques, guidelines on preparation, related medications, complications, and more. There are over 1,000 illustrations in this book. This atlas begins with a very detailed guide to equipment and examination techniques, complete with three-dimensional computerized views of scope positioning, photographs demonstrating how to apply pressure over each colon section, and illustrations demonstrating loop techniques. The following three main sections cover normal examination procedure and non-pathological findings, pathological findings, and endoscopic intervention. Topics include modern endoscopic techniques, such as magnifying or zoom endoscopy, and safety of the patient and monitoring. The *Atlas of Colonoscopy* is an essential resource for anyone working in an endoscopy unit. It is a required resource for hospital and academic libraries.

Colon & Rectal Surgery. 5th ed. Author: Marvin L. Corman. Lippincott Williams & Wilkins, 2005.
http://www.ovid.com/
ISBN: 9780781740432
Recommended for: Hospital, Academic Libraries

Colon and Rectal Surgery serves as a guide to operative procedures for diseases and injuries to the colon, rectum, and anus. It begins with general chapters on anatomy, physiology, and drugs and nutrition, then discusses general diagnostic techniques and equipment. The remainder of the 34 chapters covers specific diseases and injuries, with details of diagnosis and surgical techniques. The concluding chapter presents medico-legal aspects of colon and rectal surgery. There are over 1,300 illustrations, including drawings, photos, and radiographic and ultrasound images. Boxes highlight biographies of historical leaders in the field, which are listed in a separate index. This text would serve students, residents, and practitioners and be useful for hospital and academic libraries.

Colonoscopy: Principles and Practice. 2nd ed. Editors: Jerome D. Waye, Douglas K. Rex, Christopher B. Williams. Wiley-Blackwell, 2009.
http://onlinelibrary.wiley.com/book/10.1002/9781444316902
ISBN: 9781405175999
ISBN: 9781444316902 (Online)

Recommended for: Hospital, Academic Libraries
Doody's Core Titles Selection

The first edition of *Colonoscopy: Principles and Practice* received the 2004 BMA (British Medical Association) Medical Book Competition in Gastroenterology award. The second edition covers several different topics including virtual colonography, pathology, techniques for pediatric and adult procedures, and legal aspects. This resource is focused on clinical patient care and would be a perfect addition for any hospital or academic library that supports practitioners who work with colonoscopy and colon imaging procedures. This print resource includes a companion DVD with supplementary material including demonstrations of techniques for both common and unique cases.

Fundamentals of Anorectal Surgery. 2nd ed. Editors: David E. Beck, Steven D. Wexner. WB Saunders, 1998.
ISBN: 9780702023668
Recommended for: Hospital, Academic Libraries

Even though this print resource is somewhat dated, it continues to be used by practicing colorectal surgeons. The contributors represent many of the major colorectal centers in North America. This resource would be an excellent addition for any library that supports medical students or practitioners seeking information on diseases and therapy of the anorectal region. This resource does not include colonic disease and only focuses on anorectal disease. All surgical procedures are outlined in systematic detail.

Operative Strategies in Inflammatory Bowel Disease. Editors: Fabrizio Michelassi, Jeffrey W. Milsom. Springer, 1999.
ISBN: 9780387949666
Recommended for: Hospital, Academic Libraries

Recommended by a colorectal surgeon, this book encompasses operative techniques as well as the indications, pitfalls, strategies, timing, complications, and long-term results involved in the surgical treatment of ulcerative colitis and Crohn's Disease. This book is perfect for an academic or hospital library supporting surgeons, surgical trainees, and other practitioners who treat patients with inflammatory bowel disease. This book is illustrated with over 200 line drawings.

Principles and Practice of Surgery for the Colon, Rectum, and Anus. 3rd ed. Authors: Philip H. Gordon, Santhat Nivatvongs. Informa Healthcare, 2007.
http://online.statref.com/titleinfo/fxid-254.html
http://www.ebrary.com/
http://extranet.netlibrary.com/TitleSelect/
ISBN: 9780824729615
ISBN: 9781420017991 (Online)
Recommended for: Hospital, Academic Libraries
Doody's Core Titles Selection

This edition has been updated with the most recent information on diagnosis and therapy, including new drugs. This readable reference allows practitioners to locate needed information easily in a single chapter. Part I covers essential considerations, including anatomy, physiology, diagnosis, pre- and postoperative management, local anesthesia, pharmacology, and electrosurgery and laser surgery. Parts II and III discuss the details of anorectal and colorectal disorders, while Part IV focuses on problem-oriented approaches to colorectal disease. Part V details minimally invasive surgery. Part VI, titled "Et Cetera," covers less common disorders. Every chapter includes tables, figures, and a list of references. This work has superb color illustrations that will assist any practicing clinician in everyday practice. It would be an excellent choice for any hospital or academic library that supports colorectal surgeons.

Reoperative Colon and Rectal Surgery. Editors: Walter E. Longo, John Northover. Taylor & Francis/Informa Healthcare, 2003.
ISBN: 9781841841830
Recommended for: Hospital, Academic Libraries

This is an excellent resource for practicing surgeons who care for patients with recurrent and persistent colorectal disorders. In this edition, a team of international experts provides comprehensive coverage of colorectal diseases that require reoperation. The 23 chapters focus on surgical procedures when primary treatments have failed or when there are persistent complications. Chapter topics include recurrent surgery for acute and chronic small bowel obstruction, reoperative surgery in the HIV-positive patient, reoperative surgery for recurrent colon cancer and rectal cancer, and reoperative surgery for radiation-related complications.

Reoperative Pelvic Surgery. Editors: Richard P. Billingham, Kathleen C. Kobashi, William A. Peters. Springer, 2009.
http://www.springerlink.com/content/978-0-387-89998-5
http://www.ebrary.com/
http://extranet.netlibrary.com/TitleSelect/
ISBN: 9780387899985
ISBN: 9780387899992 (Online)
Recommended for: Hospital, Academic Libraries

Recommended by a prestigious colorectal surgeon, this book is essential for any academic or hospital library's surgical collection. Colorectal surgeons, general surgeons, and gynecologic or urologic surgeons are the main audience for this publication. *Reoperative Pelvic Surgery* has three main sections: "Decision Making," "Operative Strategies," and "Complications Management." This resource also discusses all anatomical components of the pelvic floor, including colon, rectum, anus, and gynecologic and urologic organs. This work will provide surgeons with the information needed for optimal surgical management of these difficult conditions.

Journals

Colorectal Disease. v. 1, Wiley-Blackwell for the Association of Coloproctology of Great Britain and Ireland, 1999.
http://onlinelibrary.wiley.com/journal/10.1111/(ISSN)1463-1318/issues
ISSN: 14628910
ISSN: 14631318 (Online)
Indexed in: MEDLINE
Recommended for: Hospital, Academic Libraries

Colorectal Disease is designed for physicians, nurses, surgeons, technologists, and other clinicians who are interested in diseases of the colon and rectum. The aim of this journal is to improve the clinical outcome of patients diagnosed with colorectal diseases, such as bowel cancer. This journal has an impact factor of 2.438 and is ranked twenty-seventh out of 66 gastroenterology and hepatology titles (2009 *Journal Citation Reports*). It is indexed/abstracted in multiple sources, including Current Contents/Clinical Medicine, Embase/Excerpta Medica, Health Source: Nursing/Academic, International Bibliographic Information on Dietary Supplements (IBIDS), and MEDLINE. Online access is available from volume 1, 1999.

Digestive Surgery. v. 1, Karger, 1984.
http://content.karger.com/
ISSN: 02534886
ISSN: 14219883 (Online)
Indexed in: MEDLINE
Recommended for: Hospital, Academic Libraries

Begun in 1984, this colorectal surgery journal has long been a principal resource for those who want to stay abreast of advances in the diagnosis and treatment of gastrointestinal disease. This journal not only emphasizes articles that evaluate recent clinical developments, but also relevant translational research. The target audience for this journal is abdominal surgeons. This journal is a required resource for any hospital providing colorectal surgery or for academic institutions involved with physician training. The current impact factor for this journal is 1.372 (2009 *Journal Citation Reports*). Although the journal is available in both print and online formats, all articles are published electronically ahead of the print version.

Diseases of the Colon & Rectum. v. 1, Lippincott Williams & Wilkins for the American Society of Colon and Rectal Surgeons, 1958.
http://www.ovid.com/
ISSN: 00123706
ISSN: 15300358 (Online)
Indexed in: MEDLINE
Recommended for: Hospital, Academic Libraries
Brandon/Hill Selection

The official journal of the American Society of Colon and Rectal Surgeons, *Diseases of the Colon & Rectum* ranks in the top 25% of all peer-reviewed surgery journals and was listed as a Brandon/Hill title. *DC&R* focuses on conditions affecting the colon, rectum, and anus. It publishes original articles, case reports, reviews, short communications, book reviews, and society news. General surgeons, colorectal surgeons, gastroenterologists, surgical oncologists, and general oncologists rely on this publication to stay abreast of advances in this rapidly-evolving and changing discipline. Indexing sources include MEDLINE and Scopus.

International Journal of Colorectal Disease. v. 1, Springer, 1986.
http://www.springerlink.com/content/100430/
ISSN: 01791958
ISSN: 14321262 (Online)
Indexed in: MEDLINE
Recommended for: Hospital, Academic Libraries

The *International Journal of Colorectal Disease* is the official publication of the Association of Coloproctology of Great Britain and Ireland. The journal publishes articles, symposia, and reviews of subjects that focus on reporting the progress and practice of all specialties studying and treating colorectal disease. The primary audience for this journal is gastroenterologists, surgeons, pathologists, oncologists, and other health professionals who care for patients with diseases of the lower GI tract. This journal has an impact factor of 2.102 and is ranked thirty-third out of 66 gastroenterology and hepatology titles (2009 *Journal Citation Reports*). This journal is recommended for any hospital or academic library.

Journal of Crohn's & Colitis. v. 1, Elsevier on behalf of European Crohn's and Colitis Organisation, 2007.
http://www.sciencedirect.com/science/journal/18739946

ISSN: 18739946 (Print/Online)
Indexed in: MEDLINE
Recommended for: Hospital, Academic Libraries

The *Journal of Crohn's & Colitis* is the official, peer-reviewed journal of the European Crohn's and Colitis Organisation (ECCO). The primary focus of this journal is the basic science and methods related to inflammatory bowel disease. The journal is indexed in Current Contents, Embase, Excerpta Medica, Scopus, and Web of Science. An irregular, separately titled publication, *Journal of Crohn's & Colitis Supplements* (ISSN 18739954) provides meeting coverage of the ECCO congress and other society meetings. This journal has an impact factor of 1.729 and is ranked forty-first out of 66 gastroenterology and hepatology titles (2009 *Journal Citation Reports*).This journal would be a useful addition for hospital libraries supporting colorectal surgeons.

Journal of Gastrointestinal Surgery. v. 1, Springer, 1997.
http://www.springerlink.com/content/120413/
ISSN: 1091255X
ISSN: 18734626 (Online)
Indexed in: MEDLINE
Recommended for: Hospital, Academic Libraries

The *Journal of Gastrointestinal Surgery* is the scholarly, peer-reviewed official publication of the Society for Surgery of the Alimentary Tract (SSAT). The journal includes original articles on surgery of the digestive tract, gastrointestinal images, procedural articles, book reviews, symposia, letters, conference information, and more. The journal would be most useful to surgeons and other gastroenterologists. The 2009 *Journal Citation Reports* ranks the journal thirty-ninth of 166 in the surgery subject category. The *Journal of Gastrointestinal Surgery* is indexed in multiple sources such as CAB Abstracts, Embase, MEDLINE, Science Citation Index Expanded (SciSearch), and Scopus.

JSLS: Journal of the Society of Laparoendoscopic Surgeons. v. 1, Society of Laparoendoscopic Surgeons, 1997.
http://www.ingentaconnect.com/content/sls/jsls
ISSN: 10868089
ISSN: 19383797 (Online)
Indexed in: MEDLINE
Recommended for: Hospital, Academic Libraries

This peer-reviewed publication of the Society of Laparoendoscopic Surgeons (SLS) publishes original articles on basic science and technical topics involving minimally invasive surgery or laparoendoscopy. The aim of this journal is to promote communication among laparoendoscopic surgeons to improve their technique and understanding. The journal is indexed in MEDLINE. It is not listed in *Journal Citation Reports*.

The Open Colorectal Cancer Journal. v. 1, Bentham Open, 2008.
http://www.bentham.org/open/tocolcj/index.htm
ISSN: 18768202 (Online)
Recommended for: Hospital, Academic Libraries

The Open Colorectal Cancer Journal is an open access, online journal that provides original research articles, reviews, and short articles on all aspects of colorectal cancer. This peer-reviewed journal publishes articles with a quick turnaround and makes them freely available to all. This would be a useful addition for any hospital or academic library. To date, Chemical Abstracts is the only identifiable source that offers limited content indexing for this journal.

Surgical Endoscopy. v. 1, Springer, 1987.
http://www.springerlink.com/content/100368/
ISSN: 09302794
ISSN: 14322218 (Online)
See Also Chapter 11.9. Surgery
Indexed in: MEDLINE
Recommended for: Hospital, Academic Libraries

This journal covers "the surgical aspects of interventional endoscopy, ultrasound, and other techniques in the fields of gastroenterology, obstetrics, gynecology, and urology, as well as in gastroenterologic, thoracic, traumatic, orthopedic, and pediatric surgery." This is the official journal of the Society of American Gastrointestinal and Endoscopic Surgeons (SAGES) and European Association for Endoscopic Surgery (EAES). It has a 2009 *Journal Citation Reports* impact factor of 3.307 and is ranked seventeenth out of 167 surgery titles. It is indexed in numerous sources such as Embase, MEDLINE, and Scopus.

11.2. Gynecology

The physiology and disorders primarily of the female genital tract, as well as female endocrinology and reproductive physiology.

—MeSH

Contributor: Jean E. Riedlinger

Monographs

Atlas of Pelvic Anatomy and Gynecologic Surgery. 2nd ed. Editors: Michael S. Baggish, Mickey M. Karram.

Saunders Elsevier, 2006.
ISBN: 9780721638997
Recommended for: Hospital, Academic Libraries

This surgical atlas is intended to provide "precise demonstrations of true anatomy and easy to comprehend descriptions of surgical techniques." The 2nd edition features new photographs and illustrations and has added several sections that did not appear in the first edition, including an introduction to pelvic anatomy and new chapters dealing with laparoscopic surgery. The text is heavily illustrated with color photographs of anatomy and surgical procedures using cadavers and live patients. The wording is concise, with text used primarily for technical descriptions of surgical procedures and descriptions of the anatomy involved. The book is organized into four broad units. The first unit covers abdominal surgery, including a detailed anatomy section with drawings and photographs of the bones, muscles, organs, blood vessels, and other structures in the pelvic area. Also included is a new chapter with photographs of surgical instruments. The second unit focuses on cervical, vaginal, vulvar and perineal surgery, while the third unit deals with endoscopy, including hysteroscopy, laparoscopy, and cystourethroscopy. All chapters start with a section on basic anatomy and feature detailed photographs and illustrations of specific surgical procedures by location. The fourth unit, which is entirely new to this edition, covers additional procedures involving the breast, bowel, and others. This book received five stars and a score of 97 from *Doody's Review Service*. It would be useful for gynecologic and other surgeons, and it is recommended for hospital, academic, and specialized collections.

Berek & Novak's Gynecology. 14th ed. Editor: Jonathan S. Berek. Lippincott Williams & Wilkins, 2007.
http://www.ovid.com/
ISBN: 9780781768054
Recommended for: Hospital, Academic Libraries
Brandon/Hill, *Doody's Core Titles* Selection

Long considered a standard text, *Berek and Novak's* was first published in 1941. The goal of the authors and editors is to provide a comprehensive summary of the field of gynecology, as well as the related gynecologic subspecialties. The current edition has added new sections on pelvic reconstruction and urogynecology in keeping with the expansion of this subspecialty. The book is divided into eight sections. General principles of gynecologic practice, including patient care and quality of care, are covered in sections one and two, as are basic science topics such as anatomy, physiology, embryology, and genetics. Sections three and four cover preventive and primary care and general gynecology, featuring chapters on screening, family planning, complementary therapies, benign disease, pelvic pain, infections, early pregnancy loss, breast disease, and more. The remaining sections deal with operative gynecology, urogynecology and pelvic reconstructive surgery, and reproductive endocrinology. The section on gynecologic oncology includes chapters on gynecologic cancer by location. Also included are full-color photographs and anatomical and surgical illustrations. *Berek & Novak's Gynecology* is a *Doody's Core Titles* recommendation and was listed on the final Brandon/Hill list. This book would be useful to obstetrician-gynecologists and any other physicians or researchers interested in gynecology. It is recommended as an important resource for any hospital or academic library, as well as specialized collections covering women's health.

Danforth's Obstetrics and Gynecology. 10th ed. Editors: Ronald S. Gibbs, Beth Y. Karlan, Arthur F. Haney, Ingrid E. Nygaard. Lippincott Williams & Wilkins, 2008.
See Chapter 11.4. Obstetrics

Female Urology. 3rd ed. Editors: Shlomo Raz, Larissa V. Rodriguez. Saunders Elsevier, 2008.
ISBN: 9781416023395
Recommended for: Hospital, Academic Libraries

This textbook covers the gynecologic subspecialty of urogynecology. The third edition of this book has been completely reorganized and updated, presenting comprehensive coverage of female pelvic medicine, reconstruction, and urology, including surgical and non-surgical approaches to treatment. The book is illustrated, including detailed surgical illustrations, and comes with a DVD of video clips of surgical procedures. There are twelve sections, including basic concepts and anatomy, evaluation and diagnosis, and pathophysiology of voiding dysfunction. The diagnosis, treatments, and specific surgical procedures for overactive bladder and stress incontinence are covered, as are female sexual function and dysfunction, female pelvic organ prolapse (including uterine prolapse and other types), defecatory function and dysfunction, fistulas and diverticulas, pelvic pain and inflammatory conditions, geriatric urology, and pelvic reconstruction. The primary audiences for this book are urologists, urogynecologists, and general gynecologists. *Female Urology* would be appropriate for specialized collections and libraries in hospitals and academic settings with urogynecology departments or comprehensive gynecology collections.

Guidelines for Women's Health Care: A Resource Manual. 3rd ed. American College of Obstetricians and Gynecologists, 2007.
http://www.r2library.com/
ISBN: 9781932328356
Recommended for: Hospital, Academic, Consumer Health Libraries

The American College of Obstetricians and Gynecologists' (ACOG) *Guidelines for Women's Health Care* is a "concise resource encompassing the full spectrum of policy and management issues relating to women's health care." Recommendations come from ACOG's other guideline publications, including *Committee Opinions* and *Practice Bulletins*, as well as guidelines from other organizations and government agencies. The book is organized into three broad sections. Part one, "Governance and Administration," deals with legal and ethical matters, including governance, human resources, credentials evaluation and privilege granting, continuous quality improvement, risk management, compliance with government regulations, and ethical issues. Part two covers organization of services and the physical environment, such as facilities and equipment, infection control, ancillary services (such as pharmacies, laboratories, imaging, anesthesia, and more), information management, medical records, and practice management. Part three deals with patient care. Routine patient care and the well-woman visit are covered, as well as specific gynecologic conditions such as abnormal genital bleeding, endometriosis, polycystic ovary syndrome, abnormal cervical cytology, gynecologic surgery, and many more. The intended audience is primarily physicians; however, it would also be useful for anyone involved in the delivery of women's health care, including nurses and health care administrators. This book and its companion, *Guidelines for Perinatal Care*, would be appropriate for hospital libraries, academic libraries, consumer health libraries, and any specialized collection that covers women's health.

Pediatric & Adolescent Gynecology. 5th ed. Editors: S. Jean Herriot Emans, Marc R. Laufer, Donald P. Goldstein. Lippincott Williams & Wilkins, 2005.
http://www.ovid.com/
ISBN: 9780781744935
See Also Chapter 9.1. Adolescent Medicine
Recommended for: Hospital, Academic Libraries
Doody's Core Titles Selection

Since the first edition was published in 1977, this has been the classic textbook in pediatric and adolescent gynecology and a leading contributor to the growth of this field. This illustrated text addresses gynecologic problems encountered in babies, children, and adolescents, including medical and surgical approaches to their treatment. Each chapter includes information on techniques for examination, ancillary testing, and suggested treatment plans. The book covers office evaluation of the child and adolescent, prepubertal issues, puberty, menstrual problems, androgen and structural abnormalities, gynecologic pain (including dysmenorrhea, pelvic pain, endometriosis, and premenstrual syndrome), education of children and adolescents, pediatric urology, vulvovaginal complaints, sexually transmitted infections (such as bacterial infections, HIV, and the human papillomavirus), ovarian masses, and the breast. It also discusses legal issues and sexual abuse, as well as other topics such as complementary and alternative medicine for gynecologic problems in young women. The book is intended for pediatricians and gynecologists, along with other physicians and nurses who deal with pediatric and adolescent patients. This book was selected for inclusion in *Doody's Core Titles* and is recommended for hospital and academic libraries and other specialized collections covering pediatrics or gynecology.

Principles and Practice of Gynecologic Oncology. 5th ed. Editors: Richard R. Barakat, Maurie Markman, Marcus E. Randall. Wolters Kluwer/Lippincott Williams & Wilkins, 2009.
http://www.ovid.com/
ISBN: 9780781778459
See Also Chapter 10.10.6. Medical Oncology
Recommended for: Hospital, Academic Libraries
Brandon/Hill, *Doody's Core Titles* Selection

This gynecologic oncology textbook is intended to be the definitive reference on gynecologic cancer. Due to the increased complexity of gynecologic cancers and treatment, the book has a multidisciplinary focus, with chapters on specific diseases authored by a surgeon, a medical oncologist, a radiation oncologist, and a pathologist. The basic biology, pathology, modalities of therapy, and therapeutic options by disease site are all addressed. The book is divided into four sections, with the first section focusing on epidemiology of gynecologic cancer, including genetics, biology, prevention, and imaging. Section two covers therapeutic modalities and related subjects, such as surgery, radiation, chemotherapy, and a chapter on innovative twenty-first century therapies. The third section is on specific disease sites and covers types of cancer by location. Each of the disease site chapters includes information on anatomy, diagnosis and staging, pathology, prognosis, and treatment.

Section four deals with special management topics, which include infection, pain, nutrition, quality of life, end of life care, and more. This book is designed for specialists who care for women with gynecologic cancers, including surgeons, medical and radiation oncologists, pathologists, and nurses. It would also be useful for residents and fellows who plan a career in cancer care. Appearing on the final Brandon/Hill list, this book is recommended for hospital, academic, and specialized collections with oncology and gynecology coverage.

Sexually Transmitted Diseases. 4th ed. Editors: King K. Holmes, P. Frederick Sparling, Walter E. Stamm, Peter Piot, Judith N. Wasserheit, Lawrence Corey, Myron S. Cohen, D. Heather Watts. McGraw-Hill Medical, 2008.
http://extranet.netlibrary.com/TitleSelect/
http://www.r2library.com/
http://www.ebrary.com/
ISBN: 9780071417488
ISBN: 9780071593113
See Also Chapter 10.19. Venereology
Recommended for: Hospital, Academic Libraries
Brandon/Hill, *Doody's Core Titles* Selection

This book, first published 25 years ago, contains comprehensive information on the clinical, microbiological, and public health aspects of sexually transmitted diseases (STD) and HIV infection. Recent developments in the STD field are also discussed. At the beginning of the book, there is a table summarizing the major developments in the STI (sexually transmitted infections)/HIV field since the previous edition was published. Information on the history, socioeconomic impact, and epidemiology of STDs is included, as is information on social and psychological dimensions of sexuality and profiles of vulnerable populations, such as adolescents, sex workers, and homosexual and bisexual men and women. Other parts discuss specific STDs, divided into parts on viral pathogens; bacterial pathogens; and protozoa, fungi, and ectoparasites. The book then covers treatment of STDs, STD syndromes, and dermatologic manifestations of STDs in both women and men. HIV infection is also covered. The last several sections of the book discuss other issues surrounding STD and HIV infection, including pregnancy; prevention and control; STDs and HIV in developing countries; and special medical, legal, and social issues. A reprint of the Centers for Disease Control and Prevention's 2006 *Sexually Transmitted Diseases Treatment Guidelines* is included in an appendix. The audience for this book includes reproductive health specialists as well as primary care physicians. Awarded five stars and a score of 98 by *Doody's Review Service*, it appears on *Doody's Core Titles* list and appeared on the final Brandon/Hill list. It would be appropriate for hospital and academic libraries and special collections.

Te Linde's Operative Gynecology. 10th ed. Editors: John A. Rock, Howard W. Jones III. Lippincott Williams & Wilkins, 2008.
http://www.ovid.com/
http://www.r2library.com/
ISBN: 9780781772341
Recommended for: Hospital, Academic Libraries

First published in 1947, this is the most widely read textbook on gynecologic surgery. It provides a thorough review of gynecologic surgery and discusses gynecologic problems that may require surgery, including complicated or unusual problems. The basic principles for surgical techniques are presented as are the most recent major advances in gynecologic surgery. A surgical procedure DVD is included. The book is divided into nine sections. The first covers general topics affecting gynecologic surgery practice. The book then moves onto general principles of anatomy and perioperative considerations, which is followed by principles of gynecologic surgery techniques. There are several sections on specific surgical procedures for fertility, benign gynecologic conditions, obstetrics, and correction of defects in pelvic support and pelvic fistulas. The book also includes sections on related surgery and gynecologic oncology surgery. This book is recommended for surgeons and gynecologic surgeons. It is appropriate for specialized collections as well as hospital and academic medical libraries.

Williams Gynecology. Editors: John O. Schorge, Joseph I. Schaffer, Lisa M. Halvorson, Barbara L. Hoffman, Karen D. Bradshaw, F. Gary Cunningham. McGraw-Hill Medical, 2008.
http://www.accessmedicine.com/
ISBN: 9780071472579
Recommended for: Hospital, Academic Libraries

This is a new general gynecology textbook. The first edition of *Williams Gynecology* is intended to accompany the separate textbook *Williams Obstetrics*. Beginning with benign general gynecology, which includes well-woman care, contraception, abortion, infections, and other benign conditions, the first part of this publication concentrates on general gynecology and its subspecialties. Other sections in the first half of the book cover (a) reproductive endocrinology, infertility, and menopause; (b) female pelvic medicine and reconstructive surgery (including incontinence and pelvic organ prolapse); and (c) gynecologic oncology, dealing with specific cancers and their treatment such as chemotherapy and radiation. The second half of the book focuses on gynecologic surgery. One section covers basic aspects of surgery, such as anatomy and peri- and intra-operative considerations. The final section of the book is an atlas of gynecologic surgery. The atlas section is divided into chapters on surgeries for benign gynecologic conditions, pelvic reconstruction, and gynecologic malignancies, all by specific surgical procedure. Each procedure has detailed color illustrations, information on preoperative and intraoperative issues, including surgical steps from anesthesia to incision closure, and postoperative care. As an added bonus, McGraw-Hill's online version includes short video presentations for certain procedures. This would be a valuable reference for anyone involved in women's health care as well as an appropriate addition to any hospital, academic, or specialized library collection.

Yen and Jaffe's Reproductive Endocrinology: Physiology, Pathophysiology, and Clinical Management. 6th ed. Editors: Jerome F. Strauss, Robert L. Barbieri. Elsevier Saunders, 2009.
http://www.mdconsult.com/
ISBN: 9781416049074
Recommended for: Hospital, Academic Libraries
Doody's Core Titles Selection

Intended for obstetrician-gynecologists and endocrinologists, the sixth edition of this reproductive endocrinology textbook has been thoroughly revised, including new full-color illustrations and drawings. Information is presented on the diagnosis and management of endocrine disorders affecting the reproductive systems in both men and women. The sixth edition includes several new chapters on preservation of fertility, endocrine disturbances affecting reproduction, imaging, and adolescent reproductive endocrinology. The book is divided into three broad parts. Part one covers the endocrinology of reproduction, including basic science information on the hormonal issues that affect reproduction and chapters on the structure and function of the female reproductive tract, pregnancy and fetal neuroendocrine development, the male reproductive system, menopause, and male reproductive aging. Part two deals with pathophysiology and therapy, covering conditions such as disorders of sex development, puberty, polycystic ovary syndrome, female and male infertility, endometriosis, endocrine diseases of pregnancy, and more. The final section deals with reproductive technologies, including ovarian stimulation, assisted reproduction, contraception, and other topics. The full text is searchable, and all images and hyperlinked references to MEDLINE are included. This book is an Elsevier Expert Consult title and includes online access for individual users. Institutional online access is available through the MD Consult obstetrics and gynecology e-books collection. This book is recommended for hospital, academic, and specialized collections.

Journals

Adolescent Medicine: State of the Art Reviews. v. 18, American Academy of Pediatrics, 2007.
ISSN: 19344287
ISSN: 15450058 (Online)
See Also Chapter 9.1. Adolescent Medicine
Indexed in: MEDLINE, CINAHL
Recommended for: Hospital, Academic Libraries

Adolescent Medicine: State of the Art Reviews is the continuation of *Adolescent Medicine Clinics*, which was formerly titled *Adolescent Medicine*. Published three times per year, this is the official journal of the American Academy of Pediatrics Section on Adolescent Health. While not specific to obstetrics and gynecology, many of the individually themed issues are of interest to obstetrician-gynecologists and other physicians who deal with adolescent patients. For example, recent issues have focused on adolescent sexuality; contraception; "hot topics" in adolescent medicine, including the HPV vaccine; sexually transmitted diseases; endocrinology; and female reproductive health. At this time, the journal is available in print format only. The journal is indexed in MEDLINE and is considered to be a core clinical journal. This would be an appropriate journal for hospital, academic, and specialized collections.

American Journal of Obstetrics & Gynecology. v. 1, Mosby-Elsevier, 1920.
http://www.ajog.org
http://www.sciencedirect.com/science/journal/00029378
http://www.mdconsult.com/
ISSN: 00029378
ISSN: 10976868 (Online)
See Also Chapter 11.4. Obstetrics
Indexed in: MEDLINE, CINAHL
Recommended for: Hospital, Academic Libraries
Brandon/Hill Selection

Also known as the "Gray Journal," the *American Journal of Obstetrics & Gynecology* features information on the latest diagnostic procedures, research, and expert commentary in various fields, including general obstetrics and gynecology, maternal-fetal medicine, reproductive endocrinology and infertility, and gynecologic oncology. The printed journal contains article summaries that are abbreviated versions of the research and clinical opinion articles, which are published in full on the journal's website (http://www.ajog.org). Most summaries are written by journal staff and approved by the article's authors, but some are written by the original authors. Articles going back to 1995 are available from the journal's website and Elsevier's ScienceDirect and MD Consult. Some material is free to non-subscribers. Article types include reviews, clinical opinions, research, journal club articles, imaging, and a surgeon's corner article. The journal also publishes papers presented at the annual meetings of its affiliated societies, including the Society of Maternal-Fetal Medicine and the Society of Gynecologic Surgeons. The journal is indexed in MEDLINE and Scopus and is considered to be a core clinical journal. This journal is recommended for initial purchase in the final published edition of the "Brandon/Hill Selected List of Books and Journals for the Small Medical Library." This is a recommended publication for any hospital, academic, or specialized library collection.

Best Practice & Research Clinical Obstetrics & Gynaecology. v. 13, Elsevier, 1999.
See Chapter 11.4. Obstetrics

Birth: Issues in Perinatal Care. v. 9, Wiley-Blackwell, 1982.
See Chapter 11.4. Obstetrics

BJOG: An International Journal of Obstetrics and Gynaecology. v. 107, Wiley-Blackwell, 2000.
See Chapter 11.4. Obstetrics

Clinical Obstetrics and Gynecology. v. 1, Lippincott Williams & Wilkins, 1958.
See Chapter 11.4. Obstetrics

Current Opinion in Obstetrics & Gynecology. v. 1, Lippincott Williams & Wilkins, 1989.
See Chapter 11.4. Obstetrics

Gynecologic Oncology. v. 1, Academic Press, 1972.
http://www.sciencedirect.com/science/journal/00029378
ISSN: 00908258
ISSN: 10956859 (Online)
Indexed in: MEDLINE
Recommended for: Hospital, Academic Libraries

Published monthly, *Gynecologic Oncology* is an international journal which focuses on cancers of the female reproductive tract, including their etiology, diagnosis, treatment, and prevention. The journal also presents research in the areas of cell and molecular biology, chemotherapy, clinical trials, epidemiology, genetics, quality of life, radiation, and other topics. Original research reports are grouped by type of cancer. Case reports are also included. The table of contents provides a one-sentence summary of the article. The journal is published online by Elsevier's ScienceDirect going back to the first volume in 1972. This core clinical journal is indexed and abstracted by MEDLINE, Current Contents/Clinical Medicine, Index to Scientific Reviews, Science Citation Index, and Scopus. *Gynecologic Oncology* is recommended for hospital, academic, and specialized collections covering oncology and gynecology.

Gynecological Endocrinology. v. 1, Informa Healthcare, 1987.
http://informahealthcare.com/
ISSN: 09513590
ISSN: 14730766 (Online)
Indexed in: MEDLINE
Recommended for: Hospital, Academic Libraries

Gynecological Endocrinology is the official journal of the International Society of Gynecological Endocrinology. Published monthly, it covers the experimental, clinical, and therapeutic aspects of the field. Articles focus on endocrinology topics such as the control and function of endocrine glands, "the effects of reproductive events on the endocrine system, and the consequences of endocrine disorders on reproduction." Original articles are available on conditions such as polycystic ovary syndrome, diabetes, menopause, pregnancy, and others. An online version is available through informaworld, and coverage begins with volume 1, 1987. *Gynecologic Endocrinology* is considered a core clinical journal, and is indexed in MEDLINE, Science Citation Index, BIOBASE/Current Awareness in Biological Sciences (CABS), Current Contents, and Embase. This journal would be appropriate for hospital and academic libraries as well as specialized collections.

International Urogynecology Journal and Pelvic Floor Dysfunction. v. 6, Springer-Verlag, 1995.
http://www.springerlink.com/content/0937-3462
ISSN: 09373462
ISSN: 14333023 (Online)
Indexed in: MEDLINE
Recommended for: Hospital, Academic Libraries

This is the official journal of the International Urogynecological Association and the British Society of Urogynecology. First published in 1990 as *International Urogynecology Journal*, the intended audience is urologists, gynecologists, nurses, basic scientists, and researchers.

The scope is the field of urogynecology and pelvic floor disorders, with an emphasis on the clinical approach to these topics. The journal is published monthly, and each issue contains peer-reviewed original articles, case reports, and letters on topics such as urinary incontinence, pelvic organ prolapse, and surgery. In addition to being recognized as a core clinical journal, this journal is indexed in Science Citation Index, Current Contents/Clinical Medicine, MEDLINE, and Embase. It is also abstracted in *ACOG Clinical Review*. It is published online through SpringerLink beginning with the first volume from 1990 and includes online first articles. This journal is recommended for specialized collections and libraries in hospitals and academic settings with urogynecology departments or comprehensive gynecology collections.

Journal of Lower Genital Tract Disease. v. 1, Lippincott Williams & Wilkins, 1997.
http://journals.lww.com/jlgtd/
http://www.ovid.com/
ISSN: 10892591
ISSN: 15260976 (Online)
Indexed in: MEDLINE
Recommended for: Hospital, Academic Libraries

Journal of Lower Genital Tract Disease is the official publication of the American Society for Colposcopy and Cervical Pathology (ASCCP) and several international colposcopy and cervical pathology organizations. This journal is intended for professionals involved in the prevention, diagnosis, and management of cervical cancer and other lower genital tract diseases. The journal covers colposcopy techniques, as well as cancer and benign diseases of the cervix, vulva, and vagina. It includes both human papillomavirus infection and other sexually transmitted infections. Continuing medical education credits are available for some articles. Original research, reviews, case reports, and meeting abstracts are included; the journal also publishes practice guidelines from ASCCP. Recognized as a core clinical journal, this title is indexed in MEDLINE, Embase, Science Citation Index, and Current Contents/Clinical Medicine. The publication is available online through LWW Online and Journals@Ovid from the first volume in 1997 to the present. This journal would be appropriate for academic and hospital libraries and specialized collections.

Journal of Pediatric and Adolescent Gynecology. v. 9, Elsevier, 1996.
http://www.mdconsult.com/
http://www.sciencedirect.com/science/journal/10833188
http://www.jpagonline.org/
ISSN: 10833188
ISSN: 18734332 (Online)
See Also Chapter 9.1. Adolescent Medicine
Indexed in: MEDLINE
Recommended for: Hospital, Academic Libraries

Begun in 1988 as *Adolescent and Pediatric Gynecology*, this bimonthly journal is the official journal of the North American Society of Pediatric and Adolescent Gynecology and the International Federation of Pediatric and Adolescent Gynecology. The journal is intended to be a multidisciplinary source of information for physicians and other health professionals involved with pediatric and adolescent gynecology. All aspects of research in the field are presented, including basic and clinical science and molecular biology. Articles cover the viewpoints of various disciplines such as pediatrics, reproductive and pediatric endocrinology, genetics, and molecular biology. The journal publishes original studies, literature reviews, brief communications, book reviews, and letters to the editor. It is available online from 1999 to the present and is abstracted and indexed in MEDLINE, Embase, and Scopus. This core clinical journal is recommended for hospital and academic libraries and other specialized collections.

Journal of Women's Health. v. 11, Mary Ann Liebert, 2002.
http://www.liebertonline.com/loi/jwh
ISSN: 15409996
ISSN: 1931843X (Online)
Indexed in: MEDLINE, CINAHL
Recommended for: Hospital, Academic Libraries

This is the official journal of the American Medical Women's Association, focusing on diseases and medical conditions that affect women throughout their life span. It began publication in 1992 under its former title, *Journal of Women's Health and Gender-Based Medicine*. This peer-reviewed journal includes primarily clinically-oriented articles, but it also publishes review articles and case reports with an emphasis on the clinical care of women and research, especially outcomes of clinical trials. Articles covering new diagnostic procedures, the management of diseases in women, and research in gender-based biology are included. The journal takes a multidisciplinary approach and covers advances in women's medicine in the fields of internal medicine, endocrinology, oncology, obstetrics and gynecology, urogynecology, nutrition, sex-based biology, medical education, complementary medicine, sports medicine, and public policy. Published 12 times per year, the journal is available online from 1992 forward through the publisher's website. There is an open access policy where authors can choose to pay a fee, making their articles available online for free. As a core clinical journal, the *Journal of Women's Health* is indexed by many sources, including MEDLINE, Current Contents/Clinical Medicine, Science Citation Index, Social Sciences Citation Index, Embase/Excerpta Medica, Scopus, CINAHL, PsycINFO, and others. This journal would be useful in any hospital, academic, or specialized collection that includes coverage of women's health.

Menopause. v. 1, Lippincott Williams & Wilkins, 1994.
http://journals.lww.com/menopausejournal
http://www.ovid.com/
ISSN: 10723714
ISSN: 15300374 (Online)
Indexed in: MEDLINE, CINAHL
Recommended for: Hospital, Academic Libraries

This bimonthly journal is the official journal of the North American Menopause Society (NAMS). It covers new research, applied basic science, and NAMS clinical guidelines on all aspects of menopause. The journal's coverage goes beyond gynecology to include information relevant to other disciplines, including internal medicine, family practice, epidemiology, pathology, sociology, psychology, anthropology, pharmacology, and medical subspecialties such as geriatrics and cardiology. The journal attempts to integrate these diverse topics and highlight the need for future research. *Menopause* is available online through LWW Online and Journals@Ovid from the first volume in 1994 forward. This core clinical journal is indexed in MEDLINE, Current Contents/Clinical Medicine, Science Citation Index, SciSearch, Research Alert, and CINAHL. It would be an appropriate addition to any hospital, academic, or specialized library collection.

Obstetrics & Gynecology. v. 1, Lippincott Williams & Wilkins, 1953.
http://www.ovid.com/
ISSN: 00297844
ISSN: 1873233X (Online)
See Also Chapter 11.4. Obstetrics
Indexed in: MEDLINE, CINAHL
Recommended for: Hospital, Academic Libraries
Brandon/Hill Selection

Otherwise known as the "Green Journal," *Obstetrics & Gynecology* publishes editorials, original articles, and research studies on scientific advances, new medical and surgical techniques, obstetric management, and clinical evaluation of drugs and instruments. This peer-reviewed, monthly journal is the official journal of the American College of Obstetricians and Gynecologists (ACOG) and has been published since 1953. Its goal is "to promote excellence in the clinical practice of obstetrics and gynecology." Articles cover topics such as general gynecology and obstetrics, pregnancy complications, surgery, gynecologic oncology, contraception, sexually transmitted diseases, reproductive endocrinology, and more. Continuing medical education credit is available through the journal's Clinical Expert Series articles. Full-text articles beginning with the first issue in 1953 are available online through ACOG's website for members and also through LWW Online and Journals@Ovid. Beginning in 2001, the journal has published ACOG guidelines, including Practice Bulletins and Committee Opinions, in each issue in the month they were released. This MEDLINE core clinical journal was included on the final Brandon/Hill list and would be an essential journal for any hospital or academic library, as well as specialized collections.

Obstetrics and Gynecology Clinics of North America. v. 14, Saunders Elsevier, 1987.
See Chapter 11.4. Obstetrics

11.3. Neurosurgery

The treatment of diseases and disorders of the brain, spinal cord, and peripheral and sympathetic nervous system.

—MeSH

Contributor: Tim Mason

Monographs

Handbook of Neurosurgery. 7th ed. Author: Mark S. Greenberg. Thieme Medical, 2010.
ISBN: 9781604063264
Recommended for: Hospital, Academic Libraries

This overly large pocket sized handbook, 1,337 pages, is aimed at surgery and neurosurgery residents, but is also useful to the practicing neurosurgeon. New areas covered in this edition are: blunt cervical arterial injuries; awake craniotomies; brain mapping; grading systems for cervical and thoracolumbar fractures; radiation safety for neurosurgeons; organ donation after cardiac death; and expanded discussion of endovascular techniques. Each chapter covers both the basic and clinical science of a condition, in outline form. The book is mainly text with a few tables, line drawings with color highlights, and full color inserts. References are included at the end of each chapter. The information is presented in comprehensive yet condensed format. One drawback of this format is the small print. The index is extensive which makes it ideal for quick reference. Unlike many neurosurgery books costing hundreds of dollars, this is an inexpensive book, priced below $100.00. The sixth edition was a *Doody's Core Titles* essential purchase recommendation. It is recommended for hospitals with surgical residents and practitioners, as well as large academic health science libraries.

Principles and Practice of Pediatric Neurosurgery. 2nd ed. Editors: A.L. Albright, Ian F. Pollack, P.D. Adelson. Thieme Medical, 2008.
ISBN: 9781588903952
Recommended for: Hospital, Academic Libraries
Doody's Core Titles Selection

This is the textbook for pediatric neurosurgery residents or physicians. It discusses the pediatric neurosurgical disorders often found in clinical practice. Chapters are organized in outline form, with sections including cerebral disorders, spinal disorders, neoplasms, trauma, cerebrovascular disease, functional disorders, and infectious disorders. In each section these areas are discussed: diagnostic studies, pathology and pathobiology, indications for surgery, treatment alternatives, prognostic factors, and outcomes. This second edition has commentaries from the editors at the end of each chapter, pearls of wisdom that identify critical procedures, illustrations showing disease pathology, techniques, and surgical procedures. New to this edition are chapters on ethical issues, pediatric neurosurgery in developing countries, and in-utero neurosurgery. This book is recommended for hospital libraries with pediatric surgical residents and surgeons. It is currently a *Doody's Core Titles* essential purchase recommendation.

Principles of Neurosurgery. 2nd ed. Editors: Setti S. Rengachary, Richard G. Ellenbogen. Elsevier, 2005.
ISBN: 9780723432227
Recommended for: Hospital, Academic Libraries

This introductory text, intended for medical students and residents, covers the core areas as well as newer developments in neurosurgery. The editors recruited over 250 experts to write chapters on their respective brain surgery specialties. The chapters are organized and subdivided so that it can be used as a quick reference, or to review a topic previously studied. It includes all the sub-specialty areas: neuroradiology, pediatric neurosurgery, neurovascular surgery, trauma surgery, spine surgery, cranial base neurosurgery, epilepsy surgery, pituitary adenomas, and oncology. Other areas, such as perioperative patient care, traumatic injuries, neuroimaging techniques, and minimally invasive surgery are detailed. This book is heavily illustrated with photographs, flowcharts, full color line drawings, tables, and algorithms, all of which help make the text easy to read. The book is appropriate for a hospital collection which serves surgical junior and mid-level residents as well as large academic collections.

Youman's Neurological Surgery. 5th ed. Editors: H.R. Winn, Julian R. Youmans. W.B. Saunders, 2004.
http://www.neurosurgerytext.com
ISBN: 9780721682914
Recommended for: Academic Libraries
Doody's Core Titles Selection

The editors dropped the subtitle with this edition, but it is a perfect description of this encyclopedic text: "a comprehensive reference guide to the diagnosis and management of neurosurgical problems." The editors have brought together expert contributors to write the chapters, providing not only fundamental concepts but advanced surgical procedures. The contents of each volume are discrete: volume 1, "Introduction to Neurological Surgery," and "Oncology"; volume 2, "Vascular," and "Epilepsy"; volume 3, "Functional Neurosurgery," "Pain," and "Pediatric Neurosurgery"; and volume 4, "Peripheral Nerve," "Radiation Therapy and Radiosurgery," "Spine," "Trauma," and "Special Features." This edition is heavily illustrated with radiological images, photos, and graphs, many in color. This textbook is available in three versions: four-volume set and access to the companion website, which includes the complete searchable text; website only; and four-volume set in print. This set is a must have for neurosurgeons. Because of its cost, only hospital libraries with a neurosurgical department and large health science libraries are likely to purchase this set. This title is currently a *Doody's Core Titles* purchase recommendation.

Journals

Journal of Neurosurgery. v. 1, American Association of Neurosurgeons, 1944.
http://thejns.org/
ISSN: 00223085
ISSN: 19330693 (Online)
Indexed in: MEDLINE
Recommended for: Hospital, Academic Libraries

The American Association of Neurosurgeons was founded as the Harvey Cushing Society in 1931. This journal, which it publishes, is one of the earliest journals dealing specifically with neurosurgery. It has authoritative clinical articles, laboratory research papers, case reports, technical notes, historical vignettes, and more. Some areas covered are clinical neurophysiology, organic neurology, ophthalmology, radiology and pathology. All articles are peer-reviewed. In 1999, the Association began publishing the *Journal of Neurosurgery: Spine* as a quarterly supplement. It became a bi-monthly publication in 2002. The *Journal of Neurosurgery: Pediatrics* was started in 2004 as a quarterly supplement. Both *JNS: Spine* and *JNS: Pediatrics* began monthly publication in 2005. This journal is comprehensive in that it covers all aspects of this specialty. It ranks thirty-third out of 167 surgery journals (2009 *Journal Citation Reports*). It is indexed in all the major indexing and abstracting sources. This journal is a required resource for any hospital providing neurosurgery and for large academic libraries. Full online coverage from 1944 to the present is available through the publisher.

Neurosurgery. v. 1, Lippincott Williams & Wilkins, 1977.
http://journals.lww.com/neurosurgery/
ISSN: 0148396X
ISSN: 15244040 (Online)
Indexed in: MEDLINE
Recommended for: Hospital, Academic Libraries

As the official journal of the Congress of Neurological Surgeons, this title is required reading for those in this field. It includes original, peer-reviewed research articles on the latest science, technology, and medicine in neurosurgery. Articles cover clinical and laboratory observations, reviews of clinical guidelines, and technical case reports in neurosurgery. Each issue has an article on current events in neurosurgery, as well as a calendar of events. The journal is published monthly and supplements are included with some issues. Neurosurgeons and surgeons are the main audience for this journal. It ranks twenty-fourth out of 166 surgery journals (2009 *Journal Citation Reports*). This journal is a required resource for any hospital providing neurosurgical services, as well as for academic institutions training neurosurgical or surgical residents. This title is indexed in all the major abstracting and indexing sources. Full online coverage from volume 1 is available from Lippincott Williams & Wilkins (LWW).

World Neurosurgery. v. 73, Elsevier, 2010.
http://www.worldneurosurgery.org/
http://www.sciencedirect.com/science/journal/18788750
ISSN: 18788750
ISSN: 18788769 (Online)
Indexed in: MEDLINE
Recommended for: Hospital, Academic Libraries

The scope of this journal changed in 2010 when it transitioned from *Surgical Neurology* to *World Neurosurgery: A Forum for Six Continents*. It now includes a more global view of neurosurgical practice, broadly covering politics, education, research, sociology, technology, operative techniques, and laboratory science. It addresses the latest neurosurgical developments by providing peer-reviewed articles on a range of topics: cranial base, critical care, endovascular neuroradiology, pain, pediatrics, peripheral nerve, radiosurgery, basic science, spine, sports, stereotactic, and functional trauma. It is the official international journal of the World Federation of Neurosurgical Societies. This title is indexed in all the major abstracting and indexing sources. It ranks seventy-fourth out of 167 surgery journals (2009 *Journal Citation Reports*). The title is a required resource for any hospital providing neurosurgical procedures as well as health science libraries. Full online coverage from 1981 to the present is available from Elsevier.

11.4. Obstetrics

Management and care of women during pregnancy, parturition, and the puerperium.

—MeSH

Contributor: Mary A. Hyde

Monographs

Creasy and Resnik's Maternal-Fetal Medicine: Principles and Practice. 6th ed. Editors: Robert K. Creasy, Robert Resnik, Jay D. Iams. Saunders Elsevier, 2009.
http://www.mdconsult.com/
ISBN: 9781416042242
Recommended for: Hospital, Academic Libraries
Brandon/Hill, *Doody's Core Titles* Selection

The sixth edition of *Creasy and Resnik's Maternal-Fetal Medicine* has been completely revised and updated. The new edition includes comprehensive information on the biology of pregnancy. The book is an excellent resource for all obstetrician-gynecologists studying for their subspecialty boards in maternal-fetal medicine. There is a new section on disorders at the maternal-fetal interface, and new chapters have been added on the biology of parturition and intrapartum assessment of fetal health.

This edition adds new editors and chapter authors and includes a focus toward evidence-based medicine. This publication is an essential resource for hospital and academic medical centers with maternal-fetal medicine residents and subspecialists. Previous editions were included on the Brandon/Hill list, and the current edition is a *Doody's Core Titles* recommendation. Elsevier offers online access as part of its MD Consult e-book specialty collection on obstetrics and gynecology.

Danforth's Obstetrics and Gynecology. 10th ed. Editors: Ronald S. Gibbs, Beth Y. Karlan, Arthur F. Haney, Ingrid E. Nygaard. Lippincott Williams & Wilkins, 2008.
http://www.ovid.com/
ISBN: 9780781769372
See Also Chapter 1.9. Physician Assistants
Recommended for: Hospital, Academic Libraries
Brandon/Hill, *Doody's Core Titles* Selection

Just as it has for the past 40 years, the 10th edition of *Danforth's* continues to provide authoritative coverage available to practicing obstetrician-gynecologists. This edition has been thoroughly revised and has added a new section on urogynecology. Topics address issues related to the practice of ob-gyn at both the primary care and specialist level. There are chapters covering all aspects of pregnancy, including a new chapter on stillbirth. Another new chapter addresses the topic of psychological disorders of pregnancy and the postpartum period. There are new algorithms, tables, and lists in this edition. There is a companion website available with fully searchable text for individual purchasers of the print version. Ovid also offers online access. This is an excellent resource for hospitals, specialized collections, and academic medical centers. Past editions have been listed in the Brandon/Hill list, and it is currently listed in *Doody's Core Titles* as an essential purchase.

Drugs in Pregnancy and Lactation: A Reference Guide to Fetal and Neonatal Risk. 8th ed. Editors: Gerald G. Briggs, Roger K. Freeman, Sumner J. Yaffe. Lippincott Williams & Wilkins, 2008.
http://www.ovid.com/
http://www.r2library.com/
ISBN: 9780781778763
Recommended for: Hospital, Academic, Consumer Health Libraries
Brandon/Hill, *Doody's Core Titles* Selection

The eighth edition of this very popular reference title has been updated to include 127 new drugs. It reviews 1,175 drugs commonly prescribed to pregnant and breastfeeding women. Each review summarizes the possible side effects to the fetus and breastfed infant. The Food and Drug Administration's (FDA) risk factor ratings are supplied with each drug entry. The reviews are listed in alphabetical order by the American generic drug name. The index includes generic, domestic, and foreign trade names. This edition also includes more reviews on herbals and natural supplements used by women. For individuals who purchase the print book, there is also a companion website with a link to the *Briggs Update* newsletter that provides updated, published reviews and new entries. Online access is offered by both Ovid and R2 Digital Library. A previous edition of this book was included on the Brandon/Hill list and is currently listed as a *Doody's Core Titles* essential purchase. This is a resource any hospital, academic, and consumer library should include in their collection.

Guidelines for Perinatal Care. 6th ed. American Academy of Pediatrics [and] American College of Obstetricians and Gynecologists, 2007.
http://www.r2library.com/
ISBN: 9781932328363
ISBN: 9781581102703
See Also Chapter 10.13.2. Perinatology
Recommended for: Hospital, Academic Libraries
Doody's Core Titles Selection

Guidelines for Perinatal Care is the first and best place to look for authoritative guidance on the care of pregnant women, their fetuses, and newborns. The guidelines also outline basic, specialty, and subspecialty levels of perinatal care. The sixth edition has been reorganized and provides new information on vaginal birth after cesarean, HIV, and breastfeeding. There is a new chapter on the care of the neonate, and information on maternal and newborn nutrition has been expanded. This edition is a required resource for any hospital, specialized, or academic institution providing obstetrics and neonatal care. This title is also listed in *Doody's Core Titles* as an essential purchase.

Multiple Pregnancy: Epidemiology, Gestation & Perinatal Outcome. 2nd ed. Editors: Isaac Blickstein, Louis G. Keith. Taylor & Francis, 2005.
http://extranet.netlibrary.com/TitleSelect/
ISBN: 9781842142394
ISBN: 9780203017753
Recommended for: Hospital, Academic Libraries

This edition of *Multiple Pregnancy* has been completely rewritten. As the editors stated in the preface to this work, it was essential that the first edition, which was published in 1995, be rewritten completely to address the many changes that have taken place. Since the first edition was released, an epidemic of multiple births has occurred because of newer technologies and advancing prenatal care of high-risk pregnancies. The second edition has been reorganized to include information on new technologies, prenatal diagnosis, and fetal therapy. This book is an essential resource for hospital and academic medical center collections that support Level II or higher level obstetric units.

Obstetrics: Normal and Problem Pregnancies. 5th ed. Editors: Steven G. Gabbe, Jennifer R. Niebyl, Joe Leigh Simpson. Churchill Livingstone/Elsevier, 2007.
http://www.mdconsult.com/
ISBN: 9780443069307
Recommended for: Hospital, Academic Libraries
Doody's Core Titles Selection

The fifth edition of *Obstetrics: Normal and Problem Pregnancies* is an essential resource for information on diagnosis, treatment, and management of the challenges facing an obstetrician in practice. This updated edition includes new information on placental anatomy, abnormal labor, operative vaginal delivery, and cervical incompetence. Individual purchasers of this print edition have access to a companion website with fully searchable text and illustrations that can be used in presentations. Online access is also offered through MD Consult. This publication is an excellent resource for hospitals, specialized collections, and academic medical centers. It is listed in *Doody's Core Titles* as an essential purchase.

Operative Obstetrics. 2nd ed. Editors: John P. O'Grady, Martin L. Gimovsky. Cambridge University Press, 2008.
http://www.ebrary.com/
ISBN: 9780521862486
ISBN: 9780511579073 (Online)
Recommended for: Hospital, Academic Libraries

The second edition of *Operative Obstetrics* was 10 years in the making. The editors used an evidence-based approach in rewriting this textbook, although they noted that not all practice can be based on evidence. Much of the publication focuses on general obstetrics even though the title mentions "operative" obstetrics. This edition has been fully revised and updated. There are chapters on cesarean section, birth injury, ectopic pregnancy, and surgical complications. This is an excellent resource for hospitals and academic medical centers.

Williams Obstetrics. 23rd ed. Editors: F. Gary Cunningham, Kenneth J. Leveno, Steven L. Bloom, John C. Hauth, Dwight J. Rouse, Catherine Y. Spong. McGraw-Hill Medical, 2010.
http://www.accessmedicine.com/
ISBN: 9780071497015
Recommended for: Hospital, Academic Libraries
Brandon/Hill, *Doody's Core Titles* Selection

This edition of the classic *Williams Obstetrics* provides comprehensive coverage of obstetric practice. The new edition, published in full color for the first time, has a greater emphasis on evidence-based medicine. *Williams Obstetrics* leads the practitioner through anatomy, the antepartum period, and labor and delivery. There are sections on the fetus and newborn as well as the puerperium, which includes individual chapters on contraception and sterilization. There are two sections on complications in pregnancy and medical and surgical complications. As an added bonus, McGraw-Hill's online version includes short video presentations for selected procedures. This well-written textbook is an essential reference publication for hospitals, academic medical centers, and specialized collections. It has always been included on the Brandon/Hill list and *Doody's Core Titles* identified the twenty-third edition as an essential purchase.

Your Pregnancy & Birth. 4th ed. American College of Obstetricians and Gynecologists, 2005.
ISBN: 9780696225918
Recommended for: Consumer Health Libraries

Your Pregnancy & Birth is the premier guide to information on pregnancy from the American College of Obstetricians and Gynecologists. This fourth edition covers every aspect of pregnancy from preconception care to postpartum care. The book is divided into chapters on pregnancy; labor, delivery, and postpartum care; special care (complications); and health and wellness maintenance. Each chapter is divided into sections covering specific topics, such as work and pregnancy, exercise, breastfeeding, and complications. There is also a pregnancy planner and growth charts for boys and girls. This title is an essential resource for a consumer health library.

Your Pregnancy Week by Week. 6th ed. Authors: Glade B. Curtis, Judith Schuler. Da Capo Press, 2008.
ISBN: 9780738211091
Recommended for: Consumer Health Libraries

The sixth edition of this excellent patient resource has been fully revised and updated. The format provides the pregnant woman with relevant information about the development of the fetus. Illustrations of the changes happening to the growing baby are excellent and provide perspective to the new mother. The book offers tips on nutrition, health, and how actions may affect the growth of the fetus. Information on exercise during pregnancy is included, along with information for the father-to-be. This excellent resource is an essential selection for a core consumer collection.

Journals

American Journal of Obstetrics & Gynecology. v. 1, Mosby-Elsevier, 1920.
http://www.sciencedirect.com/science/journal/00029378
http://www.mdconsult.com/
http://www.ajog.org
ISSN: 00029378
ISSN: 10976868 (Online)
See Also Chapter 11.2. Gynecology
Indexed in: MEDLINE, CINAHL
Recommended for: Hospital, Academic Libraries
Brandon/Hill Selection

This excellent obstetrics-gynecology (ob-gyn) journal has covered the specialty since 1868 under the preceding title, *The American Journal of Obstetrics and Diseases of Women and Children*, volumes 1–80, 1868–1919. This journal covers all aspects of women's health, including reproductive endocrinology and infertility, maternal-fetal medicine, gynecologic oncology, and general obstetrics and gynecology. It is the official journal of many ob-gyn societies such as the Society of Gynecologic Surgeons, the Society for Maternal-Fetal Medicine, and the Association of Professors of Gynecology and Obstetrics. This journal is one of the most referenced publications and is cited frequently in the American Board of Obstetrics and Gynecology's Annual Board Certification program. According to the 2009 *Journal Citation Reports*, this journal is ranked seventh out of 70 journals in obstetrics and gynecology. This journal is a required resource for any hospital providing care to women, as well as academic institutions involved in the education of physician trainees. This journal is cited in numerous abstracting and indexing sources such as MEDLINE and CINAHL, and the National Library of Medicine considers this journal to be a core clinical title. The journal is available in both print and online formats. Full online coverage back to volume 1, number 1, 1920 is available through Elsevier's ScienceDirect.

Best Practice & Research Clinical Obstetrics & Gynaecology. v. 13, Elsevier, 1999.
http://www.sciencedirect.com/
ISSN: 15216934
ISSN: 15321932
Indexed in: MEDLINE
Recommended for: Hospital, Academic Libraries

Best Practice & Research Clinical Obstetrics & Gynaecology continues *Baillière's Clinical Obstetrics and Gynaecology* and *Baillière's Best Practice & Research Clinical Obstetrics & Gynaecology*, which is referenced in some sources. This journal provides clinicians with current clinical practice and thinking on specific topics. Each issue focuses on a specific topic, provides questions to be addressed, and defines the knowns and unknowns about the topic. Each issue also provides clinicians with practical information on treatment and patient management. This journal is a required resource for any academic institution involved in the education of physician trainees and specialized collections. This journal is cited in numerous abstracting and indexing sources such as MEDLINE and Embase. The journal is available in both print and online formats. Full online coverage back to volume 13, 1999 is available through Elsevier's ScienceDirect.

Birth: Issues in Perinatal Care. v. 9, Wiley-Blackwell, 1982.
http://onlinelibrary.wiley.com/journal/10.1111/(ISSN)1523-536X/
ISSN: 07307659
ISSN: 1523536X (Online)
Indexed in: MEDLINE, CINAHL
Recommended for: Hospital, Academic Libraries

Birth: Issues in Perinatal Care, which continues the journal *Birth and the Family Journal* (volumes 1–8, 1973–1981), is a multidisciplinary journal in obstetrics and gynecology. The journal covers issues and practices in the care of childbearing women, infants, and families. *Birth* is a required resource for hospitals and specialized collections. This journal is cited in numerous abstracting and indexing sources such as MEDLINE and CINAHL. Full online coverage back to 1973 is available through Wiley Online Library.

BJOG: An International Journal of Obstetrics and Gynaecology. v. 107, Wiley-Blackwell, 2000.
http://onlinelibrary.wiley.com/journal/10.1111/(ISSN)1471-0528/
ISSN: 14700328
ISSN: 14710528 (Online)
Indexed in: MEDLINE, CINAHL
Recommended for: Hospital, Academic Libraries
Brandon/Hill Selection

BJOG is the independently-edited journal owned by the Royal College of Obstetricians and Gynaecologists. The journal has been in existence since 1902, but it has changed its name three times. This journal covers all areas of obstetrics and gynecology, including contraception, midwifery, and urogynecology. According to the 2009 *Journal Citation Reports*, *BJOG* is ranked sixth out of 70 journals in obstetrics and gynecology. This journal is a required resource for any hospital providing care to women, as well as academic institutions involved in the education of physician trainees. This journal is cited in numerous abstracting and indexing sources such as MEDLINE and CINAHL. The National Library of Medicine considers it to be a core clinical title. Full online coverage back to volume 1, 1902 is available through Wiley Online Library.

Clinical Obstetrics and Gynecology. v. 1, Lippincott Williams & Wilkins, 1958.
http://www.ovid.com/
ISSN: 00099201
ISSN: 15325520 (Online)
Indexed in: MEDLINE, CINAHL
Recommended for: Hospital, Academic Libraries
Brandon/Hill Selection

Clinical Obstetrics and Gynecology provides quarterly symposia on timely topics of interest to obstetrician-gynecologists. The journal provides reviews on both medical and surgical procedures, clinical problems, treatments, and diagnostic aids. This journal is a required resource for any hospital providing care to women, as well as academic institutions involved in the education of physician trainees. It is cited in numerous abstracting and indexing sources such as MEDLINE and CINAHL. Full online coverage back to volume 1, number 1, 1958 is available through Ovid.

Clinics in Perinatology. v. 1, Saunders Elsevier, 1974.
http://www.mdconsult.com/
http://www.sciencedirect.com/science/journal/00955108
ISSN: 00955108
ISSN: 15579840 (Online)
See Also Chapter 10.13.2. Perinatology
Indexed in: MEDLINE, CINAHL
Recommended for: Hospital, Academic Libraries

Clinics in Perinatology provides comprehensive reviews on timely topics of interest to obstetrician-gynecologists. The journal provides reviews on diagnosis and treatments affecting the mother, fetus, and newborn. This journal covers a single topic in maternal-fetal medicine each quarter. It is a required resource for any hospital providing care to women and infants, as well as academic institutions involved in the education of physician trainees. This journal is cited in numerous abstracting and indexing sources such as MEDLINE and CINAHL. Online coverage back to volume 27, 2000 is available through ScienceDirect.

Current Opinion in Obstetrics & Gynecology. v. 1, Lippincott Williams & Wilkins, 1989.
http://journals.lww.com/co-obgyn/
ISSN: 1040872X
ISSN: 1473656X (Online)
Indexed in: MEDLINE, CINAHL
Recommended for: Hospital, Academic Libraries

Current Opinion in Obstetrics & Gynecology provides comprehensive reviews on timely topics of interest to obstetrician-gynecologists. The journal provides reviews on such topics as gynecologic pathology, prenatal diagnosis, urogynecology, and women's health. This journal is a required resource for any hospital providing care to women and infants, as well as academic institutions involved in the education of physician trainees. This journal is cited in numerous abstracting and indexing sources such as MEDLINE and CINAHL. Full online coverage back to volume 1, 1989 is available through Lippincott Williams & Wilkins.

Journal of Maternal-Fetal & Neonatal Medicine. v. 11, Informa Healthcare, 2002.
http://informahealthcare.com/
ISSN: 14767058
ISSN: 14764954 (Online)
Indexed in: MEDLINE, CINAHL
Recommended for: Academic Libraries

The Journal of Maternal-Fetal & Neonatal Medicine is the official journal of the European Association of Perinatal Medicine, the Federation of Asia and Oceania Perinatal Societies, and the International Society of Perinatal Obstetricians. This journal publishes both review and original articles on topics in maternal-fetal and neonatal medicine. This journal is a required resource for any hospital providing care to women and infants, as well as academic institutions involved in the education of physician trainees. This journal is cited in numerous abstracting and indexing sources such as MEDLINE and CINAHL. Full online coverage back to volume 1, 1992 is available through Informa Healthcare.

Obstetrics & Gynecology. v. 1, Lippincott Williams & Wilkins, 1953.
http://www.ovid.com/
ISSN: 00297844
ISSN: 1873233X
See Also Chapter 11.2. Gynecology
Indexed in: MEDLINE, CINAHL

Recommended for: Hospital, Academic Libraries
Brandon/Hill Selection

Obstetrics & Gynecology is the official journal of the American College of Obstetricians and Gynecologists. The "Green Journal," as it is commonly known, has been continuously published since 1953. The journal's goal is to publish relevant articles that promote excellence in the practice of obstetrics and gynecology. According to the 2009 *Journal Citation Reports*, the journal is ranked second of 70 journals in obstetrics and gynecology with an impact factor of 4.357. This journal is a required resource for hospitals providing care to women, as well as academic institutions involved in the education of physician trainees. This journal is cited in numerous abstracting and indexing sources such as MEDLINE and CINAHL. The National Library of Medicine considers this journal to be a core clinical title. Full online coverage back to volume 1, 1953 is available through Lippincott Williams & Wilkins.

Obstetrics and Gynecology Clinics of North America. v. 14, Saunders Elsevier, 1987.
http://www.mdconsult.com/
http://www.sciencedirect.com/science/journal/08898545
ISSN: 08898545
ISSN: 15580474 (Online)
Indexed in: MEDLINE, CINAHL
Recommended for: Hospital, Academic Libraries

Obstetrics and Gynecology Clinics of North America provides reviews on diagnosis and treatments affecting obstetrics and gynecology. This journal covers a single topic in obstetrics and gynecology each quarter, and continuing medical education credit is available. This journal is a required resource for any hospital providing care to women, as well as academic institutions involved in the education of physician trainees. It is cited in numerous abstracting and indexing sources such as MEDLINE and CINAHL. Online coverage back to volume 23, 1996 is available through ScienceDirect and MD Consult.

11.5. Ophthalmology

The structure and function of the eye and the medical and surgical treatment of its defects and diseases.

—MeSH

Contributor: Suzanne Ferimer, Gale A. Oren, Michael E. Piorunski

Monographs

All about Your Eyes. Editors: Sharon Fekrat, Jennifer S. Weizer. Duke University Press, 2006.
ISBN: 9780822336600
Recommended for: Hospital, Consumer Health Libraries

This valuable addition to the consumer health literature was edited and written by members of the Ophthalmology staff at Duke University Medical Center. The most recently published volume of its kind, it provides a clear, concise introduction to everything related to one's eyes, from basic anatomy and ocular function to up-to-date descriptions of eye diseases and ophthalmic surgical procedures. The disease descriptions are especially noteworthy, guiding the reader through each condition in a straightforward manner. From what the disease is, to symptoms, prevention, when to seek treatment, and the likelihood of visual recovery, the information contained in this volume assists the user in making proper eye care choices for a variety of ocular disorders. There is also a glossary of technical terms and links to websites containing further information on each condition. This volume should be a required reference in a great variety of library collections, ranging from consumer health collections in public libraries to hospital libraries. Ophthalmology and optometry practices should have a copy to supplement their patient education materials.

Basic and Clinical Science Course 2010–2011. American Academy of Ophthalmology, 2010.
http://www.aao.org/bcscresearch/bcsc_rsrch_ed_of.pdf
ISBN: 9781615251452
Recommended for: Hospital, Academic Libraries

This comprehensive course (*BCSC*) is the cornerstone of ophthalmic education in the United States. The set consists of 13 sections that provide a comprehensive three-year course of study. An updated version of the course is issued annually. A master index accompanies the set. The course begins with the basics of general medicine and ophthalmology, continuing on to cover all ophthalmic subspecialties. The volumes are profusely illustrated in full color and well-referenced, with a self-assessment program contained within each volume. Each volume has a unique editorial board consisting of both academic ophthalmologists and private practitioners. The individual volumes are updated on a rotating basis, which allows for revised editions of all sections to appear every three years. All ophthalmology residents in the United States receive these volumes at the beginning of their residencies. In addition to providing a comprehensive reference text and study guide, the course helps with preparation for the yearly Ophthalmic Knowledge and Assessment Program test (OKAPs), the oral and written ophthalmology board exams, as well as the Maintenance of Certification (MOC) exam taken by all board-certified ophthalmologists. The *BCSC* has been translated into several languages and is now in use throughout the world. The set is available in print form; the entire course or individual volumes are available. DVD and online versions containing advanced search features are also available.

Clinical Ophthalmology: A Systematic Approach. 6th ed. Editor: Jack J. Kanski. Butterworth Heinemann Elsevier, 2007.
ISBN: 9780080449692
Recommended for: Hospital, Academic Libraries
Doody's Core Titles Selection

This trusted resource has been used for decades by residents and students who deal with vision and eye care. One of *Doody's Core Titles*, this book covers all of the basics and is an excellent study tool for exams. The book contains 24 chapters, starting with examination and imaging techniques, developmental malformations and anomalies, then detailing the disorders of the basic structures of the eye and subspecialties in ophthalmology. The chapters are well organized into concise outline and text format, with good use of headings to keep the topics distinct and clear and to facilitate learning. One of the best features of the book is the outstanding color and black-and-white images and diagrams. This sixth edition includes online access to http://www.kanskionline.com for individuals, which includes full-text and downloadable images, as well as self-assessment tools. This text is a required resource for hospitals and academic medical libraries where residents and students are in training.

Cornea. 3rd ed. Editors: Jay H. Krachmer, Mark J. Mannis, Edward J. Holland. Mosby Elsevier, 2011.
ISBN: 9780323063876
Recommended for: Hospital, Academic Libraries
Doody's Core Titles Selection

This review refers to the second edition. This well-respected, comprehensive two-volume set covers the broad range of conditions seen by cornea specialists. Also of use to general ophthalmologists and residents, this book is highly rated by *Doody's Core Titles*. Over 250 contributors were involved in presenting the information offered in this book. Volume 1 contains eight parts; the first three detail the basic science, examination, and differential diagnosis of cornea disease. Following are sections dealing with eye banking, the ocular adnexa, the conjunctiva, diseases of the cornea, and the sclera and anterior uvea. Volume 2 examines corneal surgical procedures and refractive surgery. Lastly, readers will find an extensive index. This edition offers a DVD with over 2,000 downloadable illustrations from the book, as well as a number of three- to four-minute video clips illustrating diagnostic techniques and surgical procedures. The book includes a liberal number of high-quality images, diagrams, and charts and tables. This work is a required resource for hospital and academic medical libraries.

Ocular Pathology. 6th ed. Authors: Myron Yanoff, Joseph W. Sassani. Mosby Elsevier, 2009.
http://www.mdconsult.com/
ISBN: 9780323042321
Recommended for: Hospital, Academic Libraries
Doody's Core Titles Selection

This classic text, intended for ophthalmology residents, ophthalmologists, and ophthalmic pathologists, is considered by many to be the leading resource in the field. First published in 1975, and now it its sixth edition, it comprehensively covers everything from the basics of eye pathology to common and rare conditions, with clinical pearls throughout. Well-respected author Myron Yanoff, MD, has been joined by his new co-author, Joseph W. Sassani, MD, another leader in the field of ophthalmic pathology. Encompassing a total of 789 pages, this book is divided into 18 chapters, each with an extensive and updated reference list at the end. Organized in an outline format, which has been found very successful throughout all six editions, chapters are color-coded and subheadings are highlighted for easy navigation. The book provides over 1,900 illustrations, 1,600 of them in color, including OCT, MRI, and CT images, all downloadable from the accompanying DVD. Also included on the DVD are virtual microscopy digitized histopathology slides. This latest edition contains numerous updates, including new sections on age-related macular degeneration and complications of refractive surgery, as well as coverage of recent advances in genetics, immunohistochemistry, and molecular biology. A *Doody's* core title, this text is essential for academic libraries, residency and clinical fellowship programs, vision science libraries, and as a good starting point for clinicians seeking an understanding of ocular pathology.

Pediatric Ophthalmology and Strabismus. 2nd ed. Editors: Kenneth W. Wright, Peter H. Spiegel. Springer, 2003.
ISBN: 0387945783
Recommended for: Hospital, Academic Libraries

The second edition of this classic textbook is intended for pediatric ophthalmologists, residents, and fellows, and any other practitioner who treats children with eye disease. The focus is on eye conditions and their manifestation in children, with an emphasis on practical aspects of pediatric ophthalmology. The book is organized into ten sections, starting with a chapter on normal development, then a second chapter on practical aspects of pediatric ophthalmology. The following sections deal with a variety of disease categories; the final section is new to this edition, covering a compendium of inherited diseases with ocular involvement. The content is covered systematically and well illustrated with images, tables, charts, and decision-making guidelines. The book is highly recommended for academic medical libraries, hospitals, and any other environment where children's eye conditions are diagnosed and treated.

Retina. 4th ed. Editors: Stephen J. Ryan, David R. Hinton, Andrew P. Schachat, Pat Wilkinson. Elsevier/Mosby, 2006.
http://www.sciencedirect.com/science/book/9780323049597
ISBN: 9780323025980
ISBN: 9780323043236 (Online)
Recommended for: Hospital, Academic Libraries
Doody's Core Titles Selection

First published in 1989 and now in its fourth edition, Ryan's *Retina* remains the most comprehensive textbook for the study of the retina. The list of chapter authors reads like a "Who's Who in Retina," basic scientists and clinicians that are internationally recognized as leaders in the field. The text is profusely illustrated, with over 3,800 illustrations, 1,300 in color. The first volume details the development, structure, and function of the retina; the second describes disease processes and medical therapy of retinal diseases; the third volume is devoted to surgery of the retina. The online version is fully searchable and regularly updated. It includes all images, video clips of retinal surgery, and also links to online source materials. This text is useful as both a starting point and also a comprehensive reference source for those seeking information on anything relating to the retina and its diseases. This resource is a *Doody's Core Titles* selection, and is an important part of ophthalmology and vision science library collections.

Shield's Textbook of Glaucoma. 6th ed. Editors: R. Rand Allingham, Karim F. Damji, Sharon Freedman, Sayoko E. Moroi, Douglas J. Rhee. Wolters Kluwer/Lippincott Williams & Wilkins, 2011.
http://www.ovid.com/
ISBN: 9780781795852
Recommended for: Hospital, Academic Libraries
Doody's Core Titles Selection

This review refers to the fifth edition. With the fifth edition of this well-respected book, Dr. M. Bruce Shield's name was added to the title, as he became an emeritus senior author and transferred editorship to other leaders in the field. A *Doody's* core title, this clinically focused book is heavily used by residents, fellows and practitioners who treat glaucoma patients. The book also covers the cellular and molecular biology, genetics, and epidemiology of glaucoma. It is used both as a textbook and as a reference resource. The text is highly practical and well organized into three main sections: basic aspects, clinical forms, and management of glaucoma. Chapters frequently begin with a section on terminology, and end with a summary of key points and an extensive bibliography. The book includes a liberal number of images, diagrams, charts, and tables throughout. A section with color photos appears at the beginning of the book. This work is a required resource for hospital and academic medical libraries.

Walsh and Hoyt's Clinical Neuro-ophthalmology. 6th ed. Editors: Neil R. Miller, Nancy J. Newman, Valerie Biousse, John B. Kerrison. Lippincott Williams & Wilkins, 2005.
http://www.ovid.com/
ISBN: 9780781748148
Recommended for: Hospital, Academic Libraries
Brandon/Hill, *Doody's Core Titles* Selection

This resource has been recognized as the most comprehensive neuro-ophthalmology text since the release of the first edition in 1947. First written by a single author, the book is now a product of multiple authors. It has been condensed from a five-volume to a three-volume set without a significant change in the quality of the material. It is a clinically focused text with each chapter covering a separate disorder from history to diagnosis through treatment. All three volumes are well-illustrated in black and white and also well-referenced, providing an encyclopedic approach to the study of neuro-ophthalmology, with deeper coverage than that of comparable neurology and neurosurgery texts. A *Doody's Core Titles* selection for many years, it is also available electronically through Ovid. This text is a required resource for all practicing neuro-ophthalmologists and ophthalmology teaching programs. Academic and hospital medical libraries that serve neurology or neurosurgery divisions, as well as optometry libraries should have access to this resource.

Wills Eye Manual: Office and Emergency Room Diagnosis and Treatment of Eye Disease. 5th ed. Editors: Justis P. Ehlers, Chirag P. Shah. Wolters Kluwer/Lippincott, Williams & Wilkins, 2008.
http://www.ovid.com/
ISBN: 9780781769624
Recommended for: Hospital, Academic Libraries
Doody's Core Titles Selection

Known in the field to be a reliable and useful resource, this quick reference guide is very easy to use, concise, yet comprehensive for its purpose. Intended for students, residents, fellows, or any clinician dealing with treatment of the eye, the guide covers over 200 ophthalmic conditions. The focus is on clinical decision making. The book is organized into 14 chapters, starting with two chapters on differential diagnosis; then the long list of conditions are arranged by main topic, such as trauma, conjunctiva/sclera/iris/external disease, eyelid, orbit, pediatrics, glaucoma, neuro-ophthalmology, retina, uveitis, and general ophthalmic problems. The final chapter covers imaging modalities in ophthalmology, and is followed by a pharmacopoeia and 16 appendixes. Each condition is organized into outline format, which include symptoms, signs, work-up and treatment. The new fifth edition provides color photos to aid in diagnosis, and is attractively presented with color headings and tabs. New clinical sections and appendixes have been added. Mobile device and Spanish language versions are also available from the publisher's website. This manual has been continually selected for the *Doody's Core Titles* list and is currently classified as an essential purchase within the ophthalmology specialty. The book is highly recommended for emergency rooms, hospitals, physicians' offices, and any other environment where eye conditions are diagnosed and treated.

Journals

American Journal of Ophthalmology. v. 1, Elsevier, 1884.
http://www.ajo.com/
http://www.sciencedirect.com/science/journal/00029394
ISSN: 00029394
ISSN: 18791891 (Online)
Indexed in: MEDLINE
Recommended for: Hospital, Academic Libraries

One of the major multi-specialty journals in ophthalmology, this journal has been published monthly since 1884. It was the first monthly ophthalmic journal in the United States, and is now in its third series. The focus is on scholarly works in ophthalmology, including clinical investigations, clinical observations, and clinically relevant research studies. Each issue contains original peer-reviewed articles, brief reports, and correspondence, with editorials and perspectives (by invitation only). There is also supplemental online content. The main audience for this journal includes ophthalmologists, vision researchers, residents and fellows, and medical students, but is also of interest to physicians in related specialties and others dealing with vision care. This international journal ranks fifth out of 49 ophthalmology journals (2009 *Journal Citation Reports*). The journal is indexed in dozens of abstracting and indexing sources, including MEDLINE, Embase, Scopus, and Biological Abstracts. It is a recommended resource for hospitals, academic institutions, and ophthalmology practices. Online coverage is available back to 1998 through Elsevier ScienceDirect.

Archives of Ophthalmology. v. 64, American Medical Association, 1960.
http://archopht.ama-assn.org/
ISSN: 00039950
ISSN: 15383601 (Online)
Indexed in: MEDLINE
Recommended for: Hospital, Academic Libraries

One of the major multi-specialty journals in ophthalmology, this journal superseded (in part) the *Archives of Ophthalmology and Otology* in 1869. It began under its current title in 1960. This monthly journal is one of the ten AMA consortium journals. It focuses on scholarly works in ophthalmology, including clinical trials, clinical sciences, laboratory sciences, epidemiology, and socioeconomics and health services. In addition to peer-reviewed articles, the journal offers editorials, case reports, letters, CME, news, and a surgeon's corner. The content covers the major subspecialties in ophthalmology. The main audience for this journal includes ophthalmologists, vision researchers, residents and fellows, and medical students, but is also of interest to physicians in related specialties, or anyone doing research in the field of ophthalmology. This journal ranks fourth out of 49 ophthalmology journals (2009 *Journal Citation Reports*). This international journal is indexed in dozens of abstracting and indexing sources, including MEDLINE, Embase, Scopus, and BIOSIS Previews. It is a recommended resource for hospitals, academic institutions, and ophthalmology practices. Online coverage is available back to 1929 through the publisher.

British Journal of Ophthalmology. v. 1, BMJ Publishing Group, 1917.
http://bjo.bmj.com/

http://www.ncbi.nlm.nih.gov/pmc/journals/152/
ISSN: 00071161
ISSN: 14682079 (Online)
Indexed in: MEDLINE
Recommended for: Hospital, Academic Libraries

The *British Journal of Ophthalmology* (*BJO*) is published by BMJ Publishing Group, a subsidiary of the British Medical Association. It was started in 1917 as the merger of three separate British ophthalmology journals. Intended for all medical professionals and trainees who deal with vision science, it covers both clinical science and laboratory science articles. A typical issue of this peer-reviewed journal includes editorials, review articles, global coverage of ophthalmic issues, innovation in ophthalmology, and educational case studies. Each issue includes an article designated as "Editor's Choice," which has been chosen to be of special interest, and is freely available online. This title ranks ninth out of 49 ophthalmology journals (2009 *Journal Citation Reports*). It is indexed in dozens of abstracting and indexing sources, including MEDLINE, Embase, Scopus, and BIOSIS Previews. It is appropriate for hospitals, academic institutions, and ophthalmology practices. The journal is available in both print and online formats. Online coverage is available back to 1917 through the BMJ website and all but the most recent four years are free of charge. It is also available online in PubMed Central from 1917 up to three years from the current year.

Focal Points: Clinical Modules for Ophthalmologists. [Unnumbered], American Academy of Ophthalmology, 1983.
http://one.aao.org/CE/EducationalProducts/FocalPoints.aspx
ISSN: 08918260
Recommended for: Hospital, Academic Libraries

First published in 1983, *Focal Points* consists of 12 individually themed modules per year. Three modules are sent four times per year. It is geared toward clinical issues faced by ophthalmologists in daily practice. A clinical description of each condition is provided along with key studies, a review of the relevant evidence, goals of therapy, and a conclusion. A clinician's corner provides additional viewpoints by consultants invited by the Editorial Review Board. A suggested reading list provides reference lists for further study on the covered topic as well as a list of relevant American Academy of Ophthalmology educational materials. *Focal Points* is also available online and includes features not available in the print edition such as video footage of surgical techniques for selected modules. Issues back to 2002 are available online. Ophthalmologists use *Focal Points* as a teaching and review tool. Primary care physicians and medical students needing to research a single topic find up-to-date, concise information here.

Investigative Ophthalmology and Visual Science. v. 16, Association for Research in Vision and Ophthalmology (ARVO), 1977.
http://www.iovs.org
ISSN: 01460404
ISSN: 15525783 (Online)
Indexed in: MEDLINE
Recommended for: Academic Libraries

Although this title began in 1977, publication of the journal actually began in 1962 under an earlier title and it has long been a well-known resource for vision science research articles. As the official journal of the Association for Research in Vision and Ophthalmology (ARVO), it is aligned with the goals of the Association to disseminate knowledge and advance the field of vision and ophthalmology. The intended audience includes scientists and students conducting basic or clinical vision research. It is highly recommended for any academic institution or research organization involved in this pursuit. The content of scholarly, peer-reviewed articles is organized into thirteen sections, which represent the thirteen research subject areas of the ARVO membership. Each monthly issue also contains a list of "Recent E-Letters to the Editor" which can be accessed from the journal's website. An ARVO abstract issue was included in the journal through 2001; in 2002 it became available through the journal's website. *Investigative Ophthalmology and Visual Science* (*IOVS*) ranks sixth out of 49 ophthalmology journals (2009 *Journal Citation Reports*). This international journal is indexed in numerous abstracting and indexing sources, including MEDLINE, Embase, Scopus, BIOSIS Previews, and Chemical Abstracts. Full online coverage is available back to 1962 through the publisher.

Ophthalmology. v. 85, Elsevier, 1978.
http://www.sciencedirect.com/science/journal/01616420
ISSN: 01616420
ISSN: 15494713 (Online)
Indexed in: MEDLINE
Recommended for: Hospital, Academic Libraries

This peer-reviewed journal is the official journal of the American Academy of Ophthalmology. Its publication history goes back to 1907 when it began under an earlier title. As one of the major multi-specialty journals in ophthalmology, it covers basic science investigations and clinical studies, including major reviews, new diagnostic and surgical techniques, treatment methods, drug findings, results of clinical trials, and the latest research findings. The main audience for this journal includes ophthalmologists, vision researchers, residents and fellows, and medical students, but it is also of interest to physicians in related specialties, or anyone doing research in the field of ophthalmology. This journal ranks second out of 48 ophthalmology journals (2008 *Journal Citation Reports*). It is indexed in dozens of abstracting and indexing sources, including MEDLINE, Embase, Scopus and BIOSIS Previews. It is a recommended resource for hospitals, academic institutions, and ophthalmology practices. Online coverage is available back to 1998 through Elsevier ScienceDirect.

Databases and Other Electronic Resources

Wills Eye Video Atlas of Ocular Surgery. Lippincott, Williams, & Wilkins, 2006.
ISBN: 9780781759779
Recommended for: Hospital, Academic Libraries

Ophthalmology residents, fellows, and medical students are the primary audience for this set of six DVDs, which serve as a valuable instructional tool to help prepare trainees in ocular surgery. This resource is also of interest to ophthalmologists and operating room nursing staff. The set covers over 100 surgical procedures with high-quality video filmed in the Wills Eye Hospital operating rooms. Voice-over comments on techniques and complications have been added to the step-by-step instructions. Each DVD covers a surgical subspecialty: "Cataract and Refractive Surgery," "Cornea," "Glaucoma," "Oculoplastics," "Pediatric Ophthalmology," and "Retina." Also included is a companion 40-page color manual which covers the DVDs' surgical steps with pearls and pitfalls in a tabular outline format. The *Video Atlas* is essential for ophthalmic residency programs, and is highly recommended for any hospital where eye surgeries are performed, as well as medical schools.

11.6. Orthopedics

Medical, surgical, and physical methods to treat and correct deformities, diseases, and injuries to the skeletal system, its articulations, and associated structures.

—MeSH

Contributors: Tim Mason, Elisabeth Rowan

Monographs

Campbell's Operative Orthopaedics. 11th ed. Editors: Terry Canale, James H. Beaty. Mosby/Elsevier, 2008.
http://www.mdconsult.com/
ISBN: 9780323033299
Recommended for: Hospital, Academic Libraries
Brandon/Hill, *Doody's Core Titles* Selection

This four-volume comprehensive textbook is the bible of orthopedic surgery. Its audience is orthopedic surgeons, surgeons, residents, and allied health personnel. This edition incorporates the use of color highlighting of techniques and procedures and bulleted summaries for quick reading. It is profusely illustrated with photographs and line drawings that emphasize structures and techniques. A DVD-ROM has been added which demonstrates complex surgeries such as elbow arthroscopy, mini-incision total knee arthroscopy, shoulder arthroscopy, and other minimally invasive techniques. Available to individual purchasers of this edition is access to the fully searchable online edition which provides updates to the text, access to an image library, and links to the references. This title is a recommended *Doody's Core Titles* essential purchase and a Brandon/Hill selection. It is recommended for all hospital and academic medical libraries.

Drennan's The Child's Foot and Ankle. 2nd ed. Editors: James J. McCarthy, James C. Drennan. Lippincott, Williams & Wilkins, 2010.
See Chapter 19. Podiatry

Essentials of Musculoskeletal Care. 4th ed. Editor: John F. Sarwark. American Academy of Orthopedic Surgeons, 2010.
ISBN: 9780892035793
Recommended for: Hospital, Academic Libraries
Brandon/Hill Selection

This textbook is intended to be a musculoskeletal reference for primary care physicians, but it is also useful for internists, pediatricians, physical therapists, allied healthcare personnel, medical students, and residents. It covers over 300 orthopedic conditions. Each chapter addresses a specific part of the body, and covers clinical symptoms, physical examination, diagnostic tests, differential diagnosis, therapy, adverse effects, and referral. This edition expands coverage to include rehabilitation exercise instructions and printable forms. The included DVD-ROM has more narrated videos and includes current injection techniques and physical exam instructions. Also included with this edition for individual purchasers is searchable full-text online. This title appeared on the final Brandon/Hill list and is recommended for all hospital and academic medical libraries.

Levin and O'Neal's The Diabetic Foot. 7th ed. Editors: John H. Bowker, Michael A. Pfeifer. Mosby/Elsevier, 2008.
See Chapter 19. Podiatry

Lippincott's Primary Care Orthopaedics. Editors: Paul A. Lotke, Joseph A. Abboud, Jack Ende. Lippincott Williams & Wilkins, 2008.
http://www.ovid.com/
ISBN: 9780781771825
Recommended for: Hospital, Academic Libraries
Doody's Core Titles Selection

This book is one of the more affordable orthopedic books, priced under $100. It is intended for the primary care physician, physician assistants, nurse practitioners, residents, and osteopathic and chiropractic physicians. Profusely illustrated with color, this text has detailed articles on diagnosing and treating musculoskeletal disorders, but can easily be used to as a quick reference. Each chapter covers an orthopedic problem, detailing the clinical presentation, physical findings, studies, treatment, clinical course, referrals, and ICD-9 codes. For quick reference each chapter contains an outline of clinical points, patient assessment, "not to be missed," and treatment. Individual purchasers also have access to a website that offers full-text search, an image bank, patient information handouts, and videos of orthopedic procedures. This title is a recommended *Doody's Core Titles* essential purchase. It is recommended for all hospital and academic medical libraries.

Orthopaedic Examination, Evaluation, and Intervention. 2nd ed. Author: Mark Dutton. McGraw-Hill, 2008.
http://online.statref.com/
http://extranet.netlibrary.com/TitleSelect/
http://www.myilibrary.com/
http://www.accessphysiotherapy.com/home.aspx
ISBN: 9780071499538
ISBN: 9780071474016 (set)
ISBN: 9780071499545 (DVD)
Recommended for: Hospital, Academic Libraries
Doody's Core Titles Selection

Written by a physical therapist, this title is a one-stop guide and reference for all orthopedic health professionals and students. It provides step-by-step methods using evidence-based practice for the examination, evaluation, and rehabilitation of orthopedic injuries. The text is divided into five sections: fundamentals of orthopedics, upper and lower extremities, the vertebral column, post-surgical rehabilitation, and pharmacology and medical imaging. The addition of a DVD provides over 500 video clips of techniques and therapeutic exercises. It also features case studies with questions and answers and guidelines from the American Physical Therapy Association (APTA). The book is extensively illustrated with over 1,500 photos and images. This title is a recommended *Doody's Core Titles* essential purchase and is recommended for all hospital and academic medical libraries.

Orthopedic Physical Assessment. 5th ed. Authors: David J. Magee. Saunders/Elsevier, 2008.
See Chapter 1.3. Physical Therapy

Rockwood and Green's Fractures in Adults. 7th ed. Editors: Robert W. Bucholz, Charles Court-Brown, James D. Heckman. Lippincott Williams & Wilkins, 2010.
http://www.ovid.com/
http://www.r2library.com/
ISBN: 9781605476773
Recommended for: Hospital, Academic Libraries
Brandon/Hill, *Doody's Core Titles* Selection

Considered the gold standard for orthopedic trauma and surgery, this two-volume set provides complete coverage of bone and joint injuries, presenting both preferred and alternative treatments. The audience for this comprehensive reference on fractures is orthopedic surgeons and residents. New topics covered in this edition are complex regional pain syndrome, psychological aspects of trauma, gunshot and wartime injuries, limb salvage reconstruction, amputations, post-traumatic infections, principles of nonunions, and principles of malunions. An integrated website is available to individual purchasers and includes a fully searchable text, image bank, and 25 videos of surgical procedures. This text is also sold as a set with *Rockwood and Wilkin's Fractures in Children*. This title is a required resource for any hospital providing orthopedic services, as well as academic institutions involved in the education of physicians. This is a *Doody's Core Titles* essential purchase and a Brandon/Hill selection. It is recommended for all hospital and academic medical libraries.

Rockwood and Wilkin's Fractures in Children. 7th ed. Editors: James H. Beaty, James R. Kasser, David L. Skaggs. Lippincott Williams & Wilkins, 2009.
http://www.ovid.com/
http://www.r2library.com/
ISBN: 9781582557847
Recommended for: Hospital, Academic Libraries
Doody's Core Titles Selection

Considered the gold standard of orthopedic trauma and surgery, this volume provides complete coverage of bone and joint injuries in children, presenting both preferred and alternative treatments. New topics covered in this volume are casting, remodeling, and what is unique about children's fractures; principles of physical examination of children with fractures; and treacherous children's fractures. The audience for this comprehensive reference is orthopedic surgeons, pediatricians, and residents. An integrated website, which is available to individual purchasers, includes fully searchable text, an image bank, and 25 videos of surgical procedures. It is also sold as a set with *Rockwood and Green's Fractures in Adults*. This title is recommended *Doody's Core Titles* essential purchase. It is recommended for all hospital and academic medical libraries.

Surgical Reconstruction of the Diabetic Foot and Ankle. Editor: Thomas Zgonis. Lippincott Williams & Wilkins, 2009.
See Chapter 19. Podiatry

Tachdjian's Pediatric Orthopaedics; from the Texas Scottish Rite Hospital for Children. 4th ed. Editor: John A. Herring. Saunders Elsevier, 2008.
ISBN: 9781416022213 (set)
Recommended for: Hospital, Academic Libraries
Brandon/Hill, *Doody's Core Titles* Selection

This three-volume textbook is an encyclopedic reference on pediatric orthopedics, now in its fourth edition. It is written for practicing pediatric orthopedists and residents learning the subspecialty. It is divided into six sections: disciplines, anatomic disorders, neuromuscular disorders, orthopedic disorders, musculoskeletal tumors, and musculoskeletal injuries. It is further divided into chapters discussing individual disorders, covering pertinent aspects such as etiology, diagnosis, imaging, nonoperative and surgical treatment, and complications. Two DVDs with 22 videos are included and a website featuring fully searchable text and images is available for individual purchasers. This title is a recommended *Doody's Core Titles* essential purchase and a Brandon/Hill selection. It is recommended for all hospital and academic medical libraries.

Journals

Clinical Orthopaedics and Related Research. Issue no. 26 [v. numbering began in 2008], Springer, 1963.
http://www.springerlink.com/content/120901/
http://www.ncbi.nlm.nih.gov/pmc/journals/592/
http://www.ovid.com/
ISSN: 0009921X
ISSN: 15281132 (Online)
Indexed in: MEDLINE, CINAHL
Recommended for: Hospital, Academic Libraries
Brandon/Hill Selection

Originally published as *Clinical Orthopaedics* beginning in 1953, this journal, commonly called *CORR*, is a monthly, peer-reviewed journal of the Association of Bone and Joint Surgeons. It is aimed toward general orthopedists, specialists, and residents. It includes original clinical and research articles. A monthly feature highlights a single topic. There is also a section reprinting historically significant articles. A useful teaching tool, the Orthopaedic-Radiology-Pathology Conference, addresses an "unknown" case report as it would present in a clinical setting. *CORR* also provides an overview of six to ten important, recently published articles in a given specialty; a section providing an annotated operative note; and a previously published manuscript related to a current article, comparing and contrasting older ideas with present practice. It is available online through SpringerLink from 2008 to the present. PubMed Central provides free online access after a twelve month delay, starting with 2008, and Ovid offers an online archive covering 1963–2007.

Foot and Ankle Clinics. v. 1, Elsevier, 1996.
See Chapter 19. Podiatry

Foot and Ankle International. v. 15, Data Trace, 1994.
See Chapter 19. Podiatry

Journal of Bone and Joint Surgery, American Volume. v. 30A, Journal of Bone and Joint Surgery, 1948.
http://www.ejbjs.org
ISSN: 00219355
ISSN: 15351386 (Online)
Indexed in: MEDLINE, CINAHL
Recommended for: Hospital, Academic Libraries
Brandon/Hill Selection

This essential, widely read journal has consistently demonstrated the highest impact factor of all general orthopedic journals. It was a Brandon/Hill medical selection, and it is also listed in the *Core Collection of Medical Books and Journals* (the Hague List). First published in 1887 as the *Transactions of the American Orthopedic Association*, it later became the *Journal of Bone and Joint Surgery*, splitting into two serials, the American and the British volumes, in 1948. The journal includes two "Surgical Techniques" supplements each year, along with occasional, additional supplements. In July 2010, the publisher moved the journal to a semimonthly publication schedule. It is the official publication of 12 orthopedic associations, including the American Academy of Orthopaedic Surgeons and the American Orthopaedic Association. This comprehensive journal is peer-reviewed and contains articles on adult reconstructive surgery, including hip and knee replacement; pediatric orthopedic conditions; and basic science as it relates to clinical practice. It is a required resource for hospitals providing orthopedic surgical care and for academic institutions training new surgeons. It is available online at the journal's website back to 1889.

Journal of Bone and Joint Surgery, British Volume. v. 30B, British Editorial Society of Bone and Joint Surgery, 1948.
http://www.jbjs.org.uk
ISSN: 0301620X (Print/Online)
Indexed in: MEDLINE, CINAHL
Recommended for: Hospital, Academic Libraries
Brandon/Hill Selection

Like its American cousin, the British volume of the *Journal of Bone and Joint Surgery* is a widely read, peer-reviewed publication. It is the official journal of 14 orthopedic associations and affiliates. Its scope deals with the latest developments in treatment, surgical techniques, and appliances within the field of orthopedic surgery. The journal is geared towards practicing surgeons and residents. The London-based British Editorial Society of Bone and Joint Surgery publishes this monthly journal, which also includes several orthopedic proceedings supplements per year. It was a Brandon/Hill medical selection and appeared on the *Core Collection of Medical Books and Journals* (Hague List). Online coverage back to 1948 is available at the journal's website.

Journal of Pediatric Orthopaedics. v. 1, Lippincott Williams & Wilkins, 1981.
http://www.ovid.com/
ISSN: 02716798
ISSN: 15392570 (Online)
Indexed in: MEDLINE
Recommended for: Hospital, Academic Libraries

Serving as the official journal of the Pediatric Orthopaedic Society of North America and the European Paediatric Orthopaedic Society, this publication is an excellent addition to the library supporting the practice of pediatric orthopedics. It provides comprehensive coverage of all aspects of traumatic musculoskeletal injuries in children, from laboratory findings and drug therapies to surgical treatment. Ovid provides electronic access, with full-text coverage from 1996 to the present.

Journal of Pediatric Orthopaedics Part B. v. 1, Lippincott Williams & Wilkins, 1992.
http://www.ovid.com/
ISSN: 1060152X
ISSN: 14735865 (Online)
Indexed in: MEDLINE
Recommended for: Hospital, Academic Libraries

Like its counterpart, the *Journal of Pediatric Orthopaedics*, this is an official journal for the Pediatric Orthopaedic Society of North America. While *JPO* focuses on pediatric orthopedic injuries, *JPO B* highlights recent developments in clinical practice and research. It publishes peer-reviewed articles on the diagnosis and treatment of pediatric orthopedic disorders. It is available online via Ovid, with full-text coverage back to 2001.

Orthopedic Clinics of North America. v. 1, Saunders/Elsevier, 1970.
http://orthopedic.theclinics.com
http://www.sciencedirect.com/science/journal/00305898
http://www.mdconsult.com/
ISSN: 00305898 (Print/Online)
Indexed in: MEDLINE, CINAHL
Recommended for: Hospital, Academic Libraries
Brandon/Hill Selection

Part of the popular *Clinics of North America* series, this journal, which has been published since 1970, contains themed, hardcover issues on subjects related to orthopedic surgery. Review articles provide current, practical information related to the diagnosis and treatment of musculoskeletal conditions. Each quarterly issue is indexed for easy access by subject. The journal is indexed in numerous sources such as MEDLINE, CINAHL, and Excerpta Medica.

Spine. v. 1, Lippincott Williams & Wilkins, 1976.
http://www.ovid.com/
ISSN: 03622436
ISSN: 15281159 (Online)
See Also Chapter 3. Chiropractic
Indexed in: MEDLINE, CINAHL
Recommended for: Hospital, Academic Libraries

Spine is the premier journal in its subspecialty of spinal disorders. This peer-reviewed, biweekly journal is aimed towards specialists treating spinal disorders. The journal accepts only original papers with the understanding that articles are contributed only to *Spine*. It does not publish articles reporting data published elsewhere. Content focuses on "new developments in the field, discussions of innovative treatments and in-depth analyses of case studies." With an impact factor of 2.624, it ranks seventh out of 56 journals in the orthopedics category in the 2009 *Journal Citation Reports*. The journal is indexed in MEDLINE, CINAHL, and Scopus.

11.7. Otolaryngology

The study and treatment of disorders of the ear, nose, and throat.

—MeSH

Contributor: Mori Lou Higa

Monographs

ABC of Ear, Nose and Throat. 5th ed. Editors: Harold Ludman, Patrick J. Bradley. Blackwell, 2007.
http://extranet.netlibrary.com/TitleSelect/
http://www.ebrary.com/
ISBN: 9781405136563
ISBN: 9781444312669
Recommended for: Hospital, Academic Libraries

This popular work is part of the *ABC Series*, which supplies up-to-date, subject-oriented guides for primary care physicians, trainees, and students. The *Ear, Nose and Throat* guide provides an essential introduction to the specialty of otolaryngology head and neck surgery and serves as a practical reference tool. Authored and edited by specialists in Great Britain, this fifth edition supplies advice on the best management techniques for patients experiencing the most common ear, nose, and throat problems. This edition has been thoroughly revised and updated and includes new chapters on facial pain, head and neck tumors, sleep apnea, and epistaxis. The book includes clinical photographs, illustrations, imaging scans, and algorithms to help identify when referrals to a specialist may be necessary. While the work is geared toward students and physician trainees, this guide would be useful to any health professional needing a practical introduction to the fundamentals of otolaryngology.

Allergy in ENT Practice. 2nd ed. Authors: Hueston C. King, Richard L. Mabry, Cynthia S. Mabry, Bruce R. Gordon, Bradley F. Marple. Thieme Medical, 2005.
ISBN: 9781588902764
Recommended for: Hospital, Academic Libraries

Over the past two decades, there has been an increased emphasis on the management of allergic aspects of otolaryngic disorders, but only recently have steps been taken to address the growing demand for improved allergy education by both practicing otolaryngologists and those involved with otolaryngology training programs. The first edition of *Allergy in ENT Practice*, 1998, effectively addressed this subspecialty area. Building upon the first edition, the authors provide an updated core textbook for those who diagnose and treat ear, nose, and throat allergies. This comprehensive yet practical guide presents otolaryngic allergy as a core component of otolaryngology. The authors combine the scientific principles upon which otolaryngic allergy is based with practical, clinical guidance that can be applied directly to the delivery of allergy care. Thoroughly revised and updated chapters include testing methods, pharmacotherapy, specific types of allergies such as those involving food and plants, allergic emergencies, and appendixes covering pollens and allergenic foods. Some of the special features include "Brief Capsules," written by an experienced otolaryngic nurse, and recommendations for incorporating allergy care into an existing ENT practice. It is recommended for institutions that support otolaryngologists and otolaryngology education, pediatricians, primary care specialists, nurses, and others involved in allergy care.

An Atlas of Head & Neck Surgery. 4th ed. Authors: John M. Loré, Jesus E. Medina. Elsevier Saunders, 2005.
ISBN: 9780721673196
Recommended for: Hospital, Academic Libraries
Doody's Core Titles Selection

While there are a number of excellent quality surgical atlases from which to choose (most notably, Myers, E.N. *Operative Otolaryngology: Head and Neck Surgery*. Elsevier Saunders, 2009 and Bailey, B.J. *Atlas of Head and Neck Surgery—Otolaryngology*. Lippincott Williams & Wilkins, 2001), Loré and Medina's *Atlas* is considered to be an outstanding selection. This fourth edition was supplied the highest possible rating by *Doody's Core Titles*, based on "authoritativeness of author and publisher; scope and coverage of the subject matter; quality of content (including timeliness); usefulness and purpose; and value for money." Thoroughly covering surgical procedures of the head and neck region, this classic atlas has been revised and expanded to address the most recent techniques and developments affecting surgeons who perform head and neck surgery. Contents include radiographic anatomy and scanning, basic considerations, emergency procedures, and chapters addressing every anatomic region of the head and neck. This edition includes over 1,400 detailed illustrations and has added new chapters on microvascular surgery, endoscopic sinus surgery, skull base surgery, and selective neck dissection. Institutions supporting trainees in the ENT field and surgeons will find the work to be of considerable value.

Ballenger's Otorhinolaryngology Head and Neck Surgery. 17th ed. Editors: James B. Snow Jr., Phillip Ashley Wackym. PMPH-USA People's Medical Publishing House, 2009.
ISBN: 9781550093377
Recommended for: Hospital, Academic Libraries

First published in 1908 by William L. Ballenger under the title *Diseases of the Nose, Throat and Ear, Medical and Surgical*, this long-standing publication has served and continues to serve as a premier, comprehensive reference for all aspects of the discipline of otorhinolaryngology head and neck surgery. This centennial edition is organized into six subspecialty sections: "Otology and Neurotology," "Rhinology," "Facial Plastic and Reconstructive Surgery," "Pediatric Otorhinolaryngology," "Laryngology and Bronchoesophagology," and "Head and Neck Surgery." Written primarily by U.S. specialists, the seventeenth edition has increased from 67 to 101 individual chapters and includes numerous clinical photographs and color illustrations. Chapters include both the underlying basic science of clinical otolaryngology and comprehensive coverage of clinical topics for practitioners. New chapters in this edition include outcomes and clinical research, stereotactic radiosurgery, robotic surgery, biofilms, and chemoradiation. Although the work is intended to serve as a complete resource for students, residents, fellows, and clinicians, those seeking greater depth of coverage of specialty areas may want to consult other subspecialty resources in addition to *Ballenger's*.

Clinical Otology. 3rd ed. Editors: Gordon B. Hughes, Myles L. Pensak. Thieme, 2007.
ISBN: 9781588903648
Recommended for: Hospital, Academic Libraries
Doody's Core Titles Selection

Addressing the subspecialty of otology, *Clinical Otology* focuses on the fundamental principles of basic science, evaluation, management, and rehabilitation of those with common otologic disorders. The work is intended to provide a foundation for successful clinical practice, and, through its lengthy chapter bibliographies, offer opportunities for more extensive investigation into specific topics. Authored by 36 surgeons and scientists based in the United States, the work contains 33 revised and updated chapters that present state-of-the-art information in the field of otology and related sciences. New chapters include those addressing molecular biology, molecular disorders, and pharmacology of otologic drugs. This comprehensive overview of otologic disease is well organized and heavily illustrated. The illustrations, in fact, are one of the work's strengths with more than 400 diagrams, radiographic images, and full-color photographs. A separate, dedicated surgical atlas, however, would still be recommended for support of surgical procedures. The book is highly recommended for libraries supporting otolaryngologists in training and students. It also serves as a solid reference tool for practicing otologists, otolaryngologists, audiologists, neurologists, and neurosurgeons. In 2008, the British Medical Association awarded this book one of its "highly commended" prizes in their annual medical book competition, which is intended to "reward excellence in medical publishing."

Cummings Otolaryngology Head & Neck Surgery. 5th ed. Editors: Paul W. Flint, Bruce H. Haughey, Valerie J. Lund, John K. Niparko, Mark A. Richardson, K. Thomas Robbins, J. Regan Thomas. Elsevier Mosby, 2010.
http://www.mdconsult.com/
ISBN: 9780323052832
Recommended for: Hospital, Academic Libraries

This extensive, four-volume set is considered to be "the" authoritative, comprehensive compendium of information addressing all areas of otolaryngology-head and neck surgery. Not intended as a surgical atlas or an introductory text, the preface states that the authors' intention was to produce an indispensable reference work that is designed for both residents and experienced practitioners. Multiple editors have consolidated contributions from more than 350 international experts. *Cummings* addresses both core knowledge within the discipline, along with new discoveries and developments within all subspecialties. The first volume includes general considerations of the head, followed by a section on the face. The next volume provides information on the nose, paranasal sinuses, salivary glands, oral cavity/pharynx/esophagus, and larynx/trachea/bronchus. The third volume includes sections on the neck, thyroid/parathyroid, vestibular system, facial nerve, infectious processes, and vestibular system. The final volume focuses on the auditory system, cochlear implants, and pediatric otolaryngology. With more than 4,500 pages, 3,200 illustrations, lengthy chapter reference lists, and clinical algorithms and staging tables to assist with patient management, both academic and hospital libraries would be well served by adding this massive reference source, although expensive, to their collections. Online access through MD Consult has been enhanced recently with the new mobile version that supports various smartphone devices. This review refers to the fourth edition. In all likelihood, the fifth edition will continue to serve as a top-tier resource.

Current Diagnosis & Treatment in Otolaryngology: Head and Neck Surgery. 2nd ed. Editor: Anil Lalwani. McGraw-Hill, 2007.
http://www.accessmedicine.com/
http://extranet.netlibrary.com/TitleSelect/
http://www.ebrary.com/
ISBN: 9780071460279
ISBN: 9780071593342
Recommended for: Hospital, Academic Libraries
Doody's Core Titles Selection

Designed to be both comprehensive and convenient, the work's stated purpose is to emphasize "the practical features of clinical diagnosis and patient management while providing a comprehensive discussion of pathophysiology and relevant basic and clinical science." *Current Diagnosis* is organized by organ and anatomic region, and its consistent chapter formatting helps simplify retrieval of practical information relating to the essentials of diagnosis, testing, disease processes, and current medical and surgical management strategies. Its concisely presented content is contributed primarily by more than 80 U.S. experts, and the text is supplemented with over 500 helpful clinical photographs and line drawings. The second edition provides new and expanded coverage in several areas, including complementary and alternative medicine in otolaryngology, the latest medical and surgical treatment options, new chapters on facial plastic surgery, and additional coverage on the use of lasers in ENT/head and neck surgery. *Doody's Review Service* rated this work as an essential, core title. This book would be useful for both hospital and academic institutions that provide services to otolaryngologists, other specialists who interact with this discipline, medical students, residents, nurses, physician assistants, audiologists, speech pathologists, and other health care professionals. This work also serves as a useful review guide for those preparing for professional board examinations.

Ear, Nose, and Throat Disorders Sourcebook. 2nd ed. Editor: Sandra J. Judd. Omnigraphics, 2007.
ISBN: 9780780808720
Recommended for: Consumer Health Libraries

From the popular Omnigraphics' *Health Reference Series*, this resource is a comprehensive source for current consumer health information addressing the most common disorders of the ear, nose, and throat. The book is organized into seven sections: disorders of the ears; hearing disorders; vestibular disorders; disorders of the nose and sinuses; disorders of the throat and vocal cords; cancers of the ears, nose, and throat; and additional help and information. Each section contains lists of professional journals and other publications for additional information. Information for this *Sourcebook* is compiled from various U.S. government agencies, such as the National Cancer Institute, the National Institute of Allergy and Infectious Diseases, the National Institutes of Health, and the National Library of Medicine. A large portion of the material uses a question-and-answer format, similar to questions patients might pose to physicians. The 659-page *Sourcebook* is intended as an informational resource—not a tool to diagnosis or prescribe treatment-for the general reader who is seeking information that avoids technical medical jargon. This work is one of numerous works in the *Health Reference Series* and serves as a solid, reliable otolaryngology resource for consumer health libraries and other library collections that support patient populations.

Essentials of Otolaryngology. 5th ed. Editors: Frank E. Lucente, Gady Har-El. Lippincott Williams & Wilkins, 2004.
http://www.ovid.com/
ISBN: 9780781747073
Recommended for: Hospital, Academic Libraries
Brandon/Hill Selection

Essentials of Otolaryngology provides fundamental information relating to the diagnosis and treatment of head and neck disorders. Primarily geared toward medical students and nonspecialists, this practical "pocket" guide is intended as a quick reference tool, helping readers to quickly gain knowledge of the anatomy and physiology of the head and neck region, to understand pathologic problems, to conduct patient workups, to learn techniques for treatment, and to understand how otolaryngology interacts with other specialties supporting the head and neck region. Following preliminary chapters on anatomy, physiology, history taking, and physical examination, the majority of the remaining chapters are organized by symptoms occurring in the head and neck region such as headache, earache, swallowing difficulties, and facial pain. The authors provide current treatment recommendations and guidance on indications for referral to specialists. This edition was expanded to include additional topics such as pain management and the use of lasers in otolaryngology. Numerous tables and figures supplement the text. *Essentials* is not a substitute for a comprehensive textbook on otolaryngology head and neck surgery; instead, it is intended to provide a concise, contemporary overview of appropriate diagnostic approaches and management of common head and neck region complaints. It is a well-established, useful resource that can help quickly familiarize readers with the specialty of otolaryngology.

Pediatric Otolaryngology. 4th ed. Editors: Charles D. Bluestone, Sylvan E. Stool, Cuneyt M. Alper, Ellis M. Arjmand, Margaretha L. Casselbrant, Joseph E. Dohar, Robert F. Yellon. Saunders, 2003.
ISBN: 9780721691978
Recommended for: Hospital, Academic Libraries
Doody's Core Titles Selection

Focusing on the subspecialty of pediatric otolaryngology, this massive, two-volume set serves as a comprehensive textbook for both specialists and physician trainees handling ear, nose, and throat problems of pediatric patients. This work began under the leadership of the pioneering pediatric otolaryngologist Dr. Bluestone, who is viewed by many as the father of modern day pediatric otolaryngology. With more than 1,800 pages and over 100 chapters, this encyclopedic work addresses the diagnosis and management of otologic disorders in children. The work is well organized into seven sections and includes black-and-white illustrations, figures, tables, extensive chapter reference lists, and a lengthy index. Multiple specialists have contributed to the various sections, which include: craniofacial growth, development and malformations; ear and related structures; nose, paranasal sinuses, face, and orbit; mouth, pharynx, and esophagus; larynx, trachea, bronci, lungs, and esophagus; neck; and communication disorders. Although this work is now somewhat dated, *Pediatric Otolaryngology* has been long recognized as one of the best in the field, with multiple reviewers referring to each succeeding edition as outstanding, a classic work, a prized tome, and "the" standard. A new edition is expected in June 2011.

Journals

American Journal of Rhinology & Allergy. v. 23, Ocean-Side, 2009.
http://oceansidepubl.com/ajr/index.htm
http://www.ingentaconnect.com/content/ocean/ajra
ISSN: 19458924
ISSN: 19458932 (Online)
Indexed in: MEDLINE
Recommended for: Hospital, Academic Libraries

First published as the *American Journal of Rhinology*, this peer-reviewed publication serves as the official journal of the American Rhinologic Society (ARS). This journal provides a unified forum that brings together multidisciplinary specialists whose focus is on the best clinical and basic research within the fields of rhinology and allergy. Founded in 1987, this journal combines the perspectives of otolaryngologists, allergy specialists, and research scientists in the treatment of nasal disease. Categories of coverage include diagnosis and treatment; surgical and procedural interventions; mechanisms of rhinosinusitis, allergy, and other rhinologic diseases; and nasal physiology. Published manuscripts from worldwide contributors include original research articles, clinical trials, and review articles. The 2009 edition of *Journal Citation Reports* indicates that the *American Journal of Rhinology & Allergy* has the third highest journal ranking in the field of otorhinolaryngology. Along with the International Rhinologic Society's journal *Rhinology*, this is one of only two highly ranked journals that focus specifically on the subspecialty of rhinology. This bimonthly publication is indexed in MEDLINE, Science Citation Index Expanded, and Scopus. *American Journal of Rhinology & Allergy* is recommended for library collections supporting otolaryngologic patient care and research. Readers will include otolaryngologists, allergists, and plastic surgeons. It should be noted that the ARS has joined with the American Academy of Otolaryngic Allergy to publish a new official society journal. *International Forum of Allergy & Rhinology* (v. 1, no. 1, Feb. 2011) is published by Wiley Blackwell.

Annals of Otology, Rhinology & Laryngology. v. 6, Annals Publishing Company, 1897.
http://www.annals.com/
http://www.ebscohost.com/
ISSN: 00034894
Indexed in: MEDLINE, CINAHL
Recommended for: Hospital, Academic Libraries

Ranked within the top 20 otorhinolaryngology journals by impact factor, this popular, peer-reviewed journal is one of the discipline's major, core publications. Addressing both general and specialty areas in the field, *Annals* provides original research in both the clinical and research arenas, covering general otolaryngology, otology, neurotology, bronchoesophagology, laryngology, rhinology, head and neck oncology and surgery, plastic and reconstructive surgery, pediatric otolaryngology, audiology, and speech pathology. International in scope, journal content includes original articles; in-depth studies, which are issued as supplements; historical papers; book and computer software reviews; imaging case studies; and pathology consultations. This official journal of the American Broncho-Esophagological Association was originally published as the *Annals of Ophthalmology and Otology* beginning in 1892. This long-standing, monthly publication is indexed in numerous sources such as CINAHL, Embase, MEDLINE, and Scopus.

Archives of Otolaryngology-Head & Neck Surgery. v. 112, American Medical Association, 1986.
http://archotol.ama-assn.org/
http://www.backfiles.org/pricing-and-ordering.html
ISSN: 08864470
ISSN: 1538361X (Online)
Indexed in: MEDLINE, CINAHL
Recommended for: Hospital, Academic Libraries
Brandon/Hill Selection

First published in 1925 as *Archives of Otolaryngology*, this monthly journal serves as the official publication for the American Head and Neck Society (AHNS), the American Society of Pediatric Otolaryngology, and the American Academy of Facial and Plastic and Reconstructive Surgery, Inc. It provides peer-reviewed, clinical and basic research focusing on diseases of the head and neck. Categories of articles include original research related to reports of clinical data, basic science data, and reviews (including meta-analyses); clinical notes and case reports; clinical problem solving; and clinical challenges relating to controversial issues in the field of otolaryngology. The journal also publishes many papers from the annual meeting of the AHNS and offers CME credits to individual subscribers and AMA members. This highly-ranked otolaryngology journal, which is based on both *Journal Citation Reports*' impact rankings and analysis by specialists within the field (Roy, D "Citation Analysis of Otorhinolaryngology Journals" *J Laryngol Otol*, 2002; 116:363–366), continues to serve as a core journal for both hospital and academic libraries supporting this discipline. It is indexed in numerous sources, including MEDLINE, Embase, and Scopus. Of special note for those interested in online backfiles, the AMA has recently begun offering a one-time backfile purchase option (with annual maintenance fee) for its complete Archives collection.

Head & Neck: Journal for the Sciences & Specialties of the Head and Neck. v. 11, Wiley Periodicals, 1989.
http://onlinelibrary.wiley.com/journal/10.1002/(ISSN)1097-0347/
ISSN: 10433074
ISSN: 10970347 (Online)
Indexed in: MEDLINE
Recommended for: Hospital, Academic Libraries

International and multi-disciplinary in scope, this peer-reviewed journal addresses both clinical and research topics addressing the diagnosis, management, and prevention of diseases of the head and neck. According to the publisher's stated scope, "this area involves the overlapping interests and expertise of several surgical and medical specialties, including general surgery, neurosurgery, otolaryngology, plastic surgery, oral surgery, dermatology, ophthalmology, pathology, radiotherapy, medical oncology, and the corresponding basic sciences." In addition to original articles, this monthly journal includes technical notes, new technology descriptions, unusual case reports, brief communications, editorials, and book reviews. Published by Wiley on behalf of the International Federation of Head and Neck Oncologic Societies, this is an essential journal for all hospital and academic institutions supporting otorhinolaryngology programs. Readers will include otolaryngologists, radiotherapists, medical oncologists, plastic surgeons, dentists, oral surgeons, and pathologists. According to the 2009 *Journal Citation Reports*, *Head & Neck* has the second highest journal impact factor in the field of otorhinolaryngology for the most current year's ranking and five-year cumulative impact ranking. Beginning with its preceding title, *Head & Neck Surgery*, this journal has been published since 1978. *Head & Neck* is indexed in numerous sources including MEDLINE, Scopus, and Embase. Through the Wiley Online Library platform, online subscribers have the option to access "full-text, peer-reviewed, copyedited articles" immediately in advance of the compiled print publication.

Journal of the Association for Research in Otolaryngology: JARO. v. 1, Springer, 2000.
http://www.springerlink.com/
http://www.ncbi.nlm.nih.gov/pmc/
ISSN: 15253961
ISSN: 14387573 (Online)
Indexed in: MEDLINE
Recommended for: Academic Libraries

This peer-reviewed, quarterly publication is the official journal of the Association for Research in Otolaryngology (ARO). With an international group of contributors,

JARO has a very specific research focus offering "original experimental and theoretical studies of evolution, development, structure, function, etiology, and intervention related to the organs of hearing, balance, and the chemical senses." Its goal is to provide a forum for a wide range of disciplines that contribute to ARO. Specifically excluded from publication are clinical case studies and pharmaceutical screens unless the underlying mechanisms are included. Papers that primarily describe research methods are also excluded unless new findings of substantial significance are included. *JARO* contains mostly original research articles, with an occasional review paper on a particular topic of interest. According to the 2009 *Journal Citation Reports*, *JARO* has the highest journal impact factor in the field of otorhinolaryngology for the most current year's ranking and the third highest five-year cumulative impact ranking. It is indexed in numerous sources such as Biological Abstracts, BIOSIS Previews, Embase, MEDLINE, Science Citation Index, and Scopus. *JARO* provides one-year embargoed access to its full content on PubMed Central beginning with volume 5, 2004, in addition to Springer online access. This journal would be required for any academic or specialized collection supporting research activities related to otolaryngology and the communications sciences.

The Laryngoscope. v. 1, American Laryngological, Rhinological, and Otological Society, 1896.
http://onlinelibrary.wiley.com/journal/10.1002/(ISSN)1531-4995/issues
ISSN: 0023852X
ISSN: 15314995 (Online)
Indexed in: MEDLINE, CINAHL
Recommended for: Hospital, Academic Libraries

Now published by Wiley on behalf of the Triological Society—which is also known as the American Laryngological, Rhinological, and Otological Society—this peer-reviewed, official Society publication has offered the most important advances relating to the diagnosis and treatment of head and neck disorders for more than 100 years. Articles focus on medical, clinical, and basic research relating to the various specialty areas within the discipline of otolaryngology: bronchoesophagology, communicative disorders, head and neck surgery, facial plastic and reconstructive surgery, oncology, and speech and hearing defects. Consistently among the highest ranked otolaryngology journals by *Journal Citation Reports*, this monthly publication offers original contributions, contemporary review articles, a "Triological Society Best Practices" section, papers presented at the annual and section meetings of the Triological Society, "How I Do It" articles offering step-by-step guidance on the "the latest tested-and-proven surgical techniques," and book reviews. It is geared toward otolaryngologists and other clinicians and researchers who have an interest in this specialty. With the new Wiley publishing partnership that began in 2009, the journal is distributed to all U.S. otolaryngology residents at no charge. *The Laryngoscope* is indexed in numerous sources including MEDLINE, CINAHL, and Scopus. Through the Wiley Online Library platform, online subscribers have the option to access "full-text, peer-reviewed, copyedited articles" immediately in advance of the compiled print publication.

Otolaryngology—Head and Neck Surgery. v. 89, American Academy of Otolaryngology—Head and Neck Surgery Foundation, 1981.
http://www.sciencedirect.com/
ISSN: 01945998
ISSN: 10858679
ISSN: 10976817
Indexed in: MEDLINE, CINAHL
Recommended for: Hospital, Academic Libraries
Brandon/Hill Selection

Published since 1896, this peer-reviewed journal serves as the official publication of the American Academy of Otolaryngology—Head and Neck Surgery Foundation (AAO-HNS). It offers clinically relevant information covering all aspects of otolaryngology—head and neck surgery (ear, nose, throat, head, and neck disorders) and reflects an international range of authorship. Journal content includes literature reviews; clinical practice guidelines; case reports; clinical techniques and technology; abstracts from the annual AAO-HNS meeting; and original research addressing general otolaryngology and the many specialty areas such as allergy, facial plastic and reconstructive surgery, otology, and pediatric otolaryngology. Published by Elsevier/Mosby on behalf of the AAO-HNS, this monthly journal is considered to be one of the essential, major otolaryngology journals. *Otolaryngology—Head and Neck Surgery* is intended for otolaryngologists, clinicians, researchers, and other specialists. It is indexed in a multitude of sources such as MEDLINE, Embase, and Scopus.

Otology & Neurotology. v. 22, Lippincott Williams & Wilkins, 2001.
http://journals.lww.com/otology-neurotology/
http://www.ovid.com/
ISSN: 15317129
Indexed in: MEDLINE
Recommended for: Hospital, Academic Libraries

Otology & Neurotology serves as the official journal of the American Otological Society and the American Neurotology Society. Originally published as the *American Journal of Otology*, this journal includes original research related to "both clinical and basic science aspects of otology, neurotology, and cranial base surgery." Published eight times a year, *Otology and Neurotology* includes original articles, review articles, research methodologies, book reviews, case studies, and letters to the editor. The contributing authors and editorial board provide a global perspective of this subspecialty and routinely offer articles in a variety of categories such as cochlear implants, vestibular disorders, middle ear and mastoid disease, and basic science research. The journal has the fourteenth highest impact ranking according to the 2009 *Journal Citation Reports* in the category of otorhinolaryngology, and it is indexed in multiple sources including MEDLINE, Embase, and Scopus. *Otology and Neurotology* is recommended for both academic and hospital collections.

Databases and Other Electronic Resources

Faculty of 1000. Faculty of 1000 Ltd, Science Navigation Group, 2002.
http://f1000.com/
See Also Chapter 26. Biology
Recommended for: Hospital, Academic Libraries

Cross-disciplinary in nature, the Faculty of 1000 (F1000) uses the expertise of over 10,000 leading clinicians and researchers to filter existing literature and provide brief evaluations of "important and influential" articles in their various fields. This unique, online service is intended to save practitioners' time and energy by "identifying the essential articles and providing expert opinions that explain the key findings and the clinical impact." Rather than relying upon traditional journal impact ratings to identify important literature, F1000 uses expert consensus on the merits and quality of individual articles, including the identification of articles that have the potential to change clinical practice. The system currently addresses 40 specialties, which are divided into over 300 subspecialties. Heads of Faculty for each specialty (referred to as a Faculty) are chosen based upon broad peer input. Heads of Faculty select Section Heads, who then identify Faculty Members using criteria that considers individual achievements, fair mindedness, peer respect and trust, diversity, and a proportionate representation of faculty to the discipline's publication record. The Otolaryngology specialty section addresses multiple subspecialties: Cosmetic & Head & Neck Reconstructive Surgery; General Otolaryngology; Head & Neck Cancers; Head & Neck Disorders; Laryngology/Phonosurgery/Speech Evaluation; Otology/Vestibular/Audiology; Pediatric Otolaryngology; and Rhinology & Paranasal Sinus Disease. The 2010 launch of a new otolaryngology faculty, headed by world-renowned otolaryngologists Patrick J. Bradley and Charles Cummings, elevates this resource as a "best" otolaryngology resource. Dr. Cummings is the Executive Medical Director at Johns Hopkins International and Senior Editor of another recommended resource, *Cummings Otolaryngology Head & Neck Surgery*. Dr. Bradley is a prolific author, serves on numerous national journal editorial boards, and coedits *ABC of Ear, Nose and Throat*. In September 2010, a beta version of a new F1000 was released, which combines the former Faculty of 1000 Medicine, Faculty of 1000 Biology, and *The Scientist*. While institutional subscriptions for specific F1000 specialties are not possible, this would be an excellent, authoritative current awareness tool for any hospital or academic library supporting physicians, researchers, nurses, allied health professionals, and students needing to keep abreast of quality medical and scientific literature. The Association of Learned and Professional Society Publishers chose its initial release, Faculty of 1000 Biology, as their most innovative publication for 2002.

11.8. Regenerative Medicine

Developing and using strategies aimed at repair or replacement of damaged, diseased, or metabolically deficient organs, tissues, and cells via tissue engineering; cell transplantation; and artificial organs and bioartificial organs and tissues.

—MeSH

Contributor: Margaret Henderson

Monographs

Foundations of Regenerative Medicine: Clinical and Therapeutic Applications. Editor: Anthony Atala. Academic Press/Elsevier, 2010.
http://extranet.netlibrary.com/TitleSelect/
http://www.ebrary.com
ISBN: 9780123750853
ISBN: 9780123785626 (Online)
Recommended for: Hospital, Academic Libraries

Regenerative medicine incorporates research from many areas, including tissue engineering; stem cells; and cell, tissue, and organ transplantation. Many books and journals cover one or two of these areas as they relate to regenerative medicine, but this book brings together all aspects of these areas to provide an excellent overview of regenerative medicine. The book begins with an introduction to the field and discusses cell-based therapies and stem cell research. Other chapters cover the cellular and molecular basis of regenerative medicine. The various areas that contribute to regenerative medicine are addressed in the next sections of the book: use of stem, bone marrow, and other cells; biomaterials; cell therapy; and tissue therapy. The tissue therapy section covers a wide range of uses, from cardiac and kidney tissue to muscles and nerves and skin. There are also chapters on ethical issues, FDA regulations, and U.S. patent law. This book is a must for any library supporting a regenerative medicine program or a program in one of the other areas that support regenerative medicine. It also supplies a good, current overview for large medical library collections. This is an update of *Principles of Regenerative Medicine* (Academic Press, 2007).

Fundamentals of Tissue Engineering and Regenerative Medicine. Editors: Ulrich Meyer, Thomas Meyer, Jorg Handschel, Hans Peter Wiesmann. Springer, 2009.
http://www.springerlink.com/
http://extranet.netlibrary.com/TitleSelect/
ISBN: 9783540777557
ISBN: 9783540777540
Recommended for: Hospital, Academic Libraries

This book is a comprehensive overview of the current state of tissue engineering as it applies to regenerative medicine. Part A begins with a history of tissue engineering and regenerative medicine, economics, decision making, ethical issues, and issues surrounding the sourcing of tissues. Part B covers biological considerations, organogenesis, cytokine signaling, and mechanical effects of the growth of tissues. Part C covers engineering strategies from the genetic and molecular level, through the cell and tissue level, to actual organs. Part D focuses on the technical aspects, including biomaterials, scaffolding, and laboratory protocols. Part E covers transplantation, including immune system issues and study design. Part F describes the clinical use of engineered tissues, in areas such as the brain, dental and general surgery, renal tissues, cardiac tissues, and skin. Regulatory issues are also covered. This is an excellent, up-to-date overview of the subject for any large academic or hospital library as well as smaller libraries that support regenerative medicine or tissue engineering programs.

Regenerative Biology and Medicine. Author: David L. Stocum. Elsevier Academic Press, 2006.
http://www.sciencedirect.com/science/book/9780123693716
http://extranet.netlibrary.com/TitleSelect/
http://www.ebrary.com/
ISBN: 9780123693716
ISBN: 9780080493022 (Online)
Recommended for: Hospital, Academic Libraries

Regenerative Biology and Medicine provides an excellent overview of basic and clinical research, including research on animal limb regeneration. After an overview of the history of regenerative biology and the theory and mechanisms of the biology of regeneration and wound repair, David Stocum covers the various tissues that have been studied. An initial chapter on regeneration studies is followed by a chapter on the application of those studies to body systems. Chapters cover the following: epidermal and dental tissues, lens and cornea; neural tissues; digestive, respiratory, and urogenital tissues; musculoskeletal tissues; and hematopoietic and cardiovascular tissues. Further chapters cover adult stem cells, appendages, and research issues. Each chapter includes figures, tables, a summary, and references. The book also includes an extensive index. This book is an excellent overview for any collection.

Stem Cells and Regenerative Medicine. Editors: Walter C. Low, Catherine M. Verfaillie. World Scientific, 2008.
http://ebooks.worldscinet.com/
http://lib.myilibrary.com/
ISBN: 9789812775764
ISBN: 9789812775771 (Online)
Recommended for: Hospital, Academic Libraries

Stem cells, like biomaterials, are one type of material being used in regenerative medicine. The ability of stem cells to differentiate into cells found throughout the body has led to research that programs stem cells to replace degenerating cells and tissues. Use of embryonic and adult stem cells is covered. Chapters in this book focus on stem cells for the heart, nervous system, liver, kidney, pancreas, and muscles. This book is useful for academic and hospital collections that support regenerative medicine research. It would also be useful for collections supporting stem cell research, as a guide to translational research.

Strategies in Regenerative Medicine: Integrating Biology with Materials Design. Editor: Matteo Santin. Springer, 2009.
http://www.springerlink.com/content/978-0-387-74659-3

http://extranet.netlibrary.com/TitleSelect/
http://www.ebrary.com/
ISBN: 9780387746593
ISBN: 9780387746609 (Online)
Recommended for: Hospital, Academic Libraries
Doody's Core Titles Selection

Strategies in Regenerative Medicine: Integrating Biology with Materials Design covers topics involving basic biology and materials science and their connection in tissue engineering. Each chapter covers the biology and materials behind different types of tissues. While this is not a comprehensive book on regenerative medicine, it does an excellent job of integrating information about biomaterials into regenerative medicine therapeutics. Chapters include questions, extensive bibliographies, top ten article lists, website suggestions, figures, tables, and photographs. An extensive index helps with the organization of the book. This is an excellent book for any collection supporting a regenerative medicine program as well as biomaterials and tissue engineering programs.

Journals

Annals of Biomedical Engineering. v. 1, Springer, 1972.
http://www.springerlink.com/content/111241/
ISSN: 00906964
ISSN: 15739686 (Online)
See Also Chapter 2. Biomedical Engineering
Indexed in: MEDLINE
Recommended for: Hospital, Academic Libraries

One of the journals of the Biomedical Engineering Society, *Annals of Biomedical Engineering* presents original research on many topics, including tissue and cellular engineering and biotechnology; and biomaterials and biological interfaces, with an emphasis on engineering approaches to provide integrated solutions to biological and biomedical problems. Regenerative medicine encompasses a wide range of fields, so a few of the journals on this topic are not specific to the specialty, such as this journal. Although *Annals of Biomedical Engineering* covers many fields, it is recommended only for academic or hospital collections that support a large regenerative medicine program or for those having a biomedical engineering program. *Annals* is ranked twentieth in biomedical engineering journals (2009 *Journal Citation Reports*). This journal is indexed by BIOSIS, CSA, Google Scholar, MEDLINE, Web of Science, and others.

Annual Review of Biomedical Engineering. v. 1, Annual Reviews, 1999.
http://arjournals.annualreviews.org/loi/bioeng
ISSN: 15239829
ISSN: 15454274 (Online)
See Also Chapter 2. Biomedical Engineering
Indexed in: MEDLINE
Recommended for: Hospital, Academic Libraries

This *Annual Review* is one of the journals that covers a broad area of research with some good coverage of aspects of regenerative medicine. This annual includes the areas of biomaterials and tissue engineering, focusing on scientific discovery and patient care. Articles are targeted towards engineers, life scientists, and clinicians. Ranked first in the biomedical engineering journals category (2009 *Journal Citation Reports*), this publication is a good addition to a large academic or hospital collection that supports regenerative medicine or biomedical engineering. This journal is indexed by BIOSIS, Embase/Excerpta Medica, MEDLINE, Web of Science, and others.

Artificial Organs. v. 1, Wiley-Blackwell, 1977.
http://onlinelibrary.wiley.com/journal/10.1111/(ISSN)1525-1594
ISSN: 0160564X
ISSN: 15251594 (Online)
Indexed in: MEDLINE
Recommended for: Hospital, Academic Libraries

Artificial Organs is the official journal of the International Federation for Artificial Organs. Articles cover all aspects of artificial organ development, from the design, performance, and evaluation of the biomaterials and devices to the research, development, and clinical application of the artificial organs. The journal also publishes articles that advance the replacement, recovery, and regeneration of organ systems. This journal is necessary for any academic or hospital library supporting a regenerative medicine collection. *Artificial Organs* ranks fifteenth in transplantation journals and twenty-seventh in biomedical engineering journals according to the 2009 *Journal Citation Reports*. It has an impact factor of 1.827. This journal is indexed by BIOSIS, CSA, Embase/Excerpta Medica, MEDLINE, Web of Science, and others.

Biomaterials. v. 1, Elsevier, 1980.
http://www.sciencedirect.com/science/journal/01429612
ISSN: 01429612
ISSN: 18785905 (Online)
See Also Chapter 2. Biomedical Engineering
Indexed in: MEDLINE
Recommended for: Hospital, Academic Libraries

One aspect of regenerative medicine is the creation of artificial and bioartificial organs and tissues, which requires advances in biomaterials. Each issue of *Biomaterials* has a section on "Biomaterials and Tissue Engineering" covering the basic science and engineering of biomaterials used in the development of organs, as well as implantable medical devices and drug delivery systems. Ranked first in biomaterials journals and second in biomedical engineering journals (2009 *Journal Citation Reports*), this publication is an excellent addition to a large academic or hospital collection that supports regenerative medicine or biomedical engineering. This journal is indexed by BIOSIS, CSA, Embase/Excerpta Medica, MEDLINE, Web of Science, and others.

Regenerative Medicine. v. 1, Future Medicine, 2006.
http://www.futuremedicine.com/page/loi/rme
ISSN: 17460751
ISSN: 1746076X (Online)
Indexed in: MEDLINE
Recommended for: Hospital, Academic Libraries

This journal publishes articles that address the challenges and advances in stem cell research and regenerative medicine. Areas covered—which lead to advances in the treatment of human diseases that cause the loss or dysfunction of specific cell types in the body, such as Parkinson's disease, diabetes, or cancer—include stem cell use, tissue engineering, medical devices, gene therapies, and drug development. Regulatory, ethical, and legal issues are also considered. Ranked twelfth in the biomedical engineering journals category (2009 *Journal Citation Reports*), this is an excellent publication for any library supporting research in regenerative medicine. It is indexed in BIOSIS, Google Scholar, MEDLINE, Web of Science and others.

Stem Cells and Development. v. 13, Mary Ann Liebert, 2004.
http://www.liebertonline.com/scd
ISSN: 15473287
ISSN: 15578534 (Online)
Indexed in: MEDLINE
Recommended for: Hospital, Academic Libraries

This journal covers the research and therapeutic applications of stem cells of all tissue types. Stem cells are one of the major areas of research for developing replacement tissues and organs in regenerative medicine. Along with peer-reviewed articles, there are editorials, comprehensive or concise reviews, technical reports, and correspondence. Development of stem cells is also considered. Ranked third in the transplant journals category with an impact factor 4.146 (2009 *Journal Citation Reports*), this publication is recommended for any academic or hospital library that supports a program in regenerative medicine or any stem cell research. *Stem Cells and Development* is indexed in BIOSIS, Embase/Excerpta Medica MEDLINE, Web of Science and others.

Tissue Engineering (Parts A, B, & C). v. 14, Mary Ann Liebert, 2008.
http://www.liebertonline.com/ten
http://www.liebertonline.com/loi/tea
http://www.liebertonline.com/loi/teab
http://www.liebertonline.com/loi/teac
ISSN: 10763279 (combined parts, 1995-2007)
ISSN: 15578690 (Online—combined parts, 1995–2007)
ISSN: 19373341 (part A)
ISSN: 1937335X (Online—part A)
ISSN: 19373368 (part B)
ISSN: 19373376 (Online—part B)
ISSN: 19373384 (part C)
ISSN: 19373392 (Online—part C)
Indexed in: MEDLINE
Recommended for: Hospital, Academic Libraries

This journal is the official publication of the Tissue Engineering International & Regenerative Medicine Society. In response to a steep increase in the amount of tissue engineering research and publication, the journal expanded into three parts beginning with 2008. *Tissue Engineering*, Part A (no subtitle), focuses on basic research in engineering and the life sciences that will provide an understanding of the structure-function relationship in all tissues with the goal of developing biological substitutes. *Tissue Engineering, Part B: Reviews*, presents critical discussions, analyses, and concise summaries of research in the field of tissue engineering and special research areas such as funding, education, or commercialization. *Tissue Engineering, Part C: Methods*, presents procedures and protocols that will be adopted to address the challenges as research is translated into clinical applications for tissue-engineered products. This journal is good for a hospital or academic library collection that supports regenerative research with a focus on tissue engineering for the creation of replacement organs and tissues. The journal is ranked nineteenth in the biotechnology and applied microbiology category (2009 *Journal Citation Reports*). It is indexed in BIOSIS, CSA, Embase/Excerpta Medica MEDLINE, Web of Science and others.

Transplantation. v. 1, Lippincott Williams & Wilkins, 1963.
http://journals.lww.com/transplantjournal/
http://www.ovid.com/
ISSN: 00411337

ISSN: 15346080 (Online)
Indexed in: MEDLINE
Recommended for: Hospital, Academic Libraries

This publication is the official journal of the Transplantation Society, covering the regenerative medicine areas of cell therapy and islet transplantation *and* experimental transplantation. Rapid communications, overviews, mini reviews, and forums complement the peer-reviewed articles in the journal. Articles are grouped into the areas of "Basic and Experimental Research" and "Clinical and Translational Research." The journal also publishes articles on ethical, social, and controversial topics associated with transplantation. Ranked sixth in the transplantation journals category (2009 *Journal Citation Reports*), this journal is useful in any academic or hospital library that supports a regenerative medicine program that includes transplantation research. It is indexed in BIOSIS, Embase/Excerpta Medica MEDLINE, Web of Science and others.

11.9. Surgery

Manual or operative procedures used in the treatment of disease, injuries, or deformities.

—MeSH

Contributor: Jie Li

Monographs

ACS Surgery: Principles and Practice. 6th ed. Editors: Wiley W. Souba, Mitchell P. Fink, Gregory J.J. Jurkovich. B C Decker, 2007.
http://www.acssurgery.com
http://online.statref.com/titleinfo/fxid-61.html
ISBN: 9781550093995
Recommended for: Hospital, Academic Libraries
Doody's Core Titles Selection

ACS Surgery: Principles and Practice is the first surgery textbook that bears the prestigious American College of Surgeons in its title. It is written by almost 200 surgeons who are recognized experts. The focus is on information essential to the practicing surgeon, particularly diagnosis and treatment of surgical disease and care of critically ill surgical patients. The book first addresses the elements of contemporary practice, such as professionalism in surgery, performance measures, benchmarking surgical outcomes, evidence-based surgery, patient safety in surgical care, preoperative testing, and operative planning. Ten chapters follow devoted to basic perioperative considerations such as bleeding and infection prevention; surgery of the head and neck; surgery of the breast, skin, and soft tissue; surgery of the alimentary tract and abdominal organs; and surgery of the vascular system. Trauma and thermal injury are covered in detail, as is critical care. The book has over 1,500 excellent illustrations, including original line drawings, color photographs, and videos. It is a *Doody's Core Titles* selection.

Ashcraft's Pediatric Surgery. 5th ed. Editors: George W. Holcomb III, J. Patrick Murphy. Saunders, 2010.
http://www.sciencedirect.com/science/book/9781416061274
ISBN: 9781416061274
Recommended for: Hospital, Academic Libraries
Brandon/Hill, *Doody's Core Titles* Selection

Ashcraft's Pediatric Surgery presents practical guidance on treating the entire range of surgical problems in infants, children, and adolescents. This fifth edition provides updated coverage of current topics such as the increased use of minimally invasive surgery (MIS) for pediatric patients, bariatric surgery in adolescents, and evidence-based treatments and outcomes in children. The book first covers general considerations of pediatric surgery. Following chapters address pediatric trauma surgery, thoracic surgery, abdominal surgery, surgery of the inguinal region and scrotum, surgical diseases in urology, neoplasms, and surgery of the skin and soft tissues. The last chapter addresses other issues in pediatric surgery, such as pediatric and adolescent gynecology, breast diseases, endocrine disorders and tumors, robotic surgery, and bariatric surgery in adolescents. The book emphasizes thoracoscopic, laparoscopic, and in utero procedures. Surgical videos demonstrate many of the new techniques and procedures from the text. This book was a Brandon/Hill recommendation for the small medical library for surgery and it is currently a *Doody's Core Titles* essential purchase recommendation for pediatric surgery.

Current Diagnosis & Treatment: Surgery. 13th ed. Editor: Gerard M. Doherty. McGraw-Hill, 2009.
http://www.accessmedicine.com
ISBN: 9780071635158
Recommended for: Hospital, Academic Libraries
Brandon/Hill, *Doody's Core Titles* Selection

Current Diagnosis & Treatment: Surgery 13th edition, which continues its previous edition's title *Current Surgical Diagnosis and Treatment*, is a ready source of information about diseases managed by surgeons. Targeted for medical students, surgical residents, surgeons, and other medical practitioners, it emphasizes quick identification of major diagnostic features and brief descriptions of disease processes, followed by approaches for definitive diagnosis and treatment. Epidemiology, pathophysiology, and pathology are discussed. In its 45 chapters, the first 14 provide general information about the relationship between surgeons and their patients, training and professionalism, preoperative and postoperative care, surgical complications, wound healing, inflammation, infection, antibiotics, fluid and electrolyte management, and surgical metabolism and nutrition. Beginning with chapter 15, the book is organized by organ system and begins with head and neck tumors and ends with a chapter on hand surgery. Further chapters on pediatric surgery, oncology, and organ transplantation complete the coverage. This comprehensive yet concise textbook delivers to-the-point information on 1,000 diseases and disorders that surgeons are most often required to treat. The book is updated frequently to include the new knowledge and techniques in surgery. It was on the Brandon/Hill list for surgery.

Current Surgical Therapy. 10th ed. Editors: John L. Cameron, Andrew M. Cameron. Mosby Elsevier, 2011.
ISBN: 9781437708233
Recommended for: Hospital, Academic Libraries
Doody's Core Titles Selection

Current Surgical Therapy started its first edition in 1985 under the editorship of John L. Cameron. It is one of the "current therapy" series that are considered by many to be basic handbooks. This review refers to the ninth edition. The book is organized by body area in 19 chapters that discuss the selection and implementation of the latest treatments for surgical diseases and what to do in specific surgical situations. This concise book provides practical advice to general surgeons as well as an effective review for American Board of Surgery examinations, especially the general surgery oral boards. With nearly 940 photographs, line drawings, and radiographs, it provides important surgical visual perspectives. It is an Expert Consult Series title which provides additional online content to individual purchasers. It is currently a *Doody's Core Titles* recommendation for general surgery.

Greenfield's Surgery: Scientific Principles and Practice. 5th ed. Editors: Michael W. Mulholland, Keith D. Lillemoe, Gerard M. Doherty, Ronald V. Maier, Diane M. Simeone, Gilbert R. Upchurch, Jr. Lippincott Williams & Wilkins, 2011.
http://www.r2library.com/ (4th ed.)
http://www.ovid.com/
ISBN: 9781605473550
Recommended for: Hospital, Academic Libraries

Greenfield's Surgery: Scientific Principles and Practice is intended for general surgeons and surgical residents for practice, board review, and teaching. The first edition was published in 1993 with Lazar J. Greenfield as the book's first editor; he continued as editor for the next two editions. This review refers to the fourth edition which provides full-color text and comprehensive coverage of all types of surgery by integrating basic science with clinical practice. The book is organized with the first 15 chapters addressing the general issues of surgery: cell structure, substrate metabolism, nutrition, wound healing, homeostasis, inflammation, infection, fluids, electrolytes, burns, anesthesiology, cancer, evidence-based surgery, and quality assessment. The next 21 sections address specific surgical diseases or surgery on the specific body parts. It is well organized, providing step-by-step descriptions of the most common surgical procedures. The illustrations are clear and informative. A companion website for individuals includes a complete image bank consisting of the full-color images and a test bank for the American Board of Surgery In-Training Examination. A fifth edition is expected in late 2010.

Mastery of Surgery. 5th ed. Editors: Josef E. Fischer, Kirby I. Bland. Lippincott Williams & Wilkins, 2007.
http://www.r2library.com/
http://www.ovid.com/
ISBN: 9780781771658
Recommended for: Hospital, Academic Libraries
Doody's Core Titles Selection

Mastery of Surgery is a comprehensive text and atlas that presents detailed, step-by-step descriptions of surgical procedures enhanced with more than 3,300 illustrations. This authoritative two-volume reference represents the core procedural knowledge taught in most surgical residency programs. The book is organized into nine sections with 239 chapters on preoperative care of the surgical patient; basic surgical skills; new and emerging techniques; head and neck; endocrine surgery; the breast, chest, and mediastinum; the diaphragm; the gastrointestinal tract; nongastrointestinal transabdominal surgery; and vascular surgery. The print book automatically comes with online access, which includes the entire text, as well as web-only chapters with additional surgery guidance for individual purchasers. Evidence-based surgery and its emphasis are apparent throughout the text. This book is essential for any general surgery resident. The book is currently a *Doody's Core Titles* selection for general surgery.

Sabiston Textbook of Surgery: The Biological Basis of Modern Surgical Practice. 18th ed. Editors: Courtney M. Townsend, Daniel R. Beauchamp, B. Mark Evers, Kenneth L. Mattox. Saunders Elsevier, 2008.
http://www.mdconsult.com/
ISBN: 9781416052333
Recommended for: Academic Libraries
Brandon/Hill, *Doody's Core Titles* Selection

Sabiston Textbook of Surgery has been published since 1936 and edited by four renowned surgeon editors. This classic reference presents an in-depth understanding of surgery. In each new edition, the editors have updated the book with new technology, techniques, and knowledge in surgery. The purpose of the book, as stated by Courtney M. Townsend, the editor of current 18th edition and previous two editions, "is to remain the most thorough, useful, readable, and understandable textbook presenting the principles and techniques of surgery." At nearly 2,400 pages, it is comprehensive and thorough. While the retained chapters have been updated, the new chapters of this edition reflect the changes in and new knowledge of surgical patient safety, dealing with bioterrorism, distance surgery, and robotic and telemonitoring technology. This edition is organized into 13 sections focused on basic principles of surgery, organ-specific general surgical care, and the surgical super-specialties. The book is full of color illustrations and fully incorporates the graphics into text. Each chapter begins with an outline and contains tables presenting checklists of key principles and practices. The book is organized in color-coded sections that are easy to use. This textbook is a long-standing Brandon/Hill recommendation and is currently a *Doody's Core Titles* essential purchase recommendation for general surgery.

Schwartz's Principles of Surgery. 9th ed. Editors: F. Charles Brunicardi, Dana K. Andersen, Timothy R. Billiar, David L. Dunn, John G. Hunter, Jeffrey B. Matthews, Raphael E. Pollock. McGraw-Hill Medical, 2010.
http://www.accessmedicine.com
ISBN: 9780071547703
See Also Chapter 1.9. Physician Assistants
Recommended for: Hospital, Academic Libraries
Brandon/Hill, *Doody's Core Titles* Selection

The prestigious *Schwartz's Principles of Surgery* began publication in 1969. It is considered by many to be the definitive textbook on the practice of surgery. Seymour I. Schwartz was the founding editor of this surgical textbook which bears his name, and served as editor-in-chief for its first seven editions. The post-Schwartz editions have preserved this historical textbook's excellent reputation. This book is organized into two parts. Part I, "Basic Considerations," with 15 chapters, covers general considerations of the Accreditation Council for Graduate Medical Education Core Competencies and basic science principles, including topics such as systemic response to injury, fluid management, surgical bleeding, shock, surgical infections, trauma, burns, wound healing, oncology, transplantation, patient safety, and cells, genomics, and molecular surgery. Part II, "Specific Considerations," with 23 chapters, covers surgical diseases and procedures in key surgical areas, such as skin, breast, head and neck, chest, heart, stomach, trauma, transplantation, and neurosurgery. In addition to preserving the old chapters, the ninth edition added two new chapters, "Accreditation Council for Graduate Medical Core Competencies," and "Ethics, Palliative Care, and Care at the End of Life." The new edition also has greater focus on evidence-based medicine. Every chapter has key points and the book has full color design. The intended audience is medical students, surgical residents, and practicing surgeons. This book is a long-standing Brandon/Hill recommendation and is currently a *Doody's Core Titles* recommendation for general surgery.

Trauma. 6th ed. Editors: David V. Feliciano, Kenneth L. Mattox, Ernest E. Moore. McGraw-Hill, 2008.
See Chapter 10.5. Emergency Medicine

Washington Manual of Surgery. 5th ed. Editors: Mary E. Klingensmith, Li Ern Chen, Sean C. Glasgow, Trudie A. Goers, Spencer J. Melby. Lippincott Williams & Wilkins, 2008.
http://www.r2library.com/
http://www.ovid.com/
ISBN: 9780781774475
Recommended for: Hospital, Academic Libraries
Brandon/Hill, *Doody's Core Titles* Selection

First published in 1996, the *Washington Manual of Surgery* was designed to complement the *Washington Manual of Medical Therapeutics*. The combination of authors who are residents assisted by faculty coauthors helps focus the chapters on issues that are particularly helpful to the trainee in surgery. The manual presents brief, rational, effective approaches to the diagnosis and management of patients with surgical problems. The fifth edition of the manual includes updates on each topic as well as substantial new material. The manual devotes the first seven chapters to issues of surgical patients, such as preoperative care, nutrition, life support, anesthesia, fluid, homeostasis, transfusion therapy, wound healing, and critical care. Then it addresses surgical diseases or surgical procedures on body parts in the following 29 chapters. The last chapter discusses common surgical procedures. This edition incorporates an evidence-based medicine approach. This manual is especially valuable to surgeons who teach and train surgical residents, as well as the residents in surgical training. This book was on the Brandon/Hill list and is currently a *Doody's Core Titles* recommendation for general surgery.

Zollinger's Atlas of Surgical Operations. 9th ed. Editors: Robert M. Zollinger Jr., E. Christopher Ellison. McGraw-Hill Medical, 2011.
http://www.accesssurgery.com/
ISBN: 9780071602266
Recommended for: Hospital, Academic Libraries
Doody's Core Titles Selection

Ever since its 1st edition which was published in 1939, *Zollinger's Atlas of Surgical Operations* has been a major atlas for surgical technique in general surgery. This review refers to the eighth edition. Using 1,461 high quality explanatory line drawing figures and concise languages, *Zollinger's Atlas of Surgical Operations* describes 113 major surgical procedures in 219 plates. The first four chapters discuss surgical technique, anesthesia, preoperative preparation and postoperative care, and ambulatory surgery. Then it covers surgical anatomy before dividing the procedures into categories: gastrointestinal, miscellaneous abdominal, vascular, gynecologic, and additional procedures. In addition to most general surgical procedures, it also includes head and neck, urological, hand, and orthopedic procedures. The eighth edition has been updated to include laparoscopic and endoscopic procedures and new surgical techniques. It is considered a must-have for surgical residents and general surgeons. It is currently a *Doody's Core Titles* recommendation for general surgery. The current edition is available electronically through *AccessSurgery* as well as for various mobile and e-book devices.

Journals

American Journal of Surgery. v. 18, Elsevier, 1926.
http://www.sciencedirect.com/science/journal/00029610
http://americanjournalofsurgery.com
ISSN: 00029610
ISSN: 18791883 (Online)
Indexed in: MEDLINE
Recommended for: Hospital, Academic Libraries
Brandon/Hill Selection

American Journal of Surgery is a monthly peer-reviewed journal intended for general surgeons. It is the official journal of eight major surgical societies: the Southwestern Surgical Congress, the North Pacific Surgical Association, the Association for Surgical Education, the Association of Women Surgeons, the American Society of Breast Surgeons, the Association of VA Surgeons, Midwest Surgical Association, and the Society of Black Academic Surgeons (SBAS). In addition to original research articles, clinical studies, editorials, reviews, brief reports, correspondence, and book reviews, it published the official papers of its surgical societies. The journal was on the Brandon/Hill list for the small medical library for surgery and a core clinical title at National Library of Medicine. It is indexed in numerous indexing and abstracting sources including CAB Abstracts, CINAHL, Embase, MEDLINE, Scopus, and Web of Science. Online access back to 1926 is available from the publisher.

Annals of Surgery. v. 1, Lippincott Williams & Wilkins, 1885.
http://www.ovid.com/
http://www.annalsofsurgery.com
http://www.ncbi.nlm.nih.gov/pmc/journals/230/
ISSN: 00034932
ISSN: 15281140 (Online)
Indexed in: MEDLINE
Recommended for: Hospital, Academic Libraries
Brandon/Hill Selection

Annals of Surgery, the monthly peer-reviewed journal that started publication in 1885, is affiliated with the American Surgical Association and the European Surgical Association. As the most highly referenced surgery journal, it achieved an impact factor of 7.9 and was ranked first out of 166 journals in the surgery category (2009 *Journal Citation Reports*). Its focus is on innovations in surgical practice and technique. In addition to original research articles, the journal includes monthly review articles and a feature, "Advances in Surgical Technique," to highlight current clinical issues. It is indexed in numerous indexing and abstracting sources including CAB Abstracts, Embase, MEDLINE, Scopus and Web of Science. The journal was on the Bandon/Hill List for the small medical library for surgery and is a core clinical title at the National Library of Medicine. Online access back to 1885 is available from Ovid. Issues from 1885 through 2007 are also available online on PubMed Central, although the publisher no longer participates.

Annals of Surgical Oncology. v. 1, Springer, 1994.
http://www.annsurgoncol.org/
http://www.springerlink.com/content/1068-9265/
ISSN: 10689265

ISSN: 15344681 (Online)
Indexed in: MEDLINE
Recommended for: Hospital, Academic Libraries

Annals of Surgical Oncology is the official journal of the Society of Surgical Oncology. This peer-reviewed monthly journal broadly covers all surgical specialties. According to its website, the journal attempts to represent and advance the surgical oncology profession; promote the highest quality patient care and practice management; provide relevant cancer education and research training materials; promote clinical and translational cancer research; facilitate the career development of surgical trainees and their transition into academic and community-based practice; and promote public policy and patient advocacy issues related to the surgical patient with cancer. It achieved an impact factor of 4.130 and ranked sixth out of 166 journals in the surgery category (2009 *Journal Citation Reports*). The journal is indexed in numerous indexing and abstracting sources including Embase, MEDLINE, Scopus, and Web of Science. Online access back to 1994 is available from the publisher.

Archives of Surgery. v. 81, American Medical Association, 1960.
http://archsurg.ama-assn.org
ISSN: 00040010
ISSN: 15383644 (Online)
Indexed in: MEDLINE
Recommended for: Hospital, Academic Libraries
Brandon/Hill Selection

Archives of Surgery is an international peer-reviewed journal. This monthly journal is the official publication of the New England Surgical Society, the Pacific Coast Surgical Association, and the Western Surgical Association. In addition to the original research articles, the journal also publishes invited critiques, resident's forum articles, technique articles, commentaries, announcements, diagnostic and case quizzes, and correspondence. The journal was on the Brandon/ Hill List for the small medical library for surgery and is a core clinical title at the National Library of Medicine. It is indexed in numerous indexing and abstracting sources including CAB Abstracts, Embase, MEDLINE, Scopus, and Web of Science. Online access back to 1920 (earlier titles) is available from the Association.

British Journal of Surgery. v. 1, Wiley Blackwell, 1913.
http://onlinelibrary.wiley.com/journal/10.1002/(ISSN)1365-2168
http://www.bjs.co.uk
ISSN: 00071323
ISSN: 13652168 (Online)
Indexed in: MEDLINE
Recommended for: Hospital, Academic Libraries
Brandon/Hill Selection

British Journal of Surgery is a peer-reviewed international journal covering all aspects of general surgery. It maintains a special relationship with several surgical associations: the Association of Surgeons of Great Britain and Ireland, Association of Surgeons of the Netherlands, Society of Academic and Research Surgery, Swedish Surgical Society and Swiss Society of Surgery. The journal is incorporated with *European Journal of Surgery* and *Swiss Surgery*. With an impact factor of 4.077, it was ranked seventh out of 166 journals in the surgery category (2009 *Journal Citation Reports*). It features clinical and laboratory-based research on all aspects of surgery and related topics, including developing areas such as minimally invasive surgery and interventional radiology. In addition to the original research articles the journal publishes reviews, abstracts from key meetings, correspondence and book reviews. The intended audience is both the general and specialty surgeon. The journal was on the Brandon/Hill list for the small medical library for surgery and is a core clinical title at the National Library of Medicine. It is indexed in numerous indexing and abstracting sources including CAB Abstracts, Embase, MEDLINE, Scopus, and Web of Science. Online access back to 1913 is available from the publisher.

Journal of Foot & Ankle Surgery. v. 32, Elsevier, 1993.
See Chapter 19. Podiatry

Journal of the American College of Surgeons. v. 1, Elsevier, 1994.
http://www.journalacs.org
http://www.sciencedirect.com/science/journal/10727515
ISSN: 10727515
ISSN: 18791190 (Online)
Indexed in: MEDLINE
Recommended for: Hospital, Academic Libraries
Brandon/Hill Selection

Journal of the American College of Surgeons is a monthly peer-reviewed journal covering all aspects of surgery. In addition to original research articles the journal publishes clinical studies, review articles, clinically relevant experimental investigations, meta-analysis reviews, history articles, letters to the editors, and CME. The journal was on the Brandon/Hill list for surgery and is a core clinical title at the National Library of Medicine. It is indexed in numerous indexing and abstracting sources including CAB Abstracts, CINAHL, Embase, MEDLINE,

Scopus, and Web of Science. Online access back to 1997 is available from the publisher.

Surgery. v. 1, Mosby Elsevier, 1937.
http://www.sciencedirect.com/science/journal/00396060
ISSN: 00396060
ISSN: 15327361 (Online)
Indexed in: MEDLINE
Recommended for: Hospital, Academic Libraries
Brandon/Hill Selection

Surgery is a long-established peer-reviewed monthly journal that covers all aspects of surgery. Over its history it has associated with several key surgical associations and it is currently sponsored by the Society of University Surgeons, the Central Surgical Association, and the American Association of Endocrine Surgeons. According to its online aims and scope statement, the journal publishes "practical, authoritative information about procedures, clinical advances, and major trends shaping general surgery." In addition to original research articles the journal also publishes clinical reports and reports from the meetings of its sponsoring societies. *Surgery* was on the Brandon/Hill list and is a National Library of Medicine core clinical title. It is indexed in several indexing and abstracting sources including CAB Abstracts, Embase, MEDLINE, Scopus, and Web of Science. Online access back to 1995 is available from the publisher.

Surgical Clinics of North America. v. 1, Saunders Elsevier, 1921.
http://www.surgical.theclinics.com
http://www.mdconsult.com/
ISSN: 00396109
ISSN: 15583171 (Online)
Indexed in: MEDLINE, CINAHL
Recommended for: Hospital, Academic Libraries
Brandon/Hill Selection

Surgical Clinics of North America is a bimonthly peer-reviewed journal that publishes comprehensive reviews by experts on the diagnosis and treatment of conditions requiring surgical intervention. Each issue, which is in hardbound format, focuses on a single topic relevant to general surgery practice. Topics of recent issues include: liver surgery; simulation and surgical competency; evidence-based management of pancreatic cancer; anorectal disease; surgical practice in rural areas; endocrine surgery; advances in cardiac and aortic surgery; surgical infections; and multidisciplinary approach to cancer care. The journal was on the Bandon/Hill list for the small medical library and is a National Library of Medicine core clinical journal. It is indexed in numerous indexing and abstracting sources including CINAHL, Embase, MEDLINE, Scopus, and Web of Science. Online access back to 1996 is available from the journal's website or MD Consult.

Surgical Endoscopy. v. 1, Springer, 1987.
http://www.springerlink.com/content/0930-2794/
ISSN: 09302794
ISSN: 14322218 (Online)
See Also Chapter 11.1. Colorectal Surgery
Indexed in: MEDLINE
Recommended for: Hospital, Academic Libraries

Surgical Endoscopy, a monthly peer-reviewed journal, is the official journal of the Society of American Gastrointestinal and Endoscopic Surgeons and European Association for Endoscopic Surgery. It is international in scope, covering the surgical aspects of interventional endoscopy, ultrasound, and other techniques in the fields of gastroenterology, obstetrics, gynecology, urology, and orthopedics in both adults and children. The journal is indexed in numerous indexing and abstracting sources including CINAHL, Embase, MEDLINE, Scopus, and Web of Science. Online access back to 1987 is available from the publisher.

World Journal of Surgery. v. 1, Springer, 1977.
http://www.springerlink.com/content/0364-2313/
ISSN: 03642313
ISSN: 14322323 (Online)
Indexed in: MEDLINE
Recommended for: Hospital, Academic Libraries

World Journal of Surgery is the official journal of the International Society of Surgery. This peer-reviewed journal is international in scope, covering both clinical and experimental surgery. The journal covers a wide array of topics related to surgery, such as surgical techniques, education for surgery, general surgical care, surgical outcome comparisons and the social and economic context of surgery within the medical care system. In addition to original research articles, the journal includes case studies, meta analyses, and book reviews, as well as a feature, "World Progress in Surgery," which explores a single current topic. It is ranked twenty-eighth out of 166 journals in surgery and has an impact factor of 2.696 (2009 *Journal Citation Reports*). The journal is indexed by numerous indexing and abstracting sources including CAB Abstracts, Embase, MEDLINE, Science Citation Index, Scopus, and Web of Science. Online access from volume 1, 1977 is available from the publisher.

Wound Repair and Regeneration. v. 1, Wiley-Blackwell, 1993.
See Chapter 11.10. Plastic Surgery

Databases and Other Electronic Resources

AccessSurgery. McGraw-Hill, 2009?
http://www.accesssurgery.com
Recommended for: Hospital, Academic Libraries

AccessSurgery is an online integrated resource that provides quick answers to surgical inquiries from McGraw-Hill's publications. This product is organized around the Accreditation Council for Graduate Medical Education (ACGME) and designed for residents in general surgery. *AccessSurgery* includes the most recent editions of 15 surgery textbooks including *Schwartz's Principles of Surgery*, *Current Diagnosis & Treatment: Surgery*, *Maingot's Abdominal Operations*, *Trauma*, *Principles of Critical Care*, *Kuerer's Breast Surgical Oncology*, *Adult Chest Surgery*, *McGraw-Hill Manual Colorectal Surgery*, *McGraw-Hill Manual Endocrine Surgery*, *Robotic Surgery*, *Obesity Surgery: Principles and Practice*, *Current Diagnosis & Treatment in Otolaryngology-Head & Neck Surgery*, and *Smith's General Urology*. The surgery textbooks are arranged into several sections: "Home/Core Curriculum," "Procedures/Operations," "Textbooks," "Videos," "Board Review," "Drugs," and "DDx" (differential diagnosis). In the "Home/Core Curriculum" section, the textbooks are arranged into 15 broad subject areas and some with subsections, which serve as a table of contents to all the textbooks. The "Textbooks" section lists books individually for those who are interested in a particular book. The "Procedures/Operations" section is arranged by regional and disease surgeries. The database's "Board Review" section includes *Schwartz's Principles of Surgery: Self Assessment and Board Review* and *Surgery Review Illustrated*. Residents may sign in to take a test and get test scores. The "Video" section currently includes 140 surgical procedure videos produced by the Columbia University College of Physicians and Surgeons and Northwestern University Feinberg School of Medicine. The surgical animations are adapted from *Zollinger's Atlas of Surgical Operations*. Symptoms or diseases maybe found in the "DDx" section. Surgery residents, students and surgeons would find this database very useful for their education and practice.

11.10. Plastic Surgery

Restoration, reconstruction, or improvement of defective, damaged, or missing structures.

—MeSH: Surgery, Plastic

Contributor: Jie Li

Monographs

Facial Plastic and Reconstructive Surgery. 3rd ed. Editors: Ira D. Papel, John L. Frodel, Richard G. Holt, Wayne F. Larrabee, Nathan E. Nachlas, Stephen S. Park. Thieme, 2009.
ISBN: 9781588905154
Recommended for: Academic Libraries
Doody's Core Titles Selection

Facial Plastic and Reconstructive Surgery, recognized as the standard reference in plastic surgery, offers a concise, yet comprehensive, single-volume overview of the field. It encompasses both cosmetic and reconstructive techniques. The book is organized into six sections. Section I, "Principles of Facial Plastic and Reconstructive Surgery," addresses anatomy and physiology of the skin, wound healing, soft tissue techniques, skin grafts, scar revision, tissue implants, engineering and adhesives, lasers, computer imaging, photography, ethics and ambulatory surgery. Section II, "Aesthetic Facial Surgery," covers aesthetic facial surgery analysis, anesthesia, and youthful aging. It also reviews aesthetic facial surgery in every part of the face, from eyelids to neck. Section III discusses the functional and aesthetic surgery of the nose. Section IV addresses the reconstructive surgery of the face and neck. Section V pays special attention to trauma, and Section VI covers congenital and pediatric facial plastic surgery. Targeted to all facial plastic surgeons, oral surgeons, otolaryngologists, dermatologists, ophthalmologists, residents, fellows, and students, the book uses 2,175 high-quality illustrations demonstrating key concepts in facial plastic and constructive surgery. This 3rd edition retains the comprehensive scope of earlier editions and features new chapters on anti-aging medicine, ambulatory surgery considerations, autologous fat augmentation, pediatric rhinoplasty, tissue engineering, and non-ablative skin resurfacing techniques. It is currently a *Doody's* core title.

Grabb and Smith's Plastic Surgery. 6th ed. Editors: Charles H. Thorne, Robert W. Beasley, Sherrell J. Aston, Scott P. Bartlett, Geoffrey C. Gurtner, Scott L. Spear. Lippincott Williams & Wilkins, 2007.
http://www.ovid.com/
ISBN: 9780781746984
Recommended for: Academic Libraries
Doody's Core Titles Selection

Grabb and Smith's Plastic Surgery is a comprehensive single-volume reference on the essential aspects of plastic surgery. The 93 chapters are grouped into eight sections covering principles, techniques, and basic science;

skin and soft tissue; congenital anomalies and pediatric plastic surgery; head and neck; aesthetic surgery; breast, trunk, and lower extremity; and hand. Each chapter starts with a review of clinical anatomy and progresses to clinical aspects of disease, historically important surgical approaches, and current techniques. It provides guidance on aesthetic and reconstructive procedures. This edition features the latest clinical recommendations and procedures, such as breast prosthetics, tissue expansion, and flexor tendon surgery. An accompanying CD-ROM provides full text and color images from the book. This book is currently a *Doody's Core Titles* essential purchase recommendation. Its intended audience is practicing surgeons and those in surgical training.

Plastic Surgery. 2nd ed. Editors: Stephen J. Mathes, Vincent R. Hentz. Saunders Elsevier, 2006.
ISBN: 9780721688114
Recommended for: Academic Libraries
Doody's Core Titles Selection

This eight-volume set of nearly 8,000 pages is a classic masterwork that is the most comprehensive collection in the field. This second edition has made major updates to reflect all of the knowledge and development of new technologies in plastic surgery since the first edition was published in 1990. It covers all pertinent subjects comprehensively: general principles; head and neck surgery; pediatric plastic surgery; tumors of the head, neck, and skin; the trunk and lower extremity; and the hand and upper limb. It contains over 10,500 illustrations, with three volumes in color. A companion website is available to individual purchasers. The book is currently a *Doody's* core title for plastic and reconstructive surgery.

Total Burn Care. 3rd ed. Editor: David N. Herndon. Saunders Elsevier, 2007.
http://www.sciencedirect.com/science/book/9781416032748
ISBN: 9781416032748
Recommended for: Hospital, Academic Libraries
Brandon/Hill, *Doody's Core Titles* Selection

Total Burn Care explains how to meet the clinical, physical, psychological, and social needs of every burn patient to achieve optimal recovery and rehabilitation. The book is organized into 66 chapters. The first four chapters discuss the history of treatments of burns; teamwork; epidemiological, demographic, and outcome characteristics of burn injury; and prevention of burn injury. Chapters 5–9 cover immediate care, with a focus on burn management in disasters, pre-hospital and emergency care, and descriptions of the pathophysiology of the early burn. Chapters 10–17 discuss the burn wound, including the evaluation of the burn wound, infection care, operative wound treatment, anesthesia, skin banks, alternative wound coverings, and alloderm. Chapters 18–21 cover inhalation injury, including pathophysiology, diagnosis and treatment of inhalation injury, and respiratory care. Chapters 22–38 focus on the response to injury, covering all aspects of the systemic response to burn injury, from metabolic and immunologic changes, to nutrition effects on wound healing. Chapters 39–44 cover nonthermal injuries such as electrical, cold-induced, chemical, and radiation injuries, and exfoliative and necrotizing diseases of the integument. Chapters 45–48 cover pathophysiology. Chapters 49–51 discuss rehabilitation. Chapters 52–59 deal with the reconstruction of various body parts. Chapters 60–63, discuss social issues such as ethical dimensions, maltreatment, functional and disability assessment, and cost control and outcome measures. Chapters 64–66, cover psychological issues, including pain and discomfort management, psychiatric disorders associated with burn injury, and psychosocial recovery of the burn patients. This third edition of this definitive reference covers all of the latest advances in the treatment of burns, with full-color layout, new color illustrations, and clinical photographs. This book was on the Brandon/Hill list and is currently a *Doody's Core Titles* essential purchase recommendation for plastic surgery.

Journals

Aesthetic Plastic Surgery. v. 1, Springer, 1976.
http://www.springerlink.com/content/0364-216X/
ISSN: 0364216X
ISSN: 14325241 (Online)
Indexed in: MEDLINE
Recommended for: Academic Libraries

Aesthetic Plastic Surgery is the official journal of the International Society of Aesthetic Plastic Surgery. This peer-reviewed journal publishes original research dealing with all aspects of aesthetic plastic surgery of all parts of the body. Its focus is on the technique of surgery, although it also covers surgical complications. The journal also includes articles on the use of aesthetic plastic surgery as the final step in the complex process of reconstructive surgeries for defects that are congenital, accidental, or disease related. Other topics that are in scope for this journal probe some of the issues surrounding the psychosocial aspects of the use of aesthetic plastic surgery. The journal is indexed by numerous abstracting and indexing sources including Current

Contents, Embase, MEDLINE, Science Citation Index, Scopus, and Web of Science. Online access from volume 1, 1976 is available from the publisher.

Annals of Plastic Surgery. v. 1, Lippincott Williams & Wilkins, 1978.
http://www.annalsplasticsurgery.com
http://www.ovid.com/
ISSN: 01487043
ISSN: 15363708 (Online)
Indexed in: MEDLINE
Recommended for: Academic Libraries

Annals of Plastic Surgery is an independent journal devoted to general plastic and reconstructive surgery. This monthly peer-reviewed journal aims to provide a forum for current scientific and clinical advances in the field, as well as ideas and perspectives on its future. The journal publishes original research articles, brief communications, case reports, and notes in areas of interest to the practicing plastic surgeon. Content also includes historical and current reviews, descriptions of surgical technique, editorials, and letters to the editor. It is indexed in numerous major indexing and abstracting sources including CAB Abstracts, Embase, MEDLINE, Science Citation Index, Scopus, and Web of Science. Online access from volume 1, 1978 is available from Ovid.

Archives of Facial Plastic Surgery. v. 1, American Medical Association, 1999.
http://archfaci.ama-assn.org
ISSN: 15212491
ISSN: 15383660 (Online)
Indexed in: MEDLINE
Recommended for: Academic Libraries

Archives of Facial Plastic Surgery is the official publication of the American Academy of Facial Plastic and Reconstructive Surgery, the European Academy of Facial Plastic Surgery, and the International Federation of Facial Plastic Surgery Societies. It is an international peer-reviewed journal published six times a year. It intends to cover all aspects of reconstructive and cosmetic surgery of the head and neck, focusing on advances in reconstructive and aesthetic procedures, while also emphasizing the basic sciences related to facial development and wound healing. The journal also publishes occasional theme issues on topics such as facial rejuvenation, biotechnology, rhinoplasty and vascular birthmarks. It is indexed in many of the key abstracting and indexing sources including Embase, MEDLINE, Scopus, and Web of Science. Online access to volume 1, 1999 is available from the publisher.

Clinics in Plastic Surgery. v. 1, Elsevier, 1974.
http://www.plasticsurgery.theclinics.com
http://www.sciencedirect.com/science/journal/00941298
http://www.mdconsult.com/
ISSN: 00941298
ISSN: 15580504 (Online)
Indexed in: MEDLINE
Recommended for: Academic Libraries

Clinics in Plastic Surgery publishes comprehensive reviews by experts in the field of plastic, reconstructive, and aesthetic surgery. This peer-reviewed journal published four issues in a year, with each issue of focusing on a single topic relevant to plastic surgery. Recent issue topics include: abdominoplasty, rhinoplasty, cutaneous melanoma, burns, aesthetic facial reconstruction, emerging techniques in aesthetic plastic surgery, and evidence-based plastic surgery. The journal is indexed by numerous indexing and abstracting sources including Current Contents, Embase, MEDLINE, Science Citation Index, Scopus, and Web of Science. Online access to volume 1, 1974 is available from several publisher products.

Journal of Plastic, Reconstructive & Aesthetic Surgery: JPRAS. v. 59, Elsevier, 2006.
http://www.sciencedirect.com/science/journal/17486815
ISSN: 17486815
ISSN: 18780539 (Online)
Indexed in: MEDLINE
Recommended for: Academic Libraries

Journal of Plastic, Reconstructive & Aesthetic Surgery: JPRAS, a monthly, peer-reviewed journal, is the official journal of the British Association of Plastic, Reconstructive, and Aesthetic Surgeons and is affiliated with the Societa Italiana di Chirurgia Plastica Ricostruttiva ed Estetica. This journal began as the *British Journal of Plastic Surgery* in 1948. This international journal covers all aspects of reconstructive and aesthetic plastic surgery. According to its website, the journal "presents the latest surgical procedures with audit and outcome studies of new and established techniques in plastic surgery including: cleft lip and palate and other head and neck surgery, hand surgery, lower limb trauma, burns, skin cancer, breast surgery and aesthetic surgery." In addition to the original research papers, the journal also publishes comprehensive review articles, letters to the editor, and book reviews. It is indexed in numerous indexing and abstracting sources including Embase, MEDLINE, Scopus, and Web of Science. Online access back to 2006 is available from the publisher.

Plastic and Reconstructive Surgery. v. 31, Lippincott Williams & Wilkins, 1963.
http://journals.lww.com/plasreconsurg/
http://www.ovid.com/
ISSN: 00321052
ISSN: 15284242 (Online)
Indexed in: MEDLINE
Recommended for: Academic Libraries
Brandon/Hill Selection

Plastic and Reconstructive Surgery is the official journal of several surgical societies including the American Society of Plastic Surgeons, the American Society of Plastic and Reconstructive Surgery, the American Society for Aesthetic Plastic Surgery and the American Society of Maxillofacial Surgeons. This monthly peer-reviewed journal publishes original clinical or laboratory research, surgical procedures, comprehensive reviews, selected ideas and innovations, letters, case reports, and symposia from its connected societies. The journal covers the latest techniques for procedures such as maxillofacial reconstruction, burn repair, and cosmetic reshaping. In addition it publishes special topics in irregular supplement issues. It is indexed in numerous indexing and abstracting sources including Embase, MEDLINE, Scopus, and Web of Science. Online access back to 1963 is available through Ovid.

Wound Repair and Regeneration. v. 1, Wiley-Blackwell, 1993.
http://onlinelibrary.wiley.com/journal/10.1111/(ISSN)1524-475X
ISSN: 10671927
ISSN: 1524475X (Online)
Indexed in: MEDLINE, CINAHL
Recommended for: Academic Libraries

Wound Repair and Regeneration, the international peer-reviewed journal, is the official journal of The Wound Healing Society, the European Tissue Repair Society, the Japanese Society for Wound Healing, and the Australian Wound Management Association. According to its web-site overview, the journal "provides extensive international coverage of cellular and molecular biology, connective tissue, and biological mediator studies in the field of tissue repair and regeneration." It achieved an impact factor of 2.781 and ranked twelfth out of 48 journals in the dermatology category and twenty-fifth out of 166 journals in the surgery category (2009 *Journal Citation Reports*). The journal is indexed in numerous indexing and abstracting sources including CAB Abstracts, CINAHL, Embase, MEDLINE, Scopus, and Web of Science. Online access back to 1993 is available from the publisher.

11.11. Thoracic Surgery

Diagnosis and treatment of disorders of the heart, lungs, and esophagus. Two major types of thoracic surgery are classified as pulmonary and cardiovascular.

—MeSH

Contributors: Esther Carrigan, Jie Li

Monographs

Difficult Decisions in Thoracic Surgery: An Evidence-Based Approach. Editor: Mark K. Ferguson. Springer, 2007.
http://www.springerlink.com/content/978-1-84628-384-0
http://www.ebrary.com/
ISBN: 9781846283840
ISBN: 9781846284748 (Online)
Recommended for: Hospital, Academic Libraries
Doody's Core Titles Selection

Difficult Decisions in Thoracic Surgery: An Evidence-Based Approach describes the recommended ideal approach, rather than customary care, in selected clinical situations. The book is organized into eight parts. Part 1, "Background," addresses evidence-based medicine and its levels of evidence, the decision analytic techniques, nonclinical components of surgical decision making, and how patients make decisions with their surgeons. Then the book devotes the following parts on the lung, esophagus, diaphragm, airway, pleura, mediastinum, and chest wall. The chapters contain both evidence-based recommendations and descriptions of surgeons' personal practices based on their experience and the published literature. Chapters are organized around clearly identified recommendations, making possible the identification of useful material at a glance. Over 50 different topics are presented, including a review of available evidence and a general discussion of recommended practice. A unique approach of this book is its emphasis on decision making based on the level of supporting evidence available in specific clinical problems in thoracic surgery. Targeted audiences are practicing thoracic and general surgeons, and thoracic and general surgeons in training. It is currently a *Doody's Core Titles* essential purchase recommendation for thoracic surgery.

General Thoracic Surgery. 7th ed. Editors: Thomas W. Shields, Joseph LoCicero III, Ronald B. Ponn, Valerie W. Rusch. Lippincott Williams & Wilkins, 2009.
http://www.ovid.com/

ISBN: 9780781779821
Recommended for: Hospital, Academic Libraries
Brandon/Hill, *Doody's Core Titles* Selection

This comprehensive two-volume textbook of thoracic surgery thoroughly covers open and endoscopic surgical technique. Written by renowned thoracic surgeons, it is considered the bible in the field. The book is divided into three parts: Part A, "The Lung, Pleura, Diaphragm, and Chest Wall," Part B, "Esophagus," and Part C, "The Mediastinum." Each part is further divided into sections and then chapters, covering specific diseases in each category in detail: anatomy and embryology, physiology, invasive and noninvasive diagnostics, therapeutic intervention, and radiological sections. Diseases covered are organized into congenital, infectious/inflammatory, and malignant conditions. There are extensive sections on lung cancer and other pulmonary tumors. Multidisciplinary contributions on medical treatment, radiation oncology, surgery, and anesthesia are included. The primary audience is the practicing surgeon treating thoracic diseases or the surgical resident. This book was on the Brandon/Hill list for the small medical library for surgery and is currently a *Doody's Core Titles* essential purchase recommendation for thoracic surgery.

Johns Hopkins Manual of Cardiothoracic Surgery. Editors: David D. Yuh, Luca A. Vricella, William A. Baumgartner. McGraw-Hill, 2007.
http://www.r2library.com/
ISBN: 9780071416528
Recommended for: Hospital, Academic Libraries

The Johns Hopkins Manual of Cardiothoracic Surgery is a comprehensive single-volume guide to adult, congenital, and general cardiothoracic surgery. It synthesizes cardiac, esophageal, and thoracic surgery into a single, accessible volume. Using Johns Hopkins surgical center's leading-edge cardiothoracic surgical training programs, this heavily illustrated reference features a highly technique-oriented and consistent approach to thoracic surgery. It contains precise information on surgical techniques and pre-and postoperative strategies for managing cardiothoracic disease. The 80 chapters of the book are organized into three chapters covering general thoracic surgery, adult cardiac surgery, and congenital cardiac surgery. It provides an in-depth look at the full spectrum of disorders and their surgical (and medical) management options, including congenital, acquired, and neoplastic diseases. Supporting this detailed coverage is an easy-to-navigate format featuring focused tables and outline-formatted bullets, along with step-by-step explanations of the most complex operations. It provides thorough coverage of all major areas of cardiothoracic surgery, which makes it a perfect resource for cardiothoracic surgery fellows getting ready for oral and written Board review exams and cardiothoracic surgeons preparing for Board certification or recertification. It also provides skill-building perspectives on open, minimally invasive, and endovascular surgical procedures, complete with relevant surgical anatomy.

Mastery of Cardiothoracic Surgery. 2nd ed. Editors: Larry R. Kaiser, Irving L. Kron, Thomas L. Spray. Lippincott Williams & Wilkins, 2007.
http://www.ovid.com/
ISBN: 9780781752091
Recommended for: Hospital, Academic Libraries
Doody's Core Titles Selection

Mastery of Cardiothoracic Surgery was modeled after the successful *Mastery of Surgery*. This book is a comprehensive, yet concise guide to all cardiothoracic surgical procedures for adults and children. More than 130 master surgeons describe their techniques step by step and explain the decision-making that is crucial to a successful outcome. The book provides a comprehensive overview of various topics related to general thoracic surgery, adult cardiac surgery, and congenital cardiac surgery. It covers preoperative diagnosis, management, innovative techniques, robotic and minimally invasive procedures, and postoperative follow-up and prognosis. The book contains more than 900 detailed drawings of key surgical procedures and over 100 photographs, scans, and radiographs. Editorial comments in each chapter provide additional or alternative views. This book provides a thorough understanding of the important principles in cardiothoracic surgery. It is currently a *Doody's Core Titles* recommendation for thoracic surgery.

Operative Thoracic Surgery. 5th ed. Editors: Larry R. Kaiser, Glyn G. Jamieson. Oxford University Press, 2006.
ISBN: 9780340759738
Recommended for: Hospital, Academic Libraries
Doody's Core Titles Selection

Previous editions of *Operative Thoracic Surgery* have established it as a key guide in the field. A comprehensive reference, the book provides clear, concise, step-by-step operative instructions for a wide range of general thoracic operations, covering both open and minimally invasive procedures. Most chapters begin with a history, then proceed to principles and justification, preoperative assessment and preparation, operation, postoperative care, and outcome. The fifth edition has been entirely updated and revised. Each operative procedure is illustrated through a series of high-quality, full-color line illustrations, with detailed notes on operative technique. Additional text describes the principles and justification of choosing each procedure, pre-operative assessment and preparation, and post-operative care and outcomes. The intended audience for this text is surgeons in training and in practice, those preparing for the U.S. Surgical Boards, or experienced thoracic and cardiothoracic surgeons approaching unfamiliar or uncommon procedures. It is currently a *Doody's Core Titles* selection.

Pearson's Thoracic and Esophageal Surgery. 3rd ed. Editors: Alexander G. Patterson, Joel D. Cooper, Jean Deslauriers, Antoon E. Lerut, James D. Luketich, Thomas W. Rice. Churchill Livingstone Elsevier, 2008.
ISBN: 9780443068614
Recommended for: Hospital, Academic Libraries
Doody's Core Titles Selection

Pearson's Thoracic and Esophageal Surgery, a comprehensive two-volume resource, covers the entire range of esophageal and thoracic surgery for adults and children. It addresses all surgical diseases of the chest wall, chest cavity, upper airway, lungs, pleura, and diaphragm and presents clinical commentary at the end of each chapter that offers a variety of viewpoints regarding the pros, cons, and complications associated with the techniques used to treat a patient. This book provides state-of-the-art, clear how-to-do-it guidance on the latest surgical techniques for the treatment of lung infections, lung cancer, benign conditions, trauma, reflux, and more. A new full-color design presents outstanding visual guidance. The book comes with access to the complete contents online as an Expert Consult series title, offering individual purchasers enhanced access to the text. It is currently a *Doody's Core Titles* essential purchase recommendation for thoracic surgery.

Sabiston & Spencer Surgery of the Chest. 8th ed. Editors: Frank W. Sellke, Pedro J. del Nido, Scott J. Swanson. Saunders Elsevier, 2010.
http://www.mdconsult.com/
ISBN: 9781416052258 (set)
Recommended for: Hospital, Academic Libraries
Doody's Core Titles Selection

Sabiston & Spencer Surgery of the Chest is the classic reference work in the field of thoracic surgery. This comprehensive, thorough two-volume set encompasses about 2,500 pages. Its 134 chapters are organized into three major sections: "Thoracic Surgery," "Adult Cardiac Surgery," and "Congenital Heart Surgery." General thoracic surgery is covered in 46 chapters. Adult cardiac surgery spans 58 chapters, while congenital heart surgery is covered in 30 chapters, making the cardiac surgery content the largest portion of the work. This eighth edition boasts nearly 1,100 illustrations to clarify procedures and concepts. New content to this edition includes coverage of technique advances in mitral valve surgery, advances in congenital heart disease treatments, minimally invasive approaches for adult and congenital cardiac and thoracic surgery, stent grafting, and cellular therapies. This classic reference is an essential purchase for any hospital, special, or academic library that supports thoracic surgery training or practice.

Thoracic Surgery Atlas. Author: Mark K. Ferguson. Saunders Elsevier, 2007.
ISBN: 9780721603254
Recommended for: Hospital, Academic Libraries
Doody's Core Titles Selection

In this highly illustrated, comprehensive review of general thoracic surgery, the author of *Thoracic Surgery Atlas* shares some of his valuable experience-based observations to help guide the practitioner through details of complex procedures, avoid common problems, and manage complications when they occur. Each chapter is liberally illustrated with original line drawings that depict the relevant anatomy and steps associated with each procedure. The book is organized in 11 chapters describing and illustrating incisions, minimally invasive approaches, lung, chest wall, mediastinum, esophagus, thoracic duct, sympathetic chain, diaphragm, major airways and pleura. It is currently a *Doody's Core Titles* selection.

Journals

Annals of Thoracic Surgery. v. 1, Elsevier, 1965.
http://sciencedirect.com/science/journal/00034975
ISSN: 00034975
ISSN: 15526259 (Online)
Indexed in: MEDLINE
Recommended for: Hospital, Academic Libraries
Brandon/Hill Selection

This peer-reviewed journal is the official publication of the Society of Thoracic Surgeons and the Southern Thoracic Surgical Association., the two largest U.S. specialty surgery associations. Its focus is recent progress in chest and cardiovascular surgery and related fields. According to its online aims and scope statement, in addition to original research articles, the journal publishes "new technology articles, case reports, "How-to-do-it" features, reviews of current literature, supplements on symposia, commentary pieces and correspondence and CMEs."

The journal was on the Bandon/Hill list for the small medical library for surgery and is a National Library of Medicine core clinical journal. It is indexed in numerous indexing and abstracting sources including CAB Abstracts, Embase, MEDLINE, Scopus, and Web of Science. Online access back to 1995 is available from the publisher.

European Journal of Cardio-Thoracic Surgery: Official Journal of the European Association for Cardio-Thoracic Surgery. v. 1, Elsevier, 1987.
http://sciencedirect.com/science/journal/10107940
ISSN: 10107940
ISSN: 1873734X (Online)
Indexed in: MEDLINE
Recommended for: Hospital, Academic Libraries

This peer-reviewed monthly journal is the official journal of the European Association for Cardio-Thoracic Surgery and the European Society of Thoracic Surgeons. It is truly international in scope, being supported by the specialty societies for cardio-thoracic surgery of Austria, Great Britain and Ireland, The Netherlands, Poland, Portugal, and Scandinavia. According to its online aims and scope statement, the journal "publishes reports of significant clinical and experimental advances related to surgery of the heart, the great vessels and the chest. Special emphasis is placed on contributions from the European countries." In addition to the original research articles the journal also publishes case reports, surgical technique reports, reviews, images, editorials, letters to the editor, and selected papers from the annual meetings of the European Association for Cardio-Thoracic Surgery. It is indexed in numerous indexing and abstracting sources including CAB Abstracts, Embase, MEDLINE, Scopus, and Web of Science. Online access back to 1987 is available from the publisher.

Journal of Thoracic and Cardiovascular Surgery. v. 1, Mosby Elsevier, 1959.
http://www.sciencedirect.com/science/journal/00225223
ISSN: 00225223
ISSN: 1097685X (Online)
Indexed in: MEDLINE
Recommended for: Hospital, Academic Libraries
Brandon/Hill Selection

The *Journal of Thoracic and Cardiovascular Surgery* is an official publication of the American Association for Thoracic Surgery and the Western Thoracic Surgical Association. According to its online aims and scope statement, this peer-reviewed journal covers "conditions of the chest, heart, lungs, and great vessels where surgical intervention is indicated." Its focus is on development in techniques and procedures for a wide array of thoracic and cardiovascular surgeries. The journal was on Bandon/Hill list for the small medical library and is a National Library of Medicine core clinical title. It is indexed in numerous indexing and abstracting sources including Embase, MEDLINE, Scopus, and Web of Science. Online access back to 1995 is available from Elsevier.

11.12. Urology

The study, diagnosis, and treatment of diseases of the urinary tract in both sexes, and the genital tract in the male. Common urological problems include urinary obstruction, urinary incontinence, infections, and urogenital neoplasms.
—MeSH

Contributor: David C. Stewart

Monographs

Campbell-Walsh Urology. 9th ed. Editors: Alan J. Wein, Louis R. Kavoussi. Saunders Elsevier, 2007.
http://www.mdconsult.com/
ISBN: 9780721607986
ISBN: 9781416029663 (Online)
Recommended for: Hospital, Academic Libraries
Brandon/Hill, *Doody's Core Titles* Selection

Campbell-Walsh Urology is the leading textbook in its field. A Brandon/Hill title first published in 1954, *Campbell-Walsh Urology* is now in its ninth edition. Every area of urology is covered in four volumes with 130 chapters written by over 150 leading international specialists. Volume one covers anatomy with emphases on clinical decision making, surgery, infections, and molecular and cellular biology. Volume two concentrates on renal physiology, renal failure, and urinary neoplasms. Volume three looks at urine transport and storage, bladder function, and the prostate, while volume four is devoted entirely to pediatric urology. Numerous photographs, other illustrations, charts, graphs, and tables are found, most in full color. An electronic version of the textbook is available through Elsevier's MD Consult. This textbook can be used by students, residents, and practicing physicians and is recommended for all medical libraries.

Diseases of the Kidney and Urinary Tract. 8th ed. Editor: Robert W. Schrier. Wolters Kluwer Health/Lippincott Williams & Wilkins, 2007.

http://www.ovid.com/
http://www.r2library.com/
ISBN: 9780781793070
Recommended for: Academic Libraries
Brandon/Hill, *Doody's Core Titles* Selection

This three-volume work continues to be one of the most comprehensive textbooks in the field of nephrology. Formerly a Brandon/Hill title as *Diseases of the Kidney*, it has also been included in *Doody's* core collection. Written for practicing and academic physicians, *Diseases of the Kidney and Urinary Tract* incorporates the latest information into 14 sections. The first section, "Biochemical, Structural, and Functional Correlations in the Kidney," concentrates on the cellular and molecular aspects of the kidney. The next 12 sections are disease-oriented with the introductory chapter to each section presenting the pathophysiologic aspects of the specific disease. The fourteenth and final section covers the effects of nutrition on kidney disease and drug dosing recommendations in kidney failure. This text would not be essential for small medical libraries but is certainly a must for large academic libraries.

Smith's General Urology. 17th ed. Editors: Emil A. Tanagho, Jack W. McAninch. McGraw-Hill, 2008.
http://www.accessmedicine.com/
ISBN: 9780071457378
Recommended for: Hospital, Academic Libraries
Brandon/Hill, *Doody's Core Titles* Selection

Smith's General Urology is one of the leading textbooks in its field and is listed as an essential purchase in *Doody's* core collection. Written for medical students, residents, as well as practicing physicians, *Smith's General Urology* provides concise information on the physiology, diagnosis and treatment of urologic disorders. Forty-five chapters written by more than 30 physicians cover a wide range of topics including female urology, the older male, skin diseases of external genitalia, and abnormalities of sexual determination and differentiation. An appendix of normal laboratory values for blood, plasma, serum, and urine should be useful to the student. This text is recommended for all medical libraries.

Journals

BJU International. v. 83, Blackwell Science, 1999.
http://onlinelibrary.wiley.com/journal/10.1111/(ISSN)1464-410X
ISSN: 14644096
ISSN: 1464410X (Online)
Indexed in: MEDLINE
Recommended for: Academic Libraries

Originally known as the *British Journal of Urology*, *BJU International* is the official publication of the British Association of Urological Surgeons, the Urological Society of Australasia, and the Urological Society of India. *Journal Citation Reports* (2009) ranks it as fifteenth out of the 63 urology/nephrology journals listed. Continuously published since 1929, *BJU International* is also available online. Besides the latest research in the field of urology, *BJU International* also has a singular feature called "Surgery Illustrated" in which a surgical step is highlighted by demonstrating the technique required and how such a step modifies an already existing procedure with examples of its benefits or complications. Indexed by the leading bibliographic databases, *BJU International* is recommended for academic medical libraries.

European Urology. v. 1, Elsevier, 1975.
http://www.europeanurology.com/
ISSN: 03022838
Indexed in: MEDLINE
Recommended for: Academic Libraries

The official publication of the European Association of Urology, *European Urology* is published in print and online every month. Its peer-reviewed articles cover oncology, impotence, infertility, and pediatrics as well as recent advances in urologic surgery. Original articles report on basic and translational research, and the epidemiology, pathophysiology, diagnosis, surgical treatment, and minimally-invasive therapies related to urologic diseases. Review articles "systematically find, select, critique, and synthesize evidence relevant to well defined questions about diagnosis, therapy, and prognosis." Specific surgical techniques are highlighted in the "Surgery in Motion" section. A unique feature is the "Resident's Corner" section where original articles written by residents are published. Three articles per issue are selected by the editor as CME credit articles. Recommended for academic medical libraries.

Journal of Urology. v. 1, Elsevier, 1917.
http://jurology.com
ISSN: 00225347
ISSN: 15273792 (Online)
Indexed in: MEDLINE
Recommended for: Hospital, Academic Libraries
Brandon/Hill Selection

The official journal of the American Urological Association, Inc., the *Journal of Urology* is the standard for physicians in the field. With an impact factor of 4.016 in the *Journal Citation Reports* 2009 rankings, the *Journal of Urology* is one of the most widely read and highly cited urology journals. A major focus of its publishing mission is to translate the latest research into clinical practice. All areas of urology are covered including pediatrics, oncology, neurology, transplantation, and infertility. A Brandon/Hill initial-purchase title, it is recommended for all medical libraries.

12. Nursing

Nursing care concerned with the promotion, maintenance, and restoration of health.

—MeSH

Contributor: Richard J. Barry

Monographs

Clinical Nursing Skills & Techniques. 7th ed. Authors: Anne G. Perry, Patricia A. Potter. Mosby Elsevier, 2010.
ISBN: 9780323052894
Recommended for: Hospital, Academic Libraries
Doody's Core Titles Selection

This text provides a clear, direct presentation of more than 250 nursing skills and procedures. At over 1,300 pages, it is comprehensive and substantive, showing the skill of the editors in digesting and organizing material for optimal learning. A student with poor study skills will learn not only the needed nursing skills, procedures, and techniques but subliminally experience well-organized presentations of pertinent information for quality patient care. Information is supplemented with clear illustrations demonstrating key steps and techniques. Basic, intermediate, and advanced skills have been incorporated with an appreciation for the application of technology to assist the nursing process. Knowledgeable practitioners use all available tools from evidence-based practice to developments in technology to optimize the applicable nursing and health care process. Guidelines for universal precautions are incorporated and age specific pediatric and geriatric guidelines are included in developmental considerations. Enhanced content is available to individuals through the Evolve companion website.

Essentials of Nursing Informatics. 4th ed. Editors: Virginia K. Saba, Kathleen A. McCormick. McGraw-Hill, 2006.
See Chapter 6.3. Informatics

Fundamental Skills and Concepts in Patient Care. 9th ed. Author: Barbara K. Timby. Wolters Kluwer Health/ Lippincott Williams & Wilkins, 2008.
ISBN: 9780781779098
Recommended for: Hospital, Academic Libraries

Basic nursing skills are presented to the student nurse in such a way that they develop a knowledge base adaptable to nursing process and the needs of the immediate patient. The connection between theory and practice is accomplished, making this a useful text to well prepare practitioners. Students are increasingly visually based, growing up in our media soaked culture. The additional new illustrations in this edition build on this while emphasizing the key terms, concepts, and skills required. The current edition has a much-needed emphasis on geriatric care, given that this is the fastest-growing segment of our population. This is a good foundational text that provides critical thinking exercises, readings for further study (which helps to train for life-long learning), and Internet resources. This text also presents nursing skills applicable to diverse settings. The presentation of information helps students organize and focus their learning habits.

Fundamentals of Nursing: Human Health and Function. 6th ed. Editors: Ruth F. Craven, Constance J. Hirnle. Wolters Kluwer Health/Lippincott Williams & Wilkins, 2009.
ISBN: 9780781780230
Recommended for: Hospital, Academic Libraries
Doody's Core Titles Selection

This text seeks to teach health in a universal context by tapping into nursing constants: promotion and maintenance of individual, family, and community health; management of a healthy environment; and care of the ill. The over 1,500 pages and 52 chapters are organized into 17 units covering: delivery of nursing; essential concepts; nursing process; human function and nursing management; assessment; nursing therapeutics; health perception and health management; activity and exercise; nutrition and metabolism; elimination; sleep and rest; cognition and perception; self-perception and self-concept; roles and relationships; coping and stress management; sexuality and reproduction; and values and beliefs. The art and science of nursing are woven into each page as students learn about the health, function, and wellness of the person. Linked with art and science are appropriate selection (critical thinking) and nursing interventions to support and assist the patient toward health. As a parallel to the nursing process focus on the whole person, this text focuses on the whole person of nursing students to help them appreciate the role they play in health care, in society, and in the nursing profession.

Fundamentals of Nursing: The Art and Science of Nursing Care. 7th ed. Authors: Carol Taylor, Carol Lillis, Priscilla LeMone, Pamela Lynn. Lippincott Williams & Wilkins, 2011.
ISBN: 9780781793834
Recommended for: Hospital, Academic Libraries

This text clearly presents basic skills and develops them with increasing complexity to accommodate a variety of learning styles. The illustrations and images enhance the student's understanding of the skill being studied. An accompanying CD-ROM provides video clips. Appropriate emphasis is placed on documentation, knowing current practice guidelines, and the essential monitoring of research and evidence-based practice as the foundations of life-long learning for successful practice and quality patient outcomes. This review refers to the sixth edition, which continues the holistic approach in nursing care, utilizing critical thinking and case study for a complete understanding. The authors work to communicate to the students the array of qualities that constitute excellence in the profession by blending theory, technology, ethics, and guidelines with their individual personal involvement for quality patient outcomes.

Health Promotion Strategies through the Life Span. 8th ed. Authors: Ruth B. Murray, Judith P. Zentner, Richard Yakimo. Pearson Prentice Hall, 2009.
http://www.R2Library.com/
http://online.statref.com/titleinfo/fxid-328.html
ISBN: 9780135138663
Recommended for: Hospital, Academic Libraries

There is a positive approach in this text about health promotion and understanding normal individuals and families in context. The concept is direct, understanding what is within normal parameters, and when needed, the exception can be managed. This text requires critical thinking on the part of the practitioner to assess the whole person in his situation and then to select and adapt appropriate nursing interventions. This is not a clinical text focused on treatment of disease but a text that takes the broad view of the physical, emotional, psychological, spiritual, and social elements that play a role in presentation of the patient for treatment. The long vision across the life span is so important, especially presenting the last phase of life, death and dying. This is a useful text for both basic and advanced nursing programs. Practicing nurses who may not have been exposed to this text previously can benefit from the life span approach to health promotion for the individual and the family in context.

Kozier & Erb's Fundamentals of Nursing: Concepts, Process and Practice. 8th ed. Authors: Audrey Berman, Barbara Kozier, Glenora Erb, Shirlee J. Snyder. Pearson Prentice Hall, 2008.
http://online.statref.com/
http://www.R2Library.com/
ISBN: 9780131714687
Recommended for: Hospital, Academic Libraries
Doody's Core Titles Selection

Nurse educators/authors present a comprehensive framework for the nursing process in a clear and concise manner. Practical applications and real-world scenarios give the entry level student appropriate orientation to the basics of the profession. The over 1,600 pages in this text are organized into 10 units and 52 chapters, which unfold the complex world of health care, communicating the need for flexibility and creativity to accomplish good patient care. A chapter on elders has been added to this edition along with a new chapter on the vital role of communications. Developments in nursing process and procedures are incorporated with each section and include advances in equipment and technology that support the nursing process. Stories from novice nurses help students begin to understand the transition from theory to the hands-on world of practice.

Lippincott Manual of Nursing Practice. 9th ed. Author: Sandra M. Nettina. Lippincott William & Wilkins, 2010.
http://www.ovid.com/
ISBN: 9780781798334
Recommended for: Hospital, Academic Libraries

Now in its ninth edition, this classic text provides demonstrated outline content presentations for comprehensive nursing education. The awareness of specialty practice areas is a unique dimension of this work. Blending of the medical model with the nursing model for organizing material results in nurses prepared to think and act toward quality outcomes. Its over 1,900 pages are organized into five sections; the entire nursing process is covered and the whole patient scenario is discussed. Extensive use is made of policies and guidelines from government and nursing professional bodies that shape clinical practice. Best practices, evidence-based care, and quality initiatives are infused into the text. There is good coverage of documentation including security for electronic medical records.

Journals

American Journal of Nursing. v. 1, Lippincott Williams & Wilkins, 1900.
http://journals.lww.com/ajnonline/
ISSN: 0002936X
ISSN: 15387488 (Online)
See Also Chapter 13.20. Practical Nursing
Indexed in: MEDLINE, CINAHL
Recommended for: Hospital, Academic Libraries
Brandon/Hill Selection

AJN has application to a variety of settings reflective of the diversity of regular important features of this evidence-based peer-reviewed journal. Value to student and clinical nurses can be found in the CE articles that instruct nurses on the theory and practice of quality patient care. Practical direction for procedures are demonstrated in the "Try This" section that is nicely complemented by an online media presentation. Keeping track of developments in the broader professional world is made possible with short news stories relevant to the professional nurse. Other features of value include the regional focus on job openings and personal contributions from nurses in the form of stories or poems. This journal is indexed in numerous indexing and abstracting sources including CINAHL, Embase, International Nursing Index, MEDLINE, Scopus, and Web of Science. It is available in both print and online formats. Online access back to 1900 is available from the publisher through Ovid, and access to issue from 1900-2002 is available through JSTOR. At present the archival database issues are not fully indexed, there are missing issues, and some citations are not correctly matched to the full text, but it is still a valuable resource for the historical dimensions of American nursing.

ANS: Advances in Nursing Science. v. 1, Lippincott Williams & Wilkins, 1978.
http://journals.lww.com/advancesinnursingscience/
ISSN: 01619268
ISSN: 15505014 (Online)
See Also Chapter 12.1. Nursing Research
Indexed in: MEDLINE, CINAHL
Recommended for: Hospital, Academic Libraries
Brandon/Hill Selection

This journal aims to contribute to the development of nursing science and the application of research and theory to practice. As a profession, nursing needs good science as a basis for practice, and this journal consistently supports the science of nursing. Each issue has a single focus topic. Recent issue topics include: emancipatory scholarship; nursing essentials; practice-based evidence; and trauma and stress. Various facets of influence on practice such as theory development, concept analysis, and studying the values and ethics influencing practice and research can be found in the journal articles. "Advance" is to move forward and this journal does take new approaches and perspectives on nursing practice today. This quarterly journal is peer-reviewed and a necessary part of any doctoral program. It is indexed in numerous indexing and abstracting sources including CINAHL, Embase, International Nursing Index, MEDLINE, Scopus, and Web of Science. Online access back to 1978 is available from the publisher.

Journal of Advanced Nursing. v. 1, Wiley Blackwell, 1976.
http://www.journalofadvancednursing.com/
http://onlinelibrary.wiley.com/journal/10.1111/(ISSN)1365-2648
ISSN: 03092402
ISSN: 13652648 (Online)
Indexed in: MEDLINE, CINAHL
Recommended for: Hospital, Academic Libraries

Advancing knowledge in nursing practice, education, management, or policy are some of the areas covered by the research and scholarship of this UK-based peer-reviewed journal. Reviews of practice protocols and issues that affect nursing and midwifery are regular features. The journal publishes original research material with good scientific basis to advance practice. This international scientific journal covers evidence-based nursing, midwifery, and health care. Practicing nurses and student nurses will learn from the theoretical, philosophical, and practical approaches to quality patient care. This journal is important for nursing collections because of the culturally diverse perspectives it presents as well as a health care context from around the world. Other topics covered include professional development, interdisciplinary collaboration, and advances in education and policy. It is indexed in numerous indexing and abstracting sources including CINAHL, Embase, International Nursing Index, MEDLINE, Scopus, and Web of Science. Online access back to 1976 is available from the publisher.

Journal of Nursing Administration. v. 1, Lippincott Williams & Wilkins, 1971.
http://journals.lww.com/jonajournal/
ISSN: 00020443
ISSN: 15390721 (Online)
Indexed in: MEDLINE, CINAHL
Recommended for: Hospital, Academic Libraries

This peer-reviewed journal is focused on management and leadership issues that involve nurses and nursing practice. Except for the May issue, which addresses theoretical research, the focus is on practical issues such as leadership development; management issues; legal, corporate, ethical and other issues with administration of resources; and advancing patient care leadership. This practical hands-on approach allows the reader to quickly evaluate the usefulness of the system, model, or theory described. Although the journal is intended for those already in leadership and administrative positions, nurses not in these roles can benefit from this journal by learning what is needed to move into a leadership role. Institutions that subscribe to *JONA* will also receive the quarterly publication *JONA's Healthcare Law, Ethics and Regulation*. It is indexed in numerous indexing and abstracting sources including CINAHL, Embase, International Nursing Index, MEDLINE, Scopus, and Web of Science. Online access back to 1971 is available from the publisher through Ovid.

Journal of Nursing Scholarship. v. 32, Wiley Blackwell, 2000.
http://onlinelibrary.wiley.com/journal/10.1111/(ISSN)1547-5069
ISSN: 15276546
ISSN: 15475069 (Online)
Indexed in: MEDLINE, CINAHL
Recommended for: Hospital, Academic Libraries

This international peer-reviewed journal is the official journal of Sigma Theta Tau International, the honor society of nursing. It provides thought-provoking articles on scholarly areas of clinical scholarship, health policy and systems, profession and society, and world health. The journal aims to reach health professionals, faculty, and students in this time of global concern regarding health issues that can have local and international impact. It ranked eleventh of 70 journals in nursing (social science) and twelfth of 72 journals in nursing (science), with an impact factor of 1.459 (2009 *Journal Citation Reports*). It is indexed in numerous indexing and abstracting sources including CINAHL, Embase, International Nursing Index, MEDLINE, Scopus, and Web of Science. Online access back to 2000 is available from the publisher and several other sources.

Nursing Research. v. 1, Lippincott Williams & Wilkins, 1952.
http://journals.lww.com/nursingresearchonline/
ISSN: 00296562
ISSN: 15389847 (Online)
See Also Chapter 12.1. Nursing Research
Indexed in: MEDLINE, CINAHL
Recommended for: Hospital, Academic Libraries

This peer-reviewed journal is the official journal of the Eastern Nursing Research Society and the Western Institute of Nursing. The science that supports the profession of nursing needs to be accessible to members; *Nursing Research* fulfills this by presenting basic and clinical research studies to understand health and illness issues of individuals, families, and communities. Research on symptom management, human response to disease, and health promotion is woven throughout the content of this bi-monthly journal. Other topics covered include working with vulnerable populations, cost-effective models of care and community-based nursing studies. It is indexed in numerous indexing and abstracting sources including CINAHL, Embase, International Nursing Index, MEDLINE, Scopus, and Web of Science. Online access back to 1952 is available from the publisher through Ovid. This journal is a long-standing pillar that supports the nursing profession through research for the practice setting.

Nursing Times. v. 1, Emap Inform, 1905.
http://www.nursingtimes.net/
ISSN: 09547762
Indexed in: MEDLINE, CINAHL
Recommended for: Hospital, Academic Libraries

This journal, widely applicable across various clinical settings, is an excellent and long-standing contribution from the United Kingdom. Original research is just part of the content along with news, best practices, and opportunities for nurses to share their experiences and opinions. Although not scholarly in nature, the articles present scholarly information in ways that make research more understandable and more readily applicable. Journal issues have a few clinical articles along with the news, opinions, and other material needed to produce a weekly journal. It is indexed in several indexing and abstracting sources including CINAHL, Embase, International Nursing Index, MEDLINE, and Scopus. This is a well-respected journal with content from known international authors; it is important for any nursing collection. Online access is available from EBSCOhost and Ovid. The Nursingtimes.net website embellishes the content of the print journal but also provides journal issue listings for full text.

Research in Nursing & Health. v. 1, Wiley Blackwell, 1978.
http://onlinelibrary.wiley.com/journal/10.1002/(ISSN)1098-240X

ISSN: 01606891
ISSN: 1098240X (Online)
See Also Chapter 12.1. Nursing Research
Indexed in: MEDLINE, CINAHL
Recommended for: Hospital, Academic Libraries

According to its aims and scope statement, this peer-reviewed journal broadly covers research and theory that impact the practice of nursing and other health disciplines. Issue content covers nursing practice, education, administration, and history. Academics will find content on research methods and techniques that contribute to our understanding of the literature. This is one of the few journals in which the synthesis of knowledge and research are presented for a general approach. Some articles reflect the testing of research findings in actual practice. Core topics of interest to advancing nursing practice are covered, providing a solid basis for the practice of nursing. This quarterly journal is indexed in numerous indexing and abstracting sources including CINAHL, Embase, International Nursing Index, MEDLINE, Scopus, and Web of Science. Online access back to 1978 is available from the publisher.

12.1. Nursing Research

Research carried out by nurses, generally in clinical settings, in the areas of clinical practice, evaluation, nursing education, nursing administration, and methodology.

—(MeSH)

Contributor: Janet G. Schnall

Monographs

Nursing Research: Generating and Assessing Evidence for Nursing Practice. 8th ed. Authors: Denise F. Polit, Cheryl Tatano Beck. Wolters Kluwer Health/Lippincott Williams & Wilkins, 2008.
ISBN: 9780781794688
Recommended for: Hospital, Academic Libraries
Doody's Core Titles Selection

Selected as a *Doody's* core title and one of the *American Journal of Nursing* Books of the Year, this well-organized, well-written text is a comprehensive guide to nursing research. It explains the research process as a part of evidence-based practice, including the use of systematic reviews. The text is organized into multiple parts covering foundations of nursing research and evidence-based practice; conceptualizing and designing a study to generate evidence for nursing; collecting, analyzing, and interpreting research data; and building an evidence base for nursing practice. Chapters include critiquing guidelines, actual research examples to reinforce the critical points, practical tips on conducting research, and descriptions of both qualitative and quantitative designs. New to this edition is an emphasis on evidence-based practice, chapters on systematic reviews and development of self-report scales, and an updated title. An accompanying *Resource Manual* includes a Toolkit CD-ROM with methodological tools and documents that can be adapted for individual research. This text is an excellent resource for graduate students learning how to do research as well as those learning to appraise research reports critically and to use research findings in practice.

Nursing Research: Methods and Critical Appraisal for Evidence-Based Practice. 7th ed. Editors: Geri LoBiondo-Wood, Judith Haber. Mosby/Elsevier, 2010.
ISBN: 9780323057431
Recommended for: Hospital, Academic Libraries
Brandon/Hill, *Doody's Core Titles* Selection

This new edition of *Nursing Research* presents a comprehensive introduction to the concepts and methods of nursing research, with an emphasis on evidence-based practice. It was a recommended title on the former Brandon/Hill nursing list, and the sixth edition was selected as one of the *American Journal of Nursing* Books of the Year. The text is divided into four parts: an overview of research and evidence-based practice, including how to develop questions and how to gather and appraise literature; the process of qualitative research, including appraising; the process of quantitative research, such as experimental designs, sampling, ethical issues, reliability, and validity; and the application of research to evidence-based practice. The primary audience for this text is undergraduate students who are learning the research process and critiquing skills; however, graduate students or practicing nurses wanting to review the basics of research and the tools for evidence-based practice will find the book to be of value as well. The seventh edition provides an increased emphasis on evidence-based practice, which addresses ways to appraise and apply research to practice; updated sample research articles; color boxes and tables highlighting key concepts; and a set of Research Appraisal Guidelines placed inside the back cover offering quick reference for evaluating research. An e-book package from Elsevier Evolve is offered for individual purchase by educators and students. This excellent text provides a good foundation for evidence-based practice.

Qualitative Research in Nursing: Advancing the Humanistic Imperative. 4th ed. Authors: Helen J. Streubert Speziale, Dona Rinaldi Carpenter. Lippincott Williams & Wilkins, 2007.
ISBN: 9780781763134
Recommended for: Academic Libraries
Brandon/Hill Selection

Selected as a recommended purchase on the former Brandon/Hill nursing list, this book serves as an introduction to qualitative research methods for the new researcher as well as a reference for the more experienced nursing researcher. It examines a range of currently used qualitative methodologies, including phenomenology, grounded theory, ethnography, historical research, and action research. The authors define the role of the researcher and provide ways to generate and manage data and insure ethical conduct of studies. Chapters present an overview of each method; provide approaches used to apply these methods to nursing practice, education, and administration; and critique guidelines for each method. This book also includes chapters on triangulation, writing a qualitative research proposal with an example of a peer-reviewed funded grant and critique, and guidelines for sharing qualitative research results. New to this edition are updated articles reflecting the latest research methods and applications, along with updated sampling tables. This instructive text provides the information needed to understand and implement qualitative research methods into nursing research.

Statistics for Nursing and Allied Health. Authors: Stacey B. Plichta, Laurel S. Garzon. Wolters Kluwer/Lippincott Williams & Wilkins, 2009.
http://www.r2library.com/
ISBN: 9780781754590
Recommended for: Academic Libraries

This introductory textbook for students focuses on the importance of organizing and describing research data using basic statistics. It explains a comprehensive range of statistical techniques based on SPSS software, with examples from nursing and other health professions. Chapters describe statistical methods, compare means and medians, examine relationships among variables using cross-tabulation tables and correlation coefficients, describe basic model building, and discuss dissemination of findings. This text is useful for students interested in knowing how to analyze data and present the results of evidence-based data analysis.

Understanding Nursing Research: Building an Evidence-Based Practice. 4th ed. Authors: Nancy Burns, Susan K. Grove. Saunders/Elsevier, 2007.
ISBN: 9781416026402
Recommended for: Hospital, Academic Libraries
Brandon/Hill, *Doody's Core Titles* Selection

A *Doody's Core Titles* selection and a recommended purchase on the former Brandon/Hill nursing list, this text, written by two leaders in the nursing research field, introduces quantitative, qualitative, and outcomes nursing research methodologies. It aims to help develop skills in finding, reviewing, and using research in order to build an evidence-based practice. The work is organized into chapters, with each providing an overview and learning outcomes. Chapters cover the following topics: quantitative and qualitative research processes; identifying research problems; purposes and hypotheses; reviewing the literature; understanding theory and research frameworks; examining ethics; clarifying research designs; outcomes research; populations and samples; measurement and data collection; understanding statistics; critiquing research for nursing practice; and how to build an evidence-based practice. The text's primary audience is undergraduate nursing students, although it also serves as a resource for practicing nurses who want to learn how to incorporate evidence into their practice. It is illustrated in color with useful charts, critiquing guidelines, and diagrams. This fourth edition includes new content such as a chapter on outcomes research and updated research examples to include recently published quantitative, qualitative, and outcomes nursing studies. An accompanying CD-ROM (included with print purchase) contains 400 interactive review questions with rationales for correct and incorrect answers and a textbook page reference. For students and educators, an additional Elsevier Evolve e-book package includes test questions for further practice, open-book quizzes, and chapter crossword puzzles. This text helps students learn how to read and critique research articles and then summarize the research evidence in order to apply changes to their clinical practice.

Understanding Nursing Research: Using Research in Evidence-Based Practice. 2nd ed. Authors: Carol L. Macnee, Susan McCabe. Wolters Kluwer Health/Lippincott Williams & Wilkins, 2008.
ISBN: 9780781775588
Recommended for: Academic Libraries
Doody's Core Titles Selection

Selected as a *Doody's* core title, the goal of this text is to help train undergraduate nursing baccalaureate students "to read and comprehend published research, so that they can make professional decisions regarding the use of research reports in evidence-based practice." This user-friendly book is focused on facts needed to use research, not conduct research. The authors' approach is based on their supposition that most nursing students and nurses will only read the abstract and conclusion of research reports. Therefore, they have arranged the book in a novel manner around the sections of a research report rather than the research process. The first two chapters supply an introduction to evidence-based practice and the components and language of research reports. The third and subsequent chapters explain each section of a typical research study, starting with the end—the discussion and conclusions; continuing with background, sampling, and the research problem; and ending with the research process and the role of research in nursing. Each chapter begins with a clinical case to answer a question from a variety of settings from acute care to public health. A discussion follows of one or two published research articles relating to the case including both qualitative and quantitative methods. Chapters conclude with a learning activity for quick review. New to this edition are actual research articles included in the appendix, student outcomes for each chapter, and out-of-class exercises.

Journals

ANS: Advances in Nursing Science. v. 1, Lippincott Williams & Wilkins, 1978.
http://journals.lww.com/advancesinnursingscience/
http://www.ovid.com/
ISSN: 01619268
ISSN: 15505014 (Online)
See Also Chapter 12. Nursing
Indexed in: MEDLINE, CINAHL
Recommended for: Hospital, Academic Libraries
Brandon/Hill Selection

The primary purpose of *ANS: Advances in Nursing Science*, a quarterly, peer-reviewed journal, is to stimulate development of nursing science and promote application in practice of emerging theories and research findings. Each issue features a single, timely research topic, such as "Informatics and Technology," "Women and Aging," and "Health, Human Rights and Poverty," with implications for patient care. Researchers, nurse executives, and graduate students are the main audience for this journal. The journal's impact factor, according to the 2009 *Journal Citation Reports* (*JCR*), is 1.414, and it currently ranks twelfth of 70 titles in the nursing category (social sciences) and thirteenth of 72 titles in the nursing category (sciences). This journal is cited in numerous abstracting and indexing sources such as MEDLINE, CINAHL, Scopus, Social Sciences Citation Index, British Nursing Index, and PsycINFO. *ANS* is a starred recommendation on the former Brandon/Hill nursing list. Full online coverage back to volume 1, 1978 is available through Journals@Ovid.

Applied Nursing Research. v. 1, Saunders/Elsevier, 1988.
http://www.appliednursingresearch.org/
http://www.sciencedirect.com/science/journal/08971897
ISSN: 08971897
ISSN: 15328201 (Online)
Indexed in: MEDLINE, CINAHL
Recommended for: Hospital, Academic Libraries
Brandon/Hill Selection

Begun in 1988, *Applied Nursing Research* is a quarterly, peer-reviewed journal presenting original research findings for clinical applications in all nursing specialties. Regular features include "Ask the Experts," research briefs, clinical methods, book reviews, news and announcements, and editorials. Currently ranked forty-first of 72 journals in the nursing category, with an impact factor of 0.871 (2009 *Journal Citation Reports*), this journal was recommended for purchase in the former Brandon/Hill nursing list. It is indexed in numerous sources such as MEDLINE, CINAHL, Scopus, and Social Sciences Citation Index. Full online coverage back to volume 1, 1988 is available through Elsevier ScienceDirect.

Biological Research for Nursing. v. 1, Sage, 1999.
http://online.sagepub.com/
ISSN: 10998004
ISSN: 15524175 (Online)
Indexed in: MEDLINE, CINAHL
Recommended for: Hospital, Academic Libraries

Begun in 1999, *Biological Research in Nursing* is a quarterly, peer-reviewed journal featuring research papers, empirical and theoretical articles, editorials, abstracts of recent dissertations, and conference summaries relating to: nursing care and normal and abnormal biological phenomena, such as pain management; improvements in health care techniques developed through biological and physiological research; new methods, instruments, and techniques for biological and physiological health research; theoretical foundations that increase understanding of biological and physiological changes in health and illness; and pathophysiology and the biological foundations of nursing practice. Nursing researchers, educators, practitioners, and graduate students are the main audience for this journal, which currently ranks thirty-sixth of 72 journals in the nursing category; it has an impact factor of 0.930 (2009 *Journal Citation Reports*). This journal is indexed by MEDLINE, CINAHL, Scopus, Social Sciences Citation

Index, and more. Full online coverage back to volume 1, 1999 is available through Sage Journals Online.

BMC Nursing. v. 1, BioMed Central, 2002.
http://www.biomedcentral.com/B mcnurs/
http://www.ncbi.nlm.nih.gov/pmc/journals/51/
ISSN: 14726955 (Online only)
Indexed in: CINAHL
Recommended for: Academic Libraries

Begun in 2002, *BMC Nursing* is an open access journal publishing peer-reviewed research articles in all aspects of nursing research, training, education, and practice. All articles are submitted and judged online and are published electronically in manuscript form immediately upon acceptance; a "fully structured web version" and accompanying PDF version are published within a few weeks of acceptance. *BMC Nursing* gives authors the opportunity to publish large data sets that allow readers to manipulate data themselves, to create relevant links to external sources such as PubMed, and to include large numbers of illustrations. This online only journal is indexed by such sources as CINAHL, Scopus, and British Nursing Index. Following publication in *BMC Nursing*, the full text of each article is immediately and permanently archived in PubMed Central and may be searched in PubMed.

Evidence-Based Nursing. v. 1, BMJ Publishing Group and the Royal College of Nursing, 1998.
http://ebn.bmj.com/
ISSN: 13676539
ISSN: 14689618 (Online)
Indexed in: MEDLINE, CINAHL
Recommended for: Hospital, Academic Libraries
Brandon/Hill Selection

Jointly published by *BMJ* and the Royal College of Nursing Publishing Company, *Evidence-Based Nursing* is a quarterly journal designed to help practicing nurses base their clinical decisions on the best clinical evidence and to alert nurses to clinically relevant advances in treatment, diagnosis, etiology, and prognosis. *Evidence-Based Nursing* scans over 50 international medical journals, applying strict criteria for the quality and validity of research. Key details of the approximately 100 essential research studies per year are presented in an informative structured abstract with a nurse-expert commentary on its clinical application. The main audience for this journal includes nurses and other health professionals interested in best practices and current research findings, educators, nurse executives, quality managers, and graduate students. This journal was recommended for purchase in the former Brandon/Hill nursing list. It is cited in numerous abstracting and indexing sources such as MEDLINE, CINAHL, Scopus, and the British Nursing Index. Full online coverage back to volume 1, 1998 is available through BMJ Journals.

Nursing Research. v. 1, Lippincott Williams & Wilkins, 1952.
http://journals.lww.com/nursingresearchonline/
http://www.ovid.com/
ISSN: 00296562
ISSN: 15389847 (Online)
See Also Chapter 12. Nursing
Indexed in: MEDLINE, CINAHL
Recommended for: Hospital, Academic Libraries
Brandon/Hill Selection

Begun in 1952, *Nursing Research* is a peer-reviewed, bimonthly official journal of the Eastern Nursing Research Society and the Western Institute of Nursing. Its mission is to report empirical findings from the highest quality basic and clinical research focused on understanding health and illness experiences and to estimate the impact of therapeutic actions and nursing systems. This journal covers the key issues in nursing research, including health promotion, human responses to illness, acute care nursing research, symptom management, cost-effectiveness, vulnerable populations, health services, and community-based nursing studies. Each issue highlights the latest research techniques, quantitative and qualitative studies, new methodological strategies, and expert commentaries. According to the 2009 *Journal Citation Reports*, it currently ranks among the top nursing journals: sixth of 70 in the nursing category (social sciences) and sixth of 72 in the nursing category (sciences). With an impact factor of 1.798, this journal was a starred recommendation for purchase in the former Brandon/Hill nursing list. It is cited in numerous abstracting and indexing sources such as MEDLINE, CINAHL, Scopus, Social Sciences Citation Index, AMED (Allied and Complementary Medicine), British Nursing Index, and PsycINFO. Full online coverage back to volume 1, 1952 is available through Journals@Ovid.

Research in Nursing & Health. v. 1, Wiley, 1978.
http://onlinelibrary.wiley.com/journal/10.1002/(ISSN)1098-240X
ISSN: 01606891
ISSN: 1098240X (Online)
See Also Chapter 12. Nursing
Indexed in: MEDLINE, CINAHL
Recommended for: Hospital, Academic Libraries
Brandon/Hill Selection

Begun in 1978, *Research in Nursing & Health* is a general, peer-reviewed research journal covering research reports on nursing practice, education, administration and history, health issues relevant to nursing, and the testing of research findings in practice. Nurse researchers, educators, advanced practice nurses, hospital administrators, and graduate students are the main audience for this bimonthly journal. According to the 2009 *Journal Citation Reports*, it currently ranks tenth of 70 journals in the nursing category (social sciences) and eleventh of 72 journals in the nursing category (science). It has an impact factor of 1.514. This journal was recommended for purchase in the former Brandon/Hill nursing list. It is cited in numerous abstracting and indexing sources such as MEDLINE, CINAHL, Scopus, Social Sciences Citation Index, British Nursing Index, and PsycINFO. Online coverage back to volume 1, 1978 is through Wiley Online Library.

Western Journal of Nursing Research. v. 1, Sage, 1979.
http://online.sagepub.com
ISSN: 01939459
ISSN: 15528456 (Online)
Indexed in: MEDLINE, CINAHL
Recommended for: Hospital, Academic Libraries
Brandon/Hill Selection

Begun in 1979, the *Western Journal of Nursing Research* provides a forum for scholarly debate and for research and theoretical papers. Each of the eight issues per year offers clinical research reports broadened by commentaries and authors' responses. Nurse researchers, educators, students, and clinical practitioners are the main audience for this journal. According to the 2009 *Journal Citation Reports*, it currently ranks twenty-second of 70 journals in the nursing category (social sciences) and twenty-third out of 72 nursing journals (science). It has an impact factor of 1.090. This journal was recommended for purchase in the former Brandon/Hill nursing list. It is cited in numerous abstracting and indexing sources such as MEDLINE, CINAHL, Scopus, Social Sciences Citation Index, and PsycINFO. Full online coverage back to volume 1, number 3, 1979 is available through Sage Journals Online.

Databases and Other Electronic Resources

CINAHL Plus (Cumulative Index to Nursing and Allied Health Literature). EBSCO, 2003.
http://www.ebscohost.com
See Also Chapter 1. Allied Health
Recommended for: Hospital, Academic Libraries
Brandon/Hill Selection

The CINAHL Plus database, acquired and distributed by EBSCO in 2003, covers nursing, biomedicine, health sciences librarianship, alternative/complementary medicine, consumer health, and seventeen allied health disciplines. It provides indexing for over 4,180 journals, with some dating back to 1937, and complete coverage of English-language nursing journals and publications from the National League for Nursing and the American Nurses Association. CINAHL Plus also offers access to health care books, pamphlets, nursing dissertations, selected conference proceedings, standards of practice, educational software, audiovisuals, and book chapters. Full-text material includes almost eighty journals plus research instruments, Evidence-Based Care Sheets, clinical innovations, critical paths, quick lessons, and clinical trials. Many of the indexed journals in CINAHL Plus have searchable cited references. Subject access is available via the CINAHL Subject Heading List. The separate CINAHL database, with indexing coverage back to 1981, is also available and covers 2,968 journals. Full-text versions, with more extensive journal coverage, are available for both the CINAHL Plus and CINAHL databases. There are several ways to limit to Research Articles in CINAHL: select Research Article in the Limit Your Results options below the search boxes to retrieve all types of research articles; limit to publication type by selecting specific research designs in the Publication Type menu such as Clinical Trial or Systematic Review; or limit by Clinical Queries (which limits search retrieval to scientifically sound and clinically relevant research studies) by selecting specific query type (therapy, prognosis, review, qualitative, or causation) and focus (high sensitivity, high specificity, or best balance).

12.2. Nursing Theory

Concepts, definitions, and propositions applied to the study of various phenomena which pertain to nursing and nursing research.

—MeSH

Contributor: Janet G. Schnall

Monographs

Conceptual Models of Nursing: Analysis and Application. 4th ed. Editors: Joyce J. Fitzpatrick, Ann L. Whall. Pearson Prentice Hall, 2005.
http://www.statref.com/
http://www.r2library.com/

ISBN: 9780130480606
Recommended for: Academic Libraries
Doody's Core Titles Selection

Selected as a *Doody's* core title, this text provides a broad range of nursing theoretical models and their role in nursing practice. The primary audience for this text is graduate nursing students and educators. The focus is on the application of nursing models to nursing practice. A consistent analysis of the major nurse theorists and models (Nightingale, Peplau, Henderson, Johnson, Orem, Roy, Leininger, Neuman, King, Rogers, Newman, Watson, and Fitzparick) follows the introductory chapters, allowing a comparison of the models for use in research, education, and practice. This edition includes a new section on nursing languages and classification systems.

Contemporary Nursing Knowledge: Analysis and Evaluation of Nursing Models and Theories. 2nd ed. Author: Jacqueline Fawcett. F.A. Davis, 2005.
http://extranet.netlibrary.com/TitleSelect/
http://www.statref.com/
http://www.ebrary.com/
ISBN: 9780803611948
ISBN: 9781429480536
ISBN: 9780803620100
Recommended for: Hospital, Academic Libraries
Doody's Core Titles Selection

Selected as a *Doody's* core title and one of the *American Journal of Nursing* Books of the Year, this book is intended for nursing undergraduate and graduate students, educators, researchers, administrators, as well as practicing nurses who are interested in the development and use of nursing models and theories to guide nursing research, education, administration, and practice. The book is divided into four parts: structure and use of contemporary nursing knowledge; analysis and evaluation of conceptual models of nursing; analysis and evaluation of nursing theories; and nursing knowledge in the twenty-first century. The nursing process format is used to discuss each nursing model and theory. Some of the models described include Johnson, King, Levine, Neuman, Orem, Rogers, and Roy; theories analyzed include Newman, Parse, Orlando, Peplau, and Watson, with direct quotes from the theorists. References at the end of each chapter are supplemented by an accompanying CD-ROM (included with the print purchase), which offers comprehensive interactive bibliographies.

Integrated Theory and Knowledge Development in Nursing. 7th ed. Authors: Peggy L. Chinn, Maeona K. Kramer. Mosby/Elsevier, 2008.
ISBN: 9780323052702
Recommended for: Academic Libraries
Brandon/Hill, *Doody's Core Titles* Selection

Selected as a *Doody's Core Title* and a recommended purchase on the former Brandon/Hill nursing list under the 5th edition title *Theory and Nursing: Integrated Knowledge Development*, this textbook, which is aimed at both undergraduate and graduate students, examines how nursing theory and patterns of knowing affect current nursing practice. It describes four interrelated spheres of knowledge development: ethical, aesthetic, empiric, and the newest, emancipatory knowing. The new chapter on emancipatory knowledge emphasizes the importance of discovering underlying issues, redefining the issues, and creating change by envisioning desired outcomes. Additional new features of this edition include reflection and discussion sections at the end of each chapter to reinforce key concepts and a review of evidence-based practice that describes how it requires integration of knowledge within each pattern of knowing to support theory development. There are activities throughout the book that help reflect on important concepts and explore how these theories can be used for evidence-based practice to improve quality of care. An accompanying Evolve website from Elsevier provides additional resources for individual purchase by instructors and students.

Nursing Theorists and Their Work. 7th ed. Editors: Ann Marriner-Tomey, Martha Raile Alligood. Mosby/Elsevier, 2010.
ISBN: 9780323056410
Recommended for: Hospital, Academic Libraries
Brandon/Hill, *Doody's Core Titles* Selection

This classic work on nursing theory provides an in-depth look at 49 nursing theorists of historical, international, and significant importance. A scholar specializing in that theorist's work writes each chapter. The scholars describe a key nursing theory or philosophy; review the theorist's important ideas, literature about the theorist's publications, and the major sources the theorists used; provide an extensive bibliography; and include a case study and critical thinking activities that help in applying theory to practice. Since each chapter follows the same format, it is easy to compare theories. Diagrams of complex theories help the reader to understand abstract concepts. New to this seventh edition is information on theorist Afaf Meleis and her Transition Theory, personal quotes from the theorists, and updated references. This work was named a *Doody's Core Titles* selection, one of the *American Journal of Nursing* Books of the Year, and a starred recommended title on the former Brandon/Hill nursing list. This book is useful for nursing students at all levels and nurses interested in nursing theory.

Nursing Theory: Utilization and Application. 4th ed. Editor: Martha Raile Alligood. Mosby/Elsevier, 2010.
ISBN: 9780323056403
Recommended for: Academic Libraries
Brandon/Hill, *Doody's Core Titles* Selection

Nursing Theory: Utilization and Application describes the development of nursing theory; the application of different nursing theories, models, and philosophies; and the expansion of these practices. It is a companion to *Nursing Theorists and Their Work* and focuses on applying theories learned from that book to actual nursing practice through a variety of practical patient scenarios. The primary audience for this book is nursing students. This book is organized into three parts: "Conceptualization" (history of nursing theory); "Application" (how to apply theory to practice); and "Expansion" (how to expand theory-based practice). A chapter titled "Philosophies, Models, and Theories: Moral Obligations" explores the ethical meaning of nursing practice and specific nursing duties. New to this edition are updated nursing application examples featuring realistic scenarios that promote evidence-based practice, with references to current literature and evidence-based clinical research.

Perspectives on Nursing Theory. 5th ed. Editors: Pamela G. Reed, Nelma B. Crawford Shearer. Wolters Kluwer Health/Lippincott WIlliams & Wilkins, 2008.
ISBN: 9780781773836
Recommended for: Academic Libraries

Selected as a *Doody's* core title, this book is an anthology of classic and contemporary nursing articles that address a variety of theoretical and philosophical perspectives on nursing theory, including reflections on the evolution of nursing, the history of nursing, and highlights of the future of nursing. It provides a comprehensive overview of the important discussions taking place regarding the structures and processes of knowledge building in nursing. This work includes 72 articles and clarifies historic and contemporary controversies in nursing theory. Graduate students, educators, and nursing researchers are the primary audience for this book.

Journals

Nursing Philosophy. v. 1, Wiley-Blackwell, 2000.
http://onlinelibrary.wiley.com/journal/10.1111/(ISSN)1466-769X
ISSN: 14667681
ISSN: 1466769X (Online)
Indexed in: MEDLINE, CINAHL
Recommended for: Academic Libraries

Begun in 2000, *Nursing Philosophy* is an international, peer-reviewed journal for nurses and health care professionals seeking a more theoretical basis for their practice. This quarterly journal, the official journal of the International Philosophy of Nursing Society, provides a unique forum for discussion of philosophical issues at the foundation of nursing theory and practice. It publishes original research papers, dialogues, critical responses, and book reviews. *Nursing Philosophy* is cited in numerous abstracting and indexing sources such as MEDLINE, CINAHL, Scopus, British Nursing Index, and Social Sciences Citation Index. Online coverage back to volume 1, 2000 is available through Wiley Online Library.

Nursing Science Quarterly: Theory, Research and Practice. v. 1, Sage, 1988.
http://www.sagepub.com/
ISSN: 08943184
ISSN: 15527409 (Online)
Indexed in: MEDLINE, CINAHL
Recommended for: Academic Libraries
Brandon/Hill Selection

Begun in 1988, *Nursing Science Quarterly: Theory, Research and Practice* is a peer-reviewed, quarterly journal covering timely and key aspects of nursing science, such as theoretical dilemmas, research issues, and practice applications. Each issue publishes original manuscripts focusing on nursing theory development, nursing theory-based practice, and quantitative and qualitative research relating to existing nursing frameworks. Regular features include "Theoretical Concerns," "Research Issues," "Practice Applications," "Ethical Issues," "Teaching-Learning Processes," "Scholarly Dialogue," book reviews and new media, and "International Perspectives." Researchers, nurse executives, and graduate students are the main audience for this journal. According to the 2009 *Journal Citation Reports*, it currently ranks fifteenth of 70 journals in the nursing category (social sciences) and sixteenth of 72 in the nursing category (science). It has an impact factor of 1.215. This journal, a recommendation on the former Brandon/Hill nursing list, is cited in numerous abstracting and indexing sources such as MEDLINE, CINAHL, Scopus, and Social Sciences Citation Index. Full online coverage back to volume 1, 1988 is available through Sage Journals Online.

13. Nursing Specialties

13.1. Community Health Nursing

General and comprehensive nursing practice directed to individuals, families, or groups as it relates to and contributes to the health of a population.

—MeSH

Contributor: Paul M. Blobaum

Monographs

Community as Partner. 5th ed. Authors: Elizabeth T. Anderson, Judith M. McFarlane. Lippincott Williams & Wilkins, 2008.
ISBN: 9780781786430
See Also Chapter 13.16. Public Health Nursing
Recommended for: Hospital, Academic Libraries
Brandon/Hill, *Doody's Core Titles* Selection

Anderson and McFarlane have updated this classic text with new chapters on informatics, infectious diseases, disasters, and introductory concepts. This text is written to serve undergraduate and graduate students alike as a framework for professional community nursing practice. A real-life urban community is used as an example throughout the book. The book is divided into three main sections: "Essential Elements for Healthy Partnerships," "The Process," and "Practicing with Diverse Communities." Each of the 21 chapters contains learning objectives, key concepts, critical thinking questions, and a bibliography of further reading and Internet resources. Community health nursing practitioners in the field will appreciate the concise updated discussion of topics by a panel of 17 experts. The text is limited only in the sparse use of color (black, white, green) and graphics, but at 488 pages, the book is a practical choice for desk reading. *Community as Partner* was designated a Brandon/Hill nursing select title, and is recommended for academic, hospital, and specialized libraries.

Community Health Nursing: Advocacy for Population Health. 5th ed. Author: Mary Jo Clark. Pearson Prentice Hall, 2008.
ISBN: 9780131709829
Recommended for: Hospital, Academic Libraries
Doody's Core Titles Selection

Clark's treatment of community health nursing focuses on advocacy, based on her qualitative research that examines the community health nursing advocacy process. Practical application of this advocacy imperative is highlighted by sections on "Advocacy in Action" and "Think Advocacy" in each chapter. General principles, theory, and historical foundations of the field are presented. This 1,064-page book uses the Dimensions Model of Community Health Nursing to structure the discussion of principles and practice. Learning objectives, key terms, case studies, self assessments, and extensive references accompany each chapter, which are also supplemented by a companion website containing an audio glossary, exam review questions, videos, and additional resources. It is recommended for hospital, academic, and special libraries.

Community Health Nursing: Promoting and Protecting the Public's Health. 7th ed. Editors: Judith A. Allender, Cherie Rector, Kristine D. Warner. Lippincott Williams & Wilkins, 2010.
ISBN: 9780781765848
Recommended for: Hospital, Academic Libraries
Brandon/Hill, *Doody's Core Titles* Selection

Considered a core nursing title by Brandon/Hill, Allender's *Community Health Nursing* is a classic text for students and practitioners who are in public or community health care settings. It is also a *Resources for College Libraries* (*RCL*) title. Allender, Rector, and Spradely define the term "community health nurse" as a "practitioner in the community whose work incorporates public health philosophy, theory, and skills with an emphasis on aggregates and populations." The book is divided into eight instructional units, and six chapters are new for the seventh edition. Health promotion, protection, disaster nursing, urban nursing, rural nursing, chronic illness, and patients with disabilities are all presented from a public health practice approach. This text is recommended for academic, hospital, and specialized libraries.

Community/Public Health Nursing Practice: Health for Families and Populations. 4th ed. Editors: Frances A. Maurer, Claudia M. Smith. Saunders/Elsevier, 2009.
ISBN: 9781416050049
Recommended for: Hospital, Academic Libraries

This community health nursing text emphasizes the application of core knowledge to nursing practice, and reflects the increasing demand for community health nursing in home health care. It is intended as a basic text for the undergraduate and for graduates who are new to community health settings. RN's without a bachelor's degree will also benefit from the text if they practice in community settings. Chapters are organized with focus questions, a chapter outline, key terms, and a summary of key ideas, study questions, links to the companion website for additional study aids, and a list of references. This 875-page text is organized into eight units with 33 chapters: unit I, "Role and Context of Community/Public Health Nursing Practice"; unit II, "Core Concepts"; unit III, "Family as Client"; unit IV, "Community as Client"; unit V, "Tools for Practice"; unit VI, "Contemporary Problems"; unit VII, "Support for Special Populations"; and unit VIII, "Setting for Community/Public Health Nursing Practice." Color graphics, photographs, and highlights of key points enhance the navigation of the material throughout the text. This book is available for individual purchase in an e-book format with user guide, and also a textbook package. It is recommended for hospital, academic, and special libraries.

Community/Public Health Nursing: Promoting the Health of Populations. 4th ed. Editors: Mary A. Nies, Melanie McEwen. Saunders Elsevier, 2006.
ISBN: 9781416028871
Recommended for: Hospital, Academic Libraries

Nies and McEwen focus on the "upstream" preventive approach to community health, unique to community health nursing textbooks. The "upstream" approach shifts the typical community health nursing approach from working with individuals on health promotion and illness prevention to working with aggregate groups in activities such as advocacy, developing health policy, and working to provide options for these communities to access education, housing, employment, food, and health care. The editors intend to shift the primary unit of care from individuals and families to the wider milieu of the community's structure, using a social justice perspective. This 738-page book is intended as a textbook, but will be appreciated and used by generalist and specialized practitioners. The book is well organized into eight units consisting of 33 total chapters. Each chapter includes learning objectives, key terms, learning activities, and also a bibliography of references for further reading. Case studies and several photo novellas add to the extensive graphic content, which is presented with multicolor highlights of the text. Each chapter contains links to additional web-based resources at Elsevier's Evolve website for further review, including quizzes, additional case studies, content updates, glossaries, and additional web links. This book is recommended for academic, special, and hospital libraries.

Disaster Nursing: Emergency Preparedness for Chemical, Biological, and Radiological Terrorism and Other Hazards. 2nd ed. Editor: Tener Goodwin Veenema. Springer, 2007.
ISBN: 9780826121448
Recommended for: Hospital, Academic Libraries

"This text is the next generation of information needed by nurses to be informed about and responsive to the needs of our citizens in a disaster" (Foreword to the second edition). Written as a textbook with learning objectives, study questions, and Internet activities, this book is an invaluable resource for emergency and community health nurses for up-to-date information on nursing issues in response to catastrophic events that affect populations. It is recommended for academic, hospital, and specialized collections.

Journals

Journal of Community Health Nursing. v. 1, Routledge/Taylor & Francis, 1984.
http://www.informaworld.com/1532-7655
ISSN: 07370016
ISSN: 15327655 (Online)
Indexed in: MEDLINE, CINAHL
Recommended for: Hospital, Academic Libraries
Brandon/Hill Selection

Journal of Community Health Nursing is a peer-reviewed, scholarly journal published quarterly. The journal publishes reports on all aspects of community health practice, including schools, nursing homes, home health, clinics, and public health administration. Book reviews and news items are also featured. It is a Brandon/Hill core nursing title, and is indexed in CINAHL and MEDLINE. Full text is available from volume 1, 1984 with a 12-month embargo. It is recommended for hospital and academic libraries serving professionals and students.

13.2. Emergency Nursing

Nursing in the care of patients admitted to the emergency department.

—MeSH

Contributor: Paul M. Blobaum

Monographs

Emergency Nursing Core Curriculum. 6th ed. Editor: Kathleen Sanders Jordan. Saunders Elsevier and ENA, 2007.
ISBN: 9781416037552
Recommended for: Hospital, Academic Libraries
Brandon/Hill Selection

The Emergency Nurses Association is the world's largest nursing organization devoted to emergency nursing practice. The *Core Curriculum's* purpose is to articulate the core knowledge of the field, including the latest research basis. The current standard of practice for diagnosis and emergency interventions is presented. The material is offered in an outline format and is organized by body system. The nursing process framework is used. This text can be used for review by emergency nurses and students at all levels of expertise.

Emergency Nursing Procedures. 4th ed. Editor: Jean A. Proehl. Saunders Elsevier, 2009.
ISBN: 9781416040989
Recommended for: Hospital, Academic Libraries
Brandon/Hill, *Doody's Core Titles* Selection

Designated a Brandon/Hill nursing select title, and also a *Resources for College Libraries* title, *Emergency Nursing Procedures* is an authoritative pictorial guide to step by step assessment and interventions in a multitude of emergency situations. Over 198 topics are covered, arranged by body system or common medication. This 936-page guide covers procedures which go beyond the basic nursing knowledge base of universal precautions, draping, etc. Each procedure is based on research and practice guidelines, and reflects the latest Joint Commission patient safety standards. This book will be a valuable resource for the new emergency nurse or technician, first responders, and all personnel managing emergency medical services. It is recommended for academic, hospital, and special libraries.

Forensic Nursing: A Concise Manual. Authors: Donna M. Garbacz Bader, Sue Gabriel. CRC Press, 2009.
See Chapter 13.4. Forensic Nursing

Forensic Nursing Science. 2nd ed. Authors: Virginia A. Lynch, Janet Barber Duval. Mosby Elsevier, 2010.
See Chapter 13.4. Forensic Nursing

Sheehy's Emergency Nursing: Principles and Practice. 6th ed. Editors: Patricia Kunz Howard, Rebecca A. Steinmann, Susan Budassi Sheehy. Mosby Elsevier, 2010.
ISBN: 9780323055857
Recommended for: Hospital, Academic Libraries
Brandon/Hill Selection

Selected as a Brandon/Hill nursing title, *Sheehy's Emergency Nursing* continues the legacy of Susan Budassi Sheehy, who co-edited the first edition with Janet Miller Barber, published in 1981. Sheehy is a giant in the field of emergency and trauma nursing and the Emergency Nurses Association, and was an early advocate for improved trauma care and networks of care in the state of Washington in the late 1980's. Now in its sixth edition, *Sheehy's Emergency Nursing: Principles and Practice* has evolved over the years to reflect changing practice and technologies that shape emergency care. With the slogan, "Written by emergency nurses, for emergency nurses!" among the 58 authors are academics and clinicians from urban, rural, and suburban practice areas. Key coverage includes clinical fundamentals, treatment for trauma and medical-surgical emergencies, the foundations of emergency nursing practice, and special populations. Chapters are organized into six sections: "Foundations of Emergency Nursing," "Professional Practice," "Clinical Foundations of Emergency Nursing," "Major Trauma Emergencies," "Medical and Surgical Emergencies," and "Special Patient Populations." Tables and boxes highlight and summarize critical information. Text and illustrations are published in black and white. Recent editions have new chapters on weapons of mass destruction, discussions of outcomes management, and triage. Pandemic flu and other public health outbreaks which impact the scope of emergency nursing practice are among the many important topics discussed. The Emergency Nurses Association is the official sponsor of this book, which is recommended for academic, hospital, and special libraries.

Journals

Annals of Emergency Medicine. v. 9, Mosby Elsevier, 1980.
http://www.annemergmed.com/
http://www.sciencedirect.com/science/journal/01960644
ISSN: 01960644
ISSN: 10976760 (Online)

See Also Chapter 10.4. Disaster Medicine, Chapter 10.5. Emergency Medicine
Indexed in: MEDLINE, CINAHL
Recommended for: Hospital, Academic Libraries
Brandon/Hill Selection

Annals of Emergency Medicine is an international peer-reviewed journal, and is the official journal of the American College of Emergency Physicians. It is considered the most important journal in the area of emergency medicine for all medical and allied health specialties. Articles are published by researchers from many medical and allied health professions. In addition to research, *Annals of Emergency Medicine* publishes educational articles, clinical reports, and opinion related to teaching and practicing emergency care. Contributions are international in scope. In the 2009 *Journal Citation Reports* it ranked first of 19 titles in the emergency medicine category with an impact factor of 4.232. Also in 2009, the journal was chosen one of the 100 most influential scientific journals of the past 100 years by the Special Libraries Association (http://www.sla.org). Studies of the mapping of emergency nursing literature also rank this journal highly in the literature of emergency nursing. The journal is available online from Elsevier, EBSCO EJS, Ovid, and MD Consult. A "must have" journal for hospital libraries serving emergency care personnel, academic libraries serving advanced practice nursing students (Master's and Doctoral), and specialized collections.

International Emergency Nursing. v. 16, Elsevier, 2008.
http://www.sciencedirect.com/science/journal/1755599X
ISSN: 1755599X
ISSN: 1878013X (Online)
Indexed in: MEDLINE, CINAHL
Recommended for: Hospital, Academic Libraries

Accident and Emergency Nursing was the title for this journal until 2008. The journal is published four times a year, and publishes research on practice focusing on nurses in emergency care, as well as other members of the emergency medical services team. With the new title change, the editor has implemented a new feature article on emergency nursing across the world for each issue. The journal ranks highly in mapping studies of emergency nursing literature and is available online from Elsevier, EBSCO EJS, Ovid, and Swetswise.

Journal of Emergency Nursing. v. 1, Mosby Elsevier, 1975.
http://www.jenonline.org/
http://www.sciencedirect.com/science/journal/00991767
ISSN: 00991767
ISSN: 15272966 (Online)
Indexed in: MEDLINE, CINAHL
Recommended for: Hospital, Academic Libraries
Brandon/Hill Selection

Journal of Emergency Nursing is the official scholarly, peer-reviewed journal of the Emergency Nurses Association. The journal is published six times a year. *JEN* publishes a wide variety of articles on any aspect of nursing as it relates to emergency care. Articles for continuing education are available for credit in each issue. *JEN* is on the Brandon/Hill core nursing list, and is indexed in CINAHL and MEDLINE. Online content begins with 1995, and it is available online from Elsevier, Ovid, and EBSCO EJS.

13.3. Family Nursing

The provision of care involving the nursing process, to families and family members in health and illness situations.
—MeSH

Contributor: Paul M. Blobaum

Monographs

Family Health Care Nursing: Theory, Practice and Research. 4th ed. Editors: Joanna Rowe Kaakinen, Vivian Gedaly-Duff, Deborah Padgett Coehlo, Shirley May Harmon Hanson. F.A. Davis, 2009.
ISBN: 9780803621664
Recommended for: Hospital, Academic Libraries
Brandon/Hill Selection

The editors intend this book to be used both as a nursing text for bachelor's and master's students, and also as a reference text. The purpose is to set forth the concepts and theories of family health care nursing, and learn how these concepts and theories are practiced within nursing specialty areas. Family nursing is seen as the "umbrella" under which all specialties should practice. This textbook is recognized internationally as a leading textbook in family nursing. It has been translated into Japanese. The book is divided into three units, unit 1, "Foundations of Family Health Care Nursing"; unit II, "Family Nursing Practice"; and unit III, "Future of Families and Family Nursing." Each chapter is prefaced by an enumeration of "critical concepts," and concludes with a bibliography for further research. This text includes discussions about home schooling, military families, transracial adoption, same sex couples, and children with incarcerated parents. Practical tools such as the Calgary Assessment Model and the Friedman Family Assessment

Model are discussed. Four theoretical models are discussed: Family Ecological Theory, Family Resiliency Model, Family Systems Model, and the Family Life Cycle Model. Two additional online chapters are available in this edition, covering research in families and family nursing, and international family nursing. An instructor's manual is published online, which includes PowerPoint slides, a bibliography of classic books and movies depicting family interactions, case studies, and other resources. A companion website is available for students who purchase the text.

Family Nursing. 5th ed. Authors: Marilyn M. Friedman, Vicky R. Bowden, Elaine G. Jones. Prentice Hall Health, 2003.
ISBN: 9780130608246
Recommended for: Hospital, Academic Libraries
Brandon/Hill Selection

These well-known educators and practitioners have updated a classic text on family nursing theory, research, and practice. The Friedman Family Assessment Model and other important nursing theories are presented as part of the theoretical underpinnings of the family nursing process. Chapters are presented with learning objectives, an outline of chapter content, and review questions. This title is designated a Brandon/Hill core nursing title.

Nurses and Families: A Guide to Family Assessment and Intervention. 5th ed. Authors: Lorraine M. Wright, Maureen Leahey. F.A. Davis, 2009.
http://extranet.netlibrary.com/TitleSelect/
ISBN: 9780803621305
Recommended for: Hospital, Academic Libraries
Brandon/Hill Selection

Wright and Leahey assert that this is a "how to" book for undergraduate, graduate, and practicing nurses, mainly, about how to involve families in their health care. Students and practitioners of community and public health nursing, maternal child nursing, pediatric nursing, mental health nursing, geriatric nursing, palliative care nursing, as well as nurse educators will find this book useful. The book gives specific guidelines for nurses to utilize when conducting family meetings, from the first interview to discharge planning. Clinical ideas are based on theory, research, and the authors' 35 years of work with family clients. The Calgary Family Assessment Model (CFAM) is used as a framework for discussion of assessments in the book, and the Calgary Family Intervention Model (CFIM), a model developed by the authors, is utilized in discussions of nursing interventions. A Brandon/Hill core nursing title, this text is recommended for academic, hospital, and specialized libraries.

Practice Guidelines for Family Nurse Practitioners. 3rd ed. Authors: Karen Fenstermacher, Barbara T. Hudson. Saunders Elsevier, 2004.
ISBN: 9780721603452
Recommended for: Hospital, Academic Libraries
Brandon/Hill Selection

Practice Guidelines for Family Nurse Practitioners is intended as a quick reference book for nursing students and practitioners. Chapters are organized by body system, and cover signs and symptoms of disease, diagnostic methods, drug therapy, and treatment. Color photographs of dermatologic signs are helpful additions to the black and white text. Designated as a Brandon/Hill select nursing title, this book is also available for handheld devices. This book is recommended for hospital, academic, and specialized collections serving advanced practice nursing professionals and students.

Journals

Journal of Family Nursing. v. 1, Sage, 1995.
http://jfn.sagepub.com/
ISSN: 10748407
ISSN: 1552549X (Online)
Indexed in: MEDLINE, CINAHL
Recommended for: Hospital, Academic Libraries

Journal of Family Nursing is a scholarly, peer-reviewed journal, publishing articles on nursing research, practice, education, and policy relating to nursing care of families. The journal is international in scope. The current editor, Jan Bell is a key leader in the International Family Nursing Association, incorporated in 2009. The journal is intended to be a forum where practitioners, researchers, and educators from a variety of disciplines can critically discuss the family in health and illness. The journal is indexed in CINAHL, MEDLINE, PsycINFO, Sociological Abstracts, and Social Science and Science Citation Indexes. The journal is published four times a year, and is available online through Sage.

13.4. Forensic Nursing

The application of nursing knowledge to questions of law. It is a specialty of nursing practice involving victims of crime which includes not only attending to the physical and emotional distress of victims, but also the identifying, collecting, and preserving evidence for law enforcement and the criminal justice system.

—MeSH

Contributors: Kristine M. Alpi and Robert Sotak

Monographs

Child Fatality Review: An Interdisciplinary Guide and Photographic Reference. Authors: Randell Alexander, Mary E. Case. GW Medical, 2008.
See Chapter 10.7.2. Forensic Pathology

Clarke's Analytical Forensic Toxicology. 1st ed. Editors: Sue Jickells, Adam Negrusz. Pharmaceutical Press, 2008.
See Chapter 17.8.2. Forensic Toxicology

Color Atlas of Forensic Medicine and Pathology. 1st ed. Editor: Charles A. Catanese. CRC Press, 2010.
See Chapter 10.7. Forensic Medicine

Death Investigation: Systems and Procedures. Author: Randy Hanzlick. CRC Press, 2007.
See Chapter 10.7. Forensic Medicine

DNA: Forensic and Legal Applications. Authors: Lawrence Kobilinsky, Thomas F. Liotti, Jamel Oeser-Sweat. Wiley, 2005.
See Chapter 10.7.1. Forensic Genetics

Effective Expert Witnessing: Practices for the 21st Century. 4th ed. Authors: Jack V. Matson, Suha F. Daou, Jeffrey G. Soper. CRC Press, 2004.
See Chapter 10.7. Forensic Medicine

Elder Abuse Detection and Intervention: A Collaborative Approach. Authors: Bonnie Brandl, Carmel Bitondo Dyer, Candace J. Heisler, Joanne Marlatt Otto, Lori A. Stiegel, Randolph W. Thomas. Springer, 2007.
http://www.r2library.com/
ISBN: 9780826131140
Recommended for: Academic, Consumer Health Libraries

Elder abuse victims are cared for by many types of clinicians. Forensic and emergency nurses will be able to apply the content about understanding and responding to elder abuse. While detection is part of the title, there are not any images of elder abuse injuries. Social workers, lawyers, law enforcement, and a physician came together to prepare this multidisciplinary work. Much of the content deals with interagency collaboration and case management teams. The content becomes more personal and touching through cases which humanize the issues. Multidisciplinary responses involving nurses, physicians, social workers, protective services, and law enforcement are given from a variety of specialties and settings. Chapters 8–13 are more about protecting victims and improving the local, state, and national legal and health system to prevent and intervene more effectively, using the expertise of geriatricians and gerontologists among other health professionals. This well-referenced and indexed volume could have a place in any public or academic library.

Forensic Entomology: The Utility of Arthropods in Legal Investigations. 2nd ed. Editors: Jason H. Byrd, James L. Castner. CRC Press, 2010.
See Chapter 10.7. Forensic Medicine

Forensic Nursing Science. 2nd ed. Authors: Virginia A. Lynch, Janet Barber Duval. Mosby Elsevier, 2010.
ISBN: 9780323066372
Recommended for: Hospital, Academic Libraries

Virginia Lynch, founding member and first president of the International Association of Forensic Nurses, and Janet Barber Duval guide nurses through applying assessment skills to identify patients who are victims of criminal events, collecting court-admissible evidence, and preparing to give accurate, reliable testimony while delivering high-quality patient care. This 2010 second edition is full color with 300+ illustrations. Twelve new chapters expand the work from the highly regarded 2005 first edition of *Forensic Nursing*: "Digital Evidence," "Medical Evidence Recovery at the Death Scene," "Asphyxia, Electrical and Thermal Injury," "Intrafamilial Homicide and Unexplained Childhood Death," "Human Trafficking," "Credential Development for Forensic Nurses," "Gangs and Hate Crimes," "Ethics Issues in Forensic Nursing," "Forensic Physics and Fracture Analysis," "Sexual Deviant Behaviors," and "Crime and Forensic Epidemiology." Almost every chapter includes an illustrated case study with critical thinking questions, and "Key Point" and "Best Practice" boxes help focus attention on important concepts and recommendations. Five appendixes include sexual assault procedures for male victims, protocols for collecting physical evidence of torture, guidelines for evidence collection in emergency rooms, nursing diagnoses, and a code of ethics.

Forensic Nursing: A Concise Manual. Authors: Donna M. Garbacz Bader, Sue Gabriel. CRC Press, 2009.
http://www.crcnetbase.com/isbn/978-1-4200-6730-9
ISBN: 9781420067309
ISBN: 9781420067316 (Online)
Recommended for: Hospital, Academic Libraries

Forensic nurses are often at the forefront of evidence collection and preservation. They also care for victims, assist victims' families, provide education on prevention and intervention, work with community and law enforcement, and testify as expert witnesses. The authors present concise and practical information on these diverse activities and offer guidelines for examining patients in light of their medical, psychological, ethical, and legal situations. In outline format, the text introduces forensic nursing and forensic science; discusses crime scene and death investigation, evidence collection, autopsies, legal issues, and ethics; and examines the nursing process as a tool for identifying both the medical needs of the victim and the legal aspects of crime scene investigation. The authors pinpoint the role of the forensic nurse in an array of incident scenarios, including blunt and sharp force injuries, gunshot wounds, asphyxia, child abuse, sexual assault, and intimate partner violence. They also explore human trafficking and the forensic nurse's role in mass disasters. Selected chapters by forensic specialists include Gary Plank's chapter on profiling, Erin Kimmerle's piece on forensic anthropology, and nursing home death and excited delirium syndrome by Theresa DiMaio, RN and forensic pathologist Dr. Vincent DiMaio. Flowcharts and references in each chapter invite further study. The text is available online via CRCnetBASE. Designed as a course text, instructor materials are available with qualifying course adoption.

Forensic Nursing: Scope and Standards of Practice. American Nurses Association and International Association of Forensic Nurses, 2009.
ISBN: 9781558102651
Recommended for: Hospital, Academic Libraries

Forensic nursing focuses on providing patient care and counseling while collecting evidence and communicating with professionals in legal systems. All institutions employing or training forensic nurses should have a copy of *Forensic Nursing: Scope and Standards of Practice.* Specialists in other areas of forensics will find it helpful in understanding the role and approach of nurses with whom they work. Developed by a panel of nurse experts convened by the American Nurses Association and the International Association of Forensic Nurses to update the 1997 *Scope and Standards of Forensic Nursing*, the 2009 guide outlines six standards for forensic nursing practice and nine standards for performance as professional nurses.

Handbook of Common Poisonings in Children. 4th ed. American Academy of Pediatrics, 2010.
See Chapter 17.8.2. Forensic Toxicology

Introduction to Environmental Forensics. 2nd ed. Authors: Brian L. Murphy, Robert D. Morrison. Elsevier, 2007.
See Chapter 10.7. Forensic Medicine

Principles and Practice of Child and Adolescent Forensic Mental Health. Editors: Elissa P. Benedek, Peter Ash, Charles L. Scott. American Psychiatric, 2010.
See Chapter 9.10.4. Forensic Psychiatry

Sexual Assault: Victimization across the Life Span, a Clinical Guide and a Color Atlas. Editors: Angelo P. Giardino, Elizabeth M. Datner, Janice B. Asher, Barbara Girardin, Diana K. Faugno, Mary J. Spencer. GW Medical Publishing, 2003.
ISBN: 9781878060471
Recommended for: Hospital, Academic Libraries

This two-volume clinical guide and color atlas contains over 1,800 images. The supplementary CD-ROM provides 130 images with case studies. This reference and learning tool will be useful for emergency medical personnel, pediatricians, child advocates, law enforcement, and legal professionals. Volume one is the clinical guide with chapters on anatomy, screening, documentation, special settings such as incarceration, disabilities, and psychosocial and legal issues. Volume two is the color atlas divided into seven age groups from infants to the elderly. The images are very graphic and intended for health and legal professionals. The editors are physicians from emergency medicine, obstetrics and gynecology, and pediatrics; and forensic nurses, including a sexual assault nurse examiner who is a Fellow of the American Academy of Forensic Science. While not as widely held as the *Color Atlas of Sexual Assault* (Mosby, 1997), this two-volume set has many more cases and illustrations and was positively reviewed in *JAMA* in 2004 (292(18):2276). The pocket size version called *Sexual Assault: Quick Reference for Healthcare, Social Service, and Law Enforcement Professionals* (Spiral-bound, GW Medical Publishing, 2003) is affordable and useful as a field reference. The reference guide is available in the Rittenhouse R2 Digital Library, but is it not clear whether the online resource includes the supplemental CD-ROM material.

Spitz and Fisher's Medicolegal Investigation of Death: Guidelines for the Application of Pathology to Crime Investigation. 4th ed. Editors: Werner U. Spitz, Daniel J. Spitz, Russell S. Fisher, Ramsey Clark. Charles C Thomas, 2006.
See Chapter 10.7. Forensic Medicine

Journals

American Journal of Forensic Medicine & Pathology. v. 1, Lippincott, Williams & Wilkins, 1980.
See Chapter 10.7. Forensic Medicine

Forensic Science International. v. 11, Elsevier, 1978.
See Chapter 10.7. Forensic Medicine, Chapter 10.7.1. Forensic Genetics

Forensic Science, Medicine, and Pathology. v. 1, Humana, 2005.
See Chapter 10.7. Forensic Medicine

International Journal of Legal Medicine. v. 104, Springer, 1990.
See Chapter 10.7. Forensic Medicine, Chapter 10.7.1. Forensic Genetics

Journal of Forensic Nursing. v. 1, International Association of Forensic Nurses/Wiley, 2005.
http://onlinelibrary.wiley.com/journal/10.1111/(ISSN)1939-3938
ISSN: 15563693
ISSN: 19393938 (Online)
Indexed in: MEDLINE, CINAHL
Recommended for: Hospital, Academic Libraries

The *Journal of Forensic Nursing* is the official journal of the International Association of Forensic Nurses. This quarterly journal covers all facets of this worldwide multidisciplinary nursing specialty and brings health care, law enforcement, legal issues, and forensic science into the patient care context. Content comes from empirical studies, review and theoretical articles, methodological papers, and case studies on topics such as interpersonal violence, death investigation, legal and ethical issues, forensic psychiatric nursing, correctional nursing, and emergency/trauma. *Journal of Forensic Nursing* is indexed by MEDLINE, CINAHL, ProQuest and PsycINFO. All issues of the journal back to 2005 are available online from Wiley Online Library, which took over publishing the journal in 2008.

On the Edge. v. 1, International Association of Forensic Nurses, 1995.
http://www.iafn.org
ISSN: None
Indexed in: CINAHL
Recommended for: Hospital, Academic Libraries

This quarterly peer-reviewed newsletter is focused on forensic nursing and its clinical application. Each issue of offers feature articles and several regular columns—letters, education and training, focus on personalities, global updates, tips and tricks, research briefs, and member news. Librarians will find its book reviews very helpful. The features cover basic topics such as grieving and death investigation as well as examine current issues such as organ donation and forensic nursing. The complete run is indexed by CINAHL with full text in EBSCOhost from March 1, 2007 to present. The newsletter website provides free full text from volume 6 (2000) onwards.

13.5. Geriatric Nursing

Nursing care of the aged patient given in the home, the hospital, or special institutions such as nursing homes, psychiatric institutions, etc.

—MeSH

Contributor: Marcia Henry

Monographs

Advanced Practice Nursing with Older Adults: Clinical Guidelines. Editors: Valerie T. Cotter, Neville E. Strumpf. McGraw-Hill, 2002.
ISBN: 9780071341578
Recommended for: Hospital, Academic Libraries
Doody's Core Titles Selection

The work's 30 contributors offer guidelines for geriatric care for the advance practice nursing student. This practical text features guidelines, strategies, protocols, and principles for working with older adults. The book, which is organized by body system, provides essential coverage of diagnosis, treatment standards, management, special concerns, judgment calls, and more. Unique coverage is provided for pain management, care for the dying, palliative care, and advance directives. The contributors offer practical assistance with the evaluation and treatment of cardiovascular, respiratory, genitourinary, gastrointestinal, thyroid, gynecological, musculoskeletal, and CNS disorders, as well as diabetes mellitus. Also provided is in-depth guidance on problems such as falls, sensory deficits, pressure injuries, and elder abuse and neglect. *Advanced Practice Nursing with Older Adults: Clinical Guidelines* is considered an essential purchase by *Doody's Core Titles.*

Elder Abuse Detection and Intervention: A Collaborative Approach. Authors: Bonnie Brandl, Carmel Bitondo Dyer, Candace J. Heisler, Joanne Marlatt Otto, Lori A. Stiegel, Randolph W. Thomas. Springer, 2007.
See Chapter 13.4. Forensic Nursing

Evidence-Based Geriatric Nursing Protocols for Best Practice. 3rd ed. Editors: Elizabeth Capezuti, DeAnne

Zwicker, Mathy Mezey, Terry T. Fulmer. Springer, 2008.
http://www.ebrary.com/
http://extranet.netlibrary.com/TitleSelect/
http://www.r2library.com/
http://www.statref.com/
ISBN: 9780826111036
ISBN: 9780826111050 (Online)
Recommended for: Hospital, Academic Libraries
Doody's Core Titles Selection

This title is a valuable resource for all nurses caring for hospitalized, older adults. It is the third edition of the book formerly titled *Geriatric Nursing Protocols for Best Practice*. The protocols address key clinical conditions and circumstances likely to be encountered by hospital nurses caring for older adults. They represent best practices for acute care of the elderly, practices that are developed by nursing experts around the country as part of the Hartford Foundation's Nurses Improving Care to the Hospitalized Elderly (NICHE) project. This third edition includes 17 revised and updated chapters and more than 15 new topics including critical care, diabetes, hydration, oral health care, palliative care, and substance abuse. Each chapter includes educational objectives, problem assessment, nursing intervention or care strategies, and references; most chapters include case studies. *Doody's Core Titles* recommends this as an essential purchase title.

Gerontologic Nursing. 4th ed. Editor: Sue E. Meiner. Mosby/Elsevier, 2011.
http://www.nursingconsult.com/
ISBN: 9780323069991
Recommended for: Hospital, Academic Libraries
Brandon/Hill, *Doody's Core Titles* Selection

With 22 contributing authors, the third edition of this valuable work covers health promotion and the most common medical-surgical problems associated with the older adult. It is divided into six parts with coverage of essential wellness and disorders information. The second edition was a Brandon/Hill geriatric nursing selection. This review refers to the third edition. A fourth edition by Sue Meiner was released in late 2010. A new chapter on "Loss and End-Of-Life Issues" has been included along with new features such as updated nursing care plans linked to NANDA-I (North American Nursing Diagnosis Association International) nursing diagnoses, NIC (nursing interventions classification) priority interventions for specific conditions, and NOC (nursing outcomes classification) suggested outcomes to guide appropriate care.

Gerontological Nursing. 7th ed. Author: Charlotte Eliopoulos. Wolters Kluwer Health/Lippincott Williams & Wilkins, 2010.
ISBN: 9780781753449
Recommended for: Hospital, Academic Libraries
Brandon/Hill Selection

The seventh edition of *Gerontological Nursing* is written by Charlotte Eliopoulos, the founder of the American Association for Long-Term Care Nursing. It is arranged into units: "Understanding the Aging Experience," "Foundations of Gerontological Nursing," "Fostering Connection and Gratification," "General Care Concerns," "Facilitating Physiologic Balance," "Multisystemic Disorders," and "Gerontological Care Issues." There are special indexes for assessment guides and nursing care plans. An earlier edition was a Brandon/Hill selection.

Gerontological Nursing: Competencies for Care. 2nd ed. Editor: Kristen L. Mauk. Jones & Bartlett, 2010.
ISBN: 9780763755805
Recommended for: Hospital, Academic Libraries

Written to help students learn about evidence-based practice in gerontological nursing, this publication was awarded the *American Journal of Nursing's* 2009 Book of the Year Award. Forty authors contributed to *Gerontological Nursing: Competencies for Care*. Key features of the text include chapter outlines, learning objectives, discussion questions, personal reflection boxes, and case studies.

Handbook of Geriatric Assessment. 4th ed. Editors: Joseph J. Gallo, Hillary R. Bogner, Terry Fulmer, Gregory J. Paveza. Jones & Bartlett, 2006.
http://extranet.netlibrary.com/TitleSelect/
http://www.r2library.com/
ISBN: 9780763730567
ISBN: 9781435603318
Recommended for: Hospital, Academic Libraries

The *Handbook of Geriatric Assessment* presents instruments for use in many aspects of geriatrics and describes how to use a team approach to manage older adults. It is not meant to be a comprehensive guide to all assessment instruments; instead, it provides instruments, questionnaires, and concepts that can be employed in designing clinical assessment procedures. The book is organized into four sections: "The Context of Assessment" (geriatric care, emergency, ethnicity, older adult driver, advance directive, mistreatment); "Domains of Assessment" (cognitive, depression, substance use and abuse, activities of daily living, social assessment, physical, pain, health promotion); "Settings of Assessment" (home, nursing home, hospitalization); and "Specialty Topics" (adherence to medical treatment, teams, disaster preparedness and response). The *Handbook of Geriatric*

Assessment won a 2006 *American Journal of Nursing* Book of the Year Award.

Handbook of Health Psychology and Aging. 1st ed. Editors: Carolyn M. Aldwin, Crystal L. Park, Avron Spiro III. Guilford Press, 2007.
See Chapter 9.4. Behavioral Medicine

Hazzard's Geriatric Medicine and Gerontology. 6th ed. Editors: Jeffrey B. Halter, Joseph G. Ouslander, Mary E. Tinetti, Stephanie Studenski, Kevin P. High, Sanjay Asthana. McGraw-Hill, 2009.
http://www.accessmedicine.com/
http://www.r2library.com/
http://www.ebrary.com/
http://extranet.netlibrary.com/TitleSelect/
ISBN: 9780071488723
ISBN: 9780071641241 (Online)
See Also Chapter 9.8. Geriatrics
Recommended for: Hospital, Academic Libraries
Brandon/Hill, *Doody's Core Titles* Selection

First published in 1985 as *Principles of Geriatric Medicine*, this work is often cited by reviewers as the best geriatrics book. *Hazzard's Principles of Geriatric Medicine and Gerontology* is now in its sixth edition, complete with updated content and a design overhaul that makes it easier to read and navigate. Its main focus of blending gerontology principles with clinical geriatrics, however, is unchanged. This brand new package, authored by the world's best geriatricians, contains a number of changes. Evidence-based medicine is emphasized through the expanded use of clinical practice guidelines, as well as references to systematic reviews and critically appraised topics. The editors have also added a new chapter on international geriatric care. Meanwhile, tables, drawings, and clinical algorithms have been enhanced by the new color format, and all content on geriatric syndromes has been placed at the front of the work. The 2003 Brandon/Hill list selected the fourth edition of *Principles of Geriatric Medicine and Gerontology* (1999) for its geriatrics category.

Matteson and McConnell's Gerontological Nursing: Concepts and Practice. 3rd ed. Authors: Adrianne D. Linton, Helen W. Lach. Saunders/Elsevier, 2007.
ISBN: 9781416001669
Recommended for: Hospital Libraries

This book provides a background on gerontology and normal aging changes, practical assessment instruments, and research-based reviews of clinical topics. It supplies evidence-based guidelines for the care of older adults. Chapters address gerontological nursing roles and leadership, including interdisciplinary collaboration, case management, end of life, and health promotion concepts. This book is a comprehensive reference for all nurses with an interest in the care of older adults.

Reichel's Care of the Elderly: Clinical Aspects of Aging. 6th ed. Editors: Christine Arenson, Jan Busby-Whitehead, Kenneth Brummel-Smith, James G. O'Brien, Mary H. Palmer, William Reichel. Cambridge University Press, 2009.
http://www.cambridge.org/
http://www.r2library.com/ [Forthcoming]
http://www.ebrary.com/
http://extranet.netlibrary.com/TitleSelect/
ISBN: 9780521869294
ISBN: 9780511508349 (Online)
See Also Chapter 9.8. Geriatrics
Recommended for: Hospital, Academic Libraries
Brandon/Hill, *Doody's Core Titles* Selection

The sixth edition of *Reichel's Care of the Elderly* offers new topics in the clinical management of the geriatric patient: hormonal therapy in postmenopausal women, drug therapy for Alzheimer sufferers, alternative medicine, the chronic understaffing of nursing homes, management of delirium, and ethical issues. The targeted audience is the geriatric specialist, as well as the medical and allied health practitioner who needs practical and relevant information in a comprehensive format.

Toward Healthy Aging: Human Needs and Nursing Response. 7th ed. Authors: Priscilla Ebersole, Patricia Hess, Theris Touhy, Kathleen Jett, Ann S. Luggen. Mosby/Elsevier, 2008.
ISBN: 9780323047302
Recommended for: Hospital, Academic Libraries
Brandon/Hill, *Doody's Core Titles* Selection

Toward Healthy Aging serves as a comprehensive resource on health promotion and maintenance for older adults, their families, and caregivers. According to the publisher's description, the book "includes the most current information you need to provide effective holistic care, promote healthy lifestyle choices, and address end-of-life issues. Grounded in the core competencies recommended by the AACN (American Association of Critical-Care Nurses) in collaboration with the Hartfound *[sic]* Institute for Geriatric Nursing and using Maslow's hierarchy of needs, this book includes complete coverage of both common and uncommon conditions in the older adult. *Toward Healthy Aging* also highlights key aging issues with sections devoted to basic physiologic needs, safety and security, the need to belong, self-esteem, and self-actualization." This best seller is a former Brandon/Hill nursing book recommendation and is currently a *Doody's Core Titles* purchase recommendation within the nursing clinical specialties geriatrics section.

Journals

Age and Ageing. v. 1, Oxford University Press/British Geriatrics Society, 1972.
http://ageing.oxfordjournals.org/
ISSN: 00020729
ISSN: 14682834 (Online)
See Also Chapter 9.8 Geriatrics
Indexed in: MEDLINE, CINAHL
Recommended for: Hospital, Academic Libraries

Age and Ageing is the medical journal of the British Geriatrics Society. It covers biological gerontology and geriatrics, including research on aging and the clinical, epidemiological, and psychological aspects of medicine in old age. Current issues include the following sections: editor's view, editorial, report, news and reviews, commentary, review, research papers, research letters, case reports, letters to the editor, and book reviews.

Archives of Gerontology and Geriatrics. v. 1, Elsevier, 1982.
http://www.sciencedirect.com/science/journal/01674943
ISSN: 01674943
Indexed in: MEDLINE, CINAHL
Recommended for: Hospital, Academic Libraries

The *Archives of Gerontology and Geriatrics* is an international journal integrating experimental, clinical, and social studies on aging. The principal aim of the journal is to facilitate the exchange of information between gerontological research specialists in experimental gerontology, clinical geriatrics, and social geriatrics. The journal accepts experimental papers dealing with the basic mechanisms of aging at the molecular, cellular, tissue, or organ levels. Also accepted are clinical papers providing new information and papers dealing with anti-aging pharmacological preparations in humans. Articles addressing the social aspects of geriatrics are accepted if they are of general interest to the epidemiology of aging and the efficiency and working methods of the social organizations for the health care of the elderly.

Geriatric Nursing. v. 1, Mosby/Elsevier, 1980.
http://www.sciencedirect.com/science/journal/01974572
ISSN: 01974572
ISSN: 15283984 (Online)
Indexed in: MEDLINE, CINAHL
Recommended for: Hospital, Academic Libraries
Brandon/Hill Selection

Geriatric Nursing offers clinical information and management advice relating to the care of older adults. The journal's peer-reviewed articles report the latest developments in the management of acute and chronic disorders and provide practical advice on the care of older adults across the long-term continuum. *Geriatric Nursing* addresses current issues related to drugs, advance directives, staff development and management, legal issues, client and caregiver education, infection control, and other topics. The journal is written specifically for nurses and nurse practitioners who work with older adults in any care setting. *Geriatric Nursing* is the official journal of the American Assisted Living Nurses Association (AALNA), National Gerontological Nursing Association (NGNA), Gerontological Advanced Practice Nurses Association (GAPNA), and the Nurses Improving Care for Healthsystem Elders (NICHE). In addition to subject-based articles written by and for practicing nurses and nursing students, there is information for the practitioner such as educational classes, financial grants, and awards. Continuing education credit exams are included in each issue, along with association news and event calendars. In addition to nurses and nurse practitioners, the journal is suitable for medical and academic libraries with nursing programs. It was an initial purchase recommendation on the Brandon/Hill nursing list.

International Journal of Older People Nursing. v. 1, Wiley-Blackwell, 2006.
http://onlinelibrary.wiley.com/journal/10.1111/(ISSN)1748-3743
http://www.ebscohost.com/
ISSN: 17483735
ISSN: 17483743 (Online)
Indexed in: MEDLINE, CINAHL
Recommended for: Hospital, Academic Libraries

Begun in 2004 as supplemental issues to the *Journal of Clinical Nursing*, this publication was issued separately beginning with volume 1 in 2006. The *International Journal of Older People Nursing* is a peer-reviewed, scholarly journal. This quarterly publication aims to "challenge assumptions and provoke new ideas" to help nurses develop and inform their practice and engage in the debates about the health and social care services for older people. The journal consists of two sections. The first part publishes scholarly, peer-reviewed original articles, and the second part forms a practice development section, which is also peer-reviewed. Within the practice development section are three commissioned scholarly papers: literature scan, application to practice, and a review paper. Each issue features practice development on a key aspect of older people nursing of relevance to all nurses. The journal is indexed by CINAHL, PsycINFO, and MEDLINE. Wiley Online Library offers the complete, full text; CINAHL Plus with Full Text offers access with a one-year embargo.

Journal of Gerontological Nursing. v. 1, SLACK, 1975.
http://www.jognonline.com/
ISSN: 00989134
ISSN: 1938243X
Indexed in: MEDLINE, CINAHL
Recommended for: Hospital, Academic Libraries

The *Journal of Gerontological Nursing* covers all aspects of gerontological nursing with original clinical articles and the latest research. The *Journal of Gerontological Nursing* is a monthly, peer-reviewed journal that publishes clinically relevant, original articles on the practice of gerontological nursing across the continuum of care in a variety of health care settings. The major sections, which are not necessarily included in every issue, are: original feature articles (clinical or review articles), continuing education, "Geropharmacology," "Assessment," "Clinical Outlook," "Genetics and Gerontology," "Geropsychiatry," "Healthy Aging," "Innovations in Community-based and Long-term Care," "Interdisciplinary Care," "Legal Issues," "Multicultural Aging," "Public Policy," "Research Briefs," and "Technology Innovations." Other regular features include news, letters to the editor, book and media reviews, future events, artwork, photos, editorials, and the continuing education quiz. The journal is cited in several abstracting and indexing services such as MEDLINE, CINAHL, AGELINE, Web of Science, Scopus, and Google Scholar.

Journal of the American Geriatrics Society. v. 1, Wiley/American Geriatrics Society, 1953.
http://onlinelibrary.wiley.com/journal/10.1111/(ISSN)1532-5415
ISSN: 00028614
ISSN: 15325415
See Also Chapter 9.8. Geriatrics
Indexed in: MEDLINE
Recommended for: Hospital, Academic Libraries
Brandon/Hill Selection

The *Journal of the American Geriatrics Society* is a peer-reviewed, monthly journal covering common diseases and disorders of older adults. Its articles are relevant to the clinical care of the elderly. It covers the principles of aging, biology, psychosocial aspects, pharmacology, legal and ethical issues, and health care finance. Articles also address the approach to the older patient: hospital-based and community-based geriatric care, nursing home care, geriatric assessment, preventive geriatrics, physical activity, rehabilitation, palliative care, and alternative medicine. The journal covers such geriatric syndromes as dementia, delirium, urinary incontinence, hearing and vision impairment, malnutrition, eating and feeding problems, osteoporosis and osteomalacia, falls and gait disturbances, dizziness and syncope, pressure ulcers, and sleep disorders. Within the area of geriatric psychiatry, it accepts articles on depression and other mood disorders, anxiety disorders, psychotic disorders, personality/somatoform disorders, substance abuse, and mental retardation. Finally, the journal addresses a wide range of geriatric diseases and disorders including cardiovascular diseases, hypertension, musculoskeletal diseases, back pain, diseases and disorders of the foot, neurologic diseases, infectious diseases, respiratory diseases, oral diseases, gastrointestinal disorders, endocrine and metabolic disorders, diabetes, hormone replacement therapy, gynecologic diseases and disorders, disorders of sexual function, hematologic diseases and disorders, oncology, renal diseases, prostate disease, and dermatologic diseases. The journal is indexed in a wide range of sources such as MEDLINE, Chemical Abstracts, AGELINE, CINAHL Plus, PsycINFO, Biological Abstracts, several social science indexing and abstracting services, Google Scholar, Scopus, and Web of Science. Wiley Online Library provides full online coverage back to volume 1.

Journals of Gerontology. Series A, Biological Sciences and Medical Sciences. v. 50A, Oxford/Gerontological Society of America, 1995.
http://Biomedgerontology.oxfordjournals.org/
ISSN: 10795006
ISSN: 1758535X
See Also Chapter 9.8. Geriatrics
Indexed in: MEDLINE, CINAHL
Recommended for: Hospital, Academic Libraries
Brandon/Hill Selection

Begun in 1946 as the *Journal of Gerontology*, the *Journals of Gerontology. Series A* started publishing peer-reviewed, original scientific and research papers on the biological and medical aspects of aging under this separate title in 1995. The pertinent "Medical Sciences" section includes "articles representing the full range of medical sciences pertaining to aging. Appropriate areas include, but are not limited to, basic medical science, clinical epidemiology, clinical research, and health services research for professions such as medicine, dentistry, allied health sciences, and nursing. It publishes articles on research pertinent to human biology and disease. The following types of articles are published: (1) articles reporting original research; (2) rapid communications; (3) review articles; (4) guest editorials." The journal is widely indexed in such databases as MEDLINE, CINAHL, AGELINE, Web of Science, Scopus, and Google Scholar.

Journals of Gerontology. Series B, Psychological Sciences and Social Sciences. v. 50B, Oxford/Gerontological Society of America, 1995.
http://psychsocgerontology.oxfordjournals.org/
ISSN: 10795014
ISSN: 17585368 (Online)
See Also Chapter 9.8. Geriatrics
Indexed in: MEDLINE, CINAHL
Recommended for: Hospital, Academic Libraries
Brandon/Hill Selection

Begun in 1946 as the *Journal of Gerontology*, the *Journals of Gerontology. Series B* began in 1995 as the companion journal to *Journals of Gerontology. Series A, Biological Sciences and Medical Sciences*. Similar to Series A, Series B is divided into two parts, each with separate pagination: "Psychological Sciences" and "Social Sciences." "Psychological Sciences" covers applied, clinical, counseling, developmental, experimental, and social psychology related to aging and the elderly. Articles are expected to demonstrate the theoretical or methodological implications of the research results reported. They may also relate psychological aspects of aging to other disciplines. Four types of articles are included: lengthy articles on original research, brief reports on original research, invited reviews and position papers, and articles on theory or methodology. The second section, "Social Sciences," covers topics related to aging in various social science disciplines, such as anthropology, demography, economics, epidemiology, geography, political science, public health, social history, social work, and sociology. Five types of articles are included in this journal: lengthy articles on original research, brief reports on original research, letters to the editor, review articles, and articles on theory or methodology. The journal is widely indexed in such databases as MEDLINE, CINAHL, PsycINFO, Web of Science, Scopus, and Google Scholar.

Nursing Older People. v. 12, RCN Publishing, 2000.
http://nursingolderpeople.rcnpublishing.co.uk
ISSN: 14720795
Indexed in: MEDLINE, CINAHL
Recommended for: Hospital, Academic Libraries

This journal began in 1981 as the *British Journal of Geriatric Nursing* and experienced multiple title changes. Currently known as *Nursing Older People*, this professional trade journal is issued 10 times a year. The publication contains news analysis, nursing practice, clinical and research articles, book and journal reviews, and conference listings. It is widely indexed in such databases as MEDLINE, CINAHL, and several EBSCOhost and Gale databases.

Research in Gerontological Nursing. v. 1, SLACK, 2008.
http://www.geronurseresearch.com
ISSN: 19382464
ISSN: 19404921
Indexed in: MEDLINE, CINAHL
Recommended for: Hospital, Academic Libraries

Research in Gerontological Nursing is a peer-reviewed, interdisciplinary gerontological nursing research journal for educators, academicians, clinicians, and policymakers involved with older adults in all health care settings. This bimonthly journal is indexed in several databases such as MEDLINE, CINAHL, and AGELINE.

13.6. Holistic Nursing

A philosophy of nursing practice that takes into account total patient care, considering the physical, emotional, social, economic, and spiritual needs of patients, their response to their illnesses, and the effect of illness on patients' abilities to meet self-care needs.

—MeSH

Contributor: Paul M. Blobaum

Monographs

Healing with Alternative and Complementary Therapies 2000. Author: Lynn Keegan. Delmar Thomson Learning, 2001.
ISBN: 076681890X
Recommended for: Hospital, Academic Libraries

Keegan has written several books on the nurse as healer since the early 1990s, and this book sets forth what she considers the most important elements of state-of-the-art healing practices today. The text is organized into six parts: Part I, "Concept of Healing," discussing the types, history, and future of healing, Part II, "Complementary and Alternative Approaches to Healing" focuses on these therapies and integrative health care; Part III, "Healing Modalities," has 10 chapters about the theory and practice of selected healing modalities such as acupuncture, herbal remedies, Chinese medicine, and manual therapies; Part IV, "Healers and the Healed," discusses the process of becoming a healer, and the dispositions required of a healer; Part V, "Body-Mind-Spirit Connection to Health and Illness," discusses the connection of the mind to stress and the immune system; and Part VI, is a directory of Internet sites, organizations, and other resources. Chapters are founded with the latest research evidence, and are supplemented with an interactive website where feedback is invited.

Holistic Nursing: A Handbook for Practice. 5th ed. Editor: Barbara Montgomery Dossey. Jones & Bartlett, 2008.
ISBN: 9780763754297
Recommended for: Hospital, Academic Libraries
Doody's Core Titles Selection

Holistic nursing is a movement in the profession to integrate nursing knowledge and skill with the art and practice of healing of persons. The holistic approach considers all the spiritual, emotional, social, and physical aspects of the nurse and patient and the power of nurses to promote health and healing. The purpose of this book is to develop the knowledge base for holistic nursing, and delineate the essence of contemporary nursing. This handbook updates the previous edition with the new status of recognition of holistic nursing as a nursing specialty by the American Nurses Association in 2006. The 2007 *Holistic Nursing: Scope and Standards of Practice* are integrated into this edition. The core values of holistic nursing provide the framework for this book. Written by holistic nursing leaders, this text is a "must have" resource for students, clinicians, educators, and researchers who seek to learn about holism and expand their knowledge.

The Holistic Nursing Approach to Chronic Disease. Author: Carolyn Chambers Clark. Springer, 2004.
http://www.ebrary.com/
ISBN: 9780826125040
Recommended for: Hospital, Academic, Consumer Health Libraries

This book is a helpful guide to the evidence-based approaches to major chronic illnesses such as diabetes, fibromyalgia, HIV, heart diseases, multiple sclerosis, gastrointestinal problems, as well as the conditions of obesity and pain. Each chapter is organized with a guide to holistic nursing assessment, treatment planning, treatment, information to share with clients (teaching resources), and a bibliography of citations to primary research resources. The sections on client information will be useful to patients as well. These discussions provide helpful bullet points on what to do and what not to do to promote healing processes. This title is recommended for all libraries.

Profiles of Nurse Healers. Authors: Lynn Keegan, Barbara M. Dossey. Delmar, 1998.
ISBN: 9780827379589
Recommended for: Academic Libraries

This book is part of the Delmar *Nurse as Healer* series. Keegan and Dossey are prominent leaders in the Holistic Nurses' Association, and have collaborated on many publishing projects. This book examines the role of nurses as healers, and the evolution of nurse healers, and provides insight as to the meaning of holistic nursing practice. Most of the book comprises profiles of nurse healers and narratives of their healing journeys. This text is useful for academic and specialized libraries.

Journals

Holistic Nursing Practice. v. 1, Lippincott Williams & Wilkins, 1986.
http://journals.lww.com/hnpjournal
http://www.ovid.com/
ISSN: 08879311
ISSN: 15505138 (Online)
Indexed in: MEDLINE, CINAHL
Recommended for: Hospital, Academic Libraries
Brandon/Hill Selection

As stated in its subtitle "The Science of Health and Healing," *Holistic Nursing Practice* is a scholarly, peer-reviewed journal focusing on holistic models of clinical nursing practice. Articles explore theoretical interventions and outcomes, research, and policy, using holistic and complementary medical approaches. The journal is indexed in CINAHL and MEDLINE, and is published six times a year. Full-text coverage beginning with 1999 is available from Ovid.

Journal of Holistic Nursing. v. 1, Sage, 1983.
http://jhn.sagepub.com/
ISSN: 08980101
ISSN: 15525724 (Online)
Indexed in: MEDLINE, CINAHL
Recommended for: Hospital, Academic Libraries

Journal of Holistic Nursing is a peer-reviewed, scholarly journal exploring the art and science of nursing, considering the wholeness of body, mind, spirit, and emotions. It is the official journal of the American Holistic Nurses Association, and is published quarterly. The journal publishes foundational articles which explore the power of healing through caring nursing practice, and the promotion of health and well-being at all levels. Each issue contains continuing education articles for CE credit. The journal is available online through Sage.

13.7. Maternal-Child Nursing

Nursing care of women throughout their pregnancy and childbirth and the care of their newborn children.

—MeSH

Contributor: Paul M. Blobaum

Monographs

Breastfeeding and Human Lactation. 4th ed. Editors: Jan Riordan, Karen Wambach. Jones & Bartlett, 2010.
ISBN: 9780763754327
See Also Chapter 10.18. Reproductive Medicine
Recommended for: Hospital, Academic Libraries

This review refers to the third edition. A lactation consultant is a specialist in maternal child nursing, trained to work with mothers and babies to promote successful infant nutrition through breast feeding. Riordan brings together the latest clinical methods and research findings to enliven evidence-based practice. The book is focused on the clinical setting. Important concepts are summarized at the end of each chapter, along with listings of related Internet resources. A CD-ROM with over 100 photos of actual breastfeeding situations may be used to develop PowerPoint presentations. This text is recommended for hospital, academic, and specialized libraries.

Impact of Birthing Practices on Breastfeeding. 2nd ed. Authors: Linda J. Smith, Mary Kroeger. Jones & Bartlett, 2010.
ISBN: 9780763763749
Recommended for: Hospital, Academic Libraries

Smith critically examines the research and evidence connecting birth practices with breastfeeding outcomes. This book reflects the "Mother Friendly Childbirth Module" of the WHO's 2009 Baby-Friendly Hospital Initiative. The consequence of hospital care is the tendency to medicalize normal births. Medical interventions such as anesthesia can impact the mother/baby relationship and successful nursing for the baby. The focus of this book is on making breast feeding a reality for mothers and their babies. At 248 pages, this book is accessible and important, written for hospital personnel such as anesthetists, managers, and quality improvement committees, who are responsible for labor and delivery care, but who are unlikely to read lactation research articles. It is recommended for hospital, academic, and specialized libraries.

Labor and Delivery Nursing: A Guide to Evidence-Based Practice. Authors: Michelle L. Murray, Gayle M. Huelsmann. Springer, 2009.
See Chapter 13.9. Obstetrical Nursing

Maternal & Child Health Nursing: Care of the Childbearing and Childrearing Family. 6th ed. Author: Adele Pilitteri. Lippincott Williams & Wilkins, 2010.
ISBN: 9781582559995
Recommended for: Hospital, Academic Libraries
Brandon/Hill Selection

Maternal & Child Health Nursing is based on the premise that these areas are part of a continuum of nursing care and not two distinct practice areas. Pillitteri has authored a classic text appropriate for the undergraduate nursing curriculum, whether these subjects are taught in one course or two. Divided into eight units of 56 chapters and 1,778 pages, Pillitteri comprehensively discusses maternal and child care from the nursing perspective from conception through adolescence, using a holistic approach. The book is limited in its treatment of non-nuclear families (husband, wife, children), although other structures such as foster, gay and lesbian, adoptive, single parent, polygamy, and polygyny families are mentioned briefly as possibilities in chapter 3. Each chapter is accompanied by extensive references for further research, summaries of key points, and critical thinking exercises. The book is extensively illustrated with color charts, photographs, and highlighted texts which facilitates navigation. This book is a Brandon/Hill core nursing title. Nursing students and practitioners wishing to have a ready book for reference and to update their knowledge will benefit from this book, which is accompanied by a CD-ROM of student learning resources. It is recommended for hospital, academic, and specialized libraries.

Maternity and Women's Health Care. 9th ed. Editors: Dietra Leonard Lowdermilk, Shannon E. Perry. Mosby Elsevier, 2007.
ISBN: 9780323043670
Recommended for: Hospital, Academic Libraries
Brandon/Hill, *Doody's Core Titles* Selection

Lowdermilk and Perry and a team of expert faculty, clinicians, and specialists from other health care areas have revised this classic text with the latest health care standards and research. This text uses the philosophy that pregnancy and childbirth and developmental changes in a woman's life are natural processes. The text uses over 750 color photographs and drawings throughout, illustrating important concepts and techniques. Each chapter begins with a section of learning objectives and references to electronic resources on the companion CD-ROM or website at http://evolve.Elsevier.com. Key terms are listed, and defined within the chapter. Each chapter also has critical thinking exercises and an extensive list of references for further reading. The ninth edition is organized into eight units: Unit 1, "Introduction to Maternity and Women's Health Care"; Unit 2, "Women's Health"; Unit 3, "Pregnancy"; Unit 4, "Childbirth"; Unit 5, "Postpartum"; Unit 6, "The Newborn"; Unit 7, "Complications of Pregnancy"; and Unit 8, "Newborn Complications." Additional instructional materials are available for the text, including the instructor's resource manual and test bank, a curriculum guide, and electronic image collection, a student study guide, and a clinical companion. The companion CD-ROM package accompanies the text book, and includes case studies, critical thinking questions, videos of assessments and births, a care plan constructor, illustrated skills, anatomy reviews, and English/Spanish guidelines and glossaries. This book is designated as a Brandon/Hill core nursing title.

Maternity Nursing. 8th ed. Editors: Deitra Leonard Lowdermilk, Shannon E. Perry, Kitty Cashion. Mosby Elsevier, 2010.
ISBN: 9780323066617
Recommended for: Hospital, Academic Libraries
Brandon/Hill Selection

Maternity Nursing is a Brandon/Hill core nursing title. Intended as a text for undergraduate nursing students, nursing care material is presented in the organizational framework of Care Management, demonstrating the nursing care process and collaboration with the health care team to provide evidence-based care. Assessment, diagnosis, interventions, and evaluation of care are highlighted; nursing plans of care, care pathways, and patient teaching components are important features of the text. The 28 chapters are fully illustrated with photographs and highlighted texts for key points. Learning objectives and key terms are defined for each chapter, and critical thinking exercises with answers are helpful for student review of learning. A companion website at http://evolve .Elsevier.com provides access to additional case studies, review questions, and web links. A companion CD-ROM contains video and animations including births and assessments, care plans, an English/Spanish audio glossary, and additional critical thinking questions and rationales. Chapters are accompanied by full bibliographies for further reading, Internet resources, and directories of organizational resources contribute to this book being a valuable resource beyond the classroom for the maternity nurse. This review refers to the seventh edition.

Medications and Mother's Milk: A Manual of Lactational Pharmacology. 13th ed. Author: Thomas W. Hale. Hale, 2008.
See Chapter 13.9. Obstetrical Nursing

Perinatal Nursing. 3rd ed. Editors: Kathleen Rice Simpson, Patricia A. Creehan. Lippincott Williams & Wilkins, 20008.
ISBN: 9780781767590
Recommended for: Hospital, Academic Libraries
Doody's Core Titles Selection

The editors' goal is to "provide perinatal nurses with the latest evidence to promote the best possible outcomes for mothers and babies." This is accomplished through integrating Association of Women's Health, Obstetric and Neonatal Nurses (AWHONN) standards and guidelines throughout the text. The majority of the chapters presented discuss the process of the transition to motherhood, from pregnancy, to labor and delivery, to the care of the the mother post-birth in the hospital setting. Hospital safety, cultural competency, and planning for parenthood are among the additional topics covered. Each topic is related to AWHONN care standards and guidelines. Over 600 review questions and answers make this book a valuable resource for reviewing knowledge for certification examinations.

Journals

Journal of Perinatal Education. v. 1, Lamaze International, 1992.
http://www.ingentaconnect.com/content/lamaze/jpe
http://www.ncbi.nlm.nih.gov/pmc/journals/359/
ISSN: 10581243
ISSN: 15488519 (Online)
Indexed in: CINAHL
Recommended for: Hospital, Academic Libraries

Published quarterly, the *Journal of Perinatal Education* is the leading peer-reviewed, scholarly journal for childbirth educators. The journal is published by Lamaze International for readers who provide parent education in the areas of childbirth, pregnancy, breastfeeding, neonatal care, postpartum, early parenting, and young family development. The journal is indexed by CINAHL, and published online by Ingenta. Full-text articles are also available through EEBSCOhost. Open access articles are available through PubMed Central, including all issues from 2000 to the present.

***MCN: The American Journal of Maternal Child Nursing*.** v. 1, Lippincott Williams & Wilkins, 1976.
http://www.mcnjournal.com
ISSN: 0361929X
ISSN: 15390683 (Online)
Indexed in: MEDLINE, CINAHL
Recommended for: Hospital, Academic Libraries
Brandon/Hill Selection

In its first issue in 1976, Editor Barbara Bishop wrote that the goal of *MCN* is to "be of help to the practicing nurse so that the care given to individuals and families during the childrearing and childbearing phases of the life cycle can be of high quality." This scholarly, peer-reviewed journal is published six times a year and among its readership are nurse midwives, and perinatal, neonatal, pediatric, and maternal-child nurses. *MCN* publishes clinically relevant practices and research manuscripts aimed at assisting nurses towards evidence-based practice, including updates on diseases and nursing care, health promotion, physiology and pathophysiology, family behavior, and research that helps nurses achieve evidence-based practice. Articles that carry CE credit are available in each issue. It is indexed in CINAHL, and MEDLINE with full text available from Lippincott and Ovid.

Databases and Other Electronic Resources

***Drugs and Lactation Database (LactMed)*.** Division of Specialized Information Services, National Library of Medicine, 2006.
See Chapter 13.9. Obstetrical Nursing

13.7.1. Neonatal Nursing

Nursing care of newborn infants during the first four weeks after birth.

—MeSH

Contributor: Paul M. Blobaum

Monographs

***Comprehensive Neonatal Care: An Interdisciplinary Approach*.** 4th ed. Editors: Carole Kenner, Judy Wright Lott. Saunders Elsevier, 2007.
ISBN: 9781416029427
Recommended for: Hospital, Academic Libraries
Doody's Core Titles Selection

This text is a comprehensive, in-depth survey of the state-of-the-art care of neonates from a physiologic and pathophysiologic approach, incorporating up-to-date standards and evidence. It provides a complete foundation for each neonatal body system, and includes medical, surgical, and psychosocial care to the newborn and family. This book incorporates the Preemie Bill of Rights, and an interdisciplinary, integrative approach to nursing care of the neonate. Intended to be a textbook as well as care manual, this book has a companion learning resource website at http://evolve.Elsevier.com/kenner, which includes case studies, animations demonstrating physiologic processes, audio pronunciations of key terms and definitions, and selected materials from *Neonatal Nursing Handbook*. It is recommended for hospital, academic, and specialized libraries.

Journals

***Journal of Perinatal & Neonatal Nursing*.** v. 1, Lippincott Williams & Wilkins, 1987-.
http://www.jpnnjournal.com
ISSN: 08932190
ISSN: 15505073 (Online)
Indexed in: MEDLINE, CINAHL
Recommended for: Hospital, Academic Libraries

The *Journal of Perinatal and Neonatal Nursing* is a quarterly, peer-reviewed scholarly journal, published in online and print formats by Lippincott Williams & Wilkins. The objective of the journal is to provide neonatal nurses with current information on perinatal and neonatal nursing. The journal advances evidence-based practice through the publication of research, editorials, expert opinions, continuing education, and legal and risk management and education articles. The journal states that "the perinatal focus of *JPNN* centers around labor and delivery and intrapartum services specifically and overall perinatal services broadly. The neonatal focus emphasizes neonatal intensive care and includes the spectrum of neonatal and infant care outcomes." *JPNN* is indexed in CINAHL and MEDLINE. Full-text articles for all issues of JPNN are available from Lippincott and Ovid, and through EBSCO's EJS and CINAHL Plus beginning with 1999.

***Neonatal Network: The Journal of Neonatal Nursing*.** v. 1, Academy of Neonatal Nursing, 1981.
http://www.neonatalnetwork.com
ISSN: 07300832
ISSN: 15392880 (Online)
Indexed in: MEDLINE, CINAHL
Recommended for: Hospital, Academic Libraries
Brandon/Hill Selection

Neonatal Network is the official journal of the Academy of Neonatal Nursing. It is a scholarly, peer-reviewed journal, and is published six times a year by the Academy. The goal of the journal is to assist nurses and other neonatal care givers to keep up-to-date with current research and practices in the field. Articles are published in the areas of neonatal clinical practice, research, education, and administration. The journal is available online from EBSCO EJS, and from the publisher beginning with 2004. The journal is indexed in CINAHL and MEDLINE.

13.8. Midwifery

The practice of assisting women in childbirth.
—MeSH

Contributor: Paul M. Blobaum

Monographs

Evidence-Based Care for Midwives: Clinical Effectiveness Made Easy. 2nd ed. Authors: Donna Brayford, Ruth Chambers, Elizabeth Boath, David Rogers. Radcliffe, 2008.
ISBN: 9781846191473
Recommended for: Hospital, Academic Libraries

Although written from a British viewpoint, this book will be a useful resource for American nurse-midwives. This practical guide to clinical effectiveness and clinical governance contains references to important evidence-based resources. The stages of the evidence-based practice process are presented, from forming a research question, gathering the evidence, reviewing published research papers, and applying the evidence in practice. This book is recommended for academic, special, and hospital libraries.

Medications and Mother's Milk: A Manual of Lactational Pharmacology. 13th ed. Author: Thomas W. Hale. Hale, 2008.
See Chapter 13.9. Obstetrical Nursing

Primary Care of Women: A Guide for Midwives & Women's Health Providers. Authors: Barbara Hackley, Jan M. Krebs, Mary Ellen Rousseau. Jones & Bartlett, 2007.
ISBN: 9780763716509
Recommended for: Hospital, Academic Libraries

The American authors are academics and certified nurse midwives. The book is heavily referenced with American literature and standards. Chapters are typically illustrated with charts and graphics to promote absorption of the material. Basic topics of health and common disease states among women are discussed in short, accessible chapters. A section is included on how midwives can be partners in assessing women and planning care with other members of the interdisciplinary team. The book, which is over 900 pages in length and illustrated in black and white, is recommended for academic, hospital, and nursing libraries.

Professional Issues in Midwifery. Author: Lynette A. Ament. Jones & Bartlett, 2007.
ISBN: 9780763728366
Recommended for: Hospital, Academic Libraries

This book provides an in-depth analysis and overview of key issues facing American midwifery today. It is designed as a handbook to the American College of Nurse-Midwives and for public programs affecting the healthcare of women and children. This book serves as a primary source of professional issues for student and professional midwives, and uses learning objectives and summaries of key points. This is a critical resource for all who need information on the relationship of midwifery to nurses and physicians in the health care system, regulatory issues, certification and licensure, competencies and standards of practice, insurance reimbursement for services, and other critical issues. It is recommended for hospital, academic, and specialized libraries.

Varney's Midwifery. 4th ed. Authors: Helen Varney, Jan M. Krebs, Carolyn L. Gegor. Jones & Bartlett, 2004.
http://extranet.netlibrary.com/TitleSelect/
ISBN: 9780763718565
Recommended for: Hospital, Academic Libraries

Varney's Midwifery covers the provision of care of women from puberty through old age, including the childbearing cycle, and care of the newborn and infant. Designated an *American Journal of Nursing* Book of the Year award winner in 2003, this text is considered a "must have" basic textbook on midwifery. Each chapter contains extensive bibliographies of journal and Internet resources. The book provides the gold standard of midwifery care in the United States and is recommended for hospital, special, and academic libraries supporting advanced practice nurses.

Journals

Evidence Based Midwifery. v. 1, Ten Alps Publishing, 2003-.

http://www.rcm.org.uk/ebm/
ISSN: 14794489
Indexed in: CINAHL
Recommended for: Hospital, Academic Libraries

Evidence Based Midwifery is the scholarly, peer-reviewed journal of the Royal College of Midwives of the United Kingdom. It is published quarterly. The current issues are published online in open-access format, while previous issues require a subscription or membership in the College. The journal is indexed in CINAHL. The journal publishes qualitative and quantitative research articles, philosophical research, action research, systematic reviews, and meta-analysis of qualitative and quantitative data. The journal aims to promote the dissemination and implementation of midwifery evidence at the local, national, and international levels.

Journal of Midwifery and Women's Health. v. 45, Elsevier, 2000.
http://www.jmwh.com/
ISSN: 15269523
ISSN: 15422011 (Online)
Indexed in: MEDLINE, CINAHL
Recommended for: Hospital, Academic Libraries

Journal of Midwifery and Women's Health is the official journal of the American College of Nurse-Midwives. The journal is a bimonthly, peer-reviewed scholarly journal. Original research and reviews that focus on midwifery and women's health, pertaining to education, evidence-based practice, policy, public health, and research are published. The journal is included in Elsevier's NursingConsult database and is also published on other Elsevier platforms. It is also available through EBSCO EJS. The journal is indexed in CINAHL, MEDLINE, and beginning in 2007, PsycINFO.

Midwives. v. 11, Redactive Pub. Ltd, 2008.
http://www.rcm.org.uk/midwives/
ISSN: 14792915
Indexed in: MEDLINE, CINAHL
Recommended for: Hospital, Academic Libraries

Midwives is the peer-reviewed magazine of the Royal College of Midwives of the United Kingdom. It is published bimonthly. The previous titles of the journal were *RCM Midwives* (2002–2007), *RCM Midwives Journal* (1998–2001), *Midwives* (1996–1997), and *Midwives Chronicle* (1888–1995). The magazine publishes reviews of research, news, expert opinions, case studies, book reviews, practice articles, and policy analysis. Full-text articles are available in EBSCO, CINAHL Plus, and also through EBSCO EJS. The current issue of *Midwives* magazine is available online in open-access format from the journal website. Prior issues require a subscription or membership in the Royal College of Midwives. The journal is indexed in CINAHL, and also MEDLINE.

Databases and Other Electronic Resources

Drugs and Lactation Database (LactMed). Division of Specialized Information Services, National Library of Medicine, 2006
See Chapter 13.9. Obstetrical Nursing

Maternity and Infant Care Source: MIDIRS (Midwives Information & Resource Service) Reference Database. MIDIRS (Midwives Information & Resource Service), 1988.
http://www.midirs.org/ols
http://www.ovid.com/
Recommended for: Hospital, Academic Libraries

First developed in 1988, this fee-based international database contains citations to "journal articles, book chapters, reports, pamphlets, news items, audio visual materials, conference proceedings and other 'grey literature' relating to the midwifery profession, pregnancy, labour, birth, postnatal care, and neonatal care extending into the first year of life." Coverage extends from 1973 to the present. With over 144,000 citations, and over 12,000 added annually, the Maternity and Infant Care Source is an important contribution to accessing midwifery knowledge. The database is also available in the United States through Ovid.

13.9. Obstetrical Nursing

Nursing care given to the pregnant patient before, after, or during childbirth.

—MeSH

Contributor: Paul M. Blobaum

Monographs

Labor and Delivery Nursing: A Guide to Evidence-Based Practice. Authors: Michelle L. Murray, Gayle M. Huelsmann. Springer, 2009.
http://www.statref.com/
http://extranet.netlibrary.com/TitleSelect/
ISBN: 9780826118035
Recommended for: Hospital, Academic Libraries

This text is intended for use during the orientation of nursing staff to the labor and delivery room, or as a review for experienced professionals. This book may also be used as a reference or study guide for nurses taking certification examination in obstetrics or labor and delivery. Each chapter includes a True or False self-assessment. Chapters are written with extensive bibliographies of the primary sources, and are illustrated with black and white photographs and illustrations.

Manual of High Risk Pregnancy and Delivery. 4th ed. Authors: Elizabeth Stepp Gilbert, Judith Smith Harmon. Mosby/Elsevier, 2007.
ISBN: 9780323040167
Recommended for: Hospital, Academic Libraries
Brandon/Hill, *Doody's Core Titles* Selection

Designated as a Brandon/Hill core nursing title, this book was written for nurses serving in clinics, emergency rooms, and primary care settings who may recognize complications of pregnancy and be in a position to provide immediate care. This book is organized around the nursing process framework for discussions of emergent care and nursing interventions. The book is designed to provide precise and comprehensive evidence-based information in a portable and accessible format. Management and intervention protocols for high risk and critical obstetrical care are discussed. Incidence, prevalence, etiology, physiology, pathophysiology, as well as advanced practice nursing protocols are presented. Complementary and integrative medical interventions are discussed. This text is recommended for hospital and specialized libraries, and academic libraries serving advanced practice nurses.

Medications and Mother's Milk: A Manual of Lactational Pharmacology. 13th ed. Author: Thomas W. Hale. Hale, 2008.
http://www.ibreastfeeding.com/
ISBN: 9780981525723
Recommended for: Hospital, Academic Libraries

This comprehensive reference book contains information on the potential impact of medicines on mother's milk, and the health of nursing infants. Over 1,000 drugs, herbs, over the counter medications, vaccines, and vitamins are listed and described, with bibliographies for further reading. This book differs from the National Library of Medicine's LactMed database by including the coverage of herbs and vitamins in its scope. Dr. Hale's thorough research and concise presentation, and its coverage of herbs and vitamins, makes this book a "must have" resource for nurses and physicians caring for nursing mothers. The book is available online for individuals or institutions by annual subscription.

Journals

Journal of Obstetric, Gynecologic, and Neonatal Nursing (JOGNN). v. 14, Wiley/Blackwell, 1985.
http://onlinelibrary.wiley.com/journal/10.1111/(ISSN)1552-6909
ISSN: 08842175
ISSN: 15526909 (Online)
Indexed in: MEDLINE, CINAHL
Recommended for: Hospital, Academic Libraries
Brandon/Hill Selection

JOGNN is the official journal of the Association of Women's Health, Obstetric, and Neonatal Nurses (AWHONN). *JOGNN* is a scholarly, peer-reviewed journal, and it is published bi-monthly in print and electronic formats. The journal's focus is on the nursing care of women and newborns. The journal publishes quantitative and qualitative research, clinical care articles on the the best supporting evidence for practice, and policy discussions. Emerging AWHONN policy statements, standards, and guidelines are published in the journal, as well as CNE articles. Current issues are published in full-text for free on the journal's website, but prior issues dating back to 1972 require a subscription. It was designated as a Brandon/Hill core nursing journal.

Databases and Other Electronic Resources

Drugs and Lactation Database (LactMed). Division of Specialized Information Services, National Library of Medicine, 2006.
http://toxnet.nlm.nih.gov/
Recommended for: Hospital, Academic, Consumer Health Libraries

LactMed is a peer-reviewed database of full-text documents, reporting data on drugs to which breastfeeding mothers may be exposed. Included in each report is a summary of use during lactation, effects in breastfed infants, possible effects on lactation, the AAP (American Academy of Pediatrics) category, alternative drugs to consider, and substance identification information. Reference to primary research articles is included in each record, and links are provided to other NLM resources. Searches can be conducted by CAS registry number, drug or chemical name, pharmacologic category, or subject term. Records are organized by the substance name. Search results may be printed, downloaded, or viewed online. LactMed has been published for free through NLM's TOXNET service since 2006 and is recommended for nurses and health professionals caring for nursing mothers as well as consumer health libraries.

13.10. Occupational Health Nursing

Nursing in the work environment.

—MeSH

Contributor: Paul M. Blobaum

Monographs

Core Curriculum for Occupational and Environmental Health Nursing. 3rd ed. Author: Mary K. Salazar. Saunders, 2006.
ISBN: 9781416023746
Recommended for: Hospital, Academic Libraries
Brandon/Hill, *Doody's Core Titles* Selection

Part I, "Foundations of Occupational and Environmental Health Nursing Practice," sets forth the history, and conceptual and theoretical foundations of the specialty. Traditions, legal and regulatory issues, leadership, management, business trends, and research foundations are also presented. Part II, "Strategies and Approaches to Occupational and Environmental Health Nursing Practice," gives a comprehensive overview of the knowledge and processes that are central to the field. This section is presented in an outline format. Competencies for job performance at each level of practice are presented within the framework of Standards of Practice. Part III, "Advancing Professionalism in Occupational and Environmental Health Nursing," presents professional development issues. This edition includes updates on the regulatory environment including HIPAA and OSHA's "Strategic Management Plan," and disaster management and planning. Designated a Brandon/Hill select nursing title, this book is an essential reference resource for libraries serving students in occupational and community health areas and is recommended for hospital, academic, and special libraries.

Hazard Recognition and Control in Institutional Settings: A Guide for Hospitals, Universities and Nursing Homes. Editor: George Byrns. American Society of Safety Engineers, 2009.
ISBN: 9781885581549
Recommended for: Hospital, Academic Libraries

This book is intended to serve as a textbook for environmental health and safety students who wish to learn about controlling hazards in institutional settings. The book is not intended to be a comprehensive treatment of all hazards these institutions may encounter, but to highlight the most significant threats and provide a framework for addressing emerging hazards. Practitioners in the field will also find the book useful. The book employs Haddon's Matrix, originally developed to improve traffic safety, and also basic tenets of industrial hygiene. A summary of the best practices for managing waste management, violence prevention, occupational hazards, emergency preparedness, and infection control are among the topics covered, using OSHA, Joint Commission, and other regulatory health and safety standards. Each chapter includes learning objectives, reference citations, classroom activities, and student learning exercises. An instructor's guide is available. It is recommended for hospital, academic, and special libraries.

Working Safely in Health Care: A Practical Guide. Author: Deborah L. Fell-Carlson. Thomson Delmar Learning, 2008.
ISBN: 9781418006235
Recommended for: Hospital, Academic Libraries

Fell-Carlson has written a comprehensive resource of workplace safety focusing on the healthcare environment. The book focuses on current best practices based on evidence. The purpose is to be an introduction to the more common safety and occupational health issues of concern to health care workers. The book can be used as a text for training workers in all health care settings. Supplementary materials include *Training Modules to Accompany Working Safely in Health Care* (ISBN 1418006246), which includes a CD-ROM and PowerPoint presentation, handouts, tests, and more. *Working Safely in Health Care: A Quick Reference* (ISBN 1418006254) is a companion resource, and contains brief synopses of key points in the text.

Journals

AAOHN Journal. v. 34, Slack, 1986.
http://www.aaohnjournal.com/
ISSN: 08910162
ISSN: 19382448 (Online)
Indexed in: MEDLINE, CINAHL
Recommended for: Hospital, Academic Libraries
Brandon/Hill Selection

AAOHN Journal is the official journal of the American Association of Occupational Health Nurses. This journal is published monthly, and is peer-reviewed. The journal publishes original articles, health updates, news, media reviews, and professional practice updates. CE credit is available in each issue. Online issues are available from 2002 to the present from Slack, and from 2003 through CINAHL and Ovid. The journal is indexed in CINAHL and MEDLINE.

13.11. Oncologic Nursing

Nursing care provided cancer patients. It includes aspects of family functioning through education of both patient and family. The specialty of oncologic nursing focuses on cancer as a major health care problem.

—MeSH

Contributor: Mark Vrabel

Monographs

Cancer Nursing: Principles and Practice. 7th ed. Editors: Connie Henke Yarbro, Debra Wujcik, Barbara Holmes Gobel. Jones & Bartlett, 2010.
ISBN: 9780763763572
Recommended for: Hospital, Academic Libraries
Brandon/Hill, *Doody's Core Titles* Selection

A *Doody's* essential purchase recommendation with its earlier editions appearing on the Brandon/Hill lists, *Cancer Nursing: Principles and Practice* is a 1,900+ page definitive text that is to oncology nurses what *DeVita Cancer: Principles and Practice of Oncology* is to oncologists. Over 90 contributors, with expertise in various specialty areas, ensure a comprehensive scope of coverage. Chapters range in topic from prevention and detection, diagnosis, and standard treatments—such as chemotherapy, radiation, and surgery—to emerging therapies and modalities such as biologic and targeted therapies, gene therapy, and complementary and alternative treatments. Also covered are bone marrow and hematopoietic cell transplantation, oncologic emergencies, supportive care, professional nursing issues, and individual cancers. All topics include extensive references, and the book is thoroughly indexed. It is a selected reference on the Oncology Nursing Certification Corporation (ONCC) Oncology Nursing Certification Test Bulletin for various certification examinations: OCN® (Oncology Certified Nurse); CBCN™ (Certified Breast Care Nurse); AOCNP® (Advanced Oncology Certified Nurse Practitioner); and AOCNS® (Advanced Oncology Certified Nurse Specialist). An essential reference for both experienced and novice oncology nurses, it would be particularly relevant in scope for hospital or other medical, nursing, and clinical library collections.

Chemotherapy and Biotherapy Guidelines and Recommendations for Practice. 3rd ed. Editors: Martha Polovich, Julie M. Whitford, MiKaela M. Olsen. Oncology Nursing Society, 2009.
http://www.statref.com/
ISBN: 9781890504816
Recommended for: Hospital Libraries
Doody's Core Titles Selection

More than 72,000 health care professionals use this 2009 *Doody's Core Titles* recommendation, which received a perfect score of 100 out of 100 in the *Doody's* reviews. The updated edition of this longtime best seller is an essential resource for oncology nurses in all practice settings. The book is used as the training material for the Oncology Nursing Society's chemotherapy courses; upon successful completion of the course, participants receive a chemotherapy provider card. It is a selected reference on the Oncology Nursing Certification Corporation (ONCC) Oncology Nursing Certification Test Bulletin for the OCN® (Oncology Certified Nurse), CBCN™ (Certified Breast Care Nurse), AOCNP® (Advanced Oncology Certified Nurse Practitioner), and AOCNS® (Advanced Oncology Certified Nurse Specialist) certification examinations. Arranged in an outline format, it covers in detail all principles of antineoplastic agent administration, from pretreatment through post-treatment care. Sections include fundamentals of administration, side effects and immediate complications, treatment schedules (including dose category and determination), safe management in the home, clinical practicum and evaluations, and more. Many detailed tables and graphics are incorporated throughout the text, and an extensive index is included. The full text of this book is available online via STAT!Ref, and individual sections and full-text versions are available via pay-per-view download at http://ons.metapress.com. For mobile, handheld technology, some of its content is incorporated into the PEPID RN ONS Platinum Suite ("The only fully integrated, comprehensive point-of-care information resource for oncology nurses") at http://www.pepid.com/iphone/ONSPlatinumdetails.asp.

Mosby's Oncology Nursing Advisor: A Comprehensive Guide to Clinical Practice. Editors: Susan Newton, Margaret Hickey, Joyce Marrs. Mosby/Elsevier, 2009.
ISBN: 9780323045971

Recommended for: Hospital Libraries
Doody's Core Titles Selection

This 2009 *Doody's Core Titles* recommendation is an update of the 1999 text *Oncology Nursing Assessment and Clinical Care*. With over 40 contributing authors, the book is organized into seven main sections: introduction, "Major Cancers," "Principles of Cancer Management," "Principles of Symptom Management," "Oncologic Emergencies/Emergent Issues," "Palliative Care and End-of-Life Issues," and "Patient Teaching." There are thorough descriptions of over 50 major cancer types and 30 common symptoms. In addition to the primary treatment modalities of chemotherapy, radiation, and surgery, there is detailed coverage of the growing fields of biological response modifiers, targeted therapies, and complementary and alternative treatments. More than 25 reproducible patient teaching handouts are included. It is a selected reference on the Oncology Nursing Certification Corporation (ONCC) Oncology Nursing Certification Test Bulletin for the OCN® (Oncology Certified Nurse) and CBCN™ (Certified Breast Care Nurse) certification examinations. The book is a useful reference tool for both experienced and novice oncology nurses. It would be particularly relevant in scope to hospital or other medical, nursing, and clinical library collections.

Oncology Nursing. 5th ed. Editors: Martha E. Langhorne, Janet S. Fulton, Shirley E. Otto. Mosby/Elsevier, 2007.
ISBN: 9780323041850
Recommended for: Hospital, Academic Libraries
Brandon/Hill, *Doody's Core Titles* Selection

This *Doody's Core Titles* recommendation, with its earlier editions appearing on the Brandon/Hill lists, offers a comprehensive but manageable overview of all elements of the oncology nursing discipline. The book is organized into five main units: "Clinical Aspects of Cancer Diagnosis," "Clinical Management of Major Cancers," "Cancer Treatment Modalities," "Cancer Care Supportive Therapies," and "Symptom Management." Chapters within these units contain information on future directions, along with graphs, tables, and charts presenting clinically relevant information. There are many references as well as five appendixes: glossary of terms, oral grading scale, Internet resources, lab values, and diagnostic tests. It is a selected reference on the Oncology Nursing Certification Corporation (ONCC) Oncology Nursing Certification Test Bulletin for the OCN® (Oncology Certified Nurse) certification examination. It is also a useful study guide with over 400 multiple-choice review questions accompanying chapter case studies. An essential reference for both experienced and novice oncology nurses, it would be particularly relevant in scope to hospital or other medical, nursing, and clinical library collections.

Putting Evidence into Practice: Improving Oncology Patient Outcomes. Editors: Linda H. Eaton, Janelle M. Tipton. Oncology Nursing Society, 2009.
http://www.statref.com
ISBN: 9781890504847
Recommended for: Hospital, Academic Libraries
Doody's Core Titles Selection

The Oncology Nursing Society (ONS) *Putting Evidence into Practice* (*PEP*) resources are designed to summarize the evidence on interventions for common cancer-related symptoms, side effects, or complications. The interventions are classified into color-coded levels of evidence: green (recommended for practice), yellow (effectiveness not established), and red (not recommended for practice). The four original topics were fatigue, chemotherapy-induced nausea and vomiting, sleep-wake disturbances, and prevention of infection, which were issued in 2006 as pocket-sized reference cards to facilitate ease of use by bedside nurses. After 12 other topics were developed and published as articles in the *Clinical Journal of Oncology Nursing* and a dedicated section of the ONS website, this book was produced to combine and update all of the existing *PEP* material and to add new sections on incidence of the problem, clinical assessment and measurement tools, and case studies on how to use the tools in practice. The full text of this book is available online via STAT!Ref, and individual sections and full-text versions are available via pay-per-view download at http://ons.metapress.com. Free updated content is available at http://www.ons.org/Research/PEP. For mobile, handheld technology, there is an iPhone application for the book and the individual *PEP* topics, and some of its content is incorporated into the PEPID RN ONS Platinum Suite ("The only fully integrated, comprehensive point-of-care information resource for oncology nurses") at http://www.pepid.com/iphone/ONSPlatinumdetails.asp. Finally, some of the *PEP* content is summarized in consumer-friendly language in a section in *The Cancer Journey* (http://www.thecancerjourney.org), a patient website designed by ONS. The book is intended for health care practitioners and is thus suitable for medical libraries or other hospital or academic health collections. *The Cancer Journey* would be useful to consumer health librarians.

Radiation Therapy: A Guide to Patient Care. 1st ed. Editors: Marilyn L. Haas, William P. Hogle, Giselle J.

Moore-Higgs, Tracy A. Gosselin-Acomb. Elsevier, 2007. *See* Chapter 10.17.2. Radiation Oncology

Journals

Cancer Nursing. v. 1, Lippincott Williams & Wilkins, 1978.
http://www.cancernursingonline.com
http://www.nursingcenter.com
http://www.ovid.com/
ISSN: 0162220X
ISSN: 15389804 (Online)
Indexed in: MEDLINE, CINAHL
Recommended for: Hospital, Academic Libraries
Brandon/Hill Selection

Cancer Nursing: An International Journal for Cancer Care is the bimonthly, official publication of the International Society of Nurses in Cancer Care. It covers delivery practices worldwide, publishing research on prevention and early detection, geriatric and pediatric cancer nursing, medical and surgical oncology, ambulatory care, nutritional support, psychosocial issues, and other nursing interventions. Its impact factor of 1.878 ranks fifth out of 72 journals in the nursing category (2009 *Journal Citation Reports*). Accepted for inclusion in *Index Medicus* in 1985, the journal is included in numerous abstracting and indexing sources deemed 2009 "Essential Nursing Resources" by the Interagency Council on Information Resources in Nursing (ICIRN), such as MEDLINE, Embase, and CINAHL. The journal publishes continuing nursing education articles and is available in both print and online formats. Full online coverage back to volume 1, 1978 is available at http://www.cancernursingonline.com, and coverage back to volume 19, 1996 is available via both Ovid and http://www.nursingcenter.com.

Clinical Journal of Oncology Nursing. v. 1, Oncology Nursing Society, 1997.
http://ons.metapress.com
http://www.ebscohost.com
http://www.ovid.com/
ISSN: 10921095
ISSN: 1538067X (Online)
Indexed in: MEDLINE, CINAHL
Recommended for: Hospital Libraries

The mission of this bimonthly official journal of the Oncology Nursing Society is to provide practical information necessary to care for patients and their families across the cancer continuum and to develop publication skills in oncology nurses. Through its feature articles and columns such as "Professional Issues," "Oncology Nursing 101," and "Evidence-Based Practice," it addresses topics such as cancer care delivery and programs, comorbidities, genomics, interventional radiology, and symptom management. The journal is included in numerous abstracting and indexing sources deemed 2009 "Essential Nursing Resources" by the Interagency Council on Information Resources in Nursing (ICIRN), such as CINAHL, PsycINFO, and MEDLINE. Full-text coverage is offered in EBSCOhost databases such as Health Source: Nursing/Academic Edition and CINAHL Plus with Full-Text, and the journal is available via Ovid. It has received numerous awards, including the 2009 American Society for Association Executives (ASAE) & the Center for Association Leadership Gold Circle Award in the Peer-Reviewed Journal category and the 2008 Society of National Association Publications (SNAP) EXCEL Silver Award in the Scholarly Journals—Feature Article category. The journal publishes continuing nursing education articles and is available in both print and online formats. Full online coverage back to volume 6, 2002 is available via MetaPress.

Oncology Nursing Forum. v. 4, Oncology Nursing Society, 1977.
http://ons.metapress.com
http://www.ebscohost.com
http://www.ovid.com/
ISSN: 0190535X
ISSN: 15380688 (Online)
Indexed in: MEDLINE, CINAHL
Recommended for: Hospital, Academic Libraries
Brandon/Hill Selection

Begun in 1974 in newsletter form before changing title and becoming the *Oncology Nursing Forum* in 1977, its mission is to convey information related to practice, technology, education, research, and leadership within the scope of the oncology nursing specialty. Accepted for inclusion in *Index Medicus* in 1990, this bimonthly, official journal of the Oncology Nursing Society includes original, peer-reviewed research articles, as well as news items and product and publication reviews. Its impact factor of 1.907 ranks fourth out of 72 journals in the nursing category (2009 *Journal Citation Reports*). The journal is included in numerous abstracting and indexing sources deemed 2009 "Essential Nursing Resources" by the Interagency Council on Information Resources in Nursing (ICIRN), such as the British Nursing Index, CINAHL, PsycINFO, and MEDLINE. Full-text coverage is offered in EBSCOhost databases such as Health Source: Nursing/Academic Edition and CINAHL Plus with Full-Text, and the journal is available via Ovid. It has received numerous awards, including the 2007 Society of National Association Publications (SNAP) EXCEL Gold Award in the Scholarly Journals—Feature Article category. The journal publishes continuing nursing education articles and is available in both print and online formats. Full online coverage back to volume 29, 2002 is available via MetaPress.

Seminars in Oncology Nursing. v. 1, Elsevier, 1985.
http://www.seminarsoncologynursing.com
http://www.sciencedirect.com/science/journal/07492081
ISSN: 07492081 (Print/Online)
Indexed in: MEDLINE, CINAHL
Recommended for: Hospital, Academic Libraries
Brandon/Hill Selection

Appearing on the Brandon/Hill lists when they were still published, this quarterly journal's mission is to disseminate knowledge in the field of cancer nursing. Each issue has its own theme and guest editor with expertise on the topic; for example, articles in the November 2009 issue are devoted to "Fertility Concerns in Young Cancer Survivors." The journal is included in CINAHL and MEDLINE. It is available in both print and online formats. Full online coverage back to volume 1, 1985 is available via ScienceDirect, and coverage back to volume 11, 1995 is available at http://www.seminarsoncologynursing.com.

13.12. Orthopedic Nursing

Nursing in the care of the orthopedic patient.
—MeSH

Contributor: Elisabeth Rowan

Monographs

Core Curriculum for Orthopaedic Nursing. 6th ed. Author: National Association of Orthopaedic Nurses. Pearson, 2007.
ISBN: 9780536386939
Recommended for: Hospital, Academic Libraries

The National Association of Orthopaedic Nurses (NAON) produces this book for nurses practicing in the area of orthopedics, nursing faculty, advanced practice nurses, nurse managers, and nursing students. It is particularly useful for those needing a comprehensive review for the Orthopaedic Nursing Certification (ONC) examination. Although the book itself is not available online, there are two sets of online review questions for almost every chapter. The second of these may be used to obtain continuing education contact hours; details may be found in the preface. The book is organized as an outline of points to remember regarding each topic, supplemented by tables. The book begins by looking at the different practice settings for orthopedic nursing and a detailed examination of anatomy and physiology follows. Steps for assessment and types of diagnostic studies are covered, along with discussions related to perioperative patient care, the effects of immobility, pain, complications, infections, and therapeutic modalities. For disorders and conditions, such areas as assessment, therapy, nursing diagnoses, outcomes, interventions, practice setting considerations, and home care considerations are all fully covered. Trauma and tumors are discussed, and then a chapter-by-chapter look at each area of the skeletal system (shoulder, hand/wrist, spine, hip/femur/pelvis, knee, and foot and ankle) is addressed in turn. The last chapter deals with preparation for the certification exam. Each chapter includes objectives, key points, and a relevant bibliography. The book is fully indexed.

Orthopaedic and Trauma Nursing. 2nd ed. Editors: Julia D. Kneale, Peter S. Davis. Churchill Livingstone, 2005.
ISBN: 9780443061820
Recommended for: Hospital, Academic Libraries

The focus of this book is on the preservation of movement and the care of patients with various musculoskeletal issues or trauma. The publication provides a good grounding on the specialty, including both the scope of care and its theory. *Orthopaedic and Trauma Nursing* also provides an overview of how the locomotor system works and why both movement and, at times, its restriction are important. Chapters cover such core areas as infections, various musculoskeletal conditions, bone tumors, and issues that are special to youth and the elderly. Special consideration is given to spine and spinal cord injuries and conditions. The work includes additional content on the importance of nutrition, planned and emergency patient admissions, and epidemiology influences. Helpful illustrations and practical suggestions in sidebars, such as exercises that will help the condition, are provided. The audience includes nurses who work or specialize in orthopedics and/or trauma, as well as students who are new to the concepts of the field.

Orthopaedic Nursing. 3rd ed. Editors: Ann Butler Maher, Susan Warner Salmond, Teresa A. Pellino. W.B. Saunders, 2002.
ISBN: 9780721693026

Recommended for: Hospital, Academic Libraries
Brandon/Hill Selection

This comprehensive text is an invaluable tool for nursing faculty, nursing students, orthopedic nurses, and other non-specialists who need a good resource for the care of patients with musculoskeletal issues. Evidence-based practice is related to the discussion at hand, and a team approach is taken throughout the text. Clear illustrations, tables, and diagrams supplement the book. The information is organized in such a way that each subject is presented consistently and analyzed in a clear fashion. The work covers core areas such as anatomy, pain management, assessment, mobilization and immobilization, disorders, sports injuries, neoplasms, amputation, and infections. Also included are helpful subjects such as genetics, ergonomics, psychosocial care, and computers as a resource for education. The book provides an all-inclusive look at the field of care.

Journals

International Journal of Orthopaedic and Trauma Nursing. v. 14, Elsevier, 2010.
http://www.sciencedirect.com/science/journal/18781241
ISSN: 18781241 (Print/Onlne)
Indexed in: CINAHL
Recommended for: Hospital, Academic Libraries

Formerly known as the *Journal of Orthopaedic Nursing*, this serves as the association journal of the Australia New Zealand Orthopaedic Nurses Association, the Canadian Orthopaedic Nurses Association, and the Royal College of Nursing Society of Orthopaedic and Trauma Nursing. It is a peer-reviewed journal that includes original research, literature reviews, international policy digests, and personal reflections on practice, education, and management issues. It is aimed at practitioners in the field of orthopedic and trauma nursing, providing tools for evidence-based practice and allowing an arena for debate on best methods. Both the current volume of the *International Journal of Orthopaedic and Trauma Nursing* and older issues of the *Journal of Orthopaedic Nursing* can be found in ScienceDirect under their respective titles.

Orthopaedic Nursing. v. 1, Lippincott Williams & Wilkins, 1982.
http://www.orthopaedicnursing.com
http://www.ovid.com/
ISSN: 07446020
ISSN: 15388654 (Online)
Indexed in: MEDLINE, CINAHL
Recommended for: Hospital, Academic Libraries
Brandon/Hill Selection

The National Association of Orthopaedic Nurses (NAON) began printing its association journal in 1982, just two years after the group's formation. The journal is international in scope, reflecting the Association's membership that includes individuals from the United States and several other countries. It has become a major publication in this specialty and the premier journal for orthopedic nursing in the United States. *Orthopaedic Nursing* is published bimonthly, providing information on activities within NAON and its departments, research, product and drug information, and items of interest in the literature. Each issue also includes continuing education opportunities. Issues often include overviews and nursing implications for disorders that may be encountered in an orthopedic environment. The journal is aimed at nurses working in the specialty of orthopedics regardless of clinical setting. It is of value to orthopedic specialty collections, academic libraries serving nursing students who may be considering the specialty, or hospital libraries that support orthopedic care. Full online coverage back to volume 1, 1982 is available through Lippincott Williams & Wilkins.

13.13. Pediatric Nursing

Nursing care of children from birth to adolescence. It includes the clinical and psychological aspects of nursing care.

—MeSH

Contributor: Paul M. Blobaum

Monographs

Pediatric Primary Care. 4th ed. Authors: Catherine E. Burns, Ardys M. Dunn, Margaret A. Brady, Nancy Barber Starr, Catherine G. Blosser. Saunders/Elsevier, 2009.
ISBN: 9781416040873
Recommended for: Hospital, Academic Libraries
Brandon/Hill, *Doody's Core Titles* Selection

The primary audience of this book is advanced practice nurses such as pediatric nurse practitioners, and family nurse practitioners. Physician assistants, pediatricians, family physicians, pediatric clinical nurse specialists, community health nurses, pediatric ambulatory care nurses, school nurses, and other primary care professionals will find this book useful. The third edition of this book received an *American Journal of Nursing* Book of the Year Award for primary care, and the first edition won an award from *Nurse Practitioner* journal. This 1,351 page text is valuable for students and professionals alike. The book is divided into five sections: introduction, "Development," "Approaches to Health Management in Primary Care," "Disease Management," and "Practice Management." New to this edition are in-depth discussions of obesity and mental health problems, complementary therapies, and discussion questions in each management chapter. The book uses a problem-oriented focus, and latest care standards and guidelines for care of children in the United States are used. It is recommended for hospital, academic, and special libraries.

Wong's Essentials of Pediatric Nursing. 8th ed. Editors: Marilyn J. Hockenberry, David Wilson. Mosby Elsevier, 2009.
ISBN: 9780323053532
Recommended for: Hospital, Academic Libraries
Brandon/Hill Selection

Named for the original co-author of the text, Donna Lee Wong, the 8th edition of this leading textbook brings rewritten or revised chapters in areas of pediatric nursing that are undergoing rapid changes. Written as a text for students, it also serves as a reference manual for practicing nurses. The latest standards of care have been included. Websites and e-mail addresses have been added for hundreds of organizations and other educational resources. This 1,245-page book is organized into nine units that comprise 32 chapters. Canadian nurses will benefit from the inclusion of Canadian health statistics and organizational resources. Key points and content are highlighted by colorful graphics and over 500 illustrations are included. A companion CD-ROM contains anatomy reviews, animations of clinical presentations, case studies, critical thinking exercises, NCLEX review questions, and pediatric assessment video clips. As with other Mosby texts, a companion student learning site at http://evolve.elsevier.com, facilitates a community of learners. Designated a Brandon/Hill select nursing title, this book will be an important addition to hospital, academic, and specialized libraries.

Journals

Journal for Specialists in Pediatric Nursing. v. 7, Wiley-Blackwell, 2002.
http://onlinelibrary.wiley.com/journal/10.1111/(ISSN)1744-6155
ISSN: 15390136
ISSN: 17446155 (Online)
Indexed in: MEDLINE, CINAHL
Recommended for: Hospital, Academic Libraries

Journal for Specialists in Pediatric Nursing is an international, peer-reviewed, scholarly journal publishing evidence-based research. The journal is interdisciplinary in scope, and publishes qualitative and quantitative research, clinical expertise, and perspectives of children and their families. The journal is published quarterly, and is indexed in CINAHL and MEDLINE. Full-text content is available from EBSCO (including EJS and CINAHL Plus), Ovid, and ProQuest.

Journal of Pediatric Nursing. v. 1, Saunders Elsevier, 1986.
http://pediatricnursing.org/
ISSN: 08825963
ISSN: 15328449 (Online)
Indexed in: MEDLINE, CINAHL
Recommended for: Hospital, Academic Libraries

Journal of Pediatric Nursing is the official scholarly, peer-reviewed journal of the Society of Pediatric Nurses and the Pediatric Endocrinology Nursing Society. The bimonthly journal publishes articles disseminating knowledge in research, clinical practice, theoretical, and policy aspects of child health and illness from infancy through adolescence, using a family perspective. Regular columns include "Child Health Policy," "International Pediatric Nursing," "Child in the Community: Nursing Makes a Difference," "Clinical Practice," "SPN News" and "PENS News." The journal is indexed in CINAHL and MEDLINE. Full-text articles are available from 1995 from Elsevier, and through Ovid from 2000.

Pediatric Nursing. v. 1, Janetti, 1975.
http://www.ajj.com/services/pblshng/pnj/
ISSN: 00979805
Indexed in: MEDLINE, CINAHL
Recommended for: Hospital, Academic Libraries
Brandon/Hill Selection

Pediatric Nursing is a scholarly, peer-reviewed clinical journal, focusing on the needs of pediatric nurses in education, administration, and clinical practice. The purpose of the journal is to reflect trends, policies, practice, and research in pediatric nursing. CE articles are included in each issue, and are published for free online. The journal is published six times a year. Full-text articles are available online through EBSCO, Ovid, and ProQuest. The journal is indexed in MEDLINE and CINAHL, and it is on the Brandon/Hill list of nursing journals.

13.14. Perioperative Nursing

Nursing care of the surgical patient before, during, and after surgery.

—MeSH

Contributor: Paul M. Blobaum

Monographs

Alexander's Care of the Patient in Surgery. 13th ed. Editors: Jane C. Rothrock, Donna R. McEwen. Mosby/Elsevier, 2007.
ISBN: 9780323039277
Recommended for: Hospital, Academic Libraries
Brandon/Hill, *Doody's Core Titles* Selection

This book has been a standard reference for perioperative care for more than 60 years, and is considered a classic. The thirteenth edition is divided into three units: "Foundations of Practice," "Surgical Interventions," and "Special Considerations." Each chapter is illustrated with charts and photographs, and an updated list of references. Chapters incorporate best practices, research highlights, sample plans of care, and patient education content. The history of perioperative nursing for the past 20 years is also discussed. It was a Brandon/Hill nursing core title, and is recommended for academic, hospital, and special libraries serving nurses.

Berry & Kohn's Operating Room Technique. 11th ed. Editor: Nancymarie Phillips. Mosby/Elsevier, 2007.
ISBN: 9780323044837
Recommended for: Hospital, Academic Libraries
Brandon/Hill, *Doody's Core Titles* Selection

Designated a Brandon/Hill nursing title, this 1,280-page book would also be beneficial to surgical technicians, and anyone who works in the perioperative environment. Chapters incorporate the AORN standards, practices, and guidelines, and are organized with objectives and an outline. Useful as a textbook, this book serves to provide a review of current practice for the expert and novice nurse alike. A supplemental website on the Elsevier Evolve platform is available for students and instructors, containing review materials, PowerPoint presentations, a glossary, images, and other materials (http://evolve.elsevier.com). This text is recommended for hospital, academic, and special libraries.

Core Curriculum for Perioperative Nursing. 4th ed. Author: Billie Fernsebner. OR Manager, 2003.
ISBN: 9780945970118
Recommended for: Hospital, Academic Libraries

Useful as a review for experienced perioperative nurses, as well as an introduction for those new to the field, this is the up-to-date guide for required knowledge and skills. It uses the AORN Standards and applies them to specific subjects in the specialty. Recommended for academic, hospital, and specialized libraries.

Essentials of Perioperative Nursing. 3rd ed. Author: Cynthia Spry. Jones & Bartlett, 2008.
ISBN: 9780763758813
Recommended for: Hospital, Academic Libraries
Brandon/Hill, *Doody's Core Titles* Selection

A Brandon/Hill Select title for nursing, this book is written to be a review of the essential knowledge and competencies necessary for perioperative nurses to effectively care for patients. Each chapter is preceded by learning objectives, and an outline of the chapter's content. Review questions for each chapter are provided. An accompanying CD-ROM contains test-bank questions. This book is recommended for hospital, academic, and special libraries.

Instrumentation for the Operating Room: A Photographic Manual. 7th ed. Author: Shirley M. Tighe. Mosby Elsevier, 2007.
ISBN: 9780323043106
Recommended for: Hospital, Academic Libraries
Brandon/Hill, *Doody's Core Titles* Selection

Designated a Brandon/Hill core nursing title, this book is accompanied by an electronic version on CD-ROM. Primarily a photographic atlas, this book goes beyond photographs to discuss utilization of instruments and their sterilization, care, handling, and storage. Chapters are procedure specific, with discussions of the latest techniques. Surgical departments may wish to adopt this text as their training resource. It is recommended for hospital, academic, and special libraries.

Review of Perioperative Nursing. Authors: Bettyann Hutchisson, Mark L. Phippen, Maryann M.P. Wells. Saunders Elsevier, 2000.
ISBN: 9780721634135
Recommended for: Hospital, Academic Libraries

This book provides an outline of essential knowledge needed to successfully pass the Certified Nurse in the Operating Room exam. Students and expert nurses alike may test their knowledge using the Q and A format. It is recommended for academic, hospital, and special libraries.

Journals

AORN Journal. v. 1, Elsevier, 1963.
http://www.aorn.org/AORNJournal/
http://www.aornjournal.org/
ISSN: 00012092
Indexed in: MEDLINE, CINAHL
Recommended for: Hospital, Academic Libraries
Brandon/Hill Selection

AORN Journal is the official journal of the Association of Perioperative Registered Nurses and is designated a Brandon/Hill core nursing journal. This peer-reviewed, scholarly journal is published monthly, and covers a wide range of issues of importance to application of research evidence and AORN standards in caring for patients before, during, and after surgery. Topics include patient education, asepsis, instrumentation, anesthesia, and communications, among others. It is indexed in CINAHL and MEDLINE. Current full-text issues are available online from Ovid, Elsevier, and EBSCO EJS. Full-text is also available in Elsevier's Nursing Consult, and CINAHL Plus with 12-month embargo. This title is recommended for academic, hospitals, and special collections.

13.15. Psychiatric Nursing

The application of psychiatric principles in caring for the mentally ill. It also includes the nursing care provided the mentally ill patient.

—MeSH

Contributor: Paul M. Blobaum

Monographs

Essentials of Psychiatric Mental Health Nursing: A Communication Approach to Evidence-Based Care. Authors: Elizabeth M. Varcarolis, Margaret Jordan Halter. Saunders Elsevier, 2009.
ISBN: 9781416000518
Recommended for: Hospital, Academic Libraries

Varcarolis and Halter distill the essentials of the psychiatric field, using many topics from their 864-page *Foundations of Psychiatric Mental Health Nursing* text, to present a 592-page text appropriate for shorter course formats. The book is accompanied by the http://evolve.elsevier.com companion website, and a CD-ROM containing an audio glossary, review questions, animations, and interactive activities. Chapters contain a listing of key terms and concepts, learning objectives, Internet references, key point summaries, critical thinking exercises, review questions, and a bibliography for further reading. The text is illustrated with drawings, and is highlighted in various colors and shaded boxes for emphasis and focus.

Foundations of Psychiatric Mental Health Nursing: A Clinical Approach. 6th ed. Editors: Elizabeth M. Varcarolis, Margaret Jordan Halter. Saunders Elsevier, 2010.
ISBN: 9781416066675
Recommended for: Hospital, Academic Libraries
Brandon/Hill Selection

This book is intended as an introductory text for undergraduate students. The sixth edition has been updated with current standards of care and is well organized with learning objectives, key terms, a review of key points discussed, critical thinking questions, additional readings, and review questions. Case studies are presented with nursing care plans. Discussions of evidence-based practice within the nursing practice framework help students relate theoretical underpinnings to clinical practice. Multimedia resources include a CD-ROM with more than 300 review questions, and online study tools, including audio chapter summaries, audio glossary and flashcards, case studies and care plans, and more. This text is recommended for hospital and academic libraries.

Lippincott's Manual of Psychiatric Nursing Care Plans. 8th ed. Authors: Judith M. Schultz, Sheila L. Videbeck. Lippincott Williams & Wilkins, 2009.
http://www.ovid.com/
ISBN: 9780781747882
Recommended for: Hospital, Academic Libraries
Brandon/Hill Selection

This manual is a learning tool, as well as a reference manual for students and professional mental health nurses. The nursing process in mental health interventions provides a foundation for planning for clients with emotional or psychiatric issues in community health and clinical settings. A CD-ROM provides resources for writing individualized patient care plans, locating drug information, and assessment tools that will be useful. It is available online through Ovid. This book is a Brandon/Hill core nursing title and is recommended for hospital, academic, and specialized libraries.

Mental Health & Mental Illness. 7th ed. Author: Patricia D. Barry. Lippincott Williams & Wilkins, 2002.
ISBN: 9780781731386
Recommended for: Hospital, Academic Libraries
Brandon/Hill Selection

This text was written for nurses training to be mental health and psychiatric nurses. The book focuses on the most frequently occurring mental disorders and the most effective nursing care. The book reflects the shift from hospital to community mental health care settings. Each chapter contains learning objectives, self-awareness activities, questions for review, and a brief bibliography for further reading. Barry's 512-page book is presented as a synopsis of the core knowledge for each topic. There are five units. Unit 1, "Patterns of Mental Health Care," is a presentation of trends in mental health care, with legal and ethical aspects. Unit 2, "Foundations of the Therapeutic Relationship," presents nurse-patient relationships; Unit 3, "Foundations of Decision-Making in the Mental Health Setting," presents a discussion of the application of knowledge in the nursing process, dealing with stress, and assessment of the patient. Unit 4, "Nursing a Client with a Mental Disorder," discusses the nursing care of clients in the framework of the most common DSM-IV disorders. Unit 5 discusses global issues of crisis intervention and milieu and group therapies, drug therapies, and other interventions. There is limited use of graphics and illustrations. The book is a Brandon/Hill nursing core title, and will be most useful for advanced practice nursing students, and professionals seeking to review their knowledge.

Principles and Practice of Psychiatric Nursing. 9th ed. Editor: Gail W. Stuart. Mosby Elsevier, 2009.
ISBN: 9780323052566
Recommended for: Hospital, Academic Libraries
Brandon/Hill Selection

Stuart's text contains many of the features of other Mosby nursing textbooks: the Evolve website (http://evolve.elsevier.com), containing supplemental materials, extensive use of photographs and graphics, illustrations, a presentation of learning objectives and key terms, chapter focus points, an extensive bibliography, and contributions by experts in the field. This comprehensive textbook discusses a variety of DSM-IV diagnoses, including gender identity disorders, eating disorders, and addictions. The text integrates a holistic biopsychosocial approach to psychiatric nursing care based on the Stuart Stress Adaptation Model, emphasizing the full continuum of care of patients and their families. This text provides the student and psychiatric mental health nurse the tools to stay up-to-date with knowledge in the specialty, and enable them to provide competent care. The six units have 39 chapters. Unit 1, "Principles of Psychiatric Nursing Care," presents the foundational knowledge of history of the specialty, laws, and current professional issues. Here, Stuart presents the Stuart Stress Adaptation Model of Psychiatric Nursing Care. Unit 2 deals with prevention, crisis intervention, and recovery and rehabilitation. Unit 3 applies nursing principles to specific disorders. Unit 4 describes evidence-based modalities of treatment. Unit 5 discusses the hospital- and community-based practice settings. Unit 6 discusses the needs of special populations, including the elderly, children, adolescents, survivors of abuse and violence, and care of persons with life-threatening illness.

Journals

Archives of Psychiatric Nursing. v. 1, Saunders Elsevier, 1987.
http://www.psychiatricnursing.org
ISSN: 08839417
ISSN: 15328228 (Online)
Indexed in: MEDLINE, CINAHL
Recommended for: Hospital, Academic Libraries
Brandon/Hill Selection

Archives of Psychiatric Nursing is the official scholarly, peer-reviewed journal of the Society for Education and Research in Psychiatric-Mental Health Nursing (SERPN) division of the International Society of Psychiatric-Mental Health Nurses. Articles considering the broadest scope of mental health nursing, including theory, research, practice, and policy discussions relating to all population groups and all practice settings are published. The journal publishes six issues a year. The journal is included in Elsevier's Nursing Consult database. Online articles are available from the publisher beginning with 2000, and from other Elsevier products. Online full text is also available through EBSCO EJS and Ovid. The journal is indexed in CINAHL and MEDLINE.

Journal of Child and Adolescent Psychiatric Nursing. v. 7, Wiley-Blackwell, 1994.
http://onlinelibrary.wiley.com/journal/10.1111/(ISSN)1744-6171
ISSN: 10736077
ISSN: 17446171 (Online)
Indexed in: MEDLINE, CINAHL
Recommended for: Hospital, Academic Libraries
Brandon/Hill Selection

This international journal is the only nursing journal devoted to child and adolescent mental health around the world. *Journal of Child and Adolescent Psychiatric Nursing* is the official journal of the Association of Child and Adolescent Psychiatric Nurses (ACAPN) division of the International Society of Psychiatric-Mental Health

Nurses (ISPN). *JCAPN* is a scholarly, peer-reviewed journal and is published quarterly. The journal publishes articles on a wide range of subjects of importance to psychiatric nursing with children and adolescents, including psychopharmacology, impact of interventions on cognitive, emotional, and social growth and development, social policy, care of disturbed children in the schools, interactions with the juvenile justice system, and nursing education and research. Conference highlights, case studies, and book reviews are among the regular columns published. The journal is indexed in CINAHL, MEDLINE, and PsycINFO. Full-text articles are available from EBSCO's CINAHL Plus and EBSCO EJS, ProQuest, as well as Wiley.

Journal of Psychosocial Nursing and Mental Health Services. v. 1, Slack, 1987.
http://www.jpnonline.com
ISSN: 02793695
ISSN: 19382413 (Online)
Indexed in: MEDLINE, CINAHL
Recommended for: Hospital, Academic Libraries
Brandon/Hill Selection

Journal of Psychosocial Nursing and Mental Health Services is a monthly, peer-reviewd journal for psychiatric and mental health nurses in all practice settings. The aim of the journal is to publish practical, up-to-date articles for today's psychosocial nurse. It publishes articles on clinical care, psychopharmacology, case studies with practical recommendations, mental health care of older adults, and child and adolescent issues. Each issue includes a clip-and-save article on current medications for psychiatric nurses, including CE credits. Available in full text from EBSCO (CINAHL Plus and EJS), ProQuest, Slack, and Ovid. The journal is indexed in CINAHL, PsycINFO, AGELINE, and MEDLINE.

Journal of the American Psychiatric Nurses Association. v. 1, Sage, 1995.
http://jap.sagepub.com/
ISSN: 10783903
ISSN: 15325725 (Online)
Indexed in: CINAHL
Recommended for: Hospital, Academic Libraries

Journal of the American Psychiatric Nurses Association is a scholarly, peer-reviewed journal published six times a year. The goal of the journal is to provide up-to-date information to promote psychiatric nursing, improve mental health care, and shape policy for the delivery of care. The journal publishes research, clinically focused articles, editorials, continuing education, and briefings from the American Psychiatric Nurses Association (APNA). The journal also publishes supplements on specific psychiatric disorders and their management. The journal is indexed in CINAHL and PsycINFO. Full-text articles are available from Sage and Ovid.

Perspectives in Psychiatric Care: Journal for Advanced Practice Psychiatric Nurses. v. 1, Wiley-Blackwell, 1963.
http://www.blackwellpublishing.com/ppc
ISSN: 00315990
ISSN: 17446163 (Online)
Indexed in: MEDLINE, CINAHL
Recommended for: Hospital, Academic Libraries

Perspectives in Psychiatric Care is the official scholarly, peer-reviewed journal of the Adult and Geropsychiatric-Mental Health Nurses (AGPN) Division of the International Society of Psychiatric-Mental Health Nurses (ISPN), and is published quarterly. It is the journal recognized specifically for advanced practice psychiatric nurses and nurse psychotherapists. It publishes interdisciplinary perspectives on clinical practice, education, or administration; evidence-based synthesis of research findings; public policy analysis; and original research. Articles are focused on practical application of knowledge, with recommendations for how to apply knowledge, and resources for further research. It is indexed in CINAHL, MEDLINE, PsycINFO, and AGELINE. Full-text articles are aviable through CINAHL Plus (EBSCO) and EBSCO EJS, Wiley, Journals@Ovid, and ProQuest.

13.16. Public Health Nursing

Nursing focusing on the health of the community through educational and preventive programs, as well as providing treatment and diagnostic services.

—MeSH

Contributor: Elizabeth Fine

Monographs

Community as Partner: Theory and Practice in Nursing. 5th ed. Authors: Elizabeth T. Anderson, Judith McFarlane. Lippincott Williams & Wilkins, 2008.
ISBN: 9780781786430
See Also Chapter 13.1. Community Health Nursing
Recommended for: Hospital, Academic Libraries
Brandon/Hill, *Doody's Core Titles* Selection

Elizabeth Anderson and Judith McFarlane's classic text focuses on the essentials of working with the community and serves as a handbook for students and practicing public health nurses. The fifth edition is updated with new chapters on introductory concepts, informatics, infectious diseases, and disasters. The book is divided into three parts: "Essential Elements for Healthy Partnerships," "The Process," and "Practicing with Diverse Communities." The book includes features such as learning objectives at the beginning of each chapter, "Take Note" boxes highlighting key concepts for readers, and critical thinking questions at the end of each chapter. These features are especially useful in educational settings. The book uses images sparsely, but the softcover 488-page volume is pleasantly readable and portable. *Community as Partner* presents essential concepts of theory and practice for the field of public health nursing. It is recommended for academic, hospital, and public health agency libraries.

***Disaster Nursing: A Handbook for Practice*.** Authors: Deborah S. Adelman, Timothy J. Legg. Jones & Bartlett, 2009.
ISBN: 9780763758448
Recommended for: Hospital, Academic Libraries

Deborah Adelman and Timothy Legg's book covers all aspects of disaster nursing and serves as a practical guide for addressing almost any disaster situation or disaster victim. The entire topic covered by the book is of broad interest to public health nurses, and the chapters on the care of vulnerable populations in disasters will be of particular interest. The book approaches disaster nursing from a leadership standpoint and helps readers develop critical thinking skills that will allow them to adapt and apply appropriate interventions in any disaster situation. Early chapters cover broad issues such as the "Nature of Disasters," "Leadership and Management in a Disaster," and "Psychology of Disaster." Several later chapters cover specific topics within burn management in a mass casualty incident. A companion website accompanies the individual purchase of the print text, where instructors may download PowerPoint slides, case studies, and disaster drills to reinforce the material covered in the book. *Disaster Nursing* is limited by sparse illustrations and blocks of text, but it is well organized for both foundational learning and quick reference. At 347 pages, this softcover book is a nicely-sized handbook for practice. The book was the winner of the *American Journal of Nursing* (AJN) Book of the Year in 2009 for the category of Community/Public Health Nursing. It is recommended for academic, hospital, and public health agency libraries.

***Public Health Nursing: Population-Centered Health Care in the Community*.** 7th ed. Authors: Marcia Stanhope, Jeanette Lancaster. Mosby/Elsevier, 2008.
ISBN: 9780323045407
Recommended for: Hospital, Academic Libraries
Brandon/Hill, *Doody's Core Titles* Selection

Marcia Stanhope and Jeanette Lancaster's respected text provides a comprehensive foundation of the theories, concepts, and interventions in the field of public health nursing. The seventh edition (previously titled *Community and Public Health Nursing*, has been updated to include new or expanded chapters on public health surveillance and outbreak, population-based public health nursing practice, forensic nursing, health education and group practices, and global health. The book comprehensively covers the many roles played by public health nurses and the varied settings and groups they encounter. The text is divided into seven sections: "Perspectives in Health Care and Population-Centered Nursing (PCN)," "Influences on Health Care Delivery and PCN," "Conceptual and Scientific Frameworks Applied to PCN," "Issues and Approaches in PCN," "Health Promotion with Target Populations across the Life Span," "Vulnerability: Issues for the Twenty-First Century," and "Nurse Roles and Functions in the Community." The use of different colors in the text is a bit distracting at times, but the book is rich with visually coded segments such as "how-to," questions, and "did you know." At 1,154 pages, the book is intended as a textbook, but it can also serve as a well-organized, comprehensive resource for professionals as well as students. It is recommended for academic, hospital, and public health agency libraries.

***Public Health Nursing: Practicing Population-Based Care*.** Editors: Marie Truglio-Londrigan, Sandra B. Lewenson. Jones & Bartlett, 2011.
ISBN: 9780763766542
Recommended for: Hospital, Academic Libraries
Doody's Core Titles Selection

Public Health Nursing: Practicing Population-Based Care, as described in the foreword, "presents a fresh examination of the influences that shaped public health nursing and offers strategies to merge national issues and health agendas into public health nursing's agenda and activities." The text ties history to current issues and practice, and each chapter begins with a quote and a photograph from nursing history. Chapters are well organized and referenced, with objectives and key terms presented at the beginning of each chapter. The interventions chapters contain case studies, and there is a glossary at the end of the book. The authors/editors designed one of the book's highlights, the third chapter's Public Health Nursing Assessment Tool, which incorporates *Healthy*

People 2010, the Minnesota Department of Health's Population-Based Public Health Nursing Practice Intervention Wheel, and nursing process. The book has a companion website for individual purchasers containing PowerPoint slides, flash cards, and critical thinking exercises to support the printed text. The book makes excellent, judicious use of color and images, and the softcover 417-page book is highly readable. It is an excellent resource for students and practicing public health nurses. It is recommended for academic, hospital, and public health agency libraries.

Journals

American Journal of Public Health. v. 61, American Public Health Association, 1971.
http://ajph.aphapublications.org/
http://www.ncbi.nlm.nih.gov/pmc/journals/258/
ISSN: 00900036
ISSN: 15410048 (Online)
See Also Chapter 9.7. Epidemiology, Chapter 10.16. Public Health
Indexed in: MEDLINE, CINAHL
Recommended for: Hospital, Academic Libraries
Brandon/Hill Selection

The *American Journal of Public Health* is a peer-reviewed, scholarly journal published monthly. By publishing original research and evaluation articles, the journal seeks to advance public health research, policy, practice, and education. The journal is indexed by MEDLINE and CINAHL, and all articles are freely available in PubMed Central 24 months after publication. The broad public health scope of this journal is highly useful to both practitioners and researchers in the field of public health nursing. The journal is recommended for hospital, academic, and public health agency libraries.

Health Education & Behavior. v. 24, Sage, 1997.
http://heb.sagepub.com/
ISSN: 10901981
ISSN: 15526127 (Online)
See Also Chapter 33. Health Education
Indexed in: MEDLINE, CINAHL
Recommended for: Hospital, Academic Libraries

The official publication of the Society for Public Health Education, *Health Education & Behavior* is a scholarly, peer-reviewed journal published bimonthly. The journal explores social and behavioral change as it affects health status and quality of life. It also examines the processes of planning, implementing, managing, and assessing health education and social-behavioral interventions. The journal provides empirical research, case studies, program evaluations, literature reviews, and discussions of theories of health behavior and health status, as well as strategies to improve social and behavioral health. Regular features include "Perspectives," which offer thoughtful insights into complex subjects, and "Practice Notes," which summarize innovative programs in health education. It is indexed by MEDLINE and CINAHL. The journal is of special interest to public health nurses in smaller agencies, where the nurse often serves as a health educator. It is also of broad interest to public health nurses in other settings. The journal is recommended for academic, hospital, and public health agency libraries.

Journal of Public Health Management and Practice. v. 1, Lippincott Williams & Wilkins, 1995.
http://journals.lww.com/jphmp/
ISSN: 10784659
ISSN: 15505022 (Online)
See Also Chapter 10.16. Public Health
Indexed in: MEDLINE, CINAHL
Recommended for: Hospital, Academic Libraries

Journal of Public Health Management and Practice is a scholarly, peer-reviewed journal published bimonthly. The journal publishes articles focused on evidence-based public health practice and research, and it is indexed by MEDLINE and CINAHL. It includes articles in a wide range of population health topics, including research to practice; emergency preparedness; bioterrorism; infectious disease surveillance; environmental health; community health assessment, chronic disease prevention, and health promotion; and academic-practice linkages. This journal is especially relevant to public health nurses because of its focus on practice in a wide range of population health topics. The journal is recommended for academic, hospital, and public health agency libraries.

MMWR. Morbidity and Mortality Weekly Report. v. 25, no. 10, U.S. Centers for Disease Control and Prevention, 1976.
http://www.cdc.gov/mmwr/
ISSN: 01492195
ISSN: 1545861X (Online)
See Also Chapter 10.16. Public Health
Indexed in: MEDLINE, CINAHL
Recommended for: Hospital, Academic Libraries

The Centers for Disease Control and Prevention (CDC) prepares the *Morbidity and Mortality Weekly Report* (*MMWR*) series. The weekly report is the CDC's primary vehicle for scientific publication of timely, reliable, authoritative, accurate, objective, and useful public health information and recommendations. *MMWR* provides provisional data, based on weekly reports to the CDC by state health departments. The reporting week concludes at close of business on Friday; compiled data on a national basis are officially released to the public on the succeeding Friday. The journal is indexed by MEDLINE, and full text back to 1982 is freely available through the CDC website. *MMWR* can also be found on Facebook and Twitter, and its presence on these social networking sites allows quick dissemination of information from the CDC, providing a venue for discussion and feedback on *MMWR* material from the public health community. The timely distribution of public health information, recommendations, reports and trends makes *MMWR* of high interest to practitioners and researchers in public health nursing. It is recommended for academic, hospital, and public health agency libraries.

Preventing Chronic Disease. v. 1, U.S. Dept. of Health and Human Services, Centers for Disease Control and Prevention, National Center for Chronic Disease Prevention and Health Promotion, 2004.
http://www.cdc.gov/pcd/
http://www.ncbi.nlm.nih.gov/pmc/journals/245/
ISSN: 15451151 (Online only)
See Also Chapter 10.16. Public Health
Indexed in: MEDLINE
Recommended for: Hospital, Academic Libraries

Preventing Chronic Disease is a scholarly, peer-reviewed journal that is published bimonthly. It is freely available in its entirety on the journal's website and PubMed Central. Both MEDLINE and CINAHL Plus index this publication. The journal brings together prevention research and public health practice and provides a forum to share research and practical experience. Articles focus on preventing diseases such as cancer, heart disease, diabetes, and stroke, which are among the leading causes of death in the United States. The educational and research roles of public health nurses are increasingly directed at preventing chronic disease, so this journal is of high interest to both practitioners and researchers. It is recommended for academic, hospital, and public health agency libraries.

Public Health Nursing. v. 1, Wiley-Blackwell, 1984.
http://onlinelibrary.wiley.com/journal/10.1111/(ISSN)1525-1446
ISSN: 07371209
ISSN: 15251446 (Online)
Indexed in: MEDLINE, CINAHL
Recommended for: Hospital, Academic Libraries
Brandon/Hill Selection

Public Health Nursing is a peer-reviewed journal that is published bimonthly. The journal publishes empirical research reports, program evaluations, and case reports focused on populations at risk across the life span. It also contains articles related to developments in practice; education of public health nurses; theory development; methodological innovations; legal, ethical, and public policy issues in public health; and the history of public health nursing throughout the world. The journal is indexed by MEDLINE and CINAHL. The primary geographic audience for the journal is North American, but the journal has recently expanded its focus to include articles of international interest. The journal is appropriate for hospital, academic, and public health agency libraries.

Public Health Reports. v. 89, Association of Schools of Public Health, 1974.
http://www.publichealthreports.org/
http://www.ncbi.nlm.nih.gov/pmc/journals/333/
ISSN: 00333549
ISSN: 14682877 (Online)
See Also Chapter 10.16. Public Health
Indexed in: MEDLINE, CINAHL
Recommended for: Hospital, Academic, Libraries
Brandon/Hill Selection

Public Health Reports is a scholarly, peer-reviewed journal that publishes six regular issues per year and at least two supplements on special topics. It is the official journal of the U.S. Public Health Service; it publishes research and presents discussions of issues of interest to the public health community. Each issue publishes viewpoint, practice, and research articles that address current problems in public health; other columns target specialized interest areas such as global health issues or news related to the Association of Schools of Public Health. It is indexed by CINAHL and MEDLINE. Articles from the journal are freely available in PubMed Central 24 months after publication. Public health nurses will appreciate the presentation of issues relevant to public health practice. The journal is recommended for hospital, academic, and public health agency libraries.

Databases and Other Electronic Resources

Canadian Best Practices Portal for Health Promotion and Chronic Diseases Prevention. Public Health Agency of Canada, 2004.
http://cbpp-pcpe.phac-aspc.gc.ca/
Recommended for: Hospital, Academic Libraries

The *Canadian Best Practices Portal* describes itself as "a compendium of community interventions related to chronic disease prevention and health promotion that have been evaluated, shown to be successful, and have the potential to be adapted and replicated by other health practitioners working in similar fields." This well organized database contains interventions and resources (such as program plans and handbooks), and both categories may be browsed or searched by keywords. The presentation is excellent, and result lists have visual cues to indicate intervention and study characteristics at a glance. The freely available database is a superb resource that allows public health nursing practitioners and researchers to access effective chronic disease prevention and health promotion interventions that have been thoroughly evaluated. When consulting resources from countries other than that in which the information will be applied, users are advised to read carefully for applicability, as the frameworks of primary care and the terminology used varies between countries. Nevertheless, public health nursing models from other countries can be a rich source of information, and the Public Health Agency of Canada has designed an outstanding resource to support evidence-based practice in public health nursing. This continually updated portal is recommended for academic, hospital, and public health agency libraries.

Centers for Disease Control and Prevention (CDC) Publications "Portal." U.S. Centers for Disease Control and Prevention, 20??
http://www.cdc.gov/Publications/
Recommended for: Hospital, Academic, Consumer Health Libraries

Public health nursing is a widely varied field, and practitioners work with many different groups. The Centers for Disease Control and Prevention (CDC) is the most important source for up-to-date public health information in the United States, and the CDC Publications "Portal" website is the access point for these full-text resources. Important titles such as *Epidemiology and Prevention of Vaccine-Preventable Diseases* ("The Pink Book") and *MMWR Morbidity and Mortality Weekly Report* can be reached through this continually updated site, as well as a wealth of other resources for professionals and consumers. The site is organized in broad topics of interest to public health nurses, such as adolescent and school health, chronic disease, diabetes, and immunization and vaccines. Each section has professional-level resources such as handbooks, guides, and reports, as well as resources appropriate for consumer education. The Publications Portal is recommended for academic, hospital, consumer health, and public health agency libraries.

Guide to Community Preventive Services (The Community Guide). Community Guide Branch, National Center for Health Marketing (NCHM), U.S. Centers for Disease Control and Prevention, 20??
http://www.thecommunityguide.org/
Recommended for: Hospital, Academic Libraries

The *Community Guide* is a database of evidence-based recommendations and findings about public health interventions and policies. The database is produced by the Centers for Disease Control and Prevention (CDC). Its content is overseen by the Task Force on Community Preventive Services (established in 1996), which is an independent, non-federal, volunteer, rotating body of experts who are renowned for their expertise in public health research, practice, and policy. The *Community Guide* conducts systematic reviews of interventions in many areas of public health, and the Task Force uses the results of the reviews to issue evidence-based recommendations and findings to the public health community. The systematic review process is described on the site. As a federally funded resource, all content on the site is freely available. The database is organized by topic, and users can browse to the desired subject and view the Task Force's recommendations and findings, rationale statement, a summary evidence table, and a list of included studies. The *Community Guide* is relevant to a wide variety of people involved with public health, and it is especially valuable to public health nurses because of the evidence summaries and recommendations on interventions. This continually updated database is recommended for academic, hospital, and public health agency libraries.

13.17. Rehabilitation Nursing

The diagnosis and treatment of human responses of individuals and groups to actual or potential health problems with the characteristics of altered functional ability and altered life-style.

—MeSH

Contributor: Paul M. Blobaum

Monographs

Comprehensive Rehabilitation Nursing. Editors: Jill B. Derstine, Shirlee Drayton-Hargrove. Saunders Elsevier, 2000.
ISBN: 9780721669779

Recommended for: Hospital, Academic Libraries
Brandon/Hill Selection

The authors designed this book to cover the basic aspects of rehabilitation nursing, including basic concepts, approaches to common rehabilitation categories, and important issues for rehabilitation nursing. It is designed to be used as a reference tool, and covers the continuum of care from hospital to community setting. Part I addresses foundational issues such as history, ethics, concepts, working with the interdisciplinary team, and cultural competency. Part II examines rehabilitation management. Part III discusses common rehabilitation diagnoses and the information the rehabilitation nurse requires to address the needs of the patient. Definitions, incidence and cost, risk factors, pathophysiology, clinical findings, diagnosis, treatment, and nursing approaches are thoroughly presented with rehabilitation principles and approaches. The book is intended for rehabilitation nursing professionals at all levels.

Rehabilitation Nursing Secrets. Editor: Jeanne Flannery. Elsevier Mosby, 2005.
ISBN: 9780323031455
Recommended for: Hospital, Academic Libraries

This book was written to provide novice and experienced nurses with the essential knowledge of rehabilitation nursing, and is published as part of the Mosby *Nursing Secrets* series. The book is divided into four sections: Section 1, "Rehabilitation Nursing Practice Issues," discusses foundational issues such as history, trends, ethics, research; definitions; philosophy; goals; and scope. Section 2, "Approaches to Improvement of Outcomes," addresses accreditation standards and quality indicators and outcome measures. Section 3, "Health Promotion: Maintenance of Health Patterns," discusses nutrition, bowel and bladder care, sleep and relaxation, activities of daily living, complementary therapy, and cultural issues. Section 4, "Rehabilitation Nursing with a Special Focus," presents the essential knowledge of rehabilitation nursing management of specific conditions such as burn care, diabetes, stroke, cardiac, and other common rehabilitation settings. While books setting forth the essential knowledge in a field often use outline format, this book uses a question and answer format. Key points are summarized and highlighted, and a bibliography provides references to the evidence-based care literature for further reading.

Restorative Care Nursing for Older Adults: A Guide for All Care Settings. Editor: Barbara Resnick. Springer, 2004.
http://extranet.netlibrary.com/TitleSelect/
ISBN: 0826124542
Recommended for: Hospital, Academic Libraries

Written for caregivers and administrators at all levels of care and practice, this book presents material that will assist readers to develop and implement successful restorative care programs. The decline of function in the activities of daily living, such as getting dressed, bathing, ambulation, and stair climbing, has a great impact on health care resources. Functional impairments have many causes, and can be amplified by encounters with the health care system. Restorative care nursing focuses on the improvement or maintenance of physical function. This book provides practical discussion of how to implement programs, train staff, and manage documentation and billing issues surrounding restorative care.

Specialty Practice of Rehabilitation Nursing: A Core Curriculum. 5th ed. Author: Kristen L. Mauk. Association of Rehabilitation Nurses, 2007.
ISBN: 9781884278136
Recommended for: Hospital, Academic Libraries

This book is a compilation of the essential knowledge in the field of advanced practice rehabilitation nursing. Written in an outline format, it includes chapters on case management, research, and evidence-based practice, as well as advanced practice material. This book is a valuable resource for certification review.

Journals

Rehabilitation Nursing. v. 6, Association of Rehabilitation Nurses, 1981.
http://www.awebsource.com/clients/arn/ws_resource/public_index.php
ISSN: 02784807
Indexed in: MEDLINE, CINAHL
Recommended for: Hospital, Academic, Libraries
Brandon/Hill Selection

This journal is the official publication of the Association of Rehabilitation Nurses (ARN). Article topics range from administration and research to clinical topics, nursing perspectives, resource reviews, CE, and product information. It is published six times a year and indexed in CINAHL and MEDLINE. Recent CE articles are published for free on the *Rehabilitation Nursing* website. It is published online through the ARN website, and available in EBSCO EJS, ProQuest Nursing and Allied Health collection, and other ProQuest databases.

13.18. School Nursing

Health and nursing care given to primary and secondary school students by a registered nurse.

—MeSH

Contributor: Paul Elliott Dahl

Monographs

Individualized Healthcare Plans for the School Nurse: Concepts, Framework, Issues and Applications for School Nursing Practice. 1st ed. Editors: Cynthia K. Silkworth, Martha J. Arnold, Judith F. Harrigan, Donna S. Zaiger. Sunrise River Press, 2005.
ISBN: 9780962481468
Recommended for: Academic Libraries

This comprehensive resource helps school nurses develop individualized healthcare plans (IHPs) for 57 common acute, chronic, or infectious conditions/diseases typically found in children and adolescents. This worthy work is organized into three sections. The first section provides the concepts, framework, and issues of IHPs in 13 chapters. The second section outlines special student issues in six chapters. The third and final section provides the elements to develop an IHP for the 57 common acute, chronic, or infectious conditions and diseases. Information on the pathophysiology and management of a condition or disease is provided and a case study is also found at the end of the chapter. The elements covered in the IHP are assessment, nursing diagnoses (commonly NANDA), goals, nursing interventions, and expected outcomes. A list of chapter references, a bibliography of additional resources, and a listing of web resources are also provided at the end of each chapter. The book contains a companion CD with an interactive software program (compatible with both Windows and Macintosh sytems) allowing the creation of IHPs with nursing diagnoses, goals, interventions, outcomes, and assessment data. Detailed student demographic information can be added, leading to the development of a comprehensive, complete student record. This resource is a required purchase for school nurses. Academic institutions with nursing programs should also purchase this book.

Manual of School Health: A Handbook for School Nurses, Educators, and Health Professionals. 3rd ed. Authors: Keeta DeStefano Lewis, Bonnie J. Bear. Saunders-Elsevier, 2009.
ISBN: 9781416037781
Recommended for: Academic Libraries

Completely updated, the third edition of this portable manual provides quick access to practical health and wellness information for youth from birth to age 21. The manual contains 12 chapters, 10 useful appendixes, a glossary, and an index in its 654 pages. Some of the topics covered in this helpful resource include growth and development, acute and chronic conditions, mental health disorders, adolescent and gender-specific issues, emergency and disaster preparedness, and first aid. One of the most useful sections of the manual is in the acute conditions chapter in which color photographs and illustrations of common dermatological conditions and skin lesions are presented. The effectively designed black-and-white illustrations throughout the book help convey information. The websites and bibliographies provided in each chapter of the manual are useful in pointing to more in-depth resources. While this resource is ideal for school nurses, it also is suitable for child care providers, community health nurses, and any person working with youth. This is a required resource for school nurses. It should also be found in academic institutions that support nursing programs.

Journals

Journal of Adolescent Health. v. 12, Elsevier, 1991.
http://sciencedirect.com/science/journal/1054139X
http://www.journals.elsevierhealth.com/periodicals/jah/issues
ISSN: 1054139X
ISSN: 18791972 (Online)
See Also Chapter 9.1. Adolescent Medicine
Indexed in: MEDLINE, CINAHL
Recommended for: Hospital, Academic Libraries

This monthly multidisciplinary scientific journal focuses on adolescent health issues and was previously known as the *Journal of Adolescent Health Care* (volumes 1–11, 1980–1990). This journal is the official publication of the Society for Adolescent Health and Medicine (SAHM). Research findings range from "basic biological and behavioral sciences to public health and policy." Besides publishing original, peer-reviewed articles in its pages, the journal also contains editorials, review articles, health briefs, and position papers. Supplement issues are also published each year. While this journal is worthy reading for a diverse group of health practitioners ranging from pediatricians to social workers, it is of particular value for school nurses. Hospitals and academic institutions would find this to be an essential resource. The impact factor for *Journal of Adolescent Health* was 3.325 in the 2009 *Journal Citation Reports* and it was ranked sixth out of 94 pediatrics journals. Full online coverage back to volume 12, 1991 is available through Elsevier ScienceDirect.

Journal of School Health. v. 7, Wiley, 1937.
http://onlinelibrary.wiley.com/journal/10.1111/(ISSN)1746-1561
ISSN: 00224391
ISSN: 17461561 (Online)
See Also Chapter 33. Health Education
Indexed in: MEDLINE, CINAHL
Recommended for: Academic Libraries

This journal is one of the two top-tier journals that school nurses will find directly related to their role of enhancing and maintaining a healthy place for students. This monthly journal published on behalf of the American School Health Association focuses on providing the programs, services, and environment leading to improved health and well-being of school-aged youth. Original, peer-reviewed research articles, a school health policy article, and a commentary are the typical items published in an issue. The *Journal Citation Reports* impact factor for this journal was 1.953 in 2009 ranking it fifty-first out of 122 journals (science) and twenty-fourth out of 95 journals (social science) in the public, environmental, and occupational health category. This journal is cited in numerous abstracting and indexing sources such as MEDLINE, CINAHL, Current Contents, and ERIC. Full online coverage back to volume 1, 1930 is available through Wiley Online Library.

Journal of School Nursing. v. 7, Sage, 1993.
http://jsn.sagepub.com/
ISSN: 10598405
ISSN: 15468364 (Online)
Indexed in: MEDLINE, CINAHL
Recommended for: Academic Libraries

This bi-monthly journal is the official journal of the National Association of School Nurses and is one of the top-tier journals specifically directed to school nurses. The mission of the journal is to be a "forum for advancing the specialty of school nursing, promoting the professional growth of school nurses, and improving the health of children in school." The journal has peer-reviewed feature and research articles in every issue. An editorial often appears in each issue. This journal is required reading for school nurses, its main audience. Academic institutions involved in the education of nurses-in-training will find this a mandatory purchase. This journal is cited in numerous abstracting and indexing sources such as MEDLINE, CINAHL, PsycINFO, and ERIC. Full online coverage back to volume 16, number 4, 2000 is available through Sage.

Pediatrics. v. 1, American Academy of Pediatrics, 1948.
http://pediatrics.aappublications.org
ISSN: 00314005
ISSN: 10984275 (Online)
See Also Chapter 10.13. Pediatrics
Indexed in: MEDLINE, CINAHL
Recommended for: Hospital, Academic Libraries
Brandon/Hill Selection

Begun in 1948, this prestigious pediatric journal is essential reading for those needing to stay knowledgeable about current pediatric medicine and child health developments. This journal is the official journal of the American Academy of Pediatrics. The vision of the journal's first editor that "the content of the journal is intended to encompass the needs of the whole child in his physiologic, mental, emotional, and social structure" continues to be successfully met. Original peer-reviewed articles, clinical observations, special feature articles, commentaries, and policy statements are the staple of this monthly journal. Supplement issues are published frequently. Even though pediatricians and other medical professionals are the target audience for the journal, school nurses and public health professionals rely on this journal time and again as they work to improve the health of children and adolescents. Hospitals and academic institutions will find that this is a required resource. This journal is the most-cited journal in pediatrics and has an impact factor of 4.687 in 2009. The journal is cited in numerous abstracting and indexing sources such as MEDLINE, CINAHL, Embase, and PsycINFO. The online format has all the print content and exclusive online only articles. Full online coverage back to volume 1, 1948 is available through American Academy of Pediatrics (HighWire Press).

13.19. Transcultural Nursing

Created to answer the need for developing a global perspective in the practice of nursing in a world of interdependent nations and people. The focus of this nursing discipline is on the integration of international and transcultural content into the training. Courses include study in the area of cultural differences, nursing in other countries, and international health issues and organizations, as an example.

—MeSH

Contributor: Paul M. Blobaum

Monographs

Cultural Diversity in Health and Illness. 7th ed. Author: Rachel E. Spector. Pearson, 2008.
ISBN: 9780135035894
Recommended for: Hospital, Academic Libraries
Brandon/Hill Selection

Rachel Spector's book has been the authoritative, go-to book for health care providers and students for developing cultural competencies, so necessary for providing care for a diverse society, for over 30 years. The purpose of the book is to increase awareness of the dimensions and complexities involved in caring for people from diverse cultural backgrounds. Spector not only discusses health beliefs and values amongst various cultural groups, but also probes the American health care system and the health disparities that exist. An instructor's resource center is available online from the freely available companion website (http://www.prenhall.com/spector), as well as online course management tools to integrate with Blackboard, Moodle, Angel, and other learning platforms. The companion website also contains test questions and additional learning activities for cultural competence. This book can be used as a course text, and is also valuable for a review of knowledge; either way, it is an essential resource for any health care professional and student.

Transcultural Health Care: A Culturally Competent Approach. 3rd ed. Editors: Larry D. Purnell, Betty J. Paulanka. F.A. Davis, 2008.
http://extranet.netlibrary.com/TitleSelect/
ISBN: 9780803618657
Recommended for: Hospital, Academic Libraries
Brandon/Hill Selection

This text presents the Purnell 12-Step Model for Cultural Competence, which has been translated into numerous languages and is recognized internationally. Cultural groups included in the book were selected based on prevalence in North America, status as new immigrants, and whether the groups have much written about them, among other factors. The book is organized according to cultural group. It will best serve as a reference book, or supplement to course textbooks. Each chapter has a bibliography of references for further reading. It is recommended for all libraries.

Transcultural Nursing: Assessment and Intervention. 5th ed. Authors: Joyce Newman Giger, Ruth Elaine Davidhizer. Mosby Elsevier, 2008.
ISBN: 9780323048118
Recommended for: Hospital, Academic Libraries
Brandon/Hill Selection

Giger and Davidhizar wrote the first edition based on their work as nursing faculty at Bethel College, Mishawaka, Indiana. The population groups chosen for discussion in the text are based on the major cultural groups now in the United States. The disabled also are identified as a cultural group for the first time in this edition. The Giger-Davidhizer Cultural Assessment model was developed as a quick reference for working with clients in diverse clinical settings, and has been cited, excerpted, and modified for inclusion in over 490 nursing texts. The model, based on Giger and Davidhizar's extensive research, is used as a framework for discussions in this text using the latest research. This book is unique in its discussion of biotechnological approach, discussing the sensitive topic of biological differences among racial and ethnic groups and influences on health status. As with other Mosby texts, a companion website is available at http://evolve.elsevier.com, containing additional review questions, case studies, and sample care plans for each cultural group. The book is written primarily for nurses and nursing students, but the authors also believe it to be applicable to other disciplines such as psychology, sociology, medicine, and anthropology, because it not only presents a nursing perspective but also a historical and biotechnological approach to transcultural health care. It is a valuable resource for the improvement of patient and client care.

Transcultural Nursing: Concepts, Theories, Research, and Practice. 3rd ed. Authors: Madeleine M. Leininger, Marilyn R. McFarland. McGraw-Hill, 2002.
ISBN: 9780071353977
Recommended for: Academic Libraries

Leininger is the founder of the Transcultural Nursing movement, and developer of the ethnonursing research method. She is recognized as the world authority on nursing cultural care. McFarland is also a transcultural nursing researcher and collaborated with Leininger on several transcultural nursing texts. This text is organized into five sections: Section 1, "Transcultural Nursing: Essential Knowledge Dimensions," discusses foundational issues; Section 2, "Special Topics in Transcultural Nursing," discusses the cultures of medical institutions and professions, American transcultural challenges in urban settings, and ethical, legal, and moral dimensions; Section 3, "Culture Care Theory, Research, and Practice in Diverse Cultures," presents research on the application of Culture Care Theory, using specific cultural health care paradigms; Section 4, "Transcultural Nursing

Teaching, Administration, and Consultation," discusses educational and administrative issues; and Section 5 concludes the text with a chapter on future directions. This text focuses on Anglo-American, Lithuanian American, Arab Muslim, Philippine American, elderly Polish, Taiwanese American, Jewish American, Native American, and Mexican American culture care. Insights into transcultural healthcare in India, Canada, Taiwan, and Australia, and among the homeless in the western United States are also discussed in this edition. Previous editions are valuable resources for discussions of additional cultural perspectives.

Databases and Other Electronic Resources

Cultural Competence Resources for Healthcare Providers. U.S. Health Resources and Services Administration, 2010.
http://www.hrsa.gov/culturalcompetence/
Recommended for: Hospital, Academic Libraries

The Health Resources and Services Administration has compiled a useful website of resources for health care professionals seeking to develop cultural competencies. Many of the resources are published by government agencies, some are from universities and non-profit organizations. The webpage is divided in the main areas of: assessment tools, culture and language specific readings, disease specific information for various cultural groups, health professions education links, research links, rural community information, special populations, technical assistance, training curricula, and web-based training tutorials.

EthnoMed. University of Washington, Library of the Health Sciences, 2010.
http://ethnomed.org
Recommended for: Hospital, Academic, Consumer Health Libraries

EthnoMed is a joint program of the University of Washington Health Sciences Libraries and Harborview Medical Center's Interpreter Services Department/Community House Calls Program (ISD/CHC). The purpose of the EthnoMed website is to provide culturally relevant information for providers and patients in the King County, Washington area (the Seattle area) served by Harborview Medical Center. The website is free. The intention is to provide health providers with information to help them understand Cambodian, Ethiopian, Hispanic, Oromo, Somali, Tigrean, and Vietnamese communities and their understandings of health and illness, and to have ready access to culturally appropriate patient education materials. These cultural groups are recent immigrants or refugees living in the Seattle area. Other ethnic groups, such as Chinese, Karen (an ethnic group from Thailand), and Hmong are being included as materials are written. To prevent duplication of efforts, EthnoMed provides links to appropriate and authoritative external websites. The website is organized in five main sections: "Cultures," "Clinical Topics," "Patient Education," "Cross-Cultural Health," and "Calendar." "Cultures" provides background information on each ethnic group, including geographical origins, history, culture, and health-related issues. "Clinical Topics" include the topics of asthma, breastfeeding, cancer, case studies, communicable diseases, culture-bound syndromes, dermatology, diabetes, domestic violence, end of life, hepatitis, hyperlipidemia, mental health, mother/child/infant care, nutrition, oral health, pharmacy, refugee health, traditional medicine, tuberculosis, and women's health. Patient education information is extensive. Printable documents in PDF and Microsoft Word format, web tutorials, and occasionally, audio files are available. In addition to the above topics, patient handouts discussing SARS, cough and cold, diaper rash, HIV/AIDS, rickets, smoking, medical tests, procedures and radiology, swine flu, vomiting, disaster preparedness, and mental health are published. "Cross Cultural Health" provides a variety of related resources and articles, including a bibliography, interpreter resources, immigration/naturalization information, and links to full-text journal articles that are re-published with permission. The "Calendar" shows daily cultural events that could affect health care delivery. EthnoMed is fully searchable, and RSS feeds are available.

Population Groups. National Library of Medicine, 2010.
http://www.nlm.nih.gov/medlineplus/populationgroups.html
Recommended for: Hospital, Academic, Consumer Health Libraries

The National Library of Medicine provides health information focusing on specific population groups through its MedlinePlus website. Topics include: African-American health; Asian-American health; children's health; gay, lesbian, and transgender health; health disparities; Hispanic-American health; men's health; Native-American health; seniors' health; teen health; veterans and military family health; and women's health.

13.20. Practical Nursing

Nursing by licensed, non-registered persons qualified to provide routine care to the sick.

—MeSH: Nursing, Practical

Contributor: Rebecca Raszewski

Monographs

Basic Concepts of Psychiatric-Mental Health Nursing. 7th ed. Author: Louise R. Shives. Lippincott Williams & Wilkins, 2008.
http://www.ovid.com/
ISBN: 9780781797078
Recommended for: Hospital, Academic Libraries
Brandon/Hill, *Doody's Core Titles* Selection

Louise Shives' book has been an important psychiatric-mental health nursing resource for nurses and practical nursing and vocational students for over 20 years. It highlights the different settings where these nurses could work, fostering the communication skills they will need in these environments. The book chapters cover psychiatric disorders and psychiatric therapies, along with how to work with clients in specific age groups or with those having specific diagnoses. The seventh edition has a new chapter on forensic nursing, new content on spirituality, and updated psychopharmacological material. The book contains a CD-ROM geared towards students, which includes NCLEX review questions, psychotropic drug monographs, and clinical simulations for depression and schizophrenia. This book would be an important purchase for academic libraries that support practical/vocational nursing. With its focus on interdisciplinary teamwork, hospital libraries should also investigate purchasing this book because of its emphasis on practical nursing skills.

Contemporary Practical/Vocational Nursing. 6th ed. Author: Corrine R. Kurzen. Lippincott Williams & Wilkins, 2009.
http://www.r2library.com/
ISBN: 9780781782692
Recommended for: Academic Libraries

Contemporary Practical/Vocational Nursing is an introductory text to the practical and vocational profession. This book is arranged into four units: getting started, understanding the profession, preparing for successful practice, and moving forward in one's career. There are several appendixes that will be helpful to students. Topics covered in these appendixes include stress management techniques, Andrews/Boyle "Transcultural Nursing Assessment Guide for Individuals and Families," standards and competencies for the profession, and a complementary and alternative medicine (CAM) dictionary of terms. The sixth edition has additional leadership and management information, new case studies, enhanced NCLEX information, material for non-traditional students, and interactive "Assess Yourself" boxes. There is also a companion website with additional content such as video clips. *Contemporary Practical/Vocational Nursing* will serve as a valuable introduction to the practical nursing field for students. Academic libraries with practical/vocational nursing programs should consider purchasing this title for their collections.

Foundations of Basic Nursing. 3rd ed. Authors: Lois White, Gena Duncan, Wendy Baumle. Delmar/Cengage Learning, 2011.
ISBN: 9781428317741
Recommended for: Academic Libraries

The *Foundations of Basic Nursing* is an introductory textbook that covers various levels of nursing procedures. Eight units in the book include topics such as communication, health promotion, nursing procedures, and infection control. Procedures covered are fully illustrated with photographs and drawings. Nursing management sections indicate the nurse's responsibilities in the nursing process sections. There are also sample nursing care plans and case studies for critical thinking. The third edition includes new chapters on bioterrorism, self-concept, and spirituality, as well as a new feature called "Memory Tricks" that provides mnemonic devices for important concepts. The appendixes contain useful information that nursing students need: NANDA Nursing Diagnoses; English/Spanish words and phrases; recommended childhood and adolescent immunization schedule; abbreviations, acronyms, and symbols; and a glossary. An accompanying CD-ROM includes quizzes, learning games, and video clips of nursing procedures. This textbook is recommended for academic libraries since it covers topics that practical and vocational nursing students need, such as study materials to prepare them for the NCLEX-PN.

Introductory Medical-Surgical Nursing. 10th ed. Authors: Barbara K. Timby, Nancy E. Smith. Lippincott Williams & Wilkins, 2010.
ISBN: 9781605470634
Recommended for: Hospital, Academic Libraries
Brandon/Hill Selection

Introductory Medical-Surgical Nursing has been published for over 30 years. The first few sections of the book cover the nurse's role and responsibility, client concerns, and the foundations of medical-surgical nursing, such as infection and pain management. The following chapters cover disorders of the body system and how to care for clients with these disorders, including those with multi-system disorders. There are over 30 care plans on various topics. A CD-ROM and a companion website accompany this book. This extra content includes a Spanish-English audio glossary, animations, review questions, and the full text of the book. *Introductory Medical-Surgical Nursing* was a Brandon/Hill selection. This book would be useful for academic libraries since it introduces students to medical-surgical nursing. Hospital libraries should also consider purchasing this book because of its patient care information aimed at nursing staff.

Maternity Nursing: An Introductory Text. 10th ed. Author: Gloria Leifer. Saunders/Elsevier, 2008.
ISBN: 9781416048701
ISBN: 9781416067535
Recommended for: Hospital, Academic Libraries
Brandon/Hill Selection

Maternity Nursing: An Introductory Text is a part of the *LPN Thread* series, which is published by Saunders. The six units of this book provide content from the development of the fetus to the newborn. It includes chapters about nursing care during labor and for the newborn. Within the chapters are clinical pathways that focus on collaborative care, nursing care plans, and critical thinking activities. This edition contains a CD-ROM of video clips of normal and caesarian births, an audio glossary, audio clips, and teaching plans in English and Spanish. A perforated self-assessment workbook is located in the back of the book, which offers clinical situations, Internet activities, and multiple-choice questions. Organization is provided by a simple-to-complex and health-to-illness continuum, making it easy to locate and access information and allowing one to see how complex content builds upon simpler concepts. Health-to-illness reflects the wellness basis for maternal and newborn care. Health Promotion and Family-Centered Care are the major themes throughout the book, which reflect *Healthy People 2010* objectives and the overall focus on wellness and illness prevention in health care. A pictorial of labor and birth includes fourteen vivid photos that support visualization of the birth experience from start to finish. This publication is sold as a print text or as a combined text and e-book package for individual use. This book was a former Brandon/Hill nursing book selection. In addition to serving as an introductory textbook for students, *Maternity Nursing* serves as a resource for nurses in hospital libraries.

Nursing Leadership, Management, and Professional Practice for the LPN/LVN: In Nursing School and Beyond. 4th ed. Author: Mary Ann Anderson. F.A. Davis, 2009.
ISBN: 9780803619449
Recommended for: Hospital, Academic Libraries

Nursing Leadership, Management, and Professional Practice for LPN/LVN: In Nursing School and Beyond advertises itself as two books in one because it provides vocational and nursing management and leadership content. The book is split into two units: the nursing profession in today's health care environment and the transition from student to nurse. The fourth edition contains a new chapter about personal and professional priority setting, new full color images, and "Focus Your Learning Charts." This book will be a valuable purchase for both academic and hospital libraries because it includes important skills for both students and nurses, such as dealing with conflict and understanding the benefits of change. Practical and vocational nurses will find this book useful, especially if they are entering a leadership role; they will learn skills such as team building and motivating employees.

Success in Practical/Vocational Nursing: From Student to Leader. 6th ed. Authors: Signe S. Hill, Helen Stephens Howlett. Saunders/Elsevier, 2009.
ISBN: 9781416056591
ISBN: 9781416064947
Recommended for: Academic Libraries
Brandon/Hill Selection

Success in Practical/Vocational Nursing is a part of the *LPN Threads* series available through Saunders. This book moves from preparing for the NCLEX-PN to interactions with patients and colleagues. The publication includes questions and quizzes for self-assessment and exercises on critical thinking. An additional section on leadership and management offers activities, management tools, and hints. A personal health promotion chapter demonstrates actions to encourage healthy behavior in patients. Students will appreciate the time-management tips to help them establish priorities. The 6th edition includes NCLEX questions with each chapter, expanded cultural content, new content related to simulation in nursing, and updated board and competencies information that are contained in the appendixes. This book will help students prepare effectively for a practical/vocational nursing career. Academic libraries should consider this book because it includes the skills students need for the future. There is also a separate text and e-book package available for individual use.

Journals

American Journal of Nursing. v. 1, Lippincott Williams & Wilkins, 1900.
http://ajnonline.com
http://www.ovid.com/
http://www.jstor.org/
ISSN: 0002936X
ISSN: 15387488 (Online)
See Also Chapter 12. Nursing
Indexed in: MEDLINE, CINAHL
Recommended for: Hospital, Academic Libraries
Brandon/Hill Selection

The *American Journal of Nursing* (*AJN*) is the oldest nursing journal in the world. *AJN* is a peer-reviewed, evidence-based journal, covering nursing from a global perspective with informative content. In addition to news and drug updates, this monthly publication contains featured articles, including *AJN* reports and continuing education. *AJN* is a required subscription for an academic or hospital library. Its content is applicable to nurses from every educational background. The journal is cited in numerous abstracting and indexing sources such as CINAHL, MEDLINE, and Scopus. The Special Library Association's BioMedical & Life Sciences Division listed this sole nursing title in their 2009 Top 100 Journals in Biology and Medicine. Full online coverage back to volume 1, 1900 is available through JSTOR and Ovid. Other vendors such as EBSCOhost EJS and Swets Information Services have online coverage from either 2002 or 2004 onward.

Journal of Practical Nursing. v. 13, no. 8, National Association for Practical Nurse Education and Service, 1963.
http://napnes.org/jpn/jpn_subscriptions.html
http://www.proquest.com/
ISSN: 00223867 (Print/Online)
Indexed in: MEDLINE, CINAHL
Recommended for: Hospital, Academic Libraries
Brandon/Hill Selection

The *Journal of Practical Nursing* (*JPN*) is a peer-reviewed journal that is published quarterly by the National Association for Practical Nurse Education and Service, Inc. (NAPNES), the oldest association in the United States for practical and vocational nurses. *JPN*, which was formerly known as *Practical Nursing*, has been the preeminent journal for practical and vocational nurses for over 50 years. The audience for this journal includes practical and vocational nursing educators, nurses, and students in practical nursing programs. The journal provides NAPNES approved contact hours of continuing education, articles on evidence-based practice, association updates, and educational and scholarship information. The journal is cited in numerous abstracting and indexing services such as AGELINE, MEDLINE, CINAHL, and Scopus. Hospitals and academic libraries with practical and vocational nursing programs should subscribe to *JPN*. It serves as a useful resource for those who need to stay abreast in this profession. Full online coverage beginning in 2004 is available through ProQuest.

LPN: The Journal for Excellence in Practical Nursing. v. 1, Lippincott Williams & Wilkins, 2005.
http://www.ovid.com/
ISSN: 15530582
ISSN: 15530590 (Online)
Recommended for: Hospital Libraries

LPN is a bimonthly, peer-reviewed publication. Published by Lippincott Williams & Wilkins, this relatively new journal claims Scopus as its only indexing source to date. *LPN* is geared toward certified practical nurses and would be a good purchase for hospital libraries. Journal content may cover basic skills, such as documenting a patient's initial assessment to transferring a patient from a bed to a stretcher. There are also articles on topics such as pain assessment, overview of diseases, and care for patients with particular conditions. Additionally, the journal includes career development information and a "This Just In..." section, which contains summaries of recent developments in various health topics along with a "Did You Know?" subsection. Full online coverage back to volume 1 is available through EBSCOhost EJS and Ovid.

14. Nutritional Sciences

The study of nutrition processes as well as the components of food, their actions, interaction, and balance in relation to health and disease.

—MeSH

Contributor: Robin Sabo

Monographs

***Biochemical, Physiological, & Molecular Aspects of Human Nutrition*.** 2nd ed. Editor: Martha H. Stipanuk. Saunders Elsevier, 2006.
ISBN: 9781416002093
Recommended for: Hospital, Academic Libraries
Brandon/Hill Selection

Included on the Brandon/Hill list as *Biochemical and Physiological Aspects of Human Nutrition*, this second edition is intended as an advanced level nutrition textbook or reference book. Per the author, upper-level undergraduate and graduate students and professionals who have completed coursework in organic chemistry, biochemistry, molecular biology, and physiology will find this book useful. Over 50 authors from academia, government, and industry have contributed to this book. It is primarily organized by nutrient classification (carbohydrates, proteins, lipids, vitamins, and minerals). In addition, there is a unit covering historical aspects, nonessential food components with health benefits, and guidelines for food and nutrient intake. Added content includes chapter outlines, references, and recommended readings and websites. Many tables, charts and boxes highlighting nutrition insights, clinical correlations, food sources; and Recommended Dietary Allowances/ Adequate Intakes are scattered throughout the book. This book is recommended for academic libraries with human nutrition and biomedical programs. Hospital libraries affiliated with medical schools will also find this to be a helpful purchase.

***Encyclopedia of Human Nutrition*.** 2nd ed. Editors: Benjamin Caballero, Lindsay Allen, Andrew Prentice. Elsevier/Academic Press, 2005.
http://extranet.netlibrary.com/TitleSelect/
http://www.sciencedirect.com/science/referenceworks/9780122266942
http://www.gale.cengage.com/
ISBN: 9780121501105
ISBN: 9780122266942 (Online)
ISBN: 9780080454283 (Online)
Recommended for: Hospital, Academic Libraries

Choice Reviews considers this reference book to be an outstanding title. This second edition has been increased by 20 percent to reflect the rapidly expanding knowledge in human nutrition. This book includes over 250 articles written by an internationally diverse group of experts from academia, government, and industry. Topics include nutrients, nutrition-related diseases and conditions, food safety, food composition, cultural influences, and eating behaviors. Some articles are from the previous edition with revisions by the editors. This title is available online through ScienceDirect and Gale Virtual Reference. In the introduction, the editors state the book is intended "for both nutrition and non-nutrition scientists." In addition, this book is a helpful reference for practicing clinicians such as physicians, nurses, and dietitians. It is recommended for academic and medical libraries; much of the material is too technical for most lay readers. Access through Gale includes the ability to select audio, which is helpful for those with vision difficulties. The print version is a four-volume set.

***The Health Professional's Guide to Popular Dietary Supplements*.** 3rd ed. Authors: Allison Sarubin-Fragakis, Cynthia Thomson. American Dietetic Association, 2007.
http://online.statref.com/
ISBN: 9780880913638
Recommended for: Hospital, Academic, Consumer Health Libraries
Doody's Core Titles Selection

Published by the American Dietetic Association, this book is co-authored by two dietitians and reviewed by multiple nutrition experts. The third edition (2007) includes over 100 of the most popular dietary supplements and summarizes more than 450 new research studies. Included as a *Doody's Core Titles* (2009), this handbook is intended as a reference for health professionals to assist them in understanding the benefits and the potential harmful effects of dietary supplements.

Content provided on each supplement includes a brief overview, a summary of media/marketing claims and efficacy, safety information, drug/supplement interactions, food sources, dosage information, and bioavailability. There are extensive references on each of the dietary supplements. Appendixes include information on government regulation of dietary supplements, ethical issues, Dietary Reference Intakes, additional resources, and sample questions to assist health professionals in assessing their clients' use of dietary supplements. This book is recommended for academic libraries, hospital libraries, and consumer health collections serving more sophisticated users.

Nutrient-Drug Interactions. Editor: Kelly Anne Meckling. CRC/Taylor & Francis, 2007.
Http://extranet.netlibrary.com/TitleSelect/
ISBN: 9781574449150
ISBN: 1420019139 (Online)
Recommended for: Academic Libraries
Doody's Core Titles Selection

This book, which appears on the *Doody's Core Titles* list, is a collection of review articles on specific topics relating to nutrient-drug interactions. It is not intended to be a comprehensive reference handbook for clinicians, but instead will be of interest to researchers and clinicians who are interested in discrete topics and gaining a better understanding of current and future research directions in this area. Examples of chapter titles include "Diabetes, Obesity, and Metabolic Syndrome," "Nutrient and Phytochemical Modulation of Cancer Treatment," "Supplements and Anesthesiology," and "Nutrients and Herbals in the Pharmacotherapy of Unipolar/Major Depression." Each chapter begins with a table of contents and finishes with extensive reference lists. Per the author, "the major focus of each section will be on the molecular mechanisms(s) by which the food or chemical is thought to modify disease process and drug behavior." This book is recommended for academic libraries with graduate programs in nutrition, pharmacy, or medicine.

Practical Sports Nutrition. Author: Louise Burke. Human Kinetics, 2007.
ISBN: 9780736046954
Recommended for: Hospital, Academic, Consumer Health Libraries
Doody's Core Titles Selection

The first sentence of this textbook, "The aim of this book is to examine sports nutrition in the context of real-life practice," explains how this book differs from others. Nutritional advice is sport-specific. Recommended in *Doody's Core Titles*, all but one chapter of this book is written by Dr. Louise Burke, a dietitian at the Australian Institute of Sport. Chapters are based on categories of athletic activities including road cycling and triathlon, running, swimming and rowing, sprinting and jumping, field-based team sports, court and indoor team sports, racket sports, strength and power sports, weight-making sports, and gymnastics and winter sports. Information on training, physiology, lifestyle and culture, dietary surveys, nutrition issues, and sport foods and supplements is included. In addition, there are general chapters on "Training and Competition Nutrition," "Practical and Cultural Factors," and "Sport Foods and Supplements." The book is well-organized and includes many tables, charts, and references. Students and practicing professionals in dietetics, exercise physiology, and athletic training are the intended audience. Academic and hospital libraries collecting in these areas will find this to be a helpful book. Consumer health libraries serving sophisticated users would also find this book to be a useful purchase.

The Vitamins: Fundamental Aspects in Nutrition and Health. 3rd ed. Author: Gerald F. Combs, Jr. Elsevier Academic Press, 2008.
ISBN: 9780121834937
Recommended for: Hospital, Academic Libraries
Doody's Core Titles Selection

This is the third edition of this book, which appears on the *Doody's Core Titles* list. In a review of the 1992 edition, *Choice Reviews* considered it as an "outstanding title." The author, Gerald Combs Jr., Cornell University Emeritus Professor of Nutrition, explains that the book is intended as a textbook for an upper-level nutrition course and a ready-reference book for nutrition and other health professionals. The book uses a concept-centered approach including chapter lists of anchoring concepts, learning objectives, vocabulary terms, study questions, and case studies. This edition includes expanded content on vitamins A, D, E, C, and folate as well as added content on "quasi-vitamins" such as lycopene, xanthophylls, and flavonoids, and information on quantifying vitamin needs. There is also an online companion site containing PowerPoint slides of graphs, tables, and charts. References include major reviews, and extensive appendixes include terminology; lists of relevant journals, books, and websites; and vitamin and mineral content of common foods. This book is recommended for academic libraries with nutrition and health-related programs and for larger hospital libraries.

Journals

Annual Review of Nutrition. v. 1, Annual Reviews, 1981.
http://www.annualreviews.org/journal/nutr
ISSN: 01999885
ISSN: 15454312 (Online)
Indexed in: MEDLINE, CINAHL
Recommended for: Hospital, Academic Libraries

Published by Annual Reviews, a nonprofit scientific publisher, the *Annual Review of Nutrition* has an impact factor of 8.783, ranking first in the nutrition and dietetics category in the 2009 *Journal Citation Reports*. Annual Reviews were founded to help scientists make an overwhelming volume of scientific research more manageable. Articles include both clinical topics such as "Pica in Pregnancy," and basic research reviews, such as "Retinoic Acid in Regulation of Apoptosis." Available as a print or online subscription, this publication is indexed in MEDLINE from 1981 (volume 1) to present. Other major databases indexing this journal are Biosis, Chemical Abstracts, CINAHL, and Embase. This annual publication is of interest to nutrition and other health researchers, practitioners, and students. Academic libraries and large hospital libraries will find this to be a useful purchase.

The Journal of Nutrition. v. 1, American Society for Nutrition, 1928.
http://jn.nutrition.org
ISSN: 00223166
ISSN: 15416100 (Online)
Indexed in: MEDLINE
Recommended for: Hospital, Academic Libraries

Published beginning in 1928 by the American Society for Nutrition, this journal is ranked ninth in "Mapping the Literature of Dietetics" (AM Smith, *Bull Med Libr Assoc* 1999 July; 87(3):292–97). *Journal Citation Reports* (2009) ranks it eighth among 66 journals in the nutrition and dietetics category. This monthly, peer-reviewed journal was the "first scientific journal created solely for the publication of nutrition research" (*Magazines for Libraries*, March 9, 2010). Content is original nutrition research including biochemical, molecular, and genetic mechanisms; nutrition physiology, metabolism, and nutrition interactions; nutrition and disease; nutrient requirements and optimal nutrition; nutritional epidemiology; community and international nutrition; nutritional immunology; and ingestive behavior and neurosciences. Added content includes symposia proceedings and supplements. The *Journal of Nutrition* is indexed in MEDLINE, Biosis, Chemical Abstracts, and Embase; and free access to full-text articles after 12 months is available on PubMed Central. The journal is essential for academic libraries with nutrition and health-related curricula and for libraries supporting teaching hospitals.

Tufts University Health & Nutrition Letter. v. 14, number 12, Tufts University, 1997.
http://www.tuftshealthletter.com
ISSN: 15260143
Indexed in: CINAHL
Recommended for: Hospital, Academic, Consumer Health Libraries

Previously published as the *Tufts University Diet and Nutrition Letter*, this eight-page, monthly newsletter has a long-standing reputation as a trustworthy source of nutrition information for consumers. Content of the newsletter is primarily drawn from the expertise of the faculty at the Gerald J. and Dorothy R. Friedman School of Nutrition Policy, including anthropologists, biomedical scientists, economists, epidemiologists, nutritionists, physicians, political scientists, and psychologists. This newsletter is indexed in well-known general and health-specific databases (for example, Factiva, Health Source, SPORTDiscus with Fulltext, Academic OneFile, and CINAHL) and was recommended for purchase by large public libraries, academic libraries with health programs and medical libraries (*Magazine for Libraries*, March 9, 2010). In a review of medical newsletters (*Wall Street Journal*, June 3, 2003), the *Tufts University Diet and Nutrition Letter* was noted to be one of the author's favorites, stating that the information is useful and practical, "and the content is often quirky and surprising."

14.1. Child Nutrition Sciences

The study of nutrition processes as well as the components of food, their actions, interaction, and balance in relation to health and disease in children, infants or adolescents.

—MeSH

Contributor: Robin Sabo

Monographs

Breastfeeding: A Guide for the Medical Profession. 6th ed. Authors: Ruth A. Lawrence, Robert M. Lawrence. Elsevier Mosby, 2005.
http://www.sciencedirect.com/science/book/9780323028233

ISBN: 9780323028233
See Also Chapter 10.18. Reproductive Medicine
Recommended for: Hospital, Academic Libraries

This book has been a premier resource on human lactation since its first publication in 1980. The sixth edition provides updates on the growing body of research in this field, including managing breastfeeding with infectious diseases, hormonal pathways, and behavioral mechanisms. In addition, updates on drugs and herbal products and their safety during lactation are included. The audience for this book includes physicians, nurses, dietitians, and lactation consultants. Especially helpful to clinicians are the materials located in the appendixes, including an extensive table on drugs in breast milk and their effect on the infant, normal serum values of breastfed infants, and information on expressing and storing of human milk. Of interest to educators is a chapter on training the medical professional. "A monumental work" and "an important reference work" are descriptions appearing in a book review from *Early Human Development* (2006: 279). This book is an essential purchase for university libraries with medical and allied health programs and for all hospital libraries.

Eating Behaviors of the Young Child: Prenatal and Postnatal Influences on Healthy Eating. Editors: Leann L. Birch, William H. Dietz. American Academy of Pediatrics, 2008.
http://www.r2library.com/
ISBN: 9781581102789
Recommended for: Hospital, Academic Libraries
Doody's Core Titles Selection

Published by the American Academy of Pediatrics, this book is listed as a *Doody's Core Titles* recommendation in the health sciences—nutrition category. Along with a summary section, the book is divided into three major sections: "Nutrition Influences on Growth and Development," "Cultural and Parenting Influences," and "Delivery Systems." This book was a product of a round table meeting sponsored by an education grant from the Johnson & Johnson Pediatric Institute. Written by pediatricians, researchers, dietitians, policymakers, and social scientists, this book focuses on promoting the development of healthy eating behaviors during the first five years of life. It is written for pediatricians and other child health professionals. A companion 24-page brochure for parents (*I Won't Eat It: Answers to Your Questions about Feeding Babies and Toddlers*) was also produced. This book is recommended for hospital libraries serving institutions that care for children and for academic libraries with medical, dietetic, and other health professions programs.

Handbook of Pediatric Nutrition. 3rd ed. Authors: Patricia Queen Samour, Kathy King. Jones & Bartlett, 2005.
ISBN: 9780763783563
Recommended for: Hospital, Academic Libraries

The 26 chapters in this reference work are written primarily by pediatric dietitians considered experts in their fields. A review of the previous edition described it as "a well-written practical book" (*Am J Clin Nutr* 2000: 1065). This updated third edition includes an expanded chapter on weight management and the new Babson and Benda's growth charts for preterm infants. Intended for healthcare practitioners and researchers, this book covers nutritional needs from the prenatal period through adolescence. In addition, normal and specialized nutrition needs in disease states and conditions are included. Other topics include enteral nutrition, parenteral nutrition, and the use of botanicals. In addition to growth charts, the appendixes include reference data for mid-upper arm circumference and skinfold measurements and for laboratory parameters. Dietitians studying for pediatric specialty exams commonly use this book. It is essential for libraries in larger hospitals that care for infants and children and for academic libraries with dietetic, medical, physician assistant, or nurse practitioner programs.

Nutrition in Pediatrics: Basic Science, Clinical Applications. 4th ed. Editors: Christopher Duggan, John B. Watkins, W. Allan Walker. B.C. Decker, 2008.
http://www.r2library.com/
ISBN: 9781550093612
Recommended for: Hospital, Academic Libraries

Edited by three professors of pediatrics from Harvard Medical School, this textbook meets their stated goal of establishing "a comprehensive and accessible approach to pediatric nutrition." This fourth edition has six additional chapters including a new section on "Obesity and Energy Balance" to reflect the current epidemic of childhood obesity. Other major sections of the book include "General Concepts," "Physiology and Pathophysiology," "Perinatal Nutrition," "Nutrition in Disease," and "Nutritional Support." Appendixes include additional information on nutritional assessment, nutritional requirements, and product information for infant formulas and enteral formulations. Useful tables, graphs, charts, and extensive reference lists populate the text. A book review of the previous edition (*Am J Clin Nutr* 2004: 1091) recommended this book for all general pediatricians, pediatric subspecialists, and pediatric nutritionists. All hospital libraries with pediatrics units and academic libraries with medical, dietetics, or nursing programs should find this book extremely useful.

Nutrition of the Preterm Infant: Scientific Basis and Practical Guidelines. 2nd ed. Editor: Reginald C. Tsang. Digital Educational, 2005.
ISBN: 9781583521007
Recommended for: Hospital, Academic Libraries

With a slight change in title from the previous edition, *Nutrient Requirements in Preterm Infants* (1993), this updated work provides a seminal resource for providing nutritional care for premature infants. Preterm births represent approximately ten percent of all births, making care of these infants a sizable issue. The book is aimed towards practicing physicians, dietitians, and nurses, and students in these fields. Fourteen chapters are authored by well-known academicians, clinicians and researchers. The content underwent peer review by both internal and external reviewers. Topics covered include nutritional needs for macronutrients, vitamins, and minerals. Additional chapters deal with enteral nutrition, human milk, follow-up care, and specialized nutritional needs of infants with complications. This book is essential for all libraries in hospitals with neonatal intensive care units. Academic libraries with programs in dietetics, nursing, and medicine will also find this book helpful.

Pediatric Nutrition Handbook. 6th ed. Editor: Ronald E. Kleinman. American Academy of Pediatrics, 2009.
ISBN: 9781581102987
Recommended for: Hospital, Academic Libraries
Doody's Core Titles Selection

From the American Academy of Pediatrics, Committee on Nutrition, this comprehensive volume includes contributions from over 70 physicians and registered dietitians who are experts in the field. First published in 1979 and now in its sixth edition, this book serves as a ready reference for clinicians and upper level health professions students. Major subjects covered in this almost 1,500 page volume are infant nutrition including breastfeeding, nutritional needs of preterm infants, inborn errors of metabolism, child and adolescent nutrition, parenteral and enteral nutrition, nutrition needs during illness, and food labeling and safety. New chapters on nutritional management of children with liver disease and inflammatory bowel disease have been added. Extensive appendixes include growth charts, food composition data, and information on infant formulas and enteral nutrition products. Included on the *Doody's Core Titles* list, this book is highly recommended for academic libraries with health professions programs and for hospital libraries.

Pediatric Nutrition in Chronic Diseases and Developmental Disorders: Prevention, Assessment, and Treatment. 2nd ed. Editors: Shirley W. Ekvall, Valli K. Ekvall. Oxford University, 2005.
ISBN: 9780195165647
Recommended for: Hospital, Academic Libraries

This volume is an important work in a frequently ignored area. In addition to covering nutrition for special-needs children, general information on pediatric growth and nutrition, topics including sports nutrition, vegetarian diets, childhood obesity, herbal supplements, and constipation are presented. The importance of teamwork in caring for these children is emphasized. A large section of this book is devoted to the nutritional needs of children with hereditary metabolic disorders. Many tools for nutritional assessment are included in the appendixes (e.g., growth charts, screening forms, anthropometric standards, and laboratory data.) The book is intended for health care professionals. A review of the first edition states, "This book should be in the library of every pediatric nutritionist and every clinic where children with chronic illness are cared for" (*N Engl J Med* 1994: 1625). Hospital libraries with pediatric populations as well as academic libraries will find this book very valuable.

Pediatric Nutrition Support. Editors: Susan S. Baker, Robert D. Baker, Anne M. Davis. Jones & Bartlett, 2007.
ISBN: 9780763731540
Recommended for: Hospital Libraries

The editors collaborated previously on *Pediatric Parenteral Nutrition* (1997, 2001) and on *Pediatric Enteral Nutrition* (1994). Both parenteral and enteral nutrition are now combined into one work. The intended audience for this book is dietitians, pharmacists, nurses, and physicians who manage nutrition support for pediatric patients. Authors of the 37 chapters were selected for their clinical expertise along with "their recognized stature in the medical and nutrition community." Topics covered include growth, nutritional assessment, and technical information on parenteral and enteral feedings in children. A number of chapters are focused on providing nutrition support to pediatric populations with particular disease states and conditions. The appendixes include an extensive listing of nutrient content for infant formulas, specialized pediatric enteral formulas, and adult enteral formulas. Especially useful are tables dealing with medications including food-drug interactions, osmolarity of selected drugs, and recommendations for administering drugs with feeding tubes. A book review calls this work "a valuable reference" (*Nutr Clin Pract* 2008: 346). This book is recommended for large hospital libraries in institutions providing pediatric care and home nutrition support. Academic libraries in universities with medical schools and those that train dietitians, pharmacists, and nurses should also consider this an important purchase.

Your Child's Weight: Helping without Harming, Birth through Adolescence. Author: Ellyn Satter. Kelcy Press, 2005.
ISBN: 9780967118918
Recommended for: Hospital, Academic, Consumer Health Libraries

As both a dietitian and social worker, Ellyn Satter provides a unique perspective on child feeding. Since the publication of her first book in 1983, *Child of Mine: Feeding with Love and Good Sense*, Satter's books have become nutrition classics. Satter emphasizes "Feeding Dynamics" and "Division of Responsibility" in the feeding relationship. The book emphasizes that parents are responsible for when and what to feed and the child decides how much and whether to eat. Separate chapters on three different age groups, "Birth through Preschool," "The School-Age Child," and "Adolescents," discuss optimizing feeding dynamics according to developmental stages. Case examples are used throughout the book to explain general principles. This book is intended for parents, but dietitians, pediatricians, and others working with child feeding issues will find this book very helpful. Recommended by the *Journal of Nutrition Education and Behavior* (2007:S198) as a resource that "dietitians and other professionals can unreservedly recommend . . . to their clients," this is an important resource for consumer health, academic, and hospital libraries.

Journals

Journal of Pediatric Gastroenterology and Nutrition. v. 1, Lippincott Williams & Wilkins, 1982.
http://journals.lww.com/jpgn/pages/default.aspx
ISSN: 02772116
ISSN: 15364801 (Online)
Indexed in: MEDLINE
Recommended for: Hospital, Academic Libraries

The specific focus on both pediatrics and nutrition makes this an important journal in the field of child nutrition. With an impact factor of 2.183 (*Journal Citation Reports*, 2009), this journal ranks thirty-first of 65 in nutrition and dietetics and twenty-third of 94 in pediatrics. This peer-reviewed publication is the official journal for the North American Society of Pediatric Gastroenterology, Hepatology and Nutrition and for the European Society for Paediatric Gastroenterology, Hepatology and Nutrition. Types of articles include original research, reviews, case reports, special reports, and rapid communication. Topics covered include infant formulas, parenteral and enteral nutrition in infants and children, nutrition needs of preterm infants, and treatment of children with gastrointestinal diseases and disorders. The journal is indexed in major databases including Biological Abstracts, Chemical Abstracts, and MEDLINE. Full-text online access is available via Ovid from 1996 (volume 22) to present. This journal is an important purchase for hospital libraries in institutions caring for pediatric patients and for academic libraries with medical schools or strong nutrition research programs.

14.2. Dietetics

The application of nutritional principles to regulation of the diet and feeding persons or groups of persons.

—MeSH

Contributor: Robin Sabo

Monographs

American Dietetic Association Complete Food and Nutrition Guide. 3rd ed. Editor: Roberta L. Duyff. John Wiley & Sons, 2006.
Http://extranet.netlibrary.com/TitleSelect/
ISBN: 9780470041154
ISBN: 9780470048429
Recommended for: Hospital, Academic, Consumer Health Libraries

A review of the first edition (1996) of this book states, "What distinguishes (this book) from other general nutrition references, is how the author translates scientific facts concerning nutrition into practical suggestions" (*J Nutr Educ* 1998 Mar–Apr; 32(2): 124). The fourth edition continues this tradition, presenting practical information in an interesting manner. Among the updated content is additional information on women's health, functional foods, phytonutrients, celiac disease, and ethnic foods. Self-quizzes, charts and quick tips populate the text. Chapters cover dining out, nutrition from infancy to geriatrics, vegetarian diets, eating to prevent and manage disease, and dietary supplements. An additional 30 pages of appendixes present information on food additives, Dietary Reference Intakes, and a listing of further resources. This book has been the recipient of the National Health Information Award and the National Federation of Press Women Award. An essential purchase for consumer health collections, this book is also a valuable addition to academic and hospital libraries.

Bowes & Church's Food Values of Portions Commonly Used. 19th ed. Authors: Judith Spungen, Jean A.T. Pennington. Lippincott Williams & Wilkins, 2010.
ISBN: 9780781781343
ISBN: 9781608313655 (CD-ROM)
ISBN: 9780781782890 (Text with CD-ROM)
Recommended for: Hospital, Academic, Consumer Health Libraries
Brandon/Hill, *Doody's Core Titles* Selection

First published in 1937, this food composition handbook remains a valuable resource. The purpose of the book as stated in the 1st edition and continuing to the present edition is "to supply authoritative data on the nutritional values of foods in a form for quick and easy reference." Nutrient information is expressed for commonly eaten portion sizes and includes information on macronutrients, fiber, minerals, vitamins, and fatty acids. Intended for dietitians, research nutritionists, and dietetic students, this book may also be useful for those in other health disciplines, for consumers following special diets, or for others interested in nutrition. The "Main Database for the Composition of Foods" is organized by various food categories, including sections on "Fast Foods and Restaurant Foods" and "Special Dietary Foods." The last section of the book contains supplementary databases that are especially useful, including sections on caffeine, gluten, and plant sterols. This book is included on *Doody's Core Titles* list (health sciences-nutrition; nursing-nutrition), and a previous edition appeared on both the last Brandon/Hill list for allied health and for the small medical library. *Bowes & Church's* is also available on CD-ROM and as a combination print and CD-ROM package. Hospital, academic, and consumer health libraries will all find this book to be a worthwhile purchase.

DRI, Dietary Reference Intakes: The Essential Guide to Nutrient Requirements. Editors: Jennifer J. Otten, Jennifer P. Hellwig, Linda D. Meyers. National Academies Press, 2006.
ISBN: 9780309157421
Recommended for: Hospital, Academic Libraries

This book summarizes the eight volume *Dietary Reference Intake* series published from 1997–2005, and replaces the previous *Recommended Dietary Allowances* (RDAs). The audience for this book from the National Academies Institute of Medicine's Food and Nutrition Board is health professionals from the United States and Canada. These guidelines are intended for planning and assessing the diets of healthy people. The *DRI* also discusses the relationship between inadequate or excessive nutrient intake and the risk of chronic disease. The book is divided into three parts: "Development and Application of the DRIs," "Energy, Macronutrients, Water, and Physical Activity," and "Vitamins and Minerals." For each nutrient, information on function, absorption, metabolism, storage and excretion, determining the DRIs, dietary sources, and adverse effects of inadequate intakes or excessive intakes are covered. Appendixes and summary tables provide additional essential information. This is a required reference for both academic and hospital libraries.

Geriatric Nutrition: The Health Professional's Handbook. 3rd ed. Editor: Ronni Chernoff. Jones & Bartlett, 2006.
ISBN: 9780763731816
Recommended for: Hospital, Academic Libraries
Brandon/Hill Selection

With publication of the first edition in 1991, this work has become a classic text. The third edition features 21 chapters written by 33 authors with expertise in the field of nutrition and aging. A review from the *Journal of Nutrition Education* (2007 May–Jun; 39(3): 179) states, "Use this handbook to deepen your understanding and appreciation for nutrition and the aging process." Several chapters deal with nutrient requirements and the effect of aging. Successive chapters cover changes in taste and smell, swallowing problems, and the effects of aging on various organ systems. The last chapters cover pharmacology, exercise, nutrition assessment, nutrition support, provision of nutrition services, and health promotion. This book includes many excellent references. As the subtitle, "The Health Professional's Handbook" implies, this book serves as a reference for practicing health professionals. In addition, classes for advanced level nutrition students would find this to be an appropriate text. This book is recommended for medical libraries and for academic libraries with nutrition, gerontology, and other health professions programs.

Krause's Food & Nutrition Therapy. 12th ed. Editors: L. Kathleen Mahan, Sylvia Escott-Stump. Saunders/Elsevier, 2008.
ISBN: 9781416034018
Recommended for: Hospital, Academic Libraries
Brandon/Hill, *Doody's Core Titles* Selection

First published in 1952, this textbook is now in its twelfth edition. It is intended to be used by dietetic, nursing, and other allied health students. Practitioners in these fields will also find this book helpful. Chapters are organized into sections that include key terms, useful websites, and pathophysiology and clinical management algorithms. New with this edition is a change in title from "diet therapy" to "nutrition therapy," aligning with changing practice. In addition, two new medical nutrition chapters have been added on psychiatric conditions and developmental disabilities. Instructor resources included with this book include over 900 PowerPoint slides and test bank questions. Color diagrams, tables, photographs, and more than 100 pages of appendixes assist with making this voluminous work more approachable. This book appears on *Doody's Core Titles* list for nutrition and the tenth edition was listed on the final Brandon/Hill list for allied health. This textbook is recommended for academic libraries with dietetics and nursing programs and for hospital libraries.

Modern Nutrition in Health and Disease. 10th ed. Editors: Maurice E. Shils, Moshe Shike, A. Catherine Ross, Benjamin Caballero, Robert J. Cousins. Lippincott Williams & Wilkins, 2006.
http://www.ovid.com/
ISBN: 9780781741330
Recommended for: Hospital, Academic, Consumer Health Libraries
Brandon/Hill, *Doody's Core Titles* Selection

This is the fiftieth anniversary edition of this classic human nutrition text. The book is divided into seven major sections: "Historical Landmarks in Nutrition," "Specific Dietary Components," "Nutrition in Integrated Biologic Systems," "Nutrition Needs and Assessment during the Life Cycle," "Prevention and Management of Disease," "Diet and Nutrition in Health of Populations," and "Adequacy, Safety and Oversight of the Food Supply." Written by leading nutrition scholars and researchers, more than half of the 116 chapters have new contributors with this edition. Growth in knowledge of the interrelationships between nutrition and disease prevention have led to expanded content. Photographs, tables, extensive references, and nearly 200 pages of appendixes complement the text. Intended for clinicians, upper level undergraduates, medical and graduate students, and nutrition researchers, this book is a mandatory purchase for both academic and hospital libraries. It is listed on the *Doody's Core Titles* list for nutrition and appeared on the final Brandon/Hill list. Larger public library systems may find it useful as well. An electronic edition is available through Ovid.

Nancy Clark's Sports Nutrition Guidebook. 4th ed. Author: Nancy Clark. Human Kinetics, 2008.
http://www.eblib.com/
ISBN: 9780736074155
ISBN: 9780736080866 (Online)
Recommended for: Consumer Health Libraries

A classic consumer-health book first published in 1990, this book is helpful for athletes and coaches as well as those interested in learning about normal nutrition. According to the book cover, over 500,000 copies have been sold. Written by a registered dietitian who is board-certified in sports dietetics, Clark's clients have included members of the Boston Red Sox, the Boston Celtics, and Olympic athletes. A review of the previous edition states, "With a motivating tone, it gives the tools, and the recipes, for readers to build their own healthy lifestyle" (*J Am Diet Assoc*, 2004 Jan; 104(1): 134). Information presented in this 4th edition includes eating to enhance performance, weight control, and the American Heart Association dietary guidelines. This book includes many tables with food composition information, dietary recommendations and sample menus. There is also a 50-page section on healthy, easy-to-prepare recipes. The extensive appendixes list additional sources of information such as journal articles, websites, and books. This book is recommended for consumer health collections. Some academic libraries and hospitals may also find it valuable.

Nutrition and Diagnosis-Related Care. 6th ed. Author: Sylvia Escott-Stump. Wolters Kluwer Health/Lippincott Williams & Wilkins, 2008.
ISBN: 9780781798457
Recommended for: Hospital, Academic Libraries
Brandon/Hill, *Doody's Core Titles* Selection

Listed as an essential purchase in nutrition (*Doody's Core Titles*) and appearing on the Brandon/Hill list for allied health, this book is now in its 6th edition. First published in 1985, it is intended for registered dietitians, dietetic students, and other health care professionals. This book covers medical nutrition therapy, normal nutrition throughout the lifecycle, religious dietary practices, and therapeutic nutrition for many disease states, conditions, and disorders. Information is presented clearly and attractively with photographs, drawings, and tables supplementing the text. Each section includes definitions, background information, nutritional interventions, commonly used medications, and sources for additional information. The book has been updated with the new Dietary Reference Intakes. Appendixes include "Dietetic

Process Forms and Counseling Tips," "Laboratory Values, Nutrition Diagnostic Labels and Definitions," and "Acuity for Dietitian Roles in Medical Diagnoses." This book is mandatory for hospital libraries and academic libraries supporting dietetics and medicine curricula.

Journals

American Journal of Clinical Nutrition. v. 2, American Society for Nutrition, 1954.
http://www.ajcn.org/
ISSN: 00029165
ISSN: 19383207
Indexed in: MEDLINE, CINAHL
Recommended for: Hospital, Academic Libraries
Brandon/Hill Selection

Rated third in nutrition and dietetics journals (2009 *Journal Citation Reports*) with an impact factor of 6.307 and second on the list of top journals from "Mapping the Literature of Dietetics" (AM Smith, *Bull Med Libr Assoc* 1999 July; 87(3): 292–97), this peer-reviewed journal reports worldwide basic and clinical research in human nutrition. Primary audiences for this journal are health care professionals, nutrition researchers, academics, and upper-level undergraduate and graduate students. Major topics covered include obesity and eating disorders, nutritional needs across the lifecycle, diabetes, cardiovascular disease, nutrition support, and dietary supplements. Periodic topical supplementary issues include selected proceedings from major conferences including Experimental Biology. Indexed and abstracted in many major scientific and medical databases (AGRICOLA, Biological Abstracts, Chemical Abstracts, CINAHL, Food Science and Technology Abstracts and MEDLINE), this journal is considered an essential resource for academic and hospital collections. Beginning as the *Journal of Clinical Nutrition*, the journal is available in from the American Society of Nutrition with full online coverage available from volume 1, 1952 to present.

Journal of Parenteral and Enteral Nutrition. v. 1, Sage, 1977.
http://www.sagepub.com/
ISSN: 01486071
ISSN: 19412444 (Online)
Indexed in: MEDLINE, CINAHL
Recommended for: Hospital, Academic Libraries

Essential to clinicians and researchers, this journal covers important, unique content on the nutritional support of critically ill patients. Sage publishes this bimonthly journal in association with the American Society for Parenteral and Enteral Nutrition (ASPEN). ASPEN was formed in 1975 as an interdisciplinary association in response to the development of a new feeding method, parenteral nutrition. Peer-reviewed research studies, review articles, brief reports, and case reports are included. *JPEN* is listed as the fifteenth most-cited journal in "Mapping the Literature of Dietetics" (AM Smith, *Bull Med Libr Assoc* 1999 July; 87(3): 292–297). Databases that index this journal include Biological Abstracts, CAB Abstracts, CINAHL, Embase, and MEDLINE. This journal is essential to hospital libraries and to academic libraries with medical, physician assistant, nursing, human nutrition, and dietetics programs. Institutional subscriptions are available in print, electronic or print + online. Full-text online subscriptions begin with 1999 and backfiles from 1977–1998 are available for purchase.

Journal of the American Dietetic Association. v. 1, Elsevier, 1925.
http://www.adajournal.org/
http://www.mdconsult.com/
http://www.sciencedirect.com/science/journal/00028223
ISSN: 00028223
ISSN: 18783570 (Online)
Indexed in: MEDLINE, CINAHL
Recommended for: Hospital, Academic Libraries
Brandon/Hill Selection

As the official journal of the American Dietetic Association, the accrediting body for Registered Dietitians in the United States, this peer-reviewed journal, begun in 1925, is a major information resource in dietetics. It is listed as the top resource in "Mapping the Literature of Dietetics" (AM Smith, *Bull Med Libr Assoc* 1999 July; 87(3): 292–297) and appears on the former Brandon/Hill lists for allied health and small medical libraries. Coverage includes nutritional sciences, medical nutrition therapy, public health nutrition, food science, food service systems, professional development, and dietetics education. Major databases indexing this journal include AGRICOLA, CAB Abstracts, CINAHL, Chemical Abstracts, Food Science and Technology Abstracts, and MEDLINE. This journal is highly recommended for academic and hospital libraries.

15. Optometry

Primary eye and vision care that includes the measurement of visual refractive power and the correction of visual defects with lenses or glasses.

—MeSH

Contributors: Suzanne Ferimer, Nicole Mitchell, Heather Stone Edmonds, Sharon Tabachnick

Monographs

Adler's Physiology of the Eye: Clinical Applications. 11th ed. Editors: Leonard A. Levin, Siv F.E. Nilsson, James Ver Hoeve, Samuel Wu, Paul L. Kaufman, Albert Alm. Mosby Elsevier, 2011.
ISBN: 9780323057141
Recommended for: Hospital, Academic Libraries
Doody's Core Titles Selection

Adler's has been the standard source on ocular function since it was first published in 1950 and continues to be the book of choice today. Its depth of analysis, detailed facts, and understanding of the structure and function of the eye have made it an important resource for the researcher, educator, or clinician who is looking for a comprehensive reference source. This review refers to the tenth edition, which added new color inserts that present full-color photomicrographs of normal and abnormal ocular physiology, anatomical illustrations, fundus photographs, and clinical-related material and also incorporated recent advances to the understanding of eye physiology such as neural control of eye movement, infant vision development, color vision, ocular circulation, and much more. It is divided into 14 sections that help the reader to better understand the basic functions of the eye and the entire visual system. At this time there is no other source that covers this material in such a detailed and comprehensive manner. The eleventh edition includes the Expert Consult online version for individual users.

Borish's Clinical Refraction. 2nd ed. Editor: William J. Benjamin. Butterworth-Heinemann/Elsevier, 2006.
http://www.sciencedirect.com/science/book/9780750675246
ISBN: 9780750675246
Recommended for: Hospital, Academic Libraries
Doody's Core Titles Selection

Borish's Clinical Refraction comprehensively covers refractive technologies and clinical applications of eye examinations. The book is divided into five sections: "Principles," "Adjunct Examinations," "The Refraction," "Analysis and Prescription of Optical Corrections," and "Special Conditions." Some of the topics covered include refractive anomalies, color vision, the physical examination, monocular and binocular subjective refraction, correction with contact lenses, patients with anisometropia and aniseikonia. Each chapter is richly illustrated with color photographs, diagrams, tables, and figures. Readers are not only provided with step-by-step instructions for performing various refraction techniques but also with the underlying theories and principles of the techniques as well. Intended for practicing optometrists and students, this text is required for optometry and ophthalmology libraries.

Clinical Decision Making in Optometry. Editors: Ellen Richter Ettinger, Michael W. Rouse. Butterworth-Heinemann, 1997.
ISBN: 9780750695718
Recommended for: Academic Libraries

The editors' goal for this title is "to examine the process of clinical decision making in vision care, in an effort to help students and optometrists develop and refine their decision-making skills" (Ettinger, 1997: xvii). Used heavily in the optometric field since it was published in 1997, the book addresses the fact that making decisions in a clinical setting can often be an uncertain and difficult process, and provides invaluable examples to assist both students new to clinical care and seasoned optometrists alike. The work is divided into two major sections, with part I focusing on the principles used in clinical decision making. The chapters in this section address clinical decision-making skills, dealing with clinical uncertainty, using epidemiology in the decision-making process, effective use of the biomedical literature, and making ethical clinical decisions. Part II provides clinical scenarios of 18 common ocular conditions, each of which includes patient background; diagnostic hypotheses, testing, and summary; treatment options; and references for further reading. The book is replete with tables, graphs, and flow charts illustrating the decision-making process for each case. This work is a required resource for academic institutions supporting optometry students and educators, and is highly recommended for practicing optometrists.

Clinical Ocular Pharmacology. 5th ed. Editors: Jimmy D. Bartlett, Siret D. Jaanus. Butterworth-Heinemann/Elsevier, 2008.
http://www.sciencedirect.com/science/book/9780750675765
ISBN: 9780750675765
Recommended for: Hospital, Academic Libraries
Doody's Core Titles Selection

Now in its fifth edition, *Clinical Ocular Pharmacology* provides a discussion of ocular drugs and the use of such drugs in primary eye care. The fifth edition addresses new research in ocular pharmacology such as new drug delivery systems and pharmacologic treatment of retinal diseases. Divided into three sections, chapter topics also include ocular hypotensive drugs, ophthalmic drug administration, nutritional agents, allergies, and adverse reactions. A selected bibliography completes each chapter. The book is illustrated with tables, charts, diagrams, and photographs. Intended for clinicians, residents, and students, this comprehensive textbook provides readers with the practical uses of pharmaceuticals in eye care.

Clinical Procedures for Ocular Examination. 3rd ed. Authors: Nancy B. Carlson, Daniel Kurtz. McGraw-Hill, 2004.
ISBN: 9780071370783
Recommended for: Academic Libraries
Doody's Core Titles Selection

The revised and updated third edition of this title is an essential resource for anyone involved in evaluating vision health. The authors' mission is "to describe how to perform a wide variety of useful tests without a large body of theory" (Carlson, 2004: xi). This practical manual covers over 125 ocular examination techniques; discusses purpose, indication, necessary equipment and set-up, examples, and expected findings; and includes detailed, step-by-step instructions for how to perform each one. Organized into eight major aspects of vision care, including refraction, ocular health assessment, and cranial nerve screening, the book is comprehensive in its coverage of the tests that address each core category. The book also features numerous charts, graphs, tables, photographs, and line drawings to support the techniques. Some of the new procedures in the third edition include corneal topography, pharmacological pupil testing, and photo stress testing. This work is a required resource for academic institutions supporting optometry students and educators, and is highly recommended for practicing optometrists and ophthalmologists.

Primary Care Optometry. 5th ed. Author: Theodore P. Grosvenor. Butterworth-Heinemann/Elsevier, 2007.
ISBN: 9780750675758
Recommended for: Academic Libraries

This book is an essential resource for optometrists and optometry students who want a comprehensive, in-depth study of the diagnosis and management of common eye and vision problems. It does not cover secondary and tertiary care areas of optometry. The book is divided into three parts: anomalies of refraction and binocular vision, where the student is provided with background information on the optical system of the eye; the optometric examination, which is broken into five areas that helps student organize the optical examination; and optometric diagnosis and management, where the student learns to formulate a treatment plan, initiate the therapy, and educate the patient. This fifth edition includes newly developed instrumentation such as autorefraction, biomicroscopy, ophthalmoscopy, visual fields, and ocular photography.

System for Ophthalmic Dispensing. 3rd ed. Authors: Clifford W. Brooks, Irvin M. Borish. Butterworth-Heinemann Elsevier, 2007.
http://www.sciencedirect.com/science/book/9780750674805
ISBN: 9780750674805
Recommended for: Academic Libraries
Doody's Core Titles Selection

This highly regarded reference work provides step-by-step instructions on properly fitting and adjusting eyewear, written in such a way that is accessible both for those new to the optometric profession and for those with years of experience. The first section of the book focuses on the mechanics of ophthalmic dispensing and selecting and fitting eyewear frames, while the second section provides a comprehensive review of various types of ophthalmic lenses and their optical properties. Each chapter includes useful diagrams, detailed illustrations, problem examples and solutions, and a proficiency test, with answers in the back of the book. This revised third edition of the textbook features color photographs throughout, and is updated with new material on progressive, aspheric, atoric, and absorbtive lenses, as well as the optical aspects of aniseikonia. This work is a required resource for academic institution supporting optometry students and educators, and is highly recommended for practicing optometrists who wish to stay current and/or train new employees in ophthalmic dispensing.

Your Eyes. 4th ed. Author: Thomas Chalkley. Charles C Thomas, 2000.
ISBN: 9780398070489
Recommended for: Consumer Health Libraries

Now in its fourth edition, this consumer resource has been educating laypeople on ocular structure, functions, and conditions since 1974. According to the author, "the purpose of this little volume is to fulfill the need for a simple, straightforward, uncomplicated book concerning your eyes" (Chalkley, 2000: ix). The book is concise, and designed in such a way that the reader can select the topic of interest and learn the basics quickly and easily. Included topics are general eye anatomy and physiology, light and vision, the conjunctiva, the cornea, cataracts, glaucoma, the uveal tract, the retina, neuro-ophthalmology, strabismus, the lids and lachrymal system, and eye changes associated with general diseases and injuries. Each chapter features detailed and well-labeled drawings of the eye and self-test questions. Also included are a general glossary of commonly used eye terms and a section on frequently asked questions. The fourth edition includes a new chapter on refractive vision correction. This title is a required resource for consumer health libraries, and is highly recommended for optometrists' waiting rooms, as well as ophthalmic and optometric assistants.

Journals

Optometry and Vision Science. v. 66, Lippincott Williams & Wilkins, 1989.
http://journals.lww.com/optvissci/
http://www.optvissci.com/
http://www.aaopt.org/section/ovs/
ISSN: 10405488
ISSN: 15389235 (Online)
Indexed in: MEDLINE
Recommended for: Academic Libraries

The official journal of the American Academy of Optometry, *Optometry and Vision Science* began in 1924 as the *American Journal of Optometry*. Published monthly, topics covered include optometry, physiological optics, eye and vision science, optometric education, public health and epidemiology, and related fields. This peer-reviewed journal includes original articles, technical reports, case reports, Academy news, product news, and a calendar of events. Practicing optometrists and eye care professionals are the primary audience for this journal, which ranked twenty-fifth of the 49 ophthalmology journals (2009 *Journal Citation Reports*). A required resource for academic health sciences and optometry libraries, this journal is indexed in numerous indexing and abstracting sources including CINAHL Plus, Embase, MEDLINE, Scopus, and Web of Science. Open access is provided to one lead article from each issue, as well as full access to journal issues published prior to the last 12 months. Online access back to volume 66, 1989 is also available through several Lippincott Williams & Wilkins collections from Ovid.

Optometry: Journal of the American Optometric Association. v. 71, Elsevier, 2000.
http://www.optometryjaoa.com/
http://www.sciencedirect.com/science/journal/15291839
ISSN: 15291839
ISSN: 15581527 (Online)
Indexed in: MEDLINE
Recommended for: Academic Libraries

Begun in 1929 as the *Journal of the American Optometric Association*, this monthly peer-reviewed publication is required reading for optometrists and optometry students wanting to keep abreast of research to improve the quality of eye and vision care. The journal covers a range of topics such as pharmaceuticals, primary care optometry, practice management, contact lenses, low vision, and current research on eye diseases. The journal regularly features book reviews, industry news, health notes, medical abstracts, historical perspectives, and case reports. It is indexed in numerous abstracting and indexing sources including CINAHL Plus, Embase, MEDLINE, and Scopus. Online access to articles back to 2004 is available through Elsevier ScienceDirect.

Databases and Other Electronic Resources

Reference Sight: Online Index to the Optometric Periodical Literature. Centre for Contact Lens Research at the University of Waterloo, Canada, 200?
http://cclr.uwaterloo.ca/ReferenceSight/References.htm
http://cclr.uwaterloo.ca/vsrd/Index.asp
Recommended for: Academic Libraries

Students, faculty, researchers, practicing optometrists, and manufacturers are the primary audience for this online index, which is one of only three existing indexes (the other two being VISIONET and VisionCite specifically dedicated to covering the optometric periodical literature. Reference Sight is produced by the Centre for

Contact Lens Research at the University of Waterloo. It provides free access to optometric, ophthalmologic, optic, medical, and vision related article citations, with a special focus on contact lenses, refractive surgery, and external ocular disease. Although there is some overlap with MEDLINE, especially in the ophthalmology literature coverage, many of the journal articles covered by this index are not indexed in MEDLINE or in any other general health-related indexes. A list of journals indexed by Reference Sight may be found at http://cclr.uwaterloo.ca/vsrd/Index.asp. Although not a full-text database, it includes full article citations and keywords that make it relatively easy to find the articles in one's own collections or to request them via interlibrary loan or document delivery services. In addition, full abstracts and links to e-text are included where possible, as well as links to publishers and reprint sites. All customers may search this index free of charge. Registration is optional, and it provides searchers with more options.

VisionCite: Online Index to the Optometric Periodical Literature. Illinois College of Optometry (ICO) Carl F. Shepard Library, 1984.
http://www.visioncite.com/
Recommended for: Academic Libraries

Students, faculty, researchers, practicing optometrists and manufacturers are the primary audience for this online index, which is one of only three existing indexes (the other two being VISIONET and Reference Sight) specifically dedicated to covering the optometric periodical literature. Started in 1984, VisonCite utilizes the entire journal collection of the Illinois College of Optometry Carl F. Shepard Library, which includes optometric, ophthalmologic, optic, medical, and vision related journals. Although there is some overlap with MEDLINE especially in the ophthalmology literature coverage, many of the journal articles covered by this index are not indexed in MEDLINE or in any other general health-related indexes. A list of journals covered by VisonCite may be found at http://www.visioncite.com/serials_indexed.pdf. Although not a full-text database, it includes full article citations and keywords that make it relatively easy to find the articles in one's own collections or to request them via interlibrary loan or document delivery services. In addition, VisonCite is open URL compliant. It is available to non-ICO customers by subscription.

VISIONET: Online Index to the Optometric Periodical Literature. Southern College of Optometry (SCO) Library, 1976.
http://www.sco.edu/library/Pages/visionet.aspx
Recommended for: Academic Libraries

Students, faculty, researchers, practicing optometrists, and manufacturers are the primary audience for this online index, which is the very first index (and one of only three existing indexes, the other two being VisionCite and Reference Sight) specifically dedicated to covering the optometric periodical literature. Produced by the Southern College of Optometry (SCO) Library since 1976, VISIONET utilizes the entire journal collection of the SCO library, which includes optometric, ophthalmologic, optic, medical, and vision related journals. Although there is some overlap with MEDLINE especially in the ophthalmological literature coverage, many of the journal articles covered by this index are not indexed in MEDLINE or in any other general health-related indexes. A list of journals covered by VISIONET may be found at http://www.sco.edu/library/Pages/journals.aspx. Although not a full-text database, it includes full article citations and keywords that make it relatively easy to find the articles in one's own collections or to request them via interlibrary loan or document delivery services. VISIONET is available to non-SCO customers by subscription.

16. Orthoptics

The study and treatment of defects in binocular vision resulting from defects in the optic musculature or of faulty visual habits. It involves a technique of eye exercises designed to correct the visual axes of eyes not properly coordinated for binocular vision.

—MeSH

Contributors: Suzanne Ferimer, Gale A. Oren, Michael E. Piorunski

Monographs

Binocular Vision and Ocular Motility: Theory and Management of Strabismus. 6th ed. Editor: Gunter K. Von Noorden. Mosby Elsevier, 2002.
http://www.cybersight.org/bins/content_page.asp?cid=1-2193
ISBN: 9780801658228
Recommended for: Hospital, Academic Libraries

In its sixth edition, this resource is recognized as a classic text on strabismology. Appropriate for medical students, residents, fellows, pediatric ophthalmologists, and anyone seeing patients with strabismus, this comprehensive and well-balanced text covers the what, how, and why of this eye condition. It provides an outstanding historical perspective with extensive reference lists following each chapter. A unique feature is its focus on theory as well as management. It is divided into four sections: "Physiology of the Sensorimotor Cooperation of the Eyes," "Neuromuscular Anomalies of the Eyes," "Clinical Characteristics of the Neuromuscular Anomalies of the Eyes," and "Principles of Therapy." The book includes some illustrations, but it is not an atlas. Academic medical and hospital libraries, as well as practitioners who treat strabismus should have access to this resource. While the print version of this book is out of print, the book in its entirety has been made available free of charge on the Internet by ORBIS's Cyber-Sight project.

Journals

American Orthoptic Journal. v. 1, University of Wisconsin Press, 1951.
http://uwpress.wisc.edu/journals/journals/aoj.html
http://aoj.uwpress.org/
ISSN: 0065955X
ISSN: 15534448 (Online)
Indexed in: MEDLINE
Recommended for: Academic Libraries

This journal is the official journal of the American Association of Certified Orthoptists and is sponsored by the American Orthoptic Council. It has been published annually since 1951. The papers presented at the previous year's joint symposium of the American Orthoptic Council, the American Association of Certified Orthoptists, and the American Academy of Ophthalmology are published in the journal. Historical vignettes, case reports, book reviews, and abstracts of orthoptic literature published in other journals are also included. This journal also includes the American Orthoptic Council Statement of Ethics and the administrative directories of both organizations. It is indexed by EBSCO's Academic Search, MEDLINE, and Scopus. Online access from 2001 is available from the publisher. The electronic version is fully searchable and includes advanced search options.

Journal of AAPOS. v. 1, Elsevier, 1997.
http://www.sciencedirect.com/science/journal/10918531
ISSN: 10918531
ISSN: 15283933 (Online)
Indexed in: MEDLINE
Recommended for: Hospital, Academic Libraries

As the official publication of the American Association for Pediatric Ophthalmology and Strabismus, this peer-reviewed journal started in 1997. It focuses on eye diseases in children and on strabismus in all age groups. Peer-reviewed articles written by experts in the field cover both clinical and research aspects of medical and surgical care. Published six times a year, each issue contains editorials, major articles, case reports, and letters. The online version includes the full text as well as supplementary materials. This journal's audience includes ophthalmologists, orthoptists, residents, and any other medical personnel who see children with eye conditions or patients with strabismus. The journal is indexed in MEDLINE, Scopus, Embase, and a number of other abstracting and indexing services. This resource is recommended for hospitals, academic institutions, and ophthalmology/optometry practices. Online coverage is available from 1997 through Elsevier ScienceDirect.

17. Pharmacology

The study of the origin, nature, properties, and actions of drugs and their effects on living organisms.

—MeSH

Contributor: Sharon Leslie

Monographs

Applied Therapeutics: The Clinical Use of Drugs. 9th ed. Editors: Mary Anne Koda-Kimble, B. Joseph Guglielmo, Lloyd Y. Young, Wayne A. Kradjan, Brian K. Alldredge, Bradley R. Williams, Robin L. Corelli. Wolters Kluwer/ Lippincott Williams & Wilkins, 2009.
ISBN: 9780781765558
See Also Chapter 17.6. Clinical Pharmacology
Recommended for: Hospital, Academic Libraries
Doody's Core Titles Selection

This well-regarded student textbook begins with general principles of therapy and medication management, laboratory tests, and drug toxicities. Clinical applications of drugs are illustrated using case studies for each disease state. The use of case studies leads the student to understand the concepts and to think about applying them in practice. The audience is pharmacy and medical students and practicing clinicians. Competently written with minimal illustrations, additional resources are available online for individuals, including quizzes, images and PowerPoint presentations. *Applied Therapeutics* is a *Doody's Core Titles* essential purchase.

Basic and Clinical Pharmacology. 11th ed. Editors: Bertram G. Katzung, Susan B. Masters, Anthony J. Trevor. McGraw-Hill Medical, 2009.
http://www.accessmedicine.com/
ISBN: 9780071604055
See Also Chapter 17.6. Clinical Pharmacology
Recommended for: Hospital, Academic Libraries
Doody's Core Titles Selection

A primary textbook for pharmacology courses, this *Doody's Core Titles* selection is in its eleventh edition. The book covers essential topics in pharmacology fundamentals. After a review section on basic principles of pharmacology, the book addresses the different drug classes such as cardiovascular-renal, chemotherapeutic, and endocrine. Each class is broken down into chemical classification, pharmacokinetics, and toxicity, with a drug summary table at the end of the chapter. Changes to the new edition include using case studies to complement chapters and expansion of sections on drug receptors and transporters. Well-illustrated with full-color diagrams and tables and written at a basic student-level, this primer is intended for students of pharmacology but is essential for hospital libraries and primary care settings. It is recommended by the American Association of Colleges of Pharmacy's *Basic Resources for Pharmacy Education* list as a core title.

Brody's Human Pharmacology: Molecular to Clinical. 5th ed. Authors: Lynn Wecker, Lynn M. Crespo, George Dunaway, Carl Faingold, Stephanie Watts, Theodore M. Brody. Mosby/Elsevier, 2010.
ISBN: 9780323053747
Recommended for: Hospital, Academic Libraries
Doody's Core Titles Selection

This *Doody's Core Titles* recommended reference text details the fundamental clinical applications of pharmacology. It is designed for all students and health professionals interested in learning or revisiting the basics. An overview of the general principles of pharmacology (pharmacokinetics, toxicology) is given and then each organ system is examined, as well as chemotherapies. All chapters contain self-assessment questions at the end for review. It is illustrated with hundreds of full-color drawings, with further animations available online for individuals through the Student Consult version. It is recommended by the American Association of Colleges of Pharmacy's *Basic Resources for Pharmacy Education* as a core title.

Drugs in Pregnancy and Lactation: A Reference Guide to Fetal and Neonatal Risk. 8th ed. Editors: Gerald G. Briggs, Roger K. Freeman, Sumner J. Yaffe. Lippincott Williams & Wilkins, 2008.
See Chapter 11.4. Obstetrics

Goodman & Gilman's The Pharmacological Basis of Therapeutics. 12th ed. Editors: Laurence L. Brunton, Bruce A. Chabner, Björn C. Knollman. McGraw-Hill, 2011.

http://www.r2library.com/ (11th ed.)
http://www.ebrary.com/ (11th ed.)
http://extranet.netlibrary.com/TitleSelect (11th ed.)
ISBN: 9780071624428
See Also Chapter 17.6. Clinical Pharmacology
Recommended for: Hospital, Academic Libraries
Brandon/Hill, *Doody's Core Titles* Selection

A classic text, *Goodman and Gilman's* is a comprehensive therapeutics primer and a "must have" for virtually all clinical health professionals. Detailing drugs, their mechanisms of action and effects in dozens of classes, it is a resource physicians expect to see on a library shelf. This review refers to the eleventh edition. A new chapter on pharmacogenetics presents individual variations in drug responses. *Goodman and Gilman's* is now available in digital format through numerous vendors for libraries or through personal subscription for individuals. The bulky size and exhaustive detail make this more than a typical student may need, but it is an outstanding reference for physician offices and hospitals. A *Doody's Core Titles* essential purchase, it is also recommended by the American Association of Colleges of Pharmacy's *Basic Resources for Pharmacy Education* as a core title.

Oral Pharmacology for the Dental Hygienist. Authors: Mea A. Weinberg, Cheryl Westphal, James Burke Fine. Pearson Prentice Hall, 2008.
See Chapter 1.8. Dental Auxiliaries

Principles of Pharmacology: The Pathophysiologic Basis of Drug Therapy. 2nd ed. Editor: David E. Golan. Lippincott Williams & Wilkins, 2008.
ISBN: 9780781783552
Recommended for: Hospital, Academic Libraries
Doody's Core Titles Selection

This textbook, although only in its second edition, has quickly become a standard in pharmacology education and is a *Doody's Core Titles* recommendation. Opening with a chapter on the fundamental principles of pharmacology, drug action, and the pathophysiology and biochemistry of drugs, the introductory chapters include pharmacodynamics, pharmacokinetics, and drug metabolism and toxicity. The book covers the basics of each physiologic system and the respective therapeutic drugs. A new chapter on principles and mechanisms of drug toxicity was added as well as a large section on drug discovery, development, and regulation. Although more difficult to read than some other pharmacology titles, it is still a recommended purchase for medical and pharmacy students, health care professionals, and pharmacists. An online text and an accompanying image bank are available on Lippincott's the Point website (http://thepoint.lww.com/) for individual purchase.

Stahl's Essential Psychopharmacology: Neuroscientific Basis and Practical Application. 3rd ed. Author: Stephen M. Stahl. Cambridge University Press, 2008.
http://stahlonline.cambridge.org/
ISBN: 9780521857024
See Also Chapter 9.10. Psychiatry
Recommended for: Hospital, Academic Libraries

This book covers the fundamentals of neuroscience, the mechanisms of neurotransmitters and receptors, and contains detailed examinations of common psychiatric illnesses and their treatments. Each chapter ends with a summary paragraph about what was covered. Excellent full-color illustrations on almost every page show the concepts in simple diagrams. It is written for both students and practicing clinicians such as physicians, pharmacists, and mental health professionals. A separate companion prescribing guide goes into greater detail about doses, adverse effects and toxicity of over 100 drugs for psychiatric disorders. The online edition includes the full text plus numerous additional resources and features. Additionally, CME credits are available through the website of the Neuroscience Education Institute.

Trease and Evans' Pharmacognosy. 16th ed. Authors: William C. Evans, Daphne Evans, George E. Trease. Saunders Elsevier, 2009.
ISBN: 9780702029332
Recommended for: Academic Libraries

This reference book, now in its sixteenth edition, covers all aspects of natural products from discovery to taxonomy to manufacturing. Traditional herbs and complementary medicines are covered, as well as non-medicinal toxic plants and pesticides. Pharmacological preparations are represented by chemical compounds and plant families in table form. The latest edition has a newly-included chapter on plant nutraceuticals to reflect the growing awareness of a public now more demanding of knowledge of the effects of food on health. This chapter covers soy, tea, and pomegranate, to name a few. The book is recommended for academic institutions supporting pharmacy schools, alternative health practitioners, and the pharmaceutical industry. This book has a five-star *Doody's Review Service* rating and is recommended by the American Academy of Pharmacy's *Basic Educational Resources for Pharmacy Education* as a first purchase title.

Journals

Annual Review of Pharmacology and Toxicology. v. 16, Annual Reviews, 1976.
See Chapter 17.8. Toxicology

Clinical Pharmacology and Therapeutics. v. 1, Nature Publishing Group, 1960.
http://www.nature.com/clpt/
ISSN: 00099236
ISSN: 15326535 (Online)
Indexed in: MEDLINE, CINAHL
Recommended for: Hospital, Academic Libraries
Brandon/Hill Selection

The official journal of the American Society for Clinical Pharmacology and Therapeutics, *CPT* ranks eleventh out of 237 pharmacology and pharmacy journals (2009 *Journal Citation Reports*) and is a core clinical journal of the National Library of Medicine. It is also recommended by the American Association of Colleges of Pharmacy's *Basic Resources for Pharmacy Education* as a core title. Published since 1960, the journal contains original peer-reviewed research on a variety of topics in clinical pharmacology and new therapies, such as pharmacokinetics and pharmacodynamics, genomics and clinical trials. This journal is intended for clinicians, pharmacists, academic organizations, and researchers. The journal is indexed in numerous indexing and abstracting sources such as Embase, International Pharmaceutical Abstracts, MEDLINE, Science Citation Index, Scopus, and Web of Science. Online access back to 1995 is available through Nature Publishing Group.

Journal of Clinical Pharmacology. v. 1, Sage, 1973.
http://jcp.sagepub.com
ISSN: 00912700
ISSN: 15524604 (Online)
Indexed in: MEDLINE, CINAHL
Recommended for: Hospital, Academic Libraries

The official journal of the American College of Clinical Pharmacology, this journal has been in print under other titles since 1961. Written for clinicians, researchers, and pharmacists, the journal publishes original, peer-reviewed articles on the safety, tolerability, efficacy, and toxicology of drugs. Contents include sections on pharmacokinetics, drug interactions, case reports, and pharmacodynamics. It is ranked fifty-seventh out of 236 journals in pharmacology and pharmacy and has an impact factor of 3.442 (2009 *Journal Citation Reports*). It is also recommended by the American Association of Colleges of Pharmacy's *Basic Resources for Pharmacy Education* as a core title. The journal is indexed in numerous indexing and abstracting sources including CAB Abstracts, CINAHL, Embase, International Pharmaceutical Abstracts, MEDLINE, Scopus, and Web of Science. It is available in print and online formats, with access back to 1973 from HighWire and to 1961 from Sage.

Journal of Pharmacology and Experimental Therapeutics. v. 1, American Society for Pharmacology and Experimental Therapeutics, 1909.
http://jpet.aspetjournals.org/
ISSN: 00223565
ISSN: 15210103 (Online)
Indexed in: MEDLINE
Recommended for: Hospital, Academic Libraries
Brandon/Hill Selection

Published monthly, according to its website, *JPET* coverage includes "all aspects of the interactions of chemicals with biological systems." Each peer-reviewed issue contains articles grouped by major topic: behavioral pharmacology; cardiovascular; cellular and molecular; chemotherapy, antibiotics, and gene therapy; drug discovery and translational medicine; endocrine and diabetes; gastrointestinal, hepatic, pulmonary, and renal; inflammation, immunopharmacology, and asthma; metabolism, transport, and pharmacogenomics; neuropharmacology; toxicology; and other. "Perspectives on Pharmacology" are occasional invited reviews on contemporary or emerging topics. *JPET* ranked thirty-seventh out of 237 pharmacology and pharmacy journals with an impact factor of 4.093 (2009 *Journal Citation Reports*). It is indexed in major sources, including BIOSIS Previews, Current Contents, MEDLINE, PsycINFO, Science Citation Index Expanded, Scopus, and Web of Science. Online full text is available back to volume 1, 1909 through the HighWire platform.

Pharmacological Reviews. v. 1, American Society for Pharmacology and Experimental Therapeutics, 1949.
http://pharmrev.aspetjournals.org/
ISSN: 00316997
ISSN: 15210081 (Online)
Indexed in: MEDLINE
Recommended for: Hospital, Academic Libraries
Brandon/Hill Selection

Pharmacological Reviews publishes invited, comprehensive reviews of the current state of innovations in pharmacology and experimental therapeutics. In addition to three to five review articles in each quarterly issue, the journal also publishes International Union of Basic and Clinical Pharmacology (IUPHAR) nomenclature reports. With an impact factor of 17.0, *Pharmacological Reviews* ranks third of 237 pharmacology and pharmacy journals in the 2009 *Journal Citation Reports*. It is indexed in many major resources, including Embase, MEDLINE, Scopus, and Web of Science. Online full text is available back to volume 1, 1949 on the HighWire platform.

Psychopharmacology. v. 47, Springer, 1976.
http://www.springerlink.com/content/0033-3158
ISSN: 00333158
ISSN: 14322072 (Online)
Indexed in: MEDLINE
Recommended for: Hospital, Academic Libraries

The journal *Psychopharmacology* publishes original, peer-reviewed research on the mechanisms of action and effects of psychopharmacologic drugs used in clinical psychiatry. Articles may include preclinical, experimental, or clinical studies in humans or animal models. The intended audience for this journal is clinicians, pharmacologists, and researchers. It has an impact factor of 4.103 (2009 *Journal Citation Reports*) and is indexed in numerous indexing and abstracting sources including CAB Abstracts, Embase, MEDLINE, Neuroscience Citation Index, Scopus, and Web of Science. It is available in both print and online formats, with online access back to 1976 available from the publisher.

Databases and Other Electronic Resources

Natural Medicines Comprehensive Database. Therapeutic Research Faculty, 1999.
See Chapter 17.2. Herbal Medicine, Chapter 17.5. Pharmacognosy

Natural Standard. Natural Standard, 200?
http://www.naturalstandard.com
See Also Chapter 10.9. Integrative Medicine
Recommended for: Hospital, Academic, Consumer Health Libraries

The Natural Standard collaboration is a subscription database which summarizes evidence-based, peer-reviewed studies on complementary and alternative therapies. Various levels of monographs are collected, including brief summaries and detailed professional monographs. Monographs generally contain a color photograph of the subject, a history and overview of conditions treated, assessment of efficacy data, dosing and toxicology information, and a summary of the product and references. Additional databases within the content allow one to assess comparative effectiveness of substances and to check drug/herb/food and laboratory interactions. Additionally, a calculators feature includes BMI, target heart rate, ovulation calendars, and more. Patient education handouts in English and Spanish are available. This highly regarded resource is also available for mobile devices in a limited fashion.

17.1. Ethnopharmacology

The actions and properties of medicinal agents, often derived from plants, indigenous to populations or ethnic groups.
—MeSH

Contributor: Sharon Leslie

Journals

Journal of Ethnopharmacology. v. 1, Elsevier, 1979.
http://sciencedirect.com/science/journal/03788741
ISSN: 03788741
ISSN: 18727573 (Online)
See Also Chapter 17.2. Herbal Medicine
Indexed in: MEDLINE
Recommended for: Academic Libraries

The *Journal of Ethnopharmacology* is the official journal of the International Society for Ethnopharmacology. According to its aim and scope statements, its purpose is to discuss "people's use of plants, fungi, animals, microorganisms and minerals" in traditional healing and contemporary medicine. The journal is multidisciplinary, covering natural and social sciences. Targeted toward a wide audience of pharmacologists, pharmacists, biochemists, ethnobotanists, and anthropologists, it is concerned with conservation of native species and with scientific analysis of known and unknown plants. The journal publishes original, peer-reviewed research on the topics of pharmacological and toxicological mechanisms of action and anthropological and ethnobotanical field studies. It is indexed by numerous indexing and abstracting sources including CAB Abstracts, CINAHL Plus, Embase, International Pharmaceutical Abstracts, MEDLINE, Scopus, and Web of Science. Online access back to 1979 is available from the publisher.

17.2. Herbal Medicine

Medicines derived from botanical sources.
—MeSH: Medicine, Herbal

Contributor: Yunting Fu

Monographs

ABC Clinical Guide to Herbs. Editor: Mark Blumenthal. American Botanical Council, 2003.
ISBN: 9781588901576
ISBN: 9783131323910
Recommended for: Hospital, Academic Libraries

The *ABC Clinical Guide to Herbs* covers 29 herbs that were selected because of their high ranking in retail sales or their popularity in the United States. Each herb chapter contains a two-page clinical overview, a one-page patient information sheet, and a comprehensive monograph. Coverage includes pharmacological actions, clinical reviews, and clinical studies, which are especially valuable as these tend to be unique in herbal reference sources published during this time period. The information on clinical studies is displayed in a series of detailed tables that can be scanned quickly. An appropriate audience for this work includes clinical practitioners, pharmacists, physicians, and dietitians. The book can serve as a valuable continuing education module for physicians and as a reference source for clinical practices or pharmacies. This publication is highly recommended for hospital library collections, and it would also offer value to academic library collections.

E/S/C/O/P Monographs: The Scientific Foundation for Herbal Medicinal Products. 2nd ed., rev. Author: European Scientific Cooperative on Phytotherapy. Thieme Medical Publishers, 2003.
ISBN: 9781588902337
ISBN: 9781901964073
ISBN: 9783131294210
Recommended for: Hospital, Academic Libraries

Unlike other U.S. herbal publications, *E/S/C/O/P Monographs* presents the work of the European national phytotherapy associations relating to European herbal medicine products. The 80 monographs contained within this work address herbal medicine products that are not commonly used in the United States, and they are formally submitted as a basis for establishing core data on the leading herbal medicinal products in Europe. Thus, they serve as a major contribution to the harmonization of standards for herbal medicines across the European Union. The monographs are organized by the pharmacopeial name, and each contains the definition, constituents, clinical particulars, pharmacological properties, and references. This work updates data provided by the Commission E (Germany). The book is recommended for academic and hospital collections and would be useful for students, researchers, and pharmacists. Thieme has recently released *E/S/C/O/P Monographs, 2nd edition: Supplement 2009* (ISBN 9783131499813) that updates the existing monographs and expands the group with the addition of 27 new monographs.

The 5-Minute Herb & Dietary Supplement Consult. Author: Adriane Fugh-Berman. Lippincott Williams & Wilkins, 2003.
ISBN: 9780683302738
Recommended for: Hospital, Consumer Health Libraries

Doody's Review Service assigned a score of 100 to this work. Author Adriane Fugh-Berman is well known in the United States as an authority on herbs and dietary supplements. This book concisely organizes information on 175 high-use herbs and dietary supplements. The content of each monograph includes a description, part of the herb used, active constituents, food sources, main functions, and pharmacokinetics. Each monograph features the "10 Second Take" section, providing concise information on how the herbs can be used; and a "Common Questions and Answers" section, offering practical answers to frequently asked questions. Another feature is the herb chart listed at the back of the book, which provides the English, Latin, Spanish, French, German, and pharmacopoeia names for each herb. This chart can help find the English equivalent for herbs known by varying cultural names. This is a very good information resource for the general public who are interested in herbs. It is also valuable for students and practitioners who need a quick reference or guide. It is recommended for consumer health and hospital library collections.

Herbal Drugs and Phytopharmaceuticals: A Handbook for Practice on a Scientific Basis. 2nd ed. Editors: Norman G. Bisset, Max Wichtl. CRC Press, 2001.
ISBN: 9780849310119
Recommended for: Hospital, Academic, Consumer Health Libraries

This book provides very practical information on 181 herbs that could be used for the preparation of teas or as components of herbal mixtures. It is particularly useful in counseling patients in use of herbal preparations. The most significant feature of the book is its colorful pictures of each herbal drug, both in the herb's natural environment and as a dried product. Because the items selected are prepared for tea making, the method of preparation is also listed. If it is available, the regulatory status in different countries will be included. The individual monographs list plant source, origin, synonyms, constituents, indications, side effects, tea making, phytomedicines, regulatory status, authentication, evaluation, quantitative standards, adulteration, and storage. It does not include information on pharmacokinetics or drug-herb interactions; and because it is confined to herbs used as teas or in other preparations, it does not cover commercial herbal products taken as pills. Physicians, herbalists, and phytotherapists are the target audience. The title is recommended for consumer health, hospital, and academic libraries. See also *Herbal Drugs and Phytopharmaceuticals: A Handbook for Practice on a Scientific Basis*, 3rd. rev. ed, 2004, CRC Press, ISBN 9780849319617.

Herbal Medicine: Expanded Commission E Monographs. Editors: Mark Blumenthal, Alicia Goldberg, Josef Brinckmann. Integrative Medicine Communications, 2000.
ISBN: 9780967077215
Recommended for: Academic Libraries
Brandon/Hill Selection

This work is an expansion of the original, 1998 publication entitled *The Complete German Commission E Monographs: Therapeutic Guide to Herbal Medicines*. Based on the original Commission E compendium, each monograph includes color pictures, in-depth overviews, chemistry and pharmacology, dosage and administration, and other information. An extensive list of references enhances each monograph. The original *Commission E* is a classic work, but dated. This updated, expanded version serves as a basic background information resource building upon *Commission E*. The target audience is general health care professionals.

Herbal Products: Toxicology and Clinical Pharmacology. 2nd ed. Editors: Timothy S. Tracy, Richard L. Kingston. Humana Springer, 2007.
See Chapter 17.8.2. Forensic Toxicology

Natural Standard Herb & Supplement Reference: Evidence-Based Clinical Reviews. Editors: Catherine E. Ulbricht, Ethan M. Basch. Mosby, 2005.
ISBN: 9780323029940
Recommended for: Hospital, Academic Libraries

Clinicians, herbalists, pharmacists, and educators are the audience for this book. The publication by more than 114 contributors covers information on 98 products, including 17 of the 20 top-selling herbs in the United States. Each monograph contains information on synonyms, the clinical bottom line, dosing and toxicology, adverse effects, interactions, mechanisms of action, tables with discussion, reviews of evidence, and brands used in clinical trials and third party testing. A significant feature of the book is the use of a grading scale to rate the quality of evidence regarding clinical efficacy for each product. This grading scale is developed by experts in primary care and prevention, and it is used to systematically review the evidence of herb and supplement effectiveness and to develop recommendations for clinical preventive services. This book is recommended as a handy reference for libraries that do not have access to the Natural Medicines Comprehensive Database.

Journals

The American Journal of Chinese Medicine. v. 7, World Scientific Publishing, 1979.
http://www.worldscinet.com/ajcm/
ISSN: 0192415X
ISSN: 17936853
Indexed in: MEDLINE, CINAHL
Recommended for: Hospital, Academic Libraries

The American Journal of Chinese Medicine is ranked seventh of 17 titles in integrative and complementary medicine (2009 *Journal Citation Reports*). The journal's aim and scope are the publication of "original articles and essays relating to traditional or ethnomedicine of all cultures." According to the journal's website, its areas of interest include: (a) basic scientific and clinical research in indigenous medical techniques, therapeutic procedures, medicinal plants, and traditional medical theories and concepts; (b) multidisciplinary study of medical practice and health care; (c) international policy implications of comparative studies of medicine in all cultures; and (d) translating scholarly ancient texts or modern publications on ethnomedicine. Researchers and educators are the target audience for this publication, which is recommended for research and academic library collections.

Journal of Ethnopharmacology. v. 1, Elsevier, 1979.
http://www.sciencedirect.com/science/journal/03788741
ISSN: 03788741
ISSN: 18727573 (Online)
See Also Chapter 17.1. Ethnopharmacology
Indexed in: MEDLINE
Recommended for: Academic Libraries

Based on *Journal Citation Reports*, the *Journal of Ethnopharmacology* ranks first by five-year impact factor and third by 2009 impact factor in the category of integrative and complementary medicine. The journal publishes original articles concerned with the observation and experimental investigation of biological activities of plant and animal substances used in traditional medicine of past and present cultures. The publisher describes this title as "dedicated to the exchange of information and understandings about people's use of plants, fungi, animals, microorganisms and minerals and their biological and pharmacological effects." It is printed 18 times a year and features abstracts and book reviews. The journal is indexed in MEDLINE and other major databases. The *Journal of Ethnopharmacology* is recommended for academic and hospital collections.

Phytomedicine: International Journal of Phytotherapy and Phytopharmacology. v. 1, Urban & Fischer, 1994.
http://www.sciencedirect.com/science/journal/09447113
ISSN: 09447113
ISSN: 1618095X (Online)
Indexed in: MEDLINE, CINAHL
Recommended for: Academic Libraries

The impact factor of *Phytomedicine* has risen from 1.403 to 2.174 in the past 5 years (2009 *Journal Citation Reports*). The journal publishes research results on phytotherapy (clinical trials), phytopharmacology, pharmacognosy, and standardization and phytotoxicology, obtained with plant extracts as well as isolated compounds from these extracts and phytopharmaceuticals. As described by the publisher, the title is published to "attract and disseminate innovative and expert findings in the fields of phytopharmacology, phytotherapy and phytotoxicology." The content consists of case reports; pharmacological and molecular biological studies; screening studies; chemical structure—activity studies; chemical analysis and standardization of plant drugs and phytopharmaceuticals; and invited reviews. The journal's target audience includes pharmacologists, toxicologists, pharmacists, pharmacognosists, and practitioners.

Planta Medica. v. 1, Georg Thieme, 1953.
http://www.thieme.de/plantamedica/index.html
https://www.thieme-connect.com/ejournals/toc/planta medica
ISSN: 00320943
ISSN: 14390221 (Online)
Indexed in: MEDLINE, CINAHL
Recommended for: Academic Libraries

As the official publication of the Society for Medicinal Plant and Natural Product Research, *Planta Medica* covers the areas of medicinal plants and natural products research. Content features pharmacology and clinical studies, natural product chemistry, analytical studies, biochemistry, and biological screening. Though the journal does not have a very high ranking in *Journal Citation Reports*, it is highly recommended by researchers in the herbal medicine field. Scientists and researchers are the target audience. *Planta Medica* is recommended for academic and research library collections.

Databases and Other Electronic Resources

Herbal Medicine: An Alternative and Complementary Medicine Resource Guide. Alternative Medicine Foundation, 1998.
http://www.amfoundation.org/herbinfo.htm
Recommended for: Hospital, Academic, Consumer Health Libraries

This herbal medicine resource guide is a service of the Alternative Medicine Foundation, which is a nonprofit organization providing reliable information about alternative medicine to the public and health professionals. The introduction states that "these resources relate mainly to Western traditions of herbal medicine (also referred to as phytomedicine, herbal medicine or botanical medicine) that rely primarily on the use of single herbs." The guide lists various types of herbal resources, including books, journals, educational and training opportunities in herbal medicine, professional and referral organizations, search services, and web resources. While the guide can serve as a useful starting point for collection specialists, it can also aid more general users with their research needs.

MedlinePlus—Drugs, Supplements, and Herbal Information. National Library of Medicine, National Institutes of Health, 1998.
http://www.nlm.nih.gov/medlineplus/druginfo/herb_All .html
Recommended for: Hospital, Academic, Consumer Health Libraries

This free, web-based database is an authoritative source for health and medical information. Developed by the National Library of Medicine, a part of the National Institutes of Health, MedlinePlus targets both consumers and health care professionals. The Drugs & Supplements section is part of the database that provides reliable information on herbs and supplements. Content is supplied by Natural Standard, which is one of the world's premier sources of information in the field of complementary and alternative therapies. The consumer health information is written in easily understandable language, and the format is designed for quick access and navigation. Users can search or browse by the product name. The content of each monograph consists of background, synonyms, evidence, dosing, safety, interactions, methodology, and selected references similar to a textbook. The most significant difference between this database and others is that the content is written for non-medical professionals. This is a great resource for the general public and is highly recommended for both consumer health and hospital libraries.

Natural Medicines Comprehensive Database. Therapeutic Research Faculty, 1999.
http://www.naturaldatabase.com
See Also Chapter 17.5. Pharmacognosy
Recommended for: Hospital, Academic Libraries

Pharmacists, practicing physicians, and researchers are the primary audience for this database. Originally released in 1999, the Natural Medicines Comprehensive Database covers evidence-based clinical information and serves as a broad-based reference text for information on herbal, vitamin, and mineral components that make up modern natural medicines. Data is compiled and analyzed by pharmacologists, dietitians, pharmacists, and physicians. Users can search by product name, natural ingredient, disease, and other items. They can also browse lists such as those for commercial products, fixed herbal combinations, alternative treatments, and modalities. For each product, the database provides comprehensive information including safety, effectiveness, and drug interactions. Physicians and pharmacists can use the patient education handouts in their daily practices, and researchers will benefit by the mechanism of action information. Natural Medicines is highly recommended for hospital and academic collections.

17.3. Neuropharmacology

The action of drugs upon various parts of the nervous system.

—MeSH

Contributor: Sharon Leslie

Monographs

The Biochemical Basis of Neuropharmacology. 8th ed. Authors: Jack R. Cooper, Floyd E. Bloom, Robert H. Roth. Oxford University Press, 2003.
http://online.statref.com/titleinfo/fxid-145.html
ISBN: 9780195140088
Recommended for: Hospital, Academic Libraries

First published in 1970, this is a classic text in the field of neuropharmacology. It covers drugs that affect the central nervous system and psychotropic drugs such as sedatives, narcotics, and analgesics. Since information about therapeutic indications is available in other books, this book focuses on the biochemistry, mechanisms of drug action, and neurotransmitters that affect brain function. As dense as the subject matter would dictate, it has two-color illustrations, a crisp format, and numerous references at the end of each chapter. The audience is clinicians and students in neuroscience, psychology, and pharmacology.

Journals

Neuropharmacology. v. 9, Elsevier, 1970.
http://sciencedirect.com/science/journal/00283908
ISSN: 00283908
ISSN: 18737064 (Online)
Indexed in: MEDLINE
Recommended for: Hospital, Academic Libraries

Neuropharmacology addresses the numerous treatments and adverse effects of drugs used to treat neurological diseases. Intended for neurological clinicians and researchers, this peer-reviewed journal publishes preclinical articles on biology, neurophysiology, behavior and virtually all aspects of neuroscience, with emphasis on neuropharmacology. According to its aim and scope statement, "each year Elsevier/*Neuropharmacology* organise a satellite symposium to the Meeting of the Society for Neuroscience. The journal publishes a Special Issue to accompany each meeting." It is recommended by the American Association of Colleges of Pharmacy's *Basic Resources for Pharmacy Education* as a core title and has an impact factor of 3.909, ranking forty-third out of 237 titles in pharmacology and pharmacy (2009 *Journal Citation Reports*). It is indexed by numerous indexing and abstracting sources including Current Contents, Embase, MEDLINE, Scopus, and Web of Science. Online access back to 1970 is available from the publisher.

17.4. Pharmacoepidemiology

The benefit and risk of drugs used in populations and the analysis of the outcomes of drug therapies. Pharmacoepidemiologic data come from both clinical trials and epidemiological studies with emphasis on methods for the detection and evaluation of drug-related adverse effects, assessment of risk vs benefit ratios in drug therapy, patterns of drug utilization, the cost-effectiveness of specific drugs, methodology of postmarketing surveillance, and the relation between pharmacoepidemiology and the formulation and interpretation of regulatory guidelines.

—MeSH

Contributor: Sharon Leslie

Monographs

Pharmacoepidemiology. 4th ed. Editor: Brian L. Strom. Wiley, 2005.
http://onlinelibrary.wiley.com/book/10.1002/9780470059876
ISBN: 9780470866818
ISBN: 9780470-866832 (Online)
Recommended for: Hospital, Academic Libraries

Written by the current editor of *Pharmacoepidemiology and Drug Safety*, the official journal of the International Society for Pharmacoepidemiology, this book is a comprehensive reference source on the subject. *Pharmacoepidemiology* helps identify drug safety issues in large patient populations. Response to global drug regulation has caused industry to conduct post-marketing drug surveillance investigating adverse drug reactions. After an introduction to the topic, subsequent chapters deal with very specific realms of consideration, such as "Pharmacoepidemiologic Studies of Devices," or "The Use of Meta-Analysis in Pharmacoepidemiology." Methodological issues including study design and bias as well as statistical analysis are also covered. This fourth edition has material for industry, academia, regulatory bodies, and public health personnel. A glossary of terms is included.

Journals

Pharmacoepidemiology and Drug Safety. v. 1, Wiley Blackwell, 1992.
http://onlinelibrary.wiley.com/journal/10.1002/(ISSN)1099-1557
ISSN: 10538569
ISSN: 10991557 (Online)
Indexed in: MEDLINE
Recommended for: Hospital, Academic Libraries

Published since 1992, *Pharmacoepidemiology and Drug Safety* is the official journal of the International Society for Pharmacoepidemiology. The journal publishes original, peer-reviewed research for clinicians, public health educators, biostatisticians, and industry. Its focus is on observation of post-marketing safety and outcomes of pharmaceuticals, biologics, and medical devices. Also covered are drug utilization and legal and economic aspects of pharmacoepidemiology. It is recommended by the American Association of Colleges of Pharmacy's *Basic Resources for Pharmacy Education* as a core title. The journal is ranked one-hundred-fifth out of 236 journals in pharmacology and pharmacy and has an impact factor of 2.527 (2009 *Journal Citation Reports*). It is indexed by numerous indexing and abstracting sources including Embase, International Pharmaceutical Abstracts, MEDLINE, Scopus, and Web of Science. The journal is available in both print and online formats, with online access back to 1992 available from the publisher.

17.5. Pharmacognosy

Drugs prepared from natural-sources including preparations from plants, animals, and other organisms as well as minerals and other substances included in materia medica.

—MeSH

Contributor: Sharon Leslie

Monographs

Medicinal Plants of the World: Chemical Constituents, Traditional and Modern Medicinal Uses. Author: Ivan A. Ross. Humana, 2003.
http://www.ellibs.com/book/9781592598878 (v. 3 only)
ISBN: 9781588292810 (v.1)
ISBN: 9781402012471 (v.2)
ISBN: 9781588291295 (v.3)
ISBN: 9781592598878 (Online v.3)
Recommended for: Hospital, Academic, Consumer Health Libraries

Written by a biologist with the U.S. Food and Drug Administration, this three-volume encyclopedia covers a total of 67 plants from all over the world and illustrates their medicinal value. Volume 1 covers 27 plants including garlic, turmeric, and lemon grass. The first chapter of this volume discusses the botanical nomenclature and contains line drawings showing the leaf, flower, fruit, seed, and stalk types that are described later in each subsequent volume. Each chapter of all three volumes contain common names the for the plant in countries around the world, a black-and-white photo of the plant, how it is prepared, the botanical description, origin and distribution, and traditional medicinal uses in many countries. This is followed by the chemical constituents and then the pharmacological activities for which the plant has been used or studied, for example, analgesic activity, embryotoxic effects, insecticide activity, carcinogenesis inhibition, etc. All data is referenced to published articles. Published over the course of several years, each volume adds to the knowledge base of medicinal plants. Each volume is cross-referenced and includes a glossary. This resource is recommended for pharmacologists involved in drug discovery, herbal practitioners, toxicologists, and consumers interested in the background of some of the medicines they may be taking.

Journals

Journal of Natural Products. v. 42, American Society of Pharmacognosy/American Chemical Society, 1979.
http://pubs.acs.org/journal/jnprdf
ISSN: 01633864
ISSN: 15206025 (Online)
Indexed in: MEDLINE
Recommended for: Academic Libraries

Co-published by the American Chemical Society and the American Society of Pharmacognosy, this peer-reviewed journal broadly covers natural products research. According to the journal scope statement, examples of specific topics include: "secondary metabolites of microorganisms, including antibiotics and mycotoxins; physiologically active compounds from terrestrial and marine plants and animals; biochemical studies, including biosynthesis and microbiological transformations; fermentation and plant tissue culture; the isolation, structure elucidation, and chemical synthesis of novel compounds from nature; and the pharmacology of compounds of natural origin." This journal had an impact factor of 3.159 in the 2009 *Journal Citation Reports* and ranked twelfth out of 46 (medicinal chemistry) and sixty-ninth out of 237 (pharmacology and pharmacy). It is indexed in numerous indexing and abstracting sources including CAB Abstracts, Embase, MEDLINE, Science Citation Index, Scopus, and Web of Science. It is available in print and online formats, with access from 1979 available from the publisher. It is recommended by the American Association of Colleges of Pharmacy's *Basic Resources for Pharmacy Education* as a core title.

Databases and Other Electronic Resources

AltCareDex (MICROMEDEX). Thomson Reuters, 19??
http://www.micromedex.com/products/altmeddex
Recommended for: Hospital, Academic, Consumer Health Libraries

Part of the MICROMEDEX system, AltCareDex offers pharmacists and clinicians extensive monographs detailing herbs, vitamins, dietary supplements, Chinese medicines, and more. Each monograph contains dosing information, synonyms, contraindications, adverse reactions, drug interactions, clinical applications and thorough references. A team of editorial writers ("physicians, clinical pharmacists, nurses, and other allied health professionals as well as medical librarians") create each monograph. Also part of the online package are complementary and alternative medicine (CAM) patient education handouts. This resource is available as a component of a MICROMEDEX subscription. It is updated quarterly.

Natural Medicines Comprehensive Database. Therapeutic Research Faculty, 1999.
www.naturaldatabase.com
See Also Chapter 17.2. Herbal Medicine
Recommended for: Hospital, Academic Libraries

Published by Therapeutic Research Faculty, the same company that publishes *Prescriber's Letter* and *Pharmacist's Letter*, this database has existed since 1999. Searches may be done by natural ingredient or supplement name or by disease or condition. Each entry contains the scientific name, alternative names, uses, safety information, mechanism of action, dosage, adverse effects, drug interactions, and a link to brand name products if relevant. All monographs are reviewed for safety, effectiveness, and interaction potential by an editorial board of practitioners from many disciplines, including pharmacy, medicine, nutrition, research, and nursing. An additional subset of "USP Verified Brands" shows dietary supplements that have passed the USP verification of quality, purity, and potency. References in each monograph link out to PubMed. Canadian products are also covered. Patient handouts are available in English and Spanish. The site also has an online message board for health care professionals to ask each other questions. The database is updated daily. Both the professional and consumer online versions are available by subscription only; the professional version is also available in print and for mobile devices. The database is well-organized and easy to use. This is a comprehensive resource for herbal and dietary supplement information that would be of great benefit to pharmacies, clinicians, and students.

Natural Standard. Natural Standard, 200?
See Chapter 10.9. Integrative Medicine, Chapter 17. Pharmacology

Review of Natural Products. Facts and Comparisons, 2001.
http://www.factsandcomparisons.com/facts-comparisons-Online.aspx

http://www.ovid.com/
http://online.statref.com/titleinfo/fxid-15.html
Recommended for: Hospital, Academic, Consumer Health Libraries

This comprehensive source was established in 1980 as a print publication and has been available in both print and online since 2001. It is available online as a database, updated monthly, from Facts and Comparisons and through Ovid and STAT!Ref. Monographs detail the common name, botany, history, chemistry, pharmacology, interactions, dosing, toxicology, and adverse effects of over 300 natural products. Sample content includes betel nut, kaolin, deer velvet, and zinc, and nutraceuticals such as soy, honey, and wine. The appendix contains information on evidence-based herb-drug interactions and the use of herbal medicinal products during pregnancy and lactation. The intended audience is all health care professionals and consumers interested in alternatives to prescription medicines.

17.6. Clinical Pharmacology

The effectiveness and safety of drugs in humans.
—MeSH

Contributor: Amy Knehans

Monographs

AHFS Drug Information: American Hospital Formulary Service. Editor: Gerald K. McEvoy. American Society of Health-System Pharmacists, 2010.
http://www.ahfsdruginformation.com/
http://www.statref.com/
ISBN: 9781585282470
Recommended for: Hospital, Academic Libraries

Also known as, "*The Big Red Book*," *AHFS DI* is a comprehensive and objective drug information reference that is standard for clinical pharmacist and health care professionals. Designated an official compendium by the U.S. Congress for Reimbursement Determinations on Unlabeled Uses, *AHFS* is a collection of drug monographs on every drug available in the United States. It is written and published by pharmacists and reviewed by hundreds of experts. It provides information on uses included in the "labeled" category and those that are "off label" uses. The drug monographs are arranged by AHFS Pharmacologic-Therapeutic Classification. Information on a particular drug can be located by several methods. It can be searched by the trade name, generic name, synonym, abbreviation, pharmacy equivalent name, or former name. Monographs include drug interactions; adverse reactions; cautions and toxicity; therapeutic perspective; specific dosage and administration information; preparations, chemistry, and stability; pharmacology and pharmacokinetics; contraindications; and more. AHFS is available in print, online and for mobile devices. "The mission of AHFS Drug Information is to provide an evidence-based foundation for safe and effective drug therapy." (ASHP American Society of Health-System Pharmacists) An additional benefit is that this essential resource can be used on the desk top or with a mobile device. For mobile device use see Lexicomplete, Epocrates Essentials, and Skyscape Mobile Medical References.

Applied Therapeutics: The Clinical Use of Drugs. 9th ed. Editors: Mary Anne Koda-Kimble, Joseph B. Guglielmo, Lloyd Y. Young, Wayne A. Kradjan, Brian K. Alldredge. Lippincott Williams & Wilkins, 2009.
ISBN: 9780781765558
See Also Chapter 17. Pharmacology
Recommended for: Hospital, Academic Libraries
Doody's Core Titles Selection

This resource is intended for health science students and clinical professionals. It was selected as a core title for *Doody's Core Titles in the Health Sciences*, with a five-star rating. This title is also an essential purchase title from the American Association of Colleges of Pharmacy's *Basic Resources in Pharmacy Education* list. The book is divided into sections according to organ system, with individual chapters addressing common diseases; all start with a basic introduction or definition. Each section is written by a leading expert and provides fine details of treatment. The text helps students develop practical problem-solving skills so that they can provide the best evidence-based drug therapy for their patients. An additional feature is the newly added culturally competent care issues which are incorporated into chapters.

Basic and Clinical Pharmacology. 11th ed. Editors: Bertram G. Katzung, Susan B. Masters, Anthony J. Trevor. McGraw-Hill Medical, 2009.
http://www.accessmedicine.com
ISBN: 9780071604055
See Also Chapter 17. Pharmacology
Recommended for: Hospital, Academic Libraries
Doody's Core Titles Selection

This is a gold standard textbook for teaching pharmacology to health professionals. It gives comprehensive, in-depth coverage of all the important topics about the science of pharmacology and its application to clinical practice. It begins with a history of pharmacology and covers every important aspect of medical pharmacology: basic principles; autonomic drugs; cardiovascular-renal drugs; drugs with important actions on smooth muscle; drugs that act in the central nervous system; drugs used to treat diseases of the blood, inflammation, and gout; endocrine drugs; chemotherapeutic drugs; and toxicology. The last sections contain evidence-based chapters on special topics such as aspects of "Perinatal & Pediatric Pharmacology," "Geriatric Pharmacology," "Dermatologic Pharmacology," and "Drugs Used in the Treatment of Gastrointestinal Diseases." It is a required textbook for many pharmacology courses. Special features include special interest boxes and lists of common preparations, as well as dosage information and critical discussions of treatment strategies and recommended drugs for all major diseases.

Brody's Human Pharmacology: Molecular to Clinical. 5th ed. Authors: Lynn Wecker, Lynn M. Crespo, George Dunaway, Carl Faingold, Stephanie Watts, Theodore M. Brody. Mosby/Elsevier, 2010.
See Chapter 17. Pharmacology

Clinical Ocular Pharmacology. 5th ed. Editors: Jimmy D. Bartlett, Siret D. Jaanus. Butterworth-Heinemann/ Elsevier, 2008.
See Chapter 15. Optometry

Goodman & Gilman's The Pharmacological Basis of Therapeutics. 12th ed. Editors: Laurence L. Brunton, Bruce A. Chabner, Björn C. Knollman. McGraw-Hill, 2011.
http://www.accessmedicine.com
ISBN: 9780071624428
See Also Chapter 17. Pharmacology
Recommended for: Hospital, Academic Libraries
Brandon/Hill, *Doody's Core Titles* Selection

This book is a comprehensive and authoritative source on the pharmacology of drugs and considered a gold standard of pharmacology textbooks. It has a five-star rating from *Doody's Review Service*. This is a highly used resource in colleges of pharmacy and a resource for all who study, research, teach, or practice clinical pharmacology. It has the reputation of being the bible of pharmacology. This is a multi-author book; expert scholars have written individual chapters. Chapters are organized consistently to make it easy for students to find the physiology and basic pharmacology set forth in regular type in each chapter. The print version comes with a non-transferable subscription to an online digital version. Each drug in the digital version is hyperlinked to Gold Standards, Clinical Pharmacology Online, an online database. Mobile device downloads are also available. This review refers to the eleventh edition.

Manual of Clinical Psychopharmacology. 7th ed. Authors: Alan F. Schatzberg, Jonathan O. Cole, Charles DeBattista. American Psychiatric Publishing, 2010.
See Chapter 17.7. Psychopharmacology

Merck Index: An Encyclopedia of Chemicals, Drugs, and Biologicals. 14th ed. Editor: Maryadele J. O'Neil. Merck & Co, 2006.
http://www.merck.com/
ISBN: 9780911910001
See Also Chapter 18. Pharmacy
Recommended for: Hospital, Academic Libraries

This is an essential reference for anyone who works with chemicals, biologicals, and pharmaceuticals. The Merck Index is a one-volume, multidisciplinary reference handbook that contains more than 10,200 monographs that describe significant chemicals, drugs, and biological substances. Chemicals are those that are commonly found in industry, medicine, and agriculture. Each monograph gives a brief description of a single substance or a small group of closely related compounds. The monographs vary in length. There are a number of monographs devoted to families of natural products or biological substances. Information is well organized. The types of information found in the monographs are monograph number, monograph title, chemical information, Chemical Abstract Registry Number, alternate names, molecular formula, literature references, biological and pharmacological information, structure, physical data, derivatives use, therapeutic category, and more. It also includes a companion CD-ROM which features 989 monographs no longer available in print, organic name reactions, and supplemental tables that have been revised to include acronyms, vaccines, and physical constants.

Pharmacotherapy: A Pathophysiologic Approach. 7th ed. Editors: Jospeph T. Dipiro, Robert L. Talbert, Gary C. Yee, Gary R. Matzke, Barbara G. Wells, Michael L. Posey. McGraw-Hill Medical, 2009.
http://www.accesspharmacy.com
http://www.ebrary.com
http://extranet.netlibrary.com/TitleSelect
ISBN: 9780071478991
Recommended for: Hospital, Academic Libraries
Brandon/Hill, *Doody's Core Titles* Selection

This is an authoritative book written by physicians and pharmacists for pharmacy students, pharmacists, and other clinical professionals. It is an easy-to-use textbook that contains detailed and comprehensive information on pharmacotherapy that takes an evidence-based approach to the drug treatment of diseases. The first section introduces some of the basic principles of clinical pharmacology followed by sections on the management of diseases, organized according to systems of the body. Each chapter deals with individual diseases through discussion of the pathophysiologic principles and an outline of the methods of drug therapy appropriate to each. Handy features include "Critical Presentation" boxes that summarize common disease signs and symptoms, the "Clinical Controversies" boxes that examine complicated issues faced when providing drug therapy. A very nice addition is the presentation of psychosocial issues that affect compliance, topics related to a patient's ability to understand and manage often complex therapy as well as lifestyle changes that may reduce the need for drug therapy or improve pharmacotherapeutic outcomes. This title is a four-star rating for *Doody's Core Titles* and was selected as an essential purchase title from the American Association of Colleges of Pharmacy *Basic Resources in Pharmacy Education* list.

Principles of Pharmacology: The Pathophysiologic Basis of Drug Therapy. 2nd ed. Editor: David E. Golan. Lippincott Williams & Wilkins, 2008.
See Chapter 17. Pharmacology

Journals

Annals of Pharmacotherapy. v. 26, Harvey Whitney Books, 1992.
http://www.theannals.com/
ISSN: 10600280
ISSN: 15426270 (Online)
Indexed in: MEDLINE, CINAHL
Recommended for: Hospital, Academic Libraries

This peer-reviewed medical journal publishes evidence-based articles on practice, research, and education in pharmacotherapy. It is an international, independent journal for pharmacists, physicians, nurses, and other healthcare professionals. Typical issues include research reports, reviews, commentaries, and case reports. The editorial board consists of clinicians, researchers, and educators with collective expertise in all areas of pharmacy. The journal emphasizes the advancement of safe, effective, and economical use of medications in patients. Some of the special article features include new drug evaluations, therapeutic controversies, recent therapeutic advances, international reports, and continuing education. Online access is available from 1998 to the present from the publisher.

Clinical Pharmacology and Therapeutics. v. 1, Nature Publishing Group, 1960.
See Chapter 17. Pharmacology

Journal of Clinical Pharmacology. v. 1, Sage, 1973.
See Chapter 17. Pharmacology

Journal of Pharmaceutical Sciences. v. 50, Wiley-Blackwell, 1961.
http://onlinelibrary.wiley.com/journal/10.1002/(ISSN)1520-6017
ISSN: 00223549
ISSN: 15206017 (Online)
Indexed in: MEDLINE
Recommended for: Hospital, Academic Libraries

This peer-reviewed journal focuses on concepts in basic pharmaceutical science spanning a variety of disciplines, including physical pharmacy, pharmaceutical engineering, materials science, pharmacokinetics/pharmacodynamics, pharmacogenomics, animal and human biopharmaceutics, cellular and molecular biopharmaceutics, drug delivery, drug metabolism, pharmaceuticals, biotechnology, analytical chemistry, computer modeling, medicinal chemistry, pro-drug developments, and targeted drug delivery. The editorial Advisory Board consists of 146 persons who collectively reflect the diversity of scientific disciplines served by the journal. The *Journal of Pharmaceutical Sciences* is a publication of American Pharmaceutical Association., published by Wiley-Blackwell. Online coverage back to volume 50, 1961 is available from Wiley Online Library.

Pharmacotherapy. v. 1, Pharmacotherapy Publications, 1981.
http://www.pharmacotherapy.org/
ISSN: 02770008
ISSN: 18759114 (Online)
Indexed in: MEDLINE
Recommended for: Hospital, Academic Libraries

This peer-reviewed journal publishes original research articles on all aspects of human pharmacology and review articles on drugs and drug therapy. It is the official journal of the American College of Clinical Pharmacy. Articles published in this journal are original research reports on pharmacokinetic, bioavailability and drug interaction studies, clinical trials and investigations of specific pharmacological properties of drugs, and related topics. Typical issue content includes original clinical research articles, research reports, brief reports, mini-reviews, practice insights, special articles, reviews of therapeutics, case reports, and alternative viewpoints. A noteworthy feature is the articles from "Pharmacy Practice Insights" and "Drug Use Insights." These articles report innovative practice guidelines and outcomes-oriented drug use studies. Online access is available from 1999 to the present from the publisher.

Databases and Other Electronic Resources

Clinical Pharmacology. Elsevier, 200?
http://www.clinicalpharmacology.com/
Recommended for: Hospital, Academic Libraries

This database provides information on FDA-approved prescription drugs, new and investigational drugs, herbal supplements, Phase 3 trials, and nutritional and over-the-counter products. It is an excellent resource for pharmacy students and pharmacists as well as all other health professionals. It can be searched by generic or brand name. The database is made up of peer-reviewed drug monographs and patient education records. Drug monographs include description, mechanism of action, and pharmacokinetics. Additional links are used to access the indications and dosage, administration, contraindications and precautions (with separate categories for pregnancy and breastfeeding), interactions, adverse reactions, patient education, costs and monitoring, how the drug is supplied and product information, classification, and chemical structures. Patient education records are available in English or Spanish. The database is updated frequently with updates highlighted in a monthly digest. Information is derived from peer-reviewed journals, standard reference texts, FDA websites, and manufacturer product labels. Features include a frequent task menu, references with links to monographs, consumer handouts, drug interaction utility, drug comparison utility, IV compatibility utility, drug patent search, and tutorials, with an index and advanced search providing different methods of finding drug information.

Embase. Elsevier, 199?
http://www.embase.com/
http://www.ovid.com/
ISBN: 1573000X
Recommended for: Hospital, Academic Libraries

Embase is an abstracting and indexing database specializing in the biomedical field with extensive coverage of pharmaceutical research. It began as a print tool and is used by a variety of biomedical scientists. It contains bibliographic records with citations and abstracts and indexing derived from biomedical articles in peer-reviewed journals. Articles usually appear in the database within two weeks of receipt of the original journal. There is a short lag time due to the extensive indexing that is done manually. It is updated daily with more than 3,000 records added every day. Each record contains the full bibliographic citation, indexing terms, and other information about the original article. The scope covers drug therapy and research, including pharmaceutics, pharmacology, and toxicology; clinical and human experimental medicine; basic biological science relevant to human medicine; biotechnology and biomedical engineering; health policy and management; public, occupational, and environmental health; psychiatry and mental health; forensic science; and alternative and complementary medicine. Unique features include coverage of the European and Japanese literature. It covers 1,800 biomedical journals that are not covered in MEDLINE and provides access to research on adverse reactions that have been reported in clinical trials. Database records are linked to full-text articles.

Facts & Comparisons eAnswers. Wolters Kluwer Health, 2011.
http://www.factsandcomparisons.com/facts-comparisons-Online.aspx
Recommended for: Hospital, Academic Libraries

Formerly known as Facts & Comparisons 4.0, Facts & Comparisons eAnswers is a browser-based electronic version of the following print publications: *Drug Facts and Comparisons*, *Drug Interaction Facts*, *Review of Natural Products*, *Nonprescription Drug Therapy*, *MedFacts*, *Drug Interaction Facts: Herbal Supplements and Food*, and *A to Z Drug Facts*. All publications can be searched at one time by a simple search or advanced search, and searches can easily be refined. Additional features include a cross-reference feature and an alternative view feature, related documents, drug news daily updates, a drug identification tool, drug interactions database, herbal information, patient handouts in English and Spanish, advanced dosing tools, and clinical calculators. Users can print sections of drug monographs or tables of drug information. This reference is also available in mobile versions.

MICROMEDEX Healthcare Series. Thomson Reuters, 2009.
http://www.micromedex.com/products/hcs/
See Also Chapter 34.2. Indexing and Database Resources
Recommended for: Hospital, Academic Libraries

MICROMEDEX Healthcare Series is a point-of-care, evidence-based resource primarily for health professionals and students working in hospitals, managed care facilities, industrial settings and health sciences academic institutions. It is a gold standard for drug information. This resource provides a wide range of information related to drugs, acute care, toxicology, and information on patient education. Modules include patient care tools. The CareNotes System can produce patient education materials in English or Spanish and are customizable. This resource is compromised of several comprehensive health databases including Martindale, the Physician's Desk Reference (PDR), DRUGDEX, DISEASEDEX, POISONDEX, and several alternative medicine databases, including information on vitamins, minerals, and other dietary supplements. It contains FDA-approved or "labeled" indications, unapproved or "off-label" indications for drug therapy as well as information on international drugs. The database incorporates extensive U.S. and state regulatory information including daily Federal Register updates. All information is updated periodically. An added bonus is free access to a mobile version for all health care professionals associated with a facility that subscribes to this online database.

17.7. Psychopharmacology

The effects of drugs on mental and behavioral activity.

—MeSH

Contributor: Sharon Leslie

Monographs

American Psychiatric Publishing Textbook of Psychopharmacology. 4th ed. Editors: Alan F. Schatzberg, Charles B. Nemeroff. American Psychiatric Publishing, 2009.
http://www.psychiatryonline.com/
ISBN: 9781585623099
ISBN: 9781585623860 (Online)
Recommended for: Hospital, Academic, Consumer Health Libraries

Over 1,600 pages long, this text has been considered the gold standard on the subject of psychopharmacology through four editions. It contains comprehensive information about current medications prescribed for patients with mental illnesses, as well as other treatments such as electroconvulsive therapy. Principles of neuroanatomy, various classes of drugs, and clinical psychobiology are detailed in color and black-and-white illustrations, and each chapter contains full references. Each drug entry reviews the history and discovery of the drug, mechanism of action, pharmacokinetics, indications, side effects and toxicology, and drug interactions. Additional chapters cover conditions such as anxiety disorders, eating disorders, and Alzheimer's disease, and are kept small enough so they do not overwhelm. The new edition has added chapters on genomics and genetics, neurobiology of childhood disorders, and chronic pain syndromes as well as an entire section on ethical issues. An online component has also been added with full access to the entire text. Written by experts in the field, it is well designed and relatively easy to read. The intended audience is clinical psychiatrists, pharmacists, physicians, and any clinicians dealing with mental health issues. This title is also recommended by the American Association of Colleges of Pharmacy's *Basic Resources for Pharmacy Education* as a core title.

Introduction to Neuropsychopharmacology. Authors: Leslie L. Iverson, Susan D. Iverson, Floyd E. Bloom, Robert H. Roth. Oxford University Press, 2009.
ISBN: 9780195380538
Recommended for: Hospital, Academic Libraries

Co-written by Floyd Bloom, a pioneer in neuropharmacology and former editor-in-chief of the journal *Science*, *Introduction to Neuropsychopharmacology* covers the basics of neuropharmacology (effect of drugs on the nervous system) and psychopharmacology (effect of drugs on behavior). Dr. Bloom was a co-author on the classic book, *The Biochemical Basis of Neuropharmacology*, which has been supplemented by this new streamlined text. Written in a conversational tone, the book reviews drugs for depression and anxiety, Alzheimer's disease, and recreational drugs that impair brain function while discussing the mechanisms of action and effects on the brain and CNS. Well illustrated, this book is for clinicians, hospitals, academic institutions and research facilities.

Manual of Clinical Psychopharmacology. 7th ed. Authors: Alan F. Schatzberg, Jonathan O. Cole, Charles DeBattista. American Psychiatric Publishing, 2010.
http://www.psychiatryonline.com/
ISBN: 9781585623778
Recommended for: Hospital, Academic Libraries

This text, in its seventh edition, offers clinical advice, evidence from scientific literature, and real-world examples of pharmacotherapy for psychiatric populations. Introductory chapters address general principles and disease diagnosis and classification. Other chapters cover all the major classes of drugs: antidepressants, antipsychotics, mood stabilizers, antianxiety agents, hypnotics and stimulants. Where relevant, issues such as withdrawal, detoxification and use in pregnancy are addressed. The remaining five chapters cover treatment-resistant disorders, emergency department treatment, substance use disorders and special situations. Two appendixes cover strengths and costs of antidepressants and antipsychotics; and suggested readings. It is written in an easy-to-read style and includes summary tables for quick reference. This book is for all clinicians treating psychiatric patients including, psychiatrists, clinical psychologists, psychopharmacologists, and practicing clinicians.

Stahl's Essential Psychopharmacology: Neuroscientific Basis and Practical Applications. 3rd ed. Author: Stephen M. Stahl. Cambridge University Press, 2008.
See Chapter 9.10. Psychiatry, Chapter 17. Pharmacology

Journals

Journal of Clinical Psychopharmacology. v. 1, Lippincott, Williams & Wilkins, 1981.
http://journals.lww.com/psychopharmacology
ISSN: 02710749
ISSN: 1533712X (Online)
Indexed in: MEDLINE
Recommended for: Hospital, Academic Libraries

This peer-reviewed journal reports on clinical and preclinical developments in psychopharmacologic drugs including biological activity, adverse effects, pharmacogenetics, pharmacokinetics, and clinical trials. The aims and scope of the journal states that "Problems of special populations (the elderly, children, adolescents, pregnant women, and minorities) are of particular concern." It is recommended by the American Association of Colleges of Pharmacy's *Basic Resources for Pharmacy Education* as a core title. Intended for clinicians, pharmacologists, and researchers, the journal is indexed in numerous indexing and abstracting sources such as CAB Abstracts, Embase, International Pharmaceutical Abstracts, MEDLINE, Neuroscience Citation Index, Scopus, and Web of Science. Online access back to 1973 is available from the publisher through Ovid.

Journal of Psychopharmacology. v. 1, Sage, 1987.
http://jop.sagepub.com
ISSN: 02698811
ISSN: 14617285 (Online)
Indexed in: MEDLINE
Recommended for: Hospital, Academic Libraries

This peer-reviewed journal is the official publication of the British Association for Psychopharmacology. It publishes original research and review articles on "preclinical and clinical aspects of psychopharmacology," as well as evidence-based guidelines and consensus statements. The intended audience for this journal is clinicians, psychiatrists, pharmacologists, and researchers. With an impact factor of 3.647, this journal is ranked thirty-first out of 167 journals in clinical neurology, forty-eighth of 236 journals in pharmacology and pharmacy and thirty-first out of 117 journals in psychiatry (2009 *Journal Citation Reports*). The journal is indexed in numerous indexing and abstracting sources including CAB Abstracts, CINAHL, Embase, International Pharmaceutical Abstracts, MEDLINE, Scopus, and Web of Science. Online access back to 1987 is available from the publisher.

Databases and Other Electronic Resources

PsycINFO. American Psychological Association, 199?
http://www.apa.org/pubs/databases/psycinfo/index.aspx
See Also Chapter 34.2. Indexes and Database Resources
Recommended for: Hospital, Academic, Consumer Health Libraries

PsycINFO is one of several databases published by the American Psychological Association that offer comprehensive coverage of clinical, social, and behavioral aspects of psychology. *PsycINFO* contains bibliographic citations and abstracts while *PsycArticles* contains full-text articles. *PsycExtra* has "gray literature including technical reports, conference presentations." Abstracts are from about 1995 with scholarly, peer-reviewed articles having preference. Subjects covered include developmental psychology, physiological psychology and neuroscience, and psychopharmacology. Designed for psychologists, psychiatrists, researchers, and students, these behavioral sciences products are available by subscription through multiple vendors including EBSCO, Ovid, and ProQuest.

17.8. Toxicology

The detection, chemical composition, and biological action of toxic substances or poisons and the treatment and prevention of toxic manifestations.

—MeSH

Contributors: Robert Sotak, Carol E. Vreeland

Monographs

Casarett and Doull's Toxicology: The Basic Science of Poisons. 7th ed. Editor: Curtis D. Klaassen. McGraw-Hill, 2008.
http://www.ebrary.com/
http://extranet.netlibrary.com/TitleSelect
http://www.r2library.com/
http://online.statref.com/titleinfo/fxid-157.html
ISBN: 9780071470513
ISBN: 9780071593519 (Online)
Recommended for: Hospital, Academic Libraries
Brandon/Hill, *Doody's Core Titles* Selection

Widely regarded as the gold standard in the field, this authoritative volume is meant to serve primarily as a textbook for graduate students in toxicology. Clear and very readable, the work of 57 contributors from universities, government agencies, and industries is organized into seven units, with an emphasis on the mechanisms of toxicity. The first unit introduces the general principles of toxicology and risk assessment. The second unit, covering the disposition of toxicants, is highlighted by a comprehensive chapter on the biotransformation of xenobiotics. Units three and four discuss the site of action of toxins in the body, while the fifth unit is organized by the type of toxin. The last two units provide an overview of environmental, food, analytic/forensic, clinical, and occupational toxicology. The major limitation of this book is its inadequate index. There may be only one page listed for a topic that is actually discussed in more than one chapter, so the reader needs to know where to look. However, each chapter does start with a brief outline. This book is one of the primary reference resources for the American Board of Toxicology certification exam. The breadth of its subject coverage also makes it a valuable reference for research scientists, graduate students, and others concerned with community health, agriculture, food technology, pharmacy, veterinary medicine, and related disciplines.

Color Atlas of Human Poisoning and Envenoming. Author: James H. Diaz. CRC Press/Taylor & Francis, 2006.
http://www.ebrary.com/
http://extranet.netlibrary.com/TitleSelect
ISBN: 9780849322150
ISBN: 9781420003963 (Online)
Recommended for: Hospital, Academic Libraries

Color Atlas of Human Poisoning and Envenoming is intended as a handy medical atlas and review outline of human poisoning, employing bulleted text, tables, and figures to cover toxic exposures in children and adults. The author has supplemented the well-indexed text with high-quality images in some, but not all, chapters. Physician specialists have contributed computerized tomograms, radiographs, and plant photographs, and biologists of the Audubon Nature Institute in New Orleans provided color photographs of venomous animals. The work is organized around clinical encounters. The first four chapters discuss general evaluation and management of the poisoned patient and useful antidotes. Chapters five through 24 cover management strategies and antidotes for specific poisonings and envenomings, grouped in categories that include over-the-counter, prescription, and illicit drugs; common household products; foods, plants, and animals; occupational exposures; and chemical and biological weapons. The twenty-fifth chapter contains a useful review of workplace substance abuse monitoring, including U.S. federal regulations. The book concludes with a chapter on epidemiological research design and analysis. Intended as a ready reference and study guide, this atlas is useful for emergency, military, and public health physicians; pediatricians; veterinarians; and current health sciences students, medical students, and graduates in training.

Computational Toxicology: Risk Assessment for Pharmaceutical and Environmental Chemicals. Editor: Sean Ekins. John Wiley & Sons, 2007.
http://onlinelibrary.wiley.com/book/10.1002/9780470145890
http://extranet.netlibrary.com/TitleSelect
http://www.ebrary.com/
ISBN: 9780470049624
ISBN: 9780470145890 (Online)
ISBN: 9780470145883 (Online)
Recommended for: Academic Libraries

Seventy international scientists with experience in academia, industry, and government agencies contributed to this volume. After a brief introductory chapter on the field of toxicology and its methods, the authors describe *in vitro* toxicological methods, such as the Ames Salmonella mutagenicity assay to determine mutagenic potential of chemicals. The authors also address physiological-based modeling and its limitations. They explain an alternative approach of biochemical reaction network modeling, methods used in toxicogenomics, and related challenges. The section on computational methods presents an overview of toxicoinformatics and provides a thorough description of quantitative structure-activity relationship (QSAR) models for toxicological studies.

Pharmaceutical applications include the prediction of physicochemical properties, such as aqueous solubility and vapor pressure. There are also computational approaches for predicting toxicity such as QSAR and expert rule-based systems. The contributors describe some approaches for use in pharmaceutical research and development, such as ADME (absorption, distribution, metabolism, and excretion) assays and *in silico* models. Computational applications to environmental toxicology include risk assessment methods for chemical mixtures, QSAR models in aquatic toxicology, and computational models to predict dermal absorption of chemicals and drugs. The last section describes some new techniques such as the use of nano- and microfabrication techniques applied to cell culture systems for toxicological study. The authors discuss potential future applications of computational toxicology. This book is recommended for pharmaceutical toxicologists, ecotoxicologists, systems biologists, statisticians, and those interested in *in silico* modeling.

Ecotoxicology: A Comprehensive Treatment. Authors: Michael C. Newman, William H. Clements. CRC Press, 2008.
http://www.crcnetbase.com/isbn/9781420005011
http://extranet.netlibrary.com/TitleSelect
http://www.ebrary.com/
ISBN: 9780849333576
ISBN: 9781420005011 (Online)
See Also Chapter 17.8.1. Ecotoxicology
Recommended for: Academic Libraries

Ecotoxicology: A Comprehensive Treatment presents a synthesis of the field of ecotoxicology, which the authors feel is necessary to bridge the gap that currently exists between textbooks and technical books that have a narrow focus. The main sections of the book are arranged in four hierarchical levels: organismal ecotoxicology, population ecotoxicology, community ecotoxicology, and ecosystem ecotoxicology. The authors explore each level in detail and then integrate ecotoxicological concepts from these four levels of biological organization. The population ecotoxicology section begins with population definitions and then proceeds to epidemiology, demographic analysis, and the population genetics of toxicant-exposed populations. The organismal ecotoxicology section covers the effects of toxicants on cells, tissues, organs and organ systems, bioaccumulation, and lethal and sublethal effects. The community ecotoxicology section addresses the ways that groups of interacting species respond to toxicants. The ecosystem ecotoxicology section provides background information on ecosystems and ecosystem processes; it also describes approaches for studying ecosystem responses to contaminants and the effect of global atmospheric stressors on ecosystems. Chapters serve as bridges for previous and succeeding chapters. Most chapters have boxes that explore topics in more detail or provide real world examples. Chapters conclude with key concepts, a summary of foundation concepts and paradigms, and a lengthy references section. Each section has a concluding chapter that highlights key concepts covered in the section. This book is appropriate for upper level undergraduates, graduate students, and academic and government agency researchers in ecotoxicology.

Fundamental Toxicology. 2nd ed. Editors: John H. Duffus, Howard G.J. Worth. Royal Society of Chemistry, 2006.
http://www.rsc.org/publishing/ebooks/2006/9780854046140.asp
ISBN: 9780854046140
ISBN: 9781847552648 (Online)
Recommended for: Hospital, Academic, Consumer Health Libraries

Twenty-five contributors, mostly Europeans and a small number of North Americans from government agencies, universities, and industry, provide a diversity of expertise and perspectives for this excellent introductory text. The first chapter provides an overview of exposure to toxic substances, toxicity testing, and epidemiology. Individual chapters cover the toxicology of organs (liver, kidney, skin, and nerves), and systems such as reproductive, respiratory, and immune. The contributors offer information about chemicals in the environment and ecotoxicology, and they briefly cover topics in toxicogenomics, such as microarrays and proteomics. The text also explains toxicodynamics, toxicokinetics, risk management and risk assessment, and carcinogenicity. It concludes with a practical chapter on the proper handling of chemicals and good laboratory practice. The appendixes contain a list of abbreviations, acronyms, and a lengthy glossary of toxicological terms. The first edition, *Fundamental Toxicology for Chemists*, 1996, was written for chemists, but this updated edition is intended for any scientist who works with chemicals. *Fundamental Toxicology* is recommended for industrial, government, or academic researchers who work with chemicals but have not received formal training in toxicology.

Goldfrank's Toxicologic Emergencies. 9th ed. Editors: Lewis Nelson, Neal Lewin, Mary Ann Howland, Robert Hoffman, Lewis Goldfrank, Neal Flomenbaum. McGraw-Hill, 2010.

http://www.r2library.com/ (8th ed.)
ISBN: 9780071605939
ISBN: 9780071605953
ISBN: 9780071605946 (Online)
Recommended for: Hospital, Academic Libraries
Brandon/Hill, *Doody's Core Titles* Selection

The eighth edition of this classic volume, to which this review refers, is still considered the definitive reference source for clinical toxicology. The work of 135 international contributors has been updated, and almost 30 chapters have been added. The six editors, affiliated with the New York City Poison Center, have maintained the book's well-known case study approach. In the primary section of the work, "Part C: The Clinical Basis of Medical Toxicology," most individual chapters begin with a case study involving the agent, followed by a discussion of history and epidemiology, pharmacology, pharmacokinetics and toxicokinetics, pathophysiology, clinical manifestations, diagnostic tests, and management, and ending with a summary. This standard format is intended to facilitate rapid information retrieval. Starting with the eighth edition, only partial content appears in the print copy of the book. Supplemental color photographs of plants and venomous animals, the traditional workbook of case studies, and study questions are only accessible at a companion website for individual purchasers of the print text and through other online providers such as STAT!Ref. A requirement for the toxicological emergency room, *Goldfrank's Toxicologic Emergencies* is intended for medical toxicologists and emergency physicians. However, it is also useful for students in medicine, nursing, and pharmacy, along with residents and physicians in internal medicine, pediatrics, and other fields where toxicology expertise is needed.

Molecular Toxicology. 2nd ed. Authors: P. David Josephy, Bengt Mannervik. Oxford University Press, 2006.
ISBN: 9780195176209
See Also Chapter 17.8.3. Toxicogenetics
Recommended for: Hospital, Academic Libraries

Molecular Toxicology is divided into three parts: "Toxicity at the Cellular Level," "Enzymology of Biotransformation," and "Molecular Principles Applied to Specific Toxicants." The first part covers covalent binding of toxicants to DNA and protein, DNA damage and various repair mechanisms, mutagenesis, types of mutations, mutation assays, and carcinogenesis including oncogenes and tumor suppressor genes. The authors address the toxicology of oxygen and the enzymes that control the toxic effects of its free radicals and anions. The second part focuses on the enzymes cytochrome P450 and glutathione transferase and conjugation reactions catalyzed by glucuronidase and sulfotransferase. The protective role of the cellular reductant, glutathione, against toxicants is well presented. The third part discusses specific toxicants, such as alkylating agents, and their role in chemical warfare and cancer chemotherapy; aromatic amines and their role in mutagenicity and carcinogenicity; and carcinogenic polycyclic aromatic hydrocarbons. Each chapter contains numerous references to original research articles. The authors bring expertise in biochemical and molecular toxicology to this text. Sidebars effectively explore some concepts in more detail such as knockout mouse technology, isotopes of hydrogen, and molecular epidemiology. The companion website provides selected, color figures from the text, which may be downloaded for personal use. The audience for *Molecular Toxicology* is graduate students, researchers, and clinicians in toxicology, pharmacology, and biochemistry.

Principles and Methods of Toxicology. 5th ed. Editor: A. Wallace Hayes. CRC Press/Taylor & Francis, 2008.
ISBN: 9780849337789
Recommended for: Hospital, Academic Libraries

This authoritative tome is intended to be used as a textbook for graduate courses in general and advanced toxicology. Its aim is to provide the reader with the understanding of the biologic mechanisms and methods needed to determine the safe use of a chemical or physical agent. The book is divided into three parts, starting with the history and principles of toxicology and the types of toxic agents. The last part is devoted to a comprehensive presentation of test methods and evaluation strategies, including many of the test protocols required to meet regulatory needs worldwide. Updates in the fifth edition include new chapters dealing with genomics, plant and animal toxins, pathology for toxicologists, toxicological information sources, and alternative methods. One of the strengths of the work is its organization. The editor has put a great deal of effort into the organization and unification of almost 100 contributors from academia, hospitals, government, and industry. Each chapter starts with a detailed, paginated table of contents and ends with review questions. Although it is not an easy read for a novice, readers new to the subject are aided by illustrations, an extensive index, and a well-developed glossary. This is an essential text for toxicology graduate students and a valuable reference resource for researchers in toxicology, public health, human or veterinary medicine, pharmacology, and other fields involved with toxicological methodology.

Principles and Practice of Toxicology in Public Health. Author: Ira S. Richards. Jones & Bartlett, 2008.
ISBN: 9780763738235
Recommended for: Hospital, Academic Libraries

Principles and Practice of Toxicology in Public Health is divided into four sections. The first section provides a brief history of toxicology beginning with the ancient world and overviews of hazardous chemicals, toxins and poisons, and environmental pollutants. The second section, "Toxicology Principles," covers dose and response, absorption and elimination of toxicants, and mutagenesis and cancer. The next section, "Systemic Toxicology," includes effects of toxicants on immune, liver, skin, and respiratory systems. The last section, "Toxicology Practice" explains regulatory issues, toxicity testing, and risk assessment. Most chapters conclude with a bibliography, while some provide a list of relevant websites. Appendixes are also found at the end of some chapters. A useful appendix is titled "Regulatory Agencies that Maintain Lists for Hazardous Materials and Regional Poison Control Centers." The glossary of terms will be helpful for novices. This book will be most useful to American public health workers who are interested in learning the basic principles of the field of toxicology.

Journals

Annual Review of Pharmacology and Toxicology. v. 16, Annual Reviews, 1976.
http://arjournals.annualreviews.org/loi/pharmtox
ISSN: 03621642
ISSN: 15454304 (Online)
Indexed in: MEDLINE
Recommended for: Hospital, Academic Libraries

Annual Review of Pharmacology and Toxicology has the highest impact factor in the subject of toxicology according to the 2009 science edition of *Journal Citation Reports*. Articles are typically written by recognized experts in their field. Toxicology is covered primarily as it relates to pharmacology. Recent reviews include articles on the interaction of engineered nanomaterials with biological systems, disruption of signaling homeostasis, and cellular response to arsenic. Articles have a large number of references that may facilitate further exploration of a topic. Articles conclude with a list of summary points and a list of future issues. *Annual Review of Pharmacology and Toxicology*, which was initially known as the *Annual Review of Pharmacology*, is indexed by BIOSIS Previews, Chemical Abstracts, MEDLINE, and Web of Science. It is available in print and online formats from Annual Reviews starting with volume 1. The journal is valuable to students trying to gain a broad overview of a field that is new to them. It is an excellent resource for a wide range of users, from upper level undergraduate students to researchers, and is recommended for toxicologists, pharmacologists, clinicians, and environmental health scientists.

Aquatic Toxicology. v. 1, Elsevier, 1981.
www.sciencedirect.com/science/journal/0166445X
ISSN: 0166445X
Indexed in: MEDLINE
Recommended for: Academic Libraries

This specialized journal occupies an important niche in the field of toxicology. Peer-reviewed and published 20 times a year, *Aquatic Toxicology* publishes original scientific papers dealing with the mechanisms of toxicity in aquatic environments and the understanding of responses to toxic agents at the community, species, tissue, cellular, and subcellular levels. Starting in 2009, one or two issues per year are themed around topics important for aquatic toxicology; special issues to date have focused on amphibian toxicology, zebrafish as a research model, and genomic methods. The journal is indexed in Aquatic Sciences & Fisheries Abstracts, BIOSIS, CAB Abstracts, Chemical Abstracts, Embase, MEDLINE, Science Citation Index, Scopus, Toxicology Abstracts, and other sources. It currently ranks twenty-second of 77 journals in toxicology and fifth of 88 journals in the marine and freshwater biology category (2009 *Journal Citation Reports*), with an impact factor of 3.124. Intended for environmental toxicologists, marine biologists, ecotoxicologists, biochemical toxicologists, and conservationists, it is available online from ScienceDirect.

Chemical Research in Toxicology. v. 1, American Chemical Society, 1988.
http://pubs.acs.org/journal/crtoec
ISSN: 0893228X
ISSN: 15205010 (Online)
Indexed in: MEDLINE
Recommended for: Academic Libraries

In addition to articles and reviews, *Chemical Research in Toxicology* publishes perspectives, communications, and chemical profiles. The monthly journal has recently added a category called "Rapid Reports," which are short articles on timely topics. It publishes new techniques that elucidate mechanisms of toxicity and the cellular responses to toxicants. An "In This Issue" section provides highlights of notable articles. "Spotlight" articles draw attention to important research findings published recently in other journals. *Chemical Research in Toxicology* is indexed in multiple sources such as CAB Abstracts, Chemical Abstracts, MEDLINE, Scopus, and Web of Science. Its editorial board represents a range of backgrounds including pharmacology, oncology, and medicinal chemistry. Online issues are available via American Chemical Society Web Editions (1996–present) and American Chemical Society Legacy Archives, (1988–1995). Topics of some recent articles are xenobiotic metabolism, biomarkers that can be used to monitor levels of isothiocyantates in humans, and the roles of drugs and chemicals in triggering autoimmune diseases. Its 2009 impact factor ranks it eighth out of 77 journals in the toxicology category. This journal is recommended for graduate students and researchers in chemistry, toxicology, pharmacology, and environmental science.

Critical Reviews in Toxicology. v. 7, Informa Healthcare, 1980.
http://informahealthcare.com/loi/txc
ISSN: 10408444
ISSN: 15476898 (Online)
Indexed in: MEDLINE
Recommended for: Hospital, Academic Libraries

This refereed journal publishes up-to-date, comprehensive reviews of research findings related to the mechanisms of action, responses, and assessment of health risks due to toxicant exposure. Toxicants of concern include commodity and specialty chemicals, including pesticides; pharmaceutical agents; consumer products; environmental agents; and occupational exposures. Reviews cover toxicological responses ranging from observations at the molecular and cellular level to physiological and pathological alterations in wildlife, laboratory animals, and human populations. Particular attention is given to cancer, reproductive, and developmental effects. Ten issues are published per year, with an occasional extra review published as a supplement. A few of the individual reviews (or supplements) are open access. Indexing coverage includes BIOSIS Previews, CAB Abstracts, Chemical Abstracts, MEDLINE, Science Citation Index, Scopus, Toxicology Abstracts, and other sources. *Critical Reviews in Toxicology* currently ranks sixth of 27 journals in toxicology (2009 *Journal Citation Reports*) and has an impact factor of 4.232. Its reviews are useful for researchers and practitioners in the life sciences, health and safety sciences, and industry. The journal, which began as *CRC Critical Reviews in Toxicology* (1971–1979), is available in both print and online formats. Full online coverage back to the first volume is available through Informa Healthcare.

DNA Repair. v. 1, Elsevier, 2002.
http://www.sciencedirect.com/science/journal/15687864
ISSN: 15687864
ISSN: 15687856 (Online)
Indexed in: MEDLINE
Recommended for: Hospital, Academic Libraries

DNA Repair covers all aspects of cellular responses to DNA damage. Articles are also found on mutagenesis, cell cycle regulation, and apoptosis, as they relate to DNA damage. The journal publishes research papers, mini-reviews, letters to the editor, brief reports, hot topics in DNA repair, commentaries, and meeting reports. "This Month in *DNA Repair*" provides a one sentence summary of important findings published that month. Online articles provide links to supplemental data. Some recent articles cover nucleotide excision repair, reactive oxygen species, and an investigation of a protein complex involved in radiation resistance. Research subjects range from bacteria cultures to mammalian cell lines, and some articles report on plant model species. The monthly journal is indexed by BIOSIS Previews, CAB Abstracts, Chemical Abstracts, MEDLINE, and Web of Science. Its 2009 impact factor of 4.199 ranks it seventh out of 77 journals in the toxicology category. *DNA Repair* is recommended for graduate students, researchers, and clinicians in molecular toxicology, cell biology, and cancer biology.

Drug Safety. v. 5, Adis International, 1990.
http://adisonline.com/drugsafety
ISSN: 01145916
ISSN: 11791942 (Online)
Indexed in: MEDLINE
Recommended for: Hospital, Academic Libraries

Drug Safety is the official journal of the International Society of Pharmacovigilance, which is published monthly by Adis, a Wolters Kluwer business. Its primary subjects are pharmacovigilance, pharmacoepidemiology, risk assessment, risk management, and adverse drug reactions. It publishes current opinions, special articles, review articles, original research articles, and correspondence. Recent articles include a review of the pulmonary toxicity of an antiarrhythmic drug, drug-induced metabolic acidosis, and a study of the reporting of adverse drug reactions in hospitals. *Drug Safety* is indexed in BIOSIS Previews, Embase/Excerpta Medica, MEDLINE, and Science Citation Index. Its 2009 impact factor of 3.522 ranks it twelfth out of 77 journals in the toxicology category of *Journal Citation Reports*. It also ranks in the top quartile of two other categories: (a) pharmacology and pharmacy, and (b) public, environmental, and occupational health. *Drug Safety* is recommended for graduate students, researchers, and clinicians in toxicology, pharmacology, and related biomedical sciences. This journal was previously known as *Medical Toxicology and Adverse Drug Experience* and *Medical Toxicology*.

Environmental Health Perspectives. v. 1, U.S. National Institute of Environmental Health Sciences, National Institutes of Health, Department of Health and Human Services, 1972.
http://ehp.niehs.nih.gov/
http://www.ncbi.nlm.nih.gov/pmc/journals/253/
ISSN: 00916765
ISSN: 15529924 (Online)
See Also Chapter 5. Environmental Health, Chapter 10.15.1. Environmental Medicine
Indexed in: MEDLINE, CINAHL
Recommended for: Hospital, Academic, Consumer Health Libraries

Environmental Health Perspectives (*EHP*) is a peer-reviewed, open access journal that serves as an important forum for the discussion of the interrelationships between the environment and human health. Published monthly, the multidisciplinary journal publishes research articles and news items covering basic research, epidemiologic studies and environmental case reports, risk assessment, policy topics, and more. A research section is devoted specifically to the environmental health of children. Additional content includes review articles, book reviews, and editorials. *EHP* also produces some special issues. The highly regarded publication currently ranks fourth of 122 journals in public, environmental, and occupational health and third of 180 journals in the environmental sciences category (2009 *Journal Citation Reports*), with an impact factor of 6.191. It is indexed in Academic Search Premier, CINAHL, MEDLINE, Scopus, and other sources. All content is free online, and issues are available immediately in PubMed Central. The journal is essential for researchers, health workers, policy makers, college students, and others interested in potential health hazards associated with elements in the environment.

Environmental Toxicology and Chemistry. v. 1, Society of Environmental Toxicology and Chemistry, 1982.
http://onlinelibrary.wiley.com/journal/10.1002/(ISSN)1552-8618
ISSN: 07307268
ISSN: 15528618 (Online)
See Also Chapter 17.8.1. Ecotoxicology
Indexed in: MEDLINE
Recommended for: Academic Libraries

Environmental Toxicology and Chemistry is published monthly by Wiley-Blackwell on behalf of the Society of Environmental Toxicology and Chemistry (SETAC). It covers a very wide range of disciplines such as environmental toxicology, chemistry and biochemistry, physiology, microbiology, genetics and genomics, environmental engineering, earth sciences, epidemiology, and modeling. It addresses the application of prediction and risk assessment of chemicals in the environment. In addition to research articles, it also publishes editorials, critical reviews, letters to the editor, and short communications. Recent articles included a study that monitored the presence of pharmaceuticals and hormones in sewage sludge, a study of the toxicity of molybdate anions in soil, endocrine disrupting effects of an antibacterial agent in a fish species, and toxic effects of leachates from furfurylated wood on a marine bacterium and the crustacean, *Daphnia*. *Environmental Toxicology and Chemistry* is indexed in BIOSIS Previews, CAB Abstracts, MEDLINE, Scopus, and Web of Science. Online issues going back to volume 1 are available via Wiley Online Library. It is recommended for upper level undergraduates, graduate students, and researchers in environmental science, environmental engineering, life science, epidemiology, toxicology, and chemistry.

Toxicological Sciences. v. 41, Oxford University Press, 1998.
http://toxsci.oxfordjournals.org/
ISSN: 10966080
ISSN: 10960929 (Online)
See Also Chapter 10.15.1. Environmental Medicine
Indexed in: MEDLINE
Recommended for: Hospital, Academic Libraries

Toxicological Sciences is the official journal of the Society of Toxicology. Published monthly, it primarily publishes original, peer-reviewed research articles in all areas of toxicology. Issues are organized into sections to facilitate the location of articles of interest; some of the 17 possible section categories include carcinogenicity, environmental toxicology, in vitro methods and alternatives to animals, and nanotoxicology. Additional journal features include reviews, a forum section for articles on policy or research issues, and editorials. Some online articles include access to supplementary data not included in the printed version. With an impact factor of 4.814 (2009 *Journal Citation Reports*), the publication currently ranks fourth of 77 journals in the toxicology category and is indexed by BIOSIS Previews, CAB Abstracts, Chemical Abstracts, Embase, MEDLINE, Science Citation Index, Scopus, Toxicology Abstracts, and many other sources.

Its audience includes researchers and specialists in agriculture, life sciences, chemistry, and health and safety sciences in academic institutions, industry, government, and the private sector. The journal was originally known as *Fundamental and Applied Toxicology* (1981–1997). Oxford provides full online coverage back to the first volume, although access to articles prior to 1996 is limited to purchasers of the digital archive. Some online articles are open access.

Toxicology and Applied Pharmacology. v. 1, Elsevier, 1959.
www.sciencedirect.com/science/journal/0041008X
ISSN: 0041008X (Print/Online)
Indexed in: MEDLINE
Recommended for: Hospital, Academic Libraries

Started in 1959, this journal publishes peer-reviewed, original scientific research articles related to the effects of chemicals, drugs, or natural products on animals and humans. Articles focus on mechanistic approaches used to understand toxicologic and pathologic lesions and the methods used to describe those responses. The journal also publishes reviews and articles discussing contemporary issues in toxicology, and it encourages papers concerned with alternatives to the use of experimental animals. Published twice a month, *Toxicology and Applied Pharmacology* currently ranks sixteenth of 77 journals in toxicology and fifty-ninth of 236 journals in pharmacology and pharmacy (2009 *Journal Citation Reports*). The journal has an impact factor of 3.359. Its intended audience is composed of toxicologists, pharmacologists, cancer researchers, epidemiologists, and molecular and cell biologists. Indexed in: BIOSIS Previews, CAB Abstracts, Chemical Abstracts, Embase, MEDLINE, Science Citation Index, Scopus, Toxicology Abstracts, and other sources, the journal is available in both print and online formats. Online access is available through ScienceDirect.

Databases and Other Electronic Resources

TOXNET. Division of Specialized Information Services, National Library of Medicine, 1998.
http://toxnet.nlm.nih.gov/
Recommended for: Hospital, Academic, Consumer Health Libraries

TOXNET (Toxicology Data Network) is a free, web-based system of databases on toxicology, hazardous chemicals, environmental health, toxic releases, consumer products, and other related areas. It is produced by the Toxicology and Environmental Health Information Program (TEHIP) in the Division of Specialized Information Services (SIS) of the National Library of Medicine (NLM). A user-friendly interface allows simultaneous searching of all TOXNET databases. ChemIDplus provides access to over 380,000 chemical structure and nomenclature authority files. Hazardous Substances Data Bank (HSDB) contains peer-reviewed content on approximately 5,000 chemicals, including information on human exposure, emergency handling procedures, environmental fate, and regulatory requirements. *Toxicology Literature Online* (TOXLINE), NLM's bibliographic toxicology database, contains over 3.5 million records from 1965 to the present. LactMed covers more than 500 drugs and other chemicals to which breastfeeding mothers may be exposed; it includes the possible adverse effects on the nursing infant and alternative drugs. Household Products Database provides human health effects information on over 9,000 brand-name consumer products, using manufacturers' Material Safety Data Sheets (MSDS). The other TOXNET databases are Chemical Carcinogenesis Research Information System (CCRIS), Developmental and Reproductive Toxicology Database (DART), Genetic Toxicology (GENE-TOX), Integrated Risk Information System (IRIS), International Toxicity Estimates for Risk (ITER), Toxics Release Inventory (TRI), TOXMAP, and Haz-Map. TOXNET contains a wealth of information, serving as an invaluable resource for toxicologists, health professionals, and researchers in related fields. Checks for new data are made weekly, if not more frequently, and databases are updated when new information becomes available.

17.8.1. Ecotoxicology

Environmental pollution and the toxic effects of environmental pollutants on the ecosystem.

—MeSH

Contributor: Stephanie Holmgren

Monographs

Ecotoxicology: A Comprehensive Treatment. Authors: Michael C. Newman, William H. Clements. CRC Press, 2008.
http://extranet.netlibrary.com/TitleSelect/
http://www.ebrary.com/
ISBN: 9780849333576
ISBN: 9781420005011
See Also Chapter 17.8. Toxicology
Recommended for: Academic Libraries

At an extensive 36 chapters, this book lives up to its subtitle. The authors seek to find a balance between a textbook and a specialized technical reference. Michael Newman, author of the undergraduate textbook, *Fundamentals of Ecotoxicology*, addresses many of the same topics but does so with a more detailed and methodological approach. As with the undergraduate book, the authors begin by establishing a foundation by looking at ecotoxicology in a hierarchical framework. The book is divided into sections, taking a progressive look at ecotoxicology from organismal, population, community, and ecosystem perspectives. Each chapter includes a summary of the "foundation concepts and paradigms." Boxes are used appropriately to expand on a concept, provide alternative thinking, or highlight examples. Given the expansive nature of this work, each section has its own conclusion to summarize the key concepts. Unusually, the book itself has a conclusion chapter that integrates the concepts and paradigms into a cohesive picture. Conventional approaches to ecotoxicology typically focus on individual species-level impacts. This textbook moves away from that tradition and includes topics not normally taught, such as the impact of species diversity on ecosystem function or the stresses brought about by global atmospheric changes on ecosystem dynamics. As stated by the authors, this book is intended for graduate-level students. *Ecotoxicology* is recommended for academic libraries and some special libraries.

Fundamentals of Ecotoxicology. 3rd ed. Author: Michael C. Newman. CRC Press, 2009.
ISBN: 9781420067040
Recommended for: Academic Libraries

This popular textbook is divided into four main sections. The first primarily reviews the need for and practice of ecotoxicology. It also includes a long chapter on the nature, cycling, and fate of key environmental contaminants such as metals; organometallic, inorganic and organic compounds; and even nutrients. Section two addresses factors associated with the uptake, biotransformation, elimination, and accumulation of contaminants. It also explores the factors that affect bioaccumulation and bioavailability through the food chain. The next seven chapters uniquely delineate the toxic effects of contaminants from a micro- to macro-level perspective. At the lower level, chapters focus on molecular effects—DNA modification and oxidative stress—and next level cytotoxic and pathological changes to cells, tissues, and organs. The author then looks at sub-lethal effects (development, reproduction, and other) along with acute and chronic lethal effects on the individual organism. Finally, the remaining chapters explore dynamics at the population community, regional, and global levels. The last chapter is devoted to the fundamentals of both human and ecological risk assessment. This third edition has removed the chapter on risks from exposure to radiation. Each chapter opens with a relevant and interesting quotation. This textbook makes use of footnotes to qualify discussion of a topic. The chapters are also interspersed with informative and descriptive vignettes written by experts in that field that deepen discussion of a topic. Suggested readings are provided at the end of each chapter. Study questions and an extensive list of references are included in the appendix. Key terms highlighted within the chapters have an entry in the glossary. This edition has brought in more international case studies and looks at legislation on a global level to counteract the North American focus of the last edition. Its strength lies in the exploration of ecotoxicology at all levels, from molecular to global. This edition does lack coverage of plants, which are quite important to ecosystems, and could benefit from a chapter dedicated to the interplay between toxicity testing and risk assessment and regulatory developments. *Fundamentals* is intended for upper-level undergraduate or graduate students and can serve as a general reference resource. It is designed to complement the author's graduate-level book, *Ecotoxicology: A Comprehensive Treatment*. This work is recommended for academic and special libraries.

Genomics in Regulatory Ecotoxicology: Applications and Challenges. Editors: Gerald T. Ankley, Ann L. Miracle, George P. Daston, Edward J. Perkins. CRC Press, 2008.
http://www.crcnetbase.com/isbn/978-1-4200-6682-1
http://extranet.netlibrary.com/TitleSelect/
http://www.ebrary.com/
ISBN: 9781420066821
ISBN: 9781420066838 (Online)
Recommended for: Academic Libraries

This book resulted from a Pellston workshop on "Molecular Biology and Risk Assessment: Evaluation of the Potential Roles of Genomics in Regulatory Ecotoxicology." A goal of the workshop was to develop a conceptual framework on how genomic data could have short- and long-term impacts on ecological risk assessment. Working groups explored how genomics could be applied to various aspects of ecotoxicology: screening, tiered testing, risk assessment for pesticides and complex mixtures, and environmental remediation. This book is the first attempt to explore the application of genomics to regulatory ecotoxicology. The results from each working group form the content of each chapter. In addition to describing the applications that toxicogenomics could have, the book also highlights the challenges of using toxicogenomics and makes recommendations for priority areas of research and setting guidelines. This book was published in collaboration with the Society of Environmental Toxicology and Chemistry and is geared towards the interests of its members—environmental scientists involved in research, management, chemical manufacturing and regulation, risk assessment, and education. It is recommended for academic and special libraries.

Handbook of Ecotoxicology. 2nd ed. Editors: David J. Hoffman, Barnett A. Rattner, G. Allen Burton Jr., John Cairns Jr. CRC Press, 2003.
http://extranet.netlibrary.com/TitleSelect/
http://www.ebrary.com/
http://www.crcnetbase.com/isbn/978-1-56670-546-2
ISBN: 9781566705462
ISBN: 9781420032505 (Online)
Recommended for: Academic Libraries

This *Handbook* provides a practical reference for quantifying and measuring ecotoxicological effects. The book is divided into five theme areas: (a) testing methods for application to aquatic or terrestrial systems; (b) contaminants, such as pesticides, petroleum, lead, dioxins, deforestation, and pathogens, and their effects; (c) real case histories that look at how contaminants impact the natural ecosystem, such as Chernobyl and radiation or Hudson River and polychlorinated biphenyls; (d) techniques used for making estimates, predictions, and models for risk assessments of potential ecotoxicological effects; and (e) new and significant issues in ecotoxicology. The latter section, despite being almost seven years old, contains numerous topics that are still critical and timely, such as endocrine disruptors, contaminant contribution to amphibian decline, and trace elements and nutrition. Each chapter starts with its own detailed table of contents that facilitates quick finding of information. As a result, the index is rather shallow. Figures and tables are not used heavily, but incorporated appropriately. More than 75 international experts contributed content, and a Technical Review Board reviewed all manuscripts for accuracy and currency. The book is targeted at students, researchers, consultants, and other professionals in the environmental sciences as well as the disciplines of toxicology, chemistry, biology, and ecology. The *Handbook* is suitable for academic, industrial, and governmental settings and is recommended for academic and special library collections.

Hot Zone Forensics: Chemical, Biological, and Radiological Evidence Collection. Author: Steven C. Drielak. Charles C Thomas, 2004.
See Chapter 17.8.2. Forensic Toxicology

Introduction to Environmental Toxicology: Molecular Substructures to Ecological Landscapes. 4th ed. Authors: Wayne G. Landis, Ruth M. Sofield, Ming-Ho Yu. CRC Press, 2011.
http://www.ebrary.com/ (3rd ed.)
ISBN: 9781439804100
Recommended for: Academic Libraries

This review refers to the third edition. This graduate-level textbook and reference provides a detailed and comprehensive review of environmental toxicology. The book begins with the usual introduction and looks at the role of environmental toxicology in the management of ecosystems. The framework for the environmental toxicology chapter looks at both the classical viewpoint for classifying toxic effects as well as the alternative complexity theory view. A fairly thorough chapter explores the design, methods, and statistics used in toxicity testing. The subsequent chapter delves into specific single-species and multi-species tests. An appendix within that chapter describes the history and utilization of selected test species in aquatic vertebrates, plus fresh and saltwater invertebrates. Two chapters discuss the routes of exposure, mechanisms of toxic action, and factors affecting the toxicity of a contaminant. The next three chapters focus on selected categories of toxic compounds: inorganic gaseous pollutants, heavy metals, and fluoride in developing economies. The remaining chapters describe the processes of biotransformation; measurement and prediction of ecological response to toxicants; and, finally, ecological risk assessment. Each chapter ends with references, suggested readings, and study questions. This textbook uniquely provides specifics associated with species toxicity testing and addresses the difficult endeavor of measuring and evaluating the impact a toxicant will have on an ecological system. Those strengths outweigh the absence of the effects from pesticides and other organic compounds. This work is recommended for academic and special libraries.

Journals

Chemosphere. v. 1, Elsevier/Pergamon, 1972.
http://www.sciencedirect.com/science/journal/00456535
ISSN: 00456535
Indexed in: MEDLINE
Recommended for: Academic Libraries

Chemosphere is both an international and multidisciplinary journal touching on all areas of environmental science. Each issue is dedicated to one of four subject areas: environmental chemistry, environmental toxicology and assessment, persistent organic pollutants and dioxins, and science for environmental toxicology. The environmental chemistry content encompasses the kinetic and dynamic processes—transport, biodegradation, deposition, adsorption—of inorganic and organic elements in aquatic, atmospheric, and terrestrial environments. Analytical methods, environmental modeling, and monitoring techniques are also included. All aspects of toxicology—adverse effects, mechanisms of action, toxicokinetics, epidemiological evidence, test validation, biomonitoring, occupational hazards, risk characterization—are incorporated in the environmental toxicology and risk assessment issues. The pollutants and dioxins section targets only those chemicals of a "persistent" nature, with emphasis on halogenated organic chemicals. The journal limits its acceptance of studies to those with a global impact. Finally, the "Science for Environmental Technology" section focuses on techniques for reduction, remediation, elimination, or treatment, including use of green chemistry. Articles may be in the form of original research, reviews, or short communications for important new findings that require immediate publication. This journal provides a breadth across varying levels of ecosystems and species and depth across all aspects of the diverse disciplines that comprise ecotoxicology. *Chemosphere* is recommended for academic and special libraries. Full online coverage is available back to volume 1, 1972 with a prolific 44 issues per year or approximately four issues per month. It is cited in the major indexes, such as BIOSIS, CSA, Embase, MEDLINE, Science Citation Index, and Scopus, and is available through Elsevier's ScienceDirect.

Ecotoxicology. v. 1, Springer Netherlands, 1992.
http://www.springerlink.com/content/0963-9292
ISSN: 09639292
ISSN: 15733017 (Online)
Indexed in: MEDLINE
Recommended for: Academic Libraries

This international journal seeks to compile research that elucidates the mechanisms and processes behind chemical effects on ecosystems. This journal does not publish articles that simply involve toxicity testing or establish levels of a contaminant in the environment. Rather, the journal emphasizes understanding of the impact of chemicals at the population or community level in all ecosystems—freshwater, marine water, or terrestrial. Therefore, individual studies must quantify population- or community-level effects. Unlike some journals, this publication invites regulatory-related articles that address methods for controlling substances or conserving threatened species. *Ecotoxicology* is composed primarily of original research papers but also includes technical notes and review articles. Some issues may be dedicated to a special topic, such as biomarkers of marine pollution or endocrine disruptors in invertebrates. Despite its broad, encompassing title, *Ecotoxicology* focuses its content compared to other journals in this field, providing a macro-level perspective of the effects of chemical contaminants in various biomes and on diverse species. The journal is recommended for academic and special libraries. Full online coverage through SpringerLink is available back to volume 1, 1992 with eight issues per year. It is cited in the major indexes, such as Biological Abstracts, CAS, Embase, MEDLINE, Science Citation Index, and Scopus.

Ecotoxicology and Environmental Safety. v. 1, Academic Press/Elsevier, 1977.
http://www.sciencedirect.com/science/journal/01476513
ISSN: 01476513
ISSN: 10902414 (Online)
Indexed in: MEDLINE
Recommended for: Academic Libraries

Ecotoxicology and Environmental Safety encompasses a range of research on short- and long-term effects of substances and mixtures on environmental systems and subsystems. The full spectrum of ecotoxicological principles is covered: bioavailability, bioaccumulation, and biotransformation in the target organism to biological and mechanistic responses. Consideration is also given to studies that highlight new methods and techniques such as biosensors, advanced computational methods, and photonic technologies. Emphasis is on identifying proven ways to prevent or ameliorate human-induced environmental damage. In addition to the regular research articles, the journal publishes "Frontier Articles," a by-invitation-only analysis of the current thinking on a timely and critical issue. Although this journal does not have a high impact factor due to the niche nature of its subject coverage, its content focus is highly relevant to environmental managers, ecology researchers, and others who need the breadth and depth of this research to undertake risk assessment, risk characterization and prediction, and ultimately risk management. It is recommended for academic and special libraries. Full online coverage through Elsevier's ScienceDirect is available back to volume 1, 1977 with eight issues per year. It is indexed in MEDLINE.

Emerging Topics in Ecotoxicology: Principles, Approaches, and Perspectives. v. 1, Springer, 2009.
http://www.springerlink.com/
ISSN: 18681344
Recommended for: Academic Libraries

This completely new monographic series that launched in 2009 seeks to keep abreast of the rapid research advances in other scientific disciplines—biology, chemistry, genomics—and their applications to the fundamental problems facing ecotoxicology. While this monographic series does not have an established history, the first two volumes have timely topics and are a good indication of the direction of the series. The first volume explores the fate and distribution of steroids and antibiotics generated from animal feeding operations through water and soil. The most recent volume covers the types, applications, and limitations of various modeling and computational methods used by ecotoxicologists to determine and/or predict the fate of chemicals. This series was written for a range of audiences, including both young and established practitioners as well as graduate and postdoctoral level researchers. The series is recommended for academic and special libraries.

Environmental Pollution. v. 43, Elsevier, 1987.
http://www.sciencedirect.com/science/journal/02697491
ISSN: 02697491
Indexed in: MEDLINE
Recommended for: Academic Libraries

Environmental Pollution focuses on the distribution and ecological effects of contaminants such as air pollutants, detergents, fertilizers, industrial effluents, metals, mining waste, oil, pesticides, plastics, radioactive materials, and sewage that man introduces into the environment. Attention is also given to research that highlights new techniques for studying and measuring pollution and its effects. Besides original research and reviews, the journal also includes short communications, which are small versions of original research; rapid communications, which are findings of considerable importance put on an accelerated publishing schedule; new initiatives or briefings on new areas of research; commentaries; and letters to the editor. The international board ensures that the published research has significance at a regional or global level. Studies conducted around the world from countries such as China, Poland, Spain, and Taiwan are well represented in the journal. Given the nature of this journal, its content encompasses a much broader treatment of the various contaminants and xenobiotics found in nature. The journal is available in both print and online formats. This title is available back to volume 43, 1987. Earlier title changes are also available online. The original volume 1, 1970 was titled *Environmental Pollution*. In 1980, the title was split into *Series A: Ecological and Biological* and *Series B: Chemical and Physical*. The separate series were merged again into *Environmental Pollution* in 1987. Full online coverage is available through Elsevier's ScienceDirect with 12 issues per year. It is cited in the major indexes such as Embase, MEDLINE, and Science Citation Index.

Environmental Toxicology and Chemistry. v. 1, Society of Environmental Toxicology and Chemistry, 1982.
http://www.setacjournals.org/
http://onlinelibrary.wiley.com/journal/10.1002/(ISSN)1552-8618
ISSN: 07307268
ISSN: 15528618
See Also Chapter 17.8. Toxicology
Indexed in: MEDLINE
Recommended for: Academic Libraries

This society-supported journal publishes papers based on original experimental or theoretical work encompassing the multidisciplinary nature of the field. Varying aspects of biochemistry, chemistry, ecology, physiology, microbiology, genetics, environmental engineering, modeling, and even earth sciences are touched upon as they relate to understanding environmental impacts. Articles are published based on their contribution to three main areas: environmental chemistry, environmental toxicology, or hazard/risk assessment. In addition, editorials, letters to the editor, and critical reviews are included occasionally. SETAC (Society of Environmental Toxicology and Chemistry) seeks to publish work that will "enhance capabilities for the prediction, measurement, and assessment of the fate and effects of chemicals in the environment." Its relatively low impact factor does not reflect the number of highly cited articles in its publication nor the strict quality guidelines for publication inclusion. Methodological papers must state how the new method differs from current practice and substantiate the importance of that difference. Field studies must also offer lessons beyond the local setting, by elucidating processes or mechanisms that operate regardless of the scale of the environmental setting (local, regional or global). This journal does not encompass studies that focus on human health, occupational exposure, remediation or environmental control. As a society publication, its content is geared towards the interests of its members who are involved in the study or practice of environmental management or environmental research. It would be suitable for an academic or special library collection. Full online coverage dates back to volume 1, 1982 with 12 issues per year. Among others, it is well indexed in CSA, MEDLINE, and Science Citation Index. It is available through the Society website and Wiley Online Library.

Journal of Environmental Science and Health, Part C: Environmental Carcinogenesis and Ecotoxicology Reviews. v. 9, Taylor & Francis, 1991.
http://www.informaworld.com/smpp/title~content=t713597270
http://www.tandf.co.uk/journals/titles/10590501.asp
ISSN: 10590501
ISSN: 15324095 (Online)
Indexed in: MEDLINE
Recommended for: Academic Libraries

Part C, one of three parts in the *Journal of Environmental Science and Health* series, focuses on publishing reviews on the toxic and carcinogenic effects of agents in the environment. Subject areas range from basic research methodology and modeling to biomarkers, host susceptibility, and risk assessment. The editors pick timely topics such as the toxicity and environmental risks of nanomaterials or effects of methylmercury in fish. Some reviews do broaden the focus outside of the pure definition of ecotoxicology and incorporate human health effects. Its slightly above the average impact factor (3.227 in 2009) ranks it twentieth in toxicology and twenty-fifth in environmental sciences. The journal is indexed in numerous sources such as Biological Abstracts, Embase, MEDLINE, and Science Citation Index. The journal is published quarterly and usually contains only a handful of reviews in each issue. The journal is of benefit to toxicologists, environmentalists, and biochemists or professionals in environmental or hazardous waste management. It would be suitable for an academic or special library collection. Full online coverage is available back to volume 1, 1983, which includes the journal's preceding title, *JESH, Part C: Environmental Carcinogenesis Reviews*, 1983–1991. It is available through Informaworld.

Reviews of Environmental Contamination and Toxicology. v. 98, Springer, 1987.
http://www.springer.com/series/398
http://www.springerlink.com/
ISSN: 01795953
Indexed in: MEDLINE
Recommended for: Academic Libraries

This monographic series has a long-standing history and reputation for thoroughly researched and comprehensive reviews on topics of interest to environmental researchers. *Reviews*, unlike other monographic series that create individual titles for each volume, maintains its series title name. Each volume publishes a handful of detailed review articles focusing on the toxicological effects of chemicals in all types of ecological systems. Recent coverage has focused on pesticides in aquatic organisms, environmental fate of polychlorinated biphenyls, and the stress effects of lead on the physio-biochemical activities of higher plants. Some of the more recent volumes are available online. The original series started in 1962 (volumes 1–97) and was published as *Residue Reviews. Residues of Pesticides and Other Contaminants in the Total Environment.*

Databases and Other Electronic Resources

ECOTOXicology Database (ECOTOX). Environmental Protection Agency, 1999.
http://www.epa.gov/ecotox/
Recommended for: Academic Libraries

Access to specific chemical toxicity data is necessary to characterize, diagnose, and predict the effects of chemicals on the environment or humans. The ECOTOXicology Database is the U.S. Environmental Protection Agency's federated search engine covering three of its ecological effects databases: AQUIRE, TERRETOX, and PHYTOTOX. Each provides information on single chemical toxicity—lethal, sublethal, and residue effects—data for aquatic, terrestrial, and plant species respectively. Starting in 1970, data was sourced from peer-reviewed literature as well as from data sets originating from France, Germany, the Netherlands, and Russia. Approximately 5,900 species and 8,400 chemicals are covered. Lately, emphasis has been placed on incorporating data for chemicals of interest to the Agency, particularly pesticides, metals, and some endocrine disrupting chemicals. This extremely searchable database allows browsing by chemicals, effects, or species, but users may also search by numerous other fields, such as endpoints (LD50, bioaccumulation, or other), exposure media (saltwater, mineral soil, or other), test location (lab, natural field, or other), and many more. Typically, the database is updated on a quarterly basis. ECOTOX offers a wealth of research data in an accessible format. The data is quality controlled and must meet minimum data requirements for inclusion. This ensures that the data can be used to conduct valid hazard and risk assessments and to set thresholds. Users are able to search on a variety of useful parameters and output results to an Excel spreadsheet. This database is primarily of use to practitioners and researchers who need access to validated data. ECOTOX is recommended for special libraries serving these user groups.

Environmental Sciences and Pollution Management Database. Cambridge Scientific Abstracts, 199?
http://www.csa.com/factsheets/envclust-set-c.php
Recommended for: Academic Libraries

The Environmental Sciences and Pollution Management (ESPM) database provides the most comprehensive coverage of the environmental sciences. This Cambridge Scientific Abstracts (CSA) database is composed of thirteen subfiles covering topics ranging from air quality and ecology to pollution and toxicology. The subfiles date back to various years. Water Resource Abstracts goes back to 1967 while the most recent subfile is Sustainability Science dating to 2003. The database currently includes over 6,000 journals, plus conference proceedings, reports, monographs, books, and government publications. The database also includes some unusual publication types such as film, map, and sound recording. It is updated monthly. Since ecotoxicology draws from diverse fields, the ability to search the ecology, pollution, and toxicology abstracts subfiles in one database is beneficial. ESPM also provides the flexibility of limiting the search to a specific subfile or searching across the whole database. CSA's Illumina platform accommodates proximity searching by using either "near" or "within x." A thesaurus allows the user to identify controlled vocabulary to retrieve more relevant results. One shortcoming of the database is the absence of the CAS number in the other 35 searchable fields. ESPM's audience includes students and practitioners in the field. The database would be useful for collections in academic and special libraries.

17.8.2. Forensic Toxicology

The application of toxicology knowledge to questions of law.
—MeSH

Contributors: Kristine M. Alpi and Robert Sotak

Monographs

Clarke's Analytical Forensic Toxicology. 1st ed. Editors: Sue Jickells, Adam Negrusz. Pharmaceutical Press, 2008.
http://www.pharmpress.com/
http://extranet.netlibrary.com/TitleSelect/
http://www.eblib.com/
ISBN: 9780853697053
ISBN: 9780853698517 (Online)
Recommended for: Hospital, Academic Libraries
Doody's Core Titles Selection

Clarke's Analytical Forensic Toxicology is a graduate level textbook written by 46 contributors mostly from U.K. and U.S. universities, industry, and government agencies. The editors wanted to make *Clarke's Analysis of Drugs and Poisons* (2004) more readily accessible and affordable. The first half of the book provides introductory material; basic pharmacokinetics and metabolism; substances encountered in toxicology; tissues, organs, and fluids used in testing; and more specific situations such as workplace drug testing and drug monitoring in clinical settings. The second half covers techniques such as types of spectroscopy and chromatography. All chapters have reference and/or further reading sections and typically contain numerous illustration and tables. Several topics have been added since the 2004 edition, such as drugs in sweat, in utero exposure to drugs, and drug-facilitated sexual assault. This title is also available online from Ebook Library and NetLibrary. Recommended for all health sciences libraries, general academic libraries, and students and practitioners of toxicology.

Color Atlas of Forensic Medicine and Pathology. 1st ed. Editor: Charles A. Catanese. CRC Press, 2010.
See Chapter 10.7. Forensic Medicine

Effective Expert Witnessing: Practices for the 21st Century. 4th ed. Authors: Jack V. Matson, Suha F. Daou, Jeffrey G. Soper. CRC Press, 2004.
See Chapter 10.7. Forensic Medicine

Forensic Entomology: The Utility of Arthropods in Legal Investigations. 2nd ed. Editors: Jason H. Byrd, James L. Castner. CRC Press, 2010.
See Chapter 10.7. Forensic Medicine

Fundamentals of Analytical Toxicology. Authors: Robert J. Flanagan, Andrew A. Taylor, Ian D. Watson, Robin Whelpton. Wiley, 2007.
http://onlinelibrary.wiley.com/book/10.1002/9780470516294
ISBN: 9780470319345
ISBN: 9789470516294 (Online)
Recommended for: Academic Libraries

Detecting, identifying, and measuring drugs and poisons in clinical and forensic cases is a function of analytical toxicology. Four UK-based authors provide a practical approach to basic analytical, statistical, and pharmacokinetic principles in toxicology with a work that assumes only a basic knowledge of analytical chemistry and laboratory operations. It follows the International Union of Pure and Applied Chemistry (IUPAC) nomenclature for chemical names. American readers will find cross referencing in the index from American to British drug names such as "Acetaminophen, See Paracetamol." The extremely detailed table of contents outlines information on sample collection, transport, storage and disposal, and preparation. Seven chapters introduce analytical techniques: color tests, spectrophotometry and luminescence measurements, various methods for chromatography and electrophoresis, mass spectrometry, and immunoassay. A chapter is devoted to the analysis of trace elements and toxic metals. The final chapters review toxicology testing at the point of care, xenobiotic absorption, distribution and metabolism, pharmacokinetics, and clinical interpretation of analytical results. *Fundamentals of Analytical Toxicology* is useful resource for students at several levels. The authors compare this to other works saying that it is not intended to provide detailed coverage such as that given in *Clarke's Analysis of Drugs and Poisons*. Supplementary materials on the open website (http://www.wiley.com/legacy/wileychi/flanagantoxicology/) include an appendix of interpretations for therapeutic and toxic concentrations of analytes with CAS registry numbers, a list of volatile compounds and conversion factors, and a glossary of commonly used terms. The full text is available online in PDF format from Wiley Online Library. For a more basic introduction to the chemistry that underlies forensic science, Dr. Suzanne Bell's *Forensic Chemistry* (Prentice Hall, 2005) brings the perspective of analytical chemistry, addressing the legal context in which forensic chemistry is conducted, types of samples and matrices, and extensive use of instrumentation. It offers a solid foundation for basic chemistry, introducing chemical concepts and practices from a forensic perspective—including multivariate statistics, quality assurance/quality control (QA/QC), and protocols used in working forensic laboratories. Public libraries note that Dr. Bell is also the author of the 2008 Facts on File title *Drugs, Poisons and Chemistry* from the *Essentials of Forensic Science* series.

Handbook of Common Poisonings in Children. 4th ed.
American Academy of Pediatrics, 2010.
ISBN: 9781581101966
Recommended for: Hospital, Academic, Consumer Health Libraries

The National Committee on Injury, Violence, and Poison Prevention of the American Academy of Pediatrics updated this manual which covers poison prevention, acute poisoning, drug abuse, toxicity calculations, and discussions of specific poisons. The fourth edition of this quick reference tool offers practitioners guidance on assessing poisoning exposure and initiating the appropriate course of action. It is also useful to forensic toxicologists trying to ascertain what may have transpired in fatal poisoning situations. The recently out-of-print *Pediatric Toxicology: Diagnosis and Management of the Poisoned Child* (McGraw-Hill, 2005) is another excellent resource for toxicologists needing information for pediatric cases.

Handbook of Forensic Toxicology for Medical Examiners.
Author: D.K. Molina. CRC Press, 2010.
http://www.crcnetbase.com/isbn/978-1-4200-7641-7
http://extranet.netlibrary.com/TitleSelect/
ISBN: 9781420076417
ISBN: 9781420076424 (Online)
Recommended for: Hospital, Academic Libraries

Part of the series *Practical Aspects of Criminal and Forensic Investigations*, this quick reference handbook brings forensic toxicology expertise in the interpretation of common toxicology results to the medical examiner and other forensic professionals. Forensic toxicology comprises the identification and quantification of drugs, and also what those drugs mean in death. The first chapter addresses specimen selection and collection, and then subsequent chapters address methodologies such as immunoassay, spectrophotometry, and testing from screening to confirmatory. The bulk of the text is an alphabetical listing of drugs including common drugs of abuse, poisons, and prescription and over-the-counter medications. Each drug has its own page with a compilation of data from the literature on therapeutic/nontoxic, toxic, and lethal concentrations. Half life and volume of distribution are also given when available. The author indicates that articles were chosen on scientific merit and the lack of confounding factors. Bexar County Medical Examiner's Office Data from 1996–2007 is listed as a source for many drugs. Five appendixes present common acetylcholinesterase inhibitors, drugs that prolong the QT interval, pharmacogenetics, and normal lab values.

Herbal Products: Toxicology and Clinical Pharmacology.
2nd ed. Editors: Timothy S. Tracy, Richard L. Kingston.
Humana Springer, 2007.
http://www.springerlink.com/content/978-1-58829-313-8
http://extranet.netlibrary.com/TitleSelect/
http://www.ebrary.com/corp/order.jsp

ISBN: 9781588293138
ISBN: 9781597453837 (Online)
Recommended for: Hospital, Academic, Consumer Health, Libraries

This second revised and expanded edition of *Toxicology and Clinical Pharmacology of Herbal Products* includes herbs based on their popularity, toxicity, and quantity and quality of evidence available. The 17 herbs are Ma huang and the ephedra alkaloids, Kava, Ginkgo biloba, Valerian, St. John's wort, Echinacea, Feverfew, Garlic, Ginger, Saw palmetto, Panax ginseng, Cranberry, Hawthorn, Evening primrose, Citrus aurantium, Vitex agnus-castus, and Bilberry. The authors give detailed technical information on the uses, efficacy, and projected safety as well as compilations of the things that have or could have happened to people taking them based on objective, peer-reviewed scientific literature. The references at the end of each chapter cover historical and current papers in many languages. The amount of information included in each of these sections varies according to what is available in the literature. The index includes commercial product names and cross-references with common and Latin names; one problem with the index is that it ignores the Greek characters at the front of terms. Forensic toxicologists and pathologists will find this book useful in situations where herbal remedies may be implicated in poisoning, as previous reported cases of toxicity and the toxicological effects of each herb are described. The "Pharmacokinetics" section of each chapter covers absorption, tissue distribution, elimination, and body fluid concentrations that may be useful in investigations. This book will also be of interest to a variety of clinicians interested in herbal medicine and the specifics of adverse effects, pharmacokinetics, and interactions with drugs or food. This volume, part of the *Forensic Science and Medicine* series, is available online via SpringerLink and through other e-book providers such as NetLibrary. There is also a companion volume, *Dietary Supplements: Toxicology and Clinical Pharmacology*, which covers nonherbal dietary supplements.

Hot Zone Forensics: Chemical, Biological, and Radiological Evidence Collection. Author: Steven C. Drielak. Charles C Thomas, 2004.
ISBN: 9780398074647
Recommended for: Hospital, Academic Libraries

Hot Zone Forensics introduces the challenges of sampling from crime scenes in hazardous situations, covering the equipment and protocols for gathering biological, chemical and radiological evidence. Dermal sampling from affected patients is relevant to all types of emergency clinicians and the larger issues are relevant to all working in crime scene investigation, public health, emergency preparedness, and hazardous materials control. Black-and-white photos, sample protocols, and chain of custody data sheets are useful. Appendixes from key organizations include a data table on chemical warfare agents and their precursors, lists of equipment for sampling, a list of extremely hazardous substances from the EPA, and the CDC's anthrax protocols. The glossary is helpful and the book is indexed, although one must look for a specific chemical under the heading "chemical agents" first, then by the first letter of the name. It is recommended for toxicologists who may be analyzing materials sampled from patients or objects exposed, or the agents themselves. A related useful free online resource from the National Association of Medical Examiners is *The Medical Examiner/Coroner's Guide for Contaminated Deceased Body Management* (2006).

Introduction to Environmental Forensics. 2nd ed. Authors: Brian L. Murphy, Robert D. Morrison. Elsevier, 2007.
See Chapter 10.7. Forensic Medicine

Karch's Pathology of Drug Abuse. 4th ed. Author: Steven B, Karch. CRC Press, 2009.
http://www.crcnetbase.com/isbn/978-0-8493-7880-5
ISBN: 9780849378805
ISBN: 9780849378812 (Online)
Recommended for: Hospital, Academic Libraries

This is the fourth edition of a work focused on the investigation of drug-related deaths and practical approaches to the detection of drug abuse. Detailed tables of contents outlining each of nine chapters provide quick reference to rich information provided on the following drugs: cocaine, natural stimulants, synthetic stimulants, hallucinogens, opiates and opioids, dissociative anesthetics, anabolic steroids, solvents, and marijuana. Four appendixes cover conversion formulas, blood alcohol concentrations, distribution calculations and normal heart weights. The book is also well indexed. With 2,000+ new citations to the literature, numerous color photos, and tables of comparative information, this is an excellent reference work. *Karch's Pathology of Drug Abuse* is available in print and online via CRCNETBase, as well as through e-book providers such as ebrary. Dr. Karch is also the editor of the comprehensive reference work *Drug Abuse Handbook*, (CRC Press, 2nd ed., 2007) and the concise *Postmortem Toxicology of Abused Drugs* (CRC Press, 2008) among many other works relevant to forensic toxicologists, pathologists, and death scene investigators.

Principles of Forensic Toxicology. 3rd ed. Editor: Barry Levine. American Association for Clinical Chemistry, 2010.
ISBN: 9781594250965
Recommended for: Academic Libraries

Dr. Barry Levine and his chapter authors are well qualified to produce this handbook which can serve as a forensic toxicology textbook, a review for those studying for toxicology board examinations, or a quick reference handbook for those who work in toxicology laboratories. The structure remains the same in the third edition which includes new chapters on non-narcotic analgesics and antihistamines, as well as updated method and drug chapters, including mass spectrometry, cannabis, and opioids. The handbook is broken into three sections. The first provides an introduction to postmortem forensic toxicology, human performance forensic toxicology, forensic drug testing, and pharmacokinetics and pharmacodynamics. Analytical principles and methodologies are the focus of the second section. The final section covers commonly encountered analytes, including drugs of abuse, classes of prescription and non-prescription drugs, as well as carbon monoxide/cyanide, inhalants, and metals—each with sections on effects, mechanism of action, pharmacokinetics, methods of analysis, and interpretation of results.

Spitz and Fisher's Medicolegal Investigation of Death: Guidelines for the Application of Pathology to Crime Investigation. 4th ed. Editors: Werner U. Spitz, Daniel J. Spitz, Russell S. Fisher, Ramsey Clark. Charles C Thomas, 2006.
See Chapter 10.7. Forensic Medicine

Journals

American Journal of Forensic Medicine & Pathology. v. 1, Lippincott, Williams & Wilkins, 1980.
See Chapter 10.7. Forensic Medicine

Analytical Chemistry. v. 19, American Chemical Society, 1947.
See Chapter 10.7. Forensic Medicine

Forensic Science International. v. 11, Elsevier, 1978.
See Chapter 10.7. Forensic Medicine, Chapter 10.7.1. Forensic Genetics

Forensic Science, Medicine, and Pathology. v. 1, Humana, 2005.
See Chapter 10.7. Forensic Medicine

Forensic Toxicology. v. 24, Springer, 2006.
http://www.springerlink.com/content/1860-8965
ISSN: 18608965
ISSN: 18608973 (Online)
Recommended for: Academic Libraries

Forensic Toxicology, the twice yearly, English language journal formerly known as the *Japanese Journal of Forensic Toxicology*, is becoming more international. Published since 1983 as the official journal of the Japanese Association of Forensic Toxicology, the approximately 100 pages per year include original articles, reviews, mini-reviews, short communications, and case reports primarily from Japanese authors on analytical methods for toxic substances, drugs of abuse, doping agents, chemical warfare agents, and their metabolisms and analyses. Forensic Toxicology is not indexed by MEDLINE, but is covered by Academic OneFile, Chemical Abstracts Service, Elsevier Biobase, Embase, EMBiology, Gale, Google Scholar, INPHARMA, OCLC, Scopus, and Web of Science.

International Journal of Legal Medicine. v. 104, Springer, 1990.
See Chapter 10.7. Forensic Medicine, Chapter 10.7.1. Forensic Genetics

Journal of Analytical Toxicology. v. 1, Preston, 1977.
http://www.jatox.com/
http://www.ingentaconnect.com/content/pres/jat
ISSN: 01464760
ISSN: 19452403 (Online)
Indexed in: MEDLINE
Recommended for: Academic Libraries

The Journal of Analytical Toxicology (*JAT*) is an international, peer-reviewed journal addressing the practical aspects of chemical analysis of potentially toxic substances such as pharmaceuticals, drugs of abuse, pesticides, industrial chemicals, poisons, and environmental toxins. Focused on state-of-the art techniques used in clinical, forensic, workplace, sports testing, and other toxicology laboratories for identifying, isolating, and quantifying substances, JAT has published methods in immunoassay testing, gas chromatography, liquid chromatography, mass spectrometry, atomic absorption spectrometry, and solid- and liquid-phase extraction techniques. In addition to original articles, toxicology developments are communicated through technical notes, case reports, and letters. The journal publishes nine issues a year; October is a special issue from the Society of Forensic Toxicologists. With a 2009 impact factor of 1.867, *JAT* ranks forty-seventh of 77 toxicology journals and thirty-second of 70 analytical chemistry journals in the science *Journal Citation Reports*. Papers are applicable to therapeutic drug monitoring, abused drugs, clinical and forensic toxicology, workplace environmental exposure, chemical warfare, and sports doping, resulting in wide indexing coverage including Agricultural Engineering Abstracts, Analytical Abstracts, Aquatic Sciences & Fisheries Abstracts, BIOBASE, CAB Abstracts, Chemical Abstracts, EBSCOhost Academic Search, Embase, Global Health, MEDLINE, OCLC Articles First, Scopus, and Web of Science. It is available online as subscription or single article purchase back to volume 1, 1977 via IngentaConnect.

Journal of Forensic Sciences. v. 1, Wiley-Blackwell, 1972.
See Chapter 10.7. Forensic Medicine

Journal of Medical Toxicology. v. 1, Springer, 2005.
http://springerlink.com/content/121536/
ISSN: 15569039
ISSN: 19376995 (Online)
Indexed in: MEDLINE
Recommended for: Hospital, Academic Libraries

Journal of Medical Toxicology is the official journal of the American College of Medical Toxicology. This quarterly international, peer-reviewed journal advances the science and practice of medical toxicology, a medical subspecialty focusing on the diagnosis, management, and prevention of poisoning and adverse health effects due to medications, chemicals, occupational and environmental substances, and biological hazards. The journal publishes original articles in basic science and clinical research, case reports, reviews, and special features such as toxicology in the news and the *CDC Tox Report* which summarizes toxicity research and activities at the CDC and the Agency for Toxic Substances and Disease Registry. This relatively new journal is not included in the 2009 *Journal Citation Reports* or indexed by Web of Science, but is covered by databases such as Expanded Academic, Google Scholar, Health Reference Center Academic, OCLC, MEDLINE, Scopus, and TOC Premier. This journal is especially important for libraries serving poison control centers. Full archives are available online via Springer with Online First Articles. Note that only one issue (December) was published with Penn Press for volume 1, 2005; quarterly publication started with 2006.

Medicine, Science & the Law. v. 1, Royal Society of Medicine Press, 1960.
See Chapter 10.7. Forensic Medicine

17.8.3. Toxicogenetics

The study of existing genetic knowledge, and the generation of new genetic data, to understand and thus avoid drug toxicity and adverse effects from toxic substances from the environment.

—MeSH

Contributor: Stephanie Holmgren

Monographs

Applications of Toxicogenomic Technologies to Predictive Toxicology and Risk Assessment. Authors: Committee on Applications of Toxicogenomic Technologies to Predictive Toxicology and Risk Assessment, National Research Council. National Academies Press, 2007.
http://www.nap.edu/catalog.php?record_id=12037
http://extranet.netlibrary.com/TitleSelect/
ISBN: 9780309112987
ISBN: 9780309112994
Recommended for: Academic Libraries

The ultimate goal of toxicogenomic research is the ability to use what is learned from model systems to predict pathogenesis, assess risk, and prevent human disease. The National Research Council assembled a committee of 16 experts from academia, industry, environmental advocacy groups, and the legal community and charged them with examining the potential applications of toxicogenomics in predictive toxicology, identifying the challenges, and making recommendations. Chapters address applications of toxicogenomics to hazard identification screening, mechanism of action studies, classification of compounds, exposure assessment, defining genetic susceptibility, and reducing the use of test animals. For each of these applications, "proof of concept studies from the published literature" were analyzed to identify limitations, challenges, and potential solutions. The remainder of the book focuses on validating toxicogenomic methods so that they can be utilized for risk assessment and on the ethical, legal, and social issues that may hinder its use. The final chapter compiles the recommendations offered at the end of each chapter and adds a few overarching suggestions not mentioned previously. This work is important because no other publication has evaluated and highlighted the future of toxicogenomics in the arena of predictive toxicity and risk assessment. The inclusion of opportunities, challenges, and detailed recommendations makes this a unique report on the topic. A broad range of parties would be interested, including researchers and practitioners, government policy makers, regulatory officials, industrial toxicologists, and even members of the public. The work is recommended for academic and special libraries.

Handbook of Toxicogenomics: A Strategic View of Current Research and Applications. Editor: Jürgen Borlak. Wiley, 2005.
http://onlinelibrary.wiley.com/book/10.1002/3527603719
http://www.ebrary.com/
http://extranet.netlibrary.com/TitleSelect/
ISBN: 9783527603718
ISBN: 9783527303427
ISBN: 9783527604517
Recommended for: Academic Libraries

Although not a handbook in the traditional sense, this publication does focus on practical rather than theoretical aspects of toxicogenomic research. The beginning chapters describe the use of different types of toxicogenomic technologies, such as various microarray platforms, mass spectrometry, chromatin immunoprecipitation, and NMR spectroscopy. The next section focuses on the application of bioinformatics tools to toxicogenomic analysis. Of special interest is a chapter devoted to the Chemical Effects in Biological Systems (CEBS) Knowledge Base. The heart of the book's content is dedicated to 11 chapters of case studies in which toxicogenomics has been applied to different types of toxicity testing, such as endocrine disruption, biomarkers, nephrotoxicity, and teratogenicity. The section ends with an interesting chapter on "How Things Could Be Done Better Using Toxicogenomics." The last few chapters provide an account of the toxicogenomic programs in the United States and Japan and discuss the need for an ICH (International Conference on Harmonisation of Technical Requirements for Registration of Pharmaceuticals for Human Use) harmonized guideline to include toxicogenomic data as part of the drug registration process. This handbook provides a detailed and practical approach to toxicogenomics. Next generation systems are mentioned within the context of the systems biology chapter, and a chapter is dedicated to the challenges that genetic variability brings to toxicogenomic analysis. Examples are well placed throughout the book. International experts from major government, industry, and academic research institutions contributed content to the book. The *Handbook of Toxicogenomics* is a Society of Toxicology "publication of interest."

An Introduction to Toxicogenomics. Editor: Michael E. Burczynski. CRC Press, 2003.
http://extranet.netlibrary.com/TitleSelect/
http://www.ebrary.com/
ISBN: 9780849313349
ISBN: 9780203504819
ISBN: 9780203611760
Recommended for: Academic Libraries

Although this book was written at the advent of this new subdiscipline, it is a useful resource for understanding the application of genomics techniques to the field of toxicology. The book is divided into six sections, starting with an overview of how to conduct expression profiling analysis. Chapters are devoted to utilizing microarrays, understanding the differences between cDNA and oligonucleotide array results, ensuring quality control of the profile data, and applying clustering algorithms to analyze the data. The next section applies expression profiling by looking at the use of transcriptional profiling in toxicology. The third theme details two model systems often used in toxicogenomic studies. The next two sections examine aspects of conducting mechanistic and predictive studies. Finally, the last chapter looks forward to the future of the subdiscipline in terms of new technologies, tools for data analysis and interpretation, and the role toxicogenomics can play in risk assessment. Each chapter is written by a set of experts to accurately and comprehensively represent that topic. Contributing authors come from government, pharmaceutical, and academic research settings representing toxicology, genetics, and drug safety. Figures and tables are used appropriately, with a special insert of color figures illuminating the expression profiles and clustering generated from an analysis. Chapter references and an index are also included. Given the rapid advances in sequencing technology, it is difficult for any book to remain current in that regard. This book does not cover the more recent next generation sequencing technology or the new upcoming single molecule real time sequencers. The intended audience is wide ranging, from undergraduates and graduate students to scientists and clinicians involved in toxicology. This work is recommended for academic and special libraries.

Molecular and Biochemical Toxicology. 4th ed. Editors: Robert C. Smart, Ernest Hodgson. John Wiley & Sons, 2008.
http://onlinelibrary.wiley.com/book/10.1002/9780470285251
http://www.ebrary.com/
http://extranet.netlibrary.com/TitleSelect/
ISBN: 9780470285251
ISBN: 9780470102114
ISBN: 9780470285244
Recommended for: Academic Libraries

The fourth edition has not only been renamed from its predecessor, *Introduction to Biochemical Toxicology*, but it has been completely revised to incorporate the increasing contributions of molecular, cellular, and genomic biology to mechanistic toxicology. At 35 chapters, this is not an introductory text. Instead, it provides a comprehensive treatment of the principles of molecular and biochemical toxicology and the complex mechanisms of toxicity. After defining molecular and biochemical toxicology and highlighting molecular techniques, the editors launch into four new chapters on toxicogenomics, proteomics, metabolomics, and bioinformatics. These are followed by several chapters dedicated to enzymatic action, metabolism, cellular transport, toxicant-receptor interaction, essential metals, and DNA damage and repair. Later content focuses on specific toxicities: genotoxicity, hepatotoxicity, neprotoxicity, immunotoxicity, reproductive, developmental, and dermal. Nine new chapters were added to cover more contemporary topics. Most chapters were significantly revised and updated. Complex and sophisticated methods are described in a straightforward, easy-to-understand style. Illustrations, figures, and tables tend to be descriptive and supportive of the explanatory text, such as the figures used to explain nuclear magnetic resonance. The comprehensive nature of the book makes it suitable for an upper-level biochemical/molecular toxicology class or as a reference book for toxicologists and health professionals. The book is recommended for academic and special libraries and is considered a Society of Toxicology "publication of interest."

Molecular Toxicology. 2nd ed. Authors: P. David Josephy, Bengt Mannervik. Oxford University Press, 2006.
ISBN: 9780195176209
See Also Chapter 17.8. Toxicology
Recommended for: Academic Libraries

Due to significant scientific and technological developments, this second edition of *Molecular Toxicology* is a major rewrite of the earlier 1997 version. In those 10 years, scientific research has been able to better elucidate how chemicals can alter the biochemical and physiological processes at the molecular level. Oxygen, the fuel of human life, is the subject of the leading chapter. The chapter explores reactive oxygen species, addressing how they interact with cellular parts and the consequences. Discussion then moves to covalent binding of xenobiotics to DNA, DNA repair mechanisms, and the role DNA damage plays in chemical mutagenesis and carcinogenesis. The fifth chapter describes how mutations in certain gene types, oncogenes, and tumor suppressor genes can promote cancer. Several subsequent chapters detail the various enzymes involved in the process of biotransformation; these include the cytochrome P450 and glutathione enzyme families. The last section applies the concepts from the earlier chapters to specific chemical groups, such as polycyclic aromatic hydrocarbons, acetaminophen, aromatic amines, and others. The emphasis in this book is primarily the effects on mammals, especially humans. The underlying theme connecting the content is that many of the same enzymes involved in the metabolism and biotransformation of endogenous substances are also used against exogenous chemicals. Each chapter begins with a historical refresher of the pioneers behind the key discoveries in biochemical and molecular toxicology. Sidebars and text boxes are used to expand on a topic or pose questions for further research; for example, do environmental chemicals cause heritable damage to the genome? The book is very detailed and completely referenced. Selected figures from the book are made available in color and can be downloaded from the book's companion website. Upper undergraduate or graduate students in toxicology or pharmacology, along with academic and industrial researchers in toxicology, will find the book useful. A basic understanding of toxicology and biochemistry principles is necessary. *Molecular Toxicology* is recommended for academic and special libraries.

Toxicogenomics: A Powerful Tool for Toxicity Assessment. Editor: Saura C. Sahu. John Wiley & Sons, 2008.
http://onlinelibrary.wiley.com/book/10.1002/9780470699638
http://extranet.netlibrary.com/TitleSelect/
http://www.ebrary.com/
ISBN: 9780470518236
ISBN: 9780470699638
ISBN: 9780470699645
Recommended for: Academic Libraries

In *Toxicogenomics*, Sahu and 59 other co-contributors utilize a practical approach to link toxicology and genetics to understanding human disease. The book begins with straightforward explanations of how to utilize microarrays and how to mine and analyze the data. Challenges associated with study design and source variability are also highlighted. The primary content focuses on the use of toxicogenomics for specific testing purposes: drug safety, carcinogenesis, hepatotoxicity, nutrigenomics, and others. Several chapters are devoted to the role toxicogenomics could play in the regulatory arena, culminating in how toxicogenomics is used by the Environmental Protection Agency. Some interesting and unique topics are incorporated in this book that others do not touch upon, such as risk assessment of natural products, principals of data mining, and use of biomarkers in work settings. The book is geared toward researchers involved in toxicology genetics, medicine, and food science, as well as regulators of drug and food products. It is recommended for academic and special libraries and is considered a "publication of interest" by the Society of Toxicology.

Toxicogenomics: Principles and Applications. Editors: Hisham K. Hamadeh, Cynthia A. Afshari. Wiley, 2004.
http://onlinelibrary.wiley.com/book/10.1002/0471669040
ISBN: 9780471434177
ISBN: 9780471669043 (Online)
Recommended for: Academic Libraries

In the spirit of the cross-disciplinary nature of the field, the authors have organized this book to reveal the interface between the concepts of toxicology and the technologies behind genomic analyses. The text begins by introducing nontoxicologists to the principles of toxicology: dose and response; adsorption, distribution, metabolism, and elimination; and acute and chronic toxicity. The next few chapters expose toxicologists to the basics of genomic technologies: microarrays, scanners, and real-time polymerase chain reaction (PCR). Further chapters detail experimental design, data interpretation, and database systems. The ninth chapter merges the two fields by exploring how toxicology and gene expression interrelate. Proteomic and metabolomic applications are also examined. The final chapter provides a useful list of toxicogenomic resources. *Toxicogenomics: Principles and Applications* is a practical guide rather than a theoretical tome. Tables and illustrations are used well to support the textual explanations. The chapters include quality references and websites when applicable. The book will be useful for toxicology graduate students, toxicologists, molecular and cellular biologists, informatics and computational scientists, and engineers involved in toxicology and risk assessment. The work is recommended for academic and special libraries.

Journals

Journal of Biochemical and Molecular Toxicology. v. 12, Wiley, 1998.
http://onlinelibrary.wiley.com/journal/10.1002/(ISSN)1099-0461
ISSN: 10956670
ISSN: 10990461 (Online)
Indexed in: MEDLINE
Recommended for: Academic Libraries

This international journal explores both exogenous and endogenous chemical effects on molecular mechanisms such as enzymes, receptors, hormones, genes, and proteins at the cellular, tissue, or organ system level. The scope also includes examining these effects throughout all stages of development. Besides agricultural, environmental, and industrial chemicals, natural products and food additives are of interest. Although broader in focus than strict toxicogenetics, this journal does indicate an interest in research focusing on the mechanistic effects of toxins on nucleic acids, gene expression, and protein synthesis. *The Journal of Biochemical and Molecular Toxicology* contains original research papers, rapid communications, mini reviews, and book reviews. Volumes 1–11 were originally titled *Journal of Biochemical Toxicology*. In 1998, the title changed to its current one to reflect the advances being made in molecular biology and their application to the field of toxicology. The journal's audience is targeted to biochemists, molecular biologists, toxicologists, and others working in the regulatory field of toxic chemicals. *Journal of Biochemical and Molecular Toxicology* is recommended for academic and special libraries. It is published bimonthly, with one volume of six issues per year. Several popular indexes cite the journal: Biological Abstracts, CAS, Embase, MEDLINE, Scopus, and Web of Science. It is available through Wiley Online Library.

Databases and Other Electronic Resources

Comparative Toxicogenomics Database. Mount Desert Island Biological Laboratory, 2004.
http://ctd.mdibl.org/
Recommended for: Academic Libraries

The Comparative Toxicogenomics Database (CTD) provides scientific data of the relationships among chemicals, genes, and human disease to advance the understanding of the molecular mechanisms behind susceptibility and environmentally-influenced disease. The chemical categories are based on NLM's (National Library of Medicine) MeSH (Medical Subject Headings) and can be accessed through a chemical browser. Chemical data includes structure, toxicity data, pathways, gene, and disease associations. A cross-species gene vocabulary—symbol, name, synonyms—is derived from the NCBI's (National Center for Biotechnology Information) Gene database. Gene information includes gene ontology, organism, and chemical and disease associations. Finally, the disease categories are extracted from the genetic disorders mentioned in the Online Mendelian Inheritance in Man (OMIM) database and the disease subset of MeSH. CTD is set up for either browsing or searching the relationships between chemicals and a gene/protein; chemical and a disease; or a gene/protein and disease. Professional PhD scientists manually curate these interactions and relationships for both vertebrates and invertebrates from the published scientific literature. A controlled "interaction" vocabulary comprises 70 terms (such as action, qualifier, or operator) used to characterize the physical, regulatory, and biochemical interactions between chemicals and genes or proteins. The data attempts to capture whether the chemical-gene/protein interaction is direct or indirect. For the gene-disease and chemical-disease relationships, the evidence is either direct or inferred. Because the database incorporates the Gene Ontology, users can also identify which cellular functions are affected by a chemical. This free database is updated monthly and currently includes curated data from 17,322 references. It has a powerful search interface, allowing users to quickly see the associated interactions and pathways when documented for each chemical, gene, or disease. A VennViewer even allows the user to see the interrelationship among three or fewer chemicals, genes, or diseases at one time. The data can also be downloaded in various formats. CCTB is recommended for academic and special libraries.

18. Pharmacy

Compounding and dispensing medicinal preparations.
—MeSH

Contributor: Jean L. Siebert

Monographs

Ansel's Pharmaceutical Dosage Forms and Drug Delivery Systems. 9th ed. Authors: Loyd V. Allen Jr., Nicholas G. Popovich, Howard C. Ansel. Lippincott Williams & Wilkins, 2010.
http://www.r2library.com/ (forthcoming)
ISBN: 9780781779340
See Also Chapter 22. Pharmaceutical Technology
Recommended for: Academic Libraries

This book is the most comprehensive source for pharmaceutical dosage forms and drug delivery systems. The content corelates with competencies from the California Accreditation for Pharmacy Education (CAPE), the American Pharmacists Association (APhA), and North American Pharmacist Licensure Examination (NAPLEX). This edition includes updated drug information and has an increased focus on physical pharmacy. Coverage incorporates all new dosage forms on the market as well as those in the current United States Pharmacopoeia-National Formulary. Updated photos are included. *Ansel's Pharmaceutical Dosage Forms and Drug Delivery Systems* is very readable, and has an excellent index and useful appendixes, charts, and photographs. This book is a starred listing in the 2009 edition of *Basic Resources for Pharmacy Education*, prepared by the Libraries/Educational Resources Section of the American Association of Colleges of Pharmacy.

Art, Science, and Technology of Pharmaceutical Compounding. 3rd ed. Author: Loyd V. Allen Jr. American Pharmaceutical Association, 2008.
ISBN: 9781582120355
See Also Chapter 22. Pharmaceutical Technology
Recommended for: Academic Libraries

Art, Science, and Technology of Pharmaceutical Compounding presents the information a pharmacist or pharmacy student needs to understand the purpose and processes of compounding, including establishing, equipping, and operating a compounding facility. The book also incorporates over 200 formulations that cover all the dosage forms and delivery systems of modern medications. The third edition has been revised and expanded to address new standards in the U.S. Pharmacopeia and to reflect new growth in compounding opportunities in geriatric, veterinary, and other special populations. It also includes chapters on compounding in the event of a natural disaster or a terrorist attack. Nine appendixes provide essential information on the compounding processes and examples of standard operating procedures. The book lacks color photographs; however, it includes a useful table of contents and excellent index. The "Sample Formulations" Index is organized by dosage form and well designed for pharmacist use. This book is listed (but not starred) in the 2009 edition of *Basic Resources for Pharmacy Education* prepared by the Libraries/Educational Resources Section of the American Association of Colleges of Pharmacy. This title is not available electronically, but is highly recommended for any library affiliated with a college of pharmacy.

Foundation in Pharmacy Practice. Authors: Ben Whalley, Kate Fletcher, Sam Weston, Rachel Howard, Clare Rawlinson. Pharmaceutical Press, 2008.
http://extranet.netlibrary.com/TitleSelect/
ISBN: 9780853697473
Recommended for: Academic Libraries

This book is designed for first-year pharmacy students in Great Britain. It is organized into 16 chapters covering the major topics in pharmacy practice, including an introduction to medication management; essential communication skills for pharmacists; types of prescriptions; legal requirements for dispensing; interpretation and understanding prescriptions; packaging and labeling of drugs; patient compliance, adherence and concordance; and the sale and supply of medications. The book contains numerous tables, charts, and diagrams which are well labeled and easy to read. Each chapter has a list of references to articles, books, and useful websites. This work is recommended for libraries supporting pharmacy students, faculty, or staff that are interested in pharmacy education in other countries. The table of contents is adequate, the glossary is helpful, and the index is very good and includes some cross references.

Handbook on Injectable Drugs. 16th ed. Author: Lawrence A. Trissel. American Society of Health-System Pharmacists, 2011.
http://online.statref.com/titleinfo/fxid-141.html
http://www.r2library.com/ (15th ed.)
ISBN: 9781585282487
ISBN: 9781585282500 (CD-ROM)
Recommended for: Academic Libraries
Doody's Core Titles Selection

This handbook presents concise information about preparing, storing, and administering 359 parenteral drugs. The drug monographs are organized alphabetically by generic name, with an index that includes brand, trade, and generic names. The monographs are also cross-referenced with AHFS drug information. All the references for the monographs are listed at the end of the handbook, which can hinder their quick use. This book is currently listed as an essential purchase in *Doody's Core Titles*. The *Handbook on Injectable Drugs* is a starred title in the 2009 edition of *Basic Resources in Pharmacy Education*, prepared by the Libraries/Educational Resources Section of the American Association of Colleges of Pharmacy. This review refers to the fifteenth edition.

The Merck Index: An Encyclopedia of Chemicals, Drugs, and Biologicals. 14th ed. Editor: Maryadele J. O'Neil. Merck, 2006.
http://www.merckbooks.com/mindex/online.html
ISBN: 9780911910001
See Also Chapter 17.6. Clinical Pharmacology
Recommended for: Academic Libraries

The Merck Index is a one-volume encyclopedia of chemicals, drugs, and biologicals that contains 10,450 monographs with 7,033 derivatives, 32 supplemental tables, and 450 organic name reactions. Each monograph concisely describes a single substance or a small group of closely related compounds. In the fourteenth edition there are 50 new approved monographs. It has excellent, unique indexes and numerous useful tables in the front of the index. The derivatives for all monographs that have them have been added to the "Basic Physical Properties" and the "Health and Safety Related Properties" tables. The properties for the substances covered by retired monographs (and their derivatives) have been added to two new tables. The electronic version, which is available through several vendors, facilitates readability by providing each monograph on a separate screen that can either be printed or saved for export. This title is starred in the 2009 edition of *Basic Resources for Pharmacy Education* prepared by the Libraries/Educational Resources Section of the American Association of Colleges of Pharmacy.

Pharmacy Practice and the Law. 6th ed. Author: Richard R. Abood. Jones & Bartlett, 2010.
ISBN: 9780763781293
Recommended for: Academic Libraries
Doody's Core Titles Selection

Targeted at U.S. pharmacy students, *Pharmacy Practice and the Law* provides background, history, and discussion of pharmacy law. Each chapter includes discussion questions and edited cases, which are particularly useful for group learning. Citations to all laws, court cases, regulations, and other documents are provided. The sixth edition includes updates on new legal, regulatory, and policy developments. Chapter 3 covers federal regulations of medications, including compounding and dispensing laws and court cases. Also included are a table of cases with page numbers, a glossary of legal terms, and a useful index. *Pharmacy Practice and the Law* is listed in *Doody's Core Titles*. The fifth edition is a starred title in the 2009 edition of *Basic Resources for Pharmacy Education* prepared by the Libraries/Educational Resources section of the American Association of Colleges of Pharmacy.

Remington: The Science and Practice of Pharmacy. 21st ed. Editors: University of the Sciences in Philadelphia. Lippincott Williams & Wilkins, 2006.
ISBN: 9780781752114
Recommended for: Academic Libraries
Doody's Core Titles Selection

This book is very comprehensive, with over 2,000 pages. It has a table of contents and is organized by disciplines within pharmacy. The target audience is pharmacy students, faculty, and practitioners. Dispensing is thoroughly covered in chapter 101, "The Prescription"; pharmacy laws are covered in chapter 111, "The Laws Governing Pharmacy"; and compounding is covered in chapter 105, "Extemporaneous Prescription Compounding." The index is well organized. The print colors of black with green highlights are more legible than previous editions, although color photographs should replace the standard black and white. It is a very worthwhile resource that is highly recommended for a library directly supporting a College of Pharmacy. *Remington* is listed in *Doody's Core Titles*. This title is starred in the 2009 edition of *Basic Resources for Pharmacy Education* prepared by the Libraries/Educational Resources Section of the American Association of Colleges of Pharmacy.

Trissel's Stability of Compounded Formulations. 4th ed. Author: Lawrence A. Trissel. American Pharmacists Association, 2009.
http://online.statref.com/titleinfo/fxid-204.html

ISBN: 9781582121253
See Also Chapter 22. Pharmaceutical Technology
Recommended for: Academic Libraries

Trissel's Stability of Compounded Formulations summarizes specific formulations and stability information on drugs in compounded oral, enteral, topical, ophthalmic, and other specialized preparations. Used to determine whether formulated compounds will remain stable for the anticipated duration of use, this publication provides guidance on properly storing and repackaging compounded formulations, preparing formulations to meet documented standards, and counseling patients on the use and storage of compounded medications. The 433 product monographs are arranged alphabetically by nonproprietary name. Each monograph provides information on properties, general stability considerations, and stability reports of compounded preparations. When available, information on compatibility with other drug products and compatibility with common beverages and foods is included. A summary of USP benchmarks for assigning beyond-use periods is contained within two appendixes. Numerous references and an index of nonproprietary and brand names enhance usability. This title is listed in the 2009 edition of *Basic Resources for Pharmacy Education* prepared by the Libraries/Educational Resources Section of the American Association of Colleges of Pharmacy.

Journals

American Journal of Health-System Pharmacy. v. 52, American Society of Health-System Pharmacists, 1995.
http://www.ajhp.org/
ISSN: 10792082
ISSN: 15352900 (Online)
Indexed in: MEDLINE, CINAHL
Recommended for: Hospital, Academic Libraries

American Journal of Health-System Pharmacy (*AJHP*) is the official publication of the American Society of Health-System Pharmacists and continues *American Journal of Hospital Pharmacy.* It publishes peer-reviewed scientific papers on contemporary drug therapy and pharmacy practice innovations in hospitals and health systems. *AJHP* is one of the most widely recognized and respected clinical pharmacy journals in the world. It has an impact factor of 2.097 and is ranked one-hundred-thirty-second of 237 pharmacology and pharmacy journals in the 2009 *Journal Citation Reports.* Articles in *AJHP* are abstracted and indexed in MEDLINE, International Pharmaceutical Abstracts, and many other scientific databases. Full text is available online back to volume 54, 1997; abstracts are available from volume 32, 1975; and tables of contents are available back to volume 22, number 9, 1965.

Hospital Pharmacy. v. 1, Thomas Land, 1996.
http://www.thomasland.com/hospitalpharmacy.html
ISSN: 00185787
ISSN: 19451253 (Online)
Recommended for: Hospital, Academic Libraries

Hospital Pharmacy provides peer-reviewed, clinical information about drug and disease state management, recent FDA approvals, medication error and adverse reaction reporting, automation, medical usage evaluation, and governmental regulation. Written for the pharmacy practitioner, it is recommended for pharmacists in all settings, including managed care practices, nursing homes, long-term care facilities, and pharmacy schools. It is specifically focused on medication error prevention. Prior to its acquisition by Thomas Land, *Hospital Pharmacy* was also known as *Lippincott's Hospital Pharmacy.* This journal is indexed in Academic Search Complete (since 2006), Biological Abstracts, and International Pharmaceutical Abstracts.

International Journal of Pharmaceutical Compounding. v. 1, International Journal of Pharmaceutical Compounding, 1997.
http://www.ijpc.com/
ISSN: 10924221
ISSN: 19435223 (Online)
Indexed in: CINAHL
Recommended for: Academic Libraries

The *International Journal of Pharmaceutical Compounding* (*IJPC*) is a peer-reviewed journal that addresses hands-on compounding techniques. With articles ranging from scientific to informational, *IJPC* is the only journal to address pharmaceutical compounding in patient care. Peer reviewers include not only practicing pharmacists but also pharmaceutical scientists and academicians, and experts in related specialties. *The International Journal of Pharmaceutical Compounding* is indexed in International Pharmaceutical Abstracts, CINAHL, SciFinder Scholar (Chemical Abstracts), and Elsevier bibliographic databases including Embase, EMNursing, and Scopus.

Journal of the American Pharmacists Association. v. 43, no. 3, American Pharmacists Association, 2003.
http://www.pharmacist.com/japha
ISSN: 15443191
ISSN: 15443450 (Online)

Indexed in: MEDLINE
Recommended for: Academic Libraries

This journal continues the *Journal of the American Pharmaceutical Association*, which began publication in 1912. The *Journal of the American Pharmacists Association* (*JAPhA*) is the official peer-reviewed journal of the American Pharmacists Association. It provides original research, reviews, case studies, and opinion articles on all aspects of pharmaceutical care, drug therapy, and trends in pharmacy practice and therapeutics. Articles in *JAPhA* are indexed in SciFinder Scholar, Excerpta Medica, International Pharmaceutical Abstracts, Iowa Drug Information Service, and MEDLINE. Online full text is provided back to volume 42, 2002.

Pharmacy Times. v. 35, no. 9, Intellisphere, 1969.
http://www.pharmacytimes.com
ISSN: 00030627
Recommended for: Hospital, Academic Libraries

Pharmacy Times provides practical clinical information on essential topics, including disease state management, patient counseling, product news, and pharmacy law. It has an occasional column called "Your Compounding Questions Answered." Most articles are one or two pages. It also provides accredited continuing education. This journal is not peer-reviewed. It is indexed in Academic Search Complete, TOC Premier, and International Pharmaceutical Abstracts. Free access to articles from issues back to 2002 can be found by article type at the publication's website.

U.S. Pharmacist. v. 1, Jobson Medical Information, 1976.
http://www.uspharmacist.com/econnect/
ISSN: 01484818
Recommended for: Academic Libraries

U.S. Pharmacist contains peer-reviewed clinical articles relevant to pharmacy practice in a variety of settings, including academia. The publication is also useful to pharmacy technicians, students, other health professionals, and individuals interested in health management. This journal has an occasional article on compounding. The electronic version is freely available and listed in the *Directory of Open Access Journals*. *U.S. Pharmacist* is indexed in International Pharmaceutical Abstracts.

19. Podiatry

The diagnosis and treatment of foot disorders and injuries and anatomic defects of the foot.

—MeSH

Contributor: Rajia Tobia

Monographs

Clinical Skills in Treating the Foot. 2nd ed. Editors: Warren A. Turner, Linda M. Merriman. Elsevier Churchill Livingstone, 2005.
ISBN: 9780443071133
Recommended for: Hospital, Academic Libraries

The second edition of this text was written as a companion to *Assessment of the Lower Limb*; however, *Clinical Skills in Treating the Foot* stands alone as an introductory text for anyone providing support to patients with foot disorders. The editors and contributing authors are from the United Kingdom; however, the information contained in the text will have applicability to treatment planning in any setting. The book is divided into three sections. Section 1, "Essential Principles of Management," concerns the general principles of managing foot disorders, including evidence-based management. Section 2, "Methods of Managing Foot Conditions," discusses clinical therapeutics including surgery, pharmacology, physical therapy, mechanical therapies, prescription devices, and footwear. Section 3, "Managing Specific Client Groups," includes information on treating adult and children's foot disorders, injuries in athletes, and tissue viability. Illustrations and photographs are in black and white. Chapters are well referenced, with some providing references for additional reading and website addresses for further reference. This text, written primarily for podiatrists, will be useful for any library serving podiatric medicine programs.

Drennan's The Child's Foot and Ankle. 2nd ed. Editors: James J. McCarthy, James C. Drennan. Lippincott, Williams & Wilkins, 2010.
ISBN: 9780781778473
Recommended for: Academic Libraries

The second, completely revised edition of Drennan's definitive text aims to serve as a single, comprehensive resource for pediatric foot and ankle disorders. In 33 chapters it provides complete information on the anatomy, etiology, clinical features and presentation, natural history, and treatment of congenital and acquired conditions and injuries. Information is included on radiographic, magnetic resonance imaging, and computed tomography evaluation of foot and ankle problems. More than 700 radiographs, black-and-white photographs, and line drawings complement the text. Information is included on casting techniques, assessment and treatment of children with cerebral palsy, fracture care, and sports injuries. Chapters are extensively referenced, with some chapters providing guides to additional readings. This book is useful for pediatrics, orthopedics, and podiatry collections.

Levin and O'Neal's The Diabetic Foot. 7th ed. Editors: John H. Bowker, Michael A. Pfeifer. Mosby/Elsevier, 2008.
ISBN: 9780323041454
Recommended for: Hospital, Academic Libraries
Brandon/Hill, *Doody's Core Titles* Selection

Fifty-eight interdisciplinary specialists contributed to the seventh edition of what has become the authoritative book on managing the patient with diabetic foot lesions. It is noted as a Brandon/Hill first-purchase selection. The book includes chapters on pathophysiology, diagnosis, and medical and surgical treatment of diabetic foot problems. The editors provide a balanced, coordinated, team-care approach with multidisciplinary perspectives from diverse health professionals who care for diabetic patients with foot problems, including orthopedists, endocrinologists, vascular surgeons, podiatrists, and wound care nurses. Chapters are included on diagnostic and procedural coding and medical-legal aspects of treating diabetic foot problems. Appendixes provide patient instructions for care of the diabetic foot and a list of useful websites. An interactive DVD developed by the International Working Group on the Diabetic Foot is included. This book is a must for both hospital and academic libraries.

Master Techniques in Podiatric Surgery: Foot and Ankle. Editor: Thomas J. Chang. Lippincott, Williams & Wilkins, 2005.

ISBN: 9780781732352
Recommended for: Hospital, Academic Libraries

This book, written for a podiatric medicine and surgery audience, focuses on techniques in foot and ankle surgery. The book is divided into 41 chapters written by a host of authors recognized for their expertise in foot and ankle surgery and for being leading educators. The book is written as a how-to manual for a variety of surgical procedures. It is profusely illustrated with color and black and white photographs as well as line drawings. Authors describe their preferred techniques, including potential pitfalls and complications that are encountered with various surgical procedures. Each chapter focuses on a specific procedure and covers indications, contraindications, preoperative planning, surgical technique, postoperative management, and complications. Chapters include clinical tips and pearls that should prove useful for podiatry students and residents as well as experienced practitioners. A list of recommended readings appears at the end of each chapter.

Merriman's Assessment of the Lower Limb. 3rd. ed. Editor: Ben Yates. Elsevier Churchill Livingstone, 2009.
ISBN: 9780080451077
Recommended for: Hospital, Academic Libraries

The intent of this book is to encompass all aspects of lower limb assessment. The audience for the book is primarily podiatrists; however, any health care practitioner needing to review assessment of the foot and lower limb will benefit from its thorough discussion of various assessment methods. The editor and contributors are from the UK, yet the information in the book is globally relevant. The third edition has been extensively revised and like its predecessors is divided into four sections. Part 1, "Approaching the Patient," provides an introduction to the assessment process, including the assessment interview, presenting problem, and outcome measures. Part 2, "Systems Examination," covers the separate components of limb assessment such as the medical and social history, and vascular, neurological, musculoskeletal, dermatological, and footwear assessments. Part 3, "Laboratory and Hospital Investigations," focuses on tests that can be performed to support the clinical examination, including blood tests, urine analysis, microbial identification, histopathology, and diagnostic imaging. Part 4, "Specific Client Groups," covers the assessment of special patient groups including pediatric, sports, and older patients. The section also discusses the painful foot, the at-risk foot, and assessment of the surgical patient. Each chapter is well referenced and some chapters include suggestions for further reading. A DVD accompanying the book includes supplementary diagnostic imaging illustrations along with dynamic ultrasound images. This book is recommended for podiatric medicine collections.

Neale's Disorders of the Foot. 8th ed. Editors: Paul Frowen, Maureen O'Donnell, J. Gordon Burrow, Donald Lorimer. Elsevier Churchill Livingstone, 2011.
ISBN: 9780702030291
Recommended for: Hospital, Academic Libraries

This review refers to the seventh edition. The editors state in the preface to the seventh edition that the purpose of this text since the first edition in 1981 has been "to act as a focus of the knowledge base of the profession while at the same time accepting that its role is within the wider medical profession, contributing to it as well as drawing from it." The editors are all from United Kingdom as are most of the contributing authors; therefore, the text emphasizes a British viewpoint. However, it is a comprehensive text relevant to podiatric practice around the world. Chapters discuss dermatology; nail disorders; circulatory, metabolic, and neurological disorders affecting the foot; leprosy; tropical diseases; and diabetic foot disorders. There are chapters describing foot disorders in the elderly and in pediatric patients; and a chapter devoted to sports medicine and injuries is included. Basic biomechanics of gait and structure and function of the foot are discussed, as are orthoses and footwear. Chapters on surgical procedures and infection control round out the text. Most illustrations are in black and white; however, a section of color plates is included at the beginning of the book. *Neale's Disorders of the Foot* provides an excellent overview of podiatric medicine and is a must for any collection serving a podiatric medicine program.

Reconstructive Foot and Ankle Surgery. 2nd ed. Author: Mark S. Myerson. Elsevier Saunders, 2010.
ISBN: 9781437709230
Recommended for: Academic Libraries

This review refers to the first edition. This book is a comprehensive guide to reconstructive foot and ankle surgery most frequently seen in practice by orthopedists and podiatrists. Although the book is authored by an MD, it has applicability to the podiatric surgical practitioner. The book contains numerous full color and black and white photographs that illustrate radiographs and surgical procedures. Each surgical procedure is accompanied by techniques, tips, and pitfalls and each chapter has references for further reading. A DVD narrated by the author accompanies the book and provides demonstrations of the surgical procedures described in the text.

Surgery of the Foot and Ankle. 8th ed. Editors: Michael J. Coughlin, Roger A. Mann, Charles L. Saltzman. Mosby/Elsevier, 2007.
ISBN: 9780323033053
ISBN: 9780323040280 (Online updated edition)
Recommended for: Academic Libraries
Doody's Core Titles Selection

This eighth edition of a classic surgical reference text originally written by Henri DuVries, who was both a podiatrist and MD, is published in two volumes, with two DVDs, and a passcode for a continually updated online edition. The text presents problems of the forefoot, neurologic disorders, arthritic conditions, postural disorders, miscellaneous disorders, sports medicine, pediatric foot and ankle problems, and trauma. It reflects major advances in ankle reconstruction, the management of foot disorders in the diabetic patient, and nerve problems in the foot. Both conservative and surgical treatment options are covered. The accompanying DVD includes 59 video clips that detail key procedures. Color photographs and drawings illustrate the surgical procedures and contribute to the overall didactic objectives of the book.

Surgical Reconstruction of the Diabetic Foot and Ankle. Editor: Thomas Zgonis. Lippincott Williams & Wilkins, 2009.
ISBN: 9780781784580
Recommended for: Hospital, Academic Libraries

This book is a comprehensive review of surgical treatment of foot disorders in persons with diabetes. The editor and contributing authors present a detailed, logical, and pragmatic methodology for evaluating and treating diabetic pathology of the foot and ankle. The book has 29 chapters authored by a multidisciplinary team representing surgery, orthopedics, and podiatry. Topics covered include surgical reconstruction of the acute and chronic Charcot foot and ankle; local random, muscle, and pedicle flaps for soft tissue coverage of the diabetic foot; equinus deformity and the diabetic foot; surgical management of malunions and nonunions; and autogeneous bone grafting and orthobiologics. The book is profusely illustrated with 1,200 illustrations including over 800 in full color. Each chapter is well referenced and some chapters have suggested readings for additional information. With diabetes being a significant health issue in many communities, this book can be recommended for hospital libraries, medical, and podiatric school collections.

Journals

Clinics in Podiatric Medicine and Surgery. v. 3, Elsevier, 1986.
http://www.podiatric.theclinics.com/
ISSN: 15596486
ISSN: 15582302 (Online)
Indexed in: MEDLINE, CINAHL
Recommended for: Academic Libraries

Published four times a year, *Clinics in Podiatric Medicine and Surgery* publishes primarily invited review articles. Each issue is devoted to a single topic. Review articles are intended to update readers on the latest trends in patient management, latest advances in podiatric medicine and surgery, and treatment options. Each focused issue is presented under the direction of an experienced guest editor. *Clinics in Podiatric Medicine and Surgery* is indexed in MEDLINE, CINAHL, and Scopus.

Foot and Ankle Clinics. v. 1, Elsevier, 1996.
http://www.foot.theclinics.com/
ISSN: 10837515
ISSN: 15581934 (Online)
Indexed in: MEDLINE
Recommended for: Academic Libraries

Foot and Ankle Clinics provides comprehensive, state-of-the-art reviews by experts in the field of orthopedics and podiatry. Published four times a year, each issue is devoted to a single topic and provides current, practical information on the diagnosis and treatment of conditions affecting the ankle and foot. Each issue is edited by a guest editor who is an expert in the topic. *Foot and Ankle Clinics* is indexed in MEDLINE, CINAHL Plus, and Scopus.

Foot and Ankle International. v. 15, Data Trace, 1994.
http://www.datatrace.com/medical/FAI_body.htm
ISSN: 10711007
ISSN: 19447876 (Online)
Indexed in: MEDLINE
Recommended for: Academic Libraries

Foot and Ankle International, published monthly, is the official publication of the American Orthopaedic Foot and Ankle Society. The journal offers peer-reviewed articles emphasizing surgical and medical management as well as basic clinical research related to foot and ankle problems. The journal focuses on the following areas of interest: surgery, wound care, bone healing, pain management, in-office orthotic systems, diabetes, and sports medicine. *Foot and Ankle International* is indexed in MEDLINE, CINAHL Plus, and Scopus.

Journal of Foot & Ankle Surgery. v. 32, Elsevier, 1993.
http://www.elsevier.com./locate/jfas
ISSN: 10672516
ISSN: 15422224 (Online)
Indexed in: MEDLINE, CINAHL
Recommended for: Academic Libraries

Journal of Foot & Ankle Surgery is the official journal of the American College of Foot and Ankle Surgeons. It is a leading source for original, clinically-focused articles on the surgical and medical management of the foot and ankle. Each bi-monthly, peer-reviewed issue addresses relevant topics to the profession of foot and ankle surgery, such as adult reconstruction of the forefoot, adult reconstruction of the hindfoot and ankle, diabetes, medicine/rheumatology, pediatrics, research, sports medicine, trauma, and tumors. *Journal of Foot & Ankle Surgery* is indexed in MEDLINE, CINAHL, and Scopus.

Journal of the American Podiatric Medical Association. v. 75, American Podiatric Medical Association, 1985.
http://www.japmaonline.org/
ISSN: 87507315
ISSN: 19308264 (Online)
Indexed in: MEDLINE, CINAHL
Recommended for: Academic Libraries

Published by the American Podiatric Medical Association, *Journal of the American Podiatric Medical Association* is the oldest and most frequently cited peer-reviewed journal in the profession of podiatry. The journal publishes research studies, case reports, literature reviews, special communications, book reviews, and other types of submissions. It is indexed in a number of sources including MEDLINE, CINAHL, and Scopus.

20. Medical Psychology

Collaboration between psychologists and physicians in the management of medical problems. It differs from clinical psychology, which is concerned with the diagnosis and treatment of behavior disorders.

—MeSH: Psychology, Medical

Contributor: Tracey Minzenmayer

Monographs

A Compendium of Neuropsychological Tests: Administration, Norms, and Commentary. 3rd ed. Authors: Esther Strauss, Elizabeth M.S. Sherman, Otfried Spreen. Oxford University Press, 2006.
See Chapter 9.4. Behavioral Medicine

Handbook of Adolescent Behavioral Problems: Evidence-Based Approaches to Prevention and Treatment. Editors: Thomas P. Gullota, Gerald R. Adams. Springer, 2005.
See Chapter 9.1. Adolescent Medicine

Handbook of Health Psychology and Aging. 1st ed. Editors: Carolyn M. Aldwin, Crystal L. Park, Avron Spiro III. Guilford Press, 2007.
See Chapter 9.4. Behavioral Medicine

Learning Cognitive-Behavior Therapy: An Illustrated Guide. 1st ed. Authors: Jesse H. Wright, Monica R. Basco, Michael E. Thase. American Psychiatric Publishing, 2006.
See Chapter 9.4. Behavioral Medicine

Journals

Behaviour Research and Therapy. v. 1, Elsevier, 1963.
See Chapter 9.4. Behavioral Medicine

British Journal of Health Psychology. v. 1, British Psychological Society, 1996.
See Chapter 9.4. Behavioral Medicine

Health Psychology. v. 1, American Psychological Association, 1982.
See Chapter 9.4. Behavioral Medicine

Journal of Behavioral Medicine. v. 1, Springer, 1978.
See Chapter 9.4. Behavioral Medicine

Journal of Clinical Psychology. v. 1, Wiley-Blackwell, 1945.
http://onlinelibrary.wiley.com/journal/10.1002/(ISSN)1097-4679
ISSN: 00219762
ISSN: 10974679 (Online)
Indexed in: MEDLINE, CINAHL
Recommended for: Hospital, Academic Libraries

With an impact factor of 1.525 (2009 *Journal Citation Reports*) and a ranking of forty-fourth out of 93 clinical psychology titles, the breadth of coverage in this peer-reviewed journal makes it an essential resource for psychologists. In addition to articles on traditional clinical psychology topics such as psychopathology and psychotherapy, the journal covers clinical outcomes and treatment effectiveness, health psychology, and behavioral medicine. The mix of topics makes this publication particularly appropriate for mental health professionals working in an interdisciplinary environment. Research studies, articles on contemporary professional issues, case reports, news, and notes are included in each issue. Occasionally, special sections focusing on a particular topic are published. This title is recommended for hospitals and academic institutions supporting medical psychologists and other mental health practitioners. Numerous indexing and abstracting sources cite the journal, including CINAHL, Embase, MEDLINE, and PsycINFO. Wiley Online Library provides online coverage starting with volume 1, 1945.

Journal of Psychosomatic Research. v. 1, Elsevier, 1956.
See Chapter 9.4. Behavioral Medicine

Psychological Medicine. v. 1, Cambridge University, 1970.
http://journals.cambridge.org/action/displayJournal?jid=PSM
ISSN: 00332917
ISSN: 14698978 (Online)
Indexed in: MEDLINE
Recommended for: Hospital, Academic Libraries

This interdisciplinary peer-reviewed journal is one of the most respected publications covering the intersection of medicine and mental health. With an impact factor of 5.012, it ranked fourth out of 93 clinical psychology journals and sixth out of 94 psychiatry journals (2009 *Journal Citation Reports*). The journal's main focus is on original research in psychiatry, medical psychology, and related aspects of the basic sciences, but each issue also includes literature reviews, editorials, and book reviews. Although the primary audience of the publication is mental health professionals, physicians will also find articles of interest. Academic libraries supporting training programs for future psychiatrists or psychologists and hospital libraries supporting mental health professionals are highly advised to add this publication to their collections. Numerous indexing and abstracting sources cite this journal, such as CINAHL Plus, MEDLINE, and PsycINFO. Online coverage is available from Cambridge Journals starting with volume 1, 1970.

Journal of Youth and Adolescence: A Multidisciplinary Research Publication. v. 1, Springer, 1972.
See Chapter 9.1. Adolescent Medicine

Psychophysiology: The International Journal of the Society for Psychophysiological Research. v. 1, Wiley-Blackwell, 1964.
http://onlinelibrary.wiley.com/journal/10.1111/(ISSN)1469-8986
ISSN: 00485772
ISSN: 14698986 (Online)
Indexed in: MEDLINE
Recommended for: Hospital, Academic Libraries

Begun in 1964 and superseding *Psychophysiology Newsletter*, this peer-reviewed journal is the oldest and one of the most respected in psychophysiology. Its broad-based coverage includes theoretical, empirical, evaluative, and methodological articles in psychology, psychiatry, neuroscience, behavioral medicine, and biomedical engineering. The main audience for this journal is practitioners and researchers interested in examining the interplay between brain and behavior from a psychophysiological perspective. The journal is published in association with the Society for Psychophysiological Research and has an impact factor of 3.926 (2009 *Journal Citation Reports*). It is highly recommended for academic institutions offering training in the health sciences or mental health fields and for hospitals supporting psychology, psychiatry, and neuroscience programs. This journal is cited in various abstracting and indexing sources, including Embase, MEDLINE, and PsycINFO. Online coverage is available through Wiley Online Library starting with volume 1, 1964.

Psychosomatic Medicine. v. 1, Lippincott Williams & Wilkins, 1939.
http://www.psychosomaticmedicine.org/
ISSN: 00333174
ISSN: 15347796 (Online)
Indexed in: MEDLINE
Recommended for: Hospital, Academic Libraries

With an impact factor of 4.236 (2009 *Journal Citation Reports*) and its status as the official journal of the American Psychosomatic Society, this publication is one of the essential journals for medical psychology and behavioral medicine. This interdisciplinary, peer-reviewed journal focuses on experimental and clinical research on the relationships among social, psychological, and behavioral factors and the physical body. Occasional supplementary issues may contain either reports of original research presented at conferences or monographs. The journal has wide appeal to specialists in behavioral medicine, psychology, psychiatry, physiology, anthropology, and clinical medicine. It is highly recommended for hospitals offering behavior therapy and preventive care and for academic institutions with programs in the behavioral and medical sciences. Numerous indexing and abstracting sources cite this journal, including CINAHL Plus, Embase, MEDLINE, and PsycINFO. Online coverage starting with volume 1, 1939 is available through the American Psychosomatic Society.

21. Medical Sociology

The social determinants and social effects of health and disease, and of the social structure of medical institutions or professions.

—MeSH: Sociology, Medical

Contributor: Christina Daley

Monographs

Medical Sociology. 11th ed. Author: William C. Cockerham. Prentice Hall, 2009.
ISBN: 9780136053101
Recommended for: Hospital, Academic Libraries

Now in its eleventh edition, *Medical Sociology* covers relevant concepts, issues, and research in the field of medical sociology. The reference incorporates the most recent U.S. health statistics, data, and research, with tables and figures reinforcing key concepts and data. The book also includes numerous websites of relevant professional associations and organizations. It is a useful reference tool for students, health care professionals, sociologists, and other individuals who are interested in medical sociology.

The New Blackwell Companion to Medical Sociology. Editor: William C. Cockerham. Blackwell, 2010.
http://www.blackwellreference.com/
ISBN: 9781405188685
Recommended for: Hospital, Academic Libraries

The *New Blackwell Companion to Medical Sociology* boasts a list of 35 respected contributors in the field of medical sociology. The foundation of the book is established in a comprehensive introductory section on the practical aspects and theory of medical sociology. The following sections include essays that address "Health and Social Inequalities," "Health and Social Relationships," "Health and Disease," and "Health Care Delivery." The final section addresses new developments in ethics, genetics and neurosciences. Unlike the previous edition, *The Blackwell Companion to Medical Sociology*, these essays do not give particular attention to regional perspectives.

Perspectives in Medical Sociology. 4th ed. Editor: Phil Brown. Waveland, 2008.
ISBN: 9781577665182
Recommended for: Hospital, Academic Libraries

Now in its fourth edition, *Perspectives in Medical Sociology* is a compendium of articles representative of a wide range of perspectives in the field of medical sociology. The book contains 38 articles covering the social context of health and illness, the state of being ill and the process associated with accessing care, and the health care system. The articles represent a variety of research methods and perspectives utilized in medical sociology. On a macro level, the compendium provides insight into the current social structure and factors impacting medicine. On a micro level, the compendium suggests the future exploration of the individual's experience within the health care system and interactions with the providers. Brown does an excellent job of integrating the classic approaches with the modern approaches, making this an essential resource for students in the health care field, professionals, and sociologists.

The Word as Scalpel: A History of Medical Sociology. Author: Samuel W. Bloom. Oxford University, 2002.
http://extranet.netlibrary.com/TitleSelect/
ISBN: 9780195149296
ISBN: 9780195072327
ISBN: 9781417587575 (Online)
Recommended for: Hospital, Academic Libraries

The Word as Scalpel: A History of Medical Sociology provides a comprehensive history of the field of medical sociology. The origin of medical sociology is traced through biographies and organizational histories. Through the process, the author provides insight into the key figures in medical sociology and the interrelationship of medicine and the social sciences. This work would be recommended for any health science library, academic library, or hospital library.

Journals

Journal of Health and Social Behavior. v. 8, American Sociological Association, 1967.
http://www.asanet.org/journals/jhsb/index.cfm
http://www.sagepub.com/
http://www.jstor.org/journals/00221465.html

ISSN: 00221465
ISSN: 21506000 (Online)
Indexed in: MEDLINE, CINAHL
Recommended for: Hospital, Academic Libraries

The *Journal of Health and Social Behavior*, published by the American Sociological Association, is a premier journal focusing on theoretical issues in medical sociology. The journal publishes empirical and theoretical articles that examine the interrelationships between social factors and health. The journal, which is published quarterly, has an impact factor of 2.350 based on the 2009 *Journal Citation Reports* and ranks ninth out of 50 in the social psychology category. As of 2010, the electronic format will be available via SAGE. It is indexed and abstracted in a variety of sources such as MEDLINE, along with EBSCOhost's SocINDEX and Academic Search Premier.

Social Science & Medicine. v. 1, Elsevier, 1967.
http://www.sciencedirect.com/science/journal/02779536
ISSN: 02779536
ISSN: 18735347 (Online)
See Also Chapter 9.11. Social Medicine
Indexed in: MEDLINE, CINAHL
Recommended for: Hospital, Academic Libraries

Social Science & Medicine is an international and interdisciplinary journal that was founded in 1967. The journal publishes original research and analytical or critical reviews relevant to health and social sciences. The intended audience is social scientists, health professionals, policy makers, and individuals interested in health and illness. According to the 2009 *Journal Citation Reports*, *Social Science & Medicine* was the fourth most cited biomedical social science journal with an impact factor of 2.710 and a five-year impact factor of 3.615. The journal is published 24 times per year and is cited in numerous abstracting and indexing sources, including Academic Search Premier, MEDLINE, and SocINDEX.

Sociology of Health & Illness. v. 1, Wiley-Blackwell, 1979.
http://onlinelibrary.wiley.com/journal/10.1111/(ISSN)1467-9566/
ISSN: 01419889
ISSN: 14679566 (Online)
Indexed in: MEDLINE, CINAHL
Recommended for: Hospital, Academic Libraries

Sociology of Health & Illness is an international, peer-reviewed journal that was founded in 1979. The journal covers issues related to health, medicine, and illness from a sociological perspective. The journal includes original research and review articles with clear empirical and theoretical relevance to the field. The electronic journal home page recently introduced a podcast feature specifically related to the field of medical sociology. The electronic journal also includes virtual special issues designed to highlight classic, relevant works in specific areas within medical sociology. Based on the 2009 *Journal Citation Reports*, the journal has the fifth highest ranking of 115 sociology journals. It has an impact factor of 2.041 and a five-year impact factor of 2.598. The journal is published six times per year with subscribers receiving an additional special issue. It is cited and indexed in numerous sources such as MEDLINE, Academic Search Premier, and SocINDEX.

Databases and Other Electronic Resources

SocINDEX with Full Text. EBSCO, 2006.
http://www.ebscohost.com/
Recommended for: Hospital, Academic Libraries

SocINDEX with Full Text is a comprehensive sociology research database. It provides coverage of sociological topics and the associated subdisciplines, including medical sociology. The database indexes and abstracts articles, books, monographs, conference proceedings, and other resources. Full-text access is provided for over 700 journals, more than 800 monographs, and over 13,000 conferences. A unique feature of SocINDEX with Full Text is the author profiles option. The profiles of over 25,000 authors are accessible in a searchable A-Z format. The listing is updated on an ongoing basis. The profiles contain credentials, contact information, associated journals, keywords, subjects, geographic areas, and people. Full-text journal coverage is available from 1908 to the present. EBSCO also offers the SocINDEX database without the full-text component.

22. Pharmaceutical Technology

The application of scientific knowledge or technology to pharmacy, pharmacology, and the pharmaceutical industry. It includes methods, techniques, and instrumentation in the manufacture, preparation, compounding, dispensing, packaging, and storing of drugs and other preparations used in diagnostic and determinative procedures and in the treatment of patients.

-MeSH

Contributor: Sharon Leslie

Monographs

Ansel's Pharmaceutical Dosage Forms and Drug Delivery Systems. 9th ed. Authors: Loyd V. Allen, Nicholas G. Popovich, Howard C. Ansel. Wolters Kluwer Health/Lippincott Williams & Wilkins, 2010.
ISBN: 9780781779340
See Also Chapter 18. Pharmacy
Recommended for: Hospital, Academic Libraries

This introductory source of pharmaceutical dosage forms and delivery is geared toward pharmacy students. The book addresses all manner of drug formulations: tablet, capsule, transdermal, suppository, injection, etc. The first five chapters cover new drug development, manufacturing standards, biopharmaceutical issues, and the role of regulatory agencies. Subsequent chapters address the manufacture of each form, including use of excipients, mode of action, doses of individual formulations, packaging, and drug stability. Each chapter includes a pharmaceutics and clinical case study, as well as teaching plans. Although well organized and easily readable, it is illustrated with dated-looking black-and-white photographs. Additional Web resources are offered with a print purchase, including a 200-question quiz bank for students. The book is a fine guide for students learning about the drug development process and good practice standards. Hopefully future editions of this *Doody's* starred source will include more modern-looking photographs.

Art, Science, and Technology of Pharmaceutical Compounding. 3th ed. Author: Loyd V. Allen, Jr. American Pharmacists Association, 2008.
ISBN: 9781582121109
See Also Chapter 18. Pharmacy
Recommended for: Hospital, Academic Libraries

Preparing drug formulations for individualized patient healthcare may not be in every pharmacist's repertoire or job description. Most drugs are mass produced by pharmaceutical manufacturing companies before being presented to consumers for use. On a smaller scale, for more personalized prescriptions, a specialty compounding pharmacy or a community pharmacy with trained pharmacists would be called upon to prepare drugs for patients. This text presents the basic technical steps of compounding various medication formulations including capsules, tablets, creams, emulsions, inhalation products, and veterinary products. The author also addresses quality control issues for compounding facilities such as equipment and the regulatory record keeping necessary for compliance. Each chapter describes historical use of the form, applications, recipes, mixing calculations, storage, labeling, stability, and patient counseling issues. The text is written at an introductory level suitable for pharmacy students and academic institutions but also appropriate for practicing compounding pharmacies and hospital libraries.

Encyclopedia of Pharmaceutical Technology. 3rd ed. Editor: James Swarbrick. Informa Healthcare, 2007.
http://www.informaworld.com/9780849393990
ISBN: 9780849393990
Recommended for: Hospital, Academic Libraries

With the third edition, this set has grown from three to six volumes covering 70 additional topics from its previous 2002 incarnation. Arranged alphabetically and illustrated with black-and-white drawings and photographs, each chapter begins with a brief introduction then delves deeper into the subject. The overall themes are drug development, manufacturing, and processing. Topics include everything from various drug delivery routes and microencapsulation technology to laminar airflow equipment, packaging, coloring, and cosmetics. In addition to technology issues it also has chapters on FDA regulations that relate to the drug approval process. Written in easy-to-read language by academics and pharmaceutical industry scientists, this reference set is for graduate students, industry professionals, and academics in pharmaceutical sciences and technology. It is also available in e-book form from the publisher.

Pharmaceutical Calculations. 13th ed. Author: Howard C. Ansel. Lippincott Williams & Wilkins, 2010.
ISBN: 9781582558370
Recommended for: Hospital, Academic Libraries

This classic textbook is used by pharmacy students and practicing pharmacists in community and hospital pharmacies as well as the pharmaceutical industry. Vastly illustrated with figures and tables, the content covers basics such as calculation of doses for pediatric and geriatric patients, intravenous infusions, pharmacokinetic and pharmacoeconomic calculations, veterinary formulas, and how to reduce and enlarge formulas. The appendixes include basic statistical concepts, a glossary, and conversion tables. An additional section provides review problems and answers. Considered the gold standard in the subject, this work is recommended by the American Association of Colleges of Pharmacy's *Basic Resources for Pharmacy Education* as a core title.

Trissel's Stability of Compounded Formulations. 4th ed. Author: Lawrence A. Trissel. American Pharmacists Association, 2009.
http://online.statref.com/titleinfo/fxid-204.html
http://www.r2library.com/
ISBN: 9781582121253
See Also Chapter 18. Pharmacy
Recommended for: Hospital, Academic Libraries

This comprehensive compilation of available drug stability data has added 78 new monographs for a total of 433 in this edition. Because drugs may be altered by heat, light, exposure to oxygen, or humidity, information on how to compound, store, repackage, and ensure stability of drugs is presented. The text includes all types of preparations, such as oral, topical, enteral, and ophthalmic. Organized alphabetically, each entry contains specifics about the drug's properties, stability considerations, compatibility with other drugs, and compatibility with common beverages and foods, with studies and references to support this information. An appendix discusses "Beyond Use" dates for both sterile and non-sterile preparations. For pharmacists in all arenas and hospitals it is also appropriate for academic institutions with schools of pharmacy. It is available in electronic format via STAT!Ref and R2 Libraries.

23. Veterinary Medicine

The prevention, diagnosis, and treatment of diseases in animals.

—MeSH

Contributors: C. Trenton Boyd and Esther Carrigan

Monographs

Georgis' Parasitology for Veterinarians. 9th ed. Author: Dwight D. Bowman. Saunders Elsevier, 2009.
ISBN: 9781416044123
Recommended for: Academic Libraries

This is the ninth edition of a well-respected classic which presents comprehensive information on all parasites found in both domestic and exotic animals. Species covered include dogs, cats, horses, pigs, ruminants, poultry, laboratory animals, and some exotic species. The text begins with an introduction and overview of parasitology, which is new to this edition. Chapters covering the parasites follow and include arthropods, protozoans, and helminths. The next chapter, also new to this edition, on vector-borne diseases, considers viruses, rickettsiae and other bacteria, protozoa, and helminths in the context of disease vectors. The remaining chapters cover antiparasitic drugs, diagnostic parasitology, and histopathological diagnosis. An appendix provides tables of parasiticides for six animal species and a table of commercially available antiparasitic vaccines. This textbook is written for veterinary students, but it would also be useful for residents or practitioners. It is highly recommended as a key resource for any academic or special library that serves a college of veterinary medicine. An online Veterinary Consult version is available for individual purchase from the publisher.

Medical and Veterinary Entomology. 2nd ed. Editors: Gary R. Mullen, Lance A. Durden. Academic Press Elsevier, 2009.
See Chapter 26.7. Parasitology

Merck Veterinary Manual. 10th ed. Editor: Cynthia M. Kahn. Merck & Co., 2010.
http://www.merckvetmanual.com/mvm/
ISBN: 9780911910933
Recommended for: Academic Libraries
Doody's Core Titles Selection

The *Merck Veterinary Manual* is the standard reference source for veterinary information. Veterinary librarians, students, and practitioners widely consider this the ideal starting point in a search for veterinary information. At 3,000 pages, it is comprehensive, thorough, and authoritative. Changes for this tenth edition include expanded and updated information on numerous species of exotic animals, zoonoses, antimicrobial resistance, animal behavior, and immunology topics. Ten new chapters cover "African Hedgehogs"; "Biology of the Immune System"; "Cloning of Domestic Animals"; "Complementary and Alternative Veterinary Medicine"; "Disorders of Potassium Metabolism"; "Equine Metabolic Syndrome"; Poisonous Mushrooms"; "Porcine Circovirus Diseases"; "Pseudopregnancy in Goats"; and "Seminal Vesiculitis in Bulls." The volume features hundreds of color illustrations, including photomicrographs, radiographs, ultrasonographs, and endoscopic images. An online version of this resource is made available free of charge by the Merck and Merial companies as a service to the veterinary profession; a PDA version is also available. The intended audience is veterinary students and practitioners worldwide. This volume is highly recommended as an essential reference for any academic or veterinary library. It would be a useful addition to medical library collections as well.

Merck/Merial Manual for Pet Health. Editor: Cynthia M. Kahn. Merck & Co., 2007.
ISBN: 9780911910995
Recommended for: Academic, Consumer Health Libraries

The *Merck/Merial Manual for Pet Health* is the premier resource for veterinary information written for consumers, i.e., pet owners. It is an animal health counterpart to the very successful and popular home edition of the *Merck Manual of Diagnosis and Therapy*. This volume is an excellent, authoritative, and comprehensive source for answers to the companion animal health and diseases questions that plague pet owners. Besides information on common diseases and disorders, emergency care and first aid, diagnostic tests, drugs and vaccines, there is also information on preventive medicine for pets, traveling with pets, and even choosing the right pet. It covers a wide range of pets: dogs, cats, horses, birds, reptiles, fishes, and other exotics. The intended audience is pet owners, but it is also a very useful reference for both veterinary students and practitioners. It is highly recommended as an essential basic reference for any academic, public, or veterinary library.

Saunders Comprehensive Veterinary Dictionary. 3rd ed. Authors: Douglas C. Blood, Virginia P. Studdert, Clive C. Gay. Saunders Elsevier Saunders, 2007.
ISBN: 9780702027888
Recommended for: Academic Libraries

This is the third edition of the classic veterinary dictionary that was first published in 1988. This dictionary is often described as premier, authoritative, massive, or encyclopedic, and all are appropriate descriptors. As would be expected, it is an excellent source for definitions of scientific and technical terms encountered in veterinary medicine and at over 2,100 pages and over 65,000 definitions, can be considered comprehensive. It also contains a multi-section appendix packed with useful information. The first appendix section presents laboratory services including the International System of Units, temperature equivalents between Celsius and Fahrenheit, and blood groups of domestic animals; the second covers anatomy, featuring the musculoskeletal, circulatory, and nervous systems; next is a clinical section that includes useful information like body temperature equivalents and important venomous snakes. The final section of the appendix is a professional directory that provides an international listing of veterinary schools, veterinary degrees, and veterinary and related organizations and programs. The intended audience for this dictionary is veterinary students, but it is an essential reference for anyone working in the field of veterinary medicine. It is highly recommended as an essential reference for any academic, medical, or veterinary library.

Veterinary Clinical Parasitology. 7th ed. Authors: Anne M. Zajac, Gary A. Conboy. Wiley-Blackwell, 2006.
See Chapter 26.7. Parasitology

Veterinary Parasitology. 3rd ed. Authors: Mike A. Taylor, R.L. Coop, Richard L. Wall. Wiley-Blackwell, 2008.
ISBN: 9781405119641
See Also Chapter 26.7. Parasitology
Recommended for: Academic Libraries

This is the third edition of a well-respected resource in veterinary parasitology. The volume begins with an overview of parasite taxonomy and morphology. The main content is arranged by species and for each species the arrangement follows organ systems. Species covered include cattle, sheep and goats, horses, pigs, dogs and cats, poultry and gamebirds, ungulates, laboratory animals, and exotics. Next are chapters on facultative ectoparasites and arthropod vectors, the epidemiology of parasitic diseases, resistance to parasitic diseases, antiparasitics, and laboratory diagnosis of parasitism. The consistent arrangement within the chapters on the various host species is an especially effective presentation for veterinary students. This third edition is a major update with thoroughly revised and restructured content. The target audience for this resource is veterinary students and researchers, as well as practitioners. It is highly recommended as a key resource for any academic library that serves a program in parasitology or a college of veterinary medicine.

Journals

American Journal of Veterinary Research. v. 1, American Veterinary Medical Association, 1940.
http://www.avma.org/journals/ajvr/ajvr_index.asp
ISSN: 00029645
ISSN: 19435681 (Online)
Indexed in: MEDLINE
Recommended for: Academic Libraries

The *American Journal of Veterinary Research* is the foremost research journal in the field of veterinary medicine. It is ranked as the number two journal in the third edition of the "Basic List of Veterinary Serials," compiled in 2009 by the Veterinary Serials Committee of the Veterinary Medical Libraries Section of the Medical Library Association. Produced by the American Veterinary Medical Association, this international peer-reviewed journal publishes very broadly in the field of veterinary medical research. The mission of this journal is "to enhance the health, welfare, and performance of animals and humans" and to "foster global interdisciplinary cooperation in veterinary medical research." Journal contents include original research articles; reviews of books, media, and software; and a veterinary research news section. It is indexed by most of the major indexing and abstracting services including Academic Search Complete, AGRICOLA, BIOSIS, CAB Abstracts, Current Contents, Embase, Index Veterinarius, ISI Web of Science, MEDLINE, Scopus, and Veterinary Bulletin. The intended audience is graduate and veterinary students, researchers, and practitioners. This title is highly recommended as an essential resource for any academic library which serves a program in animal science or college of veterinary medicine.

Journal of the American Veterinary Medical Association. v. 48, American Veterinary Medical Association, 1915.
http://avmajournals.avma.org/loi/javma
ISSN: 00031488
ISSN: 1943569X (Online)
Indexed in: MEDLINE
Recommended for: Academic Libraries

The *Journal of the American Veterinary Medical Association*, or *JAVMA*, the official publication of the association, is the premier journal in veterinary medicine. This peer-reviewed journal, probably the most widely read publication in veterinary medicine, publishes very broadly in order to encompass anything relevant to the practice of veterinary medicine. It is ranked as the number one journal in the third edition of the "Basic List of Veterinary Serials," compiled in 2009 by the Veterinary Serials Committee of the Veterinary Medical Libraries Section of the Medical Library Association. In addition to original research articles, scientific reports, and special reports, the journal contains a section of *JAVMA* news that includes current information in areas such as academia, business, global issues, government, and the veterinary community, with coming events, meeting information and reports, accolades, and obituaries; classified advertisements; continuing education listings; reviews of books, media, and software; and letters to the editor. Another journal section, "Veterinary Medicine Today," includes regular features of clinical reports such as "What Is the Evidence?," "What's Your Diagnosis?," "Pathology in Practice," and "ECG of the Month." The journal is indexed by most of the major indexing and abstracting services including Academic Search Complete, AGRICOLA, BIOSIS, CAB Abstracts, Current Contents, Embase, Index Veterinarius, ISI Web of Science, MEDLINE, Scopus, and Veterinary Bulletin. The intended audience is graduate and veterinary students, researchers, and practitioners. This title is highly recommended as an essential resource for any academic library which serves a college of veterinary medicine.

Veterinary Parasitology. v. 1, Elsevier, 1975.
http://www.sciencedirect.com/science/journal/03044017
ISSN: 03044017
ISSN: 18732550 (Online)
See Also Chapter 26.7. Parasitology
Indexed in: MEDLINE
Recommended for: Academic Libraries

Veterinary Parasitology is the official organ of the American Association of Veterinary Parasitologists, the European Veterinary Parasitology College, and the World Association for the Advancement of Veterinary Parasitology. This international peer-reviewed journal publishes original research articles, review articles, rapid communications, short communications, letters to the editor, and book reviews. According to its scope statement, the journal is concerned with those aspects of helminthology, protozoology, and entomology that are of interest to animal health investigators, veterinary practitioners, and others with a special interest in parasitology. It covers all aspects of disease prevention, pathology, treatment, epidemiology, and control of parasites in all domestic animals. The parasitology of laboratory animals is included only as a disease model for domestic animals; the parasitology of wild animals is included only where the wild animal acts as a disease or zoonotic reservoir for domestic animals. *Veterinary Parasitology* is indexed and abstracted by all of the major indexing and abstracting services including Academic Search Complete, AGRICOLA, Biological Abstracts, CAB Abstracts, Current Contents, Embase, Index Veterinarius, ISI Web of Science, MEDLINE, Scopus, and Veterinary Bulletin. This journal is highly recommended as an important resource for any academic library that serves a program in parasitology or a college of agriculture, medicine, or veterinary medicine.

Databases and Other Electronic Resources

CONSULTANT: A Diagnostic Support System for Veterinary Medicine. Cornell University, College of Veterinary Medicine, 200?
http://www.vet.cornell.edu/consultant/Consult.asp
Recommended for: Academic Libraries

This online diagnostic support system, founded by Dr. Maurice White, long-term faculty at the Cornell Veterinary College, began in the 1990s as computer discs to be loaded on a single workstation. The program has since been enhanced both technologically and in content. It is available free of charge. According to the information provided on the website, "CONSULTANT is a diagnostic support system used to suggest possible diagnoses or causes for clinical signs and to provide a brief synopsis of the diagnosis/cause including: 1) a general description, 2) species affected, 3) the signs associated with it, and 4) a list of recent literature references. CONSULTANT is supported by a database consisting of hundreds of signs, thousands of diagnoses/causes, and tens of thousands of literature references." The database can be searched by diagnosis or by clinical signs. A particular species can be indicated or the search can span eight species of domestic and wild animals. Species included are avian, canine, feline, bovine, equine, caprine, ovine, and porcine. Literature covering disease classification, diagnosis, treatment, prognosis, and prevention constitute the database that the program searches. The database is not intended to be comprehensive, but to provide the most clinically relevant articles. Recently selected citations for items included in the CONSULTANT database appear on a New and Noteworthy tab. The intended audience is veterinary students, recently qualified veterinarians, or practicing clinicians wishing assistance and confirmation in clinical situations. This very useful diagnostic support system is a required resource for any academic library that serves a school of veterinary medicine.

International Veterinary Information Service: IVIS.
International Veterinary Information Service, 2000.
http://www.ivis.org/
Recommended for: Academic Libraries

This online resource, commonly known as IVIS, is free to veterinarians, veterinary students, animal health professionals, and biomedical librarians. According to the website, "The IVIS project is supported by financial contributions from individuals and corporations that recognize the importance of this site for the veterinary profession and the improvement of animal health worldwide... IVIS was established in 1998 in Ithaca NY by academic faculty from veterinary colleges and veterinary research institutes in North America and Europe." The founding group incorporated as a non-profit organization and by 2000 their website of veterinary resources was available. This online publisher of veterinary books and proceedings also includes a calendar of veterinary meetings, classified ads, continuing education sites, as well as a veterinary drug database that covers over 3,000 products with links to manufacturers' websites and the FDA. Probably the single most useful IVIS content for librarians is the online proceedings. The coverage is international, with proceedings of dozens of international professional veterinary organizations. Although registration is required and access is single-user sign-on with password, this is a very useful resource. Any library that serves a college of veterinary medicine, an animal science program, or practitioners should advertise and promote this resource to its users and staff.

Vetmed Resource. CABI, 200?
http://www.cabi.org/VetMedResource/
Recommended for: Academic Libraries

VetMed Resource is the most comprehensive single source of information on all aspects of veterinary medicine available online. It is fueled by the database of knowledge amassed by CABI in their efforts to provide access to information and knowledge to improve the health and welfare of all species (including humans) worldwide. The foundation of the system is the indexing and abstracting citations and full-text documents from *CAB Abstracts* and the datasheets from another of their products, *Production and Health*. All contents have been chosen for their relevancy to animal diseases and pathogens. This knowledge base grows continuously; it currently numbers more than one million indexing/abstract records covering more than 3,500 journals, books, and conference proceedings; more than 30,000 full-text documents; and more than 800 datasheets. In addition to the abstracts, full-text documents, and datasheets, the resource contains prepared searches, news and reviews, and events. Prepared searches are a very helpful feature, created by expert searchers to yield the best results from the database. They are based on commonly requested topics and there is a link provided to request additional searches. The review articles are specially commissioned and peer-reviewed. The over 2,000 video clips that cover procedures and diagnostic situations would be useful in both teaching and practice environments. This is an excellent, high-quality resource, built on the *CAB Abstracts* database, the premiere index to the veterinary literature. It is highly recommended for any library that serves a college of veterinary medicine or veterinary practitioners.

23.1. Veterinary Anatomy and Physiology

Morphologic structure and normal function in animals.
—Adapted from *Stedman's Medical Dictionary*, 28th ed. (2006)

Contributors: C. Trenton Boyd and Esther Carrigan

Monographs

Anatomy and Physiology of Farm Animals. 7th ed.
Authors: Rowen D. Frandson, W. Lee Wilke, Anna Dee Fails. Wiley Blackwell, 2009.
ISBN: 9780813813943
Recommended for: Academic Libraries

This is the seventh edition of a classic anatomy and physiology text. It is comprehensive in its coverage, providing both microscopic and macroscopic anatomy and physiology, with a special emphasis on the role of cellular and molecular mechanisms in physiological processes. With the addition of a new chapter on poultry in this edition, it covers all farm animals. It receives praise for its clear presentation of the differences between farm species and its successful blending of broad scope and depth of content with clarity of presentation. The content is organized from general introductory concepts which progress through cellular and tissue anatomy and physiology and then move to a body system view. This seventh edition also has enhanced illustrations, with new line drawings and radiographs. While its intended audience is undergraduate and veterinary students, it is also an excellent reference for animal researchers and practitioners. This resource is highly recommended for any academic library that serves an animal science program or a college of veterinary medicine.

Dellman's Textbook of Veterinary Histology. 6th ed. Editors: Jo Ann Eurell, Brian L. Frappier. Wiley Blackwell, 2006.
ISBN: 9780781741484
Recommended for: Academic Libraries
Doody's Core Titles Selection

Since its first publication in 1976, this classic volume has become the leading veterinary histology text. It covers basic histology, cytology, and microscopic anatomy. The volume begins with basic cytology and progresses in 18 chapters through the histology of tissues and organ systems: epithelium, connective and supportive tissues, blood and bone marrow, muscle, nervous system tissue, cardiovascular system, immune system, respiratory system, digestive system, urinary system, male reproductive system, female reproductive system, placentation, endocrine system, integument, eye, and ear. This organization by body system enhances the comparison of different species. The accompanying CD-ROM provides more than 800 color images that include identifying labels and descriptive legends. Its concise presentation and straightforward writing makes it very accessible and a perfect match for its intended audience of first-year veterinary students, but it is also appropriate for graduate students and practicing veterinarians. This title is a required resource for any academic library which serves a college of veterinary medicine, animal science, or comparative histology program.

Dukes' Physiology of Domestic Animals. 12th ed. Editor: William O. Reece. Comstock Cornell University, 2004.
ISBN: 9780801442384
Recommended for: Academic Libraries

This is the twelfth edition and a major revision of the highly-respected classic text in veterinary physiology, *Dukes' Physiology of Domestic Animals*, which first appeared in 1933. *Dukes* is considered the gold standard of veterinary physiology texts. William Reece continues as the editor of this edition, which also employs expert section editors. This comprehensive text of over 50 chapters and 1,000 pages is arranged in six major sections: the body fluids and blood; renal and respiratory function and acid-base balance; the cardiovascular system; digestion, absorption and metabolism; endocrinology, reproduction, and lactation; and nervous system, special senses, muscle, and temperature regulation. The consistent chapter organization, which includes a content outline, study questions, and exercises, makes it well-suited for its intended audience of undergraduate and veterinary students. It is also an excellent reference for practitioners. This resource is highly recommended as an essential resource for any academic library that serves an animal science program or a college of veterinary medicine.

Functional Anatomy and Physiology of Domestic Animals. 4th ed. Author: William O. Reece. Wiley-Blackwell, 2009.
ISBN: 9780813814513
Recommended for: Academic Libraries

Functional Anatomy and Physiology of Domestic Animals is an excellent basic text and overview of structure and function in domestic animals. It covers the most important domestic animals: horses, dogs, cats, cattle, sheep, goats, pigs, and chickens. Of special note for this text is its expanded coverage of avian physiology. Chapter contents include: basics of structure and function; body water: properties and functions; blood and its functions; nervous system; sensory organs; endocrine system; bones, joints, and synovial fluid; muscle; cardiovascular system; respiratory system; urinary system; digestion and absorption; body heat and temperature regulation; male reproduction; female reproduction; and lactation. An appendix provides normal blood values for several species. This edition provides additional illustrations and enhances others through the use of a two-color system for over 350 total illustrations. The chapter design, which includes an outline, study questions, exercises, and the inclusion of clinical correlates make this text well-suited for its intended audience of undergraduate and veterinary students. It is also an excellent reference for practitioners. This resource is highly recommended for any academic library that serves an animal science program or a college of veterinary medicine.

Illustrated Veterinary Anatomical Nomenclature. 2nd ed. Editor: Oskar Schaller. Enke, 2007.

ISBN: 9783830410690
Recommended for: Academic Libraries

This essential reference work, in its second edition, presents over 1,000 illustrations for the more than 6,500 anatomical terms listed in the *Nomina Anatomica Veterinaria*, the international standard for veterinary anatomical terms. Illustrations are by Georghe M. Constantinescu. This comparative anatomy resource is arranged by regions of the body and presents gross anatomical structures. Terms are presented with brief definitions and a labeled illustration on a facing page. The focus is on the major species of domestic animals: cat, dog, pig, ox, sheep, goat, and horse. There is also a section on general anatomical terms and a comprehensive index based on Latin terminology. Contributors to this work are well-respected veterinary anatomists and educators of international stature. This is an excellent resource not only for libraries serving schools of veterinary medicine, but could also serve as a primary resource on veterinary anatomical terms for academic, medical, and public libraries.

Textbook of Veterinary Anatomy. 4th ed. Authors: Keith M. Dyce, Wolfgang O. Sack, Cornelis J.G. Wensing. Saunders/Elsevier, 2010.
ISBN: 9781416066071
Recommended for: Academic Libraries

This comprehensive, scholarly, well-respected textbook of veterinary anatomy presents basic anatomical concepts and covers all species. The work is organized into six main parts which comprise its 37 chapters. The first 10 chapters present basic concepts and the general anatomy of body systems: locomotor, digestive, respiratory, urogenital, endocrine, cardiovascular, nervous, sense organs, and common integument. Parts two through seven each focus on a particular species or class of animal: dogs and cats, horses, ruminants, pigs, and birds. The same logical approach is used to present the information for most animals: head and ventral neck; the neck, back, and vertebral column; thorax; abdomen; pelvis and reproductive organs; forelimb; and hindlimb. This fourth edition provides all color images, including dissection photographs and includes a companion website with additional images and board exam practice questions, which is available only to individual purchasers. The intended audience is the veterinary student; it is often used as a required text in the first year of veterinary school. This title is considered a required text for any academic library that serves a college of veterinary medicine or a program in animal science.

Veterinary Anatomy of Domestic Mammals: Textbook and Colour Atlas. 4th ed. Editors: Horst E. Konig, Hans-Georg Liebich. Shattauer, 2009.
ISBN: 9783794526772
Recommended for: Academic Libraries

This massive (dimensions and weight) volume meets the quality expectations for German atlases. As did earlier editions, this fourth edition English translation combines textbook and color atlas, covering all domestic animals, with special emphasis on dogs, cats, and horses. Information on the ox/cow, pig, sheep, goat, and rabbit is also included. The book begins with a section to build the foundation for the study of veterinary anatomy, covering fundamental concepts as well as the history of the science. This foundational material is followed by 19 chapters covering animal organs and organ systems. There are over 1,000 superb color illustrations, photographs, drawings, radiographs and MRIs, and sonogram and microscopic images to illustrate gross systematic and topographical anatomy. The general approach of the authors is to present the anatomy within a context of clinical conditions. The overall quality of the illustrations is exceptional and far surpasses the text. Given the size and quality of this atlas, the expensive price tag is not a surprise. It is suitable for students, practitioners, and researchers in veterinary medicine. This title is an important resource for any academic library that serves a college of veterinary medicine or with a comparative anatomy program.

Veterinary Embryology. Authors: Thomas A. McGeady, P.J. Quinn, E.S. FitzPatrick, M.T. Ryan. Wiley-Blackwell, 2006.
ISBN: 9781405111478
Recommended for: Academic Libraries

This textbook aspires to provide a thorough discussion of the cellular, molecular, and tissue changes that an animal embryo undergoes as a foundation for understanding the normal development and congenital defects that can occur. It chronicles the developing embryo through nine chapters beginning with cell division, growth, and differentiation up to the point of implantation and placentation. The next section includes twelve chapters on the origin and development of major body systems in the animal embryo. The last two chapters cover age determination of the embryo and fetus, and the genetic, chromosomal, and environmental factors that adversely affect the developing animal. This volume is the best work on animal embryology that is currently available. It is intended for veterinary students, but would be useful for animal science students as well. It is recommended for any academic library that serves a college of veterinary medicine or has an animal science program.

Journals

Anatomia, Histologia, Embryologia: Journal of Veterinary Medicine. Series C. v. 1, Wiley-Blackwell, 2000.
http://onlinelibrary.wiley.com/journal/10.1111/(ISSN)1439-0264
ISSN: 03402096
ISSN: 14390264 (Online)
Indexed in: MEDLINE
Recommended for: Academic Libraries

This premier journal is described as the journal of the World Association of Veterinary Anatomists. It was formerly Series C of the German title, *Zentralblatt fur Veterinarmedizin*, which began in 1953. As indicated by its title, the journal provides a forum for the fields of anatomy, histology, and embryology through research articles, reviews, brief communications, and book reviews. The aims and scope statement of the journal speak to its intent to emphasize the links between animal morphology and experimental and veterinary medicine and to give priority to studies on clinically relevant animal species. It is indexed and abstracted by many of the major indexing and abstracting services, including AGRICOLA, Biological Abstracts, CAB Abstracts, Current Contents, Embase, Index Veterinarius, ISI Web of Science, MEDLINE, and Veterinary Bulletin. Potential readership for this title includes professional and graduate students, faculty, researchers, and clinicians. The basic science focus and comparative species approach make this journal a valuable resource for academic, medical and veterinary libraries.

23.2. Veterinary Dentistry

The teeth, oral cavity, and associated structures, and the diagnosis and treatment of their diseases including prevention and the restoration of defective and missing tissue in animals.
—Adapted from MeSH

Contributors: C. Trenton Boyd and Esther Carrigan

Monographs

Equine Dentistry. 3rd ed. Editors: Jack Easley, Padraic M. Dixon, James Schumacher. Saunders Elsevier, 2010.
ISBN: 9780702029806
Recommended for: Academic Libraries

This review refers to the second edition of a key reference on equine dentistry that first appeared in 1999. It is comprehensive and authoritative, edited by recognized experts in the field and is often referred to as the definitive resource on the subject. A survey of some of its contents illustrates the broad coverage it provides: equine dental evolution; bits, bridles, and accessories; dental anatomy, physiology, and aging; abnormalities; management of oral and dental trauma, periodontal disease, dental decay, endodontic disease, and oral and dental tumors; dental examination and imaging; and various treatments including orthodontics and dental surgery, including equipment and supplies. It is heavily illustrated with both color and black-and-white photographs and line drawings. This edition boasts new and expanded coverage of complications in oral surgery, dental disease of miniature horses, teeth evolution, bits and biting, horse headwear, and dental equipment. The intended audience is veterinary students and practitioners with a focus on equine or mixed practices, as well as veterinary dentists. It is highly recommended as an essential reference for any academic library that serves a college of veterinary medicine.

Small Animal Dentistry: A Manual of Techniques. Author: Cedric Tutt. Wiley-Blackwell, 2007.
http://onlinelibrary.wiley.com/book/10.1002/9780470753187
http://extranet.netlibrary.com/TitleSelect
ISBN: 9781405123723
ISBN: 9781405173315 (Online)
Recommended for: Academic Libraries

This is a key resource on small animal dentistry, written as a practical manual to assist the general small animal practitioner through the routine dental procedures necessary in general practice. It is logically organized for quick consultation. An overview of the chapter content reinforces the practical, routine expectation for its coverage: tooth development, clinical examination, equipping a veterinary dental operatory, radiography, exodontics, jaw fracture repair, oral surgery, suture material, restoration, endodontic therapy, pain management, malocclusions and normal occlusion, and cases to refer to the local veterinary dentist. There are over 400 color illustrations and radiographs to clarify the textual information and to illustrate the step-by-step instructions provided. It also includes practical tips and trouble-shooting suggestions. The intended audience is general veterinary students and small animal or mixed animal practitioners. This text is recommended as an important resource for any academic library that serves a college of veterinary medicine.

Veterinary Dental Techniques: For the Small Animal Practitioner. 3rd ed. Authors: Steven E. Holmstrom,

Patricia Frost Fitch, Edward R. Eisner. Saunders Elsevier, 2004.
http://www.sciencedirect.com/science/book/9780721693835
ISBN: 9780721693835
Recommended for: Academic Libraries

This is the third edition of a key reference on veterinary dentistry in small animals that first appeared in 1992. Now at just over 700 pages, this volume continues the growth pattern seen between editions, with a third more pages than the earlier edition. It is intended to be a practical guide to dental techniques and materials for the small animal practitioner so it covers a wide array of topics. Content includes: dental records, equipment, radiology, prophylaxis and periodontal disease stages, periodontal therapy and surgery, exodontics, endodontics, restorative dentistry, orthodontics, maxillofacial fractures, pain management, regional and local anesthesia, and general health, safety and ergonomics in the veterinary dental workplace. The consistent formatting of chapters to present general comments, indications, contraindications, and advantages and disadvantages for all techniques and dental materials greatly facilitates quick consultation of this resource. An appendix provides a listing of manufacturers and sources of dental materials. In addition to the expected updating for advances in techniques and materials, this edition also includes new chapters on maxillofacial fractures and regional and local anesthesia, plus new material on periodontal disease stages. The intended audience is veterinary students, veterinary dental technicians, small animal practitioners, and veterinary dentists. It is highly recommended as an essential reference for any academic library that serves a college of veterinary medicine.

Journals

Journal of Veterinary Dentistry. v. 4, NICHEPUBS, 1987.
ISSN: 08987564
Indexed in: MEDLINE
Recommended for: Academic Libraries

The *Journal of Veterinary Dentistry* is the official publication of the American Veterinary Dental Society, the Academy of Veterinary Dentistry, and the American Veterinary Dental College. This peer-reviewed title is the primary journal in the field of veterinary dentistry. It covers general veterinary dentistry, operative dentistry, endodontics, orthodontics, periodontics, and restorative dentistry as well as general oral health. Journal content includes original articles, letters to the editor, news items, and announcements. Although online full text is not available, article citations with summaries are available online back to volume 8, 1991 at http://www.jvdonline .org/. It is indexed by most of the major indexing and abstracting services including CAB Abstracts, Embase, Index Veterinarius, ISI Web of Science, MEDLINE, Scopus, and Veterinary Bulletin. The intended audience is veterinary students, dentistry interns and residents, veterinary dental technicians, and practitioners. This title is an important resource for any academic library that serves a college of veterinary medicine or a veterinary dental technician program.

23.3. Veterinary Dermatology

The skin, its structure, functions, diseases, and treatment in animals.

—Adapted from MeSH

Contributors: C. Trenton Boyd and Esther Carrigan

Monographs

Muller & Kirk's Small Animal Dermatology. 6th ed. Authors: Danny W. Scott, William H. Miller, Craig E. Griffin. Saunders Elsevier, 2001.
ISBN: 9780721676180
Recommended for: Academic Libraries

This is the sixth edition of the classic reference on the skin diseases of small animals, which was first published in 1969. With over 1,500 pages, it is comprehensive, covering all aspects of the basic science, etiology, pathogenesis, clinical signs, diagnosis, and therapy of skin diseases in dogs, cats, pet rodents, rabbits, and ferrets. Its 22 chapters begin with the basic anatomy and physiology of the skin, diagnostic methods, and therapies. These are followed by 15 chapters organized by the etiology of the skin disorder. The final four chapters each present a specialized focus, including a chronology of key events in veterinary dermatology beginning with 1900. The text is enhanced by over 1,200 high-quality illustrations that include photographs, line drawings, and diagrams offering clinical, histological, and microscopic views. Colored illustrations are peppered across the chapters. This resource also includes extensive bibliographic chapter references as well as recommendations for client education. Expansion of this edition to present new content added over 300 pages; there are 70 newly recognized dermatologic conditions and the chapter on immunologic skin diseases has been expanded into two chapters. The intended audience is veterinary students, and general and specialty interns, residents, and practitioners. This book is highly recommended as an essential reference for any academic library that serves a college of veterinary medicine.

Pascoe's Principles & Practice of Equine Dermatology. 2nd ed. Author: Derek C. Knottenbelt. Saunders Elsevier, 2009.
ISBN: 9780702028816
Recommended for: Academic Libraries

This is the second edition of a key resource covering dermatological conditions in horses, which was first published in 1999. It is authoritative and comprehensive, yet with a practical approach to the presentation of information, covering both common and rare conditions and diseases with an international perspective. The volume begins with three general chapters on the approach to equine dermatological cases, diagnostic and investigative procedures and the principles of dermatological therapeutics. Twelve chapters on equine dermatological disorders follow, organized by etiology. The final three chapters cover injuries and diseases of the hoof, neoplastic conditions, and syndromes in equine dermatology. This edition has been extensively revised and expanded, with over 200 additional pages over the original 300-paged edition. Most notable are the extensive high-quality color images, with over 650 in the text alone, and an accompanying CD-ROM that offers more than 300 additional illustrations. The intended audience is veterinary students, general and specialty interns, residents, and equine and mixed practitioners. This volume is highly recommended as an essential reference for any academic library that serves a college of veterinary medicine.

Skin Diseases of the Dog and Cat: Clinical and Histopathlogic Diagnosis. 2nd ed. Authors: Thelma Lee Gross, Peter J. Ihrke, Emily J. Walder, Verena K. Affolter. Wiley-Blackwell, 2005.
ISBN: 9780632064526
Recommended for: Academic Libraries

This is the second edition of a highly-regarded specialized reference in small animal dermatology and dermatopathology. By focusing on diagnosis and partnering, and emphasizing the histopathological features of skin diseases along with clinical features, it fills a need in the literature of veterinary dermatology. It is comprehensive, having nearly doubled in size since the first edition was published in 1992, and is written by well-respected experts. Its 37 chapters are divided into two main sections: inflammatory, dysplastic, and degenerative diseases (21 chapters); and neoplasms and other tumors (16 chapters). The first section covers diseases of the epidermis, dermis, adnexa, and panniculus. The section on tumors covers epidermal tumors, follicular tumors, sebaceous tumors, sweat gland tumors, nailbed tumors, fibrous tumors, vascular and perivascular tumors, smooth muscle and skeletal muscle tumors, neural and perineural tumors, and melanocytic, histiocytic, mast cell and lymphocytic tumors. Information for each condition includes etiopathogenesis, clinical features, recommendations for biopsy site selection, and histopathologic features. This edition has improved the already abundant, excellent illustrations with many color images of clinical lesions. In addition, there are over three dozen new inflammatory diseases and the integration of the 1998 World Health Organization standardized tumor nomenclature in the organization and presentation of the chapters on neoplasms. It also increases the presentation of information on analogous human tumors. The intended audience is veterinary students, specialty interns and residents, veterinary dermatologists, veterinary diagnostic pathologists, and small animal practitioners. This work is highly recommended as an essential reference for any academic library that serves a veterinary diagnostic laboratory, a comparative pathology program, or a college of veterinary medicine.

Small Animal Dermatology: A Color Atlas and Therapeutic Guide. 3rd ed. Author: Keith A. Hnilica. Saunders Elsevier, 2010.
ISBN: 9781416056638
Recommended for: Academic Libraries

This third edition is intended as a pictorial companion to the classic reference, *Muller & Kirk's Small Animal Dermatology*. It follows the general organization of that text, using etiology as its chapter organizing factor. It begins with a chapter on differential diagnosis, followed by a chapter on general diagnostic techniques. The final chapter, which was added with the previous edition, presents before and after treatment images of cases. This chapter is especially useful for educating clients and encouraging compliance with treatment regimens. This volume has an abundance of high-quality color images, most notably clinical photographs that present multiple views of lesions. Along with the images, the text also presents the clinical features, differential and diagnostic signs, treatment, and prognosis for each condition. Appendixes provide a listing of available topical shampoos, topical therapeutics, otic preparations, and systemic therapeutic drugs. The intended audience is veterinary students and general and specialty interns, residents, and practitioners. This is highly recommended as an essential reference for any academic library that serves a college of veterinary medicine.

Journals

Veterinary Dermatology. v. 1, Wiley-Blackwell, 1989.
http://onlinelibrary.wiley.com/journal/10.1111/(ISSN)1365-3164
ISSN: 09594493
ISSN: 13653164 (Online)
Indexed in: MEDLINE
Recommended for: Academic Libraries

Veterinary Dermatology is published on behalf of the European Society of Veterinary Dermatology and is the official journal of several international associations: the European Society of Veterinary Dermatology, the American College of Veterinary Dermatology, the American Academy of Veterinary Dermatology, the European College of Veterinary Dermatology, the Canadian Academy of Veterinary Dermatology, the Australian College of Veterinary Scientists, and the Asian Society of Veterinary Dermatology. It is ranked as one of the top 25 journals in the third edition of the "Basic List of Veterinary Serials," compiled in 2009 by the Veterinary Serials Committee of the Veterinary Medical Libraries Section of the Medical Library Association. According to its scope statement, this peer-reviewed international journal publishes papers on all aspects of the skin and skin diseases of mammals, birds, reptiles, amphibians, and fish. The journal contains scientific research papers, clinical case reports, review articles, editorials, letters to the editor, and book reviews. It is indexed by most of the major indexing and abstracting services including AGRICOLA, CAB Abstracts, Current Contents, Index Veterinarius, ISI Web of Science, MEDLINE, Scopus, and Veterinary Bulletin. The intended audience is veterinary students and general and specialty residents, interns, and practitioners. This title is recommended as a key resource for any academic library that serves a college of veterinary medicine.

23.4. Veterinary Emergency Medicine and Critical Care

Resuscitation, transportation and care of animals from the point of injury or beginning of illness through the hospital or other emergency treatment facility.

—Adapted from MeSH

Contributors: C. Trenton Boyd and Esther Carrigan

Monographs

Small Animal Critical Care Medicine. Authors: Deborah C. Silverstein, Kate Hopper. Saunders Elsevier, 2009.
ISBN: 9781416025917
Recommended for: Academic Libraries

This is a welcome addition to the field of small animal critical care medicine. At about a thousand pages, it is a comprehensive and authoritative resource, with over 200 chapters organized into 19 major sections. Appropriately, it begins with a section on assessment and triage and one on common problems seen in intensive care medicine. Other sections that follow cover respiratory disorders; cardiovascular disorders; electrolytes and acid-base disturbances; fluid therapy; endocrine disorders; intoxications including poisoning and drug overdose as well as animal and insect bites; neurologic disorders; infectious disorders; intra-abdominal disorders; urogenital disorders; surgical and postoperative conditions; trauma; anesthesia and pain management; miscellaneous disorders; pharmacology; monitoring; and mechanical ventilation. The appendixes include conversion tables, calculations and continuous rate infusions, reference ranges, and management of the critical care unit. Both common and unusual critical care situations are covered, as well as common internal medicine problems seen from a critical care perspective. It has a clinical orientation, providing salient details in a concise and consistent format to assist the critical care practitioner. The intended audience is the veterinary student, general and specialty interns, residents, and practitioners. This volume is highly recommended as a key resource for any academic library that serves a college of veterinary medicine.

Veterinary Disaster Response. Editors: Wayne E. Wingfield, Sally B. Palmer. Wiley-Blackwell, 2009.
ISBN: 9780813810140
ISBN: 9780813807270 (Online)
Recommended for: Academic Libraries

This volume is a welcome and much-needed addition to the resources available on veterinary disasters and general disaster response. It is endorsed by the Veterinary Emergency and Critical Care Society. This volume presents its content through a question-and-answer format and is peppered with chiefly color illustrations. Its 39 chapters are organized into four main sections: training, disaster planning, preparation, and recovery. The section on training covers a wide array of topics from introducing the Incident Command System, through veterinary risk assessment, zoonotic diseases, wildlife handling, domestic animal handling, first aid, and emergency sheltering, to humane euthanasia and carcass disposal. The clear focus of the section on disaster planning is the elements of the plan from several perspectives: private practice, a community basis, the state and federal level, and the role of the military. The section on disaster preparation considers family issues, preparing a practice for an impending disaster, preparing the farm and its animals, and explores the ethics of veterinary disaster response. The recovery section covers psychological and emotional factors in veterinary disaster response, assistance for homeowners and businesses, and disaster assistance from the American Veterinary Medical Foundation. Its intended audience extends beyond the veterinary medicine sector to include anyone involved in disaster medicine. This volume is highly recommended as a key resource for any academic library that serves a program in emergency planning or a college of veterinary medicine. An e-book version is available from the publisher for individual purchasers.

Veterinary Emergency and Critical Care Procedures. Authors: Tim B. Hackett, Elisa M. Mazzaferro. Wiley-Blackwell, 2006.
ISBN: 9780813823317
Recommended for: Academic Libraries

This resource, with its emphasis on visual presentation of emergency medicine procedures, is a much-needed addition to the literature. Clearly written by experienced emergency care practitioners, it is authoritative and well organized to support its purpose. Its nine chapters cover the following: vascular access techniques, nutritional support, thoracocentesis and thoracostomy tube placement, oxygen supplementation, urinary catheter placement, abdominocentesis and diagnostic peritoneal lavage, pericardiocentesis, central venous pressure (CVP), and a listing of supplies needed. Photographs accompany each step in the instructions provided by this manual. The spiral-bound format facilitates the use of this manual for quick consultation of illustrated techniques. The intended audience is the veterinary student, and both the general practitioner and emergency care specialist. This manual is highly recommended as a key resource for any academic library that serves a college of veterinary medicine.

Journals

Journal of Veterinary Emergency and Critical Care. v. 11, Wiley-Blackwell, 2001.
http://onlinelibrary.wiley.com/journal/10.1111/(ISSN)1476-4431
ISSN: 14793261
ISSN: 14764431 (Online)
Indexed in: MEDLINE
Recommended for: Academic Libraries

The *Journal of Veterinary Emergency and Critical Care* is the official publication of the American College of Veterinary Emergency and Critical Care, the Veterinary Emergency and Critical Care Society, and the European Veterinary Emergency and Critical Care Society. According to the statement of its aims, this international peer-reviewed journal seeks to advance the international clinical standard of care for emergency and critical care patients of all species. The journal publishes basic, applied, and clinical research in the form of original research articles, clinical articles, case reports, review articles, clinical practice reviews, brief clinical communications, and letters to the editor. It is indexed by most of the major indexing and abstracting services including Academic Search Complete, CAB Abstracts, Embase, Index Veterinarius, ISI Web of Science, MEDLINE, Scopus, and Veterinary Bulletin. The intended audience is veterinary students and general and specialty residents, interns, and practitioners. This title is recommended as an important resource for any academic library that serves a college of veterinary medicine.

23.5. Veterinary Endocrinology and Reproduction

The metabolism, physiology, and disorders of the endocrine system and reproduction in animals, and the veterinary problems of fertility and lactation.
—Adapted from MeSH: Endocrinology, Reproduction

Contributors: C. Trenton Boyd and Esther Carrigan

Monographs

Canine and Feline Endocrinology and Reproduction. 3rd ed. Authors: Edward C. Feldman, Richard W. Nelson. Saunders Elsevier, 2004.
ISBN: 9780721693156
Recommended for: Academic Libraries

This is the third edition of the text that has become the gold standard reference for the field since it was first published in 1987. It continues the growth-in-pages-pattern begun with the second edition in 1996; over 300 pages have been added to this edition. This reference provides comprehensive coverage of endocrine, metabolic, and reproductive diseases in dogs and cats. It also includes material on the importance of testing procedures in endocrine and reproductive diseases, including cost-effective and expedient diagnostic protocols. The 1,100 pages of this text are organized into nine sections: pituitary gland, thyroid gland, endocrine pancreas, parathyroid gland, renal hormones, atrial natriuretic hormone, canine female reproduction, canine male reproduction, and feline reproduction. In addition to the customary updating and revisions for currency, this third edition has expanded the material on both hyperadrenacorticism and diabetes mellitus into separate chapters for the dog and cat, as well as expanding the material on canine and feline reproduction. The intended audience is veterinary students, interns and residents, and small animal practitioners. It is recommended as an essential resource for any academic library that serves a college of veterinary medicine.

Current Therapy in Large Animal Theriogenology. 2nd ed. Editors: Robert S. Youngquist, Walter R. Threlfall. Saunders Elsevier, 2007.
ISBN: 9780721693231
Recommended for: Academic Libraries

This is the second edition of the premiere text in large animal reproduction that was first published in 1997. At over a thousand pages contributed by recognized experts in the field, it is comprehensive and authoritative. Its 141 chapters are organized into seven sections by the large animal species they cover: horses, cattle, goats, sheep, swine, llamas, and various special livestock species, chiefly deer and bison. Each of these sections begins with a review of the reproductive anatomy and physiology of both the male and female. This is a research-based, practical presentation of the normal reproduction and reproductive disorders of each of these large animal species. Updates to this edition provide the latest in reproductive technologies throughout the sections, including artificial insemination, embryo transfer, and estrus synchronization. The intended audience is animal scientists, theriogenologists, veterinary students, interns, residents and large animal practitioners. It is highly recommended as a key resource for any academic library that services a program in animal science or reproductive biology, or a college of veterinary medicine.

Journals

Domestic Animal Endocrinology. v. 1, Elsevier, 1984.
http://www.sciencedirect.com/science/journal/07397240
ISSN: 07397240
ISSN: 18790054 (Online)
Indexed in: MEDLINE
Recommended for: Academic Libraries

Domestic Animal Endocrinology is an international peer-reviewed journal that publishes research on the endocrine physiology of domestic animals. Other species are included only when treated as clinical or production models for domestic animals. The journal publishes basic, applied, and clinical research in the form of both original research articles and review articles. It is indexed by most of the major indexing and abstracting services including Academic Search Complete, AGRICOLA, CAB Abstracts, Current Contents, Embase, Index Veterinarius, ISI Web of Science, MEDLINE, Scopus, and Veterinary Bulletin. The intended audience for this journal is graduate students in animal science, physiology, and reproductive biology, as well as veterinary students and general and specialty residents and interns. It is also an excellent resource for researchers and practitioners in animal science, endocrinology, physiology, and veterinary medicine. This title is recommended as an important resource for any academic library that serves a program in animal science or reproductive biology or a college of veterinary medicine.

Theriogenology. v. 1, Elsevier, 1974.
http://www.sciencedirect.com/science/journal/0093691X
ISSN: 0093691X
ISSN: 18793231 (Online)
Indexed in: MEDLINE
Recommended for: Academic Libraries

Theriogenology is an international, well-respected, peer-reviewed journal that focuses on reproduction in animals. Classes of animals covered include domestic and non-domestic mammals, birds, reptiles, and fish. This journal covers a wide range of reproductive biology topics by publishing both basic and applied research in original articles, review articles, and technical notes. It is indexed by most of the major indexing and abstracting services including Academic Search Complete, AGRICOLA, CAB Abstracts, Current Contents, Embase, Index Veterinarius, ISI Web of Science, MEDLINE, Scopus, and Veterinary Bulletin. The intended audience for this journal is graduate students in animal science and reproductive biology, as well as veterinary students and general and specialty residents and interns. It is also an excellent resource for researchers, industry professionals, and practitioners in animal science, reproductive biology, and veterinary medicine. This title is recommended as a key resource for any academic library that serves a program in animal science or reproductive biology or a college of veterinary medicine.

23.6. Veterinary Internal Medicine

The diagnosis and treatment of diseases of the internal organ systems of animals.

—Adapted from MeSH

Contributors: C. Trenton Boyd and Esther Carrigan

Monographs

Clinical Avian Medicine. Editors: Greg J. Harrison, Teresa L. Lightfoot. Spix Publishing, 2006.
ISBN: 9780975499405
Recommended for: Academic Libraries

This resource is a key reference in avian medicine. With two volumes spanning over a thousand pages, it is comprehensive and authoritative, written and edited by international avian experts. It is highly illustrated, predominantly with excellent color photographs, many of which present step-by-step instructions for procedures; there are numerous tables and line drawings as well to summarize and clarify key information. Its 42 chapters cover the basics of clinical avian practice, companion birds, avian behavior and behavior modification, metabolism and nutrition in health and disease, the physical examination, emergency and critical care, drug and other therapies, pain management, preventive medicine, surgery, various diagnostic techniques, toxicology, and infectious diseases. There are several chapters on evaluating and treating disorders of different body systems and several chapters on the management of different avian species. Appendixes include tables of avian hematologic reference ranges and avian biochemistry reference ranges. This resource, with limited availability, can be ordered from the Iowa State University Extension Online Store (http://www.extension.iastate.edu/store/) and the IVIS website (http://www.ivis.org/avianmedicine.asp) in either a print or DVD format. Its intended audience is veterinary students, general and specialty interns, residents, and practitioners. This work is highly recommended as an essential resource for any academic library that serves an avian biology program or a college of veterinary medicine.

Diseases of Poultry. 12th ed. Editor: Y.M. Saif. Wiley-Blackwell, 2008.
ISBN: 9780813807188
ISBN: 9780813807232
Recommended for: Academic Libraries

This is the twelfth edition of the gold standard classic and definitive reference on poultry diseases that was first published in 1943. It is comprehensive and authoritative, covering the topic from a global perspective with international experts as chapter authors. Its 33 chapters are organized into five main sections, based on the etiological disease agent: viral, bacterial, fungal, parasitic, and other causes. The work begins with two general chapters: one on the principles of disease prevention, control, therapy and diagnosis, and a second on host factors for disease resistance. The section on diseases of other causes includes nutritional diseases, developmental and metabolic diseases, toxins and poisons, mycotoxins, and emerging diseases and diseases of complex or unknown etiology, such as multi-causal respiratory and enteric diseases. The disease chapters follow a consistent format to include information on history, etiology, pathobiology, diagnosis, therapy, and prevention and control strategies. Since poultry are chiefly food animals, most of these chapters also include an economic and public health perspective. The intended audience is broad and includes veterinary students, specialist researchers, and practitioners, as well as veterinary pathologists and poultry health workers. This work is highly recommended as an essential resource for any academic library that serves a program in poultry science or a college of veterinary medicine. An e-book is available from the publisher for individual purchase.

Diseases of Swine. 9th ed. Editors: Barbara E. Straw, Jeffery J. Zimmerman. Wiley-Blackwell, 2006.
ISBN: 9780813817033
Recommended for: Academic Libraries

This is the ninth edition of a well-respected classic in swine medicine that was first published in 1958. It is comprehensive and authoritative, covering basic swine health and production as well as swine diseases in over 1,150 pages and 71 chapters. Content progresses from the basics of herd examination, diagnosis, and the immune system, through a general discussion of diseases by body system, specific viral and bacterial diseases, miscellaneous conditions, and finally on to husbandry related topics and the delivery of veterinary services. Discussions of specific diseases follow a standard organization that presents historical perspectives on the disease, etiology, epidemiology, clinical signs, pathogenesis, lesions, diagnosis, immunology, and prevention and control, including vaccines. In addition to the expected revision and updating to reflect developments in the field, this edition boasts several new and expanded disease chapters such as swine fever and West Nile viruses. The intended audience is students in animal husbandry and veterinary medicine as well as large animal or mixed practice veterinarians. This volume is highly recommended as an essential reference for any academic library that serves a program in animal husbandry or a college of veterinary medicine.

Equine Internal Medicine. 3rd ed. Editors: Stephen M. Reed, Warwick M. Bayly, Debra C. Sellon. Saunders Elsevier, 2010.
ISBN: 9781416056706
Recommended for: Academic Libraries

This is the third edition of the premier resource on the practice of equine medicine. With over 1,450 pages of content written by expert contributors, it is comprehensive and authoritative. Its 22 chapters are organized into two main sections: mechanisms of disease and principles of treatment, and disorders of specific body systems. The volume ends with a chapter on disorders in foals and one on toxicologic problems. There is also an accompanying DVD which includes more than 120 high-quality video clips for cardiovascular and neurologic procedures. Using a problem-based approach, it focuses on applying clinical evidence to equine problems and conditions. This edition has been extensively reorganized and updated, adding more than 400 pages to the size of the second edition. New additions to this third edition include new information on changes in body weight, expanded and reorganized coverage of critical care, and new material on inborn errors of metabolism and acquired myopathies. The intended audience is veterinary students, specialty residents, and equine or large animal practitioners. It is highly recommended as an essential resource for any academic library that serves a college of veterinary medicine.

Infectious Diseases of the Dog and Cat. 3rd ed. Editor: Craig E. Greene. Saunders Elsevier, 2006.
ISBN: 9781416036005
Recommended for: Academic Libraries

This is the third edition of the definitive reference on small animal infectious diseases which was first published in 1990. At over 1,400 pages, it is comprehensive and authoritative, written by well-respected content experts. The extensive updating of the third edition can be seen in the over 50 percent increase in size beyond the 1998 second edition. Its 100 chapters are organized into five sections based on etiologic agent: viral, rickettsial, chlamydial and mycoplasmal diseases (32 chapters); bacterial diseases (23 chapters); fungal diseases (14 chapters); protozoal diseases (15 chapters); and clinical problems (16 chapters). Each of the sections on etiologic agents begins with a chapter on diagnostic techniques for that organism, including information on interpreting test results. The last section covers infections of specific body systems and organs, immunodeficiencies and infectious diseases, fever, prevention and management of infectious diseases in multi-cat environments, prevention and management of infection in kennels, immunocompromised people and shared human and animal infections, and immunoprophylaxis. There are nine useful appendixes presenting information such as vaccination recommendations for dogs and cats, manufacturer listings, and an antimicrobial drug formulary. The work is peppered with full-color illustrations, tables, and diagrams and there is an accompanying CD-ROM with extensive reference listings for further study and research. The intended audience is veterinary students, specialty interns and residents, veterinary infectious disease specialists, and small animal practitioners. This work is highly recommended as an essential resource for any academic library that serves a college of veterinary medicine.

Kirk's Current Veterinary Therapy. 14th ed. Editor: John D. Bonagura. Saunders Elsevier, 2009.
ISBN: 9780721694979
Recommended for: Academic Libraries
Doody's Core Titles Selection

This fourteenth edition of a classic resource in veterinary medicine has been long awaited, since the nine-year gap between this and the last edition is three times the accustomed pacing of editions. This is the premiere resource for diseases and therapies in dogs and cats. The work is the product of the collaboration of numerous leading experts in small animal medicine. Spanning over 1,400 pages, its 285 chapters are organized into 13 sections, beginning with critical care situations, toxicologic disorders, 10 sections that organize disorders by body system, and a closing section on infectious diseases. Appendixes are dense with useful information, including reference values, various diagnostic and function tests, nutrient profiles, and a table of common drugs. A companion CD-ROM provides information from the earlier edition that is still considered current therapy. Most chapters follow an established format in presentation: clinical features, basis for therapy, practical hints for treatment, and pending innovations in therapy; this consistency is especially helpful for quick consult situations. It also boasts an extensive index. The intended audience is both the veterinary student and practitioner. It is highly recommended as an essential reference for any academic library that services a college of veterinary medicine.

Large Animal Internal Medicine. 4th ed. Editor: Bradford P. Smith. Mosby Elsevier, 2009.
ISBN: 9780323042970
Recommended for: Academic Libraries

This is the fourth edition of a highly-respected resource on large animal medicine. It is the most current text available on large animal medicine covering equine and ruminant medicine with an international perspective, although it does not cover swine. At over 1,800 pages, it is comprehensive and authoritative, written by experts in the field. Its 54 chapters are organized into seven parts: history, physical examination and medical records; manifestations of disease; disorders and management of the neonate; collection of samples and interpretation of laboratory results; disorders of the organ systems; preventive and therapeutic strategies; and congenital, hereditary, immunologic, and toxic disorders. This work employs a problem-based approach, presenting clinical symptoms and laboratory test results to reach a diagnosis. New content for this edition includes expanded coverage for diagnostic testing, critical care and fluid therapy, biosecurity and infection control, and genetic disorders. The intended audience is veterinary students and large animal or mixed animal practitioners. This volume is highly recommended as an essential resource for any academic library that serves a college of veterinary medicine.

Large Animal Neurology. 2nd ed. Author: Joe Mayhew. Wiley-Blackwell, 2009.
ISBN: 9781405154932
Recommended for: Academic Libraries

This is the long-awaited second edition of the classic reference on the neurologic diseases and disorders of horses, ruminants and swine. Since the earlier edition was published in 1989, this second edition is considerably enhanced over the earlier work. Its 37 chapters are organized into four main parts: the evaluation of large animal neurologic patients; clinical problems in large animal neurology; mechanisms and specific diseases; and the video library. The first part covers neuroanatomy, neurologic evaluation, diagnostic aids, and neuropathology. The clinical problems presented in part two span a wide range including behavior disorders, seizures, sleep disorders, blindness, facial paralysis, disorders of posture and movement, diffuse weakness, and self-mutilation. The varied content of the third part includes congenital, genetic, and familial disorders; infectious, inflammatory, and immune diseases; physical and chemical causes; toxic diseases; nutritional diseases; metabolic diseases; neoplasms and other tumors; and, multifactorial and idiopathic disorders. Part four is the video clip library contained on two accompanying DVDs which illustrates actions, movements, postures, and syndromes that are correlated to the chapter where descriptions occur in the text. The volume is peppered throughout with high-quality color photographs and line drawings. The intended audience is veterinary students, general and specialty interns and residents, veterinary neurologists and large animal practitioners. This work is highly recommended as an essential resource for any academic library that serves a college of veterinary medicine.

Manual of Canine and Feline Cardiology. 4th ed. Editors: Lawrence P. Tilley, Francis W.K. Smith Jr., Mark Oyama, Meg M. Sleeper. Saunders Elsevier, 2008.
ISBN: 9781416023982
Recommended for: Academic Libraries

This is the fourth edition of the highly respected classic text in small animal cardiology; the lead editor is widely considered to be one of the premier experts in the field. It covers all the major areas of cardiology with a comprehensive yet concise and practical approach, distilling complex concepts into quick reference summaries such as bulleted lists, highlighted text boxes, and flowcharts. Its 21 chapters are organized into three main sections covering the diagnosis of heart disease, cardiovascular diseases, and treatment of cardiovascular diseases. There are four very useful appendixes presenting a canine breed listing for predilection for heart disease, common cardiovascular drugs, echocardiographic normals by body weight and breed, and a classification system for canine heart failure. The diagnosis section covers general history and physical examination, and the radiology, electrocardiography, and Doppler ultrasound of the heart, as well as special diagnostic techniques. Specific diseases covered in the next section include valve disease, cardiomyopathy, heartworm disease, cardiac tumors, pericardial disease, congenital disorders, and hypertension. Treatment coverage includes heart failure, arrhythmias and conduction disturbances, cardiopulmonary arrest and resuscitation, emergencies and critical care, and anesthesia. New to this edition are chapters on cor pulmonae and pulmonary thromboembolism, cardiac surgery, and pacemaker therapy. The intended audience is veterinary students, general and specialty interns and residents, veterinary cardiologists, and small animal practitioners. This is highly recommended as an essential resource for any academic library that serves a college of veterinary medicine.

Small Animal Internal Medicine. 4th ed. Editors: Richard W. Nelson, C. Guillermo Couto. Mosby Elsevier, 2009.

ISBN: 9780323048811
Recommended for: Academic Libraries

This is the fourth edition of a highly-respected reference on the internal medicine of small animals that was first published in 1992. At 1,500 pages, it is a comprehensive and authoritative resource on the diseases of dogs and cats, with focused sections written by content experts. Its 104 chapters are organized around the disorders of body systems and etiological agents. A practical diagnostic approach guides the presentation of information throughout this resource, moving from clinical signs and diagnostic testing to therapies and management of the disorder. The work is peppered with chiefly color illustrations to clarify the clinical presentation of diseases and disorders and to visually explain step-by-step procedure guidelines. Summary boxes and tables are provided throughout the work to provide quick reference displays of clinical and differential diagnostic signs and therapies. This fourth edition boasts the addition of many new color photographs and tables, fully updated drug and treatment guideline tables, and the expansion of content on immune-mediated disorders into its own separate section. The intended audience is veterinary students, general and specialty interns and residents, and small animal practitioners. This work is highly recommended as an essential resource for any academic library that serves a college of veterinary medicine.

Textbook of Veterinary Internal Medicine: Diseases of the Dog and the Cat. 7th ed. Editors: Stephen J. Ettinger, Edward C. Feldman. Elsevier Saunders, 2010.
ISBN: 9781416065937 (set)
Recommended for: Academic Libraries

This is the seventh edition of the gold standard classic in small animal medicine that was first published in 1975. Since that first edition, *Ettinger* has been a massive two-volume work, considered the most comprehensive and encyclopedic resource in internal medicine; this seventh edition has 333 chapters and over 2,300 pages. Content begins with the general topics such as physical examination and progresses through diseases and disorders of all body systems and etiological agents. Quite literally, *Ettinger* guides the student or practitioner from the first encounter (physical examination) with canine and feline patients through the last (euthanasia). This work also deals with communicating with clients and owners, including the use of patient information sheets. It is peppered with chiefly color illustrations. In addition to the expected updating to incorporate new developments since the 2005 edition, a scan of the table of contents identifies well over 100 new chapters. The intended audience is veterinary students, general and specialty interns and residents, and small animal practitioners. This work is highly recommended as an essential resource for any academic library that serves a college of veterinary medicine.

Veterinary Medicine: A Textbook of the Diseases of Cattle, Horses, Sheep, Pigs, and Goats. 10th ed. Editors: Otto M. Radostits, Clive C. Gay, Kenneth W. Hinchcliff, Peter D. Constable. Saunders Elsevier, 2007.
ISBN: 9780702027772
ISBN: 9780702039911 (Online)
Recommended for: Academic Libraries
Doody's Core Titles Selection

This is the tenth edition of the highly regarded classic reference on farm animal veterinary medicine that was first published in 1960. It covers all major species of farm animals and covers their diseases from an international perspective. At over 2,100 pages, more than twice the size of the original edition, it is comprehensive and authoritative. Its 35 chapters are organized into two main sections: general medicine, which is chiefly organized around body systems, and special medicine, which is primarily organized by etiology of the disease or condition. The appendixes include conversion tables, reference laboratory values, and a table on drug doses and intervals for horses and ruminants with a separate table for swine. In addition to the expected updating for currency, this edition includes new chapters on diseases caused by prions and emerging diseases. There is expanded coverage of pig diseases, toxicological diseases, and parasitic diseases caused by arthropods. Its intended audience is veterinary students and large animal or mixed animal practitioners. This volume is highly recommended as an essential resource for any academic library that serves a college of veterinary medicine. An electronic Veterinary Consult package is available from the publisher for individual purchasers.

Veterinary Neuroanatomy and Clinical Neurology. 3rd ed. Authors: Alexander DeLahunta, Eric Glass. Saunders/Elsevier, 2009.
http://www.sciencedirect.com/science/book/9780721667065
ISBN: 9780721667065
Recommended for: Academic Libraries

This is the long-awaited third edition of an authoritative reference in veterinary neuroanatomy and neurology. First published in 1977, with a second edition in 1983, this edition has been over 25 years in the making. It is comprehensive, covering all aspects of neuroanatomy, neurophysiology, neuropathology, and clinical neurology, and including both small and large animals. Its 25 chapters are organized by functional neurologic system, with general chapters on neuroanatomy, development of the nervous system, the neurologic examination and case descriptions. The emphasis throughout the work is on diagnosis and development of effective treatment strategies. This third edition boasts over 600 color photographs, line drawings, magnetic resonance brain images, and other radiographs. This text also comes with free access to 370 video clips on Cornell University's website that illustrate the case studies presented in the text. The intended audience is veterinary students, general and specialty interns, residents, and practitioners. This work is highly recommended as an essential resource for any academic library that serves a college of veterinary medicine.

Zoo and Wild Animal Medicine: Current Therapy. 6th ed. Editors: Murray E. Fowler, R. Eric Miller. Saunders Elsevier, 2007.
http://www.sciencedirect.com/science/book/9781416040477
ISBN: 9781416040477
Recommended for: Academic Libraries
Doody's Core Titles Selection

This is the sixth edition of the primary reference in zoo and wild animal medicine, which was first published in 1978. It is comprehensive and international in scope, both in terms of the representation of contributors and content perspective. Its 57 chapters are organized into four main sections based on species: conditions affecting multiple species, poikilotherms, avian, and mammals. The section on conditions affecting multiple species is especially timely, with chapters on West Nile virus, avian influenza, and other emerging diseases which move between wild and domestic species and humans, as well as several chapters on conservation medicine. The section on poikilotherms covers fish, amphibians, and reptiles. Chapters in the mammals section cover chiroptera, rodents, primates, carnivores, marine mammals, elephants, and artiodactyls. Of special note for this edition is its coverage of new and emerging wild animal diseases, the integration of a conservation biology approach to consider the effects of habitat loss on animal populations, and new approaches to monitoring possible zoonotic diseases. The intended audience is veterinary students, general and specialty interns and residents, and exotic animal practitioners, as well as students and researchers in conservation biology. This work is highly recommended as an essential resource for any special library that serves a zoo, or any academic library that serves a program in conservation biology or a college of veterinary medicine.

Journals

Avian Diseases. v. 1, American Association of Avian Pathologists, 1957.
http://www.aaap.info/mc/page.do?sitePageId=57336
ISSN: 00052086
ISSN: 19384351 (Online)
Indexed in: MEDLINE
Recommended for: Academic Libraries

This international peer-reviewed journal is the official publication of the American Association of Avian Pathologists. With a mission to promote avian health, the journal covers all aspects of avian disease from diagnosis through prevention and control. Although the content focus tends to emphasize diseases of poultry, pet and wild birds are also included. Content includes regular research articles, research notes, and case reports. The journal is ranked in the top 20 journals in the third edition of the "Basic List of Veterinary Serials," compiled in 2009 by the Veterinary Serials Committee of the Veterinary Medical Libraries Section of the Medical Library Association. It is indexed by most of the major indexing and abstracting services including AGRICOLA, BIOSIS, CAB Abstracts, Current Contents, Embase, Index Veterinarius, ISI Web of Science, MEDLINE, Scopus, and Veterinary Bulletin. The intended audience is graduate and veterinary students, interns and residents in avian medicine, avian researchers, and practitioners. This title is highly recommended as an essential resource for any academic library that serves a poultry science program, a veterinary diagnostic laboratory, or a college of veterinary medicine.

Equine Veterinary Journal. v. 1, British Equine Veterinary Association, 1968.
http://www3.interscience.wiley.com/journal/123209721/home
ISSN: 04251644
ISSN: 20423306 (Online)
Indexed in: MEDLINE
Recommended for: Academic Libraries

This international peer-reviewed journal is the official journal of the British Equine Veterinary Association. It is the premier journal in equine medicine and is ranked in the top ten journals in the 3rd edition of the "Basic List of Veterinary Serials," compiled in 2009 by the Veterinary Serials Committee of the Veterinary Medical Libraries Section of the Medical Library Association. The journal publishes research that is clinically relevant in the fields of equine and comparative physiology, pathology, medicine, or surgery. It includes original research articles, clinical evidence articles, short communications, and case reports, as well as review articles. The journal also publishes a number of special issues or supplements that focus on a specific topic. It is indexed by most of the major indexing and abstracting services including AGRICOLA, BIOSIS, CAB Abstracts, Current Contents, Embase, Index Veterinarius, ISI Web of Science, MEDLINE, Scopus, and Veterinary Bulletin. The intended audience is graduate and veterinary students, researchers, and practitioners. This title is highly recommended as an essential resource for any academic library that serves a program in equine science or college of veterinary medicine.

Journal of the American Animal Hospital Association. v. 39, American Animal Hospital Association, 2003.
http://www.jaaha.org/
ISSN: 15473317 (Online)
Indexed in: MEDLINE
Recommended for: Academic Libraries

This peer-reviewed journal is the primary scientific and educational publication of the American Animal Hospital Association. It publishes broadly in all areas of small animal medicine and surgery, with a focus on clinically relevant articles. This online-only journal was issued in print from 1965 through December 2003. The journal includes original research articles, retrospective studies based on longitudinal reviews of patient records, case series with a specific disease or syndrome focus, case reports, review articles, and letters to the editor. It is ranked in the top 10 journals in the third edition of the "Basic List of Veterinary Serials," compiled in 2009 by the Veterinary Serials Committee of the Veterinary Medical Libraries Section of the Medical Library Association. The journal is indexed by most of the major indexing and abstracting services including AGRICOLA, BIOSIS, CAB Abstracts, Current Contents, Embase, Index Veterinarius, ISI Web of Science, MEDLINE, Scopus, and Veterinary Bulletin. The intended audience is the practicing veterinarian, but it is also suitable for graduate and veterinary students, small animal medicine interns and residents, and researchers. This title is highly recommended as an essential resource for any academic library that serves an animal technology program or a college of veterinary medicine.

Journal of Veterinary Cardiology. v. 1, Elsevier, 1999.
http://www.sciencedirect.com/science/journal/17602734
ISSN: 17602734
ISSN: 18750834 (Online)
Indexed in: MEDLINE
Recommended for: Academic Libraries

This international peer-reviewed journal is the official journal of the European Society of Veterinary Cardiology. The journal publishes very broadly in the field to cover all aspects of basic, clinical, and translational research in cardiovascular disease. There is no limit on species or classes of animals covered. In addition to original research and clinical studies, the journal often includes sections of cardiovascular images, case reports, and clinical vignettes. One very interesting special feature of the journal is its integration of additional web-based images to provide enhanced detail for procedures and diagnostics beyond that which is possible with traditional print-based graphics. It is indexed by many of the major indexing and abstracting services including CAB Abstracts, Embase, Index Veterinarius, MEDLINE, Scopus, and Veterinary Bulletin. The intended audience is graduate and veterinary students, cardiology or internal medicine interns and residents, researchers, and practitioners. This title is recommended as an important resource for any academic library that serves a college of veterinary medicine.

Journal of Veterinary Internal Medicine. v. 1, Wiley-Blackwell, 1987.
http://onlinelibrary.wiley.com/journal/10.1111/(ISSN)1939-1676
ISSN: 08916640
ISSN: 19391676 (Online)
Indexed in: MEDLINE
Recommended for: Academic Libraries

This peer-reviewed journal is the official publication of the American College of Veterinary Internal Medicine, the European College of Veterinary Internal Medicine, the European College of Veterinary Neurology, and the European College of Equine Internal Medicine. Clearly international in scope, it publishes broadly in the internal medicine field of small and large animals. The journal is ranked as the number three journal in the 3rd edition of the "Basic List of Veterinary Serials," compiled in 2009 by the Veterinary Serials Committee of the Veterinary Medical Libraries Section of the Medical Library Association. In addition to original research articles it publishes review articles, case reports, brief communications, and letters to the editor. The editorial policy of the journal is to continuously improve the standards of evidence found in its articles through a clearly defined prioritization of articles accepted for publication, with the top three being meta-analyses of common conditions, prospective and randomized clinical trials, and retrospective case series that include a control population. The journal is indexed by most of the major indexing and abstracting services including Academic Search Complete, AGRICOLA, BIOSIS, CAB Abstracts, Current Contents, Embase, Index Veterinarius, ISI Web of Science, MEDLINE, Scopus, and Veterinary Bulletin. The intended audience is graduate and veterinary students, researchers, and practitioners. This title is highly recommended as an essential resource for any academic library that serves a college of veterinary medicine.

Journal of Wildlife Diseases. v. 6, Wildlife Disease Association, 1970.
http://www.jwildlifedis.org/
ISSN: 00903558
ISSN: 19433700 (Online)
Indexed in: MEDLINE
Recommended for: Academic Libraries

This international peer-reviewed journal is the official journal of the Wildlife Disease Association. The journal has a broad scope in order to cover wildlife diseases and management topics worldwide. It describes its scope as "dealing with all aspects of infectious, parasitic, toxic, nutritional, physiologic, developmental and neoplastic diseases, environmental contamination, and other factors impinging on the health and survival of free-living or captive populations of wild animals, including fish." The journal also covers zoonoses involving wild animals as well as the chemical immobilization used for them. It includes original research articles, selected case reports and survey reports, review articles, and book reviews. This journal is ranked in the top 15 journals in the third edition of the "Basic List of Veterinary Serials," compiled in 2009 by the Veterinary Serials Committee of the Veterinary Medical Libraries Section of the Medical Library Association. It is indexed by most of the major indexing and abstracting services including AGRICOLA, BIOSIS, CAB Abstracts, Current Contents, Embase, Index Veterinarius, ISI Web of Science, MEDLINE, Scopus, and Veterinary Bulletin. The intended audience is graduate and veterinary students, researchers, and practitioners. This title is highly recommended as a key resource for any special library that serves a zoo, or any academic library that serves a program in wildlife sciences or a college of veterinary medicine.

Journal of Zoo and Wildlife Medicine. v. 20, American Association of Zoo Veterinarians, 1989.
http://www.bioone.org/loi/zamd
ISSN: 10427260
ISSN: 19372825 (Online)
Indexed in: MEDLINE
Recommended for: Academic Libraries

This international peer-reviewed journal is the official publication of the American Association of Zoo Veterinarians and the European Association of Zoo and Wildlife Veterinarians. The journal aims to support the basic purpose of the American Association of Zoo Veterinarians, "to increase knowledge and understanding of captive and free-ranging wildlife species and to improve the husbandry, preventive medicine, and research required to preserve these animals." Its coverage is worldwide. The journal publishes original research articles, case reports, clinical observations, brief communications, special reports, and review articles. It also includes abstracts from selected articles published elsewhere, book reviews, editorials, and member news. It is indexed by most of the major indexing and abstracting services including AGRICOLA, BIOSIS, CAB Abstracts, Current Contents, Embase, Index Veterinarius, ISI Web of Science, MEDLINE, and Veterinary Bulletin. The intended audience is graduate and veterinary students, researchers, and practitioners. This title is highly recommended as a key resource for any special library that serves a zoo, or any academic library that serves a program in wildlife sciences, marine sciences, or a college of veterinary medicine.

Veterinary Clinics of North America: Equine Practice. v. 1, Saunders Elsevier, 1985.
http://www.vetequine.theclinics.com/
ISSN: 07490739
ISSN: 15584224 (Online)
Indexed in: MEDLINE
Recommended for: Academic Libraries

Veterinary Clinics of North America: Equine Practice is one of several species-specific journal titles that are patterned after the well-known *Clinics of North America* human medicine series. It follows the familiar pattern of that series, using expert guest editors and a featured topic for each volume. This peer-reviewed journal publishes broadly on the diagnosis and treatment of diseases in horses. Examples of recent issue topics include practice management, new perspectives in equine colic, clinical nutrition, performance horse lameness and orthopedics, and evidence-based veterinary medicine. The journal is ranked in the top 10 journals in the third edition of the "Basic List of Veterinary Serials," compiled in 2009 by the Veterinary Serials Committee of the Veterinary Medical Libraries Section of the Medical Library Association. It is indexed by most of the major indexing and abstracting services including AGRICOLA, CAB Abstracts, Current Contents, Embase, Index Veterinarius, ISI Web of Science, MEDLINE, Scopus, and Veterinary Bulletin. The intended audience is graduate and veterinary students, researchers, and practitioners. This title is highly recommended as an essential resource for any academic library that serves a program in animal science, equine science or a college of veterinary medicine.

Veterinary Clinics of North America: Exotic Animal Practice. v. 1, Saunders Elsevier, 1998.
http://www.vetexotic.theclinics.com/
ISSN: 10949194
ISSN: 15584232 (Online)
Indexed in: MEDLINE
Recommended for: Academic Libraries

Veterinary Clinics of North America: Exotic Animal Practice is one of several species-specific journal titles that are patterned after the well-known *Clinics of North America* human medicine series. It follows the familiar pattern of that series, using expert guest editors and a featured topic for each volume. This peer-reviewed journal publishes broadly on the diagnosis and treatment of diseases and disorders in exotic animals. Examples of recent issue topics include geriatrics, bacterial and parasitic diseases, nutrition and behavior of uncommon species, cardiology, hematology and related disorders, toxicology, endocrinology, neuroanatomy and neurodiagnostics, and emergency and critical care. The journal is indexed by many of the major indexing and abstracting services including CAB Abstracts, Embase, Index Veterinarius, MEDLINE and Veterinary Bulletin. The intended audience is graduate and veterinary students, researchers, and practitioners. This title is recommended as an essential resource for any academic library that serves a program in wildlife sciences or a college of veterinary medicine.

Veterinary Clinics of North America: Food Animal Practice. v. 1, Saunders Elsevier, 1985.
http://www.vetfood.theclinics.com/
ISSN: 07490720
ISSN: 15584240 (Online)
Indexed in: MEDLINE
Recommended for: Academic Libraries

Veterinary Clinics of North America: Food Animal Practice is one of several species-specific journal titles that are patterned after the well-known *Clinics of North America* human medicine series. It follows the familiar pattern of that series, using expert guest editors and a featured topic for each volume. This peer-reviewed journal publishes broadly on the diagnosis and treatment of diseases in food animals. Examples of recent issue topics include emerging, reemerging, and persistent infectious diseases of cattle; bovine ultrasound; alpaca and llama health management; bovine neonatology; field surgery of cattle; dairy heifer management; and ruminant diagnostic medicine. The journal is ranked in the top ten journals in the third edition of the "Basic List of Veterinary Serials," compiled in 2009 by the Veterinary Serials Committee of the Veterinary Medical Libraries Section of the Medical Library Association. It is indexed by most of the major indexing and abstracting services including AGRICOLA, CAB Abstracts, Current Contents, Embase, Index Veterinarius, ISI Web of Science, MEDLINE, Scopus, and Veterinary Bulletin. The intended audience is graduate and veterinary students, researchers, and practitioners. This title is highly recommended as an essential resource for any academic library that serves a program in animal science, food animal medicine, or a college of veterinary medicine.

Veterinary Clinics of North America: Small Animal Practice. v. 9, Saunders Elsevier, 1979.
http://www.vetsmall.theclinics.com/
ISSN: 01955616
ISSN: 18781306 (Online)
Indexed in: MEDLINE
Recommended for: Academic Libraries

Veterinary Clinics of North America: Small Animal Practice is one of several species-specific journal titles that are patterned after the well-known *Clinics of North America* human medicine series. It follows the familiar pattern of that series, using expert guest editors and a featured topic for each volume. This peer-reviewed journal publishes broadly on the diagnosis and treatment of diseases in small animals, primarily dogs and cats. Examples of recent issue topics include obesity, diabetes, and adrenal disorders; diseases of the brain; small animal parasites; endoscopy; new concepts in diagnostic radiology; and emerging and reemerging viruses in dogs and cats. The journal is ranked as number five in the third edition of the "Basic List of Veterinary Serials," compiled in 2009 by the Veterinary Serials Committee of the Veterinary Medical Libraries Section of the Medical Library Association. It is indexed by most of the major indexing and abstracting services including AGRICOLA, BIOSIS, CAB Abstracts, Current Contents, Embase, Index Veterinarius, ISI Web of Science, MEDLINE, Scopus, and Veterinary Bulletin. The intended audience is graduate and veterinary students, researchers, and practitioners. This title is highly recommended as an essential resource for any academic library that serves a college of veterinary medicine.

23.7. Veterinary Microbiology and Immunology

Microorganisms such as fungi, bacteria, algae, archaea, and viruses that cause diseases in animals and the hypersensitivity of animals to foreign substances and protection from the resultant infection or disorder.

—Adapted from MeSH: Microbiology, Immunology

Contributors: C. Trenton Boyd and Esther Carrigan

Monographs

Veterinary Immunology: An Introduction. 8th ed. Author: Ian R. Tizard. Saunders Elsevier, 2009.
ISBN: 9781416049890
Recommended for: Academic Libraries

This is the eighth edition of the classic reference in veterinary immunology which was first published in 1977. It covers both general and applied immunology, providing both an introduction to the basic principles of immunology and comprehensive coverage of the immunological diseases and responses which occur in domestic animals. The presentation of this information across species of mammals (horse, cattle, sheep, pig, dog, cat, mouse, human) underscores the intention to help veterinary and immunology students understand the immunological differences between species, and how some animals develop specialized immune systems. The work is peppered with high quality charts, photographs, and graphics to illustrate and clarify complex immunological concepts. In addition to the standard updating required for a rapidly evolving discipline, this edition boasts a new appendix with a comprehensive list of cytokines. Some other notable enhancements include coverage of new discoveries on the receptors of NK cells, newly identified cytokines, CD molecules, and IgA receptors, as well as coverage of emerging diseases such as Stevens-Johnson syndrome and autoimmune sarcolemmal disease in dogs. The intended audience is veterinary students, interns and residents, and practitioners, but it would also be a useful reference for general students of immunology. It is highly recommended as a key resource for any academic library that service a program in immunology or a college of veterinary medicine.

Veterinary Microbiology. 2nd ed. Editors: Dwight C. Hirsh, Nigel J. MacLachlan, Richard L. Walker. Wiley-Blackwell, 2004.
ISBN: 9780813803791
Recommended for: Academic Libraries

This is the second edition of a key resource in veterinary microbiology that was first published in 1999. It is comprehensive, providing an introduction to veterinary microbiology as well as coverage of the bacteria, fungi, and viruses that cause disease in animals. Its 74 chapters are organized into four sections; the six introductory chapters cover concepts involved in infectious diseases including host-parasite relationships, laboratory diagnosis, antimicrobial treatment, and prevention and control. The next two sections present the bacterial and fungal (42 chapters) and viral (18 chapters) disease agents that affect animals. The last section (eight chapters), which is new to this edition, provides a clinical perspective, covering these disease agents from the perspective of the animal host; these chapters are organized around the organ system. Besides the enhancement of this edition with the fourth section, the second and third sections have been revised and reorganized consistently by morphology and taxonomy. Interestingly, the preface to this edition also states that references at the ends of chapters have been eliminated since "almost universal access to the Internet and virtual libraries make such references redundant." The intended audience is veterinary students. It is highly recommended as a key resource for any library that serves a college of veterinary medicine.

Journals

Veterinary Immunology and Immunopathology. v. 1, Elsevier, 1979.
http://www.sciencedirect.com/science/journal/01652427
ISSN: 01652427
ISSN: 18732534 (Online)
Indexed in: MEDLINE
Recommended for: Academic Libraries

Veterinary Immunology and Immunopathology is an international peer-reviewed journal of comparative immunology. It is ranked as one of the top 15 journals in the third edition of the "Basic List of Veterinary Serials," compiled in 2009 by the Veterinary Serials Committee of the Veterinary Medical Libraries Section of the Medical Library Association. The journal publishes basic, comparative, and clinical immunology research in a wide array of topics such as the basic biology of the immune system, immunochemistry, immunogenetics, the immunology of infectious disease and tumors, vaccine development, the immunological aspects of pregnancy, and transplantation immunology. Classes of animals covered include companion animals, farm animals, and wild animals. It includes original research articles, short communications, technical reports, review articles, meeting reports, and book reviews. The journal is indexed by many of the major indexing and abstracting services including BIOSIS, CAB Abstracts, Current Contents, Index Veterinarius, ISI Web of Science, MEDLINE, Scopus, and Veterinary Bulletin. The intended audience for this journal is graduate students in immunology and infectious diseases, as well as veterinary students, research scientists, and practitioners. This title is recommended as an important resource for any academic library that serves a program in immunology or infectious diseases or a college of veterinary medicine.

Veterinary Microbiology. v. 1, Elsevier, 1976.
http://www.sciencedirect.com/science/journal/03781135
ISSN: 03781135
ISSN: 18732542 (Online)
Indexed in: MEDLINE
Recommended for: Academic Libraries

Veterinary Microbiology is an international peer-reviewed journal that is ranked as one of the top 25 journals in the third edition of the "Basic List of Veterinary Serials," compiled in 2009 by the Veterinary Serials Committee of the Veterinary Medical Libraries Section of the Medical Library Association. The journal broadly defines its scope as the microbial diseases of domestic animals that supply food, other useful products, or companionship. It also covers zoonotic diseases in wild animals that may spread to humans or domestic animals. Studies of antimicrobial resistance are also considered in scope. The journal includes original research articles, review articles, short communications, letters to the editor, and book reviews. It is indexed by most of the major indexing and abstracting services including Academic Search Complete, AGRICOLA, CAB Abstracts, Current Contents, Embase, Index Veterinarius, ISI Web of Science, MEDLINE, Scopus, and Veterinary Bulletin. The intended audience for this journal is graduate students in microbiology and infectious diseases, as well as veterinary students, research scientists, and practitioners. This title is recommended as an important resource for any academic library that serves a program in microbiology or infectious diseases or a college of veterinary medicine.

23.8. Veterinary Nutrition Sciences

The study of nutrition processes as well as the components of food, their actions, interaction, and balance in relation to health and disease in animals.

—MeSH: Nutrition Sciences, Animal

Contributors: C. Trenton Boyd and Esther Carrigan

Monographs

Animal Feeding and Nutrition. 10th ed. Editors: Marshall H. Jurgens, Kristjan Bregendahl. Kendall Hunt, 2007.
ISBN: 9780757531767
Recommended for: Academic Libraries

Now in its tenth edition, *Animal Feeding and Nutrition* has become one of the important reference sources for animal nutrition. It is written in a concise outline format, an effective approach for consolidating all the information required to cover the topics for students. The volume begins with a review of nutrients and digestion, including characteristics and recommended levels of nutrients. Feedstuffs and feed additives are covered next, including evaluating feedstuffs for livestock, feed formulation, and the laws and regulations governing commercial feeds. The next several chapters present feeding guides and nutrition requirement tables for swine, beef and dairy cattle, sheep, horses, poultry, dogs and cats. Tables in the volume present nutrient requirements, net energy requirements, and feedstuff composition. The intended audience is undergraduate students in animal science or nutrition. This resource is recommended as a solid introductory text on animal nutrition for any academic library that serves a program in animal science, animal nutrition, or a college of veterinary medicine.

Animal Nutrition Science. Author: Gordon Dryden. CABI, 2008.
ISBN: 9781845934125
Recommended for: Academic Libraries

Animal Nutrition Science presents a wide range of nutrition topics with a focus on land-dwelling animals, including domestic and wild animals. It covers both monogastric and ruminant digestion. Early chapters provide introductory concepts and explore how animals obtain and use foods and nutrients. Much of the text covers how to quantify nutrient requirements in animals and how various nutrients are used by animals. The volume closes with an exploration of how nutrient use can affect the environment through environmental pollution from animal wastes. This textbook is written for undergraduate and graduate students, but would also be useful to veterinary students interested in large animal or wild animal medicine. This resource is recommended as a solid introductory text on animal nutrition for any academic library that serves a program in animal science, animal nutrition, or a college of veterinary medicine.

Livestock Feeds and Feeding. 6th ed. Authors: Richard Kellems, D.C. Church. Prentice Hall, 2010.

ISBN: 9780131594753
Recommended for: Academic Libraries

Livestock Feeds and Feeding, well-established in its sixth edition, is recognized as one of the key resources in animal nutrition sciences. The focus of this textbook is applying the principles of nutrition in the real world context of producing commercially viable livestock that is both safe for consumption and does not harm the environment. The volume begins with a discussion of nutrition, digestive physiology, and nutrient utilization. Next it explores livestock feeds, including supplementation, roughages, mineral and vitamin supplements, feed additives, feed laws and labeling, feed processing, and ration formulation. Several chapters concentrate on the management and feeding practices of a wide array of domestic animals: swine, poultry, dairy cows, dairy calves and heifers, beef cows and beef cattle, horses, sheep, goats, companion and zoo animals, and rabbits. Besides the expected updating based on new scientific nutrition knowledge, this edition also attempts to revise the international framework for livestock production. While the challenge and goal for efficient livestock production remain the provision of a safe, affordable, nutritious food supply, the international context has changed considerably between editions. The intended audience is undergraduate and graduate students in animal science or nutrition. This text is recommended as an important resource on animal nutrition for any academic library that serves a program in animal science, animal nutrition, or a college of veterinary medicine.

Nutrient Requirements of Animals. Author: National Research Council. Committee on Animal Nutrition. National Academy of Sciences, 2007.
ISBN: 9780309105071
Recommended for: Academic Libraries

This is a 10-book set of the most recent editions of the classic *Nutrient Requirements of Domestic Animals* series that began publication in 1944. This set includes individual volumes that cover the nutrient requirements of horses; small ruminants (sheep, goats, cervids, and new world camelids), dogs and cats, nonhuman primates, beef cattle, dairy cattle, swine, laboratory animals, poultry, and fish. These handbooks provide the most comprehensive data available on nutrient requirements; they have been issued by various subcommittees and panels of the Committee on Animal Nutrition of the National Research Council. Several handbooks include either a disk or CD-ROM which provides the opportunity for users to predict nutrient requirements of the particular animal under different situations and varying stages of life. These handbooks are suitable reference tools for veterinary students, as well as undergraduate and graduate students in animal science or nutrition. This resource is recommended for any academic library that serves a program in animal science, animal nutrition, or a college of veterinary medicine.

Journals

Animal Nutrition Series (Washington, D.C.). v. 1, National Academies Press, 2006.
ISSN: none
Recommended for: Academic Libraries

This resource continues the *Nutrient Requirements of Domestic Animals* series. Like its predecessor, it is a series of species reports which are issued by various subcommittees and panels of the Committee on Animal Nutrition of the National Research Council. They are the foundation for animal feed formulas in the United States. Each species handbook is issued in successive editions. Over its history, the series has issued both numbered and unnumbered handbooks. These handbooks provide the most comprehensive data available on nutrient requirements. The National Academies website (http://www.nap.edu) offers free full-text for many of the handbooks and partial content for some of the most recently issued volumes. These handbooks are suitable reference tools for veterinary students, as well as undergraduate and graduate students in animal science or nutrition. This resource is highly recommended for any academic library that serves a program in animal science, animal nutrition, or a college of veterinary medicine.

Animal: The International Journal of Bioscience. v. 1, Cambridge University, 2007.
http://journals.cambridge.org/action/displayJournal?jid=ANM
ISSN: 17517311
ISSN: 1751732X (Online)
Recommended for: Academic Libraries

This international journal of animal biosciences is a multi-national joint venture of the British Society of Animal Science, the Institut National de la Recherché Agronomique, and the European Association of Animal Production. According to its aims and scope statement, "*Animal* aims to publish original, cutting-edge research and horizon-scanning reviews on animal-related aspects of the life sciences at the molecular, cellular, organ, whole animal and production system levels." While emphasis is placed on farm animals, laboratory animal models related to livestock and human health are also in scope. *Animal* strives to emphasize the integrative nature of biological systems. It is sub-divided into several sections: breeding and genetics; nutrition; physiology and functional biology of systems; behavior, health and welfare; livestock farming systems, environmental impact and climate change; and product quality and human health and well-being. This broad scope suits its intended readership of all animal scientists interested in biochemistry, microbiology, nutrition, physiology, modeling, genetics, behavior, immunology, epidemiology, engineering, economics, sociology, food science and technology, human health, farming and land-use management, and policy makers who need information on environmental impact, climate change and food quality, safety and security. *Animal* is indexed and abstracted by all the major abstracting services, including AGRICOLA, Biological Abstracts, BIOSIS Previews, CAB Abstracts, Current Contents, Index Veterinarius, and ISI Web of Science. This journal is recommended for any academic or special library providing support to animal or life science researchers.

Journal of Animal Physiology and Animal Nutrition. v. 85, Wiley-Blackwell, 2001.
http://onlinelibrary.wiley.com/journal/10.1111/(ISSN)1439-0396
ISSN: 09312439
ISSN: 14390396 (Online)
Indexed in: MEDLINE
Recommended for: Academic Libraries

The *Journal of Animal Physiology and Animal Nutrition*, a recent change in title, began publication in 1859 in German. This international peer-reviewed journal publishes original research papers in the fields of animal physiology, physiology and biochemistry of nutrition, animal nutrition, feed technology, and feed preservation. Because it includes both basic and applied research, it is an excellent source for both research findings and more practical information related to methods and techniques. It also publishes review articles on important specialized topics. The *Journal of Animal Physiology and Animal Nutrition* is indexed and abstracted by all the major abstracting services, including AGRICOLA, Biological Abstracts, BIOSIS Previews, CAB Abstracts, Current Contents, Index Veterinarius, ISI Web of Science, and MEDLINE. The intended readership includes biochemists, chemists, engineers, food scientists, geneticists, molecular biologists, nutritionists, physiologists, and others with an interest in animal science. This journal is recommended for any academic or special library providing support to animal researchers.

Journal of Animal Science. v. 1, American Society of Animal Science, 1942.
http://http://jas.fass.org/
ISSN: 00218812
ISSN: 15253163 (Online)
Indexed in: MEDLINE
Recommended for: Academic Libraries

The journal of the American Society of Animal Science is considered the premier journal for animal science. It is the leading source of new knowledge and perspectives in this area. A supplement volume includes meeting abstracts of the society. According to the purpose and scope statement, the journal encompasses a broad range of research topics in animal production and fundamental aspects of genetics, nutrition, physiology, and preparation and utilization of animal products. The journal publishes peer-reviewed research articles, invited reviews, technical notes, and letters to the editor. The *Journal of Animal Science* is indexed and abstracted by all the major abstracting services, including AGRICOLA, Biological Abstracts, BIOSIS Previews, CAB Abstracts, Current Contents, Excerpta Medica, Index Veterinarius, ISI Web of Science, and MEDLINE. The intended readership includes biochemists, animal breeders, economists, embryologists, engineers, food scientists, geneticists, microbiologists, nutritionists, physiologists, processors, public health professionals, and others with an interest in animal production and fundamental aspects of animal sciences. This journal is recommended for any academic or special library providing support to animal researchers.

Journal of Dairy Science. v. 1, American Dairy Science Association, 1917.
http://http://jds.fass.org/
ISSN: 00220302
ISSN: 15253198 (Online)
Indexed in: MEDLINE
Recommended for: Academic Libraries

Published by the American Dairy Science Association, this top-ranked, peer-reviewed journal comprehensively covers dairy cattle research. It presents current technical and scientific information on a wide variety of topics, including nutrition, physiology, feeding, genetics, breeding, and dairy foods. The annual proceedings of the American Dairy Science Association are published jointly with the *Journal of Animal Science*. The *Journal of Dairy Science* is indexed and abstracted by all the major abstracting services, including AGRICOLA, Biological Abstracts, BIOSIS Previews, CAB Abstracts, Current Contents, Index Veterinarius, ISI Web of Science, and

MEDLINE. The intended readership includes biochemists, animal breeders, economists, embryologists, engineers, food scientists, geneticists, microbiologists, nutritionists, physiologists, processors, public health professionals, and others with an interest in dairy science and dairying. This journal is recommended for any academic or special library providing support to animal researchers, especially cattle research.

Nutrient Requirements of Domestic Animals. v. 1, National Academy of Sciences, 1944.
http://www.nap.edu
ISSN: 01480952
Recommended for: Academic Libraries

This resource is actually a series of species reports which began publication in 1944 and have been issued irregularly. These handbooks have been issued by various subcommittees and panels of the Committee on Animal Nutrition of the National Research Council. They are the foundation for animal feed formulas in the United States. Each species handbook is issued in successive editions. Over its history, the series has issued both numbered and unnumbered handbooks. All begin with the title, "The Nutrient Requirements of," which is completed by the species name. These handbooks provide the most comprehensive data available on nutrient requirements. Several handbooks include either a disk or CD-ROM which provides the opportunity for users to predict nutrient requirements of the particular animal under different situations and varying stages of life. The National Academies website (www.nap.edu) offers free full text for many of the handbooks and partial content for some of the most recently issued volumes. While the most recent editions of a few of these species reports have been issued in the new series, *Animal Nutrition Series*, many of the most recent species handbooks available still come from this series. These handbooks are suitable reference tools for veterinary students, as well as undergraduate and graduate students in animal science or nutrition. This resource is highly recommended for any academic library that serves a program in animal science, animal nutrition, or a college of veterinary medicine.

23.9. Veterinary Oncology

The study of neoplasms in animals.
—Adapted from MeSH

Contributors: C. Trenton Boyd and Esther Carrigan

Monographs

Cancer Management in Small Animal Practice. Editors: Carolyn J. Henry, Mary Lynn Higginbotham. Saunders Elsevier, 2010.
ISBN: 9781416031833
Recommended for: Academic Libraries

This is a welcome addition to the veterinary oncology literature. It fills a gap by providing the general practice veterinarian with organized information to support a logical approach to cancer diagnosis and management of their small animal patients. Its 26 chapters are organized into five main parts: cancer principles and concepts; evidence-based approaches to cancer in companion animals; cancer diagnosis and staging; management of cancer; and specific tumors—a head-to-tail approach. The principles and concepts section discusses the various etiologies of veterinary cancers and carcinogenesis. The evidence-based section provides information on epidemiology and statistics, clinical trials, and access to clinical research studies. Cancer diagnosis and staging covers biopsy techniques, histopathology and tumor grading, and imaging modalities from radiographs to advanced magnetic resonance imaging. The management of cancer section discusses chemotherapy, surgery, radiation therapy, immunotherapy, photodynamic therapy, oncologic emergencies, and supportive care. The specific tumors section follows a body system and organ arrangement; each chapter follows a consistent format to cover incidence, etiology and risk factors, clinical features, diagnosis and staging, metastasis, treatment modalities, and prognosis. It also provides drug safety guidelines for safe handling and administration of cancer drugs, and drug information about available formulations, recommended dosages, toxicities, and relative costs. The intended audience is the general veterinary practitioner, but this is also a useful reference for veterinary students, interns, and residents, guiding the non-oncologist from initial diagnosis to end-of-life care. This work is highly recommended as a key resource for any academic library that serves a college of veterinary medicine.

Tumors in Domestic Animals. 4th ed. Editor: Donald J. Meuten. Iowa State Press, 2002.
ISBN: 9780813826523
ISBN: 9780470376928 (Online)
Recommended for: Academic Libraries

This is the fourth edition of a well-respected classic on neoplasms in domestic animals that was first published in 1961. It is comprehensive and authoritative, written by experts in the field. This edition continues the growth pattern exhibited between the earlier editions of this work, the size of the text of each edition increasing with the expansion of knowledge in this field. The work begins with an overview of cancer pathogenesis, diagnosis, and management, and then progresses through 14 chapters of tumors of various tissue, organs, and body systems: skin and soft tissue, hemolymphatic system, joints, bones, muscle, respiratory tract, alimentary tract, liver and gall bladder, urinary system, genital system, mammary gland, endocrine glands, nervous system, and the eye. While the chapter arrangement of earlier editions is maintained, both the text and illustrations have been significantly revised. This work attempts to provide all the clinical information needed to reach an accurate diagnosis and treatment plan for patients. The typical information provided to aid diagnosis of each type of tumor includes clinical information, prevalence data, biological behavior, and information about gross and microscopic lesions. The intended audience for this reference includes veterinary students, specialty interns and residents, veterinary pathologists, and practitioners. This work is highly recommended as an essential reference for any academic library that serves a college of veterinary medicine. An e-book version is available from Wiley at http://www.wiley.com for individual purchasers.

Withrow and MacEwen's Small Animal Clinical Oncology. 4th ed. Editors: Stephen J. Winthrow, David M. Vail. Elsevier Saunders, 2007.
http://www.sciencedirect.com/science/book/9780721605586
ISBN: 9780721605586
Recommended for: Academic Libraries

This is the fourth edition of a classic reference on small animal oncology that was first published in 1989. As indicated by the title, its focus is cancer in the dog and cat. Its 32 chapters are organized into four sections: the biology and pathogenesis of cancer, diagnostic procedures, therapeutic modalities, and specific malignancies, arranged by body system. A comparison of the contents between this edition and the last reveals that there has been extensive updating to reflect the latest advances in diagnosis and therapy. The first general section includes new chapters on the etiology and epidemiology of cancer. A new chapter on molecular diagnostics enhances the diagnostic procedures section in this fourth edition. In the therapeutic modalities section there is a new chapter on molecular targeted therapy as well as one on supportive cancer care. The last section on specific malignancies employs a very helpful, consistent presentation format: incidence and risk factors, pathology, natural behavior of tumors, history and clinical signs, diagnostic techniques, treatment options, and prognosis. There are many full color illustrations throughout. The intended audience is veterinary students, veterinary oncology interns and residents, researchers, specialists, and general practitioners. It is highly recommended as a key resource for any academic library that serves a college of veterinary medicine.

Journals

Veterinary and Comparative Oncology. v. 1, Wiley-Blackwell, 2003.
http://onlinelibrary.wiley.com/journal/10.1111/(ISSN)1476-5829
ISSN: 14765810
ISSN: 14765829 (Online)
Indexed in: MEDLINE
Recommended for: Academic Libraries

Veterinary and Comparative Oncology is the official journal of the Veterinary Cancer Society, the European Society of Veterinary Oncology, the Japanese Veterinary Cancer Society, and the British Veterinary Oncology Study Group. It is an international, peer-reviewed journal that publishes broadly in all aspects of oncology in domestic animals, including research on diagnosis, treatment, and prevention. The journal includes original research articles, brief communications, review articles, carefully selected case reports, solicited editorials, clinical papers, letters to the editor, and abstracts from the published literature. It is indexed by many of the major indexing and abstracting services including Academic Search Complete, AGRICOLA, CAB Abstracts, Embase, Index Veterinarius, ISI Web of Science, MEDLINE, Scopus, and Veterinary Bulletin. The intended audience for this journal is graduate and veterinary students, oncology interns and residents, research scientists, and veterinary practitioners. This title is recommended as an important resource for any academic library which supports an oncology program or a college of veterinary medicine.

23.10. Veterinary Ophthalmology

The structure and function of the animal eye and the medical and surgical treatment of its defects and diseases.
—Adapted from MeSH

Contributors: C. Trenton Boyd and Esther Carrigan

Monographs

Equine Ophthalmology for the Equine Practitioner. 2nd ed. Author: Dennis E. Brooks. Teton Newmedia, 2008.
ISBN: 9781591610403
Recommended for: Academic Libraries

This is the second edition of an important quick consult reference to eye problems in the horse. It is intended to be an "in the field" tool and its organization and outline presentation of information successfully achieves that purpose. With over 600 high-quality clinical photographs, over 550 of those in full color, and its step-by-step diagnosis and treatment protocols, it is an effective aid to both diagnosis and therapy. Specific contents of its eight sections include: general anatomy and physiology of the horse eye; examination of the eye; the equine orbit; eyelids, conjunctiva, nictitans, and nasolacrimal system; corneal ulceration; other corneal problems; cataracts, glaucoma, and uveal tract disease; and retinopathies. It has four appendixes on electroretinography in horses, lavage treatment systems, a glossary of selected veterinary ophthalmic terms, and a listing of drugs. In addition, there is an accompanying CD-ROM containing 29 videos which present specific diagnostic and treatment procedures. Besides the expected updating, this edition has expanded coverage of infectious diseases and expanded information on alternative therapies, retinopathy, virectomy, and ocular manifestations of systemic diseases. The intended audience, as the title indicates, is the equine practitioner; it is also intended for veterinary ophthalmologists and ophthalmology interns and residents. It is highly recommended as a key resource for any academic library that serves a college of veterinary medicine.

Slatter's Fundamentals of Veterinary Ophthalmology. 4th ed. Editors: David J. Maggs, Paul E. Miller, Ron Ofri. Saunders Elsevier, 2008.
ISBN: 9780721605616
Recommended for: Academic Libraries

This is the fourth edition of a highly respected classic in veterinary ophthalmology that was first published in 1981. This text has earned its reputation based on its coverage of a wide range of species, its logical organization, and its precise, detailed original figures. It begins with an overview of the structure and function of the eye, congenital abnormalities, pharmacology and therapeutics, and diagnostic techniques. The bulk of the chapters are ocular tissue-focused, with each chapter presenting the anatomy, physiology, pathophysiology, diseases, diagnostic tests, drug therapy, and new surgical techniques of the particular ocular tissue. Appendixes cover breed predispositions to eye disorders and a glossary of terms. In addition to extensive updating of content, new to this edition are chapters on ocular manifestations of systemic diseases, the ophthalmology of exotic pets, and the addition of color to almost all of the illustrations. The intended audience is veterinary students and practitioners, as well as ophthalmology interns and residents. This text is highly recommended as a key resource for any academic library that serves a college of veterinary medicine.

Veterinary Ophthalmology. 4th ed. Editor: Kirk N. Gelatt. Wiley-Blackwell, 2007.
ISBN: 9780781766579
Recommended for: Academic Libraries
Doody's Core Titles Selection

This is the fourth edition of the highly respected gold standard text in veterinary ophthalmology. It provides comprehensive coverage of the diseases of the animal eye and their medical and surgical treatment. Domestic, exotic, and laboratory animals are all included. Its nearly 1,700 pages are spread over two volumes, which are organized into four major sections: basic vision sciences (four chapters), foundations of clinical ophthalmology (five chapters), canine ophthalmology (14 chapters), and special ophthalmology (seven chapters). The basic vision science section covers ocular embryology, congenital malformations, anatomy, physiology and optics. Its clinical ophthalmology section includes immunity, microbiology, pharmacology and therapeutics, pathology and ophthalmic examination, and diagnosis. Section three provides in-depth coverage of the canine, while the final special ophthalmology section covers cats, horses, food animals, laboratory animals, exotics, and a chapter each on comparative neuro-ophthalmology and ocular manifestations of systemic diseases. New to this edition is coverage of noninvasive imaging technology and DNA tests for inherited retinal degenerations. In addition, the chapters on equine and feline ophthalmology, neuro-ophthalmology, and ophthalmic manifestations of systemic disease have been significantly expanded. The intended audience is veterinary students, general and specialist interns, residents and practitioners, vision scientists, and other scientists interested in comparative ophthalmology. It is highly recommended as a key reference for any academic library that serves a college of veterinary medicine.

Journals

Veterinary Ophthalmology. v. 1, Wiley-Blackwell, 1998.
http://onlinelibrary.wiley.com/journal/10.1111/(ISSN)1463

-5224
ISSN: 14635216
ISSN: 14635224 (Online)
Indexed in: MEDLINE
Recommended for: Academic Libraries

Veterinary Ophthalmology is the official journal of the American College of Veterinary Ophthalmologists and is sponsored by 11 international ophthalmology organizations which have home bases in North and Latin America, United Kingdom, continental Europe, Japan, and Australia. The sponsoring organizations alone are a testimony to its international scope and stature. The intent of this peer-reviewed journal is to broadly cover veterinary and comparative ophthalmology from both a clinical and investigational viewpoint. It publishes original research articles, invited review articles, patient-based case studies and reports, viewpoint articles (usually invited), short communications, and letters to the editor. The journal is indexed by many of the major indexing and abstracting services including Academic Search Complete, AGRICOLA, BIOSIS, CAB Abstracts, Current Contents, Embase, Index Veterinarius, ISI Web of Science, MEDLINE, Scopus, and Veterinary Bulletin. The intended audience for this journal is graduate and veterinary students, ophthalmology interns and residents, research scientists, and practitioners. This title is recommended as an important resource for any academic library that serves a program in comparative or veterinary ophthalmology or a college of veterinary medicine.

23.11. Veterinary Pathology

The causes of and changes produced in the body by disease.
—MeSH: Pathology, Veterinary

Contributors: C. Trenton Boyd and Esther Carrigan

Monographs

Clinical Biochemistry of Domestic Animals. 6th ed. Editors: J. Jerry Kaneko, John W. Harvey, Michael L. Bruss. Academic Press Elsevier, 2008.
http://www.sciencedirect.com/science/book/9780123704917
http://extranet.netlibrary.com/TitleSelect
http://www.ebrary.com/
ISBN: 9780123704917
ISBN: 9786611795382 (Online)
Recommended for: Academic Libraries

This is the sixth edition of a widely respected, standard text in the field. It covers both fundamental and clinical approaches to the diagnosis of disease. Contents include: concepts of normality in clinical biochemistry; DNA technology; carbohydrate metabolism and diabetes; lipids and ketones; proteomics; clinical immunology; the erythrocyte; the porphyrins; iron metabolism; hemostasis; the leukocytes; clinical enzymology; liver function; pancreatic function; gastrointestinal function; skeletal muscle function; kidney function; fluid, electrolyte and acid-base balance; pituitary function; adrenocortical function; thyroid function; reproductive hormones; clinical nutrition; calcium, phosphorus, and magnesium metabolism; trace minerals; vitamins; tumor markers; lysosomal storage diseases; cerebrospinal fluid; clinical toxicology; clinical biochemistry of laboratory rodents and rabbits; and clinical biochemistry of avians. Appendixes include clinical laboratory reference values in a number of animal species. The intended audience for this text is veterinary students, animal science students, researchers, and laboratory technicians at all levels in the health sciences wherever animals are being studied or are patients. It is recommended as an essential reference for any academic or special library that serves a program in animal science, laboratory animal science, a college of veterinary medicine, or a medical school.

Fundamentals of Veterinary Clinical Pathology. 2nd ed. Authors: Steven L. Stockham, Michael A. Scott. Wiley-Blackwell, 2008.
ISBN: 9780813800769
ISBN: 9780470626429 (Online)
Recommended for: Academic Libraries

This book provides in-depth information about common clinical laboratory assays that are used to evaluate domestic mammals. It covers all aspects of clinical pathology, including what assays measure, sample or assay conditions that affect results, and what results indicate about the physiologic or pathologic condition of a patient. Whenever possible, diseases and conditions are grouped by common mechanisms or processes to promote a conceptual understanding of laboratory data that can be generally applied across many species. Understanding physiologic and pathologic processes is emphasized throughout the work. It follows a modified outline format, which increases ease of use. Notable additions to the second edition include increased illustrations, especially color plates, coverage of bone marrow examination, and additional disorders and diagnostic tests. The intended audience is veterinary students, residents, clinical pathologists, and general practitioners. It is recommended as a key resource for any academic or special library that serves a college of veterinary medicine. An electronic version may be purchased by individuals from the publisher's website.

Pathologic Basis of Veterinary Disease. 4th ed. Editors: M. Donald McGavin, James F. Zachary. Mosby Elsevier, 2007.
ISBN: 9780323028707
Recommended for: Academic Libraries
Doody's Core Titles Selection

This comprehensive veterinary pathology textbook, now in its 4th edition, presents both general pathology concepts as well as the pathology of organ systems. This edition begins with six new chapters that provide a discussion of general pathology, covering topics such as cellular and tissue response to injury, vascular disorders, inflammation, wound healing, immunity, and tumor biology. The remaining 14 chapters cover the pathology of organ systems. Illustrative matter is mostly color and of high quality. Emphasis throughout the work is on mechanisms of disease and the disease process. For microbes and injurious agents, the focus is on portals of entry and defense mechanisms. This textbook is written for veterinary students, but would also be useful for pathology residents. It is highly recommended for any academic or special library that serves a college of veterinary medicine.

Schalm's Veterinary Hematology. 6th ed. Editors: Douglas J. Weiss, K. Jane Wardrop. Wiley-Blackwell, 2010.
ISBN: 9780813817989
ISBN: 9780813808963 (Online)
Recommended for: Academic Libraries

This sixth edition of the classic *Schalm's Veterinary Hematology* was 10 years in the making and long-awaited. With over 1,300 pages and nearly 150 chapters in 10 sections, it has been revised and reorganized. Each chapter begins with a content outline. More than 100 clinical cases are also included. The sections present hematopoiesis, hematotoxicity, erythrocytes, leukocytes, hematologic neoplasia, platelets, hemostasis, transfusion medicine, species specific hematology, and quality control and laboratory techniques. This in-depth text covers over 30 species. The sixth edition features a new section on the application of hematology in drug and implant device industry pre-clinical toxicity studies. The intended audience for this textbook is veterinary students, internists, and clinical hematologists. It is highly recommended as an essential reference for any academic or special library that serves a college of veterinary medicine. An e-book option is available for individual purchasers.

Veterinary Hematology: Atlas of Common Domestic and Non-domestic Species. 2nd ed. Authors: William J. Reagan, Armando R. Irizarry Rovin, Dennis B. DeNicola. Wiley-Blackwell, 2008.
ISBN: 9780813828091
Recommended for: Academic Libraries

This second edition of the widely acclaimed *Veterinary Hematology* was long awaited since the first edition appeared 10 years ago. The volume covers hematopoiesis, normal and abnormal red cell morphology, red cell inclusions and parasites, normal and abnormal white cell morphology, white cell inclusions and parasites, lymphoproliferative and myeloproliferative disorders, avian hematology, and reptilian hematology. Besides the typical updating of chapter content, this second edition has added coverage of laboratory animals and pocket pets, two new chapters on avian and exotic animals, and a PC-compatible CD-ROM that provides additional hematological images. Expanding the species covered in the original edition (dogs, cats, horses, ruminants, and llamas), the new edition also covers rats, mice, nonhuman primates, ferrets, rabbits, guinea pigs, avians, and reptiles. The resource, although a slim 128 pages, includes 171 full-color photomicrographs with short morphological descriptions. In addition, the accompanying CD-ROM contains over 2,000 images that can be searched and viewed. The intended audience includes veterinary students, veterinary technicians, and veterinary practitioners. It is highly recommended as a key resource for any academic or special library that serves a college of veterinary medicine.

Journals

Journal of Veterinary Diagnostic Investigation. v. 1, American Association of Veterinary Laboratory Diagnosticians, 1989.
http://jvdi.org/
ISSN: 10406387
ISSN: 19434936 (Online)
Indexed in: MEDLINE
Recommended for: Academic Libraries

The *Journal of Veterinary Diagnostic Investigation* is the official publication of the American Association of Veterinary Laboratory Diagnosticians. It is a key resource in veterinary pathology, having been ranked in the top 15 journals in the third edition of the "Basic List of Veterinary Serials," compiled in 2009 by the Veterinary Serials Committee of the Veterinary Medical Libraries Section of the Medical Library Association. It covers all aspects of veterinary diagnostic science. This international, peer-reviewed journal publishes review articles that cover subjects of current and broad interest to veterinary laboratory diagnosticians, full scientific reports, brief research reports, and case reports. According to the journal scope statement, the major disciplines covered are anatomical pathology, bacteriology and mycology, clinical pathology, epidemiology, immunology, laboratory information management, molecular biology, parasitology, public health, toxicology, and virology. The journal is indexed and abstracted by many of the major indexing and abstracting services including AGRICOLA, CAB Abstracts, Current Contents, Index Veterinarius, ISI Web of Science, MEDLINE, Scopus, and Veterinary Bulletin. It is highly recommended for any academic or special library that serves a program in animal science, a veterinary diagnostic laboratory, or a college of veterinary medicine.

Veterinary Clinical Pathology. v. 6, Wiley-Blackwell, 1977.
http://onlinelibrary.wiley.com/journal/10.1111/(ISSN)1939-165X
ISSN: 02756382
ISSN: 1939165X (Online)
Indexed in: MEDLINE
Recommended for: Academic Libraries

Veterinary Clinical Pathology is the official journal of the American Society for Veterinary Clinical Pathology and the European Society of Veterinary Clinical Pathology. The journal's mission is to provide an international forum for communication and discussion of scientific investigations and new developments that advance the art and science of laboratory diagnosis in animals. This peer-reviewed journal publishes original experimental research and clinical contributions in areas such as biomarkers, clinical chemistry, coagulation and hemostasis, cytopathology, education in clinical pathology, endocrinology, hematopathology, immunohematology and transfusion medicine, experimental and investigative clinical pathology, laboratory management, molecular diagnostics, pathophysiology, quality assurance, and toxicologic clinical pathology. Species covered include domestic, laboratory, avian, and wildlife. The journal is indexed and abstracted by many of the major indexing and abstracting services including AGRICOLA, CAB Abstracts, Current Contents, Index Veterinarius, ISI Web of Science, MEDLINE, Scopus, and Veterinary Bulletin. Online access from volume 1 is available from Wiley-Blackwell. It is highly recommended for any academic or special library that serves a veterinary diagnostic laboratory or a college of veterinary medicine.

Veterinary Pathology. v. 8, Sage, 1971.
http://vet.sagepub.com/
ISSN: 03009858
ISSN: 15442217 (Online)
Indexed in: MEDLINE
Recommended for: Academic Libraries

This key resource for veterinary pathology is the official journal of the American College of Veterinary Pathologists. It is ranked as one of the top 10 journals in the third edition of the "Basic List of Veterinary Serials," compiled in 2009 by the Veterinary Serials Committee of the Veterinary Medical Libraries Section of the Medical Library Association. *Veterinary Pathology* is the premier international journal for basic and applied research involving domestic, laboratory, wildlife, marine and zoo animals, and poultry. This peer-reviewed journal publishes research articles, in-depth reviews, diagnostic investigations of natural and emerging diseases of animals, and reports of experimental studies and animal models of human disease. Typical content headings used regularly to group articles cover topics such as wildlife, marine and zoo animals; laboratory animals; animal models of human disease; oncology; metabolic disease; environmental pathology; infectious disease; diagnostic pathology; and pharmaceutical pathology. The journal is indexed and abstracted by many of the major indexing and abstracting services including AGRICOLA, CAB Abstracts, Current Contents, Index Veterinarius, ISI Web of Science, MEDLINE, Scopus, and Veterinary Bulletin. Online access is available back to volume 1 through Sage. The intended audience includes veterinary students, veterinary pathologists, veterinary diagnostic laboratory staff, comparative pathologists, medical pathology researchers, environmental scientists, and others involved in veterinary diagnosis and animal research across animal species. It is highly recommended for any academic or special library that serves a program in animal science, a veterinary diagnostic laboratory, a college of veterinary medicine, or a medical school.

23.12. Veterinary Pharmacology and Toxicology

The origin, nature, properties, and actions of drugs and their effects on animals, and the detection, chemical composition, and biological action of toxic substances or poisons on animals and the treatment and prevention of toxic manifestations.

—Adapted from MeSH: Pharmacology, Toxicology

Contributors: C. Trenton Boyd and Esther Carrigan

Monographs

Plumb's Veterinary Drug Handbook. 6th ed. Author: Donald C. Plumb. Wiley Blackwell, 2008.
ISBN: 9780813810973
ISBN: 9780813820569 (pocket edition)
ISBN: 9780813821726 (mobile version)
Recommended for: Academic Libraries

This is the sixth edition of a veterinary drug handbook that has become a classic since it first appeared in 1991. New editions are issued about every three years. The main arrangement of this reference is systemic monographs, plus an index. In addition to updated dosages and information for older monographs, and updated information on ophthalmic drugs and small animal therapeutic diets, this sixth edition includes over 70 new drug monographs, a separate section on topical medications, new overdose information from the ASPCA® Animal Poison Control Center on 50 of the drugs most commonly associated with animal overdoses, and a new appendix on overdose decontamination. The intended audience is veterinary students and practitioners as well as veterinary technicians, veterinary pharmacologists, and animal research scientists. This title is highly recommended as an essential reference for any special library that serves a zoo, or any academic library that serves animal researchers, a college of pharmacy, or a college of veterinary medicine. A mobile version is available from the publisher's website.

Small Animal Toxicology. 2nd ed. Editors: Michael E. Peterson, Patricia A. Talcott. Saunders Elsevier, 2006.
ISBN: 9780721606392
Recommended for: Academic Libraries

This is the second edition of a well-respected, comprehensive text on the diagnosis and treatment of poisoning in small animals. The content has been considerably expanded, with over 400 additional pages beyond the 1st edition published in 2001. Some of the new topics covered in this edition include: toxicodynamics and toxicokinetics; effective use of a diagnostic laboratory; considerations in pregnant or lactating poisoned patients; disaster management; house or fire by-products; and, accidental poisoning in non-traditional pets. Toxicants added to this edition include amitraz, anticonvulsants, "Christmas time" plants, grapes and raisins, lilies, macadamia nuts, mercury, metronidazole, oxalate-containing plants, ricin, sodium, and vitamin A. The 84 chapters in this volume are arranged into three sections covering basic toxicologic concepts (12 chapters), general exposures (14 chapters), and the largest section (59 chapters) covering specific toxicants, from acetaminophen to zinc. The consistent organization of the toxicant chapters reinforces the use of this resource in clinical toxicology situations where quick reference is essential. Each toxicant chapter begins with an overview provided in a summary chart; the textual material covers sources, toxicokinetics, mechanisms of action, toxicity ratings, clinical signs, histopathological lesions, diagnostic testing, treatment, prognosis, and prevention. There are also quick reference charts for toxic plants, one of the more common types of poisonings in animals. The intended audience is the small animal practitioner, veterinary interns and residents, and students of veterinary medicine and toxicology. This title is highly recommended as an essential resource for any academic library that serves a program in toxicology or a college of veterinary medicine.

Veterinary Pharmacology and Therapeutics. 9th ed. Editors: Jim E. Riviere, Mark G. Papich. Wiley-Blackwell, 2009.
ISBN: 9780813820613
Recommended for: Academic Libraries
Doody's Core Titles Selection

This is the ninth edition of the classic reference on veterinary pharmacology and therapeutics that first appeared in 1954. Long considered to be the gold standard for the subject, it is comprehensive and has expanded to cover this continuously evolving field. This edition has added another 25 percent in page count over the earlier edition and has greatly expanded the number of contributors, including experts from outside the U.S. Examples of new chapter content include an expansion of the information on the FDA Center for Veterinary Medicine regulatory processes and on veterinary drug compounding. Its over 1,500 pages are organized into 12 sections which begin with principles of pharmacology. This introductory section is followed by nine chapters that are organized around either the target body organ or system, by the type of drug, or by the particular disease therapy. The final two sections cover specialty areas of pharmacology and regulatory considerations. The intended audience is veterinary students and practitioners, interns and residents, as well as animal research scientists. This title is highly recommended as a key title for any academic library that serves programs involved in animal research, a college of pharmacy, or a college of veterinary medicine.

Veterinary Toxicology: Basic and Clinical Principles. Editor: Ramesh C. Gupta. Elsevier/Academic, 2007.
http://www.sciencedirect.com/science/book/9780123704672

ISBN: 9780123704672
Recommended for: Academic Libraries

Although still in its first edition, this sizable (over 1,200 pages), well-respected source is considered the most comprehensive veterinary toxicology reference available, approaching toxicology from a broad, international perspective, and covering both large and small animal species. A survey of the approach taken in the general introductory section illustrates the broad coverage of this text: principles of veterinary toxicology, pharmacokinetics, toxicity testing, modeling, epidemiology of poisoning cases, chemical terrorism, and regulatory, legal, and ethical considerations. The remaining 18 sections cover organ toxicity; nervous system toxicity; nanoparticles, radiation, and carcinogenesis; drugs of use and abuse; metals and micronutrients; insecticides; rodenticides; herbicides and fungicides; toxic gases and smoke; industrial toxicants; environmental toxicology; bacterial toxins; poisonous and venomous organisms; estrogenic toxicants; poisonous plants; mycotoxins; feed and water contaminants; diagnostic toxicology; and therapeutic measures, covering both the prevention and treatment of poisonings. The intended audience includes veterinary students, interns and residents, faculty and practitioners, veterinary toxicologists, poison control centers, animal scientists, marine biologists, and environmental scientists. It is highly recommended as a key resource in animal toxicology for any library that serves a poison control center or any academic library that serves programs in toxicology, environmental sciences, animal science, or a college of veterinary medicine.

Journals

Compendium of Veterinary Products: CVP. v. 1, North American Compendiums, 1991.
http://vetpharm.naccvp.com/?u=vetpharm&p=pharm
ISSN: 10936327
Recommended for: Academic Libraries

This resource is actually a biennially issued publication which is the gold standard handbook for veterinary drugs. The 2008 edition, with over 2,400 pages and listings of over 5,000 pharmaceutical, biological, feed medication, and parasiticides monographs, is the most complete veterinary drug reference available. These entries are arranged by: trade name (alphabetically); manufacturer (products listed alphabetically under each); product category (by species or all species combined); product use (by species); and trade name/ingredient (all species). There is a trade name ingredient index and product category index. Also included is an alphabetical listing of manufacturers and distributors and their contact information. Species specific charts which include anthelmintics and parasiticides, biologicals, and withdrawal times are very useful and accessible. This handbook employs color-coded sections for quick reference consultations. Its intended audience is veterinary students, interns and residents, and practitioners, but it could also be of use to animal owners. This title is highly recommended as an essential resource for any library that serves a program in animal science or a college of veterinary medicine.

Journal of Veterinary Pharmacology and Therapeutics. v. 1, Wiley-Blackwell, 1978.
http://onlinelibrary.wiley.com/journal/10.1111/(ISSN)1365-2885
ISSN: 01407783
ISSN: 13652885 (Online)
Indexed in: MEDLINE
Recommended for: Academic Libraries

The *Journal of Veterinary Pharmacology and Therapeutics* is an international peer-reviewed journal that is published on behalf of several international pharmacological associations: American Academy of Veterinary Pharmacology and Therapeutics, American College of Veterinary Clinical Pharmacology, Association for Veterinary Clinical Pharmacology and Therapeutics (UK), European Association for Veterinary Pharmacology and Toxicology, and the Chapter of Veterinary Pharmacology of the Australian College of Veterinary Scientists. It is ranked as one of the top 20 journals in the third edition of the "Basic List of Veterinary Serials," compiled in 2009 by the Veterinary Serials Committee of the Veterinary Medical Libraries Section of the Medical Library Association. The journal scope covers both the basic and clinical research aspects of veterinary pharmacology, therapeutics, and toxicology. It includes original research articles, review articles, short communications, letters to the editors, and book reviews. The journal is indexed by many of the major indexing and abstracting services including Academic Search Complete, AGRICOLA, BIOSIS, CAB Abstracts, Current Contents, Embase, Index Veterinarius, ISI Web of Science, MEDLINE, Scopus, and Veterinary Bulletin. The intended audience for this journal is graduate students in veterinary pharmacology and toxicology as well as veterinary students, research scientists, and practitioners. This title is recommended as a key resource for any academic library that serves a program in veterinary pharmacology or toxicology or a college of veterinary medicine.

23.13. Veterinary Public Health

The prevention and control of disease and disability in animal populations.

—Adapted from MeSH

Contributors: C. Trenton Boyd and Esther Carrigan

Monographs

Human-Animal Medicine: Clinical Approaches to Zoonoses, Toxicants, and Other Shared Health Risks. Authors: Peter M. Rabinowitz, Lisa A. Conti. Saunders Elsevier, 2010.
ISBN: 981416068372
Recommended for: Academic Libraries

This important new addition to the literature of veterinary and human public health is notable for its novel holistic approach across human and animal species in a shared environment. A review of its contents underscore this unique approach: the convergence of human and animal medicine; legal and ethical issues in human-animal medicine; establishing a new approach to clinical health history; sentinel disease signs and symptoms; psychosocial and therapeutic aspects of human-animal interaction; the built environment and indoor air quality; allergic conditions; toxic exposures; zoonoses; food-borne illness; occupational health of animal workers; public health and human-animal medicine; and shared strategies to maximize human and animal health. This work emphasizes the increased professional communication and collaboration necessary between animal and human health workers to accomplish this integrated approach. It also provides practical guidelines and specific protocols for prevention and management of diseases and environmental health risks. As could be anticipated, the intended audience is health care students and professionals in human medicine, public health, and veterinary medicine. This work is highly recommended as an essential resource for any academic library that serves a public health program or a college of medicine or veterinary medicine.

Understanding Zoonotic Diseases. Author: Janet Amundson Romich. Thomson/Delmar Learning, 2008.
ISBN: 9781418021030
Recommended for: Academic Libraries

This is a basic textbook covering zoonotic diseases written for human and animal health care students and practitioners. Its contents begin with a general discussion of a history of zoonotic diseases, the principles of immunity, and diagnostic techniques. The remainder of its content covers specific zoonoses of different origins: bacteria, tick-borne bacteria, fungi, parasites, viruses, and prions. Coverage of each disease includes its pathogenesis, transmission, clinical signs, diagnostic tests, therapy, and prevention. The text is effectively illustrated, including photographs and tables. There is a consistent format for each chapter that includes an overview, summary, and review questions. Written in a clear and concise manner, it is an effective introduction to zoonotic diseases for both veterinary and human health professionals. This text is recommended as an important resource for any library that serves a health professions school or a college of medicine or veterinary medicine.

Veterinary Clinical Epidemiology. 3rd ed. Author: Ronald D. Smith. CRC Taylor & Francis, 2006.
ISBN: 9780849315664
Recommended for: Academic Libraries

This is the third edition of a key resource in veterinary epidemiology. Its intent to focus on the application of epidemiology to problems faced in general veterinary practice is unique. As such, it provides an important foundation and knowledge base to support evidence-based veterinary medicine. Examples include both companion and food animals, and are international in scope. This integration of epidemiology into practice is applied to patients as individuals, herds, or other defined populations. Topics covered include: an introduction with definitions; epidemiological approaches and applications of epidemiology in veterinary practice; defining the limits of normality; use and evaluation of diagnostic tests; measuring the commonness of disease, risk assessment and prevention; measuring and communicating prognoses; design and evaluation of clinical trials; statistical significance; medical ecology and outbreak investigation; measuring and expressing occurrence; establishing cause; source and transmission of disease agents; and the cost of disease. The preface to this third edition enumerates "increased coverage of hypothesis testing, survey design and sampling, and epidemiologic concepts related to the practice of evidence-based medicine." The intended audience is the veterinary student and practitioner, as well as animal health workers. This text is highly recommended as an important resource for any library that serves a program in animal science or a college of veterinary medicine.

Veterinary Epidemiology. 3rd ed. Author: Michael Thrusfield. Wiley-Blackwell, 2007.

ISBN: 9781405156271
Recommended for: Academic Libraries
Doody's Core Titles Selection

This is the third edition of a key resource in veterinary epidemiology, providing a comprehensive introduction to the field. Topics covered include: a general introduction to the scope of epidemiology; causality; disease occurrence; disease determinants; transmission and maintenance of infection; ecology of disease and disease patterns; the nature of data; surveillance; data collection and management; numerical data presentation; surveys; demonstrating association; observational studies; clinical trials; diagnostic testing; comparative epidemiology; disease modeling; the economics of disease; health schemes; and the control and eradication of disease. Examples are taken from both large and small animals and from both developed and developing nations. It includes 23 appendixes with useful information from a glossary of basic terms to tables of statistical calculations. This edition has been expanded and revised considerably over the second edition, increasing its page count by over 25 percent. The third edition was originally published in 2005; an expanded third edition paperback version was published in 2007 to provide a new section on risk analysis. The intended audience is veterinary students and practitioners, as well as epidemiology students. It is highly recommended as a key resource for any academic library that serves a program in epidemiology or a college of veterinary medicine.

Zoonoses and Communicable Diseases Common to Man and Animals. 3rd ed. Authors: Pedro N. Acha, Boris Szyfres. Pan American Health Organization, 2001.
http://www.ingentaconnect.com/content/paho/paho580
ISBN: 9789275119914 (Online)
Recommended for: Academic Libraries

This is the 3rd edition of the comprehensive resource on communicable and zoonotic diseases that is considered the gold standard text in veterinary public health. It is issued in three volumes; the first covers bacterial and fungal diseases; the second covers chlamydial, rickettsial, and viral diseases; the third volume covers parasitic zoonoses. Diseases within each volume are arranged in alphabetical order. Discussion of each disease includes etiology, geographic distribution, symptoms and occurrence in man and animals, source of infection and mode of transmission, role of animals in its epidemiology, diagnostic techniques, and methods of prevention and control. The amount of coverage provided for each disease is based on its prevalence and pathogenicity. A new edition to include recently emerging communicable and zoonotic diseases is much needed. As a basic text in communicable and zoonotic diseases, its intended audience is students, researchers, and practitioners in the fields of medicine, public health, and veterinary medicine. It is highly recommended as a key resource for any academic library that serves a school of public health or a college of medicine or veterinary medicine.

Journals

Preventive Veterinary Medicine. v. 1, Elsevier, 1982.
http://www.sciencedirect.com/science/journal/01675877
ISSN: 01675877
ISSN: 18731716 (Online)
Indexed in: MEDLINE
Recommended for: Academic Libraries

Preventive Veterinary Medicine is the leading journal in the field of veterinary public health. This peer-reviewed journal is international in scope, reporting research and programs in animal health, animal disease prevention, control and eradication, the economic cost of animal disease epidemics, and the maintenance of health and management of diseases in animal populations. It covers both domestic and wild animals. The journal publishes original research articles, review articles, short communications, letters to the editor, and book reviews. It is ranked as one of the top 30 journals in the 3rd edition of the "Basic List of Veterinary Serials," compiled in 2009 by the Veterinary Serials Committee of the Veterinary Medical Libraries Section of the Medical Library Association. *Preventive Veterinary Medicine* is indexed by most of the major indexing and abstracting services including Academic Search Complete, AGRICOLA, BIOSIS, CAB Abstracts, Current Contents, Embase, Index Veterinarius, ISI Web of Science, MEDLINE, Scopus, and Veterinary Bulletin. The intended audience is graduate students, veterinary students, researchers, and practitioners in the field of veterinary epidemiology, preventive medicine, and animal health. This title is recommended as a key resource for any academic library that serves a program in animal health or a college of veterinary medicine.

Zoonoses and Public Health. v. 54, Wiley-Blackwell, 2007.
http://onlinelibrary.wiley.com/journal/10.1111/(ISSN)1863-2378
ISSN: 18631959
ISSN: 18632378 (Online)
Indexed in: MEDLINE
Recommended for: Academic Libraries

Zoonoses and Public Health is the latest title change of a German publication that began in 1953. According to the aims and scope statement, this international peer-reviewed journal seeks to provide an opportunity for increased collaboration between veterinary and human health researchers and policy makers by fostering an integrated and global approach to zoonoses and public health issues. The journal publishes original research articles, review articles, and short communications. It is ranked as one of the top 35 journals in the third edition of the "Basic List of Veterinary Serials," compiled in 2009 by the Veterinary Serials Committee of the Veterinary Medical Libraries Section of the Medical Library Association. It is indexed by most of the major indexing and abstracting services including Academic Search Complete, AGRICOLA, BIOSIS, CAB Abstracts, Current Contents, Embase, Index Veterinarius, ISI Web of Science, MEDLINE, and Veterinary Bulletin. Given the interdisciplinary nature of public health and the study of zoonotic diseases, the intended audience for this publication is broad, including graduate students in any of the basic sciences that support the study of diseases and their transmission, veterinary students, researchers, and practitioners in the field of veterinary epidemiology, preventive medicine, and animal and public health. This title is recommended as a key resource for any academic library that serves a program in animal health, public health, or a college of veterinary medicine.

23.14. Veterinary Radiology

The use of x-ray and other forms of radiant energy in the diagnosis and treatment of disease in animals.

—Adapted from MeSH

Contributors: C. Trenton Boyd and Esther Carrigan

Monographs

Diagnostic Radiology and Ultrasonography of the Dog and Cat. 5th ed. Authors: J. Kevin Kealy, Hester McAllister, John P. Graham. Saunders Elsevier, 2010.
ISBN: 9781437701500
Recommended for: Academic Libraries

This is the fifth edition of the classic text in small animal imaging techniques and interpretation. The same general chapter content outline is followed as with the fourth edition, beginning with a discussion of the radiograph and progressing anatomically through the abdomen, thorax, bones and joints, skull and vertebral column, and soft tissues. The basic approach this text uses is to present normal anatomy and then the radiologic signs of abnormalities. As would be expected, much of the updating from the earlier 2005 edition centers on improved illustrations with high-quality images, improved line drawings and diagrams, color flow and Doppler images, and expanded magnetic resonance, computed tomography and digital images. Other enhancements in this edition include expanded coverage of computer tomography, magnetic resonance imaging, and scintigraphy, and an updating on new soft tissue conditions. The intended audience is veterinary students, general and specialty interns and residents, and practitioners. It is highly recommended as an essential resource for any academic library that serves a college of veterinary medicine.

Textbook of Veterinary Diagnostic Radiology. 5th ed. Author: Donald E. Thrall. Saunders Elsevier, 2007.
ISBN: 9781416026150
Recommended for: Academic Libraries
Doody's Core Titles Selection

This is the fifth edition of the classic reference for veterinary radiology that was first published in 1986. It is a comprehensive resource for radiological diagnosis and interpretation for the dog, cat, and horse, which includes radiologic imaging (including digital radiographs), ultrasound, computed tomography, and magnetic resonance imaging. Its 47 chapters are organized into five main sections beginning with the physics of imaging and principles of interpretation, and moving anatomically from the skeleton to soft tissue imaging. Chapters in anatomical sections typically present normal anatomy, general radiographic changes, and the most common abnormalities for the structure, organ, or system. New content in this edition includes a new chapter on digital imaging, expanded coverage of the imaging of the brain and spinal cord, and more than 500 additional high-quality images. The intended audience is veterinary students, general and specialty interns and residents, and practitioners. It is highly recommended as an essential resource for any academic library that serves a college of veterinary medicine.

Journals

Veterinary Radiology & Ultrasound. v. 33, Wiley-Blackwell, 1992.
http://onlinelibrary.wiley.com/journal/10.1111/(ISSN)1740-8261
ISSN: 10588183
ISSN: 17408261 (Online)
Indexed in: MEDLINE
Recommended for: Academic Libraries

Veterinary Radiology & Ultrasound is the official journal of the American College of Veterinary Radiology, the European College of Veterinary Diagnostic Imaging, the European Association of Veterinary Diagnostic Imaging, and the International Veterinary Radiology Association. Clearly international in scope, it is a peer-reviewed journal that attempts to publish broadly in veterinary imaging since it is the only journal in the field. Content covers techniques in radiology and ultrasound, radiologic diagnosis and therapy, and ultrasonography. According to its scope statement, the journal publishes articles reporting results of original investigations, clinical reports, case-history reports, review articles, and letters to the editor. It is indexed by many of the major indexing and abstracting services including AGRICOLA, BIOSIS, CAB Abstracts, Current Contents, Embase, Index Veterinarius, ISI Web of Science, MEDLINE, Scopus, and Veterinary Bulletin. The intended audience for this journal is graduate students in veterinary radiology and imaging as well as veterinary students, radiology interns and residents, research scientists, and practitioners. This title is recommended as an important resource for any academic library that serves a college of veterinary medicine.

23.15. Veterinary Surgery

Manual or operative procedures are used in the treatment of disease, injuries, or deformities in animals.

—Adapted from MeSH

Contributors: C. Trenton Boyd and Esther Carrigan

Monographs

Equine Surgery. 3rd ed. Editors: Jorg A. Auer, John A. Stick. Saunders Elsevier, 2006.
ISBN: 9781416001232
Recommended for: Academic Libraries
Doody's Core Titles Selection

With over 1,400 pages, this third edition of the classic *Equine Surgery* is undeniably the most comprehensive equine surgery textbook available. Its 104 chapters are organized into 12 sections. The first three sections provide an introduction by covering surgical biology, surgical methods, and advances in anesthesia. The remaining nine sections all focus their chapters on the surgery of a particular organ or body system in the equine. As would be expected, an extended focus and coverage is provided for the equine musculoskeletal system. According to the publisher, this text attempts to prepare the veterinary surgeon for managing each surgical condition by understanding its pathophysiology and evaluating alternative surgical approaches. Besides the expected updating for new techniques and drugs, changes to this edition include the reinstatement of chapters on anesthesiology and pain management, increased coverage of joint disorders and joint trauma, and expansion of the material on minimally invasive surgical techniques. The intended audience is veterinary students, surgical interns and residents, and equine practitioners and surgeons. It is recommended as an essential resource for any academic library that serves a college of veterinary medicine.

Handbook of Veterinary Anesthesia. 4th ed. Authors: William W. Muir, John A.E. Hubbell, Richard M. Bednarski, Roman T. Skarda. Mosby Elsevier, 2007.
ISBN: 9780323046787
Recommended for: Academic Libraries

The *Handbook of Veterinary Anesthesia*, now in its fourth edition, continues to provide the best compact package of complete information necessary for safe and effective anesthetic administration to both large and small animals and exotics. This handbook is recognized for its excellent presentation and organization of information, using a bulleted approach with clear instructions and diagrams, which makes it an effective quick anesthesia reference for both students and practitioners. The resource provides chapters on patient evaluation and preparation, pre-anesthetic medications, several chapters by species for local anesthesia, several chapters on general anesthesia, anesthetic toxicity and drug interactions, equipment, patient monitoring, acupuncture, several chapters by species for anesthetic procedures and techniques, fluid administration during anesthesia, shock, respiratory and cardiac emergencies, and euthanasia. In addition to the expected updating for new anesthesia drug information, this fourth edition boasts new information on pain management and local anesthesia, expanded coverage of post-anesthetic care, a new chapter on anesthetics in cats, anesthetic protocols for each species, and expanded coverage of euthanasia including current guidelines for euthanasia techniques recommended by the American Veterinary Medical Association. This text is a useful reference for veterinary students, anesthesia residents, interns, and practitioners. It is recommended as an essential resource for any academic library that serves a college of veterinary medicine.

Lumb & Jones' Veterinary Anesthesia and Analgesia. 4th ed. Editors: William J. Tranquilli, John C. Thurmon,

Kurt A. Grimm. Wiley-Blackwell, 2007.
ISBN: 9780781754712
Recommended for: Academic Libraries

This is the fourth edition of the highly respected classic text, *Veterinary Anesthesia and Analgesia*, originally authored by Lumb and Jones in 1973. With over 1,000 pages and 53 chapters, this text is often referred to as the comprehensive, gold standard anesthesia resource. It covers all aspects of anesthesia in both large and small animals, including laboratory, exotic and zoo animal species, aquatic mammals, and fish. The volume is organized into multi-chaptered sections on general topics such as an overview and general principles of veterinary anesthesia and analgesia; the physiology of various organ systems; the pharmacology of anesthetics; equipment and monitoring; selected anesthetic and analgesic techniques in chapters by species; anesthesia, analgesia, and immobilization in chapters by species and classes of animals; anesthesia and analgesia of patients with specific diseases in chapters by body system; and anesthesia and analgesia for selected patients and procedures in chapters by disease or condition. In addition to the expected updating for new anesthetic drugs and procedures, this edition boasts expanded coverage of pain and pain management, including new chapters on pain physiology, analgesic medications, acupuncture, physical rehabilitation, and palliative analgesia. The intended audience is veterinary students, anesthesia residents and interns, and practitioners. It is recommended as an essential resource for any academic library that serves a college of veterinary medicine.

Small Animal Surgery. 3rd ed. Author: Theresa W. Fossum. Mosby Elsevier, 2007.
ISBN: 9780323044394
ISBN: 9780323044400 (Online)
Recommended for: Academic Libraries
Doody's Core Titles Selection

This classic textbook, now in its third edition, serves as a comprehensive resource to all aspects of small animal surgery. It is organized into four parts covering general surgical procedures, soft tissue surgery, orthopedics, and neurosurgery. Advanced procedures are indentified for possible referral to a specialist. The format of the presentation of information in the specific surgery sections is consistent across all chapters, making the volume easy to consult for quick reference or detailed study. There are over 1,500 color illustrations detailing anatomy and surgical techniques and over 600 color photographs and radiographs, which present disorders, diseases, and procedures. New content in this edition includes added chapters on the fundamentals of physical rehabilitation following surgery, principles of minimally invasive surgery, and surgery of the eye. This is a valuable reference for veterinary surgery students, residents, and practitioners who deal with small animals. It is an essential resource for any academic library that serves a college of veterinary medicine. An e-book version is available from the publisher for individual purchasers.

Techniques in Large Animal Surgery. 3rd ed. Editor: Dean A. Hendrickson. Blackwell, 2007.
ISBN: 9780781782555
Recommended for: Academic Libraries

In the 25 years between the first edition and this third edition, this text has become a classic. It has built a solid reputation for clearly illustrated, step-by-step techniques for the surgery of any large domestic animal. It uses both color illustrations and black-and-white diagrams and sketches. The early chapters cover presurgical considerations, anesthesia and fluid therapy, surgical instruments, suture materials and needles, knots and ligatures, suture patterns, principles of wound management and the use of drains, and reconstructive surgery of wounds. Species covered include horses, cattle, swine, goats, and some exotic species, with greater emphasis on horses. In addition to the basic surgical procedures, the author also provides a review of the clinical indications for the surgery, lists of equipment needed for the procedure, and known complications. This new edition incorporates the changes in antibiotics and anesthetics since the second edition was published in 1989, as well as new material on minimally invasive techniques, laser surgery, and laparotomy. This text is a useful reference for surgery students as well as mixed and large animal practitioners. It is recommended as an essential resource for any academic library that serves a college of veterinary medicine.

Textbook of Small Animal Surgery. 3rd ed. Editor: Douglas Slatter. Saunders, 2003.
ISBN: 9780721686073
Recommended for: Academic Libraries

This two-volume comprehensive reference presents all areas of small animal surgery. It begins with two general sections: a surgical overview of topics such as shock, wound repair, nutritional support, trauma, and implants, and a discussion of surgical methods, which range from basic topics such as sterilization and instruments to more specialized topics such as cryosurgery and surgical lasers. The next 13 sections cover surgery of anatomical systems and regions, with final sections on surgical oncology, anesthesia, and dental surgery. It is nicely illustrated throughout with photographs and line drawings to present clear images of anatomy, diagnostic features, and operative procedures. A handy appendix of normal laboratory values for the dog and cat is also included. This third edition boasts an expanded section on critical care, over 30 new chapters, and an increased emphasis on surgical decision-making algorithms. At nearly 3,000 pages, this is the most extensive small animal surgery reference available. It is an excellent resource for veterinary students, small animal practitioners, and surgeons. It is an essential resource for any academic library that serves a college of veterinary medicine.

Journals

Veterinary Anaesthesia and Analgesia. v. 27, Wiley-Blackwell, 2000.
http://onlinelibrary.wiley.com/journal/10.1111/(ISSN)1467-2995
ISSN: 14672987
ISSN: 14672995 (Online)
Indexed in: MEDLINE
Recommended for: Academic Libraries

Veterinary Anaesthesia and Analgesia is the official journal of the Association of Veterinary Anaesthetists, the American College of Veterinary Anesthesiologists, the European College of Veterinary Anaesthesia, the Veterinary Technician Anaesthesia Society, the Academy of Veterinary Technician Anaesthetists, and the International Veterinary Academy of Pain Management. It is international in scope and covers both large and small animals as well as domestic, wild, and exotic species. The journal publishes peer-reviewed original research articles, review articles, special articles, short communications, case reports, and book reviews. Its scope covers all aspects of anesthesia and pain management in animals in the broadest sense, including the chemical restraint of animals and the animal welfare issues which arise in dealing with pain and distress in animals. The journal is indexed and abstracted by all of the major indexing and abstracting services including AGRICOLA, CAB Abstracts, Current Contents, Index Veterinarius, ISI Web of Science, MEDLINE, and Scopus. Potential readership for this journal includes professional students, surgical residents, and veterinary surgeons and practitioners. Its special focus makes it a recommended resource for all veterinary libraries.

Veterinary Surgery. v. 7, Wiley-Blackwell, 1978.
http://onlinelibrary.wiley.com/journal/10.1111/(ISSN)1532-950X
ISSN: 01613499
ISSN: 1532950X (Online)
Indexed in: MEDLINE
Recommended for: Academic Libraries

This key resource for animal surgery and anesthesia is the official journal of the American College of Veterinary Surgeons and the European College of Veterinary Surgeons. It is one of the top 10 journals in the third edition of the "Basic List of Veterinary Serials," compiled in 2009 by the Veterinary Serials Committee of the Veterinary Medical Libraries Section of the Medical Library Association. It continues the earlier title, *Journal of Veterinary Surgery* and absorbed *Veterinary Anesthesia* in 1985. Coverage includes surgical and anesthetic techniques, surgical diagnosis, care of surgical infections, and care of the surgical patient. The journal covers both large and small animals, and presents both the clinical and research perspective. It contains original, peer-reviewed articles, case reports, and review articles, as well as scientific abstracts from the associations' annual meetings. The aims and scope statement of the journal speak to its intent to put "new developments in perspective and to provide a forum for new concepts and a peer commentary to help better understand and evaluate the surgical patient." It is indexed by several agricultural and veterinary indexing and abstracting services including AGRICOLA, Biological Abstracts, CAB Abstracts, Current Contents, Index Veterinarius, ISI Web of Science, MEDLINE, Scopus, and Veterinary Bulletin. Potential readership for this journal includes professional students, surgical residents, and veterinary surgeons and practitioners. Its special focus makes it a recommended resource for all veterinary libraries.

24. Anatomy

The morphologic structure of an organism.
—*Stedman's Medical Dictionary*, 28th ed. (2006)

Contributor: Craig S. Elam

Monographs

Atlas of Anatomy: General Anatomy and Musculoskeletal System. Authors: Michael Schuenke, Erik Schulte, Udo Schumacher, Lawrence M. Ross, Edward D. Lamperti. Thieme, 2006.
See Chapter 24.4. Regional Anatomy

Atlas of Human Anatomy. 5th ed. Author: Frank H. Netter. Saunders/Elsevier, 2010.
ISBN: 9781416059516
ISBN: 9781437709704
See Also Chapter 1. Allied Health
Recommended for: Hospital, Academic Libraries
Doody's Core Titles Selection

Based on the classic illustrations of Frank H. Netter, this best seller remains the gold standard for human anatomy atlases. The book excels in its comprehensive, accurate, high-quality color drawings in Netter's uniquely accessible style. Brightly colored for maximum contrast and profusely labeled, the illustrations aim for a balance between simplicity and realism. For the fifth edition, a team of editors has updated the radiologic images and added both new and updated illustrations from Carlos Machado, MD, a worthy artistic successor to Dr. Netter. The plates in each section have been reorganized to proceed logically from superficial to deeper structures in order to reflect the dissection process more accurately. Although clear and detailed, this atlas is insufficient in itself for the student of anatomy. It lacks any descriptive text and has limited examples of correlating anatomical information to clinical situations. However, it serves as an ideal companion to a more comprehensive resource, such as *Grant's Atlas* or *Gray's Anatomy* for students. Individuals who purchase the print edition can access the companion website, http://www.studentconsult.com/, which contains over eighty of the most important illustrations, interactive videos, clinical images, and test questions. The website http://netterreference.com provides other purchase options, with online access to selected or additional images. This is a *Doody's Core Titles* essential purchase selection.

Color Atlas of Anatomy: A Photographic Study of the Human Body. 7th ed. Authors: Johannes W. Rohen, Chihiro Yokochi, Elke Lütjen-Drecoll. Lippincott Williams & Wilkins, 2011.
ISBN: 9781582558561
Recommended for: Hospital, Academic Libraries
Brandon/Hill, *Doody's Core Titles* Selection

First published in 1983, the latest edition of this outstanding atlas continues to present human anatomy using over 1,200 color photographs of professional cadaver dissections. Many of the photographs have been updated with higher-resolution images in this edition, and the black-and-white dissection photos of earlier editions have been replaced by color. The aim of the book is to provide first-year medical students a realistic view of the spatial relationships of anatomical structures that will improve their understanding. This atlas can be used in lieu of, or as a supplement to, laboratory dissections. Each chapter first describes the anatomical structures in a systemic manner and then depicts the regional anatomy, progressing from the surface to sequentially deeper layers as in a dissection. Although schematic drawings, radiographs, CT scans, and MRI images are used, the crisp, clear photographs are the focus of the book. Structures are identified with an unobtrusive line and number, which correlates to a numbered list on the same or opposing page. This arrangement is excellent for self-testing. Although not as comprehensive as *Netter's Atlas*, this book shows complex structures from multiple angles and planes and also identifies anatomical variations. By its realistic portrayal of anatomical dissections, this atlas is very useful in supplementing the student's learning of anatomical concepts as described in a conventional textbook or illustrated atlas. Individuals who purchase the print edition can access the companion website, http:// thepoint.lww.com/, which includes an image bank, interactive software and the full text. A version of this title appeared on the final Brandon/Hill list and it is included in *Doody's Core Titles*.

Gray's Anatomy: The Anatomical Basis of Clinical Practice. 40th ed. Editor: Susan Standring. Churchill

Livingstone/Elsevier, 2008.
ISBN: 9780443066849
ISBN: 9780808923718
Recommended for: Hospital, Academic Libraries
Brandon/Hill Selection

Celebrating the 150th anniversary of this iconic text, the fortieth edition continues to set the world standard for a comprehensive, authoritative anatomical resource. This magnificent book completes the revision begun by Dr. Standring in the previous edition. As indicated by the new subtitle, "The Anatomical Basis of Clinical Practice," the book has undergone a total reorganization from a systemic to a regional format, transforming an authoritative compendium of systemic anatomy into a more practical and accessible work relevant to modern medical curricula and practicing professionals. This reorganization is fully realized in the current edition with 2,000 new or revised illustrations. Retaining Gray's reputation for clarity and accuracy, images are now all in full color and include over 200 new diagnostic and clinical imaging studies to relate anatomical structures to clinical applications. The book integrates the full range of anatomical knowledge, from the subcellular to the regional and includes sections on histology, embryology, and neuroanatomy. To enhance its reference value, each chapter contains a brief list of valuable and current citations to the literature. The success of these efforts can be seen in its being "Highly Commended" in the 2009 British Medical Association's Medical Book Competition, where it was cited for the excellence of its updated content, readability, accuracy, and reliability as a comprehensive anatomical reference source. For the first time, online, passworded access to the complete content of the book is also made available to individual purchasers of the print book. An earlier version of the book was an initial purchase title in the last Brandon/Hill list.

Sobotta Atlas of Human Anatomy: Head, Neck, Upper Limb, Thorax, Abdomen, Pelvis, Lower Limb. 14th ed. Editors: Reinhard Putz, Reinhard Pabst, Renate Putz. Urban & Fischer/Elsevier, 2008.
See Chapter 24.4. Regional Anatomy

Journals

The Anatomical Record. v. 290, Wiley-Blackwell, 2007.
http://onlinelibrary.wiley.com/journal/10.1002/(ISSN)1097-0185
ISSN: 19328486
ISSN: 10970185 (Online)
Indexed in: MEDLINE
Recommended for: Academic Libraries

The Anatomical Record is the oldest American journal of anatomy, first issued by the Wistar Institute of Anatomy and Biology in 1906 as an official publication of the American Association of Anatomists (AAA). Its current subtitle—*Advances in Integrative Anatomy and Evolutionary Biology*—conveys its broad scope. From 1998 to 2006, the journal was published in two parts: *The Anatomical Record, Part A: Discoveries in Molecular, Cellular, and Evolutionary Biology* and *The Anatomical Record, Part B: The New Anatomist*, which provided articles of a broader scope reflecting anatomy's connections to other scientific disciplines, curricular evolution, and public policy issues. Prior years reflected the journal's original title, *The Anatomical Record*. This is a core journal in the field, providing papers on the functional morphology of vertebrate organ systems, including descriptive studies of normal and abnormal development. Review articles related to anatomy and its subdisciplines are regularly included, along with abstracts and proceedings of the annual meeting of the AAA. The journal has long held its top 10 journal impact factor ranking in its category and is one of the top five journals visited by AAA members. It is indexed by all major biomedical indexing and abstracting services.

Cells Tissues Organs. v. 164, Karger, 1999.
http://www.karger.com/CTO
ISSN: 14226405
ISSN: 14226421 (Online)
Indexed in: MEDLINE
Recommended for: Academic Libraries

Reflecting the multidisciplinary nature of modern research—where distinctions between the traditional fields of morphology, physiology, and biochemistry have greatly diminished—*Acta Anatomica*, founded as a morphological journal in 1945, reinvented itself as *Cells Tissues Organs* in 1999. While retaining its exquisite reproduction quality, the new journal presents an emphasis in modern functional morphology, seeking to bridge the gap between cell biology and developmental biology and the emerging fields of regenerative medicine, such as stem cell biology, tissue engineering, artificial organs, in vitro systems, and transplantation biology. The journal also features a section listing and briefly describing new patent submissions and patents granted. According to the 2009 *Journal Citation Reports*, *Cells Tissues Organs* has the second highest impact factor in anatomy and morphology, and is one of the top five journals visited by American Association of Anatomy members. It is indexed by all major biomedical indexing and abstracting services.

Journal of Anatomy. v. 51, Wiley-Blackwell, 1916.
http://onlinelibrary.wiley.com/journal/10.1111/(ISSN)1469-7580
http://www.ncbi.nlm.nih.gov/pmc/journals/265/
ISSN: 00218782
ISSN: 14697580 (Online)
Indexed in: MEDLINE
Recommended for: Academic Libraries

For over 150 years, the *Journal of Anatomy* has been a leading journal in the field. Published monthly by Wiley on behalf of the Anatomical Society of Great Britain and Ireland, it covers all aspects of normal human and comparative anatomy. Aspects include applied anatomy, functional imaging, physical anthropology, neuroanatomy, endocrinology, embryology, stereology, histology, histochemistry, and electron microscopy, with special emphasis on experimental morphology. The journal's impact factor has consistently ranked in the top ten in its category, and it was recently named by the Special Libraries Association as one of the 100 most influential journals in biology and medicine over the past 100 years. It is also one of the top five journals visited by American Association of Anatomy members. All review articles are free, and all content since the journal's inception in 1867 (including coverage of the preceding title, *Journal of Anatomy and Physiology*, 1867–1916) is accessible in PubMed Central after a 24-month embargo period. It is included in all the major biomedical indexing and abstracting services.

Databases and Other Electronic Resources

Anatomy.tv. Primal Pictures, 200?
http://www.anatomy.tv/
http://www.statref.com/
http://www.ovid.com/
Recommended for: Academic Libraries

Primal Pictures, Ltd. produces the online version of the interactive 3-D anatomy DVDs under the name Anatomy.tv, which is a collection of high-resolution, three-dimensional interactive models of human anatomy. Users can rotate, zoom, add, and remove layers to examine anatomical structures more effectively. The resource provides a wealth of highly detailed anatomy and clinical text, with supporting media, MRIs, X-rays, live-action movies, and animations. The content is continuously updated. This unique resource is available from STAT!Ref in several packages of regional and systemic anatomy, including both basic and all-inclusive collections. While Anatomy.tv is an excellent tool for supplemental study and presentations in anatomical instruction for medical and dental students, it is especially valuable in physical therapy and other health professions education programs where students may have limited access to cadaver material. OvidSP offers other package/module variations of this Primal Pictures resource, which Ovid refers to as Primal Pictures on OvidSP.

24.1. Artistic Anatomy

The study of anatomy for artistic purposes, as applied to painting, drawing, or sculpture.
—*Stedman's Medical Dictionary*, 28th ed. (2006)

Contributor: Craig S. Elam

Monographs

Anatomy for the Artist. Authors: Sarah Simblet, John Davis. DK, 2001.
ISBN: 9780789480453
Recommended for: Academic Libraries

Written by an artist who teaches anatomy through drawing and accompanied by photographs by John Davis, this large format book focuses on the interrelationship between external artistic form and internal structures, not detailed scientific nomenclature. This is a beautiful photographic work, presenting more than 250 black-and-white and color photos of the nude human body with transparent overlays that superimpose drawings of underlying muscle and bone. Chapters examine the muscle groups, skeletal strength, balance, poise, and grace. Highlights are 10 "Master Classes," which analyze masterworks by classical artists from Hans Holbein to Edward Hopper, with a photo of a model in the same pose as the painting for comparison. Included are a list of key terms used in the book and a glossary of anatomical terminology.

Atlas of Human Anatomy for the Artist. Author: Stephen R. Peck. Oxford University Press, 1982, 1951.
ISBN: 9780195030952
Recommended for: Academic Libraries

A classic work that has been in print for over 60 years, the *Atlas* remains unsurpassed for students of the human form. It is very comprehensive and detailed, showing anatomical structures from all angles. It includes sections on bones, muscles, surface anatomy, proportion, equilibrium, and locomotion. Of particular value are the sections on anatomical variations due to human physique, age, race, gender, and analysis of facial expressions. While some photographs are provided for general reference, it is Peck's drawings and sketches that are the most useful. Anatomical nomenclature and pronunciations are provided for the bones and muscles.

Human Anatomy for Artists: The Elements of Form. Author: Eliot Goldfinger. Oxford University Press, 1991.
ISBN: 9780195052060
Recommended for: Academic Libraries

Five years in the making by a renowned sculptor and lecturer in anatomy, this is one of the most comprehensive and best illustrated guides for artists available. It features hundreds of photos and two-color labeled illustrations detailing the surface structures of the human body. In addition, numerous cross sections—made with reference to CT scans, magnetic resonance imaging, and cut cadavers—outline the forms of all body regions and individual muscles. Extensive and detailed information, with precise scientific terminology for each structure, is located on facing pages for ease of reference. Although it has become a standard reference for artists and art students, it is valuable for all interested in the human form, including students of other branches of anatomy, physical therapists, and athletic trainers. The work is recommended for libraries supporting art or medical illustration programs.

24.2. Comparative Anatomy

The comparative study of animal structure with regard to homologous organs or parts.

—MeSH

Contributor: Craig S. Elam

Monographs

Comparative Anatomy of the Vertebrates. 9th ed. Authors: George C. Kent, Robert K. Carr. McGraw-Hill, 2001.
ISBN: 9780073038698
Recommended for: Academic Libraries

This classic text is known for its readability and high-quality illustrations, which are ideal characteristics for introducing comparative anatomy to undergraduate students. For the ninth edition, George Kent is joined by new coauthor Bob Carr. Their work presents functional and comparative morphology within a developmental and evolutionary framework, reflecting current advances in research. Early chapters cover major organ systems, evolutionary concepts, protochordates, craniates, and early morphogenesis. It is well organized, with chapter outlines and summaries, links to websites, questions, and a glossary. It presents updated information on systematic relationships and taxonomy. The text is recommended for biology majors and pre-professional students in medicine, dentistry, and the allied health fields.

Functional Anatomy of the Vertebrates: An Evolutionary Perspective. 3rd ed. Authors: Karel F. Liem, Warren F. Walker, William Bemis, Lance Grande. Harcourt College, 2001.
ISBN: 9780030223693
Recommended for: Academic Libraries

This is a standard text for undergraduate comparative anatomy courses, introducing students to the anatomical evolution of vertebrates and the functional interrelationships of organs and adaptive environments. This edition has two new coauthors, resulting in a new emphasis on current research in cladistics and placing functional anatomy in a phylogenetic context. Three chapters on the sense organs and the nervous system reflect advances in comparative vertebrate neurobiology. The text is illustrated liberally, with sources noted and extensive references to the original research literature. Overall, this is an excellent text that is recommended for biology majors and pre-professional students in medicine, dentistry, and the allied health fields.

Vertebrates: Comparative Anatomy, Function, Evolution. 5th ed. Author: Kenneth V. Kardong. McGraw-Hill Higher Education, 2009.
ISBN: 9780073040585
Recommended for: Academic Libraries

This textbook on vertebrate morphology is designed for upper-level undergraduate students in a one-semester comparative anatomy course. The first four chapters introduce the field, the origin and development of chordates, and the evolution and taxonomy of vertebrates. A new section on evolution and development, based on molecular embryology, has been added to the fifth chapter. The remaining chapters develop each major organ system, following a consistent organization comprised of basic morphology, function, and evolution. Boxed essays are included in most chapters, presenting interesting subjects or historical events. For this edition, new, neglected, or competing views on function and evolution, mostly from Europe, are also presented.

24.3. Cross-Sectional Anatomy

Descriptive anatomy based on three-dimensional imaging of the body, organs, and structures using a series of computer multiplane sections, displayed by transverse, coronal, and sagittal analyses. It is essential to accurate interpretation by the radiologist of such techniques as ultrasonic diagnosis, magnetic resonance imaging, and computed tomography.

—MeSH

Contributor: Craig S. Elam

Monographs

Basic Atlas of Sectional Anatomy with Correlated Imaging. 4th ed. Authors: Walter J. Bo, J. Jeffrey Carr, Wayne A. Krueger, Neil T. Wolfman, Robert L. Bowden. Saunders Elsevier, 2007.
ISBN: 9781416001218
Recommended for: Hospital, Academic Libraries
Brandon/Hill Selection

Primarily designed as a companion to dissection for students of gross anatomy, this atlas correlates color photographs of cadaver sections with corresponding CT, MRI, and ultrasound images on the facing pages. Its chapters are organized by regions of the body, each with sections in cross, coronal, and sagittal planes. Each section is very detailed, with extensive labels and a short description of its location and orientation. The introduction presents a comprehensive review of the physics of CT, MRI, and ultrasound imaging. This is a highly recommended resource, with a four-star review from *Doody's*. Additionally, earlier editions have appeared on the Brandon/Hill medical list.

Human Sectional Anatomy: Atlas of Body Sections, CT and MRI Images. 3rd ed. Authors: Harold Ellis, Bari M. Logan, Adrian K. Dixon. Hodder Arnold, 2007.
ISBN: 9780340912225
Recommended for: Hospital, Academic Libraries

This superb atlas presents high-quality color photographs of cadaver sections, accompanied by corresponding CT and occasional MRI images. Extensively labeled line drawings identify anatomical structures, and notes highlight key anatomical or radiological features. Many of the radiological images have been updated to represent the latest technology, including multi-detector CT and 3D-rendered CT images. This is an essential resource for medical students, as well as postgraduate physicians, radiologists, and surgeons, learning to interpret sectional images.

Introduction to Sectional Anatomy. 2nd ed. Author: Michael E. Madden. Lippincott Williams & Wilkins, 2008.
ISBN: 9780781763424
Recommended for: Hospital, Academic Libraries
Brandon/Hill Selection

This is an introductory text developed to provide radiologic technology students with a better understanding of sectional anatomy and its use in clinical imaging. Chapters on each body region begin with an anatomical overview, followed by labeled CT and MRI images presented in sequence though sagittal, coronal, and axial planes. Selected clinical cases are illustrated with CT, MRI, ultrasound, 3D, and PET/CT images. Images from several patients are included to provide students with a better understanding of normal anatomic variations. Line drawings help locate the section planes and anatomical features. Each chapter ends with review questions. This text is highly recommended in *Doody's*, and its earlier edition appeared on the Brandon/Hill list.

24.4. Regional Anatomy

An approach to anatomic study based on regions, parts, or divisions of the body (e.g., the foot or the inguinal region), emphasizing the relationships of various systemic structures (e.g., muscles, nerves, and arteries) within that area.

—*Stedman's Medical Dictionary*, 28th ed. (2006)

Contributor: Craig S. Elam

Monographs

Atlas of Anatomy: General Anatomy and Musculoskeletal System. Authors: Michael Schuenke, Erik Schulte, Udo Schumacher, Lawrence M. Ross, Edward D. Lamperti. Thieme, 2006.
ISBN: 9781588903877
ISBN: 9781588903587
Recommended for: Hospital, Academic Libraries

Eight years in the making, this first volume in the three-volume *Atlas of Anatomy* series is impressive for its stunning quality, detailed illustrations, and unique organization.

Revised and translated from the original German, this atlas surpasses its goal to guide students in their initial study of anatomy and to serve as a reliable reference for experienced students and professionals. The original and innovative illustrations have extensive and informative legends, clear and accurate labels, and many unique views to emphasize clinical applications. The illustrations are also published separately on DVD, making them available for presentations or lectures. The book is divided into four sections, starting with general anatomical concepts and followed by the musculoskeletal system of the trunk wall and upper and lower limbs. The general anatomy section covers human phylogeny and prenatal development, body proportions, surface anatomy, and general information on bones, joints, muscles, blood vessels, lymphatics, and basic neuroanatomy. Each of the three regional anatomy sections is organized into chapters covering the skeletal, muscular, and neurovascular systems. The musculature and neurovascular systems, which are unique to this atlas, are further examined in terms of their functional groups and topographical anatomy, thus providing access to these structures from multiple points of view. Especially valuable for students are the numerous summary boxes that provide detailed information such as muscle origins, insertions, innervations and actions, arterial branches, and nerve distributions in accessible schematic format. Radiographs and CT and MRI images that illustrate clinical correlations of anatomical concepts, structures, and functions are provided throughout the book. This is an essential work for any anatomy collection, especially those supporting medical and physical therapy programs.

Atlas of Anatomy: Head and Neuroanatomy. Authors: Michael Schuenke, Erik Schulte, Udo Schumacher, Lawrence M. Ross, Edward Lamperti, Ethan Taub, Juergen Rude. Thieme, 2007.
ISBN: 9781588904416
ISBN: 9781588903617
Recommended for: Hospital, Academic Libraries

Head and Neuroanatomy is the third and final volume in the *Atlas of Anatomy* series. In keeping with the high standards set by the other volumes, it presents stunning illustrations, succinct summary tables of valuable information, and concise explanatory text with numerous clinical applications. The book follows the series' unique organizational structure by integrating functional units with topographical viewpoints. There are two main sections, "The Head" and "Neuroanatomy." The first section opens with chapters on the cranial bones, muscles, blood vessels, and nerves arranged systemically; these are followed by chapters on topographical anatomy, the four sensory organs, and sectional anatomy. The "Neuroanatomy" section is divided into chapters on the major neural structures, such as the meninges, ventricular system, spinal cord, and areas of the brain; but, these are interspersed with systemic chapters on blood vessels, autonomic nervous system, and various functional systems—such as sensory, motor, visual, and auditory. The series continues its innovative format, with each specific topic concisely and clearly presented in a single, two-page spread along with hallmark, in-depth clinical correlations. The comprehensive coverage, combined with beautiful illustrations of unprecedented detail and clarity, make this an essential text for medical and professional students.

Atlas of Anatomy: Neck and Internal Organs. Authors: Michael Schuenke, Erik Schulte, Udo Schumacher, Juergen Rude, Lawrence M. Ross, Edward D. Lamperti. Thieme, 2006.
ISBN: 9781588903600
ISBN: 9781588904430
Recommended for: Hospital, Academic Libraries

This is the second volume of the impressive *Atlas of Anatomy* series. The authors' goal to produce an "ideal" atlas for students is especially evident in this volume, with stunning illustrations "revealing the underlying simplicity of the logic and order of human anatomy without sacrificing detail or aesthetics" (Preface). The book is divided into four sections: "Neck," "Thorax," "Abdomen," and "Pelvis." Similar to the first volume, *General Anatomy and Musculoskeletal System* (2006), each section is broken into functional units—spaces, organs, blood vessels, lymphatics, and nerves. An integrated topographic view is also supplied. A final section, "Neurovascular Supply to the Organs," is an extremely valuable summary for students, with unique, one-page schematic illustrations of the arterial supply, venous drainage, lymphatic circulation, and innervation for each organ. The superb illustrations are accompanied by extensive explanatory text, schematic drawings, and tables. Examples of clinical applications of anatomical concepts are outstanding, with clinically important anatomical variations covered in more depth than in most atlases. Very unique views of anatomy are illustrated to present clinically relevant information. Embryological development is also included for many systems. Another innovation is the unprecedented format, whereby each specific topic is concisely and clearly presented in a single, two-page spread. Due to translation from the original German, the atlas has a few, scattered differences in terminology from that found in American texts, but they do not detract from its value. The illustrations are also published separately in DVD format for use in instruction or presentations.

Basic Atlas of Sectional Anatomy with Correlated Imaging. 4th ed. Authors: Walter J. Bo, J. Jeffrey Carr, Wayne A. Krueger, Neil T. Wolfman, Robert L. Bowden. Saunders Elsevier, 2007.
See Chapter 24.3. Cross-Sectional Anatomy

Clinical Anatomy by Regions. 8th ed. Author: Richard S. Snell. Lippincott Williams & Wilkins, 2008.
ISBN: 9780781764049
Recommended for: Hospital, Academic Libraries

The latest edition of this standard text has been slightly re-titled and streamlined to fit the compressed anatomy courses being taught currently. The book's 12 chapters follow the typical sequence of a human dissection. Each chapter opens with a short clinical vignette, chapter outline, clinical objectives, basic clinical anatomy, radiographic anatomy, surface anatomy, clinical problems with questions and answers, and review questions in American National Board format. Scattered throughout are brief "Clinical Notes." New to this edition are "Embryological Notes," providing developmental anatomy and anomalies. The clearly labeled illustrations have been recolored for clarity, and some drawings are unique compared to other texts, although their quality is not as good. Clearly organized, well written, and updated with clinical information and diagnostic images, this remains a useful book for its target audience: medical, dental, allied health, or nursing students. For individual purchasers of the print book, a companion website offers the book's fully searchable text.

Clinically Oriented Anatomy. 6th ed. Authors: Keith L. Moore, Arthur F. Dalley, Anne M.R. Agur. Wolters Kluwer Health/Lippincott Williams & Wilkins, 2010.
See Also: Chapter 1. Allied Health
ISBN: 9780781775250
Recommended for: Hospital, Academic Libraries
Brandon/Hill, *Doody's Core Titles* Selection

The latest edition of this classic regional anatomy text retains its clear organization and excellent readability. Adding Dr. Agur as a new coauthor reflects the increased sharing of materials from *Grant's Atlas*, which she authors. The book continues to emphasize anatomy "important in physical diagnosis for primary care, interpretation of diagnostic imaging, and . . . anatomical basis of emergency medicine and surgery" (Preface). Divided into 10 color-coded sections, this edition boasts new and improved art work. An introductory chapter provides a brief systemic overview and basic anatomical terminology, followed by regional chapters heavily illustrated in color and accompanied by detailed text and color-coded tables. Surface anatomy and medical imaging, formerly separate, are now incorporated into the chapter content. Clinical correlations of important concepts are highlighted in "Blue Boxes," now categorized and grouped at the end of each chapter to improve comprehension. Each chapter concludes with a "Bottom Line" summary of key facts. This is an authoritative work whose organization and readability make it an excellent choice for its intended audience, the beginning health professions student. However, its comprehensiveness and detail may be excessive for beginning students, who may prefer *Gray's Anatomy for Students*. Opportunities for further improvement include stronger neuroanatomy material and a more thorough revision of clinical content. The book includes access to http://thepoint.lww.com, a companion website for individual purchasers of the print edition, which offers fully searchable text and access to USMLE-style case studies and quizzes. A version of this title appeared on the final Brandon/Hill list, and it is a *Doody's* essential purchase title.

Grant's Atlas of Anatomy. 12th ed. Authors: Anne M.R. Agur, Arthur F. Dalley II. Wolters Kluwer Health/Lippincott Williams & Wilkins, 2009.
ISBN: 9780781796040
ISBN: 9780781770552
Recommended for: Hospital, Academic Libraries
Brandon/Hill, *Doody's Core Titles* Selection

Originally published in 1943 with drawings of actual cadaver dissections, *Grant's Atlas* has served for many years as an essential adjunct to dissection. This latest edition is the furthest yet removed from its original intent, as seen in the tremendous increase in explanatory clinical text, diagrams, diagnostic images, and surface anatomy illustrations. Many of the illustrations have been recolored, with new tables of routine information relating to muscles, nerves, and blood vessels. Designed for health care students and professionals, the book now presents much more clinical information, often highlighted in blue boxes next to the relevant illustrations. Each of the nine chapters progresses logically from photographs of surface anatomy (many new to this edition) to the bones, detailed regional anatomy, and finally cross-sectional and diagnostic images. However, instruction on how to interpret such images is lacking. With a common author, many of the new images in *Grant's* can also be found in Moore and Dalley's *Clinically Oriented Anatomy*, a very popular anatomy book for medical professionals. For the first time, "a wide range of electronic ancillaries for both student and teacher" are accessible at the companion website, http://thepoint.lww.com, which is included when individuals purchase the print book. An earlier edition of this title appeared on the final Brandon/Hill list, and it is included in *Doody's Core Titles.*

Gray's Anatomy for Students. 2nd ed. Authors: Richard L. Drake, Wayne Vogl, Adam W.M. Mitchell. Churchill Livingstone/Elsevier, 2010.
http://www.mdconsult.com/
ISBN: 9780443069529
Recommended for: Hospital, Academic Libraries
Doody's Core Titles Selection

First published in 2005 as a "Student-oriented companion text for *Gray's Anatomy*" (Preface), the second edition of this already popular text has improved its reputation for being both fairly complete and easy to understand. Designed to teach anatomy to a variety of health professional students, the book's excellent readability makes it suitable for advanced undergraduates. It follows the trend in anatomy instruction toward a regional approach with a strong emphasis on correlating anatomy to clinical problems. Over 1,000 clearly labeled color anatomical illustrations by Richard Tibbitts and Paul Richardson and 300 clinical photographs and diagnostic images enhance the text. New to this edition is an introductory overview chapter, which provides valuable information on body systems, modern imaging technology, and applications to common clinical problems. Chapters on each body region follow, beginning with the back since it is usually the first region a student encounters in dissection. Each chapter presents a conceptual overview, detailed regional anatomy, and a very useful section on surface anatomy. Numerous "In the Clinic" boxes summarize clinical concepts and applications. Closing each chapter are several clinical cases highlighting the relevance of anatomical knowledge to injuries and disease; the cases are liberally illustrated with radiographs, CT, MRI, and other diagnostic images. Readability is increased with the addition of color coding of the top edges of the chapters and a revised index. In addition to institutional access through the MD Consult Basic Science Collection, student purchasers of the print version can access the STUDENT CONSULT website, which is unlocked by an accompanying PIN. This book is highly recommended, being a *Doody's Core Titles* recommendation and BMA (British Medical Association) 2009 Book Award winner, whose judges found it to be "a really helpful resource for any medical student."

Sobotta Atlas of Human Anatomy: Head, Neck, Upper Limb, Thorax, Abdomen, Pelvis, Lower Limb. 14th ed. Editors: Reinhard Putz, Reinhard Pabst, Renate Putz. Urban & Fischer/Elsevier, 2008.
ISBN: 9780702033230
Recommended for: Academic Libraries

Published for over a century, this classic atlas continues to be unequalled, with almost 2,000 beautiful, high-quality illustrations, clear organization, comprehensive coverage of subject, and precise attention to detail. The latest edition has added 200 figures, including many new clinical images—from X-ray, CT, and MRI images to endoscopic and intra-operative color photographs of inner organs. The atlas is organized by body region, corresponding to the standard sequence of topics in dissection and thus facilitating the reader's understanding of the clinical applications of anatomical structures. New introductions and general overviews for complex topics are helpful for the student. While more expensive than some other texts, this is a superb atlas suitable for all types of modern anatomy courses, and it also serves as an excellent reference work.

24.5. Cytology

The structure and function of cells.
—MeSH

Contributor: Cotina M. Jones

Monographs

Cytology: Diagnostic Principles and Clinical Correlates. 3rd ed. Authors: Edmund S. Cibas, Barbara S. Ducatman. Saunders/Elsevier, 2009.
http://www.sciencedirect.com/science/book/9781416053293
ISBN: 9781416053293
Recommended for: Hospital, Academic Libraries
Doody's Core Titles Selection

The authors focus on the current diagnostic techniques for a variety of cell specimens. The revised edition of this textbook includes over 700 full-color illustrations as well as updated diagnostic terminology and clinical management information. Individuals who purchase the print book are provided with online access to the entire textbook through the Expert Consult platform, allowing images from the book to be downloaded for personal use. Institutional online access is available through Elsevier's

ScienceDirect platform. This book is an excellent review source for practicing pathologists and should be included in the reference collection of hospital libraries. Postgraduate students will find this resource useful as an introduction to cytopathology.

Essential Cell Biology. 3rd ed. Authors: Bruce Alberts, Dennis Bray, Karen Hopkin, Alexander Johnson, Martin Raff, Keith Roberts, Julian Lewis, Peter Walter. Garland Science/Taylor & Francis, 2010.
ISBN: 9780815341291
Recommended for: Academic Libraries
Doody's Core Titles Selection

This text provides the reader with an introduction to cell biology. The third edition has been revised to include a DVD-ROM that provides the reader with access to over 130 videos, illustrations, and animations that help them learn cell biology. A quiz is also included that the reader can utilize to test understanding of the concepts that are presented. A glossary located at the end of the book defines relevant terms introduced to the reader throughout the textbook. This text would be an excellent addition to academic libraries that support undergraduate life science students.

Medical Cell Biology. 3rd ed. Editor: Steven R. Goodman. Elsevier, 2008.
ISBN: 9780123704580
Recommended for: Hospital, Academic Libraries
Doody's Core Titles Selection

The revised edition of this textbook is relevant for both undergraduate and graduate students in medical, dental, veterinary, and pre-health majors. Color illustrations are included that help students understand cell biology as it relates to human and animal disease. This book can be utilized as an introductory resource to learning cytology principles as they correlate to organ systems and disease. It is also effective as a review source for those students that are preparing for their National Board exams. A CD-ROM with 200 sample test questions is included to assist students with their exam preparation. This book is an appropriate addition for the reference collections of both hospital and academic libraries.

Journals

The Journal of Cell Biology. v. 12, The Rockefeller University Press, 1962.
http://jcb.rupress.org/
http://www.ncbi.nlm.nih.gov/pmc/journals/482/
http://www.jstor.org/
ISSN: 00219525
ISSN: 15408140 (Online)
Indexed in: MEDLINE
Recommended for: Academic Libraries

The Journal of Cell Biology continues *The Journal of Biophysical and Biochemical Cytology*, which was in publication from 1955 until December 1961. This journal publishes original research on topics such as cell adhesion and motility; cellular communication; cell cycle and division; cell growth, survival, and death; cell structure and dynamics; and cellular disease mechanisms. With an impact factor of 9.575 it ranked fifteenth of 162 journals in cell biology in the 2009 *Journal Citation Reports*. It is cited in many abstracting and indexing sources such as Biological Abstracts, General Science Index, MEDLINE, and Chemical Abstracts. This journal is a useful resource for academic libraries that support clinical laboratory science and medical technology programs. Online coverage back to 1962 is provided through JSTOR.

24.6. Embryology

The development of an organism during the embryonic and fetal stages of life.

—MeSH

Contributor: Peggy Cruse

Monographs

The Developing Human: Clinically Oriented Embryology. 8th ed. Authors: Keith L. Moore, T.V.N. Persaud, Mark G. Torchia. Saunders/Elsevier, 2008.
http://www.mdconsult.com/
ISBN: 9781416037064
Recommended for: Academic Libraries
Brandon/Hill Selection

This is an excellent resource for first and second-year medical students. Moore and Persaud are professors as well as physicians, and they ensure the content is clinically applicable and the organization is pedagogically conscious. The first six chapters offer an overview of fetal development. The remaining chapters focus on the development of different body systems, including the most common complications and development abnormalities for each system. The final chapter, new to this edition, explains recent discoveries in common molecular signaling pathways. Clinical content is highlighted in boxes, enabling quick reference. The book is designed to help students learn and master concepts, and they will surely appreciate chapter summaries, clinically-oriented questions, and a list of resources for further reading. Over 1,800 detailed color diagrams, illustrations, and images help readers visualize the development process. For individual purchasers of the print textbook, all content is available online through STUDENT CONSULT, along with 18 annotated animations of major fetal development processes. Institutional online access is provided through MD Consult's basic science collection. This textbook has received positive feedback from students and instructors alike and should be a staple in libraries serving first and second-year medical students. In 2008, it was highly commended by the British Medical Association as an "extremely accessible book that has a lot more clinical correlation than its previous editions." *Before We Are Born: Essentials of Embryology and Birth Defects* (2008), an abbreviated version of this text, is also available from the authors.

Developmental Biology. 9th ed. Author: Scott F. Gilbert. Sinauer, 2010.
ISBN: 9780878933846
ISBN: 9780878935642
See Also Chapter 26.2. Developmental Biology
Recommended for: Academic Libraries
Doody's Core Titles Selection

This comprehensive book is recommended primarily for undergraduate students. It would also be a helpful resource for beginning graduate and medical students, as well as a reference for developmental biology researchers. In clear and detailed writing, the book covers all essential aspects of early developmental biology, including experimental embryology, ethical considerations (a topic seldom covered in medical texts), genetic and environmental impacts, and current research and clinical applications. This text covers embryonic development in multiple animal and plant species. Numerous pictures, images, charts, and graphs compliment the text, making difficult topics easier to grasp. The book was positively reviewed in several journals, including *The Quarterly Review of Biology*, which stated, "Gilbert's publication remains the standard against which other developmental textbooks must measure themselves" (2006 Dec; 81(4):401). This textbook is also included in the *Doody's Core Titles* list for anatomy/embryology. This review refers to the eighth edition.

Human Embryology and Developmental Biology. 4th ed. Author: Bruce M. Carlson. Mosby/Elsevier, 2009.
ISBN: 9780323053853
Recommended for: Academic Libraries

As he states in the preface, Bruce Carlson's text is meant to "serve as a gateway for the uninitiated and a falling-back place for the narrow specialist who wishes to look at his or her system in a broader developmental context." The book received a positive review from a judge at the British Medical Association's 2009 Book Awards, who stated that it is "an excellent content bridge between anatomy and clinical practice." The textbook provides up-to-date explanations of key advances in mechanistic and molecular biology that have reshaped classic embryology as a discipline. It is divided into two sections: "Early Development and the Fetal-Maternal Relationship" and "Development of Body Systems." Chapters include clinical vignettes, summaries, review questions, and detailed color images. Individual purchasers of the print textbook receive online access to STUDENT CONSULT, where they may view all text and images in the book, as well as answer review questions and watch embryology animations. This book is recommended for libraries serving preclinical medical students.

Langman's Medical Embryology. 11th ed. Author: Thomas W. Sadler. Lippincott Williams & Wilkins, 2010.
ISBN: 9780781790697
Recommended for: Academic Libraries
Doody's Core Titles Selection

Now in its eleventh edition, *Langman's Medical Embryology* has become a fixture in many medical school anatomy and development curricula. It is recommended for libraries serving first and second-year medical students. Understanding the incredible volume of information that medical students must master, the author's goal is to balance thoroughness with brevity. This is accomplished by combining clear text with nearly 400 images, including diagrams, scanning electron micrographs, and clinical pictures. In fewer than 400 pages, the book describes normal and abnormal development of the embryo and fetus, molecular biology, genetics, key signaling pathways, and clinical correlates. It is divided into two sections: general embryology, from gametogenesis to birth, and the development of each body system. All book content, as well as USMLE prep questions and several animations, are available online through Lippincott's "thePoint" website for individuals who purchase the print edition. Due to the text's brevity, some students may find explanations too abrupt and choose to use this book as a review source in tandem with a more detailed text such as *Larsen's Human Embryology*. *Langman's* is a *Doody's Core Titles* selection in anatomy/embryology.

Larsen's Human Embryology. 4th ed. Authors: Gary C. Schoenwolf, Steven B. Bleyl, Philip R. Brauer, Philippa H.

Francis-West. Churchill Livingstone/Elsevier, 2009.
http://www.mdconsult.com/
ISBN: 9780443068119
Recommended for: Hospital, Academic Libraries
Brandon/Hill, *Doody's Core Titles* Selection

Now in its fourth edition, *Larsen's Human Embryology* remains committed to the original mission: "to meet the needs of first-year medical students ... and to offer them a glimpse of some of the exciting applications that are currently in use or on the horizon." In addition to serving medical students, this would be an excellent reference for practitioners who wish to see how current advances in the field are being taught. Schoenwolf has done an excellent job revising and updating this edition, which now includes: an introduction, visual organization of chapter headings and subheadings for easy reference, "Clinical Taster" sections to whet students' curiosity at the start of each chapter, and updates of all references. The book also includes "In the Clinic" and "In the Research Lab" sections that relate chapter concepts to real world applications. This is one of the most substantial embryology textbooks available, with clear writing from area experts and numerous color images. A final mark of the book's excellence, which should make librarians happy, is its introductory section titled "Want to Learn More," which offers students subject-specific research tips to develop their information literacy skills. Individual purchase of the print text comes with online access to STUDENT CONSULT. Institutional online access can be obtained through MD Consult's basic science specialty collection. *Doody's* has given this title a score of 95 and placed it on their *Core Titles* list for anatomy/embryology.

Journals

***Annual Review of Cell and Developmental Biology*.** v. 11, Annual Reviews, 1995.
http://arjournals.annualreviews.org/loi/cellbio
ISSN: 10810706
ISSN: 15308995 (Online)
Indexed in: MEDLINE
Recommended for: Hospital, Academic Libraries

This serial provides annual reviews of primary research in the fields of cellular and developmental biology. The publisher, Annual Reviews, is a non-profit group whose goal is to "provide the worldwide scientific community with a useful and intelligent synthesis of primary research literature." Each year, a panel of area experts selects topics for review, and distinguished scholars are then invited to contribute articles that review and synthesize primary research conducted within the field. It originated in 1985 under the title *Annual Review of Cell Biology* and has since become one of the most cited publications for developmental biology. According to the 2009 *Journal Citation Reports*, this publication is ranked number one out of 36 developmental biology journals. Each issue contains a subject and author index for quick reference. This serial is recommended for institutions that serve cellular and molecular biologists concerned with plant and animal development, as well as academic libraries serving graduate biology students.

***Development*.** v. 99, The Company of Biologists, 1987.
http://dev.biologists.org/
ISSN: 09501991
ISSN: 14779129 (Online)
See Also Chapter 26.2. Developmental Biology
Indexed in: MEDLINE
Recommended for: Hospital, Academic Libraries

Originating in 1953 under the title *Journal of Embryology and Experimental Morphology*, *Development* is the official journal of The Company of Biologists, a non-profit organization of biologists committed to advancing communication and research in the developmental biology community. All articles are peer-reviewed, providing up-to-date, high quality research in the field. Content also includes review and hypothesis articles, educational primer articles, and meeting reviews. The journal covers a wide range of topics, "from stem cells and nuclear reprogramming, to evolutionary developmental and systems biology, from neurobiology to regional specification, morphogenesis and organogenesis, and from epigenetics to the aetiology of disease." Print and online issues are published every two weeks. This journal is an essential addition to hospitals and academic libraries serving clinicians and research specialists in a wide range of biological science realms, from obstetricians and geneticists to teratologists. The journal is indexed in BIOBASE, CAB abstracts, CSA, Current Contents, Embase, Web of Science, MEDLINE, and Scopus. Special Library Association's BioMedical and Life Sciences Division listed *Development* as one of the top 100 most influential journals for 2009. According to the 2009 *Journal Citation Reports*, it is ranked fourth out of 36 developmental biology journals, with an impact factor of 7.194.

***Developmental Biology*.** v. 1, Elsevier, 1959.
http://www.sciencedirect.com/science/journal/00121606
ISSN: 00121606 (Print/Online)
See Also Chapter 26.2. Developmental Biology
Indexed in: MEDLINE
Recommended for: Hospital, Academic Libraries

Developmental Biology is the official journal of the Society for Developmental Biology. In 2009, the Special Libraries Association's BioMedical and Life Science Division voted *Developmental Biology* as one of the century's top 100 Biology and Medicine journals. *Developmental Biology* releases 24 issues a year; and, with a 2009 impact factor of 4.379 according to *Journal Citation Reports*, it is ranked seventh out of 36 developmental biology journals. The journal publishes original research articles pertaining to the development and growth of plants and animals. "Areas of particular emphasis include transcriptional control mechanisms, embryonic patterning, cell-cell interactions, growth factors and signal transduction, and regulatory hierarchies." This highly ranked journal is recommended for all health sciences collections that serve students and researchers studying molecular, cellular, and genetic aspects of development in animal and plant species. *Developmental Biology* is currently abstracted and indexed in 13 major science databases.

Developmental Dynamics. v. 193, Wiley-Liss, 1992.
http://onlinelibrary.wiley.com/journal/10.1002/(ISSN)1097-0177
ISSN: 10588388
ISSN: 10970177 (Online)
Indexed in: MEDLINE
Recommended for: Hospital, Academic Libraries

Originally titled *The American Journal of Anatomy*, *Developmental Dynamics* is an official journal of the American Association of Anatomists. It is published monthly and covers the latest research in the field of developmental biology, from the molecular to the organismal level. It focuses on "tissue, cellular, and molecular-genetic mechanisms of morphogenesis." In addition to reporting peer-reviewed research articles and topic reviews, the journal also publishes book reviews, a useful inclusion for instructors and collection development specialists. This journal would be suitable for institutions that serve developmental and cellular biologists, geneticists, biochemists, and anatomists. It is also recommended for graduate students studying within the above fields. According to the 2009 *Journal Citation Reports*, *Developmental Dynamics* has an impact factor of 2.833, third of 16 anatomy and morphology journals; it also ranks sixteenth out of 36 developmental biology journals. It is abstracted and indexed in over two dozen general and health science databases.

Mechanisms of Development. v. 33, Elsevier, 1990.
http://www.sciencedirect.com/science/journal/09254773
ISSN: 09254773 (Print/Online)
Indexed in: MEDLINE
Recommended for: Hospital, Academic Libraries

This monthly serial is the official publication of the International Society of Developmental Biologists. It was previously titled *Cell Differentiation and Development* (1988–1990) and *Cell Differentiation* (1972–1988). Content focuses on the molecular mechanisms involved during the development of vertebrates and invertebrates, such as embryogenesis, cell determination and differentiation, and signal transduction. The publication's aim is to "provide a unique forum for comparing and contrasting strategies of development among a wide spectrum of organisms." According to the 2009 *Journal Citation Reports*, this title has an impact factor of 2.827 and a five-year impact factor of 3.195. It is recommended for hospital and academic libraries serving molecular and cell biologists studying development.

Databases and Other Electronic Resources

Human Embryology Animations. Indiana University, 2001–2009.
http://www.indiana.edu/~anat550/embryo_main/
Recommended for: Academic, Consumer Health Libraries

Professor Valerie O'Loughlin created this collection of online embryology animations to help her undergraduate anatomy students understand the process of human development. All animations are accurate, detailed, and free to anyone with an Internet connection. The 16 animations are divided into five sections: general embryology, cardiovascular embryology, development of the head and neck, gastrointestinal embryology, and urinary and reproductive embryology. At the time of this writing, animations for the development of the limbs are still in process. Animations can be played, paused, and rewound. They are colored to aid comprehension of different structures and are accompanied by detailed explanations. Each contains a one millimeter scale reference. In addition, pre- and post-quizzes are available for students who wish to test their comprehension. According to a 2007 Indiana University-Bloomington news article, the animations have been viewed on every continent except Antarctica. In 2007, O'Loughlin received the Basmajian Award for excellence in teaching, research, and scholarship from the American Association for Anatomists. This resource is recommended for any instructor or student involved with introductory anatomy courses.

The Multi-Dimensional Human Embryo. Bradley R. Smith, 2009.
http://embryo.soad.umich.edu/

Recommended for: Hospital, Academic, Consumer Health Libraries

This collection of three-dimensional magnetic resonance images details the development of the human embryo from the 13th to 23rd Carnegie stages and is available for free to anyone who has an Internet connection. This project was funded by the National Institute of Child Health and Human Development (NICHD) in an effort to support the educational and research needs of clinicians, students, laboratory specialists, and the general public. Images for each of the ten stages were rendered using magnetic resonance microscopy (MRM). Perhaps the most noteworthy aspect of the collection is the number and variety of images at each stage. Color photographs; coronal, sagittal, and axial cross-section images; time-lapse videos; brief explanations; and rotating black-and-white QuickTime videos that highlight different organs are available for each Carnegie stage. This free resource would be valuable to anyone studying or instructing lessons in human embryo development or imaging. The website also contains a complete list of references and links to related resources and tools.

24.7. Histology

The anatomical study of the microscopic structure of animal and plant tissues.

—MeSH

Contributor: Cotina M. Jones

Monographs

diFiore's Atlas of Histology with Functional Correlations. 11th ed. Author: Victor P. Eroschenko. Lippincott Williams & Wilkins, 2008.
ISBN: 9780781770576
Recommended for: Academic Libraries
Brandon/Hill, *Doody's Core Titles* Selection

Previous editions of this textbook have been included on the Brandon/Hill list and this edition is a selection in *Doody's Core Titles*. It is an excellent resource for academic libraries that support upper-level undergraduate, graduate, and medical students. The author explains histology concepts by using full-color illustrations. The drawings are incredibly detailed, which allow the reader to view the functions of the cells and to understand how they function. The first section of this two-part book explains tissues and their relationships to their systems, and the second section explains organs and their relationships to their systems. An online component is included for individuals who purchase the print book, providing student and instructor access to all of the book's images.

Junqueira's Basic Histology: Text and Atlas. 12th ed. Editor: Anthony L. Mescher. McGraw-Hill, 2010.
http://www.accessmedicine.com/
ISBN: 9780071630207
Recommended for: Academic Libraries
Doody's Core Titles Selection

The twelfth edition of this textbook continues *Junqueira's* tradition of providing effective and comprehensive coverage of basic histology. Upper-level undergraduate, graduate, and postgraduate students will find this book useful as a primary resource to learn about histological structure and function. This edition has been updated to include over 1,000 images. The work would be a worthwhile addition for academic library collections and the reference collection of histology professionals. An introductory chapter on laboratory methods for studying tissue samples is included in this revised edition. A CD-ROM accompanies the print textbook, which contains all of the book's images.

Journals

Blood. v. 1, American Society of Hematology, 1946.
See Chapter 10.12. Pathology

Journal of Molecular Histology. v. 35, Springer Netherlands., 2004.
http://www.springerlink.com/content/111649/
ISSN: 15672379
ISSN: 15672387 (Online)
Indexed in: MEDLINE
Recommended for: Academic Libraries

The *Journal of Molecular Histology* continues *The Histochemical Journal*, which was in publication from 1968 until 2003. This journal publishes original research on topics such as cell-cell and cell extracellular matrix interactions; cellular cytoskeleton and receptor dynamics and functions; cell and tissue differentiation and remodeling; genetically engineered cells and tissues; three-dimensional reconstructions; cell cycle and cell lineage analysis involving gene expression profiles; apoptosis; gene expression analysis from histological preparations; functional genomics and proteomics; new and improved techniques; and critical reports on existing techniques used in molecular histology. It is cited in many abstracting and indexing sources such as Chemical Abstracts, Biochemistry and Biophysics Citation Index, BIOBASE, MEDLINE.

25. Biochemistry

The chemistry of living organisms and of the chemical, molecular, and physical changes occurring therein.
—*Stedman's Medical Dictionary*, 28th edition (2006)

Contributor: Susan K. Kendall

Monographs

Biochemistry. 7th ed. Authors: Jeremy M. Berg, John L. Tymoczko, Lubert Stryer. W.H. Freeman, 2011.
ISBN: 9781429229364
Recommended for: Academic Libraries
Doody's Core Titles Selection

This is a classic undergraduate biochemistry text. The emphasis is on biochemistry with physiological relevance and clinical applications. New information gained from recent gene sequencing and analysis projects keeps the book current, and there is a molecular evolutionary perspective. Discussion of many recent advances since the previous edition have been added, and now all molecular structures are available for viewing in 3D on the book's companion website. Three chapters focus solely on the tools and techniques of biochemistry and molecular biology. The fifth edition of the text is available for searching electronically on the NCBI bookshelf (http://www.ncbi.nlm.nih.gov/books) for free. This review refers to the sixth edition.

Biochemistry. 4th ed. Authors: Donald Voet, Judith G. Voet. Wiley, 2011.
ISBN: 9780470570951
ISBN: 9780470917459
Recommended for: Academic Libraries
Doody's Core Titles Selection

This comprehensive biochemistry text is more advanced, in-depth, and more chemistry oriented than the Lehninger or Berg/Stryer texts, which have a biological/medical focus. Students and researchers with a strong chemistry background find that this text better correlates biochemistry with general and organic chemistry and that it provides much more detail on mechanisms. A CD-ROM accompanies the book with animated interactive exercises and guided explorations, as well as computer-animated images of proteins and nucleic acids. The last chapter is only available on the web, and, fortunately for libraries, it is free and does not involve login or proof-of-purchase information. This review refers to the third edition.

Lehninger Principles of Biochemistry. 5th ed. Authors: David L. Nelson, Michael M. Cox, Albert Lehninger. W.H. Freeman, 2008.
ISBN: 9781429224161
Recommended for: Academic Libraries

This classic textbook was originally authored by the American biochemist, Albert L. Lehninger (1917–1986) and continues to bear his name. Major recent advances are included, and there is information on newer biochemical techniques and methods. Medically relevant examples are highlighted throughout the book, and diabetes/obesity is an integrating theme throughout the chapters devoted to metabolism. The text is also available as an e-book for individual instructors and students to purchase, although not as a purchase for institutions or libraries.

Journals

Biochemical Journal. v. 1, Portland Press, 1906.
http://www.biochemj.org/
http://www.ncbi.nlm.nih.gov/pmc/journals/74/
ISSN: 14708728 (Online)
ISSN: 02646021
Indexed in: MEDLINE
Recommended for: Academic Libraries

Published on behalf of the Biochemical Society (Great Britain) by Portland Press, this international peer-reviewed journal includes papers from all areas of biochemistry and cellular and molecular biology. The focus is on experimental research and primary articles, but each issue may also contain one or two review articles or commentary. The journal is selective, and papers are expected to promote "the development of biochemical concepts rather than the mere recording of facts." The website for the journal does more than just list available issues. It tries to be a "knowledge environment" for topical subject areas such as plant, disease, cell, gene, and metabolism, and arranges content into these environments by spotlighting relevant newly published papers from the *Biochemical Journal*, reviews, commentaries, and information on upcoming meetings. It has an impact factor of 5.155 and ranks fiftieth out of 283 journals in biochemistry and molecular biology (2009 *Journal Citation Reports*). It is indexed by numerous indexing and abstracting sources including CAB Abstracts, Embase, MEDLINE, Scopus, and Web of Science. Online access is available through PubMed Central from volume 1, 1906 through three years prior to current.

Biochemistry. v. 1, American Chemical Society, 1962.
http://pubs.acs.org/journal/bichaw
ISSN: 00062960
ISSN: 15204995 (Online)
Indexed in: MEDLINE
Recommended for: Academic Libraries

The American Chemical Society is the leading publisher of research journals in the chemical sciences, and their journals are well read, respected, and cited by chemists and biochemists. With an impact factor of 3.226 (2009 *Journal Citation Reports*), *Biochemistry* is one of the top-ranked journals in biochemistry. It also includes articles in biophysics, cellular and molecular biology, chemical biology, proteomics, and computational chemistry. In addition to peer-reviewed original research articles, the journal publishes accelerated publications, new concepts, current topics, and rapid reports. The journal is indexed in numerous indexing and abstracting sources including AGRICOLA, CAB Abstracts, Embase, MEDLINE, Scopus, and Web of Science. Online access back to v. 1, 1962 is available from the publisher.

Biochimica et Biophysica Acta. v. 1, Elsevier, 1947.
http://www.sciencedirect.com/science/journal/03044165
ISSN: 00063002
ISSN: 00052728
ISSN: 00052736
ISSN: 15709639
ISSN: 03044165
ISSN: 13881981
ISSN: 09254439
ISSN: 01674889
ISSN: 18749399
ISSN: 0304419X
Indexed in: MEDLINE
Recommended for: Academic Libraries

The first international journal in the field of biochemistry and biophysics and the first ever international journal launched by Elsevier, *Biochimica et Biophysica Acta* (*BBA*) is probably one of the only journals to have had a history written about it (*Biochimica et Biophysica Acta: The Story of a Biochemical Journal*, by E.C. Slater, Elsevier Science, 1986). It is published in topical sections whose titles and content focus changes over time to keep up with trends in the field. Currently there are nine sections: "Bioenergetics," "Biomembranes," "Gene Regulatory Mechanisms," "General Subjects," "Molecular and Cell Biology of Lipids," "Molecular Cell Research," "Proteins and Proteomics," "Molecular Basis of Disease," and "Reviews on Cancer." It remains a well-respected and high-ranking journal in the field (each section has its own *JCR* impact factor) and a very prolific one since it has so many sections. BBA is available in both print and online formats, with online access back to 1947 available from the publisher.

Cell. v. 1, Cell Press, 1974.
http://www.cell.com
http://www.sciencedirect.com/science/journal/00928674
ISSN: 00928674
ISSN: 10974172 (Online)
Indexed in: MEDLINE
Recommended for: Academic Libraries

The top ranked journal, *Cell*, was founded in 1974, and it published significantly in the areas of molecular and cellular biology throughout the eighties and nineties. In the late 1990s, a number of daughter journals were split off from the flagship journal, with each retaining editorial independence. *Cell* continues to publish research in any area of biology, although it is often ranked as a molecular biology or genetics journal due to its content. Publishing 26 peer-reviewed issues per year, *Cell* includes "findings of unusual significance in any area of experimental biology, including but not limited to cell biology, molecular biology, neuroscience, immunology, virology and microbiology, cancer, human genetics, systems biology, signaling, and disease." With an astounding impact factor of 31.152, it ranks first of 283 journals in biochemistry and molecular biology and second of 162 journals in cell biology in the 2009 *Journal Citation Reports*. It is indexed in all the major indexing and abstracting services. Online access back to volume 1, 1974 is available from both Cell Press and ScienceDirect. The Cell Press site includes a variety of additional features, including "Graphical Abstracts," "Cell Picture Show," "Paper Flicks," and podcasts.

Journal of Biological Chemistry. v. 1, American Society for Biochemistry and Molecular Biology, 1905.
http://www.jbc.org/
http://www.ncbi.nlm.nih.gov/pmc/journals/567/
ISSN: 00219258

ISSN: 1083351X (Online)
Indexed in: MEDLINE
Recommended for: Academic Libraries

One of the oldest and most respected journals in the field of biochemistry, this weekly peer-reviewed journal publishes a very large number of articles. The majority of the journal is made up of original research articles. In addition, the journal publishes invited mini-reviews to provide a concise summary of research in a particular field to assist biochemists working in any area to keep current, invited "Reflections" by major biochemists and molecular biologists who have significantly affected the field, as well as varied content from selected relevant meetings. It is ranked forty-eighth of 283 journals in biochemistry and molecular biology with an impact factor of 5.328 (2009 *Journal Citation Reports*).The journal is indexed in numerous indexing and abstracting sources including CAB Abstracts, Embase, MEDLINE, Scopus, and Web of Science. Online access back to 2905 is available from the publisher. Online access to issues from 2008 to one year prior to current is also available on PubMed Central.

Methods in Enzymology. v. 1, Elsevier, 1955.
http://www.sciencedirect.com/science/journal/00766879
ISSN: 00766879
ISSN: 15577988 (Online)
Indexed in: MEDLINE
Recommended for: Academic Libraries

This well-respected and cited monographic series now consists of over 480 volumes. Several volumes come out each year on discrete molecular and biochemical topics. Subjects covered in recent volumes include: biothermodynamics, angiogenesis, microRNA methods, nuclear magnetic resonance and chromatin. Each volume has its own editor, and the individual chapters or articles are written by different authors or groups of authors. These peer-reviewed articles focus on new experimental methodologies for researchers as well as background information about their topic. Although often considered a monographic series, this resource is indexed by numerous indexing and abstracting sources including Chem Abstracts, Embase, MEDLINE, Scopus, and Web of Science. Individual volumes are available for purchase and the series is available as a subscription either in print or online, with online access to volume 1, 1955 available from the publisher.

Trends in Biochemical Sciences. v. 1, Elsevier, 1976.
http://www.cell.com/trends/biochemical-sciences/
http://sciencedirect.com/science/journal/09680004
ISSN: 09680004
ISSN: 01677640 (Online)
Indexed in: MEDLINE
Recommended for: Academic Libraries

TiBS is the leading monthly review-only journal in biochemistry and was the first journal in the well-known *Trends in...* series. This peer-reviewed journal is published for the International Union of Biochemistry and Molecular Biology. Each issue contains four to six significant reviews of cutting edge subjects and may also contain opinion articles, historical reviews, and a research focus or update section. Like other important review journals, this is essential reading for students and researchers to keep current in the field. It ranks twelfth of 286 journals in biochemistry and molecular biology with an impact factor of 11.572 (2009 *Journal Citation Reports*). It is indexed in numerous indexing and abstracting sources including CAB Abstracts, Embase, MEDLINE, Scopus, and Web of Science. Online access back to 1976 is available from the publisher.

Databases and Other Electronic Resources

Current Protocols. Wiley, 2000.
See Chapter 26.6. Molecular Biology

25.1. Proteomics

The complete complement of proteins (proteome) of organisms.
—MeSH

Contributor: Susan K. Kendall

Systems Biomedicine: Concepts and Perspectives. Editors: Edison T. Liu, Douglas A. Lauffenburger. Academic Press Elsevier, 2010.
See Chapter 26.10. Systems Biology

Journals

Molecular and Cellular Proteomics. v. 1, American Society for Biochemistry and Molecular Biology, 2002.
http://www.mcponline.org/
http://www.ncbi.nlm.nih.gov/pmc/journals/569/
ISSN: 15359476
ISSN: 15359484 (Online)
Indexed in: MEDLINE
Recommended for: Academic Libraries

The field of proteomics is new and growing, and a number of journals specifically devoted to it have sprung up in the last ten years. This is one of the most cited and well-known and is published by the main society for biochemistry in the United States, the American Society for Biochemistry and Molecular Biology. The journal publishes three types of peer-reviewed research articles: research papers, database articles, and technology development articles. It also publishes mini-reviews and invited perspective articles on important unresolved issues. According to its scope statement, the journal is "open to contributions that describe the structural and functional properties of proteins and their expression, particularly with respect to developmental time courses. Emphasis will be placed on determining how the presence or absence of proteins affects biological responses, and how the interaction of proteins with germane cellular partners allows them to function." The online version of the journal includes the substantive supporting databases that are generated by the research reported in the issue. It is indexed in numerous indexing and abstracting sources including CAB Abstracts, Embase, MEDLINE, Scopus, and Web of Science. Access to the online version of the journal back to 2002 is available from the publisher. Issues from 2008 to one year prior to current are also available in PubMed Central.

Molecular Systems Biology. v. 1, Nature Publishing Group and European Molecular Biology Organization, 2005.
See Chapter 26.6. Molecular Biology

Proteomics. v. 1, Wiley-Blackwell, 2001.
http://onlinelibrary.wiley.com/journal/10.1002/(ISSN)1615-9861
ISSN: 16159853
ISSN: 16159861 (Online)
Indexed in: MEDLINE
Recommended for: Academic Libraries

With an impact factor of 4.426 (2009 *Journal Citation Reports*), this peer-reviewed journal is one of the top journals focusing on new applications and technologies in this expanding field. Whole proteome analyses of organisms as well as papers focusing on disease studies or biotechnological applications of proteomics technologies are accepted. Besides research articles there are other sections in the issues with a more technical focus: technical briefs, dataset briefs, and standardization and guideline articles. Each year also has special issues, such as a whole issue of proteomics reviews or yeast proteomics. It is international in scope and was recently endorsed as the official journal of the Human Proteome Organization. This journal is indexed in numerous indexing and abstracting sources including CAB Abstracts, Embase, MEDLINE, Scopus, and Web of Science. Online access back to volume 1 is available from the publisher.

26. Biology

The origin, structure, development, growth, function, genetics, and reproduction of animals, plants, and micro-organisms.

—MeSH

Contributor: Heather Cunningham

Monographs

Biology. 9th ed. Authors: Peter Raven, George Johnson, Kenneth A. Mason, Jonathan B. Losos, Susan Singer. McGraw-Hill Higher Education, 2011.
ISBN: 9780077350024
Recommended for: Academic, Consumer Health Libraries

This review refers to the eighth edition of *Biology*, which was extensively revised to integrate new research, including developments within the rapidly advancing fields of molecular biology and genomics. The authors have a wealth of experience in teaching undergraduate biology and this is reflected in the clear explanations of advanced concepts as well as the overall engaging text. The focus of this textbook is on modern biology and it connects the different areas of biology through the unifying themes of evolutionary theory and the experimental framework through which knowledge is gained. This textbook is extensively and beautifully illustrated by a team of medical and scientific illustrators, and includes color photographs as well as realistic 3-D and multi-layered figures. Great care and attention to detail went into page design and layout which clearly highlight the important concepts. This publication is divided into 59 chapters, each of which begins with a concept outline and concludes with a concept review and questions. Answers to these questions, as well as animations, videos, and other additional material on the subjects, can be found at the Assessment Review and Instruction System (ARIS) website. Also available on the ARIS website is a freely-available, full-text electronic copy of the book. The print version of this resource is available as one complete volume or divided into three separate volumes to further increase flexibility in purchasing. This textbook is highly recommended for academic libraries as well as for consumer health collections.

Dictionary of Biology. 6th ed. Editor: Robert S. Hine. Oxford University, 2008.
http://www.oup.com/online/us/oro/?view=usa
ISBN: 9780199204625
Recommended for: Hospital, Academic, Consumer Health Libraries

The sixth edition of the *Oxford Dictionary of Biology* has been revised to include 400 additional terms, many of which come from the rapidly changing fields of molecular evolution and systematics, genomics, bioinformatics, and immunology. This resource features several general appendixes on simplified plant and animal classification tables as well as a geologic timescale and a table of mass extinctions. Appendixes relevant to medical researchers include model organisms and their genomes as well as the Nobel prizewinners for medicine and physiology. This publication includes 5,500 terms, and complements the 22,000 terms included in Henderson's *Dictionary of Biology* through additional content such as the "relevant features" articles which provide two pages of coverage on timely topics such as bioinformatics or microarray. Also, both the print and online versions of the *Oxford Dictionary of Biology* contain numerous illustrations and direct the user to websites for entries requiring more in-depth information. For example, a link to the complete works of Charles Darwin is included after his brief biographical entry. This dictionary is highly recommended by the American Library Association for all university and public libraries. The online version is part of the *Oxford Reference Online* collection.

Frontiers of Life. Editors: David Baltimore, Renato Dulbecco, Francoise Jacob, Rita Levi-Montalcini. Academic, 2002.
ISBN: 9780120773404 (set)
ISBN: 9780120773411 (v.1)
ISBN: 9780120773428 (v.2)
ISBN: 9780120773435 (v.3)
ISBN: 9780120773442 (v.4)
Recommended for: Academic Libraries

Frontiers of Life is unique in its approach to the topic of modern biology in that instead of attempting to be comprehensive of such a broad topic, this work focuses on subjects considered to be of the greatest theoretical and practical importance in the biological sciences and their new fields of research and opportunity. Lengthy, detailed and thought-provoking entries, often between 15–20 pages in length with detailed bibliographies, have been compiled by eminent researchers from all fields of biology as well as physics, mathematics, chemistry, and other cross-disciplines; and the four editors of this work are all Nobel laureates. Spanning almost 200 articles over 3,000 pages and across four volumes, it has been described as "remarkable" by *Choice* and "magnificent" by *American Reference Books Annual*. The first volume explores the encompassing topic of the origin and evolution of life as well as the genetic code. The second volume expands upon this with in-depth treatises on cell development. Volume three focuses on the remarkable development and capacity of the human brain as well as the newer emerging field of artificial intelligence. The last volume then explores humanity's place and activities on earth and the bioethical issues arising from it. Originally titled *Frontiere della Vita* in Italian in 2000, this set's target audience is researchers as well as advanced students. It is highly recommended for academic libraries.

Henderson's Dictionary of Biology. 14th ed. Editor: Eleanor Lawrence. Pearson/Benjamin Cummings, 2008.
ISBN: 9780321505798
Recommended for: Hospital, Academic, Consumer Health Libraries

The fourteenth edition of this classic dictionary is an essential reference source for any library collection. The content is comprised of over 22,000 entries and has been updated to include new terms from fields such as bioinformatics, genomics and proteomics. The dictionary covers all aspects of biology and contains eight appendixes comprised of classification tables of living organisms. To further define concepts such as meiosis or to explain biologically important chemical compounds, a limited number of entries include illustrations. This publication would be a good complement to the *Oxford Dictionary of Biology*, as it contains more entries, although it lacks the links to web pages and in-depth features that are provided in the *Oxford Dictionary of Biology*. *Henderson's Dictionary of Biology* has been recommended by the *American Library Association Guide*. This dictionary is recommended for all hospital, academic, and consumer health libraries.

Synopsis and Classification of Living Organisms. 1st ed. Editor: Sybil P. Parker. McGraw-Hill, 1982.
ISBN: 978-0070790315 (set)
Recommended for: Academic Libraries

This is the first comprehensive classification scheme of all living organisms, excluding fossils, presented in one reference source in the English language. Prior to this publication, information concerning the classification of organisms was only available in disperse journal articles, many of which were obscure and published in languages other than English. The backbone of the classification system is the division of living organisms into two superkingdoms of Prokaryote and Eukaryote, which then sub-divide into four kingdoms: Virus, Monera, Plantae, and Animalia. Explanatory articles describe the characteristics, biology, ecology, and distribution for each taxa and the systematic positions of organisms down to the family level, with the number of genera and species also indicated. Cited references for each article include principal publications as well as works of historical significance. The two volumes include hundreds of illustrations and photographic plates. The appendix has a brief article on the history and role of nomenclature as well as a comprehensive article regarding biological classification. A review from *Quarterly Review of Biology* describes this work as "obviously indispensable" (1983 Dec; 58(4): 551–552). This publication is considered to be a classic biology text and is recommended for all academic institutions. The set appears to be out of print; however, it may be purchased through out-of-print book dealers.

Journals

Advances in Experimental Medicine and Biology. v. 1, Springer, 1967.
http//www.springer.com/series/5584
ISSN: 00652598
Indexed in: MEDLINE
Recommended for: Hospital, Academic Libraries

Commencing in 1967, *Advances in Experimental Medicine and Biology* is a significant monographic series covering the subject areas of neuroscience, microbiology, immunology, biochemistry, biomedical engineering, and cancer research. Each volume is dedicated to a specific theme or topic of papers presented at various international medical or scientific conferences and meetings. Sample topics include arterial chemoreceptors (Proceedings of the XVIIth International Society for the Advancement of Cytometry [ISAC] Meeting held in Valladolid, Spain, July 1–5, 2008) or progress in motor control (based on the conference Progress in Motor Control V-A Multidisciplinary Perspective held at Pennsylvania State University in 2005). These volumes present excellent state-of-the-art papers with contributions from an international body of researchers. Each volume has a large editorial board of respected professional researchers. The intended audience is medical and biological researchers and graduate students. This series is available online and also in print, though published irregularly. Academic libraries would benefit from subscribing to the entire series; however, hospital libraries would benefit from purchasing individual relevant volumes. *Advances in Experimental Medicine and Biology* is indexed in BIOSIS, MEDLINE, Embase, Scopus, and Web of Science.

Biological Reviews. v. 10, Wiley-Blackwell, 1935.
http//onlinelibrary.wiley.com/journal/10.1111/(ISSN)1469-185X
ISSN: 14647931
ISSN: 1469185X (Online)
Indexed in: MEDLINE
Recommended for: Academic Libraries

Begun in 1923, *Biological Reviews* is published quarterly on behalf of the Cambridge Philosophical Society. This publication covers the full gamut of the biological sciences with both researchers and non-specialists as the target audience. The articles, often with detailed bibliographies, present comprehensive overviews defining the current state of knowledge on a topic. *Biological Reviews* is indexed in many abstracting services such as MEDLINE, Embase, BIOSIS, Web of Science, Scopus, and Chemical Abstracts. This journal ranks second out of 76 biology journals in all three categories of impact factor, five-year impact factor, and article influence score in the 2009 *Journal Citation Reports*. This journal is required for academic institutions, but may not be suitable for hospitals due to the broad nature of biological articles covered and the small number of articles with clinical or medical bearing. Full coverage back to volume 1, 1923, is available through Wiley Online Library.

FASEB Journal. v. 1, Federation of American Societies for Experimental Biology, 1987.
http//www.fasebj.org/
ISSN: 08926638
ISSN: 15306860 (Online)
Indexed in: MEDLINE
Recommended for: Hospital, Academic Libraries

Begun in 1987, *FASEB Journal* is a monthly publication from the Federation of American Societies for Experimental Biology. Contents include review articles, research communications across disciplines, interpretive overviews of novel hypotheses, and book reviews. This peer-reviewed journal is indexed in many abstracting services such as MEDLINE, Embase, BIOSIS, Scopus, and Chemical Abstracts. This journal ranks third out of 72 biology journals in impact factor in the 2009 *Journal Citation Reports*. It is recommended for academic institutions and hospitals as it contains a high number of medically and clinically relevant articles that are available for those wishing to stay abreast of new and significant experimental findings. Scientific disciplines covered by this journal include developmental biology, nutritional sciences, molecular biology, immunology, and clinical investigation. Full coverage back to volume 1, 1987, is available through Stanford's HighWire Press.

Journal of Experimental Biology. v. 7, The Company of Biologists, 1930.
http//jeb.biologists.org/
ISSN: 00220949
ISSN: 14779145 (Online)
Indexed in: MEDLINE
Recommended for: Academic Libraries

Established in 1923, the *Journal of Experimental Biology* is published by The Company of Biologists, a charity and not-for-profit publisher with the aims of promoting research and study across all branches of biology. This semimonthly, peer-reviewed journal specializes in comparative physiology from the molecular level to the whole animal with a focus on evolutionary and environmental context. Content includes research articles, reviews, commentaries, book reviews, historical articles, and obituaries. There is an "Outside *JEB*" section, which briefly discusses articles published in other journals. The online version contains supplemental data such as figures, tables, audio files, and movie clips. The intended audience is researchers, although authors are advised to write for a wide readership. This journal is cited in many abstracting services such as BIOSIS, MEDLINE, Scopus, Chemical Abstracts, and Web of Science; Embase ceased indexing in 1991. This journal ranks nineteenth out of 76 biology journals in the 2009 *Journal Citation Reports*. It also ranks in the top 100 most influential journals for biology and medicine compiled in 2009 by the Special Libraries Association's BioMedical and Life Sciences Division. The journal is available online back to volume 1, 1923, by The Company of Biologist and HighWire Press. Content older than six months is freely available online. This journal is considered essential for academic libraries but not recommended for hospital libraries due to the many non-human and non-clinically relevant articles.

Nature. v. 1, Nature Publishing Group, 1869.
http//www.nature.com

ISSN: 00280836
ISSN: 00280836 (Online)
Indexed in: MEDLINE
Recommended for: Hospital, Academic Libraries

This peer-reviewed journal, published by Nature Publishing Group, began publication in 1869. *Nature* has the highest impact factor of all 50 multidisciplinary science journals in the 2009 *Journal Citation Reports*. It also ranks in the top 10 most influential journals for biology and medicine compiled in 2009 by the Special Libraries Association's BioMedical and Life Sciences Division. Although encompassing all fields of science, *Nature* publishes a significant amount of content about the life sciences. It features original research articles, reviews, commentaries, brief reports, and book reviews, and also contains advertisements and trade information. The online version incorporates a plethora of additional material such as podcasts, videos, and news features, as well as supplemental data relating to published articles. Rapid communication of the results of scientific research is obtained through its weekly publication schedule. Readership consists of a wide scholarly audience. *Nature* is cited in many abstracting services such as BIOSIS, MEDLINE, Embase, Scopus, and Web of Science. *Nature* is highly recommended for academic libraries as well as for hospital libraries due to its rapid publication of leading research articles from all aspects of the life sciences including the health sciences. The journal is available online back to volume 1, 1869 on the Nature Publishing Group website.

Philosophical Transactions of the Royal Society. Series B, Biological Sciences. v. 224, Royal Society, 1934.
http//rstb.royalsocietypublishing.org/
ISSN: 09628436
ISSN: 14712970 (Online)
Indexed in: MEDLINE
Recommended for: Academic Libraries

Philosophical Transactions of the Royal Society. Series B, Biological Sciences, which began publication in 1665 under the title *Philosophical Transactions*, is the longest-running scientific journal. The monthly issues are devoted to a specific theme that is either specially commissioned, such as brainstem neural networks vital for life, or resulting from papers presented at Royal Society Discussion Meetings. Audio files of the Discussion Meetings are included with the online journal. All aspects of biology are covered in this peer-reviewed journal, and are divided into four clusters: cell and development, health and disease, environment and evolution, and neuroscience and cognition. Only invited papers are considered; this journal is complementary to *Proceedings B*, which considers unsolicited papers in the same subject areas. *Philosophical Transactions B* is indexed in many sources such as BIOSIS, MEDLINE, Embase, Scopus, and Chemical Abstracts. It ranks sixth out of 76 biology journals in impact factor in the 2009 *Journal Citation Reports*. This journal is available in print and online formats, although it has modified its name several times. Full coverage back to 1888 is available through Royal Society Publishing. After one year, the content back to 2001 is free to access online. The Royal Society also provides online coverage back to 1665 for *Philosophical Transactions*, the original title before it merged with another publication. Intended for biological researchers, this publication is essential for academic libraries; however, due to its high subscription cost, hospital libraries may not wish to subscribe considering the content is not entirely focused on clinical or medical findings and it also includes ecological and evolutionary articles.

PLoS Biology. v. 1, Public Library of Science, 2003.
http//biology.plosjournals.org
ISSN: 15449173
ISSN: 15457885 (Online)
Indexed in: MEDLINE
Recommended for: Hospital, Academic, Consumer Health Libraries

PLoS Biology, which began in 2003, was the first open-access peer-reviewed journal published by the Public Library of Science (PLoS) under the Creative Commons Attribution License. It covers all aspects of general biology "from molecules to ecosystems," with an emphasis on the following areas: evolutionary, cellular, molecular, developmental, and computational, as well as the neurosciences. Primary research articles are supplemented by magazine-style content such as: synopses (digests of research articles aimed at non-specialists); community pages (forum for societies); unsolved mysteries (topics requiring further research); primers (concise introduction to a topic covered by a current research article); and various opinion pieces including essays, news, and book reviews. The intended audience is specialists as well as non-specialists. New articles are published online weekly and issues are published monthly. *PLoS Biology* is indexed in many abstracting services, which include MEDLINE, Embase, Web of Science, Scopus, Chemical Abstracts, and PsycINFO, as well as archived via PubMed Central. This journal ranks first out of 76 biology journals impact factor in the 2009 *Journal Citation Reports*. PLoS journals allow registered users (anyone can register) to employ social Web 2.0 functionality by adding notes, comments, corrections, and ratings to articles. *PLoS Biology* can be recommended for any hospital, academic, or consumer health library since the open-access model makes its high quality content freely available.

Proceedings of the Royal Society B: Biological Sciences. v. 241, Royal Society, 1990.
http//rspb.royalsocietypublishing.org
ISSN: 09628452
ISSN: 14712954 (Online)
Indexed in: MEDLINE
Recommended for: Academic Libraries

Proceedings of the Royal Society of London: Biological Sciences or *Proceedings B* is the Royal Society's flagship research journal. It covers the full spectrum of the biological sciences with an emphasis on ecology and behavioral and evolutionary biology, and also contains a number of articles that may be of interest to medical researchers in the fields of epidemiology, molecular biology, neuroscience and cognition, and biomechanics. Published every two weeks, concise, high quality peer-reviewed research articles are the mainstay of this journal. Review articles, which have a mandate to be about novel or testable theories, are available free online. This journal is indexed in many sources such as BIOSIS, MEDLINE, Embase, Scopus, and Chemical Abstracts. This journal ranks seventh out of 76 biology journals in impact factor in the 2009 *Journal Citation Reports.* It also ranks in the top 100 most influential journals for biology and medicine compiled in 2009 by the Special Libraries Association's BioMedical and Life Sciences Division. This journal is required for academic institutions, but may not be suitable for hospitals due to the broad nature of biological articles covered. This journal is available in both print and online formats, although it has modified its name several times. Full coverage back to 1905 is available through Royal Society Publishing. After one year, the content back to 2001 is free to access online.

Science. v. 1, American Association for the Advancement of Science, 1880.
http//www.sciencemag.org/
ISSN: 00368075
ISSN: 10959203 (Online)
Indexed in: MEDLINE
Recommended for: Hospital, Academic Libraries

Founded in 1880 by Thomas Edison, *Science* is published by the American Association for the Advancement of Science (AAAS). It is a highly cited and prestigious international weekly journal covering all fields of science with the majority of articles focusing on the biological sciences. A wide range of content, such as original research articles, reviews, comments, news, book reviews, and discussions of science policy, is included in this journal. The online version has additional material including podcasts, streaming media, interviews, and supplementary data to research articles. The target audience is researchers, educators, advanced students, policy makers, and the public. *Science* is cited in many abstracting services such as BIOSIS, MEDLINE, Embase, Scopus, and Web of Science. It is second out of 50 multidisciplinary sciences journals in the 2009 *Journal Citation Reports* in impact factor, five-year impact factor, and article influence. It also ranks in the top 10 most influential journals for biology and medicine compiled in 2009 by the Special Libraries Association's BioMedical and Life Sciences Division. *Science* is highly recommended for both academic and hospital libraries, as it provides frequent publication of articles concerning all aspects of the life sciences, with a focus on health sciences. The journal is available online back to volume 1, 1880 through JSTOR or Science Classic from the AAAS.

Databases and Other Electronic Resources

BIOSIS Previews. Thomson Reuters, 1926.
http://scientific.thomson.com/products/bp/
Recommended for: Academic Libraries

BIOSIS Previews provides indexing services for over 5,000 journals as well as conference proceedings. It combines both Biological Abstracts and Biological Abstracts RRM (Reviews, Reports, and Meetings). Coverage includes the full range of life science research from the traditional areas such as botany, zoology, and ecology to the multidisciplinary biotechnology, biochemistry, and the preclinical medical sciences often used to locate research on alternatives to animal testing. Updated weekly it contains more than 15 million records from 1926 to the present. Detailed indexing is available for fields such as methods and equipment, gene name, sequence data, taxonomic information, and MeSH disease terms. BIOSIS Previews complements MEDLINE in giving the researcher truly comprehensive access to the most current or retrospective life science and medical research literature. Backfiles to 1926 are available online.

Encyclopedia of Life Sciences. Wiley-Blackwell, 20??
http://www.els.net
http://onlinelibrary.wiley.com/book/10.1002/047001590X/
ISBN: 9780470066515
Recommended for: Academic Libraries

This is an online subscription-based resource with sections covering the following broad subjects: biochemistry, cell biology, developmental biology, ecology, evolution and diversity of life, genetics and disease, genetics and molecular biology, immunology, microbiology, neuroscience, plant science, science and society, structural biology, and virology. The largest section is science and society, which includes many articles about the history and philosophy of the life sciences, as well as a large bioethics sub-section. *American Reference Books Annual* describes this resource as "the most ambitious single source reference source ever produced in the biological sciences," as it spans more than 4,000 peer-reviewed articles from over 5,000 authors. *Microbiology Today* adds that the "scientific accuracy is remarkable" (Siddell S. https://www.sgm.ac.uk/pubs/micro_today/book_reviews/MTAUG02/MTA02_27.cfm). The articles are tagged as introductory or advanced and target undergraduates or non-specialists and graduate students respectively, with keynote articles focusing on controversial or topical issues. Each article, available in HTML or PDF, is detailed, thoughtful, and accompanied by illustrations, cited references, and a glossary. The print counterpart of this resource was originally published in 2002 by Nature Publishing Group as a 20-volume set. This was acquired by Wiley in 2004, and in 2007, the set was supplemented by six additional volumes to incorporate online material which made a 26-volume print set. However, since the online version is updated at a frequency of approximately 400 articles per year, the print version will always be incomplete. The online version is recommended for academic institutions and any specialized collection supporting life science research.

Faculty of 1000. Science Navigation Group, 2003.
http://f1000.com/
ISBN: 17404118
See Also Chapter 11.7. Otolaryngology
Recommended for: Academic Libraries

Faculty of 1000, which merged its Medicine and Biology sections in 2010, is a unique resource highlighting the most interesting papers in biology, based on the recommendations of over 2000 leading scientists. All aspects of biology are covered from cell biology to ecology to neuroscience. Reviewers tag their comments with a ranking based on how important they think each paper is: "Must read," "Recommended," and "Exceptional." Papers are also classified as "New finding," "Technical advance," "Interesting hypothesis," "Important confirmation," and "Controversial." Articles are evaluated on the basis of their scientific merit rather than the journal in which they appear, which complements the indirect assessment provided by journal impact factor. This resource can be used as a novel approach to keep current with the literature in a researcher's field as well as adjacent or interdisciplinary areas. Papers can be sorted to view the top 10 papers ranked in various subject categories or the "Hidden Jewels" category that highlights important articles published in less widely read journals. PubMed's linkout system makes it possible to search PubMed while displaying links to Faculty of 1000 for any article that has been evaluated. This resource is highly recommended for academic libraries and collections that support biological research.

26.1. Computational Biology

The development of techniques for the collection and manipulation of biological data, and the use of such data to make biological discoveries or predictions. This field encompasses all computational methods and theories applicable to molecular biology and areas of computer-based techniques for solving biological problems including manipulation of models and datasets.

—MeSH

Contributors: Kristine M. Alpi and Robert Sotak

Monographs

Bioinformatics: A Practical Guide to the Analysis of Genes and Proteins. 3rd ed. Editors: Andreas D. Baxevanis, B.F. Francis Ouellette. Wiley, 2005.
ISBN: 9780471478782
Recommended for: Hospital, Academic Libraries

The third edition of this popular introductory text is in a larger format to better showcase the many color screen shots and data tables. It is organized into five sections based on bioinformatics functions: biological databases, which introduces resources and how to retrieve the information contained within; analysis at the nucleotide level; analysis at the protein level; inferring relationships; and developing tools. The book contains six new chapters on genomic databases, RNA prediction techniques, sequence polymorphisms, intermolecular interactions, proteomics, and comparative genomics. The editors have added text boxes, appendixes on techniques and a more robust set of problems that have data available on the book's companion website (http://www.wiley.com). The glossary is helpful and the book is well-indexed with figures and tables indicated. This text is recommended for all libraries serving life and health sciences students and practitioners.

Building Bioinformatics Solutions: With Perl, R and MySQL. 1st ed. Authors: Conrad Bessant, Ian Shadforth, Darren Oakley. Oxford University Press, 2009.
ISBN: 9780199230198
ISBN: 9780199230235
Recommended for: Academic Libraries

Building Bioinformatics Solutions: With Perl, R and MySQL presents a relatively easy to understand text for approaching a bioinformatics project and was intentionally written to reflect the steps involved in such a project. It provides the basic knowledge for learning how to use open source, platform independent tools in order to organize, analyze, and visualize data. Although it is written at the level of graduate students and researchers it is aimed at the reader with a biological sciences background but with minimal computational skills. Chapter 1 describes how to use the book including tools, operating systems, and a companion website. Applications of bioinformatics such as microarray data analysis and proteomics and publicly available data and analysis tools are also presented. Designing a relational database, installing and configuring a MySQL server, and querying the database with SQL are all carefully explained. The basics of programming with Perl, using the Perl database interface module for accessing relational databases, and alternatives to Perl are all discussed. Chapter 4 describes how to install R, its syntax, and how R can be used to analyze and visualize biological data. In the final chapter all of the tools presented in the three previous chapters are brought together to make data and analysis tools available on the web. It also gives background information about HTML and XHTML, how to do CGI programming, plus other techniques. There is one appendix which is a tutorial for using command line interfaces. This book is highly recommended for graduate students and researchers involved with bioinformatics projects.

Clinical Bioinformatics. Editor: Ronald J.A. Trent. Springer/Humana Press, 2008.
http://www.springerlink.com/content/978-1-58829-791-4
ISBN: 9781588297914
ISBN: 9781603271486 (Online)
Recommended for: Academic Libraries

Clinical Bioinformatics is volume 141 of the series *Methods of Molecular Medicine*. It presents clinical bioinformatics applications across six themes: gene discovery, gene function, DNA mutation analysis, proteomics, online approaches, and informatics in clinical practice. The 40+ authors from basic science departments; genetics, preventive medicine, and other clinical departments in schools of medicine; centers for genetic epidemiology; virus research; and other institutes bring diverse perspectives. The format is typical of *Methods* series—each section of each article is numbered and has a descriptive heading. There are many clear figures and although the images are all black and white, the microarray data shown uses greyscale patterns so no information is lost. Chapters range from step-by-step scientific method examples such as "Microarrays for the Study of Viral Gene Expression during Human Cytomegalovirus Latent Infection" to general overviews such as the closing chapter on e-consulting. Each chapter ends with a reference list. This well-indexed volume is a useful introduction to clinical information for all health sciences libraries whose users need to have an understanding of bioinformatics as applied to clinical practice in diagnostics, therapeutics, etiology, prognosis, and epidemiology. As part of the series, this volume is indexed by MEDLINE at the chapter article level as *Methods in Molecular Medicine*. The online version of *Clinical Bioinformatics* can be purchased article by article using *Springer Protocols*, but as a complete title seems to be available only through the Springer e-books package. Another relevant title available in this manner is *Bioinformatics Methods in Clinical Research* edited by Rune Matthiesen (*Methods in Molecular Biology*, volume 593, 2009).

Computational Genome Analysis: An Introduction. Authors: Richard C. Deonier, Simon Tavaré, Michael S. Waterman. Springer, 2005.
ISBN: 9780387987859
Recommended for: Academic Libraries

This textbook provides a sound foundation in computational molecular biology, discussing and illustrating the computational and statistical principles applied to genomes. Topics are organized around biological problems, such as sequence alignment and assembly, DNA signals, analysis of gene expression, and human genetic variation. As a title in the series *Statistics for Biology and Health*, it introduces mathematics and statistics fundamentals such as probability and algorithms. Examples are based on the open source R statistical package. More than 100 illustrations and diagrams (some in color) reinforce concepts. A supporting website (http://www.cmb.usc.edu/deonier/deonier.html) provides corrections, data for exercises, and code for examples.

Genomics and Proteomics Engineering in Medicine and Biology. Editor: Metin Akay. IEEE Press/Wiley & Sons,

2007.
http://onlinelibrary.wiley.com/book/10.1002/0470052198
http://why.knovel.com/
ISBN: 9780471631811
ISBN: 9781601195043 (Online)
Recommended for: Academic Libraries

More than 30 experts from computer science, electrical engineering, and biology have contributed their expertise to this volume. Its focus is on system structure and dynamics more than individual genes and proteins. It stresses the importance of mathematical and computational tools to improve our understanding of biological systems and describes genomics and proteomics engineering as an emerging field. The intended audience is not only students in biology and biomedical engineering but also researchers in genomics, proteomics, and systems biology. The text covers construction of models to predict pathological phenotypes and also various ways to analyze microarray data such as adaptive quality-based clustering and nonlinear system identification. *In silico* approaches to modeling tumor growth and response to radiation are well described. Construction of a dictionary model to identify motifs such as binding sites in regulatory regions of genes is explained. An overview of computational analysis of proteins is presented such as sequence alignment, modeling of the three dimensional structure, classification, and prediction, as is the use of natural language processing for knowledge extraction. One chapter addresses the issue of querying multiple databases in the life sciences and efforts to integrate them. Each chapter concludes with a list of references. *Genomics and Proteomics Engineering in Medicine and Biology* is sponsored by the IEEE Engineering in Medicine and Biology Society and is available online via Wiley Online Library and Knovel. It is recommended for upper level undergraduates and graduate students and researchers interested in the interdisciplinary field of genomics and proteomics engineering.

Introduction to Bioinformatics. 3rd ed. Author: Arthur M. Lesk. Oxford University Press, 2008.
ISBN: 9780199208043
Recommended for: Hospital, Academic, Consumer Health Libraries

Each chapter of *Introduction to Bioinformatics* begins with a list of learning goals and ends with recommended reading, exercises, problems, and "weblems," which involve web-based tools. High-quality color plates are included at the end of the book. An Online Resource Centre, which is an associated website to supplement the text, has hints to help solve the end of chapter problems and also has all links referenced in the text. There is a heavy emphasis on websites since many bioinformatics resources are web accessible. Key features of the genomes of prokaryotes and eukaryotes are well presented. Chapters on scientific publications and archives include sections on databases, programming language and tools, and information retrieval. Various methods for performing amino acid and nucleotide sequence alignments and constructing phylogenetic trees are explained. The chapter on structural bioinformatics includes methods for predicting protein structure and function and developments in drug discovery. The concluding chapter describes methods used in proteomics research such as DNA microarrays and mass spectrometry, and presents some topics in systems biology such as regulatory networks. This is an excellent textbook for anyone beginning to learn about bioinformatics and is recommended for all types of libraries.

An Introduction to Systems Biology: Design Principles of Biological Circuits. Author: Uri Alon. Chapman & Hall/CRC, 2006.
See Chapter 26.10. Systems Biology

Knowledge Discovery in Bioinformatics: Techniques, Methods, and Applications. Editors: Xiaohua Hu, Yi Pan. John Wiley & Sons, 2007.
http://onlinelibrary.wiley.com/book/10.1002/9780470124642
http://extranet.netlibrary.com/TitleSelect/
ISBN: 9780471777960
ISBN: 9780470124642 (Online)
Recommended for: Academic Libraries

The aim of this text is to enable collaboration between researchers in the fields of data mining and bioinformatics. More than 50 authors, mostly from departments of computer science, information systems, and information science, contributed to this volume. Tiling arrays, which use non-overlapping or partially overlapping probes and can cover the entire genome, are described, as are its advantages over microarrays. There is an assessment of methods for mining hidden links and relationships among medical concepts found in the literature. The connection uncovered between fish oil and Reynaud's disease from complementary and non-interactive sets of articles is cited as an early example of mining hidden links. Machine learning techniques and the challenges in predicting protein secondary structure from amino acid sequence data are discussed. Mechanisms of RNA interference and computational issues related to specificity of RNAi and off-target effects, such as the knocking down of nontarget genes, are explained. Gene selection methods based on microarrays for identification of marker genes for cancer classification are compared. Use of microarrays to identify genes which can be useful for predicting survival of cancer patients is explained well. *Knowledge Discovery in Bioinformatics* is recommended for graduate students and researchers in the fields of data mining and bioinformatics.

Principles of Computational Cell Biology: From Protein Complexes to Cellular Networks. Author: Volkhard Helms. Wiley-VCH, 2008.
ISBN: 9783527315550
Recommended for: Academic Libraries

The author contends that it is not necessary to know computer science to read this book, but it does require knowledge of basic mathematics. Mathematical concepts are explained, however, in order to understand their use in specific chapters. The text is derived from a course for first-year bioinformatics graduate students and uses a network based approach. The first two chapters provide an introduction to mathematical networks and basic cell biology, mathematical graphs, algorithms, and data structures. Subsequent chapters describe protein interaction networks, gene regulatory networks, and metabolic networks using mathematical models. The remaining chapters describe modeling of time-dependent cellular phenomena, and methods for determining the three-dimensional structures of protein complexes. It concludes with a brief outlook for research in cellular networks. Although this is a fairly slim volume it covers a lot of topics with a very logical approach. It has a well-designed layout, and there is an ample number of figures, some in color, to supplement the text. Chapters end with a brief summary and a further reading section. Some chapters have study exercises. This concise book is highly recommended for anyone interested in computational biology and cellular systems.

Structural Bioinformatics. 2nd ed. Editors: Jenny Gu, Philip E. Bourne. Wiley-Blackwell, 2009.
ISBN: 9780470181058
Recommended for: Academic Libraries
Doody's Core Titles Selection

The new edition of *Structural Bioinformatics* adds Jenny Gu as an editor, replacing Helga Weissig from the 2003 edition. With intense interest in proteomics and drug development, this updated text is a welcome application of bioinformatics knowledge to questions of macromolecular structure, such as the prediction of protein structure, how proteins carry out cellular functions, and how knowledge of proteins can accelerate drug discovery and development. Eleven new chapters include sampling and search techniques, structural annotation of genomes, studying evolution using protein structure, prediction of protein-nucleic acid interactions, ligand design and docking methods, more on structure prediction, therapeutic discovery, and future challenges such as protein motion, protein conformation disorders, and protein engineering. Visualization of structures is enhanced by many color images. As of late 2010, only the first edition is available from Wiley Online Library.

Journals

Bioinformatics. v. 14, Oxford University Press, 1998.
http//bioinformatics.oxfordjournals.org/
ISSN: 13674803
ISSN: 14602059 (Online)
See Also Chapter 28. Biotechnology
Indexed in: MEDLINE
Recommended for: Academic Libraries

Bioinformatics is an official journal of the International Society for Computational Biology. All years are available online. Issues are free 12 months after publication going back to January 1996. Volumes prior to 1996 are available to purchasers of the digital archive. The main focus of the journal is recent developments in genome bioinformatics and computational biology. Besides original research papers *Bioinformatics* also contains reviews, discovery notes, applications notes, and letters to the editor. Shorter papers are published in discovery notes, which report biologically interesting discoveries using computational methods, and application notes, which are related to applications used for experiments. Some articles have links to supplemental data. A list of the 50 most frequently cited articles is updated monthly. *Bioinformatics* had the second highest impact factor, 4.926, for 2009 in the mathematical and computational biology category of *Journal Citation Reports*. It is indexed by CAB Abstracts, BIOSIS Previews, MEDLINE, Scopus, and Science Citation Index. It is an essential journal for computational biologists and researchers as well as bioinformaticians. Oxford University Press also provides free access to the annual Database and Web Server issues of *Nucleic Acids Research* (http://nar.oxfordjournals.org/) that describe biological data sources and tools for bioinformatics, many of which have clinical relevance.

Biostatistics. v. 1, Oxford University Press, 2000.
http://biostatistics.oxfordjournals.org/
ISSN: 14654644

ISSN: 14684357 (Online)
Indexed in: MEDLINE
Recommended for: Academic Libraries

Computational biology relies heavily on statistics. The quarterly journal *Biostatistics* focuses on innovative statistical methods or the creative application of statistical methodologies to biomedical problems. Ranked fifth in the mathematical & computational biology category of the 2009 *Journal Citation Reports* with an impact factor of 3.246, *Biostatistics* is a highly relevant title for many health and life science disciplines that rely on statistical methods. Indexing coverage includes MEDLINE from volume 4, Science Citation Index, CAB Abstracts, and a variety of ProQuest products. Full online coverage back to volume 1, 2000 is available through Oxford Journals.

BMC Bioinformatics. v. 1, BioMed Central, 2000.
http//www.biomedcentral.com/bmcbioinformatics
ISSN: 14712105 (Online)
Indexed in: MEDLINE
Recommended for: Hospital, Academic, Consumer Health Libraries

BMC Bioinformatics is an open access, online-only journal published by BioMed Central. It publishes articles that cover a broad range of applications of computational and statistical methods. In addition to research articles, it has methodology articles and software articles. The online format allows video and large datasets to be published as supplemental data. Each abstract is composed of condensed versions of the background, results, and conclusion. Supplements are usually based on conference materials. Lists of most viewed articles in the past 30 days and for all time are provided. Highly accessed articles are also easily identified. Readers can post comments about articles and receive alerts for new articles. Related literature provides links to articles citing the article being read, other articles by the authors, and related articles or webpages on Google, Google Scholar, and PubMed. The webpage for the journal also posts the latest relevant articles from other BioMed Central journals. The 2009 impact factor of 3.428 ranks the journal fourth out of 29 in the mathematical & computational biology category. *BMC Bioinformatics* is indexed by BIOSIS Previews, CAB Abstracts, MEDLINE, and Scopus. This is one bioinformatics journal that all libraries can afford.

Briefings in Bioinformatics. v. 1, Oxford University Press, 2000.
http//bib.oxfordjournals.org/
ISSN: 14675463
ISSN: 14774054 (Online)
Indexed in: MEDLINE
Recommended for: Academic Libraries

A segment of the intended audience for this journal includes researchers who do not specialize in bioinformatics but need to use or create bioinformatics tools. DNA sequencing, alignment methods, gene expression studies, metabolic and signaling pathways, and structure and function prediction are some of the subjects covered. Reviews of databases and analytical tools are emphasized. Out of six issues per year, several are on specific topics such as critical technologies for bioinformatics, computational proteomics, and database integration in life sciences. The journal is indexed by BIOSIS Previews, CAB Abstracts, Embase, MEDLINE, and Science Citation Index Expanded. *Journal Citation Reports* ranks it seventh out of 150 journals in biotechnology and applied microbiology and fourth out of 65 journals in biochemical research methods based on its 2009 impact factor. It was actually ranked number one in 2006 for both categories based on one very highly cited article published in 2004. *Briefings in Bioinformatics* is recommended for students of all levels, educators, and researchers who have an interest in bioinformatics and computational biology and wish to stay up to date. All articles are free after 24 months at the journal's website.

Bulletin of Mathematical Biology. v. 35, Springer, 1973.
http//www.springerlink.com/content/0092-8240
ISSN: 00928240
ISSN: 15229602 (Online)
Indexed in: MEDLINE
Recommended for: Academic Libraries

With eight issues a year, *Bulletin of Mathematical Biology* (formerly *Bulletin of Mathematical Biophysics*) offers substantial computational biology content. Articles at the junction of theoretical and experimental biology connect the disciplines of applied mathematics and biology. The official journal of the Society for Mathematical Biology, it ranks fourteenth in the mathematical and computational biology category of the 2009 *Journal Citation Reports* with an impact factor of 1.873. Indexing coverage includes Biological Abstracts/BIOSIS Previews, CAB Abstracts, Chemical Abstracts Service (CAS), Mathematical Reviews, MEDLINE, Science Citation Index, Scopus, and Zoological Record. Full online coverage back to volume 1, 1939 is available through Springer. The complete backfile is not included with a current subscription.

Journal of Computational Biology. v. 1, Mary Ann Liebert, 1994.

http//www.liebertpub.com/products/product.aspx?pid=31
ISSN: 15578666 (Online)
Indexed in: MEDLINE
Recommended for: Academic Libraries

An international group of associate editors and editorial board members from academia, medical centers, national laboratories, and industry brings broad expertise to *Journal of Computational Biology*. It is primarily focused on the latest methods for analysis, management, and visualization of cellular information at the molecular level. Quality of color and black-and-white images is acceptable. The journal is monthly for 2009 and 2010, although publication frequency increased over time, starting as quarterly in 1994, going bi-monthly in 2001 and then to 10 issues a year for 2005–2008. With its impact factor of 1.694, it ranks nineteenth in the mathematical and computational biology category of the 2009 *Journal Citation Reports*; however, it is one of the few titles in that group focused on computational biology methods and statistics. It is indexed in numerous science abstracting and indexing sources such as MEDLINE, Web of Science, Biological Abstracts/BIOSIS Previews, Embase/Excerpta Medica, Scopus, CAB Abstracts, and MathSciNet. Journal references at the end of articles link to PubMed and CrossRef. The journal is available online only starting in 2010. Full online coverage back to volume 1, 1994 is available through Mary Ann Liebert, Inc.

Molecular Systems Biology. v. 1, Nature Publishing Group and European Molecular Biology Organization, 2005.
See Chapter 26.6. Molecular Biology

PLoS Computational Biology. v. 1, Public Library of Science, 2005.
http//www.ploscompbiol.org/
ISSN: 1553734X (Online)
Indexed in: MEDLINE
Recommended for: Hospital, Academic, Consumer Health Libraries

PLoS Computational Biology is a monthly, open-access journal and is an official journal of the International Society for Computational Biology. It is described by the editors as a community journal. Articles typically employ computational methods to enhance the understanding of living systems. Articles can be browsed by issue, publication date, or subject. Subjects include biophysics, evolutionary biology, mathematics, neuroscience, and science policy. All research articles have a 150–200-word non-technical summary that aids in accessibility. In addition to research articles there are also perspectives, reviews, tutorials, editorials, education articles, and announcements. Collections are created in order to bring articles together on a topic of interest, such as biocuration. The journal makes very good use of Web 2.0 tools which allow readers to make notes or comments and rate articles. It features article level metrics, such as article views, citations, and other indicators of impact, including user ratings, reader comment, and blog coverage. A tab for related content shows related articles on the web and related blog posts. Articles are available in HTML, PDF, and XML formats. *PLoS Computational Biology* had a *Journal Citation Reports* impact factor of 5.759 for 2009, which places it first in the mathematical and computational biology category. It is essential for graduate students and researchers in computational biology and related fields.

26.2. Developmental Biology

The process of the growth and differentiation of an organism.
—MeSH

Contributor: Susan K. Kendall

Monographs

Developmental Biology. 9th ed. Authors: Scott F. Gilbert, Susan R. Singer. Sinauer, 2010.
ISBN: 9780878933846
ISBN: 9780878935642
See Also Chapter 24.6. Embryology
Recommended for: Academic Libraries
Doody's Core Titles Selection

This leading textbook in developmental biology covers basic principles like gene expression and cell-cell communication, early embryological development, later embryological development, and finally, the ramifications of developmental biology, including medical implications and genetic errors. All of the classic animal models are included: sea urchins, C. elegans (worms), drosophila (fruit fly), amphibians, fish, birds, and mammals. A companion website to the book adds supplementary material and more information for advanced students, the full set of references, and historical, philosophical, and ethical perspectives. Also included with the book is the CD-ROM, *Vade Mecum2: An Interactive Guide to Developmental Biology* by Mary Tyler and Ronald N. Kozlowski. This has videos and photographs and slides of chick embryos in whole mount and serial sections. It also contains Mary Tyler's laboratory manual, *Developmental Biology: A Guide for Experimental Study*, third edition, in electronic (PDF) format. The sixth edition of the textbook is available for searching electronically on the NCBI bookshelf (http://www.ncbi.nlm.nih.gov/ books) for free. This review refers to the eighth edition.

Journals

Cold Spring Harbor Protocols. v. 4, Cold Spring Harbor Laboratory Press, 2006.
http//cshprotocols.cshlp.org/
ISSN: 19403402
ISSN: 15596095 (Online)
Indexed in: MEDLINE
Recommended for: Academic Libraries

Cold Spring Harbor Laboratory, a private, non-profit institution focused on research in cancer, neuroscience, cell and developmental biology (plants and animals), genomics, and bioinformatics, is well known for its workshops and courses that teach new research techniques to scientists. Many of these workshops have focused on techniques in molecular, cellular, and developmental biology of various model organisms including bacteria, drosophila (fruit flies), arabidopsis (plants), zebrafish, xenopus (frog), and mice. For years, Cold Spring Harbor Laboratory Press published laboratory protocol manuals arising out of information from these workshops and detailing the methods developed by the pioneering scientists who taught the classes. Classics like *Molecular Cloning, A Laboratory Manual* or *Manipulating the Mouse Embryo* were on the bookshelves of every laboratory that worked in those areas. *Cold Spring Harbor Protocols* now provides access to those protocols and methods online. More than simply a journal, the product also includes all the content from those classic books, which are no longer being updated regularly in printed form. Instead, new issues of this online journal provide multiple new, as well as established, techniques from the Cold Spring Harbor courses and other author submissions. Protocols are searchable or browsable by topic or organism. There is also a separate section for recipes. *Cold Spring Harbor Protocols* is indexed in MEDLINE.

Development. v. 99, The Company of Biologists, 1987.
http//dev.biologists.org/
ISSN: 09501991
ISSN: 14779129 (Online)
See Also Chapter 24.6. Embryology
Indexed in: MEDLINE
Recommended for: Academic Libraries

The Company of Biologists is a nonprofit charitable organization established in the United Kingdom to promote and advance research in all areas of biology. It publishes four journals, of which *Development* (previously *Journal of Embryology and Experimental Morphology* from 1953–1986) is the most highly regarded. This peer-reviewed journal publishes primary research focused on the cellular and molecular mechanisms of both animal and plant development. This can include embryonic development, as well as evolution, stem cells, or developmental studies that lead to insight about the etiology of disease. According to its website, in addition to original research articles, the journal also publishes "Review and Hypothesis articles, educational primer articles, and reviews of meetings in the field, all of which are commissioned from leading developmental biologists." It is indexed in numerous indexing and abstracting sources including CAB Abstracts, Embase, MEDLINE, Scopus, and Web of Science. Online access back to 1987 is available from the publisher. Online access to issues from 2009 up to six months prior to current is also available on PubMed Central.

Developmental Biology. v. 1, Elsevier, 1959.
http//www.sciencedirect.com/science/journal/00121606
ISSN: 00121606
ISSN: 1095564X (Online)
See Also Chapter 24.6. Embryology
Indexed in: MEDLINE
Recommended for: Academic Libraries

This peer-reviewed journal is the official journal of the Society for Developmental Biology. It publishes original research papers in all areas of plant and animal development, including the molecular genetics of development, oncogenes, stem cells, cell interactions, and evolution. This journal achieved an impact factor of 4.379 in 2009 and it ranks with the other journals listed here as one of the top ten journals in this subject area by numbers of citations (2009 *Journal Citation Reports*). It is indexed in numerous indexing and abstracting sources including CAB Abstracts, Embase, MEDLINE, Scopus, and Web of Science. Online access back to 1959 is available from the publisher.

Developmental Cell. v. 1, Cell Press/Elsevier, 2001.
http//www.cell.com/developmental-cell
http://www.sciencedirect.com/science/journal/15345807
ISSN: 15345807
ISSN: 18781551 (Online)

Indexed in: MEDLINE
Recommended for: Academic Libraries

A very recently split-off daughter journal from the flagship journal *Cell*, which publishes research of "exceptional significance" in any area of biology, *Developmental Cell* publishes the best papers in cell biology and developmental biology. Like some of the other Cell Press journals, it has rapidly risen to a high prestige level, likely due to its association with the top tier journal, *Cell*. This peer-reviewed journal includes both original research articles as well as reviews. The Cell Press journals are editorially independent of each other, but manuscript transfer is possible such that an author can ask that a paper rejected as not appropriate for one Cell Press journal be considered for publication in a different one. It is indexed in numerous indexing and abstracting sources including Embase, MEDLINE, Scopus, and Web of Science. Online access back to 2001 is available from the publisher or on ScienceDirect.

Genes and Development. v. 1, Cold Spring Harbor Laboratory Press, 1987.
http//genesdev.cshlp.org/
http://www.ncbi.nlm.nih.gov/pmc/journals/101/
ISSN: 08909369
ISSN: 15495477 (Online)
Indexed in: MEDLINE
Recommended for: Academic Libraries

From the independent Cold Spring Harbor Laboratory Press and published in association with The Genetics Society, *Genes and Development* is considered one of the top journals in both developmental biology and genetics/molecular biology. It achieved a five-year impact factor of 14.198 and was ranked first among developmental biology journals, second out of 144 journals in genetics and heredity, and sixth out of 161 journals in cell biology (2009 *Journal Citation Reports*). Longer research papers and short communications as well as reviews and perspectives are all published in this peer-reviewed journal. More than 100 years old and boasting a distinguished history, Cold Spring Harbor Laboratory is a private, non-profit institution focused on research in cancer, neuroscience, plant biology, genomics, and bioinformatics. It also sponsors meetings, workshops and courses for the education of scientists. The journal is indexed in numerous indexing and abstracting sources including CAB Abstracts, Embase, MEDLINE, Scopus, and Web of Science. Online access back to 1987 is available from the publisher. Online access to issues from 1987 through six months prior to current is also available on PubMed Central.

26.3. Ecology

The interrelationship of organisms and their environment, especially as manifested by natural cycles and rhythms, community development and structure, interactions between different kinds of organisms, geographic distributions, and population alterations.

—MeSH

Contributor: Tracey Minzenmayer

Monographs

Ecology: From Individuals to Ecosystems. 4th ed. Authors: Michael Begon, Colin A. Townsend, John L. Harper. Wiley-Blackwell, 2006.
ISBN: 9781405111171
Recommended for: Academic Libraries

Called "a forerunner in the science of ecology" by the *Journal of Biological Education* (2006 Fall; 40(4):187), this book and its previous editions have been considered the standard advanced ecology textbook for the past 20 years. This edition premiers a title change; previous editions were known as *Ecology: Individuals, Populations and Communities*. The authors present a comprehensive coverage of the field of ecology through clear examples, illustrations, and the discussion of relevant field and laboratory studies. The text consists of 22 chapters divided into three sections: "Organisms," "Species Interactions," and "Communities and Ecosystems." The fourth edition includes three new chapters on applied ecology, a particularly vital concept for students to understand as environmental concerns become more prominent, and integrates over 800 new studies into the text. This modern classic is highly recommended for all academic libraries to support students from undergraduate to graduate levels, as well as researchers who want a comprehensive but accessible ecology text.

Foundations of Ecology: Classic Papers with Commentaries. 1st ed. Editors: Leslie A. Real, James H. Brown. University of Chicago Press, 1991.
ISBN: 9780226705941
Recommended for: Academic Libraries

This textbook gathers 40 classic papers that laid the intellectual and conceptual foundations of the field of ecology into a single volume. Spanning 1887 to 1974, the papers are divided into six sections: foundational papers, theoretical advances, synthetic statements, methodological advances, case studies, and ecological experiments.

Each section begins with an original essay by current researchers that discusses the historical context and continued relevance of the selected papers. Published with the approval of the Ecological Society of America, the papers were chosen by a committee of distinguished professionals. The level of material is appropriate for advanced undergraduate students, graduate students, and professionals wishing to learn more about the history of the field. Although published 20 years ago, this book is still often required reading in graduate ecology programs. This book is highly recommended for any academic library supporting an ecology program and any well-rounded science library.

Principles of Conservation Biology. 3rd ed. Authors: Martha J. Groom, Gary K. Meffe, C.R. Carroll. Sinauer Associates, 2006.
ISBN: 9780878935185
Recommended for: Academic Libraries

The major themes and concepts of conservation biology are explained by the authors and their many contributors in 18 chapters divided into three sections: foundations of the field, threats to biodiversity, and approaches to solving conservation problems. Both the biological and social issues involved in conservation issues are highlighted throughout the text. The organization of the third edition has been revised to emphasize various categories of threat and approaches to conservation. In addition, coverage has expanded to include both terrestrial and marine conservation issues and efforts in the United States and the international community. The companion website adds study questions, essays, case studies, suggested readings, and more to this extensive resource. The third edition *Instructor's Resource CD-ROM* contains illustrations and tables from the textbook and ready-to-use presentations. The CD-ROM is available to faculty members using the book in their classes. This textbook is highly recommended for academic institutions as a comprehensive introduction to conservation biology for advanced undergraduate students, graduate students, and researchers who have at least a basic background in biology and ecology.

Sustaining Life: How Human Health Depends on Biodiversity. Editors: Eric Chivian, Aaron Bernstein. Oxford University Press, 2008.
ISBN: 9780195175097
Recommended for: Academic, Consumer Health Libraries

Winner of the Gerald L. Young 2009 Book Award in Human Ecology and named one of the best sci-tech books of 2008 by *Library Journal*, this book is an essential purchase for all academic institutions and a highly recommended addition to consumer health collections. Led by Eric Chivian, winner of the 1985 Nobel Peace Prize, more than 100 leading scientists contributed to this comprehensive examination of the potential threats to human health from the reduction of biodiversity. The book was co-sponsored by the United Nations to raise awareness of how much biomedical and pharmaceutical research, food production, and the epidemiology of infectious diseases are affected by biodiversity. Detailed case studies of seven groups of endangered organisms are included to discuss the contributions they have already made to humans and the future benefits they are expected to yield if they are preserved. The 10 chapters of this book are richly illustrated with color photographs and charts, and are prefaced by a foreword by E.O. Wilson and a prologue by Kofi Annan, 2001 Nobel Peace Prize Laureate. Written to be accessible to the general public, this book is highly recommended for consumers, undergraduate and graduate students, public health policymakers, researchers, and physicians.

Journals

Annual Review of Ecology, Evolution, and Systematics. v. 34, Annual Reviews, 2003.
http//arjournals.annualreviews.org/loi/ecolsys
ISSN: 1543592X
ISSN: 15452069 (Online)
Recommended for: Academic Libraries

Begun in 1970 under the title *Annual Review of Ecology and Systematics* (ISSN 00664162), the journal changed to its current name in 2003 to reflect its coverage of evolutionary research. Commissioned by the editors and then peer-reviewed, the articles discuss significant developments through the full spectrum of the ecology, evolutionary biology, and systematics fields. Topics include phylogeny, molecular evolution, evolutionary physiology, population dynamics, ecosystem processes, invasion biology, and conservation. This journal ranked third out of 129 ecology journals for impact factor in 2009, and it consistently places as one of the top journals in this field (*Journal Citation Reports*). Academic institutions will find this journal an invaluable resource for ecologists and biologists. It is cited in many science abstracting and indexing sources such as AGRICOLA, BIOSIS Previews, Chemical Abstracts, and Scopus. Full online coverage back to volume 1, 1970 is available through Annual Reviews.

Ecological Monographs. v. 1, Ecological Society of America (ESA), 1931.

http//esapubs.org/esapubs/journals/monographs.htm
ISSN: 00129615
ISSN: 15577015 (Online)
Recommended for: Academic Libraries

Published by the Ecological Society of America, this title began in 1931, and is still one of the most influential journals in the field. It consistently ranks among the ecology journals with the highest impact factor, coming in tenth out of 129 titles (2009 *Journal Citation Reports*). The journal publishes observational, experimental, or theoretical studies, as well as comprehensive reviews focused on developing new insights or benchmarks in the field. It also includes concept papers that advance current knowledge in new directions and invited papers by established ecologists that provide critical commentary or historical perspective. This journal is highly recommended to any academic institution with an ecology program for its thoughtful and in-depth coverage of the field. It is cited in various abstracting and indexing sources such as AGRICOLA, Chemical Abstracts, and Scopus. Early coverage from volume 1, 1931 up to two years before the current year is available online from JSTOR. More recent online coverage is available from ESA from volume 67, 1997 to the present.

Ecology. v. 1, Ecological Society of America, 1920.
http//esapubs.org/esapubs/journals/ecology.htm
ISSN: 00129658
ISSN: 19399170 (Online)
Indexed in: MEDLINE
Recommended for: Academic Libraries

This title consistently receives the highest number of citations of any ecology journal, making it a widely read and valuable addition to any academic library serving ecologists, biologists, or science students. The journal ranked seventeenth out of 129 ecology journals in impact factor (2009 *Journal Citation Reports*). The content is primarily concise research articles on ecological concepts and techniques, including mathematical, statistical, and interdisciplinary approaches. Particular preference is given to research and review articles that lead to generalizations potentially applicable in many contexts. Published by the Ecological Society of America, this journal is included in a wide variety of abstracting and indexing sources, such as AGRICOLA, Chemical Abstracts, and MEDLINE. With over 40,000 citations in 2009 alone (*Journal Citation Reports*), this resource is a necessity for academic institutions. Early online coverage from volume 1, 1920 up to two years before the current year is available from JSTOR. More recent online coverage is available from ESA, starting with volume 78, 1997 and continuing to the present.

Ecology Letters. v. 1, Wiley-Blackwell, 1998.
http//onlinelibrary.wiley.com/journal/10.1111/(ISSN)14 61-0248
ISSN: 1461023X
ISSN: 14610248 (Online)
Indexed in: MEDLINE
Recommended for: Academic Libraries

Rapid publication of novel ecological research makes this journal one of the most influential in the field. Published in association with the Centre National de la Recherché Scientifique, it consistently ranks as one of the top four ecology journals in terms of impact factor (*Journal Citation Reports*). The focus is on concise, original papers of general interest on the cutting edge of ecological advancement. Topics may be core areas of ecology or underrepresented subdisciplines. The speed of publication makes this journal a vital tool for researchers in ecology and biology who need to stay abreast of new developments; high quality peer-reviewed articles can be made available online within weeks. All academic institutions should consider adding this title for their biology and ecology programs. This journal is cited in a variety of abstracting and indexing sources, including AGRICOLA, MEDLINE, and Scopus. Full online coverage back to volume 1, 1998 is available through Wiley Online Library.

Trends in Ecology & Evolution. v. 1, Elsevier, 1986.
http//www.cell.com/trends/ecology-evolution
http://www.sciencedirect.com/science/journal/01695347
ISSN: 01695347
ISSN: 18728383 (Online)
Indexed in: MEDLINE
Recommended for: Academic Libraries

With a journal impact factor of at least 10 from 2001 to 2008 and 11.564 in 2009 (*Journal Citation Reports*), this influential peer-reviewed journal is indispensable for researchers, faculty, and students in ecology and biology. Editor-commissioned reviews, opinions, and letters covering every area of ecology and evolutionary biology from theoretical concepts to applied research are included. The scope of the research ranges from microbiology to global environmental problems. Each issue consists predominantly of review articles detailing recent and important developments in ecological research. Opinion pieces offer a subjective look at historical, rare, or contemporary topics. Book reviews, letters, short articles on the interface of science and society, and a section summarizing recent important research papers round out each issue. The journal is cited in numerous abstracting and indexing sources such as BIOSIS Previews, Scopus, and MEDLINE. Any academic institution supporting programs in biology, ecology, environmental science, or microbiology will find this journal a valuable addition to its collection. Online coverage from volume 10, 1995 onward is available through Elsevier ScienceDirect.

26.4. Laboratory Animal Science

The procurement, breeding, care, health, and selection of animals used in biomedical research and testing.

—MeSH

Contributor: Susan K. Kendall

Monographs

Guide for the Care and Use of Laboratory Animals. 8th ed. Author: Committee for the Update of the Guide for the Care and Use of Laboratory Animals, Institute for Laboratory Animal Research and Division on Earth and Life Studies, National Research Council. National Academies Press, 2011.
http://books.nap.edu/catalog.php?record_id=12910
ISBN: 9780309134000
ISBN: 9780309154017 (Print + PDF)
Recommended for: Academic Libraries

Now in its first edition in 15 years, this guidebook, put out by the Institute for Laboratory Animal Research (ILAR), National Research Council, has been updated to reflect new scientific evidence, current guidelines from professional organizations, and U.S. federal regulations for optimal animal welfare. Its use in animal facilities is required by U.S. Public Health Service Policy. Its purpose is "to provide information that will enhance animal well-being, the quality of research, and the advance of scientific knowledge that is relevant to both human and animals" (Chapter 1). It provides information on institutional policies and responsibilities, the creation of Institutional Animal Care and Use Committees (IACUCs), protocols for animal use, guidelines for animal husbandry and management, veterinary care for laboratory animals, and animal facility design and regulations. It would be of particular use to administrators, facilities managers, animal researchers and animal care personnel. The *Guide* is available for purchase either as a bound book or as a PDF download from the National Academies site.

Handbook of Laboratory Animal Science. 3rd ed. Editors: Jann Hau, Steven J. Schapiro. CRC Press, 2003–2005.
http://www.crcnetbase.com/isbn/978-1-4200-8455-9 (v.1)
http://www.crcnetbase.com/isbn/978-0-8493-1084-3 (v.2 2nd ed.)
http://www.crcnetbase.com/isbn/978-0-8493-1893-1 (v.3 2nd ed.)
ISBN: 9781420084559 (v.1)
ISBN: 9781420084573 (v.2)
ISBN: 9780849318931 (v.3)
Recommended for: Academic Libraries

This three-volume set is an essential reference for laboratory animal science. This review refers to the second edition. Unlike some other monographs recommended here that focus on United States regulations, this work is international in focus and coverage. Volume 1 is subtitled *Essential Principles and Practices*, and it covers all of the basics: reasons for using animals, animal research ethics, overview of global legislation and regulations, assessment of animal care and use programs, education and training, animal facilities and equipment, genetic quality control, health status and monitoring, nutrition, experimental design, common techniques and procedures, anesthesia and euthanasia, surgery, postmortem, and animal alternatives. References to the primary literature and scientific studies support the information provided. Volumes 2 and 3 are subtitled *Animal Models*. The term "animal models" refers to models of human functions or disease and the focus of this book is on mammalian species. It details the different types of models (rat, mouse, guinea pig, rabbit, etc.) available for different types of studies, whether pharmacological, psychological, neuroscience, cancer research, skeletal disease, or others. It explains the considerations involved in choosing an animal model, for instance, when and why one might choose a rat over a mouse for a specific type of study. It also describes genetic models of specific diseases such as the diabetic mouse. Some non-laboratory animals used in studies, such as sheep, are also included. Ethical concerns are always taken into account, and references to the primary literature follow each chapter. Volume 3 presents animal models of specific diseases. This resource is also available online through CRCnetBASE. Volumes 1 and 2 of the third edition were published in 2011.

IACUC Handbook. 2nd ed. Editors: Jerald Silverman, Mark A. Suckow, Sreekant Murthy. CRC Press, 2006.
ISBN: 9780849340109
Recommended for: Academic Libraries

This essential handbook is for administrators and laboratory animal professionals who need to know the rules and policies regulating the establishment of an IACUC (Institutional Animal Care and Use Committee) at their institution and the use of animals for laboratory research. According to United States federal law, IACUCs are required at each institution that uses laboratory animals to oversee their welfare, care, and treatment. Comprehensive information on creation and composition of an IACUC, conduct of meetings, and formatting and reporting of protocols for compliance with current laws is included. Later chapters offer more information as answers to "commonly asked questions" about the regulations and best practices in areas ranging from animal surgery procedures, pain and distress concerns, animal acquisition, housing, cage enrichment, and veterinary care.

Journals

Comparative Medicine. v. 50, American Association for Laboratory Animal Science, 2000.
http//aalas.publisher.ingentaconnect.com/content/aalas/cm
http://www.ncbi.nlm.nih.gov/pmc/journals/833/
ISSN: 15320820
Indexed in: MEDLINE
Recommended for: Academic Libraries

The official peer-reviewed publication of the American Association for Laboratory Animal Science, *Comparative Medicine* focuses more on original research, whereas *JAALAS* has association news and briefer reports. Articles about laboratory animal models, biology, medicine, pathology, behavior, and biotechnology are all in scope. Article types include case studies, reports, reviews, clinical investigations, and basic and applied laboratory investigations. Research articles are organized by animal model: fish, mouse, rat, rabbit, hamster, swine, canine, nonhuman primate, etc. It is indexed by numerous indexing and abstracting sources including CAB Abstracts, Embase, MEDLINE, Scopus, and Web of Science. Online access back to issues from 2008 through six months prior to current is available in PubMed Central.

ILAR Journal. v. 37, National Research Council, Institute for Laboratory Animal Research, 1995.
http//dels.nas.edu/ilar_n/ilarjournal/journal.shtml
ISSN: 10842020
ISSN: 19306180 (Online)
Indexed in: MEDLINE
Recommended for: Academic Libraries

The Institute for Laboratory Animal Research (ILAR) is a component of the National Research Council of the National Academies of Sciences, U.S.A., and it provides advice to the federal government, the international biomedical research community, and the public through this quarterly journal, the web, and committee reports. The mission of ILAR is "to evaluate and disseminate information on issues related to the scientific, technological, and ethical use of animals and related biological resources in research, testing, and education. Using the principles of refinement, reduction, and replacement (3Rs) as a foundation, ILAR promotes high-quality science through the humane care and use of animals and the implementation of alternatives." The *ILAR Journal* is the only peer-reviewed journal to specifically address issues relating to Institutional Animal Care and Use Committees (IACUCs) that must, by law, be established at institutions that do research on animals. The journal publishes themed issues, in which all articles are centered on one topic, such as "Type 2 Diabetes and Obesity," "Pain and Distress in Fish," "Gene Therapy in Large Animal Models," or "One Medicine." A companion, the *ILAR e-Journal*, supplements the print (plus online) journal with extra online-only peer-reviewed articles.

Journal of the American Association for Laboratory Animal Science (JAALAS). v. 1, American Association for Laboratory Animal Science, 2006.
http//aalas.publisher.ingentaconnect.com/content/aalas/jaalas
http://www.ncbi.nlm.nih.gov/pmc/journals/817/
ISSN: 15596109
Indexed in: MEDLINE
Recommended for: Academic Libraries

JAALAS is the official communication vehicle of the American Association for Laboratory Animal Science. It publishes case reports, reviews, and peer-reviewed articles on laboratory animal biology, technology, experimental technique, facilities operations and management, compliance, and other topics of interest to those who work with or care for laboratory animals. It also publishes association news. Briefer case reports and manuscripts that are more technology or management oriented are accepted here rather than *Comparative Medicine*, the Association's other journal. It is indexed in numerous indexing and abstracting sources including CAB Abstracts, Embase, MEDLINE, Scopus, and Web of Science. Issues back to 2008 through six months prior to current are also available in PubMed Central.

Lab Animal. v. 1, Nature Publishing Group, 1972.
http//www.labanimal.com/laban/index.html
ISSN: 00937355
ISSN: 15484475 (Online)
Indexed in: MEDLINE
Recommended for: Academic Libraries

A print subscription to *Lab Animal* (North America) or *Lab Animal* (Europe) is provided free of charge to anyone who is involved with laboratory animal science in those regions. The online version requires a subscription, however, for individuals or institutions. *Lab Animal* is a monthly peer-reviewed journal publishing articles on "all aspects of laboratory animal science, including animal care and husbandry; disease diagnosis and treatment; facility planning, design, and management; staff training and education; and updates and information on regulations." Several different types of articles can be found: reviews, opinions, technique articles, resource articles, research notes, and product information. Two special columns offer feedback for readers: a diagnosis/case study section allows readers to contribute a case study for diagnosis by experts; a "Protocol Reviews" section invites several experts to address a submitted question or dilemma regarding a protocol for animal use and give an answer as to legality and appropriateness. A buyer's guide and jobs listings are also provided online. The journal is indexed in numerous indexing and abstracting sources including Embase, MEDLINE, Scopus, and Web of Science.

Laboratory Animals. v. 1, Royal Society of Medicine, 1967.
http//la.rsmjournals.com/
ISSN: 00236772
ISSN: 17581117 (Online)
Indexed in: MEDLINE
Recommended for: Academic Libraries

This peer-reviewed journal is published by the Royal Society of Medicine on behalf of Laboratory Animals Limited, a registered charity in the U.K. whose aims are to promote education and training in laboratory animal science. The journal is international in scope and has been adopted as the official journal of the Federation of Laboratory Animal Science Associations and Laboratory Animal Science Associations in several countries, including the U.K., Germany, the Netherlands, Israel, Switzerland, Spain and Portugal. *Laboratory Animals* publishes papers on the use of animals in biomedical research and laboratory animal care and management. Articles reporting on the "3R's" (replacement, reduction, and refinement) in the use of animals for research are a general focus, but particularly those that report findings that "either refine protocols involving animal models or can improve future experimental designs." Both review articles and original research articles on laboratory animal facilities, clinical case reports or studies, microbiology, toxicology, and biology of laboratory animals are all in scope. The journal is indexed in numerous indexing and abstracting source including CAB Abstracts, Embase, MEDLINE, Scopus, and Web of Science. Online access from 1967 is available from the publisher.

26.5. Microbiology

Microorganisms such as fungi, bacteria, algae, archaea, and viruses.

—MeSH

Contributor: Susan K. Kendall

Monographs

Brock Biology of Microorganisms. 12th ed. Authors: Michael T. Madigan, John M. Martinko, Paul V. Dunlap, David P. Clark. Pearson Benjamin Cummings, 2009.
ISBN: 9780132324601
Recommended for: Academic Libraries

This textbook has been the authoritative text for introductory general microbiology for almost 40 years, and it includes bacteriology, genetics, molecular biology, biotechnology, virology, and basic immunology. It has been praised for its clarity and accessibility, and there is an emphasis on evolution and ecology throughout. Extensive revisions have been made to incorporate new findings, such as those in microbial genomics. A companion website offers supplementary material for individuals who purchase the text.

Manual of Clinical Microbiology. 9th ed. Editors: Patrick R. Murray, Ellen Jo Baron, James H. Jorgensen, Marie Louise Landry, Michael A. Pfaller. ASM Press, 2007.
ISBN: 9781555813710 (set)
See Also Chapter 10.12.1. Clinical Pathology
Recommended for: Hospital, Academic Libraries
Brandon/Hill, *Doody's Core Titles* Selection

A former Brandon/Hill pick and now a *Doody's* core title, this classic set from the American Society for Microbiology is the definitive reference for diagnostic laboratories. The first part of volume one has practical information about setting up and managing a laboratory, including laboratory design, budgets, compliance, and personnel issues. It also discusses specimen collecting, disinfection, microbial identification systems, procedures, and microscopy. Later sections focus on information about all the various clinically relevant microorganisms: bacteria, viruses, fungi, and parasites. The focus is always on understanding the organism, its life cycle, description, and taxonomy, with an eye to clinical significance, epidemiology, detection, diagnosis, and therapeutics.

Journals

Cell Host and Microbe. v. 1, Cell Press/Elsevier, 2007.
http//www.cell.com/cell-host-microbe/
http://www.sciencedirect.com/science/journal/19313128
ISSN: 19346069 (Online)
ISSN: 19313128
Indexed in: MEDLINE
Recommended for: Academic Libraries

This relatively new monthly peer-reviewed journal has risen quickly to the top of impact factor charts, probably because of its association with the high quality Cell Press (from Elsevier) journals, which include the leading journal, *Cell*. It achieved an impact factor of 13.021 and ranked first out of 94 journals in the microbiology category (2009 *Journal Citation Reports*). Only papers of exceptional significance are considered for publication, and both research and review articles are included. The scope of the journal is the integrated study of microbes (of any sort) in relationship with each other, their environment, and with their hosts, whether human, invertebrate or vertebrate animal, or plant. Therefore, it stands at the intersection of immunological, cellular, and microbiological studies. It is indexed by numerous indexing and abstracting sources including CAB Abstracts, Embase, MEDLINE, Scopus, and Web of Science. Online access back to 2007 is available from the publisher.

Journal of Clinical Microbiology. v. 1, American Society for Microbiology, 1975.
http//jcm.asm.org/
http://www.ncbi.nlm.nih.gov/pmc/journals/81/
ISSN: 00951137
ISSN: 1098660X (Online)
Indexed in: MEDLINE
Recommended for: Academic Libraries

The *Journal of Clinical Microbiology* publishes current research papers on microbiological infections of humans and animals, emphasizing etiology, diagnosis, and epidemiology. All areas of microbiology are covered: bacteriology, virology, parasitology, and mycology. In addition to peer-reviewed original research articles, commentaries, mini-reviews, case reports, a point-counterpoint feature and editorials are also included. It is published by the American Society for Microbiology and maintains their high quality standards. The journal achieved an impact factor of 4.162 and ranked eighteenth out of 94 journals in the microbiology category (2009 *Journal Citation Reports*). It is indexed by numerous indexing and abstracting sources including CAB Abstracts, Embase, MEDLINE, Scopus, and Web of Science. Online access back to 1975 is available from the publisher. Access to issues from 1975 through six months prior to current is also available in PubMed Central.

Microbiology. v. 140, Society for General Microbiology, 1994.
http//mic.sgmjournals.org/
ISSN: 13500872
ISSN: 14652080 (Online)
Indexed in: MEDLINE
Recommended for: Academic Libraries

This peer-reviewed journal is published by the Society for General Microbiology (Great Britain). It has been a leader among microbiology journals. The journal publishes original research articles, reviews, and mini-reviews about both eukaryotic and prokaryotic microorganisms and viruses that infect them. Papers on viruses of higher organisms are not in scope. All aspects of microorganisms are considered including genetics, genomics, biochemistry, physiology, pathogenicity, cell biology, and evolutionary and environmental biology. It is indexed by numerous indexing and abstracting sources including CAB Abstracts, Embase, MEDLINE, Scopus, and Web of Science. The journal is available in both print and online formats, with online access back to volume 1, 1947 of its original title, *Journal of General Microbiology*, available from the publisher.

Microbiology and Molecular Biology Reviews. v. 61, American Society for Microbiology, 1997.
http//mmbr.asm.org/
http://www.ncbi.nlm.nih.gov/pmc/journals/90/
ISSN: 10922172
ISSN: 10985557 (Online)
Indexed in: MEDLINE
Recommended for: Academic Libraries

This is the top-ranked, definitive review journal in the subject areas of microbiology, immunology, and molecular biology. It is published by the American Society for Microbiology and well-maintains the standards expected of their publications. All reviews are invited and peer-reviewed, although authors may submit suggestions for a review topic. As do many review journals, *Microbiology and Molecular Biology Reviews* attempts to make connections between related fields and for both non-specialists and specialists, and to explore the potential impact and relationships of research findings across different, but related fields. It achieved an impact factor or 12.585 and ranked fifth out of 94 journals in the microbiology subject category (2009 *Journal Citation Reports*). The journal is well-established and well-respected, having begun publication in 1937 under another title. It is indexed in numerous indexing and abstracting sources including CAB Abstracts, Embase, MEDLINE, Scopus, and Web of Science. Online access back to 1997 is available through the publisher. Issues back to 1937 through one year prior to current are also available in PubMed Central.

Molecular Microbiology. v. 1, Wiley-Blackwell, 1987.
http//onlinelibrary.wiley.com/journal/10.1111/(ISSN)1365-2958
ISSN: 0950382X
ISSN: 13652958 (Online)
Indexed in: MEDLINE
Recommended for: Academic Libraries

A leading primary peer-reviewed research journal in the fields of microbiology, molecular biology, and biochemistry, *Molecular Microbiology* reports on all types of microorganisms and viruses and related cellular and molecular studies. Unlike some other microbiology journals, it does not focus on the host response or immunological studies (these are published in its sister journal, *Cellular Microbiology*). Some issues also may contain "MicroReviews," "MicroCommentaries," or "MicroMeeting Reports." It achieved an impact factor of 5.361 and ranked forty-seventh out of 283 journals in the biochemistry and molecular biology category and fourteenth out of 97 journals in the microbiology category in the 2009 *Journal Citation Reports*. The journal is indexed by numerous indexing and abstracting sources including CAB Abstracts, Embase, MEDLINE, Scopus, and Web of Science. Online access back to 1987 is available from the publisher.

PLoS Pathogens. v. 1, Public Library of Science, 2005.
http//www.plospathogens.org
http://www.ncbi.nlm.nih.gov/pmc/journals/349/
ISSN: 15537366 (Online)
See Also Chapter 26.7. Parasitology
Indexed in: MEDLINE
Recommended for: Academic Libraries

PLoS Pathogens is an open access peer-reviewed journal that publishes research articles covering all kinds of microbiological pathogens (bacteria, fungi, parasites, prions, and viruses) important in medicine and agriculture. Furthermore, these studies often lead to insights into the cellular and molecular biology of the hosts and would be of interest to immunologists and others as well. The Public Library of Science (PLoS), which publishes this journal, is a non-profit organization of scientists and physicians committed to making scientific and medical literature freely available to the public. All articles are available free upon publication. The PLoS journals use a business model of charging author publication fees, and the authors retain ownership of the copyright for their articles. Under the Creative Commons Attribution License anyone may download, reuse, reprint, modify, distribute, and/or copy articles in PLoS journals, so long as the original authors and source are cited. The PLoS journals have risen to the top of impact factor lists, presumably because articles freely available tend to be highly cited. The PLoS journals also have maintained high standards of quality. It is indexed in numerous indexing and abstracting sources including Embase, MEDLINE, Scopus, and Web of Science. Although the journal began with both print and online formats, the print format ceased in 2008 and it is now only available online.

Databases and Other Electronic Resources

Current Protocols. Wiley, 2000.
See Chapter 26.6. Molecular Biology

26.5.1. Bacteriology

The study of bacteria.
—MeSH

Contributor: Susan K. Kendall

Monographs

Bergey's Manual of Systematic Bacteriology. 2nd ed. Editors: George M. Garrity, David R. Boone, Richard W. Castenholz. Springer, 2001.
ISBN: 9780387987712 (v.1)
ISBN: 9780387241432 (v.2A)
ISBN: 9780387241449 (v.2B)
ISBN: 9780387241456 (v.2C)
ISBN: 9780387950419 (v.3)
ISBN: 9780387950426 (v.4)
Recommended for: Academic Libraries
Doody's Core Titles Selection

Bergey's Manual of Systematic Bacteriology has been an essential bacterial systematics reference for microbiologists and students of microbiology since the publication of the first edition in four volumes in 1984. That first edition expanded on many editions of the one-volume *Bergey's Manual of Determinative Bacteriology*, originally published in 1923, and an independent Bergey's Manual Trust was set up in 1936 to fund and direct publication of these manuals. The second edition of *Bergey's Manual of Systematic Bacteriology* is still in process and will consist of five volumes when finished, with volume 2 so large that it appeared three parts: A, B, and C. The 2nd edition has brought a complete rearrangement of the taxa by phylogeny, based on the latest data from molecular evolutionary studies. The publisher notes that this information is not static, and that, during the preparation of the second edition, revisions have even been made from one volume to the next in the taxonomic outline presented in the "road map to the manual." They also note the growth in the field resulting in over "2200 new species and 390 new genera" since 1984. Each genus is presented with descriptive information, enrichment and isolation procedures, taxonomic comments, and references to the primary literature. There are extensive black-and-white photomicrographs throughout.

Molecular Genetics of Bacteria. 3rd ed. Authors: Larry Snyder, Wendy Champness. ASM Press, 2007.
ISBN: 9781555813994
Recommended for: Academic Libraries
Doody's Core Titles Selection

This is a popular American Society of Microbiology textbook in bacterial molecular genetics for advanced courses. It focuses on the two most-studied bacteria, *Escherichia coli* and *Bacillus subtilis*, but also includes examples from other bacteria with medical, ecological, or biotechnological significance. It has been updated to include new developments in the field and related fields of genetics, biotechnology, and bioengineering. The book takes an experimental approach to the material, including methods and interpretation, along with the conclusions, to focus the reader on how molecular genetic approaches can be used to solve biological problems.

The Prokaryotes. 3rd ed. Editors: Martin Dworkin, Stanley Falkow, Eugene Rosenberg, Karl-Heinz Schleifer, Erko Stackebrandt. Springer, 2006.
http://www.springerlink.com/
ISBN: 9780387254999
Recommended for: Academic Libraries

The third edition of *The Prokaryotes*, a classic reference in the field, has been published in print format, although it is also available as an e-book on the SpringerLink platform. After the 1992 second edition, the publisher planned to make future updates of *The Prokaryotes* into "an evolving electronic resource for the microbiological community" that would be continually updated on an irregular basis. This online version was made available in 1999, but the plan seems to have been abandoned to go back to a more traditional edition approach, although the website entry for this new edition boasts a "new, searchable online version." *The Prokaryotes* has expanded from four volumes (in the second edition) to seven. Organized phylogenetically, it contains articles by world experts on bacterial taxa that have medical, ecological, or industrial relevance and is useful not only for identification and classification but as a treatise on comparative bacteriology. The third edition adds much updated data from such studies as those in bacterial genomics and also color illustrations.

Journals

Journal of Bacteriology. v. 1, American Society for Microbiology, 1916.
http//jb.asm.org/
http://www.ncbi.nlm.nih.gov/pmc/journals/88/
ISSN: 00219193
ISSN: 10985530 (Online)
Indexed in: MEDLINE
Recommended for: Academic Libraries

The American Society for Microbiology is the oldest and largest single life science membership organization in the world, and this is their oldest journal. ASM journals have a reputation for high quality and good value. *Journal of Bacteriology* publishes basic research on bacteria and other microorganisms in all their aspects, including biochemistry, metabolism, genetics, molecular biology, enzymology, and structure/function. Besides peer-reviewed research articles, there are also mini-reviews, meeting reviews, commentary, and genome announcements. With an impact factor of 3.94 (2009 *Journal Citation Reports*), the journal is indexed in numerous indexing and abstracting sources including AGRICOLA, CAB Abstracts, Embase, MEDLINE, Scopus, and Web of Science. It is available in both print and online formats, with online access to volume 1, 1916 available from the publisher and through PubMed Central.

Databases and Other Electronic Resources

EcoSal. American Society for Microbiology, 200?
http://www.ecosal.org/
Recommended for: Academic Libraries

EcoSal is a continually updated and revised web resource based on the classic 1996 print reference book, *Escherichia coli and Salmonella: Cellular and Molecular Biology*. A project of the American Society for Microbiology, it is intended to be a comprehensive archive of knowledge about the enteric bacterial cell for both researchers and students in microbiology, cellular, and molecular biology, but particularly for the E. coli/Salmonella research community. It is also intended to be a teaching tool. While the resource is still a work in progress, lacking content for many of the proposed chapters (modules), the modules that are included are written by international experts with extensive references, images, and outside links to provide access to such information as large datasets or sequences. This reference has added value as an electronic resource. Searching is available by keyword, title, or author, and users can register to create their own profiles, bookmarks, and saved searches. Included in the resource is also the complete 1996 edition of the book in searchable PDF format.

26.5.2. Virology

The study of the structure, growth, function, genetics, and reproduction of viruses, and virus diseases.

—MeSH

Contributor: Susan K. Kendall

Monographs

Fields' Virology. 5th ed. Editors: David M. Knipe, Peter M. Howley. Lippincott Williams & Wilkins, 2007.
http://www.ovid.com/
http://www.r2library.com/
ISBN: 9780781760607
Recommended for: Academic Libraries
Doody's Core Titles Selection

Co-edited by a PhD and an MD, the two-volume *Fields' Virology*, now in its fifth edition since 1980, is the definite reference textbook for virology, combining the molecular and genetic aspects of virus research with clinical aspects related to viral infections and pathogenesis. The emphasis is on viruses of medical interest, however, and the new edition stresses clinical relevance. Extensive editing and updating has been done since the fourth edition. Some especially timely updated areas include viruses and biodefense, and emerging and re-emerging viruses. A CD-ROM viral image bank accompanies the print version. The book is available in printed format or electronically through some of Ovid's Lippincott Williams & Wilkins electronic book collections.

Journals

Journal of Virology. v. 1, American Society for Microbiology, 1967.
http//jvi.asm.org/
http://www.ncbi.nlm.nih.gov/pmc/journals/89/
ISSN: 0022538X
ISSN: 10985514 (Online)
Indexed in: MEDLINE
Recommended for: Academic Libraries

A top quality journal from the American Society of Microbiology and a good value as well, *Journal of Virology* publishes original research on everything concerning viruses. Studies from biochemistry, biophysics, cell biology, genetics, immunology, molecular biology, morphology, physiology, and pathology are all welcome. Also included are sections for commentary and mini-reviews. With an impact factor of 5.15 (2009 *Journal Citation Reports*), the journal is ranked fourth out of 30 journals in the virology category. It is indexed in numerous indexing and abstracting sources including CAB Abstracts, Embase, MEDLINE, Scopus, and Web of Science. Online access back to volume 1, 1967 is available from the publisher and PubMed Central.

Virology. v. 1, Elsevier, 1955.
http//www.sciencedirect.com/science/journal/00426822
ISSN: 00426822
ISSN: 10960341 (Online)
Indexed in: MEDLINE
Recommended for: Academic Libraries

Virology competes with *Journal of Virology* for ranking among primary research journals in this field. It has an impact factor of 3.042 (2009 *Journal Citation Reports*). This peer-reviewed journal covers viruses of all organisms: vertebrates, invertebrates, plants, bacteria, and fungi, and draws on research in many disciplines including molecular genetics, molecular biology, biochemistry, biophysics, structural biology, cell biology, immunology, and morphology. Short communications and preliminary reports are welcome to highlight important results of work in progress. It is indexed in numerous indexing and abstracting sources including CAB ABSTRACTS, Embase, MEDLINE, Scopus, and Web of Science. Online access back to volume 1 is available from the publisher.

26.6. Molecular Biology

Biological phenomena in terms of the chemical and physical interactions of molecules.

—MeSH

Contributor: Susan K. Kendall

Monographs

Lewin's Genes X. 10th ed. Editors: Jocelyn E. Krebs, Elliott S. Goldstein, Stephen T. Kilpatrick. Jones &

Bartlett, 2011.
ISBN: 9780763766320
Recommended for: Academic Libraries

Benjamin Lewin is the well-known founder of the journal *Cell*, one of the most prestigious journals in cellular and molecular biology. His upper level textbook is now a classic in the field of modern molecular biology and molecular genetics; the first edition was published in 1983. The latest edition, issued by a new author team, has enlisted 21 scientists to provide revisions and content updates in their individual fields of expertise. It has been thoroughly revamped to keep pace with this rapidly changing field and to remain on the cutting edge. A website that contains animations and 3D pictures of molecules as well as other supplementary material accompanies the book.

Molecular Biology of the Cell: Reference Edition. 5th ed. Authors: Bruce Alberts, Alexander Johnson, Julian Lewis, Martin Raff, Keith Roberts, Peter Walter. Garland Science, 2008.
ISBN: 9780815341116
Recommended for: Academic Libraries

The bible of cellular and molecular biology, this advanced textbook has been the premier reference in this field since the first edition in 1983 and has consistently been called "excellent" and "superb" by both students and professors alike. This recommendation is for libraries for the "reference edition," which contains the textbook in printed format in its entirety. A student edition also exists, which is smaller, because Chapters 21–25, covering multicellular systems, are provided as PDF files on the DVD-ROM that accompanies the book. Much new and updated material has been added since the last edition. The fourth edition of the text is available for searching electronically on the NCBI bookshelf (http://www.ncbi.nlm.nih.gov/books) for free.

Molecular Cell Biology. 6th ed. Authors: Harvey F. Lodish, Arnold Berk, Chris A. Kaiser, Monty Krieger, Matthew P. Scott, Anthony Bretscher, Hidde Ploegh, Paul Matsudaira. W.H. Freeman, 2008.
ISBN: 9780716776017
Recommended for: Academic Libraries
Doody's Core Titles Selection

This is an authoritative, advanced textbook in cellular and molecular biology, with a focus on clinical applications. This edition is completely updated with expanded coverage of developmental biology and immunology as well as new discoveries and methodologies. The book also has an experimental emphasis, incorporating both classic and recent experiments into the explanations. A companion website includes podcasts, animations, and other supplementary material. The complete book is also available for purchase by individuals (but not institutions) as an e-book. The fourth edition of the text is available for searching electronically on the NCBI bookshelf (http://www.ncbi.nlm.nih.gov/books) for free.

Molecular Genetics of Bacteria. 3rd ed. Authors: Larry Snyder, Wendy Champness. ASM Press, 2007.
See Chapter 26.5.1. Bacteriology

Journals

Cold Spring Harbor Protocols. v. 4, Cold Spring Harbor Laboratory Press, 2006.
See Chapter 26.2. Developmental Biology

EMBO Journal. v. 1, Nature Publishing Group, 1982.
http//www.nature.com/emboj/index.html
http://www.ncbi.nlm.nih.gov/pmc/journals/78/
ISSN: 02614189
ISSN: 14602075 (Online)
Indexed in: MEDLINE
Recommended for: Academic Libraries

The field of molecular biology really grew in the 1980s, and this journal owned and run by the European Molecular Biology Organization was one of the first to focus on publishing papers of general interest to molecular biologists. This peer-reviewed journal remains one of the most highly regarded biology journals worldwide, with an impact factor of 8.993 (2009 *Journal Citation Reports*) and publishes primarily original research. It is indexed in numerous indexing and abstracting sources including CAB Abstracts, Embase, MEDLINE, Scopus, and Web of Science. It is available in both print and online formats, with access back to 1997 available from its current publisher, Nature Publishing Group. Online access to issues from 1982 up to one year prior to current is also available on PubMed Central.

Journal of Molecular Biology. v. 1, Academic Press/Elsevier, 1959.
http//www.sciencedirect.com/science/journal/00222836
ISSN: 00222836
ISSN: 10898638 (Online)
Indexed in: MEDLINE
Recommended for: Academic Libraries

A weekly journal with comprehensive coverage of the field of molecular biology from molecular genetics to protein structure in all kinds of organisms, *JMB* is older than most other journals in its field, having celebrated its 50th anniversary in 2009. It consistently continues to be one of the most highly regarded journals in this subject area; it achieved an impact factor of 3.871 in 2009 (2009 *Journal Citation Reports*). According to its online aims and scope statement, *JMB* covers "gene structure, expression, replication, and recombination in both eukaryotic and prokaryotic organisms; structure, function, chemistry, and in vivo modification and processing of proteins, nucleic acids, and other biologically important macromolecules; cellular and developmental biology; and genetics, structure, and growth cycles of viruses and bacteriophages." It is indexed in numerous indexing and abstracting sources including CAB Abstracts, Embase, MEDLINE, Scopus, and Web of Science. Online access back to 1959 is available from Elsevier.

Methods in Enzymology. v. 1, Elsevier, 1955.
See Chapter 25. Biochemistry

Methods in Molecular Biology/Springer Protocols. v. 1, Springer, 1984.
http//www.springerprotocols.com/
ISSN: 10643745
ISSN: 19406029 (Online)
Indexed in: MEDLINE
Recommended for: Academic Libraries

The *Methods in Molecular Biology* series comes out irregularly, with around 50–60 titles per year on different topics. Each book presents peer-reviewed and researched protocols and laboratory techniques. They range from the broad and popular *Genomic Protocols*, *Basic Cell Culture Protocols*, or *PCR Protocols*, to the more specialized *Retinoid Protocols*, *Bioluminescence Methods and Protocols* or *Type 2 Diabetes Methods and Protocols*. All of the latest research methods are represented in this series, and the books are well-used and popular with laboratory researchers. Although a monographic series, these are indexed in several of the standard indexing and abstracting sources including Chem Abstracts, Embase, MEDLINE and Scopus. Recently, electronic versions of these books have been packaged into a product to make an online, searchable protocols resource. This was initially done by Humana Press in their *BioMed Protocols* product. When Springer took over Humana Press, they completely revamped the interface and functionality and have now packaged the product as *Springer Protocols*. *Springer Protocols* contains the full text of more recent editions in this series; all of the newly published books are on the platform. While there are a few issues with the online product, one being that both old and new editions of books are included on the site so that one could be finding out-of-date results from a search, in general, having the books online is a plus. A site license for *Springer Protocols* will cost a library quite a bit more than merely buying the book series in print, so the amount of usage should be taken into consideration.

Molecular and Cellular Biology. v. 1, American Society for Microbiology, 1981.
http//mcb.asm.org/
http://www.ncbi.nlm.nih.gov/pmc/journals/91/
ISSN: 02707306
ISSN: 10985549 (Online)
Indexed in: MEDLINE
Recommended for: Academic Libraries

Begun in the early 1980s when molecular biology was beginning to come to the forefront of biology research, this peer-reviewed journal is consistently one of the top ranked journals in molecular biology by several different measurements. It achieved an impact factor of 6.057 and was ranked thirty-fourth out of 161 journals in the cell biology category and fortieth out of 283 journals in the biochemistry and molecular biology category (2009 *Journal Citation Reports*). The American Society for Microbiology is the oldest and largest single life science membership organization in the world and retains its own control over the publishing of its journals. According to the journal's online scope statement, it covers "gene expression, chromosome structure and dynamics, signal transduction, intracellular trafficking and mammalian genetic models." It is indexed in numerous indexing and abstracting sources including CAB Abstracts, Embase, MEDLINE, Scopus, and Web of Science. Online access back to 1981 is available from the publisher. Online access to issues from 1981 through six months prior to current is also available on PubMed Central.

Molecular Biology and Evolution. v. 1, Oxford University Press, 1983.
http//mbe.oxfordjournals.org/
ISSN: 07374038
ISSN: 15371719 (Online)
Indexed in: MEDLINE
Recommended for: Academic Libraries

This peer-reviewed journal is published on behalf of the Society for Molecular Biology and Evolution. It is also sponsored by the American Society of Naturalists. Its scope includes "investigations of molecular evolutionary patterns and processes, tests of evolutionary hypotheses that use molecular data, and studies that use molecular evolutionary information to address questions about biological function at all levels of organization." The journal publishes only original research articles and letters (short communications about research findings). It achieved an impact factor of 9.872 and was ranked seventeenth out of 283 journals in the biochemistry and molecular biology category, second out of 44 journals in the evolutionary biology category, and ninth out of 144 journals in the genetics and hereditary category (2009 *Journal Citation Reports*). The journal is indexed in numerous indexing and abstracting sources including CAB Abstracts, Embase, MEDLINE, Scopus, and Web of Science. Online access back to 1983 is available from the publisher.

Molecular Cell. v. 1, Cell Press/Elsevier, 1997.
http//www.cell.com/molecular-cell/home
ISSN: 10972765
ISSN: 10974164 (Online)
Indexed in: MEDLINE
Recommended for: Academic Libraries

The top ranked journal, *Cell*, was founded in 1974, and it published significantly in the areas of molecular and cellular biology throughout the 1980s and 1990s. In the late 1990s, daughter journals were split off from the flagship journal, and *Molecular Cell* was born. *Cell* continues to publish research of "exceptional significance" in any area of biology, although it is often ranked as a molecular biology or genetics journal due to its content. *Molecular Cell* publishes only articles that focus at the molecular level, both peer-reviewed original research and reviews. It has rapidly risen to a high prestige level, likely due to its association with the top-tier journal that it came from, achieving an impact factor of 14.608 (2009 *Journal Citation Reports*). It is indexed in numerous indexing and abstracting sources including Embase, MEDLINE, Scopus, and Web of Science. Online access back to 1997 is available through the publisher.

Molecular Systems Biology. v. 1, Nature Publishing Group and European Molecular Biology Organization, 2005.
See Chapter 26.6. Molecular Biology

Nucleic Acids Research. v. 1, Oxford University Press, 1974.
http//nar.oxfordjournals.org/
http://www.ncbi.nlm.nih.gov/pmc/journals/4/
ISSN: 03051048
ISSN: 13624962 (Online)
Indexed in: MEDLINE
Recommended for: Academic Libraries

Nucleic Acids Research publishes both original research and review papers on all aspects of nucleic acids and proteins. Popular special issues every year are devoted to reviewing biological databases and web-based software resources for biologists. It has been an established and respected journal in the field for many years; it achieved an impact factor of 7.479 and ranked twenty-seventh out of 283 journals in biochemistry and molecular biology (2009 *Journal Citation Reports*). The journal is indexed in numerous indexing and abstracting sources including CAB Abstracts, Embase, MEDLINE, Scopus, and Web of Science. It is available in both print and online formats. This peer-reviewed journal has been one of Oxford's experiments with open access and author-side payment for publication, having become completely available for free online since 2005. Online access back to 1974 is available from the publisher and on PubMed Central.

Databases and Other Electronic Resources

Current Protocols. Wiley, 2000.
http://www.currentprotocols.com/
Recommended for: Academic Libraries

Wiley's *Current Protocols* is the "largest collection of authoritative and regularly-updated step-by-step research techniques and procedures available." At present, 17 different titles make up the complete *Current Protocols* collection. *Current Protocols in Molecular Biology* was the first, and it is the best-known. Some of the other titles in this series: *Current Protocols in Protein Chemistry*, *Current Protocols in Bioinformatics*, *Current Protocols in Microbiology*, *Current Protocols in Neuroscience*, *Current Protocols in Cell Biology*, *Current Protocols in Human Genetics*, and *Current Protocols in Stem Cell Biology*. The *Current Protocols* title previously existed only as looseleaf binders, with updates arriving quarterly as part of a subscription. They are still available in that format, but the electronic version is much more convenient and easily updated. Individual *Current Protocols* titles or all of them together are available for subscription either for individuals or for institutions as a site license. Many researchers find the *Current Protocols* title for their subject area to be a must-have resource for laboratory methods. They are a widely recognized and respected series.

26.7. Parasitology

The study of the structure, growth, function, genetics, and reproduction of parasites, and parasitic diseases.

—MeSH

Contributor: C. Trenton Boyd, Esther Carrigan

Monographs

Diagnostic Medical Parasitology. 5th ed. Author: Lynne Shore Garcia. ASM (American Society for Microbiology), 2007.
http://online.statref.com/titleinfo/fxid-272.html
ISBN: 9781555813802
Recommended for: Academic Libraries
Doody's Core Titles Selection

This is the fifth edition of a major reference in diagnostic parasitology, authored by one of the foremost experts in the field, and considered by many to be the gold standard text. It covers both general information on medical parasitology and detailed information on relevant diagnostic methods. While this edition both updates and expands content, the logical organization of the earlier editions is maintained. It begins with a philosophy and approach to diagnostic parasitology and then presents comprehensive information on specific parasites including structure, life cycles, disease signs and symptoms, diagnosis, treatment, epidemiology, and prevention. The remainder of the volume covers complete diagnostic procedures used for parasite detection and identification. New to this edition is a section on medical case histories with methods used for diagnosis. This fifth edition also provides updated and enhanced tables and illustrations, and an expanded section on histological diagnosis. It incorporates newly recognized parasites and new diagnostic methods. This volume is highly recommended for any academic or special library that serves a college of medicine or diagnostic laboratory science, or a program in parasitology, microbiology, or public health.

Georgis' Parasitology for Veterinarians. 9th ed. Author: Dwight D. Bowman. Saunders Elsevier, 2009.
See Chapter 23. Veterinary Medicine

Markell and Voge's Medical Parasitology. 9th ed. Authors: David T. John, William A. Petri, Jr. Saunders Elsevier, 2006.
ISBN: 9780721647937
Recommended for: Academic Libraries

This is the ninth edition of a long-established and well-respected classic parasitology textbook. It is a comprehensive parasitology resource, covering all the animal agents which cause diseases in humans, in both tropical and temperate climates. The content includes parasites, parasitism, and host relations; protozoa; malaria; trematodes; cestodes; intestinal nematodes; arthropods as parasites and disease vectors; parasitic infections in immunocompromised hosts; signs and symptoms of parasitic diseases; pseudoparasites; and examination of specimens, including immunodiagnostic techniques. Along with the descriptions of these parasites, the text provides information on the diseases they cause, and the epidemiology, transmission, pathogenesis, diagnosis, prevention, and treatment of those diseases. In addition to the usual updating to integrate recent research and changes in techniques, this edition boasts completely redrawn line drawings and improved illustrations, using a two color design. Drawings and color plates depict the life cycle of parasites and their global distribution. The intended audience is advanced graduate and medical students. It is highly recommended as a key resource for any academic library that serves a parasitology program or college of medicine.

Medical and Veterinary Entomology. 2nd ed. Editors: Gary R. Mullen, Lance A. Durden. Academic Press Elsevier, 2009.
ISBN: 9780123725004
Recommended for: Academic Libraries

This second edition of a highly-respected textbook is an important resource on insects and arachnids of medical and veterinary importance. It begins with a general introduction and chapters to cover the structural adaptations of parasitic arthropods, epidemiology of vector-borne diseases, and forensic entomology. The next 22 chapters each focus on a different group of insects or arachnids. These chapters are consistently organized to present taxonomy, morphology, life history, behavior and ecology, public health and veterinary importance, and prevention and control. The final chapter presents molecular tools in medical and veterinary entomology. An appendix provides arthropod-related viruses of medical and veterinary importance, and a glossary and taxonomic subject index. New to this edition are the chapters on parasitic arthropod structural adaptations, forensic entomology and molecular tools, the glossary, and appendix. New full-color illustrative matter and maps have been added throughout the text. The scope of this resource makes it a valuable text for medical, veterinary and public health students, as well as graduate students in entomology. It is highly recommended for any academic library that serves a program in entomology, or a college of medicine or veterinary medicine.

Medical Parasitology. Editors: Abhay R. Satoskar, Gary Simon, Peter J. Hotez, Moriya Tsuji. Landes Bioscience, 2009.
ISBN: 9781570596957
Recommended for: Academic Libraries

This concise book, part of the publisher's *Vademecum Medical Handbook* series, fully meets the handbook expectation of providing a dense compilation of information, well-organized for quick consultation, in a small package. It is arranged in five sections: "Nematodes (Enterobiasis, Trichuriasis, Ascariasis, Hookworm, Strongyloidiasis, Trichinellosis, Onchocercosis, Loiasis, Dracunculiasis, Cutaneous Larva Migrans, Baylisascariasis and Toxocariasis, Lymphatic Filariasis)"; "Trematodes (Clonorchiasis and Opisthorchiasis, Liver Fluke: Fasciola hepatica, Paragonimiasis, Intestinal Trematode Infections, Schistosomiasis: Schistosoma japonica, Schistosomiasis: Schistosoma mansoni, Schistosomiasis: Schistosoma haematobium)"; "Cestodes (Taeniasis and Cysticercosis, Hydatid Disease)"; "Protozoans (American Trypanosomiasis [Chagas Disease]), African Trypanosomiasis, Visceral Leishmaniasis, Cutaneous Leishmaniasis, Toxoplasmosis, Giardiasis, Amebiasis, Cryptosporidiosis, Trichomoniasis, Pneumocystis Pneumonia, Malaria)"; and "Arthropods (Clinically Relevant Arthropods)." An appendix provides tables on "Drugs for Parasitic Infections" and "Safety of Antiparasitic Drugs," and a listing of "Manufacturers of Drugs Used to Treat Parasitic Infections." Each chapter follows the same general topic outline: background/introduction, life cycle, disease signs and symptoms, diagnosis, treatment, and prevention and prophylaxis. The preface describes this book as "a perfect companion for primary care physicians, residents, nurse practitioners, medical students, paramedics, other public health care personnel and as well as travelers." It is recommended as an excellent resource for any academic or special library serving students in any of the health professions or practitioners.

Veterinary Clinical Parasitology. 7th ed. Authors: Anne M. Zajac, Gary A. Conboy. Wiley-Blackwell, 2006.
ISBN: 9780813817347
Recommended for: Academic Libraries

This is the seventh edition of an essential resource on veterinary parasitology. It was prepared under the auspices of the American Association of Veterinary Parasitologists and is intended to be a quick reference. Its focus is on the detection and identification of parasites of domestic animals in North America, providing diagnostic laboratory procedures available in most veterinary practices. There are over 400 color photographs to aid in parasite identification. Contents include: detection of parasites in feces, detection of protozoan and helminth parasites in the urinary, reproductive and integumentary systems and in the eye, detection of parasites in the blood, diagnosis of arthropod parasites, and parasites of fish. Each chapter begins with a review of diagnostic techniques, information to assist in the choice of a technique, any diagnostic limitations, sensitivity and specificity concerns for a technique, and then step-by-step presentation of protocols with recipes included. This edition includes coverage of additional foreign parasites as well as expanded material to present the distribution, life cycle, and importance of each parasite. The intended audience is veterinary students, veterinary technicians and practitioners. It is highly recommended as a key resource for any academic library that serves a program in parasitology, veterinary technicians, or a college of veterinary medicine.

Veterinary Parasitology. 3rd ed. Authors: Mike A. Taylor, R.L. Coop, Richard L. Wall. Wiley-Blackwell, 2008.
ISBN: 9781405119641
See Also Chapter 23. Veterinary Medicine
Recommended for: Academic Libraries

This is the third edition of a well-respected resource in veterinary parasitology. The volume begins with an overview of parasite taxonomy and morphology. The main content is arranged by species chapters and for each species the arrangement follows organ systems. Species covered include cattle, sheep and goats, horses, pigs, dogs and cats, poultry and gamebirds, ungulates, laboratory animals, and exotics. Next are chapters on facultative ectoparasites and arthropod vectors, the epidemiology of parasitic diseases, resistance to parasitic diseases, antiparasitics, and laboratory diagnosis of parasitism. The consistent arrangement within the chapters on the various host species is an especially effective presentation for veterinary students. This third edition is a major update with thoroughly revised and restructured content. The target audience for this resource is veterinary students and researchers, as well as practitioners. It is highly recommended as a key resource for any academic library that serves a program in parasitology or a college of veterinary medicine.

Journals

Advances in Parasitology. v. 1, Academic-Elsevier, 1963.
http://www.sciencedirect.com/science/bookseries/0065308X
ISSN: 0065308X
Indexed in: MEDLINE
Recommended for: Academic Libraries

Advances in Parasitology is an irregularly issued serial that is issued as a bound volume. Editor(s) and specific topic focus varies with each volume. Volumes issued most recently also carry individual titles, such as *Important Helminth Infections in Southeast Asia*, *Parasitoids of*

Drosophila, and *Natural History of Host-Parasite Interactions*. This suggests that it is undergoing a transformation into more of a book series than a serial journal. It is, however, indexed and abstracted by many of the major indexing and abstracting services including AGRICOLA, BIOSIS, CAB Abstracts, Current Contents, Embase, Index Veterinarius, MEDLINE, ISI Web of Science, Scopus, and Veterinary Bulletin and has earned the second highest impact factor ranking of titles in parasitology (2009 *Journal Citation Reports*). Online full text of its volumes is available through ScienceDirect beginning with content from 2000. This title is highly recommended as a key resource for any academic library that serves a program in parasitology or a college of agriculture, medicine, or veterinary medicine.

International Journal for Parasitology. v. 1, Elsevier, 1971.
http//www.sciencedirect.com/science/journal/00207519
http://www.ingentaconnect.com/content/els/00207519
ISSN: 00207519
ISSN: 18790135 (Online)
Indexed in: MEDLINE
Recommended for: Academic Libraries

The *International Journal for Parasitology* is a peer-reviewed, well-respected journal that is sponsored by and published for the Australian Society for Parasitology. It covers all areas of basic and applied parasitology, including parasites, host-parasite relationships, and the social and economic aspects of parasites considered important to human and veterinary medicine and agriculture. The journal publishes both full-length research papers and rapid communications, which are designed to provide a medium for the transmission of highly significant original findings. It also publishes thematic issues and commissions review articles. A current opinion section is included to encourage critical comment and debate on matters of current controversy in parasitology. The journal is indexed and abstracted by many of the major indexing and abstracting services including Academic Search Complete, AGRICOLA, BIOSIS, CAB Abstracts, Current Contents, Embase, Index Veterinarius, ISI Web of Science, MEDLINE, and Veterinary Bulletin. This title is highly recommended as an important resource for any academic library that serves a program in parasitology or a college of agriculture, medicine, or veterinary medicine.

Molecular and Biochemical Parasitology. v. 1, Elsevier, 1980.
http//www.sciencedirect.com/science/journal/01666851
ISSN: 01666851
ISSN: 18729428 (Online)
Indexed in: MEDLINE
Recommended for: Academic Libraries

Molecular and Biochemical Parasitology is an important peer-reviewed international journal that focuses on the molecular biology and biochemical aspects of parasites and parasite-host interactions. According to its scope statement, the main subject areas covered by the journal are: the chemical structure, biosynthesis, degradation, properties and function of DNA, RNA, proteins, lipids, carbohydrates and small molecular-weight substances; intermediary metabolism and bioenergetics; molecular and biochemical studies on the mode of action of antiparasitic drugs; molecular and biochemical aspects of membrane structure and function; molecular and biochemical aspects of host parasite relationships including analysis of parasitic escape mechanisms; characterization of parasite antigens and of parasite and host cell surface receptors; analysis of gene structure, function and expression; and mechanism of genetic recombination. The journal publishes full-length original articles, short communications, technical reports, and mini-review articles. *Molecular and Biochemical Parasitology* is indexed and abstracted by most of the major indexing and abstracting services including Academic Search Complete, AGRICOLA, BIOSIS, CAB Abstracts, Current Contents, Embase, Index Veterinarius, ISI Web of Science, MEDLINE, Scopus, and Veterinary Bulletin. This title is highly recommended as an important resource for any academic library that serves a program in parasitology or a college of agriculture, medicine, or veterinary medicine.

Parasitology. v. 1, Cambridge University, 1908.
http//journals.cambridge.org/action/displayJournal?jid=PAR
ISSN: 00311820
ISSN: 14698161 (Online)
Indexed in: MEDLINE
Recommended for: Academic Libraries

Parasitology is a peer-reviewed international journal which defines its scope as all aspects of pure and applied parasitology, including biochemical, immunological, physiological, and ecological topics. Special emphasis is placed on parasites and their control. The journal publishes original research articles as well as appropriate review articles. Two special issues are published annually; one is the proceedings of the annual Symposia of the British Society for Parasitology and the second is commissioned by the editors and the editorial board to focus on an area of significant interest to readers of the journal. *Parasitology* is indexed and abstracted by all of the major indexing and abstracting services including Academic Search Complete, AGRICOLA, Biological Abstracts, CAB Abstracts, Current Contents, Embase, Index Veterinarius, ISI Web of Science, MEDLINE, and Veterinary Bulletin. This journal is highly recommended as an important resource for any academic library that serves a program in parasitology or a college of agriculture, medicine, or veterinary medicine.

Parasitology International. v. 46, Elsevier, 1997.
http//www.sciencedirect.com/science/journal/13835769
ISSN: 13835769
ISSN: 18730329 (Online)
Indexed in: MEDLINE
Recommended for: Academic Libraries

Parasitology International is the official international journal of the Japanese Society of Parasitology. This peer-reviewed journal publishes research in all areas of the fields of human and animal parasitology, including morphology, immunology, cell biology, biochemistry, molecular biology, and systematics. The journal contains original research papers, rapid communications, mini-reviews, original case reports, and letters to the editor. *Parasitology International* is indexed and abstracted by all of the major indexing and abstracting services including Academic Search Complete, Biological Abstracts, CAB Abstracts, Embase, Index Veterinarius, ISI Web of Science, MEDLINE, Scopus, and Veterinary Bulletin. This journal is highly recommended as an important resource for any academic library that serves a program in parasitology or a college of agriculture, medicine, or veterinary medicine.

PLoS Pathogens. v. 1, Public Library of Science, 2005.
http//www.plospathogens.org/
ISSN: 15537366
ISSN: 15537374 (Online)
See Also Chapter 26.5. Microbiology
Indexed in: MEDLINE
Recommended for: Academic Libraries

PLoS Pathogens is an open-access, peer-reviewed journal published monthly by the Public Library of Science, a non-profit organization. It began in 2005, primarily as an online open-access journal, although a print version was also made available. *PLoS Pathogens* has built a solid following of both contributors and readers; its impact factor, although a more traditional measure, attests to its success and places it as the highest ranked journal in parasitology (2009 *Journal Citation Reports*). From its scope statement, the journal seeks to publish "outstanding original articles that significantly advance the understanding of pathogens and how they interact with their host organisms." *PLoS Pathogens* publishes peer-reviewed articles, opinions, reviews, and editorials. It employs online tools to facilitate scholarly discussion about its articles including comments, notes, and ratings. The journal is indexed and abstracted by all of the major indexing and abstracting services including Biological Abstracts, Current Contents, Embase, ISI Web of Science, MEDLINE, and Scopus. The intended audience is medical and parasitology students, researchers, and practitioners. It is highly recommended as a key resource for any academic library that serves a program in parasitology or a college of agriculture, medicine, or veterinary medicine.

Trends in Parasitology. v. 17, Cell-Elsevier, 2001.
http//www.cell.com/cellpress/trends
ISSN: 14714922
ISSN: 14715007 (Online)
Indexed in: MEDLINE
Recommended for: Academic Libraries

Trends in Parasitology is a peer-reviewed, well-respected, review journal in parasitology with an international scope. It provides broad coverage of the field and commissions review articles by experts that are written to be accessible to those who are not parasitology experts. *Trends in Parasitology* covers parasites of both medical and veterinary importance around the world. In addition to review articles, the journal publishes opinion (trends and innovative ideas) and research articles, and includes an update section and book reviews. Its aim is "to provide a point of access for communication between workers in all disciplines, both in the field and laboratory." The journal is indexed and abstracted by most of the major indexing and abstracting services including Academic Search Complete, BIOSIS, CAB Abstracts, CINAHL Plus, Current Contents, Embase, Index Veterinarius, ISI Web of Science, MEDLINE, Scopus, and Veterinary Bulletin. This title is highly recommended as a key resource for any academic library that serves a program in parasitology or a college of agriculture, medicine or veterinary medicine.

Veterinary Parasitology. v. 1, Elsevier, 1975.
http//www.sciencedirect.com/science/journal/03044017
ISSN: 03044017
ISSN: 18732550 (Online)
See Also Chapter 23. Veterinary Medicine
Indexed in: MEDLINE
Recommended for: Academic Libraries

Veterinary Parasitology is the official organ of the American Association of Veterinary Parasitologists, the European Veterinary Parasitology College and the World Association for the Advancement of Veterinary Parasitology. This international peer-reviewed journal publishes original research articles, review articles, rapid communications, short communications, letters to the editor, and book reviews. According to its scope statement, the journal is concerned with those aspects of helminthology, protozoology, and entomology which are of interest to animal health investigators, veterinary practitioners, and others with a special interest in parasitology. It covers all aspects of disease prevention, pathology, treatment, epidemiology, and control of parasites in all domestic animals. The parasitology of laboratory animals is included only as a disease model for domestic animals; the parasitology of wild animals is included only where the wild animal acts as a disease or zoonotic reservoir for domestic animals. *Veterinary Parasitology* is indexed and abstracted by all of the major indexing and abstracting services including Academic Search Complete, AGRICOLA, Biological Abstracts, CAB Abstracts, Current Contents, Embase, Index Veterinarius, ISI Web of Science, MEDLINE, Scopus, and Veterinary Bulletin. This journal is highly recommended as an important resource for any academic library that serves a program in parasitology or a college of agriculture, medicine, or veterinary medicine.

26.8. Radiobiology

The scientific principles, mechanisms, and effects of the interaction of ionizing radiation with living matter.

—MeSH

Contributor: Debra R. Berlanstein

Monographs

Basic Clinical Radiobiology. 4th ed. Editors: Albert van der Kogel, Michael Joiner. Hodder Arnold, 2009.
ISBN: 9780340929667
Recommended for: Hospital, Academic Libraries

This is a concise but comprehensive text aimed at those seeking accreditation in radiation oncology, clinical radiation physics, and radiation technology. Beginning with the basic principles of radiation biology, this work expands to discuss the biological underpinnings of how radiation is used to manage cancer. New authors added since the last edition address new topics such as cell death, biological response modifiers, and biological image guided radiotherapy. Also revised are sections on the molecular basis of the radiation response, tumor hypoxia, and the dose-rate effect. This is a shorter and less in-depth work than Hall's *Radiobiology for the Radiologist*, but the audience is different, since *Basic Clinical Radiobiology* is aimed more at support personnel.

Essentials of Radiation, Biology and Protection. 2nd ed. Author: Steve Forshier. Cengage Learning, 2008.
ISBN: 9781428312173
Recommended for: Hospital, Academic Libraries

This second edition focuses on teaching the basic principles of radiation biology and safety to all students working in the various divisions of radiology and radiation oncology. The author has directed a radiology technology program for over 30 years and has written a concise, practical book that sets out to ensure safe use of radiation in the practice of radiology. Enhanced by excellent photos, this very readable work contains the essentials that the practicing radiologist and technician need to master in radiobiology.

Radiobiology for the Radiologist. 6th ed. Authors: Eric J. Hall, Amato J. Giaccia. Lippincott Williams & Wilkins, 2006.
ISBN: 9780781741514
Recommended for: Hospital, Academic Libraries
Doody's Core Titles Selection

This book is often the first choice for radiologists wanting to understand the effects of radiation on the human body. It focuses on clinical applications and is written in an easy-to-read style with chapter summaries for review. The first section covers diagnostic radiology, nuclear medicine, and radiation oncology. The second section is more focused on the needs of radiation oncologists. This edition also includes updated information about dosimetry and risks associated with interventional radiology and cardiology, as well as a chapter on the techniques of molecular biology as it relates to radiation biology.

Journals

BMC Medical Physics. v. 1, BioMed Central, 2001.
http://www.biomedcentral.com/bmcmedphys/
ISSN: 17566649 (Online)
Indexed in: MEDLINE
Recommended for: Hospital, Academic Libraries

BMC Medical Physics is a multi-disciplinary, peer-reviewed, open access online journal that spans all areas of medical physics, including radiobiology, nuclear medicine, and radiation therapy. Since this is a completely online journal, publication is variable but articles are high quality and the format makes it possible to offer more visuals, data sets, and even video. This is an excellent addition to the collection that complements the traditional journals in this field.

International Journal of Radiation Biology. v. 1, Informa Healthcare, 1959.
http://informahealthcare.com/journal/rab
ISSN: 09553002
ISSN: 13623095 (Online)
Indexed in: MEDLINE
Recommended for: Academic Libraries

The *International Journal of Radiation Biology* is published monthly and includes original papers, reviews, technical notes/reports, and meeting reports on the effects of all types of radiation on the human body. This includes ionizing, UV and visible radiation, accelerated particles, microwaves, ultrasound, heat, and related modalities. Focusing on the biological effects of radiation, topics include genetic abnormalities, repair phenomena, cell death, and tissue. Also covered are problems involving adjuvants and radiation in cancer therapy and hazards of low dose treatment. This is a major journal in the field of radiobiology.

Nuclear Medicine and Biology. v. 1, Elsevier, 1973.
http://www.nucmedbio.com/
ISSN: 09698051
ISSN: 18729614 (Online)
Indexed in: MEDLINE
Recommended for: Hospital, Academic Libraries

Nuclear Medicine and Biology publishes original research related to radiopharmaceutical science, and bridges the fields of nuclear medicine and radiation biology. The emphasis is on original biomedical research but the journal also addresses radiopharmacy practice, quality control, dispensing, and regulation. This is the official journal of the Society of Radiopharmaceutical Sciences and is published eight times a year.

26.9. Sociobiology

Social organization in animals including humans, especially with regard to its genetic basis and evolutionary history.
—MeSH

Contributor: Holly E. Phillips

Monographs

Defenders of the Truth: The Sociobiology Debate. Author: Ullica Segerstrale. Oxford University Press, 2001.
ISBN: 9780192862150
Recommended for: Academic Libraries

The author earned her PhD in Sociology at Harvard at the same time E.O. Wilson published and then became a lightning rod of controversy because of his book *Sociobiology: The New Synthesis*. Her PhD dissertation in the area of sociology of science focused on the sociobiology controversy. Through information from more than a decade of interviews and literature surrounding the debate, the author presents a rare and thorough argument by recounting of the sociobiology controversy through the eyes of the participants. The author does not define sociobiology or its underlying concepts. Therefore the reader should have a grasp of sociobiology before undertaking this greatly entertaining book. In three parts over 20 chapters, the book covers what happened in the sociobiology debate, attempts to make sense of the debate, and then broadens out to consider the cultural meaning of the battle for science. Well written and meticulously researched, this book is a great addition to any academic library.

On Human Nature. Revised ed. Author: Edward O. Wilson. Harvard University Press, 2004.
ISBN: 9780674016385
Recommended for: Academic Libraries

Winner of the 1979 Pulitzer Prize for Non-Fiction, *On Human Nature* is E.O. Wilson's response to criticisms stemming from the author's treatment of the basis of human sociality in the final chapter, "Man: From Sociobiology to Sociology," in the book *Sociobiology: The New Synthesis*. *On Human Nature* succeeds in this by expanding upon the rationale for relating biological principles to human behavior and how human sociobiology can help answer important questions about human instincts and nature. The nine chapters explain the relationship between the natural and human world in terms of heredity, aggression, sexual behavior, altruism, and religion. In the final chapter, "Hope," the author shares his vision of a future where science and culture meet to create a "biology of ethics" that will make the best use of our discoveries. Researchers and students of evolutionary psychology and those with a general interest in the link between biology and social sciences will enjoy this wonderfully engaging and readable book. The 2004 Harvard University Press revised edition includes a new preface in which the author reflects on the rationale for writing this work.

Selfish Gene: 30th Anniversary Edition. 3rd ed. Author: Richard Dawkins. Oxford University Press, 2006.

ISBN: 9780199291144
Recommended for: Academic Libraries

In a conversational tone aimed at lay readers, yet still of substantial interest to experts, the author sets about the task of convincing the reader that "we, and all other animals, are machines created by our genes." To substantiate a gene-centered view of evolution the author, over the course of 13 chapters, presents ideas and examples from the natural world that range from how genes arose to be the center of evolution by being "selfish" to how the resultant "survival machines" compete and populations ultimately reach an "evolutionarily stable strategy" of existence. When considering humans, the author coins the term "meme," a unit of human cultural evolution, to differentiate humans from other social species in their unique ability to counter the demands of our genes to be selfishly motivated for survival and become altruistic. The book is a readable introduction to a controversial view that has shaped social and evolutionary research. The 30th Anniversary Edition includes a new introduction in addition to the prefaces for the first and second editions. This is an essential purchase for academic libraries but could also be at home in a large hospital library.

Sociobiology: The New Synthesis, Twenty-Fifth Anniversary Edition. Author: Edward O. Wilson. Belknap Press of Harvard University Press, 2000.
ISBN: 9780674000896
Recommended for: Academic Libraries

With this groundbreaking work, the author introduced the new, and often controversial, theory of sociobiology. According to the author, sociobiology "is defined as the systematic study of the biological basis of all social behavior." The work is organized into three parts: social evolution, social mechanisms, and the social species. The first part sets the foundation of sociobiological theory and makes the case for its classification as a branch of evolutionary and population biology. The second part details the variety of mechanisms that influence social behavior. The final part covers the application of the theory to the analysis of four social species: colonial invertebrates, social insects, nonhuman mammals, and man. Each chapter contains numerous figures, tables, and photographs to aid the presentation and explanation of this complex theory. The 1975 edition was voted by the officers and fellows of the international Animal Behavior Society as one of the most important books on animal behavior of all time. In the introduction to the twenty-fifth anniversary edition, released in 2000 by Harvard University Press, the author reflects on the significance of this text and how it shaped the next 25 years of scientific research in the field. This is required reading for students and scholars interested in evolutionary psychology, genetic adaptation, and behavioral neuroscience.

Triumph of Sociobiology. Author: John Alcock. Oxford University Press, 2001.
ISBN: 9780195143836
Recommended for: Academic Libraries

Triumph of Sociobiology is a thorough, yet defensive, rebuttal of the numerous attacks lodged at sociobiology since its introduction as a discipline in 1975. As the author argues the benefit, practice, and broad scope of sociobiology, he offers a contemporary view of how the field has defined itself over the years and how it has responded to criticism. Further, while not a textbook in the strictest sense, a lot of basic information is provided. The book consists of 10 chapters covering the definition of sociobiology, how scientists practice in the field, what has been discovered, and the practical application of the findings. The author also defends the most controversial part of sociobiology, that it is deterministic in nature and that humans lack control over their own genes. This book is of interest to students and researchers in the biological and behavioral sciences and those who have an interest in how a sociobiologist defends the many and varied assaults on a relatively new discipline. This work is recommended for academic libraries or large hospital libraries with a browsing collection.

Journals

Behavioral and Brain Sciences. v. 1, Cambridge University Press, 1978.
http//journals.cambridge.org/action/displayJournal?jid=BBS
ISSN: 0140525X
ISSN: 14691825 (Online)
Indexed in: MEDLINE
Recommended for: Academic Libraries

Started in March of 1978, this bi-monthly journal utilizes "open peer commentary" to publish refereed articles in the areas of psychology, neuroscience, behavioral biology, and other related topics. Open peer commentary means each article unit consists of the original article, a number (10–25) of 1,000-word commentaries from subject specialists, and the author's response to each commentary. While not devoted to sociobiology in the 1975 sense of explaining social behavior in animals, it services sociobiology offshoots like evolutionary psychology, which analyzes psychological adaptations that, like bodily organs, may have evolved over time as a result of natural selection pressures. Researchers in the neurosciences and behavioral disciplines are the main audience of this journal, which is ranked first out of 47 behavioral sciences journals with a five-year impact factor of 23.548 (2009 *Journal Citation Reports*). The journal is cited in numerous abstracting and indexing sources such as Biological Abstracts, MEDLINE, PsycINFO, Science Citation Index, and Sociological Abstracts. Online access back to volume 1, 1978 is available from the publisher.

Behavioral Ecology and Sociobiology. v. 1, Springer, 1976.
http//www.springerlink.com/content/0340-5443
ISSN: 03405443
ISSN: 14320762 (Online)
Recommended for: Academic Libraries

Started in 1976, one year after publication of E.O. Wilson's *Sociobiology: The New Synthesis*, which created the field of sociobiology, this journal is still central to the study of the evolution and ecological adaption of behavior. The journal presents reviews, original peer-reviewed research papers, method papers, and commentaries on prior articles. Researchers and upper-level students interested in intraspecific behavioral interactions and mechanisms as well as behavioral ecophysiology and evolutionary and functional theory are the main audience. The journal ranks twenty-fifth out of 49 behavioral sciences journals (2009 *Journal Citation Reports*). It is essential for an academic library serving a wide range of behavioral and biological research. The journal is cited in SocIndex, Environment Index, PsycINFO, and Science Citation Index. Online access to volume 1, 1976 is available from the publisher. Number of issues per volume varies from 4 per volume (v. 1–17) to 6 per volume (v. 18–60) to 12 per volume (v. 61–current).

26.10. Systems Biology

Comprehensive, methodical analysis of complex biological systems by monitoring responses to perturbations of biological processes. Large scale, computerized collection and analysis of the data are used to develop and test models of biological systems.

—MeSH

Contributor: Diane C. Rein

Monographs

Handbook of Research on Systems Biology Applications in Medicine. Editor: Andriani Daskalaki. Medical Information Science Reference/IGI Global, 2009.
http://www.igi-global.com/
http://extranet.netlibrary.com/TitleSelect/
http://www.ebrary.com/
ISBN: 9781605660769
ISBN: 9781605660776 (Online)
Recommended for: Academic Libraries

This two-volume handbook of 45 chapters organized into 14 sections comprehensively compiles the many different facets of systems biology as it applies specifically to medical research. The *Handbook* takes the interesting approach of viewing systems biology as a series of research protocols. By providing specific examples that use well-established techniques, readers can directly test and apply the concepts discussed in the *Handbook* to their specific research efforts. The early sections define the basic concepts of medical systems biology that lead into sections dealing with the more traditional biological aspects of systems biology: computational methodologies, genomics, bioinformatics, proteomics, molecular network analyses, biochemistry, and various forms of data mining, all under the umbrella of a medical science context. Specific chapters relate to a systems biology approach to aging, infectious diseases, pathological fungal infections, complex diseases, and drug design. Processing of histopathological data has been synthesized for the first time in this work. Although biomedical computational biologists, statisticians, and computer scientists already engaged in some aspect of systems biology research will probably appreciate this work the most, the scope of the work is sufficiently broad and comprehensive that many biomedical researchers will also find some items of interest. Part handbook and part laboratory idea manual, the editor has effectively created a new genre in biomedical texts that has the potential to translate into new biomedical research initiatives and treatments. It is an important contribution to scholarly communications in biomedical research.

An Introduction to Systems Biology: Design Principles of Biological Circuits. Author: Uri Alon. Chapman & Hall/CRC, 2006.
ISBN: 9781584886426
Recommended for: Academic Libraries

This well-organized, concisely and artfully written book assumes no prior knowledge of biology, making it essential for cross-disciplinary reading by the many nonbiologists that are active or interested in systems biology research. As an equally important work for biologists and biomedical researchers, the author offers a novel perspective on biological processes by taking an engineering circuit design view of what governs the structure, function, and behavior of biological pathways and networks. The first chapter effectively introduces the mathematical and theoretical principles of biological network design that continue to be integrated throughout the remaining work. Subsequent chapters examine specific topics of increasing biological network complexity governing development, signal transduction, and neuronal pathways. As the chapters progress in biological complexity, the author effectively and seamlessly transcends from biological systems to engineering principles. He sets aside the various mathematical formulas, equations, and datasets as a set of appendixes, which are valuable in their own right, providing readers with a collated set of reference material that has been dispersed and fragmented in the scholarly literature for several decades. The author covers networks that are primarily protein in nature. As a consequence, this particular text does not cover the design principles of all types of cellular networks. The topics also concentrate primarily on the individual components and sub-components of cellular networks. It does not consider networks of larger scales, such as those found in organ systems and at the organismal level. Nevertheless, this work remains an important foundational and timely work in systems biology.

Systems Biology: A Textbook. Authors: Edda Klipp, Wolfram Liebermeister, Christoph Wierling, Axel Kowald, Hans Lehrach, Ralf Herwig. Wiley-VCH, 2009.
ISBN: 9783527318742
Recommended for: Academic Libraries

This monograph has an interesting genesis. Although the authors are pioneers in the field of systems biology and experienced systems biology educators, *Systems Biology: A Textbook* incorporates the feedback and suggestions of lecturers in systems biology worldwide following the release of an earlier 2005 version titled *Systems Biology in Practice.* Intended for an audience of advanced graduate students, postgraduate students, or postdoctoral fellows in the biological, engineering, and computer sciences, this 2009 version will find practical use for cross-disciplinary educational or training needs of professional level bioresearchers from many different disciplines who are interested in systems biology. The authors have distilled systems biology to its biochemical, bioinformatics, mathematical modeling, and computational biology components. The book is divided into two main sections. The first section introduces the concept of systems biology with chapters on biochemical systems and their modeling, gene expression, and network structures and function. In this first section, the authors also introduce important engineering concepts of systems design optimization and evolution. It is this mix of the systems biology elements of modeling, engineering, and biological systems that make this work particularly useful to bioresearchers of all levels and disciplines. The second section focuses on biological methods and their mathematical foundations, including chapters on mathematics, statistics, modeling tools, and higher order biological systems in cell biology. There are two chapters dealing specifically with data analyses, locating databases relevant to systems biology and retrieving their datasets, which are important topics usually overlooked in other systems biology texts.

Systems Biomedicine: Concepts and Perspectives. Editors: Edison T. Liu, Douglas A. Lauffenburger. Academic Press Elsevier, 2010.
http://www.sciencedirect.com/science/book/9780123725509
http://www.ebrary.com/
http://extranet.netlibrary.com/TitleSelect
ISBN: 9780080919836 (Online)
Recommended For: Academic Library

Although systems biology remains in an emerging phase both as a discipline and experimental approach, the authors of this work have made a serious and largely successful attempt to adopt and identify systems biology methodologies and approaches specific to human medical concerns. The work is divided into three main sections, each effectively illustrated with color diagrams and illustrations. Particularly valuable are the topically related online databases and tools that are regularly compiled into tables throughout the book. The first section focuses on those biological systems components that support systems biomedicine: genomics, proteomics, and both cellular and protein networks. This thoughtful section of the book is well written, carefully and accurately detailing the core sustaining genomic, proteomic, and biochemical methods and techniques. This is augmented with specific topical examples related to biomedicine: stem cells, microRNAs, biological fluids, and specific genes known to be regularly involved in pathological processes. Particularly useful are the sections on microRNAs, known to be key players in human pathologies, which currently are covered minimally, if at all, in other systems biology works. This first section provides a strong foundation for the second section, which deals with the computational and mathematical modeling facet of systems biology. While the first section will attract an audience trained in the biological disciplines, the second section will attract readers who deal with the physical and chemical sciences aspects of systems biomedicine. In this second section, the authors demonstrate that they have a strong concept of their audience's reading and information needs. By largely avoiding mathematical equations and complex formulas, they impart to their readers the value of mathematical and computational modeling to systems biology. This second section also provides chapters that either illuminate or are topically related to systems biology computational modeling, including the Virtual Cell Project, systems biology software tools, molecular or cellular processes, and the physicochemical interactions within molecules and between atoms. Finally, in the third section of the work, the authors conceptualize early applications of systems biology to the biomedical and pharmaceutical sciences in such areas as normal and abnormal physiological processes, drug discovery, cancer, and clinical trials. This section uniquely translates possible roles of systems biology, and its impact, to current aspects of pre-clinical and clinical medical practice. Attracting a wide range of expertise in biomedical research at all skill levels, this work represents, in its totality, a conceptualization of how systems biology can be mapped to current and emerging areas of the biomedical disciplines.

Journals

BMC Systems Biology. v. 1, BioMed Central, 2007.
http//www.biomedcentral.com/bmcsystbiol/
http://www.ncbi.nlm.nih.gov/pmc/journals/475/
ISSN: 17520509 (Online)
Indexed in: MEDLINE
Recommended for: Academic Libraries

Viewing biological systems holistically, as opposed to the individual molecular and cellular components, *BMC Systems Biology* is an open access, peer-reviewed journal that publishes original articles on the experimental and theoretical aspects of the function of biological systems. This online-only journal specifically seeks articles that address biosystems engineering and mathematical modeling, as well as those that transcend one or more biosystems level from atoms up through ecosystems. It publishes considerably on the quantitative analyses of network and pathway biosystems, including metabolic, regulatory, protein, neuronal, cellular signaling, and physiological networks. Most articles have supplementary information that can include gene lists, multimedia and data files, tutorials to new databases and software, and complex tables and figures. Its extensive editorial board has successfully integrated the disparate disciplines that constitute systems biology. Its audience focuses on those researchers active in systems biology primary research or those in academic environments who need peripheral reading knowledge in systems biology, including genomics and proteomics bioresearchers, physiologists, developmental biologists, neuroscientists, mathematicians, cell biologists, and computer scientists. The expansion of the journal in 2009 to include sections on reviews, databases, and software biotool design and implementation can be expected to expand its readership to those who desire a reading or peripheral knowledge of systems biology. Since the launch of its first issue in 2007, *BMC Systems Biology* has been rapidly recognized as the journal to publish systems biology primary research and related methodologies. It currently ranks third out of 29 journals in the 2009 *Journal Citation Reports* mathematics and computational biology section.

IET Systems Biology. v. 1, Institution of Engineering and Technology, 2007.
http//www.ietdl.org/IET-SYB
http://ieeexplore.ieee.org/
ISSN: 17518849
ISSN: 17518857 (Online)
Indexed in: MEDLINE
Recommended for: Academic Libraries

Systems biology views biological systems as an integrated and interactive network of biomolecules and structural components. At this higher level of organization, molecules and cells can be seen as circuits and relay boards that come under the paradigm of engineering principles, particularly design optimization and evolution. *IET Systems Biology* incorporates these concepts through its focus on primary research, which integrates cellular networks, pathways, and interactions with mathematical analyses, modeling, and simulation from the engineering disciplines. The journal accepts articles for peer review, including those from the genomics and proteomics research communities if authors can provide a basis for mathematical modeling and simulation between or within cells. Topical areas cover the range of the biomedical sciences, including molecular biology, cell biology, genomics, proteomics, metabolomics, metabolism, molecular networks, pathways, and cell signaling, as well as articles supporting methodologies, databases, tools, and algorithms in these areas. The majority of articles published are primary research articles, many involving the genes and pathways related to human health issues, particularly cancer. The journal also uniquely covers various symposia and conferences related to systems biology and engineering. It fills the gap in interdisciplinary knowledge among the science, medicine, and engineering disciplines, supporting biomedical researchers working in interdisciplinary, multidisciplinary, and cross-institutional research groups. Reflecting its true interdisciplinary nature, it is indexed in MEDLINE, Ei Compendex, and Inspec. 2008 was the first year the journal could be fully evaluated by *Journal Citation Reports* due to title and coverage changes, and by 2009, it ranked eighth of 29 journals in the mathematics and computational biology section. The journal has had several title changes since its launch in 2004 due to various mergers and acquisitions involving the IEE Proceedings suite of journals. Subscribers have access to the full backfile issues beginning with its original release as *Systems Biology* in 2004 (volume 1 and 2), through its title and volume issue change as *IEE Proceedings Systems Biology* in 2005 (volumes 152 and 153), and its relaunch in 2007 as *IET Systems Biology* starting again with volume 1.

Molecular Systems Biology. v. 1, Nature Publishing Group and European Molecular Biology Organization, 2005.
http//www.nature.com/
http://www.ncbi.nlm.nih.gov/pmc/journals/387/
ISSN: 17444292 (Online)
Indexed in: MEDLINE
Recommended for: Academic Libraries

Co-published by the Nature Publishing Group and the European Molecular Biology Organization (EMBO) since its inception in 2005, this premier, peer-reviewed journal seeks to explain complex biological systems in terms of their molecular components and interactions. This open access, online-only journal's scope is extensive, publishing articles in two dozen disciplines under the umbrella of systems biology, including bioinformatics, proteomics, functional genomics, regulatory networks, metabolomics, molecular biology of diseases, signal transduction, and structural biology. The journal is divided into primary research articles, reviews, reports, perspectives, commissioned news and views, and a particularly unique editorial section that focuses on emerging trends and applications of systems biology. Each of these sections, as well as each article's set of subject index terms, are separately archived providing multiple access points to content for both expert and novice systems biology readers. The journal provides an unusually rich, hyperlinked access to supplemental datasets, figures, multimedia files, and interactive models and figures. The journal also leads community efforts in setting systems biology data standards. Through the efforts of its world-class editors and editorial board, the journal is ranked tenth of the 283 journals in the highly competitive biochemistry and molecular biology section of the 2009 *Journal Citation Reports*. This journal is a core holding in systems biology for academic institutions, reaching a wide-ranging audience of expert level primary systems biology researchers, those involved with cross-disciplinary systems biology data, and faculty and graduate students seeking to increase their knowledge and education.

27. Genetics

The means and consequences of transmission and generation of the components of biological inheritance.

—MeSH

Contributor: Susan K. Kendall

Monographs

Human Molecular Genetics. 4th ed. Authors: Tom Strachan, Andrew P. Read. Garland Science/Taylor & Francis Group, 2011.
ISBN: 9780815341499
Recommended for: Academic Libraries

This book is considered an excellent and proven advanced textbook for students of genetics or a reference for researchers who need more background information on this subject area. The over 800 pages of this fourth edition are organized into five sections: "The Basics of DNA," "Chromosomes, Cells and Development," "Analyzing the Structure and Expression of Genes and Genomes," "Investigating the Human Genome and its Relationship to Other Genomes," "Human Genetic Variation and Diseases," and "Applied Human Molecular Genetics." Updated genomic technologies and sequencing are integrated throughout this new edition, which has added a new "Key Concepts" feature to each chapter. Some of the many areas that have been expanded and updated to keep pace with scientific developments and new knowledge include: stem cells, gene therapy, comparative genomics, and epigenetics. The second edition of the text (1999) is available for searching electronically on the NCBI bookshelf (http://www.ncbi.nlm.nih.gov/books) for free.

Lewin's Genes X. 10th ed. Editors: Jocelyn E. Krebs, Elliott S. Goldstein, Stephen T. Kilpatrick. Jones & Bartlett, 2011.
See Chapter 26.6. Molecular Biology

Molecular Genetics of Bacteria. 3rd ed. Authors: Larry Snyder, Wendy Champness. ASM Press, 2007.
See Chapter 26.5.1. Bacteriology

Journals

American Journal of Human Genetics. v. 1, Cell Press/Elsevier, 1949.
http://www.cell.com/AJHG/
http://www.ncbi.nlm.nih.gov/pmc/journals/203/
ISSN: 00029297
ISSN: 15376605 (Online)
Indexed in: MEDLINE, CINAHL
Recommended for: Academic Libraries

Currently published by Cell Press, an imprint of Elsevier, this peer-reviewed journal is still owned and controlled by the American Society of Human Genetics, as it has been since its inception. The society makes the journal available for free online six months after publication, unlike the policy for other Elsevier journals. Articles in this journal cover all topics in human genetics and heredity including behavioral genetics, cytogenetics, gene therapy, immunogenetics, molecular genetics, and population genetics. Information related to public policy in human genetics matters is also covered. In addition to research articles, the journal also publishes review articles, book reviews, reports, and society news. It is indexed in numerous indexing and abstracting sources including CAB Abstracts, CINAHL, Embase, MEDLINE, Scopus, and Web of Science. The journal is available in both print and online formats. Access to issues from 1949 until six months prior to current is available on PubMed Central.

Genes and Development. v. 1, Cold Spring Harbor Laboratory Press, 1987.
See Chapter 26.2. Developmental Biology

Genetics. v. 1, Genetics Society of America, 1916.
http://www.genetics.org/
http://www.ncbi.nlm.nih.gov/pmc/journals/301/
ISSN: 19432631 (Online)
Indexed in: MEDLINE
Recommended for: Academic Libraries

An old and well-respected publication from the Genetics Society of America, *Genetics* publishes articles covering all organisms from bacteria to humans. Primarily a research article publication, this peer-reviewed journal also publishes shorter contributions called "Notes," invited "Review" and "Perspective" articles, and commentaries. It is indexed in numerous indexing and abstracting sources including CAB Abstracts, Embase,

MEDLINE, Scopus, and Web of Science. The print version ceased in December 2009. Online access is available through the publisher and other vendors. Online access to issues from 1916 through six months prior to current is available on PubMed Central.

Human Molecular Genetics. v. 1, Oxford University Press, 1992.
http://hmg.oxfordjournals.org/
ISSN: 09646906
ISSN: 14602083 (Online)
Indexed in: MEDLINE
Recommended for: Academic Libraries

Human Molecular Genetics publishes top-quality original research papers on the molecular basis for human genetic disease, including such areas as cancer genetics, neurogenetics, chromosome structure and function, gene therapy, stem cell therapy, developmental genetics, and functional and computational genomics. Papers on other model organisms such as mice are also accepted if they represent models of human disease or have relevance to human genetics. Two special issues a year are devoted to review articles. With an impact factor of 7.386, it is ranked twenty-eighth out of 283 journals in the biochemistry and molecular biology category and thirteenth out of 144 journals in the genetics and heredity category (2009 *Journal Citation Index*). It is indexed in numerous indexing and abstracting sources including CAB Abstracts, Embase, MEDLINE, Scopus, and Web of Science. Online access back to volume 1 is available from the publisher.

Nature Genetics. v. 1, Nature Publishing Group, 1992.
http://www.nature.com/ng/
ISSN: 10614036
ISSN: 15461718 (Online)
Indexed in: MEDLINE
Recommended for: Academic Libraries

One of the first journals to branch off from the original journal, *Nature*, *Nature Genetics* has risen to the top of the most important journals in the area of genetics. It achieved an impact factor of 34.284 and ranked first out of 144 journals in the genetics and heredity category (2009 *Journal Citation Reports*). The scope of the journal includes both genetic and functional genomic studies in humans and other organisms, including gene therapy, genetics of complex diseases, and cancer genetics. While the *Nature* journals are editorially independent, an author can request that an article rejected from one journal be transferred to be submitted to a different *Nature* journal. Each issue contains news, research highlights, and brief communications, as well as peer-reviewed research articles. The journal is indexed in numerous indexing and abstracting sources including CAB Abstracts, Embase, MEDLINE, Scopus, and Web of Science. Online access back to 1996 is available from the publisher.

PLoS Genetics. v. 1, Public Library of Science, 2005.
http://www.plosgenetics.org/home.action
http://www.ncbi.nlm.nih.gov/pmc/journals/331/
ISSN: 15537390
ISSN: 15537404 (Online)
Indexed in: MEDLINE
Recommended for: Academic Libraries

A newcomer to the scene of genetics journals, *PLoS Genetics* is an open-access, peer-reviewed weekly journal. It publishes on both human genetics and genetics of other organisms, including cytogenetics, genomics, medical genetics, complex traits, evolution, and population genetics. The Public Library of Science (PLoS), which publishes this journal, is a non-profit organization of scientists and physicians committed to making scientific and medical literature freely available to the public. All articles are available free upon publication. The PLoS journals use a business model of charging author publication fees, and the authors retain ownership of the copyright for their articles. Under the Creative Commons Attribution License anyone may download, reuse, reprint, modify, distribute, and/or copy articles in PLoS journals, so long as the original authors and source are cited. The PLoS journals, and *PLoS Genetics* is no exception, have risen to the top of impact factor lists, presumably because articles freely available tend to be highly cited and they have also maintained high standards of quality. It is indexed in numerous indexing and abstracting sources including CAB Abstracts, Embase, MEDLINE, Scopus, and Web of Science. The print version ceased in 2008. Online access to this journal is available from a variety of sources, including PubMed Central.

Trends in Genetics. v. 1, Elsevier, 1985.
http://www.cell.com/trends/genetics
ISSN: 01689525
ISSN: 13624555 (Online)
Indexed in: MEDLINE
Recommended for: Academic Libraries

Part of the well-known *Trends in...* series so valuable to scientists, this monthly peer-reviewed journal focuses solely on review articles. Each issue contains three to five significant reviews and a "Research Focus" section for comments on new developments. A "Genome Analysis" section contains articles on the function, organization, and evolution of genomes. Some issues may also contain opinion articles and a "Science and Society" section. This journal achieved an impact factor of 8.689 (2009 *Journal Citation Reports*) and it is indexed in numerous indexing and abstracting sources including CAB Abstracts, Embase, MEDLINE, Scopus, and Web of Science. Online access back to 1985 is available from the publisher.

Databases and Other Electronic Resources

Current Protocols. Wiley, 2000.
See Chapter 26.6. Molecular Biology

27.1. Medical Genetics

The reliable prediction of certain human disorders as a function of the lineage and/or genetic makeup of an individual or of any two parents or potential parents.

—MeSH

Contributor: Susan K. Kendall

Monographs

Smith's Recognizable Patterns of Human Malformation. 6th ed. Author: Kenneth L. Jones. Elsevier/Saunders, 2006.
See Chapter 10.13. Pediatrics

Thompson & Thompson's Genetics in Medicine. 7th ed. Authors: Robert L. Nussbaum, Roderick R. McInnes, Huntington F. Willard. Saunders/Elsevier, 2007.
ISBN: 9781416030805
Recommended for: Academic Libraries
Doody's Core Titles Selection

Now in its seventh edition, *Thompson & Thompson's Genetics in Medicine* continues the framework established by James and Margaret Thompson in 1966, when they wrote a text specifically for medical students to give them a basis for the clinical application of recent genetic discoveries. The field has continued to burgeon since the completion of the human genome sequencing; this text skillfully presents the most recent information in molecular genetics by building on classic genetic principles. The first half of the text provides the foundation to move into a discussion of the tools used for research and diagnosis in human molecular genetics. The latter portion of the book presents mutation and disease at the molecular level with chapters on hemoglobinopathies, developmental disorders and birth defects, and cancer genetics. Final chapters address genetic counseling and risk assessment, molecular diagnostics, prenatal diagnosis, and genetics and society. Case studies enhance the learning process. This text's clearly written style and in-depth explanations recommend it to students and residents, but it would also be a useful reference for practitioners who see genetic disorders, particularly pediatricians and primary care specialists.

Journals

Journal of Medical Genetics. v. 1, BMJ Group, 1964.
http://jmg.bmj.com/
http://www.ncbi.nlm.nih.gov/pmc/journals/169/
ISSN: 00222593
ISSN: 14686244 (Online)
Indexed in: MEDLINE
Recommended for: Hospital, Academic Libraries

This is one of the top, international, peer-reviewed journals covering original research in human genetics. Articles can range from basic research on the molecular basis of human disease, human cancer genetics, and the like, to studies on the application of molecular genetics to medical practice. Issues usually contain research articles, letters, short reports, online mutation reports, and a review article. The journal's website indicates that interested readership would include clinical and laboratory geneticists, genetic counselors, fertility experts, physicians and scientists interested in molecular medicine, and clinical researchers. It is indexed in numerous indexing and abstracting sources including CAB Abstracts, Embase, MEDLINE, Scopus, and Web of Science. Online access back to volume 1, 1964 is available from the publisher. Issues from volume 1 through three years from current are available in PubMed Central.

Databases and Other Electronic Resources

Online Mendelian Inheritance in Man (OMIM). National Center for Biotechnology Information and Johns Hopkins University Press, 1987.
http://www.ncbi.nlm.nih.gov/omim/
Recommended for: Hospital, Academic Libraries

Dr. Victor McKusick was originally a cardiologist who became interested in genetic diseases and became the founder of medical genetics as a field of study. In the 1960s he created the original *Mendelian Inheritance in Man: Catalogs of Human Genes and Genetic Disorders* to be a comprehensive catalog of what is known about hereditary diseases and Mendelian genetic traits in humans. The book went through 12 editions up until 1998, but is now available only on the web for free from the National Center for Biotechnology Information as part of their suite of databases searchable from one interface. This is considered the authoritative source on human genes associated with genetic phenotypes; it is updated daily. Entries for each gene include all known cloning, mapping, function, biochemical and molecular genetic information with linked references to other genes and the primary literature. While freely available to anyone, the site notes that the information is intended for physicians, researchers, genetic counselors or students in medicine or genetics.

27.2. Genomics

The systematic study of the complete DNA sequences (genome) of organisms.

—MeSH

Contributors: Susan K. Kendall, Diane C. Rein

Monographs

Bioinformatics and Functional Genomics. 2nd ed. Author: Jonathan Pevsner. Wiley-Blackwell, 2009.
http://www.eblib.com/
http://www.ebrary.com/
ISBN: 9780470085851
ISBN: 9780470451489
Recommended for: Academic Libraries

The primary audiences for this "all-in-one" hybrid bioinformatics/genomics textbook are those researchers from the broad array of disciplines who use bioinformatics and genomics tools in their research programs. The book focuses on studies aimed at understanding the genomic basis of human disease. It covers the genomes of human pathogens as well as the human genome. In the first section of the book, the author introduced the fundamental bioinformatics tools needed to perform the DNA, RNA, or protein sequence searching and alignment that underpins all genomics studies. In the second section, he applies these tools to the rapidly emerging genome-wide association studies used to identify and track the genetics elements involved in disease. The final section of the book summarizes the findings and data from genome studies of human bacterial, viral, and parasitic pathogens, as well as the human genome itself. Throughout, the author avoids the use of computational and mathematical formulas and concentrates on the language and research needs of those who use bioinformatics as a tool. Consequently this work is particularly useful for medical and clinical researchers, as well as to advanced undergraduates and medical students. Chapters contain exercises, recommend free bioinformatics software, are amply illustrated, and integrate auxiliary bioinformatics topics as needed. A companion website organized by chapter and available at http://www.bioinfbook.org/ contains a mix of supporting resources including PowerPoint slides from the author's current Genomics course, exercises, downloadable datasets, hyperlinks and more.

Computing for Comparative Microbial Genomics: Bioinformatics for Microbiologists. Authors: David W. Ussery, Trudy M. Wassenaar, Stefano Borini. Springer, 2009.
http://springerlink.com/content/978-1-84800-254-8/
ISBN: 9781848002548
ISBN: 9781848002555
Recommended for: Academic Libraries

Understanding the genomics and biology of the microbial population that inhabits humans is as important an area of biomedical research as studying the human genome itself. In addition, the modern clinic now routinely screens patient tissues and specimens bioinformatically, performing DNA sequence and protein profile analyses for diagnostic and treatment purposes. Practically, the physician must be certain that the results originate from the patient and not from bacterial and microbial contaminates at the DNA and protein level. Screening of human tissue specimens for microbial sequence contamination is a requirement. Conversely, microbial communities in the human oral cavity, skin, and intestinal tract are important in both health and disease. As a result, microbial genomics and the requisite supporting tools and databases are rising rapidly in research importance and have applications in modern medical practice. *Computing for Comparative Microbial Genomics* fills a significant gap that currently exists in the study of microbial genomes as related to health and disease. Its 12 chapters, divided into four major parts, encompass a wide-ranging review of basic comparative microbial genomics topics, including the processing and comparing of a large amount of microbial genomic datasets simultaneously and visualizing data results. The first five chapters are a very basic introduction to bioinformatics for microbiologists. The next three chapters cover the fundamentals of comparative genomics, followed by another three chapters on the functional genomics of microbial RNA, gene expression, and proteomic comparisons. The last four chapters address microbial communities, metagenomics, and the identification and analysis of all microbes living in communities. The authors' target audiences are the microbiologist studying the genomic biology of microbes, as well as those professionals who create the software and tools needed to study and compare microbial genomes on a large scale. Although the authors focus on microbial organisms, many of the topics and technologies discussed are relevant to the study of other genomes, including human, and reach a wider professional research audience than microbiologists.

Dictionary of Genomics, Transcriptomics, and Proteomics. 4th ed. Author: Günter Kahl. Wiley-VCH, 2009.
ISBN: 9783527320738
Recommended for: Hospital, Academic Libraries

This three-volume reference set contains over 12,000 alphabetically arranged entries, in three separate areas of contemporary research: genomes, gene expression (including RNA transcriptomics), and proteomics. It is a greatly expanded version of the original edition, titled *Dictionary of Gene Technology*: genomics, transcriptomics and proteomics. The author includes chemical formulas and structures, with cross-referencing. The entries are often illustrated, and there are several appendixes covering units and conversions, restriction nucleases, databases, and journals. The dictionary terms range from chemical structures, through biological molecules to complex biological terms and processes. The work reaches a wide audience of all skill levels, including secondary education through post-graduate college studies, journalists, lay public, professional researchers, and the medical disciplines.

Essentials of Medical Genomics. 2nd ed. Author: Stuart M. Brown. Wiley-Blackwell, 2009.
http://www.ebrary.com
http://www.ebl.com
http://extranet.netlibrary.com/TitleSelect/
ISBN: 9780470140192
ISBN: 9780470334492
Recommended for: Hospital, Academic Libraries

Essentials of Medical Genomics concisely overviews the science and practice of genomics, proteomics, and bioinformatics topics relevant to the current and near term practice of medicine. The author writes for medical students, physicians, and other medical professionals close to clinical practice, as well as to consumers of health care. The book begins with five chapters introducing the science behind medical genomics. These include an introduction to molecular genetics, molecular biology techniques encompassing gene cloning and sequencing, and sequence comparison and alignment. A background chapter on genome databases covers genome sequencing projects, genome browsers, relevant bioinformatics databases and tools, genome annotation, and comparative genomics. After laying the scientific and bioinformatics foundations, the author moves into increasingly complex topics, writing in a practical, "just what you need to know" style. Three chapters cover the inherited and molecular basis of human disease, bringing together an interesting mix of topics which include bioinformatics tools, the genomic basis of inherited and acquired sequence variations, the bioinformatics resources that hold these data, and genomic diversity and ethnicity. Other chapters focus on clinical practice in the medical genomics era, presenting of clinical proteomics topics (biomarkers and protein drug targeting as examples), genetic testing, clinical research informatics, cancer genomics, nutrigenomics, and consumer genealogy. In an equivalent manner, the authors develop chapters that concentrate on the rapidly emerging genomics and bioinformatics research studies just beginning to affect medical practice: microarray studies of gene expression in normal and diseased processes; interference RNA and disease; pharmacogenomics; and toxicogenomics. One entire section is devoted to the ethics of medical genomics. Throughout the book, the author and his supporting contributors develop a writing style that is readily understood, making an easy read for practitioners to acquire a working knowledge of medical genomics.

A Primer of Genome Science. 3rd ed. Authors: Greg Gibson, Spencer V. Muse. Sinauer, 2009.
ISBN: 9780878932368
Recommended for: Academic Libraries

Completely updated in methodologies and new content to keep pace with the rapid change in genomics knowledge and techniques, the third edition of this work continues to uniquely bridge the gap between traditional molecular genetics textbooks and the advanced level genomics methods publications created for the highly specialized genomics researcher. The book is divided into six broad genomic divisions: genome projects, sequencing and annotation, genomic variation, gene expression, proteomics and functional genomics, and integrative genomics. Several chapters have a separate section that covers the important bioinformatics databases in the area. New topics include NextGen resequencing, genome-wide association studies, and metabolomics. Liberally illustrated with original color graphics and actual experimental data, each chapter contains a least one "Box" that explains the statistical and bioinformatics principles underlying the genomics topic under discussion. Also present within each chapter are a set of practice exercises (complete with answers), and a "Literature Cited" section of primary research articles. In keeping with the trend of genomics research metamorphosing to manipulating large amounts of data, the authors have provided access to more complicated exercises involving large datasets that can be downloaded and analyzed at will from the companion website found at http://www .sinauer.com/genomics. Also found at the companion website is a compendium of hyperlinks, organized by chapter, to resources covered in the work. Through a combination of text, graphics, and hands-on practical exercises, readers can self-pace themselves to develop research skills in genomics. The work is applicable to readers of all level of skills and professional development, including researchers not familiar with the biological science disciplines.

Systems Biomedicine: Concepts and Perspectives. Editors: Edison T. Liu, Douglas A. Lauffenburger. Academic Press Elsevier, 2010.
See Chapter 26.10. Systems Biology

Journals

BMC Medical Genomics. v. 1. BioMed Central, 2008.
http://www.biomedcentral.com/bmcmedgenomics
http://www.ncbi.nlm.nih.gov/pmc/journals/573/
ISSN: 17558794 (Online)
Indexed in: MEDLINE
Recommended for: Academic Libraries

BMC Medical Genomics is a complement to *Genome Medicine*, also published by BioMed Central. It considers primarily research articles on all aspects of functional genomics, genome structure, genome-scale population genetics, epigenomics, proteomics, systems analysis, and pharmacogenomics in relation to human health and disease, while *Genome Medicine* concentrates on overarching reviews in emerging technology areas of genomic medicine with clinical implications. The journal began publication in 2008 and has garnished a significant impact factor already in a competitive JCR subject area, ranking seventy-second out of 146 titles in genetics and heredity. It publishes one volume a year with a "rolling" publication cycle, rapidly reviewing and adding articles to each annual volume as authors submit them. It publishes occasional articles on new databases containing bioinformatics and genomics data related to human diseases and on software developed to handle biological and medical data. This peer-reviewed research journal is available online only and is indexed in MEDLINE and other major indexing and abstracting tools.

Genome Biology. v. 1, BioMed Central, 2000.
http://genomebiology.com/
http://www.ncbi.nlm.nih.gov/pmc/journals/7/
ISSN: 14656906
ISSN: 14656914 (Online)
Indexed in: MEDLINE
Recommended for: Academic Libraries

Now only available electronically, *Genome Biology* strives to be an international forum for dissemination, discussion and review of information related to genomic research. All aspects of molecular, cellular, organismal, or population biology studied from a genomic perspective are in scope, as are studies in genomics, proteomics, bioinformatics, computational biology, sequence analysis, comparative biology, and evolution. Large datasets and analysis of primary data, including data that can be read by others' software packages, would not be possible in printed journals but are available on this journal's website. These accompany the primary research articles, which are open access and available for free to anyone. Other articles focus on new technologies or methods or review the latest software, and these also appear to be open access. Mini-reviews, research news and reports and commentary articles are only available to subscribers. BioMed Central, now owned by Springer, is a publisher that has experimented with open access and hybrid journals like this one (with open access for primary research, but not reviews). Articles are continuously published online but are collated into discrete journal issues after a period of time. Issues from 2001 are available online from the publisher; PubMed Central includes issues back to 2000.

Genome Medicine. v. 1, BioMed Central, 2009.
http://genomemedicine.com/
http://www.ncbi.nlm.nih.gov/pmc/journals/863/
ISSN: 1756994X (Online)
Recommended for: Academic Libraries

Published since 2009, this open access journal, part of the Biomed Central family of journals, publishes research in all areas of medicine studied from a genomic viewpoint. In particular, it publishes research, meeting reports, and commentaries that focus on the latest technologies and data that impact the management of human health and disease at its point of practice by physicians and other healthcare providers. Of particular value is the large number of reviews and mini reviews that integrate advances in genomic research with human diseases such as arthritis, diabetes, and cancer; vaccination development; prenatal diagnostics; and more. Available only online, it is not yet ranked in *Journal Citation Reports*, and is indexed in PubMed but not MEDLINE.

Genome Research. v. 5, Cold Spring Harbor Laboratory Press, 1995.
http://genome.cshlp.org/
http://www.ncbi.nlm.nih.gov/pmc/journals/102/
ISSN: 10889051
ISSN: 15495469 (Online)
Indexed in: MEDLINE
Recommended for: Academic Libraries

A newer field than genetics, genomics is the study of the sum total of an organism's genes rather than individual genes, and new journals focusing solely on this field have appeared in the last 10–15 years. This international peer-reviewed journal publishes research on the genome biology of all organisms, including advances in genomic medicine. Comparative genomics, proteomics, genome structure and function, and more technical reports on new methodologies are all themes. Several different types of articles can be found: research articles, letters, methods or resource reports, reviews, perspectives, and commentary. Genome data sets can be found on the journal's website. More than 100 years old and boasting a distinguished history, Cold Spring Harbor Laboratory is a private, non-profit institution focused on research in cancer, neuroscience, plant biology, genomics, and bioinformatics. It also sponsors meetings, workshops and courses for the education of scientists. The journal is indexed in numerous indexing and abstracting sources including CAB Abstracts, Embase, MEDLINE, Scopus, and Web of Science. Online access to 1995 is available from the publisher. PubMed Central contains issues from 1997 to current.

Molecular Systems Biology. v. 1, Nature Publishing Group and European Molecular Biology Organization, 2005.
See Chapter 26.6. Molecular Biology

Pharmacogenomics Journal. v. 1, Nature Publishing Group, 2001.
http://www.nature.com/tpj/
ISSN: 1470269X
ISSN: 14731150 (Online)
Indexed in: MEDLINE
Recommended for: Academic Libraries

Inherently multidisciplinary, pharmacogenomics is an emerging area of translational medicine. It integrates gene-drug-human disease data together with the aim of personalizing drug therapy based upon an individual patient's genetic inheritance patterns and genomic organization. Published by the Nature Group since 2001, it has rapidly risen in impact factor, 4.398 in 2009, ranking twenty-eighth out of 146 in genetics and heredity and thirtieth out of 237 in pharmacology and pharmacy. *Pharmacogenomics Journal* was established, and remains unique in intent, as a vehicle dedicated to the biomedical and clinical progress in pharmacogenomics. The journal publishes articles pertaining to primary research, reviews, editorials, news and commentaries, ethical considerations and clinical implications related to the effects of genetic variability on drug toxicity, characterization of genetic variations relevant to drug action and the identification of genomic targets for drug development. It is valued reading for geneticists, molecular biologists, clinicians and pharmacologists, as well anyone working in biotechnology, drug discovery and drug development. It is indexed in a variety of sources and is available online back to 2001 through the publisher, as well as Academic Search Complete and Health Reference Center Academic, both with a one-year embargo.

28. Biotechnology

The use of organisms, cells or cell-derived constituents for the purpose of developing products which are technically, scientifically and clinically useful. Alteration of biologic function at the molecular level (i.e., genetic engineering) is a central focus; laboratory methods used include transfection and cloning technologies, sequence and structure analysis algorithms, computer databases, and gene and protein structure function analysis and prediction.

—MeSH

Contributor: Susan K. Kendall

Monographs

Molecular Biotechnology: Principles and Applications of Recombinant DNA. 4th ed. Authors: Bernard R. Glick, Jack J. Pasternak, Cheryl L. Patten. ASM Press, 2010.
ISBN: 9781555814984
Recommended for: Academic Libraries
Doody's Core Titles Selection

While any textbook in biotechnology is apt to go very quickly out of date, this book provides a broad background for those wanting to understand the basics before moving on to review articles and primary articles in the scientific literature. It is issued by the American Society for Microbiology. Molecular biotechnology and methods (nucleic acids and proteins), microbial systems, eukaryotic systems, and regulation and patenting are the larger subject areas included, as well as the genetic engineering of plants and animals. It has been thoroughly revised from the previous edition and includes expanded coverage of transgenics, therapeutics, and vaccines.

Journals

Bioinformatics. v. 14, Oxford University Press, 1998.
http://bioinformatics.oxfordjournals.org/
ISSN: 13674803
ISSN: 13674811 (Online)
See Also Chapter 26.1. Computational Biology
Indexed in: MEDLINE
Recommended for: Academic Libraries

Bioinformatics is a field combining computer science with biology. Computers and computer algorithms are used to collect and analyze genetic and protein sequence information. Large datasets such as those generated by proteomic and genomic studies require computers for manipulation, which is the reason that bioinformatics has grown to become so highly visible as a field in the last ten years. This peer-reviewed journal was one of the first and remains the leading one in this field. With an impact factor of 4.926, it ranks second out of 29 journals in the mathematical and computational biology category (2009 *Journal Citation Reports*). It publishes both original research and review articles. "Discovery Notes" and "Application Notes" are sections publishing shorter papers, the first describing biologically interesting discoveries and the other describing new software, databases, or similar computer applications. The journal is indexed in numerous indexing and abstracting sources including CAB Abstracts, Embase, MEDLINE, Scopus, and Web of Science. Online access back to 1998 is available from the publisher. Content from 2008 is also available in PubMed Central.

Molecular Therapy. v. 1, Nature Publishing Group, 2000.
http://www.nature.com/mt/index.html
http://www.ncbi.nlm.nih.gov/pmc/journals/902/
ISSN: 15250016
ISSN: 15250024 (Online)
Indexed in: MEDLINE
Recommended for: Academic Libraries

The official journal of the American Society for Gene Therapy, *Molecular Therapy* is the leading journal in this subject area, covering research in "gene transfer, vector development and design, stem cell manipulation, development of gene-, peptide and protein-, oligonucleotide- and cell-based therapeutics to correct genetic and acquired diseases." All stages of biotechnological development are covered, from pre-clinical studies to clinical trials, including safety and efficacy studies. Besides original articles, issues may contain reviews, meeting reports, or commentaries. It has an impact factor of 6.239 and ranked eleventh out of 150 journals in the biotechnology and applied microbiology category, and sixth out of 92 journals in the research and experimental medicine category (2009 *Journal Citation Reports*). This journal is indexed in numerous indexing and abstracting sources including Embase, MEDLINE, Scopus, and Web of Science. Content from 2009 to current is available in PubMed Central. Issues from 2000 are available from the publisher, with issues 12 months prior to current available as open access content.

Nature Biotechnology. v. 14, Nature Publishing Group, 1996.
http://www.nature.com/nbt
ISSN: 10870156
ISSN: 15461696 (Online)
Indexed in: MEDLINE
Recommended for: Academic Libraries

This journal has the highest impact factor among biotechnology journals, 29.5 (2009 *Journal Citation Reports*), and is probably the journal a library should purchase if only subscribing to one journal in this subject area. Unlike many journals in biotechnology areas that are more narrowly focused on topics such as drug discovery, gene therapy, or tissue engineering, this journal covers all of biotechnology from agricultural and environmental to the biomedical. Like some other *Nature* journals, the first part of the journal is devoted to news, essays, comments, and articles covering the societal, ethical, and legal aspects of current topics in biotechnology. Regular columns focus on the business aspects of biotechnology, such as biotechnology companies and patents. The second half of the journal contains peer-reviewed scientific research papers, both short and long contributions. It is indexed in numerous indexing and abstracting sources including CAB Abstracts, Embase, MEDLINE, Scopus, and Web of Science. Online access back to 2006 is available from the publisher.

Stem Cells. v. 11, AlphaMed Press with Wiley-Blackwell, 1993.
http://stemcells.com/
ISSN: 10665099
ISSN: 15494918 (Online)
Indexed in: MEDLINE
Recommended for: Academic Libraries

Published originally by AlphaMed Press alone, now co-published with Wiley-Blackwell and available electronically on both the HighWire and Wiley-Blackwell platforms, this peer-reviewed journal covers all aspects of stem cell research from pre-clinical to clinical studies. It would be of interest to both basic and clinical scientists. Most articles are original research, but there are occasional reviews. Although a specialty journal, it is highly cited and ranked, with an impact factor of 7.747 and a ranking of second out of 11 journals in the cell and tissue engineering category and sixth out of 150 journals in the biotechnology and applied microbiology category (2009 *Journal Citation Reports*). Article topics include embryonic and adult stem cells, cancer stem cells, proteomics, genomics, and development of new technologies. The journal is indexed in numerous indexing and abstracting sources including Embase, MEDLINE, Scopus, and Web of Science. It is available back to 1993 from Wiley-Blackwell.

Trends in Biotechnology. v. 1, Elsevier, 1983.
http://www.cell.com/trends/biotechnology/
ISSN: 01677799
ISSN: 18793096 (Online)
Recommended for: Academic Libraries
Indexed in: MEDLINE

Another journal in the well-known *Trends in*... series of review-only journals so valuable to scientists, *Trends in Biotechnology* contains three to five significant reviews per issue and a "Research Focus" section for comments on new developments. Opinion articles are another significant part of this journal and they often, but not always, focus more on political, ethical, and regulatory concerns. Given the interdisciplinary nature of this subject and the role a *Trends* journal could play, it is no surprise that this peer-reviewed journal achieved an impact factor of 6.909 (2009 *Journal Citation Reports*). It is indexed in numerous indexing and abstracting sources including CAB Abstracts, Embase, MEDLINE, Scopus, and Web of Science. Online access back to 1983 is available from the publisher.

Databases and Other Electronic Resources

Current Protocols. Wiley, 2000.
See Chapter 26.6. Molecular Biology

29. Physiology

The functions of the living organism and its parts, and of the physical and chemical factors and processes involved.
—MeSH

Contributor: Marcy L. Brown

Monographs

Ganong's Review of Medical Physiology. 23rd ed. Authors: Kim E. Barrett, Susan M. Barman, Scott Boitano, Heddwen Brooks. McGraw-Hill, 2009.
http://accessmedicine.com/
http://www.r2library.com/
ISBN: 9780071605670
ISBN: 9780071605687 (Online)
Recommended for: Hospital, Academic Libraries
Brandon/Hill, *Doody's Core Titles* Selection

A staple in the medical student's diet, *Ganong's Review of Medical Physiology* offers concise information on all aspects of human physiology. The twenty-third edition is the first for which William Ganong did not serve as an editor. This work is truly intended to be a review volume rather than an introductory textbook, so it should not serve as a student's first introduction to medical physiology or a library's sole physiology title, even in a small collection. Ganong really shines when used as a study guide for board examinations or when a clinician needs a memory jog or a clear explanation of a concept. The new edition incorporates recent findings in cellular physiology as well as updates in most of the other chapters. New features for this edition include: full color illustrations, boxed clinical cases illustrating physiological principles, and both multiple choice and short answer review questions useful for USMLE preparation. This edition also includes test questions in a format that can be downloaded to an iPod or other mobile device, and access to a companion website available at LangeTextbooks.com. The companion site offers additional cases and questions. *Ganong* is also available in searchable digital format through STAT!Ref and the Rittenhouse R2 Digital Library. It is recommended for academic collections supporting medical students, and teaching hospital libraries supporting residency programs.

Human Reproductive Biology. 3rd ed. Authors: Kristin H. Lopez, Richard E. Jones. Elsevier, 2006.
ISBN: 9780120884650
Recommended for: Academic Libraries
Doody's Core Titles Selection

This *Doody's* core title, with five stars and a whopping score of 97, provides a comprehensive overview of reproductive system anatomy and physiology. In addition to updates to existing chapters, this new edition for the first time incorporates content on aging and reproduction. *Human Reproductive Biology* explains the biological aspects of human reproduction, discusses emerging reproductive technologies, and offers information about procreation from across various cultures. The text should appeal to audiences of all levels—from undergraduate biology students to medical students to allied health professionals. The text is organized into sections including anatomical systems; sexual differentiation and development; fertility; procreation; and special topics. Each chapter contains related sidebar topics (such as Chapter 4's "Why a Scrotum?"), a concise summary, and reference lists for further and advanced reading. The text is visually appealing, with a readable font size, useful section heads, and clear and colorful illustrations and figures. A companion website offers current information related to pregnancy, fertility, and other reproductive topics. A robust glossary and an index are included. It is recommended for academic libraries that support undergraduate biology programs as well as medical, nursing, and allied health programs.

Medical Physiology: Principles for Clinical Medicine. 3rd ed. Editors: Rodney A. Rhoades, David R. Bell. Lippincott Williams & Wilkins, 2009.
ISBN: 9780781768528
Recommended for: Hospital, Academic Libraries

This volume focuses on the clinical presentation of important physiological processes. Now in its third edition, *Medical Physiology* is an excellent resource for medical students but also useful for early-career clinical practitioners. Each chapter now offers "Active Learning Objects" that apply principles to practical problems. Readers will also appreciate "Clinical Focus" sidebar boxes, in which physiology is discussed relevant to a patient or patients; and the "From Bench to Bedside" feature in which research is translated to practice. Both help students visualize the actual effects of various physiological phenomena. The book is organized by system, with sections devoted to respiratory physiology, cardiovascular physiology, and reproductive physiology, among others, and a chapter on immunology and organ function is new in the third edition. Case studies, bulleted chapter summaries, a substantive glossary, an index, and online review questions in USMLE format round out the features for *Medical Physiology*. The companion website offers the text in fully searchable format, case studies with practice questions, animations, a question bank, and web resource links. Rhoades' *Medical Physiology* is a *Doody's Core Titles* selection with a score of 91. This title is highly recommended for academic libraries that support medical or nursing schools, and is also recommended for teaching hospitals.

Physiology of the Heart. 4th ed. Author: Arnold M. Katz. Lippincott Williams & Wilkins, 2006.
ISBN: 9780781755016
Recommended for: Hospital, Academic Libraries
Doody's Core Titles Selection

This acclaimed work by renowned cardiologist Arnold Katz is now in its fourth edition. Eugene Braunwald states in this edition's foreword that "landmark improvements in cardiac care result directly from the advances in cardiovascular physiology and pathophysiology" of the past few decades. These advances include the study of the heart at cellular and molecular levels, so this volume incorporates much new knowledge about molecular cardiology. *Physiology of the Heart* also features new "Clinical Applications" sections in order to explore the clinical impact of new research findings. Dr. Katz starts with an overview of cardiac structure and function, signal transduction, and normal physiology, and then moves on to the biochemistry, biophysics, and pathophysiology of arrhythmias, ischemia, and heart failure. Readers will find a concise but well-written chapter on electrocardiography, over 400 diagrams, a substantive index, and a very accessible writing style. This *Doody's* core title is recommended for both hospital and academic health science collections.

Respiratory Physiology: A Clinical Approach. 1st ed. Authors: Richard M. Schwartzstein, Michael J. Parker. Lippincott Williams & Wilkins, 2006.
ISBN: 9780781757485
Recommended for: Hospital, Academic Libraries
Doody's Core Titles Selection

This 2006 volume was the first in the Lippincott Williams & Wilkins *Systems Physiology* series. It presents respiratory physiology from an integrated systems approach, combining functional anatomy, physiology, and pathology with the intent that the reader will learn to manage clinical respiratory problems. In addition to standard chapters on ventilation, gas exchange, and respiratory control, the authors include unique material on the physiology of respiratory sensations and also exercise physiology. Each chapter begins with detailed learning objectives and contains cases, called "Putting It Together," that illustrate the clinical application of each physiological principle. Scattered throughout the text are "Thought Questions" designed to test a reader's understanding, and "Quick Checks" to summarize important points. Answers to the thought questions are provided after each chapter summary, where the reader will also find USMLE-style review questions. An appendix provides the answer key for the review questions. The illustrations are simple and clear, and the writing is crisp and concise. *Respiratory Physiology* includes online access to interactive animations as well as a CD-ROM with supplemental information. This indexed text is a 2009 *Doody's* core title (five stars) and is highly recommended for academic collections as well as hospital libraries that provide support to residency programs.

Respiratory Physiology: The Essentials. 8th ed. Author: John B. West. Lippincott Williams & Wilkins, 2008.
ISBN: 9780781772068
See Also Chapter 10.10.8. Pulmonary Disease
Recommended for: Academic Libraries
Doody's Core Titles Selection

The *Doody's* review for *Respiratory Physiology* designates it an essential purchase for both respiratory therapy and pulmonology. It is a surprisingly slim volume, coming in under 200 pages, but it packs an incredible amount of information into its relatively small space and truly covers "the essentials." After introductory chapters on lung structure and function, ventilation, and diffusion, Dr. West moves into gas transport, the mechanics of breathing, ventilation control, and adaptations to stress. The final chapter details pulmonary function tests. Now in its eighth edition, *Respiratory Physiology* has added some student-friendly features. Each chapter closes with boxed Key Points to further summarize essential knowledge. Readers will also find USMLE-style review questions, and a detailed answer key at the end of the text with full explanations for correct answers. The companion website offers the text in a fully searchable format, as well as animations that help explain various physiological concepts. *Respiratory Physiology* is recommended for libraries that support nursing and medical students as well as allied health programs in respiratory therapy.

Textbook of Medical Physiology. 11th ed. Authors: Arthur C. Guyton, John E. Hall. Saunders, 2005.
ISBN: 9780721602400
Recommended for: Hospital, Academic Libraries
Brandon/Hill Selection

This classic physiology text continues its tradition of quality with the eleventh edition. The *Textbook of Medical Physiology* covers all anatomical systems, with emphasis on interactions between systems as well as pathophysiology. This edition features clinical vignettes that illustrate physiological principles with actual scenarios, concise summary tables for quick review, and full color including figures, charts and graphs, line drawings, and ECGs. A perennial inhabitant of *Doody's* "Essential Purchases" list, the 11th edition offers many value-added features for students and residents. The *Textbook of Medical Physiology* is available in a Student Consult edition, which offers online access to the text on Elsevier's Student Consult site. Student Consult provides the full, searchable text of the book; links to related material from other Student Consult titles; a database of linked images; a question bank of USMLE-style questions; the ability to take online notes; and the ability to download information to a mobile device. This well-indexed volume, which has become the workhorse of physiology textbooks, is recommended for both academic and clinical collections.

Journals

American Journal of Physiology. Cell Physiology. v. 1, American Physiological Society, 1977.
http://ajpcell.physiology.org/
ISSN: 03636143
ISSN: 15221563 (Online)
Indexed in: MEDLINE
Recommended for: Academic Libraries

Like a few other highly rated physiology journals, *AJP—Cell Physiology* focuses on cellular and molecular physiology, but not to the exclusion of systems and organism physiology. Papers published include the use of cellular and molecular techniques to shed light on problems at the systems or organism level. The current editor has expressed great interest in publishing cellular studies of developmental physiology, stem cell biology research, and neurophysiology, among other areas. The format mirrors that of other American Physiological Society journals, with review articles, historical articles, "Perspectives," "Translational Physiology," and "Innovative Methodology" articles in addition to original research. Translational Physiology articles either test clinical hypotheses through laboratory studies, or apply laboratory findings to clinical practice. Articles published under the Innovative Methodology heading describe new methods of data collection and analysis. Regardless of article type, content is always classified and appears in one of 10 subject-based sections such as cellular and mitochondrial metabolism, receptors and signal transduction, and protein and vesicle trafficking. Ranked thirteenth in physiology in the 2009 *Journal Citation Reports*, this title is recommended for academic and research collections that support programs in biochemistry and cellular and molecular biology.

Annual Review of Physiology. v. 1, Annual Reviews, 1939.
http://arjournals.annualreviews.org/loi/physiol
ISSN: 00664278
ISSN: 15451585 (Online)
Indexed in: MEDLINE
Recommended for: Hospital, Academic Libraries

Intended for physiologists and academic physicians, each annual volume contains "diverse yet complementary reviews representing a wide range of issues and questions pertaining to the biochemical, cellular, organismal, and behavioral aspects of physiology." The volume is organized into sections which include cardiovascular physiology, cell physiology, ecological, evolutionary, and comparative physiology, endocrinology, gastrointestinal physiology, neurophysiology, renal physiology, and respiratory physiology. Each year offers a "Special Topics" section designed to cover interrelated research from both the basic and clinical sciences. Recent special topics have included asthma, obesity, TRP channels, and beta-arrestins. Most volumes include a special perspectives paper, a first person article written by a physician or researcher, although this feature is missing from the 2009 volume. Papers are invited by the journal's editorial committee and therefore do not undergo blind review. The journal ranks second in physiology in the 2009 *Journal Citation Reports* and is a strongly recommended resource for academic collections that serve medical schools and basic and applied science researchers. This title is also recommended for teaching hospital collections.

Journal of Applied Physiology. v. 1, American Physiological Society, 1948.
http://jap.physiology.org/
ISSN: 87507587

ISSN: 15221601 (Online)
Indexed in: MEDLINE
Recommended for: Hospital, Academic Libraries

The *Journal of Applied Physiology* (*JAP*), like other key physiology journals published today, focuses on molecular and cellular mechanisms that underlie physiological occurrences. Unlike many of the other journals in the American Physiological Society stable—of which this is one—*JAP* focuses on applied physiology. Journal editors are interested in papers that focus on "adaptive" mechanisms, such as any biological adaptations made by organisms in relation to development, aging, or disease, as well as to external phenomena such as exercise, altitude, or temperature. The journal also focuses on integrative mechanisms across organ systems or from molecule to cell to organ. The *Journal of Applied Physiology* views physiology in the broadest possible light, and associate editors have wide and varying expertise in multiple physiological disciplines: muscle physiology, respiratory physiology, mathematical modeling, cardiovascular mechanisms, and the physiology of aging, among others. In addition to research articles, including theoretical research, types of articles published include "Viewpoint" pieces, which give a personal yet documented approach to a topic or problem; "Point/Counterpoint" articles which offer a debate between experts; "Innovative Methodology" articles that detail new methods of data collection and analysis; review articles, which are generally invited and peer-reviewed; historical articles focusing on the history of physiology; and "Translational Physiology" papers that bridge the gap between basic physiology and patient care. This last section, in addition to the journal's emphasis on adaptive physiology, broadens the audience for *JAP* to clinicians in addition to physiology researchers. The *Journal of Applied Physiology* is appropriate for most academic and research collections, as well as larger hospital collections.

Journal of Cellular Physiology. v. 1, Wiley, 1932.
http://onlinelibrary.wiley.com/journal/10.1002/(ISSN)1097-4652
ISSN: 00219541
ISSN: 10974652 (Online)
Indexed in: MEDLINE
Recommended for: Academic Libraries

Unlike many other leading physiology journals, the *Journal of Cellular Physiology* (*JCP*) does not accept papers on systems or organism-level physiology. Rather, it publishes research findings in cellular biology and physiology, with an emphasis on the use of molecular investigative approaches. The appropriate audience for the journal includes molecular and cell biologists, biochemists, immunologists, geneticists, cancer biologists, and cellular physiologists. In addition to original research related to growth factors, cytokines, cell adhesion molecules, signal transduction, and cell cycle progression, *JCP* publishes review articles, rapid communications, and short (<600 word) articles in its "Perspectives" series. Wiley's Online Open program allows journal authors to pay Open Access fees and make their work available to the public immediately upon publication. Article supplementary materials, such as images and video files, are freely available online. Review articles are also freely available to non-subscribers. Monthly issues are substantive, generally holding 15 to 20 research articles and one or more review or "mini-review" articles. *JCP*'s 2009 *Journal Citation Reports* impact factor places it seventh among physiology journals. Recommended for academic and research collections that support programs in molecular and cell biology, biochemistry, and cancer genetics.

Journal of General Physiology. v. 1, Rockefeller University, 1918.
http://jgp.rupress.org/
ISSN: 00221295
ISSN: 15407748 (Online)
Indexed in: MEDLINE
Recommended for: Academic Libraries

The mission statement posted on the website of the *Journal of General Physiology* (*JGP*) defines general physiology as "the study of biological mechanisms through analytical investigations, which decipher the molecular and cellular mechanisms underlying biological function." The journal serves as the official publication of the Society of General Physiologists. The focus on cellular and molecular physiology indicates that the target audience includes academic, government, and industry researchers rather than clinical professionals. The Society itself is known for promoting and disseminating research related to membrane structure, transport, and dynamics; ion channels; cellular contractility; and molecular motors. This peer-reviewed journal presents original research in these and related areas. *JGP* held the tenth-highest impact factor among all physiology journals in the 2009 *Journal Citation Reports*. Contents generally include five to eight research articles, with occasional editorials, commentaries, or tutorials. Other occasional features of interest to cell physiologists include "From the JCB" and "Perspectives." "From the JCB" summarizes research findings from the *Journal of Cell Biology*, while "Perspectives" offers two contrasting, expert points of view on emerging or controversial topics in cellular physiology.

Journal of Physiology. v. 1, Wiley-Blackwell, 1878.
http://onlinelibrary.wiley.com/journal/10.1111/(ISSN)1469-7793
ISSN: 00223751
ISSN: 14697793 (Online)
Indexed in: MEDLINE
Recommended for: Hospital, Academic Libraries

Published on behalf of Great Britain's Physiological Society, the *Journal of Physiology*'s 2009 *Journal Citation Reports* impact factor places it sixth among physiology journals and forty-third in the neurosciences. Original research includes papers on both cellular and systems physiology, with emphases in human and mammalian research. The *Journal of Physiology* also publishes "Rapid Reports," emerging research that merits rapid acceptance and publication. Another value added component is the journal's sponsorship of symposia on various topics suggested by editorial board members and held at major international meetings. Symposia in 2009 included such topics as physical activity and health; estrogen action; and intestinal microbiota. A new feature introduced in 2008 is "Techniques in Physiology," comprising short papers that introduce new methods and techniques in physiological research. Also introduced in 2008 was the "Clinical Perspectives" section of the journal. These invited commentaries review new research presented in a particular issue and discuss the potential applications to clinical therapeutics. Other article categories include topical reviews and journal club articles. Authors can choose to pay open access fees and make their work immediately available. The *Journal of Physiology* is highly recommended for academic collections and larger hospital collections.

Psychophysiology: The International Journal of the Society for Psychophysiological Research. v. 1, Wiley-Blackwell, 1964.
See Chapter 20. Medical Psychology

Physiological Reviews. v. 1, American Physiological Society, 1921.
http://physrev.physiology.org/
ISSN: 00319333
ISSN: 15221210 (Online)
Indexed in: MEDLINE
Recommended for: Academic Libraries

Published since 1921 by the American Physiological Society, *Physiological Reviews* offers broad coverage geared toward physiologists, neuroscientists, cell biologists, biophysicists, and clinicians. Reviews are invited, with eight to 10 reviews published in each quarterly issue. With an impact factor that has risen over the past decade—reaching the number one position in physiology in the 2009 *Journal Citation Reports*—the journal offers important contributions to all subfields of physiology, including computational biology. Because the reviews are invited and screened by editorial board members, blinded peer review is not a factor in article selection. However, the editorial board is diverse, international, and highly credentialed. Reviews summarize existing research and recent developments in articles that range from 10,000 to 25,000 words. *Physiological Reviews* is most appropriate for academic and research collections. The broad and comprehensive aspects of the reviews make them suitable for use in teaching or background research, but they offer limited clinical applicability. Any given issue will have only one or two articles of direct clinical interest, rendering the journal a low-priority selection for hospital settings. *Physiological Reviews* is available in both print and online formats. Legacy content—from 1921 to 1997—can be purchased from the American Physiological Society for a one-time fee.

Physiology. v. 19, International Union of Physiological Sciences; American Physiological Society, 2004.
http://physiologyonline.physiology.org/
ISSN: 15489213
ISSN: 15489221 (Online)
Indexed in: MEDLINE
Recommended for: Hospital, Academic Libraries

The bi-monthly *Physiology* publishes invited but peer-reviewed articles that summarize important developments in various physiological fields. Published jointly by the American Physiological Society and the International Union of Physiological Sciences, *Physiology* was published as *News in Physiological Sciences* from 1986 through June of 2004. The journal underwent a major redesign with its new format in 2004 and now has a strong focus on artwork and accompanying visuals. In addition to short, scholarly review articles, each issue offers "Highlights from the Literature," short summaries of important research. Occasional features include "Emerging Tools and Technologies," descriptions of technologies and methods of interest to physiologists; "Emerging Topics," brief discussions of new physiology concepts; "Point/Counterpoint" presenting opposing views on controversial topics; and "Timelines" which are brief historical articles. In an editorial published in June 2005, Ulrich Pohl pointed out that only 30 percent of authors published in the new format were affiliated with physiology departments, indicating the broad range of interests covered by the field of "physiology." For this reason the journal appeals to a wide audience, and is recommended for both academic and clinical collections.

30. Analytical, Diagnostic, and Therapeutic Techniques

30.1. Anesthesia

A state characterized by loss of feeling or sensation. This depression of nerve function is usually the result of pharmacologic action and is induced to allow performance of surgery or other painful procedures.

—MeSH

Contributor: Joanne Rich

Monographs

Anesthesia and Uncommon Diseases. 5th ed. Author: Lee A. Fleisher. Saunders/Elsevier, 2006.
http://www.mdconsult.com/
ISBN: 9781416022121
Recommended for: Hospital, Academic Libraries

This fifth edition updates the previous edition from 1998. Chapters are arranged primarily by organ system with new topics such as mitochondrial diseases and bioterrorism. Drawing on the expertise of 45 U.S. contributors, this highly regarded text provides authoritative summaries for the practicing anesthesiologist or anesthetist encountering patients with uncommon disorders. Helpful design features, such as summary tables, simple diagrams, and black-and-white images, make the content more easily readable.

Clinical Anesthesia. 6th ed. Editors: Paul G. Barash, Bruce F. Cullen, Robert K. Stoelting, Michael K. Cahalan, M. Christine Stock. Wolters Kluwer/Lippincott Williams & Wilkins, 2009.
http://www.ovid.com/
http://www.r2library.com/
ISBN: 9780781787635
Recommended for: Hospital, Academic Libraries
Doody's Core Titles Selection

A popular favorite since 1989 that balances didactic and clinical content, this sixth edition remains a mainstay in the anesthesiology library. Editors are primarily U.S. based. Topics are comprehensive and provide overviews from basics to specific areas of clinical practice and practice settings. Each chapter outlines numbered key points that are highlighted in the text using consistent numbering so readers can easily jump to specific sections. Institutional online access is offered through Ovid and R2 Library. Unfortunately, Ovid's interface does not offer the useful navigation features offered in the print publication. Individual purchasers of the print edition obtain access to a companion website that provides access to downloadable podcasts on specific topics, full-text searching with a superior results display (versus Ovid's platform), corrections reflected on the website, image bank, and interactive quiz bank.

Miller's Anesthesia. 7th ed. Editors: Ronald D. Miller, Lars I. Eriksson, Lee A. Fleisher, Jeanine P. Wiener-Kronish, William L. Young. Churchill Livingstone/Elsevier, 2010.
http://www.mdconsult.com/
ISBN: 9780443069598
Recommended for: Hospital, Academic Libraries
Brandon/Hill Selection

This is the seventh edition of *Miller's Anesthesia* since its first appearance in 1981. The number of authors continues to grow from the initial 31 in 1981 to over 200 in this current edition. International contributors represent 20 countries other than the United States. The content also continues to grow with the profession, with new chapters such as "Anesthesia for Bariatric Surgery" and an updated focus on emerging trends such as modern technology in anesthesia practice. This comprehensive and very thorough textbook continues to be the standard for anesthesiology.

Stoelting's Anesthesia and Co-Existing Disease. 5th ed. Editors: Roberta L. Hines, Katherine E. Marschall. Saunders/Elsevier, 2008.
http://www.mdconsult.com/
ISBN: 9781416039983
Recommended for: Hospital, Academic Libraries
Doody's Core Titles Selection

With the fifth edition of this title since its inception in 1983, editorship passes from Robert Stoelting and Stephen Dierdorf to a new generation. The book's original intent remains: "to provide a concise description of the pathophysiology of disease states and their medical management that is relevant to the care of the patient in the perioperative period." Decreased depth of coverage is provided for pediatric and geriatric diseases and topics of less common diseases. Content is arranged by chapters on varying disease groupings such as "Heart Failure and Cardiomyopathies," "Respiratory Diseases," and "Hematologic Disorders." Each chapter presents summaries of specific diseases within these groupings followed by summaries of "Management of Anesthesia." The content is supplemented with simple illustrations and many summarizing tables and charts. Each chapter includes references and a helpful "Key Points" section.

Journals

Acta Anaesthesiologica Scandinavica: An International Journal of Anaesthesiology and Intensive Care, Pain and Emergency Medicine. v. 1, Wiley-Blackwell Munksgaard/Acta Anaesthesiologica Scandinavica Foundation, 1957.
http://onlinelibrary.wiley.com/journal/10.1111/(ISSN)1399-6576
ISSN: 00015172
ISSN: 13996576 (Online)
Indexed in: MEDLINE
Recommended for: Hospital, Academic Libraries

As the official publication of the Scandinavian Society of Anaesthesiology and Intensive Care Medicine, this journal publishes ten issues per year (every month except June and December). In addition to original research articles and case reports, *Acta Anaesthesiologica Scandinavica* includes a calendar of events from around the world and special supplements on congresses from various conferences and meetings. It is well indexed in standard databases such as BIOSIS, Current Contents, Embase, MEDLINE, and Science Citation Index. The 2009 edition of *Journal Citation Reports* provides an impact factor of 2.260 and ranks this title eleventh in the anesthesiology journals subset.

Anaesthesia. v. 1, Wiley-Blackwell/The Association of Anaesthetists of Great Britain and Ireland, 1946.
http://onlinelibrary.wiley.com/journal/10.1111/(ISSN)1365-2044
ISSN: 00032409
ISSN: 13652044 (Online)
Indexed in: MEDLINE, CINAHL
Recommended for: Hospital, Academic Libraries
Brandon/Hill Selection

This monthly publication serves as the official Journal of the Association of Anaesthetists of Great Britain and Ireland. In addition to original research articles on general and regional anesthesia *and* intensive care and pain therapy, the journal includes research on equipment and apparatus along with abstracts from various meetings. It is well indexed in standard databases such as BIOSIS, Current Contents, Embase, MEDLINE, and Science Citation Index. The 2009 edition of *Journal Citation Reports* provides an impact factor of 2.855 and ranks this title eighth in the anesthesiology subset of journals.

Anaesthesia and Intensive Care. v. 1, Australian Society of Anaesthetists, 1972.
http://www.aaic.net.au/
ISSN: 0310057X
ISSN: 14480271 (Online)
Indexed in: MEDLINE
Recommended for: Hospital, Academic Libraries

This bimonthly publication serves as the official journal of the Australian Society of Anaesthetists, Australian and New Zealand Intensive Care Society, and New Zealand Society of Anaesthetists. In addition to original articles on anesthesia, intensive care, and pain, the journal publishes issues on symposia, review articles, historical articles, book reviews, and upcoming meetings. The 2009 *Journal Citation Reports* lists an impact factor of 1.108, which places it eighteenth among the anesthesiology subset of journals.

Anesthesia and Analgesia. v. 36, International Anesthesia Research Society, 1957.
http://www.anesthesia-analgesia.org
http://www.ovid.com/
ISSN: 00032999
ISSN: 15267598 (Online)
Indexed in: MEDLINE, CINAHL
Recommended for: Hospital, Academic Libraries

Anesthesia and Analgesia is the official journal of several societies: International Anesthesia Research Society, the Society of Cardiovascular Anesthesiologists, the Society for Pediatric Anesthesia, Society for Ambulatory Anesthesia, the International Society for Anaesthetic Pharmacology, the Society for Technology in Anesthesia, the Anesthesia Patient Safety Foundation, the American Society of Critical Care Anesthesiologists, and the Society for Obstetric Anesthesia and Perinatology. The diversity of these organizations is reflected in the contents sections: cardiovascular anesthesiology, pediatric anesthesiology, ambulatory anesthesiology, anesthetic pharmacology, technology, computing and simulation, patient safety, critical care and trauma, obstetric anesthesiology, neurosurgical anesthesiology and neuroscience, general articles, and analgesia. Other content includes book reviews, multimedia, and meetings. The Accreditation Council for Continuing Medical Education (ACCME) offers continuing medical education credit with membership in the International Anesthesia Research Society. This monthly journal was first published as *Current Researches in Anesthesia and Analgesia* between 1920 and 1956. The 2009 *Journal Citation Reports* impact factor is 3.083, which ranks this publication sixth in the anesthesiology journals subset.

Anesthesiology. v. 1, Lippincott Williams & Wilkins/American Society of Anesthesiologists, 1940.
http://www.ovid.com/
ISSN: 00033022
ISSN: 15281175 (Online)
Indexed in: MEDLINE, CINAHL
Recommended for: Hospital, Academic Libraries
Brandon/Hill Selection

This monthly publication is the official journal of the American Society of Anesthesiologists (ASA). Content includes research, reviews, and case reports pertaining to clinical practice in perioperative care, critical care, and pain medicine. The journal also includes reviews of educational material and ASA approved continuing medical education credit. The 2009 *Journal Citation Reports* impact factor is 5.354, which places this title at the number two spot for the anesthesiology journals subset.

British Journal of Anaesthesia: BJA. v. 1, Oxford University Press, 1923.
http://bja.oxfordjournals.org/
ISSN: 00070912
ISSN: 14716771 (Online)
Indexed in: MEDLINE
Recommended for: Hospital, Academic Libraries

This official journal of the Royal College of Anaesthetists includes research and reviews on many subspecialty areas, including cardiovascular, critical care, neurosciences and neuroanesthesia, obstetrics, pediatrics, pain, regional anesthesia, and respiration and the airway. The monthly journal also publishes abstracts from various meetings. The 2009 *Journal Citation Reports* provided an impact factor of 3.827, ranking this title fourth among the anesthesiology journals subset.

Canadian Journal of Anaesthesia. v. 34, Springer New York, 1987.
http://www.cja-jca.org/
http://springerlink.com/content/0832-610X/
ISSN: 0832610X
ISSN: 14968975 (Online)
Indexed in: MEDLINE
Recommended for: Hospital, Academic Libraries

Founded in 1954 as the *Canadian Anaesthetists' Society Journal*, this publication merged together the *News Letter* and the *Proceedings of the Canadian Anesthesiologists' Society*. The monthly publication offers research articles, reviews, and case reports covering many areas such as general anesthesia, regional anesthesia, pain, obstetrical and pediatric anesthesia, cardiothoracic anesthesia, respiration and airway, and neuroanesthesia and intensive care. Other content includes new media and book reviews and Continuing Professional Development (CPD) approved by the Royal College of Physicians and Surgeons of Canada. The journal is partially bilingual with English articles supplemented with French abstracts and vice versa. The 2009 *Journal Citation Reports* impact factor of 2.306 ranks this title tenth in the anesthesiology journals subset.

Journal of Clinical Anesthesia. v. 1, Elsevier, 1988.
http://www.sciencedirect.com/science/journal/09528180
ISSN: 09528180
ISSN: 18734529 (Online)
Indexed in: MEDLINE
Recommended for: Hospital, Academic Libraries

This is the official journal of the American Association of Clinical Directors, the Society for Airway Management, the Society for Education in Anesthesia, and the Orthopedic Anesthesia Pain Rehabilitation Society. Published eight times per year, it includes research, reviews, case reports, and case conferences in all areas of anesthesiology, including anesthetic administration, pharamcokinetics, preoperative and postoperative issues, coexisting disease, and cost issues. The 2009 *Journal Citation Reports* impact factor of 1.324 puts this title in the seventeenth spot of the anesthesiology journals subset.

Journal of Neurosurgical Anesthesiology. v. 1, Lippincott Williams & Wilkins, 1989.
http://www.jnsa.com/
http://www.ovid.com/
ISSN: 08984921
ISSN: 15371921 (Online)
Indexed in: MEDLINE
Recommended for: Hospital, Academic Libraries

This is the official journal of a number of international neuroanesthesia organizations: the Society of Neurosurgical Anesthesia and Critical Care, Neuroanaesthesia Society of Great Britain and Ireland, Association de Neuro-Anesthésiologie Réanimation de langue Française, Wissenschaftlicher Arbeitskreis Neuroanästhesie der Deutschen Gesellschaft fur Anästhesiologie und Intensivmedizen, Arbeitsgemeinschaft Deutschsprachiger Neuroanästhesisten und Neuro-Intensivmediziner, Korean Society of Neuroanesthesia, Japanese Society of Neuroanesthesia and Critical Care, Neuroanesthesiology Chapter of the Colegio Mexicano de Anesthesiología, and Indian Society of Neuroanesthesiology and Critical Care. This title is published four times per year and is aimed at all neurosurgical intensive care unit personnel, including neuroanesthesiologists, neurosurgeons, and neurosurgical support staff. Articles cover research, reviews, journal club synopses, debates, book reviews, and abstracts from affiliated neuroanesthesiology societies. The 2008 *Journal Citation Reports* impact factor of 2.412 ranks this title ninth in the anesthesiology subset of journals.

Pediatric Anesthesia. v. 1, Wiley-Blackwell, 1991.
http://onlinelibrary.wiley.com/journal/10.1111/(ISSN)1460-9592
ISSN: 11555645
ISSN: 14609592 (Online)
Indexed in: MEDLINE
Recommended for: Hospital, Academic Libraries

Alternatively known as *Paediatric Anaesthesia*, this monthly journal includes research, commentaries, case presentations, book reviews, reports of meetings, and a calendar of events pertaining to anesthesia and intensive care in newborns, infants, and children. The 2009 *Journal Citation Reports* impact factor of 2.149 ranks this title twelfth among the anesthesiology subset of journals.

30.2. Medical Decision Making

Application of knowledge to making informed choices.
—MeSH

Contributor: Stephen P. Bartold

Monographs

Clinical Decision Support: The Road Ahead. Editor: Robert A. Greenes. Elsevier Academic Press, 2007.
http://www.sciencedirect.com/science/book/9780123693778
http://extranet.netlibrary.com/TitleSelect
http://www.ebrary.com/
ISBN: 9780123693778
ISBN: 9780080467696
Recommended for: Hospital, Academic Libraries

This extensive, multi-author textbook emphasizes the implementation of decision support systems. The editor R.A. Greenes is a long-standing and prolific author about medical decision making (MDM) and contributes extensively to the body of the text by authoring single chapters. His perspective and command of the topic contribute to the coherence and quality of the book. The many other authors he has recruited are recognized experts with proven accomplishments in the field of MDM. These authors give descriptions of their experiences prototyping and maintaining the most successful large institutional and limited domain decision-making systems yet formulated. Nevertheless, the book is not encyclopedic. The computers, networks, logistics, organizational factors, and issues of implementation are emphasized over fundamental scientific and statistical methodologies. A noteworthy addition to the text is the final summary chapter written by Dr. Greenes, "A Proposed Strategy for Overcoming Inertia," that realistically describes the current state of MDM and his opinions about how to proceed. Extensive bibliographies accompany each chapter further expanding on the origins, history, and evolution of this nascent discipline. This is the single best textbook for a thorough reference to the topic of MDM known to this contributor and author.

Decision Making in Medicine: An Algorithmic Approach. 3rd ed. Editors: Stuart B. Mushlin, Harry L. Greene II. Mosby/Elsevier, 2010.
http://greenecology.org/science/book/9780323041072
ISBN: 0323041078
ISBN: 9780323041072
Recommended for: Hospital, Academic Libraries

This book continues as part of a series of textbooks encompassing over a dozen different specialties ranging from anesthesia to urology. The book pertaining specifically to medicine contains several hundred simple algorithms. The authors are almost exclusively from a single institution. The algorithms do not appear to be rigorously peer reviewed and are written by many authors. This work is included because it provides a quick, simple, and frequently helpful way to review or double check what is a reasonable approach to common problems encountered in the clinic or hospital. It may be especially helpful to trainees or experienced practitioners confronted by problems outside their usual repertoire. If used with caution, egregious errors of omission or commission are less likely. After personal use for many years, this contributor has yet to identify any obvious mistakes, although considerable anecdotal and personal experience influence the suggested diagnostic and management schemes. It is not a definitive resource for any of the topics covered.

Encyclopedia of Medical Decision Making. Editors: Michael W. Kattan, Mark E. Cowen. Sage, 2009.
ISBN: 9781412953726
Recommended for: Academic Libraries

This recently published book is a very welcome contribution to the body of the medical decision making (MDM) literature. It is a multi-authored collection of essays presented as topics, which, at first glance, appears to be arranged in a haphazard and illogical "topical" alphabetical order. Fortunately, the editors and a panel of distinguished experts offer an additional organizational approach using the following topical groupings: (a) biostatistics and epidemiology; (b) decision analysis...and models; (c) health outcomes and measurement; (d) measures of...possible options; (e) other techniques...; (f) perspective of the decision maker; and (g) psychology underlying MDM. These broad areas are further organized to cover the specific topics in the preface. The book consists of two volumes totaling 1,239 pages. Very importantly, the index is quite extensive but somewhat deficient in cross referencing related material in the topical groupings. The index appears only in the second volume, which is inconvenient. Despite these arbitrary organizational issues, it is a wealthy collection of well-written material unlike any other reference this contributor is aware of or could recommend. The essay topics cover a majority of the still rapidly evolving body of MDM. Given the recent incorporation of MDM into medical practice, the nomenclature has yet to be well standardized. The authors and editors have obviously wrestled with the difficulty of presenting all MDM as a comprehensive entity. It is apparent that considerable thought has gone into how and what to write, and attempts have been made to be both specific and comprehensive. To date, this is the most consolidated book for the experienced practitioner who may seek such a unified and comprehensive reference book. Almost all of the specialized and technical concepts are included, as well as "buzzwords" that typify such an immature discipline. It would be useful for this extraordinary book to offer future editions and a resolution of the cacophonous organization. Again, it is rich in content and highly recommended for those who use the tools of MDM regularly. In the interim, a searchable CD-ROM of free text would be a welcome addition.

The Logic of Medicine. 2nd ed. Author: Edmond A. Murphy. Johns Hopkins University Press, 1997.
ISBN: 9780801855382
Recommended for: Academic Libraries

It is always a delight to encounter a book that achieves the author's stated goal, which is to present the "rules of evidence" and logic behind our actions in medicine. In less than 500 pages, Murphy presents the fundamentals of medical decision making (MDM) exactly as the title implies. For those readers unfamiliar with the language of formal logic, it may be more difficult to read than some, but it is an elegant exposition. A reader who is not intimidated by the writing style of the text according to the principles of formal logic will be amply rewarded. Although written as a textbook, it is also an excellent reference to the primary literature of the subject as of 1997. While the material may seem dated, little has changed over the ensuing years at this fundamental level, rendering it adequate compared to more contemporary works. Actually, it is unique because of the emphasis on logic as taught in mathematics, philosophy, and related disciplines. Treatment of the ontology of medicine precedes an examination of epistemology of the subject. These concepts may be new to many medical and even scientific readers, making the assimilation of its content a little awkward for the novice accustomed to the more casual approach taken by most authors. Nevertheless, it is refreshing and well done. It presents a somewhat different and more rigorous approach to the disorderly subject of MDM. Almost all of the major topics of the field are covered with admirable clarity, which is no small task. That such a book has evolved with the production of a second edition is testimony to the author's success. Any health care professional can comprehend the material as presented if trouble is taken to familiarize oneself with the vernacular of logic. Of course, as alluded to earlier, any attempt to formulate the subject of MDM in rigorous fashion requires compromise that may be awkward or unacceptable to a few serious scholars. The author achieves his goal admirably, and this book is sufficiently unique to merit a "top 10" rating.

Medical Decision Making. Authors: Hal Sox, Marshal A. Blatt, Michael C. Higgins, Keith I. Marton. American College of Physicians, 2007 (Reprint of original, Butterworth-Heinemann publ., c1988.).
ISBN: 9781930513792

Recommended for: Hospital, Academic Libraries
Doody's Core Titles Selection

Hal Sox and others have written one of the "grandfather" introductory texts about medical decision making (MDM). The treatise is best directed to physicians and health care providers early in training or to those who need only a passing familiarity with the subject. It is a simple, clear, and very readable overview of the field. Having endured since 1988, the book is now being reprinted by the ACP. Throughout the intervening years, it retains the fundamental concepts and goals of the authors under the realistic constraints imposed by brevity, the chaotic status of our medical environment, and unprecedented progress in the knowledge base of medical science. The book has matured gracefully and is still contemporary for its intended audience. Standard topics, such as the following, are covered in an elementary, orderly, and clear exposition: basic probability and statistics; the appropriateness and quantification of diagnostic tests; modeling; decision trees; expected value (EV, essentially synonymous with UV in the recommended reference by Eeckhoudt); decision analysis; and cost effectiveness/benefit analyses with their various measures. Further, practical and utilitarian topics such as DRGs (diagnosis related groups), coding, optimization, and the interplay of economic, social, and insurance/finance are briefly introduced. They acknowledge the difficulty of formulating public policy versus decision under unique circumstance(s) applicable to an individual. All of this is packaged in a "no frills" book with adequate graphics, bibliographies, and indexing given its 1988 unrevised content. By using simple reasoning and a common sense approach, the authors do not overwhelm the intended audience. Practical clinical scenarios accompany conceptual material, illustrating the usefulness of the methods employed. Early in the book, the authors list a few common clinical aphorisms that are likely to be familiar to all practitioners and students. The authors then suggest that it is their goal to formulate these in a more fundamental or general way using the basic analytic methods they succinctly describe. They do so adequately, even admirably. In summary, the book is highly recommended as an introductory text to MDM.

Medical Uses of Statistics. 3rd ed. Editors: John C. Bailar III, David C. Hoaglin. Wiley, 2009.
ISBN: 9780470439531
ISBN: 9780470439524
Recommended for: Hospital, Academic Libraries

This is the third edition of the classic text first published in 1986. The authors and the several coauthors of various chapters are acknowledged experts with extensive experience in their topics. The differences between this book and the similar title by Alvan R. Feinstein, *Principles of Medical Statistics*, are substantial. This book is a "must have, bread & butter" reference for virtually any medical library. The chapters capture almost all of the common statistical methods found in the general medical literature. Many examples are taken from articles published in the *New England Journal of Medicine*. The book is fairly comprehensive in clinical applications but not technical content, and little or no explicit didactic material is included. It is a "plug & play, down & dirty" work, focusing on how to do or understand a specific topic or how to address a timely question. The references that accompany each chapter are ample for those who may require additional information. The text could be used as an introductory textbook if the instructor diligently complemented the material and presented it well. Since the most common use of the book is likely the exposition of a specific topic by any non-technical health care worker with a "need to know," it is well matched to the intended audience. Its content is elementary and accessible to any and all who have a command of their specialty and a little arithmetic accompanied by common sense. Usually, a statistical background is not assumed.

Principles of Biomedical Informatics. Author: Ira J. Kalet. Academic Press/Elsevier, 2009.
http://www.sciencedirect.com/science/book/9780123694386
http://extranet.netlibrary.com/TitleSelect
http://www.ebrary.com/
ISBN: 9780123694386
ISBN: 9780080557946
Recommended for: Academic Libraries

This single author text purports to enumerate "Methods of data collection, encoding, standardization, exchange, and interpretation . . . model construction, validation, and analysis." Given such an ambitious set of objectives, skepticism is warranted, but the author has achieved this goal. It is in an admirable treatise worthy of inclusion here. The book is interdisciplinary and only addresses quantitative or heuristic systems that can be modeled by computable methods. It is written at a level best for experts and serious researchers who are familiar with computer science or systems, knowledge engineering, artificial intelligence, and related disciplines. The emphasis is theoretical, but it includes many specific procedures and methods accompanied by pseudo code or examples written in the LISP programming language.

Although not comprehensive, it covers an extensive subset of biomedical problems that are not all strictly clinical applications. It is an excellent choice for a one or two semester, graduate-level course for the serious student of medical decision making (MDM). The intent is to illustrate how to understand and develop automated systems for biomedical applications. It is not suitable as an introductory text unless the reader has previous exposure to relevant material and an appropriate technical background. For such an audience, it is a very good synopsis of current methods and models in MDM.

Principles of Medical Statistics. Author: Alvan R. Feinstein. Chapman & Hall/CRC, 2001.
http://www.crcnetbase.com/isbn/978-1-58488-216-9
http://www.ebrary.com/
http://extranet.netlibrary.com/TitleSelect
ISBN: 9781584882169
ISBN: 9781420035681
Recommended for: Academic Libraries

Alvan Feinstein was one of the most gifted biostatisticians of the twentieth century. This textbook was his last major publication prior to his death in 2003. He also authored or coauthored two other statistical textbooks and hundreds of journal articles. He distinguished himself not so much by being prolific as profound. One cannot do justice to this single book without acknowledging his many contributions. This book is a "one of a kind" reference to the broad field of biomedical statistics. It is supplemented by over 600 references to the statistical and biomedical literature. The only small irritation noted is a rather sketchy index. While it would not be possible to produce an exhaustive or encyclopedic single book, this moderately comprehensive work offers lucid explanations of almost all major biostatistical topics with sufficient detail and coherence as only a master can do. It is not the most comprehensive, easily readable, or even definitive work on any specific topic; but, overall, it is possibly the best. *Principles of Medical Statistics* is written at an intermediate level accessible for all who have a modest command of basic statistics. In addition to being an excellent text for such an audience, it is written in the style of a basic graduate level text. The book is accompanied by exercises with solutions, examples, and an instructor's guide with additional materials. Additionally, it is an excellent reference for those who require occasional reminders about basic methodology to interpret biostatistical data. It is not likely to serve well as an introductory text except for more advanced or sophisticated students beyond their initial medical/scientific studies. Aside from the accolades above, it ought to be acknowledged that on a few topics in biostatistics—such as qualitative methods and conduct of clinical trials—Dr. Feinstein expressed unique and controversial views not always comfortably accepted by all experts. A few vocal detractors have accused him of serious bias or just plain being wrong. His more philosophic views in these areas are notably minimal in this straightforward and essentially non-controversial book. With his targeted focus on agreeable topics and a precise presentation, he mollifies some of those critics.

Rational Medical Decision Making: A Case-Based Approach. Author: Goutham Rao. McGraw-Hill Medical, 2007.
http://www.statref.com/
ISBN: 9780071463973
Recommended for: Academic Libraries

This single author, short monograph is one of the better of several recently published elementary but good, readable, comprehensive, and practical teaching texts about medical decision making (MDM). The book is written for medical students. It requires only familiarity with elementary probability and statistics, arithmetic, algebra, and set theory. It is suitable for any interested health care provider. The appeal of this book is the concise, coherent, and orderly treatment of the subject given its brevity. In 10 chapters, the author introduces almost all of the major subjects composing MDM. This exposition should allow any novice to critically evaluate most of what appears in the general medical literature according to "evidence-based" methodology. The arrangement of chapters evolves in logical order, and each is accompanied by very few references to cases germane to the topic. Each chapter lists discrete objectives, and the index is adequate but short. A final annotated bibliography citing a few of the important references to the major corpus of MDM is included. The bibliography is minimal and uneven. The book is in its first edition, and such blemishes could be easily rectified or supplemented by individuals using the text for teaching purposes. This book is recommended for those naïve to the subject of MDM.

Risk and Medical Decision Making. Author: Louis Eeckhoudt. Kluwer Academic, 2002.
ISBN: 9781402070075
Recommended for: Academic Libraries

This short, single-author monograph is written by an economist. It is an excellent, simple, and concise description of the basic principles of the Expectation-Utility

(EU) method dominant in medical decision making (MDM). It is written in the language of statistics. It requires some familiarity with logic, probability theory, and a little calculus with differential equations. Such rigor does not exceed the undergraduate level of sophistication. It also includes limited exercises qualifying it as a bona fide textbook suitable for teaching. If most medical professionals assimilated these concepts, a deeper understanding of both diagnostic and therapeutic MDM ought to result. Such methods are common in the general medical literature although usually employed by researchers or statisticians. These methods are usually ignored with some "hand waving" gesticulation by clinicians who are naïve of the underlying assumptions. The writing style is accessible and does not wander into unnecessary complexity or pedantry. The sparse index and highly truncated list of references cite most of the major concepts of the discipline. This short book is a simple mathematical exposition of the dominant paradigm of MDM. As such, it is highly recommended.

Shared Decision Making in the Patient-Physician Relationship: Challenges Facing Patients, Physicians, and Medical Institutions. Author: Dennis J. Mazur. American College of Physician Executives, 2001.
ISBN: 9780924674808
Recommended for: Hospital, Consumer Health Libraries

This is a single-author book written for and primarily from the perspective of the patient. It is not unique but different from most of the other recommended references. The author is an established expert in medical decision making (MDM). He writes well and the text is appropriate to the target audience, assuming the lay reader has a modest degree of familiarity and sophistication. The index is especially thorough. The topics covered are quite comprehensive and encompass much of the methodology of contemporary MDM. The emphasis is on methods and generic topics without much reference to disease specific entities. There are coherent explanations of ethical, technical, social, and practical aspects of the subject in a style consistent with the intended audience. The book can easily be read by an expert or health care professional in a single sitting. It makes for a pleasant overview of the topic, although there is no new or unique technical content. Achieving an appropriate level of explanation without oversimplification of the material is commendable. It is written skillfully and this book is recommended. The accompanying CD-ROM is simply a PDF of the text verbatim.

Journals

BMC Medical Informatics and Decision Making. v. 1, BioMed Central, 2001.
See Chapter 6.3. Informatics

Medical Decision Making. v. 1, Sage, 1981.
http://mdm.sagepub.com/
ISSN: 0272989X
ISSN: 1552681X (Online)
Indexed in: MEDLINE, CINAHL
Recommended for: Academic Libraries

Medical Decision Making is the official journal of the Society for Medical Decision Making and the only U.S. publication devoted to the methodologies in this field. Although relatively obscure and limited in dissemination and readership, this unique and probably foremost of the few other journals that address MDM or similar topical material is the "flagship" journal for the subject, ranking in the top five medical informatics journals as defined by the 2009 *Journal Citation Reports*. As a family of methods, MDM is relatively new, dating back approximately 50 years in its current form and only becoming a well recognized and distinguishable discipline within the last half of the twentieth century. The emergence of a special society dedicated journal, accompanied by very high quality literature and the rapidly expanding utilization of decision-support systems, guarantee this publication a secure niche for the limited number of dedicated practitioners or researchers devoted to the field. Still in progress are responses to the most challenging problems, such as support of evidence-based medicine tools; incorporation of the electronic medical record; evolving pattern recognition methods for speech, images, and test results; and the evolution toward more automation via Decision Support/Artificial Intelligence (AI) algorithms. The broad mission of the journal is to solicit and publish papers emphasizing methodological and technical issues relating to: (a) decision analysis and cost effectiveness analysis; (b) patient preferences and quality-of-life research; (c) decision psychology; and (d) outcomes research. However, coverage is more eclectic than these four categories suggest. For example, recent issues contain well-written papers on varied topics such as judgment, risk assessment, socioeconomic issues, and financial analyses of specific public policy or individual decisions. Virtually any methodology—statistical or otherwise—applied usefully in a medical context such as game theory, reliability analysis, multisensor signal detection and analysis, risk analysis, and many other methodologies from technology and engineering are applicable to MDM. The difficult task of assessing objective, measurable, and appropriate utility measured in dollars, years of life, quality of life, and competing societal, political, and technical capabilities of our medical ministrations are "hot button" applications awaiting further study. Models are central to the development of MDM, and the journal devotes significant concern for and coverage of this process. As the journal and subject have evolved, the number and selectiveness of its content have increased and improved respectively. There is significant overlap with *JAMIA* and *BMC Medical Informatics and Decision Making*, but the subject is sufficiently broad to support all these publications. Finally, the methods of MDM are deeply embedded in the entire medical literature, although this is not acknowledged as a primary topic since it is simply part of the methodology of many studies and experiments. Thus, *MDM* is highly recommended and a "must have" for the academic and very large health care facilities libraries.

Journal of the American Medical Informatics Association: JAMIA. v. 1, AMIA and BMJ Group, 1994.
See Chapter 6.2. Medical Records, Chapter 6.3. Informatics

30.3. Diagnosis

The determination of the nature of a disease or condition, or the distinguishing of one disease or condition from another. Assessment may be made through physical examination, laboratory tests, or the likes. Computerized programs may be used to enhance the decision-making process.
—MeSH

Contributor: Jackie Davis

Monographs

2010 Current Medical Diagnosis & Treatment. 49th ed.
Editors: Stephen J. McPhee, Maxine A. Papadakis.
McGraw-Hill, 2009.
http://www.accessmedicine.com/
http://www.r2library.com/
ISBN: 9780071624442
Recommended for: Hospital, Academic, Consumer Health Libraries
Brandon/Hill, *Doody's Core Titles* Selection

The editors have been providing information for the practice of general medicine for 49 years. With this 2010 edition, there are 41 chapters as well as four online-only chapters offered at no additional cost. Prominent physician and pharmaceutical experts authored the different chapters, which address over 1,000 diseases and conditions and provide evidence-based research. New and timely chapters include H1N1; vaccine safety; updated information on cancer, HIV, and AIDS; drug information; websites; and references to PubMed articles with PMID numbers. The chapters are organized in a uniform manner, and there are hundreds of tables (focusing on causes, drugs, and therapeutic interventions), a 24-page color insert, and a comprehensive index. Each clinical topic begins with the basic "Essentials of Diagnosis." These lists are the foundation for directing laboratory tests; analyzing the findings; and determining the treatment, prognosis, and recommendations for referrals of patients to specialists. The book is included in McGraw-Hill's online e-book package, *AccessMedicine*, and various third-party platforms after a publisher embargo. The book is appropriate for public and medical libraries, students, practitioners, and interested individuals.

Bates' Guide to Physical Examination and History Taking.
10th ed. Authors: Lynn S. Bickley, Peter G. Szilagyi.
Wolters Kluwer/Lippincott Williams & Wilkins, 2009.
ISBN: 9780781780582
See Also Chapter 9.5 Clinical Medicine
Recommended for: Hospital, Academic Libraries
Brandon/Hill, *Doody's Core Titles* Selection

As an internal medicine physician, Dr. Lynn Bickley writes for primary care medical education. The *Bates' Guide* (named for Barbara Bates, the original author) reflects this as she specifically addresses students in learning basic diagnostic assessment. In the introduction, Bickley encourages readers to use other resources, as well as *Bates'*, to obtain the depth necessary to understand patients' health concerns. Additionally, the author recommends using the *Bates' Pocket Guide to Physical Examination and History Taking*, 6th edition, 2008, as an abbreviated, convenient review guide. The text is divided into three units, subdivided by chapters that focus on regional systems. The first two chapters address initial assessment techniques, history taking, physical exam, recording of results, and treatment planning. There are numerous colored line drawings and photographs throughout the text, as well as tables and extensive bibliographies establishing the evidence-based research used. The text of the tenth edition includes a CD-ROM with a variety of videos and a website containing student and instructor resources. These items correspond with the written guide and demonstrate exam procedures (i.e., listening to the sounds of the heart and breath) and assessment. This edition incorporates psychosocial factors that impact health with additional issues that special populations face. *Bates' Guide* is considered a classic in the field and is recommended for medical students, nursing students, and new practitioners.

DeGowin's Diagnostic Examination. 9th ed. Editors: Richard F. LeBlond, Donald D. Brown, Richard L. DeGowin. McGraw-Hill, 2009.
http://www.accessmedicine.com/
http://extranet.netlibrary.com/TitleSelect/
ISBN: 9780071478984
ISBN: 9780071605748
See Also Chapter 9.5. Clinical Medicine
Recommended for: Hospital Libraries
Brandon/Hill, *Doody's Core Titles* Selection

"Not only to perceive the thing sharply, but to perceive the relationships between many things sharply perceived"—Theodore Roethke. Drawing connections between the truth of the whole person and the detail of the variety of physical signs and symptoms, *DeGowin's Diagnostic Examination* is peppered with various quotes giving context to the medical material. In the first chapter, the contributors cite the need for excellent differential diagnostic skills, which are often missing in an era of technology. Ensuing chapters cover, in a sequential manner, the examination by bodily systems, regions, and the psycho-social contribution to health. This new version features updated, evidence-based content, additional color photographs, and enhanced line drawings. This classic manual is almost pocket-sized, with 914 small-print pages. The eighth edition was completely reorganized for user-friendly reference, and the ninth edition includes the option to download the information to hand-held devices, thereby eliminating the need for the print manual at the bedside or examination room. The breadth and depth of this book makes it a vital addition to medical libraries and the hip pocket of medical professionals.

Diagnostic and Statistical Manual of Mental Disorders: DSM-IV-TR. 4th ed., text revision. American Psychiatric Association, 2000.
http://www.psychiatryonline.com/
ISBN: 0890420246
ISBN: 0890423342 (Online)
See Also Chapter 9.10. Psychiatry
Recommended for: Hospital, Academic Libraries
Brandon/Hill, *Doody's Core Titles* Selection

First published in 1952 and most recently revised in 2000, the next updated version of the *Diagnostic and Statistical Manual of Mental Disorders* (*DSM*) is not expected until at least 2012. The *DSM* first standardized the nomenclature of mental and behavioral syndromes and patterns. It is used widely across disciplines as a method for consistently identifying, referencing, and researching psychological issues. The *DSM-IV-TR* (text revision) is divided into the list of classifications, the five axes used for assessment, and the descriptions of the sixteen major diagnostic groups. Also included are an excellent glossary and appendixes. Appendix D identifies the specific changes that were made to the text of this edition. The application of the *DSM* as a tool has been linked with controversy. Diagnoses are tied to insurance reimbursement for the professional and also to whether clients or patients would be able to obtain future health and life insurance based on the criteria used to assess their mental state. Additionally, the American Psychiatric Association has been accused of adjusting the definition of normative versus disorder based on contemporary political issues. The authors acknowledge multiple limitations of categorizing and applying human mental conditions for diverse cultural populations and particularly for the "nonclinical decision makers." Appendix I speaks to some particularly difficult cultural concerns. The *DSM-IV-TR* is recommended for all libraries and medical professionals.

Health Assessment & Physical Examination. 4th ed. Author: Mary Ellen Z. Estes. Cengage Learning, 2010.
http://www.r2library.com/
ISBN: 9781435427563
Recommended for: Hospital, Academic Libraries
Brandon/Hill Selection

Focused on the nursing profession, this book is a guide for assessment of the whole person—physical, psychosocial, and spiritual. The author assumes that users have studied anatomy, physiology, and basic nursing skills previously. She intends to build on this knowledge to assist nurses in becoming active problem solvers in the clinical setting. The strengths of this edition are the additions of cultural factors that impact evaluation, a geriatric health chapter, extra drawings and photographs, and new content in each chapter. A CD-ROM is included that demonstrates sounds for assessments, activities, and an English-Spanish glossary. There are supplemental online products for students and instructors that can enhance and interconnect the print content. The 26 chapters are written for ease of use, beginning with a list of competencies, side boxes with alerts, advanced techniques, checklists, and tips. Chapters end with scenarios, review questions, and NANDA

(North American Nursing Diagnosis Association) diagnoses, which emphasize the science of examination. Featured in each section is an additional side box for reflective, critical thinking issues that support the development of the art of assessment. The author includes references, bibliographies, and websites for further study of the topics covered in the chapter. The nursing field has several tools for holistic documentation such as ENAP (Examination, Normal Findings, Abnormal Findings, and Pathophysiology), IPPA (Inspection, Palpation, Percussion, and Auscultation), and NANDA. This edition has added the Minimum Data Set and OASIS-B1 (Outcome and Assessment Information Set) systems for across-the-discipline relevance. *Health Assessment & Physical Examination* is recommended for nursing at every level of practice.

Mosby's Manual of Diagnosis and Laboratory Tests. 4th ed. Authors: Kathleen D. Pagana, Timothy J. Pagana. Mosby Elsevier, 2010.
ISBN: 9780323057479
Recommended for: Hospital, Academic, Consumer Health Libraries

Though carried in public and consumer health libraries, this well-respected book is geared toward medical students and professionals. The authors' intent, as stated in the preface, is to provide a convenient, standard, easy-to-use and easy-to-understand manual for reference. With a nod to health care economics, they aim for timely and accurate testing through proper preparation and procedures. Each chapter is differentiated with a colored tab, which indicates the category of study. The appendixes list additional options for locating specific tests within the manual. The first page of each chapter lists the tests alphabetically. The following pages address the "why," the "how," and reporting of results. Using a consistent design, individual test descriptions supply the following information: normal findings; indications; test explanation; procedure and patient care at different stages of the procedure (with icons highlighting patient teaching priorities); test results and clinical significance; and related tests. Included are colored feature boxes focusing on clinical priorities, age-related concerns, and home care responsibilities. The authors have succeeded in their intent to provide an inclusive and convenient reference since 1998. In this fourth edition, outdated tests have been deleted, and 30 new tests have been added. There are new, as well as enhanced, photographs and illustrations in this edition. This indispensable reference manual is a must-have for medical libraries and medical offices.

Sapira's Art & Science of Bedside Diagnosis. 4th ed. Author: Jane M. Orient. Wolters Kluwer/Lippincott Williams & Wilkins, 2009.
ISBN: 9781605474113
Recommended for: Hospital, Academic Libraries

Dr. Joseph D. Sapira authored the first edition of this book, and he set the tone for all ensuing revisions in the preface, emphasizing the "artful science of clinical examination." His bias, and that of Dr. Orient in this fourth edition, is that technology and managed care have weakened the quality of care that physicians brought to their professions previously. They argue that the clinician—with the proper training, sensitivity, and curiosity—can complete a differential diagnosis faster than employing the technology that is now used for this purpose. The text does not address individual medical specialties (e.g., psychiatry); instead, it encourages a broader, whole patient-centered approach. The first five chapters focus extensively on the interview and history taking, building the record, and assessment of outward appearance. The ensuing chapters continue the assessment of the body with appendixes and references for each section. "Pearls" of wisdom are noted with a symbol, as well as flags for probable emergency situations that necessitate immediate consultation. New to this edition are revisions based on new research findings, appropriate use of the benefits and pitfalls of evidence-based medicine, and more than 300 questions accompanied by answers and discussion. Written in a conversational manner, this book should not be considered elementary. It is intended for use by both beginning practitioners and seasoned physicians who are committed to learning more about this art form. *Sapira's* is recommended for medical libraries, students, and individual doctors.

Databases and Other Electronic Resources

Isabel PRO. Isabel Healthcare, 2002.
http://www.isabelhealthcare.com
Recommended for: Hospital Libraries

After evaluating the near fatal illness of their daughter Isabel, the Maude family determined that the failure of accurate and appropriate treatment could be traced to missed, alternative diagnoses that would have aided the physicians in understanding her deteriorating health. In 2001, the Maudes, with pediatrician Joseph Britto, created the Isabel diagnosis decision support web-based system, which is sold on a subscription basis. The goal of the system is to support physicians who are expected to remember a growing body of information, which creates unrealistic expectations. The founders of the system contend that premature closure in analysis and treatment (and physician overconfidence) leads to incorrect, missed, or delayed diagnoses, which accounts for 25 percent of all malpractice suits. Isabel serves as a reminder, not a determinant of the possible diagnoses available. After taking the initial history and examination, the system displays electronic checklists that assist in organizing and managing disparate information for a more complete differential diagnosis, thus improving patient safety. Isabel PRO can be used as a stand-alone system, or it can interface with electronic medical records (such as partners Cerner, NextGen, and Allscripts) for point-of-care use. Benefits include the recognition of natural language, the capability to download to mobile devices that are Internet connected, and the offer of a free trial. The AMA has selected Isabel PRO for AMA's new web-based physician's portal. Time and further research are needed to determine the value of Isabel's innovative approach to knowledge management and patient care. Recommended for physicians.

30.4. Evidence-Based Practice

A way of providing health care that is guided by a thoughtful integration of the best available scientific knowledge with clinical expertise. This approach allows the practitioner to critically assess research data, clinical guidelines, and other information resources in order to correctly identify the clinical problem, apply the most high-quality intervention, and re-evaluate the outcome for future improvement.

—MeSH

Contributors: Donna F. Timm, Laura Wilder

Monographs

Evidence-Based Medicine: How to Practice and Teach EBM. 4th ed. Editors: Sharon E. Straus, W. Scott Richardson, Paul Glasziou, R. Brian Haynes. Elsevier/Churchill Livingstone, 2011.
ISBN: 9780702031274
Recommended for: Hospital, Academic Libraries
Brandon/Hill, *Doody's Core Titles* Selection

Now in its fourth edition, this ground-breaking book by David L. Sackett introduced the basic teachings of evidence-based medicine to physicians, students, and librarians 35 years ago. This review refers to the third edition. The clear explanation of EBM concepts found in the first two books remains in the third; however, it has been revised by Sackett's colleagues with special focus on "how EBM can be practiced in real-time in a variety of clinical settings." Other new features include an expanded section on the limitations of EBM and how to overcome them, fresh clinical examples, discussion of the problems of web-based CAT (Critically Appraised Topic) databases, and an expanded section on diagnostic decision rules. As with the second edition, *Evidence-Based Medicine* includes an interactive CD-ROM with additional material and downloadable EBM resources for mobile devices. A supporting website (http://www.cebm.utoronto.ca) provides current examples and updates. The second edition of *Evidence-Based Medicine* was included in the final Brandon/Hill list, tagged as a "minimal core list" book. The third edition is included in *Doody's Core Titles*. Written expressly for practicing clinicians, policy makers, and teachers, this classic textbook is a required purchase for hospital libraries and academic medical libraries.

How to Read a Paper: The Basics of Evidence-Based Medicine. 4th ed. Authors: Trisha Greenhalgh. Wiley-Blackwell/BMJ Books, 2010.
http://www.netlibrary.com/
http://www.ebrary.com/
http://www.eblib.com/
ISBN: 9781444334364
ISBN: 9781444323184 (Online)
Recommended for: Hospital, Academic Libraries
Brandon/Hill, *Doody's Core Titles* Selection

A classic EBM guide, *How to Read a Paper* is an engaging introduction to evidence-based medicine that explains why a paper should be read, how to find a paper worth reading, how to understand what is being read, and how to incorporate what was read into clinical practice. Written for anyone in the health professions seeking a greater understanding of the concepts of evidence-based medicine, it covers types of research, literature searching, critical appraisal of medical literature, and statistical methods used in clinical trials. Many chapters remain unchanged from the earlier editions, while the chapters on searching, qualitative research, systematic reviews, and implementing evidence-based practice have been greatly revised. The author has added two new chapters: one on quality improvement and the other on complex interventions. A best-selling text used by clinicians and students worldwide, the second edition of *How to Read a Paper* was listed in the final Brandon/Hill list. The fourth edition is included in *Doody's Core Titles* and is highly recommended for hospital and academic medical libraries.

Users' Guides to the Medical Literature: A Manual for Evidence-Based Clinical Practice. 2nd ed. Editors: Gordon Guyatt, Drummond Rennie, Maureen O. Meade, Deborah J. Cook. McGraw-Hill Medical, 2008.
http://www.jamaevidence.com/resource/520
http://www.ebrary.com/
ISBN: 9780071590365
ISBN: 9780071590341 (Print + pocket cards)
ISBN: 9780071590358 (Online)
Recommended for: Hospital, Academic Libraries
Doody's Core Titles Selection

Continuing the excellence of the highly acclaimed first edition, this version of *Users' Guides to the Medical Literature* has been completely revised and updated to reflect the evolution of medical research and evidence-based resources. *Users' Guides* is an extremely useful and well-written reference, filled with illustrations of principles and pitfalls when using clinical research in patient care decisions. Based on Guyatt's 25 influential *JAMA* articles published from 1993 to 2000, this is a guide for "any clinician who wishes to understand the medical literature and to use it more effectively in solving patient problems." Divided into seven sections ("The Foundations," "Therapy," "Harm," "Diagnosis," "Prognosis," "Summarizing the Evidence," and "Moving from Evidence to Action"), the authors "start with the assumption that the medical literature is the single most powerful resource in medicine, moving on to clearly explain the principles of EBM and guidelines for accessing and evaluating scientific articles." All sections, except the introduction to evidence-based medicine (EBM), cover the basics as well as more advanced topics, making *Users' Guides* appropriate for all readers, from beginning students to experienced clinicians and teachers. Online versions of the second edition of *Users' Guides to the Medical Literature* are found in ebrary and JAMAevidence. An essential purchase title in *Doody's Core Titles, Users' Guides* is recommended for academic medical libraries and hospital libraries that support residency programs or medical research. A second, similarly titled publication by Guyatt, *Users' Guide to the Medical Literature: Essentials of Evidence-Based Clinical Practice*, contains a condensed version of this guide, focusing primarily on practicing clinicians. (2nd ed., 2008, ISBN 9780071590389).

Journals

ACP Journal Club (within ***Annals of Internal Medicine***). v. 148, n. 3, American College of Physicians, May 2008.
http://www.acpjc.org/
ISSN: 10568751
ISSN: 15398560 (Online)
See Also Chapter 10.10. Internal Medicine
Indexed in: MEDLINE, CINAHL
Recommended for: Hospital, Academic Libraries
Brandon/Hill Selection

Published by the American College of Physicians *ACP Journal Club* provides the best new clinical evidence for internal medicine and related specialties from over 130 clinical journals. The content presentation encourages rapid understanding and practical assimilation by clinicians. *ACP Journal Club* identifies high-quality, original studies and systematic reviews using defined criteria and clinical ratings. Structured abstracts summarize the most important articles, and clinical experts offer commentary. Published initially as a bimonthly, stand-alone journal (v. 114, suppl, 1991–v. 148, n.2, Mar/Apr 2008), it became a monthly feature of *Annals of Internal Medicine* in 2008. Each issue of the online version includes an editorial with 12 abstracts and their commentaries. Citations and references provide links to the PubMed entries and full text of the primary source when available. The online version from the American College of Physicians contains a searchable 10-year full-text archive with useful filters such as treatment, diagnosis, prognosis, and etiology. Indexed in MEDLINE beginning with v. 116, 1992, *ACP Journal Club* is also found in EBSCOhost and ProQuest databases and in Embase. Most online vendors provide full text from 2002 to the present. Ovid MEDLINE includes it as a resource in its Evidence-Based Medicine Reviews. Listed in the final Brandon/Hill list, this is the prototypical EBM journal and is included in lists of top ranked EBM resources. It is an essential journal for hospital and academic libraries.

Evidence-Based Medicine. v. 1, BMJ Group, 1995.
http://ebm.bmj.com/
http://www.ovid.com/
ISSN: 13565524
ISSN: 14736810 (Online)
Indexed in: MEDLINE, CINAHL
Recommended for: Hospital, Academic Libraries

The main purpose of *Evidence-Based Medicine* is to select, summarize, and critique important articles that are judged relevant for clinical practice. Written expressly for practicing clinicians, *EBM* reports important advances in internal medicine, general and family practice, surgery, psychiatry, pediatrics, and obstetrics and gynecology. About 50,000 articles from over 100 peer-reviewed journals are scanned yearly, but *EBM* selects only those that meet strict criteria for their quality and validity of research. *Evidence-Based Medicine's* EBM Roundup section is intended for "those who teach, study, and practice EBM" and includes articles on concepts, resources, research, and teaching. Published bimonthly by BMJ, *Evidence-Based Medicine* is indexed in major databases, including MEDLINE, CINAHL, Embase, and Scopus. *EBM* is available in both print and online formats. The online archive from 2000–2005 is freely available to all with free online registration at the BMJ website. Current online access is available from BMJ Journals and Journals@Ovid. Considered an important evidence-based resource for practicing clinicians, *Evidence-Based Medicine* is recommended for hospital and academic medical libraries.

Databases and Other Electronic Resources

ACP-PIER. American College of Physicians, 2009.
http://pier.acponline.org/index.html
http://online.statref.com/
Recommended for: Hospital, Academic Libraries

ACP-PIER stands for "American College of Physicians-Physicians' Information and Education Resource." It is an evidence-based decision support tool designed for locating clinical answers at the point of care, and it is made available to ACP members by subscription and to institutions through STAT!Ref. It is available both on the web and for mobile devices. There are two ways of finding information: (1) enter search terms and click "Search" or (2) browse the "Disease" modules in the table of contents. Each disease module presents guidance statements and graded recommendations developed from information found in peer-reviewed journals and textbooks. Each recommendation contains the following: "Rationale," "Evidence," and "Comments." Every guideline or recommendation receives a rating from A to C, and each citation referenced in a module receives an evidence rank from level 1 to 3. All studies referenced in the database must meet specific criteria for a given study type, increasing the validity and applicability of studies for clinical practice. PIER also links the user to drug information from the AHFS DI Essentials database. Editorial consultants update the disease modules continually, and new modules are added monthly. When warranted, more frequent updates are made based on the release of important new studies, drug therapies, and practice guidelines. The new modules are located at the top of the table of contents in the "What's New" section. Since each disease module is formatted with headings similar to chapters in a book, it is simple for the searcher to locate information and easy for the instructor to teach students how to use this evidence-based resource. In addition, point-of-care continuing medical education credits are offered in accordance with the American Medical Association's limit of 20 credits per year.

Cochrane Database of Systematic Reviews. Cochrane Collaboration, 2010.
http://www.cochrane.org/reviews/index.htm
Indexed in: MEDLINE
Recommended for: Hospital, Academic Libraries

The Cochrane Database of Systematic Reviews is the gold standard for evidence-based systematic reviews. It is part of the Cochrane Library, a regularly updated collection of evidence-based databases. Access to the full text of the Cochrane Reviews is available on a pay-per-view basis or through institutional subscription. The reviews are published quarterly, providing the best available evidence on drugs, interventions, and therapies applicable to specific circumstances. The purpose of the reviews is to facilitate health care decisions made by clinicians, patients, and policy makers. While most Cochrane Reviews are based upon randomized controlled trials (RCTs), other types of information may be taken into consideration when appropriate. Each systematic review identifies specific diseases or health care problems, determining which interventions work. Authors pose a specific clinical question, formulate inclusion and exclusion criteria, extract and combine data from as many relevant scientific studies (RCTs) as possible, and draw conclusions based on that data. Systematic reviews adhere to a methodologically rigorous design to minimize bias and ensure reliability. The authors' conclusions are subdivided into "Implications for Practice" and "Implications for Research." In addition, a plain-language statement summarizing the review is provided for the benefit of patients and consumers. After a Cochrane Review is published, the authors are responsible for regularly updating their review, usually about once a year. Furthermore, the Cochrane editorial team and external referees check each systematic review at all stages of the process to ensure the highest quality.

DynaMed. EBSCO, 2010.
http://www.ebscohost.com/dynamed/
Recommended for: Hospital, Academic Libraries

DynaMed is a clinical reference tool that is part of EBSCO Publishing's suite of products. It is fee-based, available online, and provides online support for mobile devices such as the iPhone and iPod Touch. DynaMed is an evidence-based clinical reference tool designed for use at the point of care. It contains over 3,000 clinical topics, and the database is updated daily. Medical experts monitor 500 clinical journals, evaluating articles for clinical relevance and scientific validity. Special features include: (1) a seven-step protocol for evaluating the medical literature, (2) graded recommendations based on studies and practice guidelines evaluated by a panel of medical experts, and (3) a free weekly e-newsletter that highlights one article of clinical significance most likely to change clinical practice. There are three ways to find information: (1) browse by topic, using the A to Z index; (2) browse topics by category; and (3) search for specified terms. Evidence reports are labeled as level 1 (likely reliable evidence), level 2 (mid-level evidence), or level 3 (lacking direct evidence). Recommendations are labeled as grade A recommendation (consistent high-quality evidence), grade B recommendation (inconsistent or limited evidence), or grade C recommendation (lacking direct evidence). Recommendations provided by the U.S. Preventive Services Task Force have a more complex rating scheme that is explained in detail on DynaMed's website. Each disease summary hyperlinks the user to resources such as the Cochrane Library and provides LinkOut to PubMed and EBSCO ejournals. Bibliographic references are provided as well.

PubMed. National Library of Medicine, 2010.
http://www.pubmed.gov
http://www.ncbi.nlm.nih.gov/pubmed/
See Also Chapter 1. Allied Health, Chapter 32. History of the Health Sciences, Chapter 34.2. Indexing and Database Resources
Recommended for: Hospital, Academic Libraries

PubMed is both an interface and a tool for searching the medical literature. It provides access to MEDLINE, the premier biomedical research database, indexing over 5,500 journals published in 70 countries from 1966 to present. PubMed is a free resource developed and maintained by the National Center for Biotechnology Information (NCBI) at the U.S. National Library of Medicine (NLM). A unique feature of PubMed is its controlled vocabulary, also known as "Medical Subject Headings" (MeSH). In addition to MEDLINE, PubMed offers in-process citations that have not been indexed with MeSH, OLDMEDLINE (pre-1966) citations, citations to articles from general science and general chemistry journals (for which the life sciences articles are indexed with MeSH for MEDLINE) and citations to articles submitted by authors of NIH-funded research. PubMed provides special search options found on the "PubMed Clinical Queries" page. From this page, the user can take an evidence-based approach to searching the literature by entering a topic, selecting the clinical question type, and targeting specific publication types. Through PubMed's "LinkOut" feature, the user can access a wide array of full-text publications, biological databases, consumer health information, and research tools. Approximately 40 percent of PubMed is linked to full-text articles on publishers' websites. The user may be required to register or pay a fee for access to the full text, unless the user's institution subscribes to the journal in which a selected article appears.

31. Ethics

The philosophy or code pertaining to what is ideal in human character and conduct. Also, the field of study dealing with the principles of morality.

—MeSH

Contributor: Margie Garner

Monographs

Bi-Annual DeVos Medical Ethics Colloquy Series. Various authors. DeVos Medical Ethics Colloquy, 2005.
http://www.devoscolloquy.org/
Recommended for: Hospital, Academic, Consumer Health Libraries

The *Bi-Annual DeVos Medical Ethics Colloquy Series* is a forum started in 2005 in Grand Rapids, Michigan, at the Cook-DeVos Center for Health Sciences of Grand Valley State University, to bring the medical community and the public together to closely examine a current hot topic in medical ethics. Two scholars considered "national experts in the field" are invited to speak at each Colloquy. Following each speaker is a question-and-answer session that provides interaction—one of the pillars of the Colloquy format—between members of the audience and the speakers. The currency of each topic, coupled with the frequency of the Colloquy, keeps this resource fresh and up-to-date. According to Dr. Luis Tomatis, Director of Medical Affairs for the DeVos Family, this free event is "...open to everyone...a conversation, not a lecture. It is important that all different people come together, ask questions, and discuss these important issues." Each Colloquy is recorded, transcribed, edited, and published for distribution free of charge in a softbound edition or PDF file. Print copies are also available through several vendors, each setting their own price. Free print copies or PDF files can be obtained through the Devos Medical Ethics Colloquy website. Topics of Colloquy to date include the following: *Disparities in Healthcare in the USA*; *The Human Genome and Genetic Intervention: Stem Cells, Embryos and Ethics—Is There a Way Forward?*; *End-of-Life Care*; *The Beginning of Life*; *Gene Ownership & Patents*; *Universal Health Care*; *Public Policy vs. Personal Choice: The HPV Vaccine Debate*; *Patient Rights vs. Doctor Conscience*; *The Mental Health Challenge: Treating Patients and Protecting Society*; *Nature and Nurture: Their Contributions to Behavior*; *Rationing vs. Rationalizing Healthcare*; and *Vaccinations: Individual Responsibility or Societal Obligation?*

Code of Medical Ethics of the American Medical Association: Current Opinions with Annotations. 2010–2011 ed. Author: Council on Ethical and Judicial Affairs (AMA). American Medical Association Press, 2010.
http://www.ama-assn.org/ama/pub/physician-resources/medical-ethics/code-medical-ethics.shtml
ISBN: 9781603592093
Recommended for: Hospital, Academic Libraries
Brandon/Hill Selection

Based on the American Medical Association's *Principles of Medical Ethics*, this tool for medical professionals addresses over 200 issues in the ethical realm of medical treatment. Although this body of work is divided into nine sections that specifically address each principle, the *Code* is to be viewed and practiced as a whole. Published every two years, the 2010–2011 edition comprises the 2001 revision of the Principles, and Opinions issued through 2009. Annotations provide summarized court decisions and some state attorney general opinions that make significant reference to a principle or opinion; summaries of selected articles from the literature are provided as well. The *Principles of Medical Ethics* may be viewed online or purchased from the AMA website.

Intervention and Reflection: Basic Issues in Bioethics. 9th ed. Author: Ronald Munson. Wadsworth/Cengage, 2011.
ISBN: 9781111186562
Recommended for: Hospital, Academic Libraries

This text's currency and comprehensive scope sets *Intervention and Reflection* apart from other books. The longevity of this work speaks to its quality and timeliness. This textbook continues to be the choice for ethics/philosophy courses in medical curricula. With each edition, the author revises the material to ensure and sustain currency until a newer edition might be produced. This review refers to the eighth edition, which is presented in five parts: "Rights," "Controls," "Resources," "Terminations," and "Foundations of Bioethics: Ethical Theories, Moral Principles, and Medical Decisions." Consistent with earlier editions, each chapter provides case presentations, social contexts, chapter introductions, and decision scenarios. Significantly revised in this edition is the chapter on reproduction control, addressing "genetic testing that may lead to too much prevention; the growing acceptance and practice of sperm shopping; and 'savior' siblings through assisted reproduction." Undergraduate and graduate students alike will find this text appropriate for their level of study, whether introductory or professional.

Journals

BMC Medical Ethics. v. 1, BioMed Central, 2000.
http://www.biomedcentral.com/bmcmedethics/
http://www.ncbi.nlm.nih.gov/pmc/journals/39/
ISSN: 14726939 (Online Only)
Indexed in: MEDLINE
Recommended for: Hospital, Academic Libraries

Founded in 2000, this peer-reviewed, open access journal is a product of BioMed Central, a membership-based publisher and repository established to make research freely accessible to all. Original research accepted for publication addresses ethical issues relevant to "biomedical research and clinical practice, including professional choices and conduct, medical technologies, healthcare systems and health policies." The unique quality of an online-only journal is that large amounts of data, in a variety of media, can be published and then manipulated by the reader for observation from a number of perspectives. Authors also have the option of including links to other relevant sources. Upon publication, each article is permanently maintained in PubMed Central, the National Library of Medicine's repository for life science literature. MEDLINE, CINAHL Plus, and PsycINFO are some of the major indexes that include *BMC Medical Ethics*.

Journal of Medical Ethics. v. 1, BMJ Publishing /Institute of Medical Ethics, 1975.
http://jme.bmj.com/
http://www.ncbi.nlm.nih.gov/pmc/journals/168/
ISSN: 03066800
ISSN: 14734257 (Online)
Indexed in: MEDLINE, CINAHL
Recommended for: Hospital, Academic Libraries

This peer-reviewed, international journal for health care professionals and researchers in medical ethics was founded in 1975 by the Institute of Medical Ethics (IME), which now shares ownership of the journal with BMJ Publishing Group, a subsidiary of the British Medical Association. The mission of the Institute—founded in 1972 as the Society for the Study of Medical Ethics—and thus the mission of the *Journal of Medical Ethics* is to promote and inspire debate and high academic standards in this continually evolving field, to involve all disciplines, and to stimulate research in specific areas, while promoting ethical reflection and conduct in scientific research and medical practice. By 1989, the IME had such a strong influence that ethics was introduced into medical school curricula. The international reach and scope of *JME* is maintained through the appointment of an International Editorial Advisory Board. The monthly journal provides original research, articles, case reports, book reviews, editorials, correspondence, and news. "Online First" articles have been peer-reviewed and accepted for publication, but these are not yet part of an issue. "Editor's choice" articles are designated by a logo and are freely accessible. Authors may make their work open access from date of publication, if they so choose, through an "Unlocked service" option, which is also designated by a logo. Another significant feature is that subscribers are provided a free full archive back to volume 1, and non-subscribers who register have free access to all issues from volume 1 through 2005. PubMed Central also offers restricted access to some of the content.

32. History of the Health Sciences

A record of earlier events, usually with some sort of analysis and interpretation.

—*Stedman's Medical Dictionary*, 28th ed., "History" (2006)

Contributors: Patricia E. Gallagher, Stephen J. Greenberg

Monographs

American Medical Association (AMA) Deceased Physicians Masterfile 1906–1969. American Medical Association, 1906-1969.
http://www.nlm.nih.gov/hmd/manuscripts/ead/ama556.html *[Finding Aid only]*
ISBN: none
Recommended for: Academic Libraries

This unique collection consists of professional and biographical information for AMA member and nonmember physicians that died before 1969, with a total of approximately 350,000 entries. Handwritten and typed cards were created by the AMA, which began collecting information in 1906. Information was gathered from licensing authorities, medical schools, AMA's membership records, obituaries in AMA publications and elsewhere, and local medical societies. No family or detailed health information is included, although cause of death is noted occasionally. Many, but not all, cards show education, year of graduation, and the state and year of licensure. The cards are in one long alphabetical sequence, with no other internal breakdown or organization. It is a resource of enormous value to genealogists and other researchers, especially once its strengths and weaknesses are understood. It would be an attractive proposition to have the information on the cards placed in a database, but the utter lack of uniformity makes this a daunting task. The data would need to be keyboarded manually. It is clear that the information was updated (by hand, in ink, and pencil) on an ongoing if somewhat haphazard basis. Some of the cards contain basic, factual data only; others include notations scribbled on every blank bit of real estate. Information from the cards can be obtained upon request from the History of Medicine Reference Division of the National Library of Medicine (NLM), where the collection is maintained.

Chiropractic: An Illustrated History. Editors: Dennis Peterson, Glenda Wiese. Mosby, 1995.
See Chapter 3. Chiropractic

A Doctor of Their Own: The History of Adolescent Medicine. Author: Heather Munro Prescott. Harvard University Press, 1998.
See Chapter 9.1 Adolescent Medicine

The DOs: Osteopathic Medicine in America. 2nd ed. Author: Norman Gevitz. Johns Hopkins University Press, 2004.
See Chapter 9.9. Osteopathic Medicine

Familiar Medical Quotations. Editor: Maurice B. Strauss. Little, Brown, 1968.
ISBN: 9780700001231
ISBN: 9780316819152
Recommended for: Hospital, Academic Libraries

Modeled on *Bartlett's Familiar Quotations*, this 1968 work is the most extensive of the available medical quotation guides. It is organized by broad subject word, but contains a detailed word index, and an author index. The only "authors" not listed in the author index are the Bible and Shakespeare, ostensibly because of the number of references attributed to them. Since it has not been revised, late twentieth-century references are lacking; however, it is far more extensive and better indexed than more recent publications of this genre.

The Greatest Benefit to Mankind: A Medical History of Humanity from Antiquity to the Present. Author: Roy Porter. HarperCollins, 1997.
ISBN: 9780002151733
Recommended for: Hospital, Academic, Consumer Health Libraries

For those times when a single volume narrative history of medicine is required, this book is the best choice. It was never designed for light summer reading, but one can easily pick it up and read cover to cover or select a specific topic from its excellent index. Ray Porter was a prolific writer who utilized armies of researchers, but his narrative style is compelling, readable, and informative. One of the book's many strengths is the excellent suggestions for further reading that follow each chapter. It is, however, mainstream medicine; fields such as dentistry and nursing are not broadly explored. Another of this book's charms is its availability in a reasonably priced paperback edition.

Osteopathic Medicine: A Reformation in Progress. Editors: R. Michael Gallagher, Frederick J. Humphrey II, Marc S. Micozzi. Churchill Livingstone, 2001.
See Chapter 9.9. Osteopathic Medicine

Morton's Medical Bibliography: An Annotated Check-List of Texts Illustrating the History of Medicine (Garrison and Morton). 5th ed. Editor: Jeremy M. Norman. Scolar Press, 1991.
ISBN: 9780859678971
Recommended for: Hospital, Academic Libraries

Although it is not getting any younger and there is no new edition on the horizon, *Morton's Medical Bibliography*, which is also known as *Garrison and Morton*, is still the first stop for history of medicine citations. Indexed by subject and author, it provides the benchmark list of historically significant books and articles along with brief notes explaining the significance of each entry. The book is organized using a broad array of subject areas: complete works, diseases, and medical specialties, following a chronological arrangement of materials within each area. It is the only truly indispensable book in the field. It is most useful for material published before 1980.

Journals

Bulletin of the History of Medicine. v. 7, Johns Hopkins University Press, 1939.
http://muse.jhu.edu/journals/bhm/
ISSN: 00075140
ISSN: 10863176 (Online)
Indexed in: MEDLINE
Recommended for: Hospital, Academic Libraries

Begun in 1933 as the *Bulletin of the Institute of the History of Medicine* and a mere "supplement" to the *Johns Hopkins Hospital Bulletin* (which became known as the *Bulletin of the Johns Hopkins Hospital*), this is one of two great American journals devoted solely to the subject. Now jointly published by the Institute and the American Association for the History of Medicine (AAHM), it is arguably the most prestigious journal in the field. Its pages are full of valued works by the great practitioners: Henry E. Sigerist was its first editor, and the initial volume contained articles by Fielding H. Garrison, John Ruhräh, Owsei Temkin, and William Wilmer. An article by Garrison appeared in volume 1, part 2—Revised Students' Checklist of Texts Illustrating the History of Medicine, with References for Collateral Reading—which is the grandfather of the formidable *Garrison and Morton's Medical Bibliography*. In fact, it is Garrison's last published work on the subject. He died in 1935, and the burden fell to Leslie T. Morton. The *Bulletin* is a perquisite of membership in AAHM, and it is available online through Project MUSE. It is peer reviewed and indexed in MEDLINE.

Index Medicus. v. 1, F. Leypoldt, 1879-1927.
ISSN: 08913986
Recommended for: Hospital, Academic, Libraries
Brandon/Hill Selection

First published in 1879 as a supplement to the *Index-Catalogue of the Library of the Surgeon-General's Office, United States Army*, this great-granddad of medical bibliographies provides the best access to the journal literature for the period from 1879 to 1927. More information on the history of the index in its various formats can be located at the National Library of Medicine's FAQ: *Index Medicus* Chronology: http://www.nlm.nih.gov/services/indexmedicus.html. Indexed by author and by subject, the volumes are broken by years or, in some cases, into two or three volumes per year. For complete research on a topic, researchers need to understand that the subject must be examined in every volume for this period.

Isis. v. 1, University of Chicago Press for the History of Science Society, 1913.
http://www.journals.uchicago.edu/toc/isis/current
http://www.jstor.org/journals/00211753.html
ISSN: 00211753
ISSN: 15456994 (Online)
Indexed in: MEDLINE
Recommended for: Hospital, Academic Libraries

The journal's subtitle succinctly explains the publication's focus: "An International Review Devoted to the History of Science and Its Cultural Influences." Begun in 1912 by George Sarton in Belgium, *Isis* became the official publication of the History of Science Society (HSS) when that group was founded in 1924, largely to secure the future of *Isis*. Early issues are primarily in French, along with some German, Italian, and English. It contains peer-reviewed articles and news from the field, but it is perhaps best known for its book reviews. An average issue will have 60 or 70 reviews. *Isis* is indexed in MEDLINE. As a history of science—not history of medicine—journal, its scope is considerably broader than that of the other recommended journals. *Isis* is edited in

Canada, but published by the University of Chicago Press. A subscription is a perquisite of membership in HSS, and it is available online.

Journal of the History of Medicine and Allied Sciences. v. 1, Oxford University Press, 1946.
http://jhmas.oxfordjournals.org/
ISSN: 00225045
ISSN: 14684373 (Online)
Indexed in: MEDLINE
Recommended for: Hospital, Academic Libraries

The *Journal of the History of Medicine and Allied Sciences* (*JHMAS*) has evolved in a different manner than *Isis* or the *Bulletin of the History of Medicine* (*BHM*). Never the official organ of an intellectual society, it has had a rather peripatetic existence since its first issue in 1946. It has lived with its editor of the moment and has had a string of publishers. It has found a home at Yale, the University of Minnesota, the Uniformed Services University of the Health Sciences, and Duke University. Since 1997, it has been published by the Oxford University Press, although it has always been edited in the United States. *JHMAS* also has some claims to fine presswork; for a number of years it was printed by the Stinehour Press. As befits its title, *JHMAS* features a somewhat broader approach than *BHM* (though not as broad as *Isis*). There are peer-reviewed articles, book reviews, and occasional exchanges of letters. It is indexed in MEDLINE. Subscriptions are available through the Oxford University Press in both print and online formats.

Databases and Other Electronic Resources

History of the Health Sciences Section/MLA Web Links. History of the Health Sciences Section of the Medical Library Association, 2002, updated 2010.
http://www.mla-hhss.org/histlink.htm
Recommended for: Hospital, Academic Libraries

This list of web links is a quality-filtered guide to websites devoted to the broad history of the health sciences. The site attempts to guide users to the best that is available, using broad categories such as associations, museums, biography and full-text historical books, databases, websites for children, history of diseases, general chronologies and histories, listservs, journals, history of health sciences libraries, and archives and educational programs.

Images from the History of Medicine (IHM). U.S. National Library of Medicine, Accessed: 03/08/2010.
http://www.ihm.nlm.nih.gov/
Recommended for: Hospital, Academic Libraries

Images from the History of Medicine is a free database of over 70,000 images from the History of Medicine Division of the National Library of Medicine. Included here are portraits, photographs, caricatures, and posters from the fifteenth to the twenty-first century. The database was totally redesigned in 2009 and now includes many enhancements, including a personalized workspace and higher-resolution, downloadable images (zipped JPEG format). The workspace allows the user to simultaneously display images from multiple searches. Metadata has also been enhanced, including more detail on image copyright status. Keyword searching is the most effective means of accessing the database. Displayed images show metadata along with the image, allowing the searcher easier access to the search terms available. Links are provided to NLM copyright information and a source for publication-quality reproductions. Free registration is required to "save, manage, use, and share images."

IndexCat. U.S. National Library of Medicine, 2004.
http://www.indexcat.nlm.nih.gov/
Recommended for: Hospital, Academic Libraries

IndexCat is the online version of the *Index-Catalogue of the Library of the Surgeon-General's Office, United States Army.* The Army Surgeon-General's Library, predecessor to NLM, eventually published 61 volumes in three complete and two partial series between 1880 and 1961, making it the first comprehensive catalog of what would become the world's largest medical library. *Index Catalogue* was not conceived as an attempt to index the history of the health sciences, but, as time passed, it became just that through its coverage of books, dissertations, journal titles and selected articles, portraits, obituaries, and myriad other types of materials found in this vast resource. This database maintains the volume/series concept. Searches reveal results by book series, which can be searched together or independently. Both simple text word and advanced search features are available, allowing the searcher to use Boolean combinations, phrase searches, or limit to specific fields, such as author, title, journal title, and subject.

PubMed. National Center for Biotechnology Information (NCBI), 1996.
http://www.ncbi.nlm.nih.gov/pubmed/
See Also Chapter 1. Allied Health, Chapter 30.4. Evidence-Based Practice, Chapter 34: 34.2. Indexing and Database Resources
Recommended for: Hospital, Academic Libraries
Brandon/Hill Selection

With article citations going back to 1947 (as well as to even older PubMed Central articles) and an extensive indexing of secondary resources about the history of medicine, MEDLINE—with free access through PubMed—is an essential resource for any researcher in the history of the health sciences. The MeSH thesaurus provides several access points for effective searching and retrieval precision: the "history" subheading; "history" subject headings; and "historical article," "biography," "classical article," and "festschrift" publication types. Also available through the PubMed search interface is the History of Medicine subset. All can be used to retrieve secondary resource articles discussing the history of medicine. Citations to important primary resources in the history of twentieth-century medicine are also available; examples include the 1953 Watson and Crick article in *Nature* along with Salk's and Sabin's original articles on polio vaccination. As the OLDMEDLINE subset of the database grows, so too will the usefulness of this already invaluable resource.

33. Health Education

Education that increases the awareness and favorably influences the attitudes and knowledge relating to the improvement of health on a personal or community basis.
—MeSH

Contributors: Amber Burtis, Mary K. Taylor

Monographs

Coalitions and Partnerships in Community Health. Author: Frances D. Butterfoss. Jossey-Bass, 2007.
ISBN: 9780787987855
Recommended for: Academic Libraries

This highly acclaimed resource achieves the author's goal for this book to be a "one-stop shop for the tools needed to be successful in collaborative work." Building on her 15 years of experience in the field as a practitioner, consultant, and academic, Butterfoss successfully blends analysis, theory, and practice. The book is divided into four sections. The first part presents historical foundations, principles and definitions of coalitions, and theoretical models and frameworks including Community Coalition Action Theory (CCAT). The second section discusses the roles and responsibilities of coalition leaders and members, essential processes (communication, decision making, conflict resolution), and coalition infrastructures. Part Three deals with marketing coalitions, funding, and sustainability. The fourth section covers community assessment, planning, activities and interventions, evaluation, and future trends. The book contains useful tables, figures, charts, and exhibits. Each chapter concludes with review questions, and where appropriate, a "Coalition Spotlight" in which the principles of the chapter are illustrated in a case involving a real coalition. This resource is appropriate for both practitioners and for use as a course textbook. It is highly recommended as a purchase for academic libraries supporting health education programs, and is an essential resource for libraries serving community health MPH programs.

Community-Based Participatory Research for Health: From Process to Outcomes. 2nd ed. Editors: Meredith Winkler, Nina Wallerstein. Jossey-Bass, 2008.
ISBN: 9780470260432
Recommended for: Academic Libraries
Doody's Core Titles Selection

By identifying a community's issues of concern and engaging them in working for social change, community-based participatory research (CBPR) has received increasing attention as a promising approach to addressing health disparities and social problems. A *Doody's* core title, the second edition of this work is one of the most respected overviews of the theory and application of CBPR. Organized into six broad sections with 21 chapters, topics include: trends; theoretical, historical, and practice roots of CBPR; experimental design; working with diverse communities; selecting issues and evaluating outcomes with CBPR; methodological and ethical considerations in planning and conducting CBPR; and the future of CBPR. A bonus feature of the book is the 12 appendixes that provide a plethora of tools and applications, including sample protocols, recommendations for completing Institutional Review Board proposals, reliability-tested guidelines for assessment of CBPR research, and listings for CBPR networks in North America. Contributors to this work are community partners, academic researchers, and practitioners. A key resource for students, practitioners, and researchers conducting research in communities affected by health disparities, this book is highly recommended for academic library collections that support health education and public health programs.

Designing Health Messages: Approaches from Communication Theory and Public Health Practice. Editors: Edward W. Maibach, Roxanne L. Parrott. Sage, 1995.
ISBN: 9780803953987
Recommended for: Academic Libraries

This text successfully demonstrates the use of communication and health behavior change theory and research to create effective health education and health promotion campaigns. Part I focuses on theory, Part II on "audience-centered strategies," and Part III includes chapters dealing with policy, administration, and the market when designing health messages. Individual chapters include types of appeals (decision making, risk reduction, fear and persuasive), market and audience segmentation research, gatekeeping, and database marketing. The blend of theory, research, and practice makes this a valuable text for its intended audience of undergraduates and graduate students in health communication and social marketing courses, and also for health education and public health students. This book is an important resource for academic libraries serving health education programs.

Health Behavior and Health Education: Theory, Research, and Practice. 4th ed. Editors: Karen Glanz, Barbara K. Rimer, Kasisomayajula Viswanath. Jossey-Bass, 2008.
ISBN: 9780787996147
Recommended for: Academic Libraries

This preeminent text in the health education field was the first to provide an in-depth and comprehensive look at health behavior theories in one volume. First published in 1990, it remains an essential title for graduate students, practitioners, and researchers interested in health behavior. Contributors are some of the best-known academics and practitioners in the field. Made up of 22 chapters in five parts, topics include the theory and practice of health education, models of individual and interpersonal health behavior, community and group models of health behavior change, and the application of theory to research and practice. Now in its fourth edition, the text includes expanded coverage of health disparities, social marketing, health communication, and e-health. This book is highly recommended for academic library collections that support health-related programs, including health education, public health, health care management, and psychology.

Health Education Evaluation and Measurement: A Practitioner's Perspective. 2nd ed. Authors: Robert J. McDermott, Paul D. Sarvela. McGraw-Hill, 1999.
ISBN: 9780697223227
Recommended for: Academic Libraries

Recognized as one of the best books on evaluation for health educators, the text is arranged in 16 chapters that cover the following topics: models for conducting program development, the politics and ethics of program evaluation, type of measures, reliability and validity of measurement, pilot testing, needs assessment and strategic planning, quantitative evaluation design, qualitative evaluation design, survey methods, sampling, statistical analysis of data, assessing program cost and effects, and preparing an evaluation report. Now in its second edition, the work includes updated and expanded learning tools in the form of detailed chapter objectives, essential key terms, and relevant case studies. Also useful are the recommended readings at the end of each chapter and a glossary of key terms. A key resource for students, practitioners, and researchers during all stages of program planning and research, this book is recommended for academic library collections that support health education and public health programs.

Health Program Planning: An Educational and Ecological Approach. 4th ed. Authors: Lawrence W. Green, Marshall W. Kreuter. McGraw-Hill, 2005.
ISBN: 9780072556834
Recommended for: Academic Libraries

First published in 1980, the "precede-proceed" model outlined in this text has become a core model in health education program planning. Written by the creators of the model, and taking an educational and ecological approach to program planning, this is the most comprehensive text to outline the principles and processes associated with this model. Divided into nine chapters, topics include social assessment; participatory planning and situation analysis; epidemiological diagnosis; health, behavioral, and environmental assessments; ecological and educational diagnosis; and the application of the model to community, occupational, educational, and health care settings. The fourth edition expands the "scope of application and range of potential users" to include public health and population health planning. Features include a companion website (http://www.lgreen.net) that provides full citations and links to PubMed abstracts for published articles that use the model, and a supplementary Instructor's Resource CD with a test bank and PowerPoint presentations for each chapter of the book. It is an essential resource for students, practitioners, and researchers involved with program planning in health education or public health. This book is recommended for academic library collections that support health education and public health programs.

Principles & Foundations of Health Promotion and Education. 4th ed. Authors: Randall R. Cottrell, James T. Girvan, James F. McKenzie. Pearson Benjamin Cummings, 2008.
ISBN: 9780321532350
Recommended for: Academic Libraries

Written by leaders in the field, this text introduces students to "the emerging profession of health education" by presenting factual information while inculcating professional values. The work is divided into ten chapters. Topics include underlying concepts, goals, and objectives of the profession; history of health education;

philosophical and theoretical foundations; ethics; credentialing and standards; roles and responsibilities; work settings; the literature of health education; and future trends. There are useful tables, charts, and diagrams. Each chapter ends with "Critical Thinking" questions, a case study, and links to related Internet sites. Scattered throughout the book are "Practitioner's Perspectives," in which the insights of health educators working in the field are given on the topic under discussion, as well as presenting information about their education, their current position, and how they obtained their job. This book is highly recommended for academic institutions supporting health education and public health programs.

Social Foundations of Thought and Action: A Social Cognitive Theory. Author: Albert Bandura. Prentice-Hall, 1985.
ISBN: 9780138156145
Recommended for: Academic Libraries

This classic text is an exposition of Social Cognitive Theory, a model of behavior change and learning developed by the author. The theory is driven by reciprocal determinism: a reciprocal, dynamic interaction takes place between a triad of personal factors (cognitive, affective, and biologic), a person's own behavior, and environmental factors. Vicarious learning, modeling, and self-efficacy, the individual's belief that he or she can change, are additional aspects in how people function, learn, and change. Chapters discuss other behavior models, "observational learning," forethought, diffusion of innovations, motivators, self-and cognitive regulators, and self-efficacy. The book is a core resource for academic libraries serving health education and health behavior programs.

Understanding Attitudes and Predicting Social Behavior.
Authors: Icek Ajzen, Martin Fishbein. Prentice-Hall, 1980.
ISBN: 9780139364358
Recommended for: Academic Libraries

This classic text is considered by many to be a core resource for students in graduate health education programs and health education faculty. The authors' Theory of Reasoned Action (TRA) is a behavior change model that deals with the relationship between beliefs, attitudes, intentions, and behavior. The book is divided into two parts. The first section is a multi-chapter exposition of TRA. The second section consists of several chapters, coauthored with other experts, demonstrating the practical applications of TRA in several areas, including weight loss, occupational choices, family planning behaviors, consumer behavior and marketing research, voting behavior, and alcoholism. Both theories have been heavily used by health educators. This text includes several helpful figures and tables. The appendixes are useful, including both a sample questionnaire and a step-by-step demonstration of the construction of a questionnaire based on TRA. It is highly recommended for academic libraries serving health education and health behavior graduate programs.

Journals

American Journal of Health Behavior. v. 20, PNG, 1996.
http://www.ajhb.org/
ISSN: 19457359 (Online)
Indexed in: MEDLINE, CINAHL
Recommended for: Academic Libraries

Begun in 1977 under the title, *Health Values*, this peer-reviewed journal is the official publication of the American Academy of Health Behavior. The publication focuses on multidisciplinary, original research exploring the factors that affect health behavior and the design and implementation of effective health promotion programs. The journal has an article acceptance rate of approximately 19 percent. It is ranked thirty-eighth out of 95 public, environmental, and occupation health journals (2009 *Journal Citation Reports*). It is covered by many indexing and abstracting services, including MEDLINE, CINAHL, Scopus, PsycINFO, and Social Sciences Citation Index. The journal is a required resource for academic libraries serving health behavior and health education programs, students, and faculty. Beginning in January 2010 the publication will only be available online. Articles are available at no charge with a one-year embargo for non-subscribers beginning with volume 23 (1999) at the journal's website.

American Journal of Health Education. v. 32, American Alliance for Health, Physical Education, Recreation, and Dance, 2001.
http://www.aahperd.org/aahe/publications/ajhe/
ISSN: 19325037
Indexed in: CINAHL
Recommended for: Academic Libraries

Sponsored by the American Association for Health Education (AAHE), the journal publishes peer-reviewed articles on original research, application of theory, systematic reviews, commentaries, and case studies from a variety of settings, including community, health care, occupational, and education. Special columns include "Teaching Ideas and Community," "Care Setting," and "Worksite Initiatives." The journal is geared towards health education professionals, including Certified Health Education Specialists (CHES) who have the opportunity to earn CE credit through self-study articles included in each journal issue. This is also a key resource for health educators in a variety of settings (i.e., local, state, federal agencies, community organizations, schools, and university health centers), and highly recommended for academic library collections supporting health education or public health programs, as well as libraries supporting health education professionals. The journal is indexed in Education Resources Information Center (ERIC) and CINAHL. The journal is available in print and recently became available online, beginning with volume 37, 2006.

Global Health Promotion. v. 16, Sage, 2009.
http://ped.sagepub.com/
ISSN: 17579759
ISSN: 17579767 (Online)
Indexed in: MEDLINE, CINAHL
Recommended for: Academic Libraries

Formerly known as *Promotion & Education*, this journal recently changed its name to more accurately represent its global focus. As an official journal of the International Union for Health Promotion and Education, the journal seeks to promote global health equity among the rich and poor nations of the world. *Global Health Promotion* is a multilingual (English, French, and Spanish) publication that aims to "ensure wide geographical coverage" with articles that are of "general interest to an international readership." The journal publishes peer-reviewed articles based on original research, practical applications, and reviews. The focus of articles is on health promotion, health education, and public health theory. An important resource for health education professionals throughout the world and researchers and students studying global health, the journal is appropriate for academic library collections supporting health education or public health programs. Journal indexing is covered by both MEDLINE and CINAHL. Online access back to volume 1, 1994 is available through Sage Journals Online.

Health Education & Behavior. v. 24, Sage, 1997.
http://heb.sagepub.com/
ISSN: 10901981
ISSN: 15526127 (Online)
See Also Chapter 13.16. Public Health Nursing
Indexed in: MEDLINE, CINAHL
Recommended for: Academic Libraries

Formerly known as *Health Education Quarterly* (1980–1996) and *Health Education* (1974–1979), this official publication of the Society for Public Health Education (SOPHE) publishes original research articles, reviews, case studies, strategies, program evaluations, and commentary. Topics are united by "discussions of theories of health behavior and health status, as well as strategies to improve social and behavioral health." Articles include both theoretical and practical approaches to topics as diverse as HIV/AIDS, stress, social support, and international health. In 2009 the journal had an impact factor of 2.194 and ranked eighteenth out of 95 in the public, environmental, and occupational health category (2009 *Journal Citation Reports*). A key resource for practitioners, researchers, and students interested in health behavior and health education, the journal is highly recommended for academic library collections supporting health education or public health programs, as well as libraries supporting health care professionals. The journal is covered by the following major indexing services: CINAHL, MEDLINE, PsycINFO, Scopus, and Social Sciences Citation Index. Online access starting with volume 2, 1974 is available through Sage Journals Online.

Health Education Research. v. 1, Oxford University Press, 1986.
http://her.oxfordjournals.org/
ISSN: 02681153
ISSN: 14653648 (Online)
Indexed in: MEDLINE, CINAHL
Recommended for: Academic Libraries

This internationally focused, peer-reviewed research journal publishes original theoretical and practice-based articles on all aspects of health education and health promotion. It also includes book reviews. Authors may upload post-prints into institutional repositories one year after publication, or may pay a fee for immediate open access at the journal's website. This publication is covered by several education and health sciences indexing and abstracting resources such as CINAHL, Education Abstracts, Embase, MEDLINE, Scopus, and Social Sciences Citation Index. Begun in 1986, the journal currently ranks eighth out of 139 education and education research titles and twentieth out of 95 titles in public, environmental, and occupational health titles (2009 *Journal Citation Reports*). This journal is an essential resource for academic libraries serving health education and public health programs. Full online coverage back to volume 1, 1986 is available through Oxford Journals.

Health Promotion International. v. 5, World Health Organization, 1990.

http://heapro.oxfordjournals.org/
ISSN: 09574824
ISSN: 14602245 (Online)
Indexed in: MEDLINE, CINAHL
Recommended for: Academic Libraries

Published in association with the World Health Organization, this journal is an official journal of the International Union for Health Promotion and Education. The journal is peer reviewed and publishes original research articles, reviews, and commentary on topics related to the following: education, health services, employment, government, the media, industry, environmental agencies, and community networks. Articles take both theoretical and practical approaches to the subject matter. Well respected in the public health field, in 2009 the journal had an impact factor of 1.544 and ranked thirty-sixth out of 95 in the public, environmental, and occupational health category and twenty-third out of 49 in the health policy and services category (2009 *Journal Citation Reports*). An important resource for health education professionals throughout the English-speaking world and researchers and students studying global health, the journal is appropriate for academic library collections supporting health education or public health programs. The journal is covered by the following major indexing services: MEDLINE, Social Sciences Citation Index, and CINAHL. Online access back to volume 1, 1986 is available through Oxford University Press.

Health Promotion Practice. v. 1, Sage, 2000.
http://hpp.sagepub.com/
ISSN: 15248399
ISSN: 15526372 (Online)
Indexed in: MEDLINE, CINAHL
Recommended for: Academic Libraries

The journal publishes peer-reviewed articles on topics related to the practice of health education and is "unique in its focus on critical and strategic information for professionals engaged in the practice of developing, implementing, and evaluating health promotion and disease prevention programs." Article types include original research, as well as articles on evaluation, policy, health care setting, career development, racial and ethnic health disparities, teaching methods, needs assessment tools and methodologies, and educational intervention strategies. Articles also deal with a variety of settings: community, health care, work site, educational, and international. The journal seeks to "promote linkages between researchers in the academic and private sectors with health promotion and education practitioners" and "address the health issues of ethnic and racial minority populations." A key resource for practitioners, researchers, and students interested in health behavior and health education, the journal is highly recommended for academic library collections supporting health education or public health programs, as well as libraries supporting health care professionals. The journal is covered by the following major indexing services: CINAHL, MEDLINE, and PsycINFO. Online access back to volume 1, 2000 is available through Sage Journals Online.

The International Electronic Journal of Health Education. v. 1, American Association for Health Education, 1998.
http://www.aahperd.org/aahe/publications/iejhe/
ISSN: 15291944 (Online)
Indexed in: CINAHL
Recommended for: Academic Libraries

The articles in this scholarly peer-reviewed, open access journal focus on health education and promotion research, theory, and programs around the world, immigrant communities in the U.S., and other areas and topics of interest to the international health education community. The journal accepts articles written in Chinese, French, and Spanish, although most articles are in English. Authors are encouraged to include supporting electronic material (streaming media, computer software, etc.). There is a "New Resources" section presenting reviews of books and other professional media. CINAHL indexes the journal back to 1998. Recent indexing coverage is provided by ERIC, Education Abstracts, and Physical Education Abstracts. This an important resource for academic libraries serving health education programs at all levels. The journal is available online only. All volumes are available at no charge via the journal's home page at the American Association for Health Education's website.

Journal of American College Health. v. 30, Routledge, 1982.
http://www.tandf.co.uk/journals/titles/07448481.asp
ISSN: 07448481
ISSN: 19403208 (Online)
See Also Chapter 9.1. Adolescent Medicine
Indexed in: MEDLINE, CINAHL
Recommended for: Academic Libraries

Formerly titled *Journal of the American College Health Association* (1952–1982), this journal is published in cooperation with the American College Health Association. It is the only American journal that focuses solely on the health of college students, and is the preeminent journal for health care providers, health educators, and student health center administrators who are involved with college students, as well as academic researchers and students interested in the field of college health. The journal is peer reviewed and publishes original research articles, clinical and program notes, commentary, and articles grounded in practice. Topical articles include drug and tobacco use, binge drinking, sexual health, eating disorders, and mental health, but also approach college health issues from a variety of fields, such as preventive medicine, environmental health, and sports medicine. This journal is recommended for academic library collections that support student health centers and health education, public health, and psychology programs. The journal is indexed in MEDLINE. Online access starting with volume 30, 1982 is available through the Informaworld website.

Journal of School Health. v. 7, Wiley-Blackwell, 1937.
http://onlinelibrary.wiley.com/journal/10.1111/(ISSN)1746-1561
ISSN: 00224391
ISSN: 17461561 (Online)
See Also Chapter 13.18. School Nursing
Indexed in: MEDLINE, CINAHL
Recommended for: Academic Libraries

Begun in 1930 as the *Bulletin* (American Association of School Physicians) and immediately preceded by *School Physicians' Bulletin* (1930–1936), this peer-reviewed official publication of the American School Health Association presents essential material for educators, health professionals, and administrators working to improve the health of the pre-kindergarten through grade 12 population and their families while providing a healthy school environment. Articles focus on original research and scholarly literature reviews in addition to ongoing columns. There are occasional theme issues. Continuing education credit for certified health education specialists and nurses is available. The journal is covered by several indexing and abstracting services including CINAHL, ERIC, MEDLINE, Science Citation Index Expanded, Social Sciences Citation Index, and Scopus. It ranks fourth out of 27 education, scientific discipline journals; eleventh out of 139 education and educational research journals; twenty-seventh out of 69 health care sciences and services journals; and twenty-fourth out of 95 public, environmental, and occupational health journals (2009 *Journal Citation Reports*). It is a core resource for academic libraries serving health education and allied health programs. Online coverage back to volume 1, 1930, is available via Wiley Online Library.

33.1. Consumer Health Information

Information intended for potential users of medical and healthcare services. There is an emphasis on self-care and preventive approaches as well as information for community-wide dissemination and use.

—MeSH

Contributor: Barbara M. Bibel

Monographs

Complete Guide to Prescription & Non-Prescription Drugs. Rev. ed. Authors: H. Winter Griffith, Stephen Moore. Penguin Group, 2009.
ISBN: 9780399534638
Recommended for: Consumer Health Libraries

This annual publication contains a wealth of information about medications. It covers over 5,000 brand-name and 800 generic drugs. The book includes the latest information from the FDA. It provides the necessary information that patients need to take medication safely. The easy-to-use chart format includes the reason for using the drug, dosage, how to take the drug, and information about side effects and interactions with other drugs, herbs, and foods. It includes information about using medications safely, buying drugs online, compliance with doctors' instructions, substance abuse, and pregnancy risk categories. There is also a section on medical conditions and the drugs commonly used to treat them. This hefty (1,120 pages), reasonably priced paperback will be very helpful for consumers because it is easy to understand and full of objective information.

Consumer Health Informatics: Informing Consumers and Improving Health Care. Editors: Deborah Lewis, Gunther Eysenbach, Rita Kukafka, P. Zoe Stavri, Holly Jimison. Springer, 2005.
See Chapter 6.3. Informatics

Gale Encyclopedia of Alternative Medicine. 3rd ed. Editor: Jacqueline L. Longe. Gale, 2008.
http://www.gale.cengage.com/
ISBN: 9781414448725
ISBN: 9781414448770 (Online)
Recommended for: Consumer Health Libraries
Doody's Core Titles Selection

The third edition of this comprehensive guide to complementary and alternative therapies contains over 875 entries. Fifty are new and 300 have been revised and updated. The entries cover 150 types of alternative medicine ranging from acupuncture to herbal medicine to yoga and osteopathy. The entries cover recommended alternative treatments for specific diseases and conditions as well as articles about herbs, types of body work, and biographies of prominent practitoners such as Deepak Chopra, David Palmer, and Edward Bach. The encyclopedia includes information about the training and certification requirements for practitioners and evidence-based information about the efficacy of the treatments. It also has a glossary, a resource guide of print and online information, a directory of alternative medicine organizations, and a comprehensive index. The text is augmented with 450 color illustrations, including charts and pictures of medicinal plants. The accessible language and evidence-based information make this an outstanding resource for all collections. It is also available as an e-book in the Gale Virtual Reference Library. This is a *Doody's* core title.

Gale Encyclopedia of Medicine. 3rd ed. Editor: Jacqueline L. Longe. Gale, 2006.
http://www.gale.cengage.com/gvrl
ISBN: 9781414403687
ISBN: 978141440851 (Online)
See Also Chapter 1. Allied Health
Recommended for: Consumer Health Libraries

The third edition of this comprehensive, authoritative medical encyclopedia contains over 1,750 articles on diseases and conditions, treatments, drugs, anatomy and physiology, tests, and disease prevention. It also has historical and biographical information in sidebars. Nearly 700 color illustrations and a resource guide of books, periodicals, organizations, and websites supplement the text. Key medical terms are defined in text boxes within the articles. A detailed table of contents, ample cross-referencing, and a subject index make information easy to find. The reading level is high school and the language is accessible to lay readers. This edition includes more than 100 new articles and 250 updated entries. It bridges the gap between single-volume medical guides and professional clinical textbooks. This is an excellent resource for public and consumer health libraries. It is also available electronically as part of the Gale Virtual Reference Library.

Gale Encyclopedia of Mental Health. 2nd ed. Editors: Laurie J. Fundukian, Jeffrey Wilson. Gale, 2007.
http://www.gale.cengage.com/
ISBN: 9781414429878
ISBN: 9781414429908 (Online)
Recommended for: Consumer Health Libraries

This encyclopedia provides a comprehensive, accessible overview of mental health for lay readers. The 450 entries cover all of the 150 conditions included in the American Psychiatric Association's *Diagnostic and Statistical Manual* (DSM-IV-TR) as well as prescription and non-prescription drugs used to treat mental illness, diagnostic procedures, types of therapy, alternative therapies, and topics such as crisis housing and neurotransmitters. Biographies of key people in the mental health field appear, also. The articles include text boxes with definitions of key terms and resource lists with books, websites, and organizations. The coverage here is concise, well written, and thorough. The reading level is high school. This is an excellent resource for public and consumer health libraries. It is also available as an e-book in the Gale Virtual Reference Library.

Gale Encyclopedia of Surgery and Medical Tests. 2nd ed. Editor: Brigham Narins. Gale, 2008.
http://www.gale.cengage.com/
ISBN: 9781414448448
ISBN: 9781414448893 (Online)
Recommended for: Consumer Health Libraries

The second edition of this comprehensive encyclopedia for consumers and allied health students covers approximately 450 surgical procedures, medical tests, and related topics. Entries include information about common laboratory tests, anesthetics, medications, and postoperative care as well as specific surgical procedures. It also covers topics such as adult day care and Do Not Resuscitate (DNR) orders. All articles have bibliographies and key terms are defined in text boxes. They also include lists of questions to ask physicians and information about who performs the procedures. One hundred seventy-five color illustrations and photographs augment the text. The encyclopedia also has a glossary, a directory of national organizations and support groups for patients, and a list of the top medical centers for specific surgical procedures. Patients facing surgery and their families will appreciate this resource. This work is also available as an e-book through the Gale Virtual Reference Library.

Healthy Child, Whole Child: Integrating the Best of Conventional and Alternative Medicine to Keep Your Kids Healthy. 2nd ed. Authors: Stuart H. Ditchek, Russell H. Greenfield. Collins Living/HarperCollins, 2009.
ISBN: 9780061685989.
Recommended for: Consumer Health Libraries

At a time when parents wonder whether vaccines are safe and worry about the impact of video games on their children, Dr. Ditchek (New York University) and Dr. Greenfield (University of Arizona) offer a welcome new edition of their child care guide. They feel that conventional and alternative medicine are complementary and that both offer tools for promoting health. First published in 2001, the revised edition has the latest information on immunization, nutrition, stress management, and dealing with popular culture. The doctors stress the importance of good nutrition, exercise, and protection from environmental hazards. They discuss the proper use of antibiotics, treatment for specific conditions such as asthma, digestive disturbances, and skin conditions, and the use of alternative therapies (massage, Chinese medicine, guided imagery, and botanicals). Their sound advice and supportive tone as well as their useful resource guide will help parents care for their children in a complex world. This is an excellent source for public and consumer health libraries.

The Merck Manual Home Health Handbook. 3rd ed. Editor: Robert S. Porter. Merck, distributed by Simon & Schuster, 2009.
ISBN: 9780911910308
Recommended for: Consumer Health Libraries

The third edition of this lay version of the *Merck Manual* covers almost everything in the professional version in accessible language. It includes general topics such as preventing disease, disability, exercise and fitness, rehabilitation, and death and dying. There is a page explaining the structure of medical terms with prefixes and suffixes as well as a section on injuries and poisoning with first aid information. Sections on organs and organ systems and the diseases affecting them as well as sections on men's, women's, children's, and senior's health and on topics such as imaging studies, clinical trials, medical decision making, and travel health make this a very useful resource. Color illustrations, charts, and a four-page anatomy atlas, a list of drugs by generic and brand name, and a directory of organizations provide further information. This is a reasonably priced source for public and consumer health libraries.

Mosby's Dictionary of Medicine, Nursing & Health Professions. 8th ed. Elsevier, 2008.
ISBN: 9780323049375
See Also Chapter 1. Allied Health
Recommended for: Consumer Health Libraries

This dictionary for allied health students and workers is also an excellent source for consumers. With over 51,000 definitions and 2,400 color illustrations, it includes encyclopedia entries with in-depth explanations of difficult concepts. The book also has 12 appendixes with units of measurement, French and Spanish translations of common medical terms, American Sign Language communication, normal reference values, health promotion, nutrition, pharmacology and clinical calculations, infection control, diagnosis related groups, nursing interventions classification, nursing outcomes classification, and nursing diagnosis. The language is simpler than that in *Dorland's* or *Stedman's* medical dictionaries, making it more user friendly for a wide range of readers.

Shared Decision Making in the Patient-Physician Relationship: Challenges Facing Patients, Physicians, and Medical Institutions. Author: Dennis J. Mazur. American College of Physician Executives, 2001.
See Chapter 30.2. Medical Decision Making

Teen Health & Wellness: Real Life, Real Answers. Rosen Publishing Online, 2007.
See Chapter 9.1. Adolescent Medicine

Journals

Consumer Reports on Health. v. 1, Consumers Union, 1993.
http://www.consumerreports.org/health
ISSN: 10443193
Indexed in: CINAHL
Recommended for: Consumer Health Libraries

Consumer Reports on Health carries no advertising. It provides objective information about doctors, hospitals, health insurance, drugs, and natural remedies. The articles about patient safety in the hospital, best buys on prescription drugs, how to choose insurance and what to do when one has lost insurance or has none are extremely valuable. *Consumer Reports on Health* also rates fitness equipment and health devices such as treadmills, blood pressure monitors, and condoms, so that consumers can make informed choices and get the most for their money. Their website, available by subscription only, is also accessible to those who subscribe to *Consumer Reports Magazine. Consumer Reports on Health* is a useful resource for consumer health collections.

Coping with Cancer. v. 1, Media America, 1986.
http://copingmag.com
ISSN: 10438637
ISSN: 15445488
Indexed in: CINAHL
Recommended for: Consumer Health Libraries

Coping with Cancer provides support for patients and their families. It has a wide range of articles: interviews with celebrity cancer survivors; medical information; resources for financial, legal, and insurance issues; wellness information; resources for caregivers; spiritual and inspirational content; and resources for further information and support. Patients, health professionals, caregivers, and representatives of relevant organizations may publish news stories, personal stories, or inspirational material in the magazine. The website has useful information about topics such as coping with chemotherapy side effects and clinical trials. This is a popular resource for cancer patients.

Diabetes Self-Management. v. 1, Rapaport Publishing, 1983.
http://www.diabetesselfmanagement.com
ISSN: 04716253
Indexed in: MEDLINE, CINAHL
Recommended for: Consumer Health Libraries

Diabetes Self-Management provides diabetics with the tools that they need to take control of their condition. The magazine provides information about the types of diabetes, the medications used to manage the disease, instruments such as glucose monitors and injection devices for insulin delivery, nutrition and recipes, complications, and alternative therapies. Articles on practical topics such as monitoring glucose levels, meal planning, and tips such as making sure to wear a medical alert bracelet help diabetics with daily living. The website features daily news and tips, a blog, an e-mail newsletter, and resources, including an "ask an expert" feature. This is a useful resource for diabetics.

Duke Medicine Health News. v. 1, Belvoir Media Group, 1994.
ISSN: 10815880
Indexed in: MEDLINE
Recommended for: Consumer Health Libraries

Physicians from Duke University Medical Center provide commentary about current medical news in this informative newsletter. The major stories on topics such as the Mediterranean diet and its role in the reduction of heart disease, dementia, and depression include fact boxes labeled "the view from Duke" with explanations by physicians who are members of the medical school faculty. There are also news briefs and a question/answer column dealing with common health concerns. The newsletter has no advertising. It is easy to understand and provides relevant, current information for consumers.

Harvard Mental Health Letter. v. 1, Harvard Medical School, 1995.
ISSN: 08843783
Indexed in: MEDLINE, CINAHL
Recommended for: Consumer Health Libraries

The *Harvard Mental Health Letter* provides current information about mental health research, new drugs and treatments for mental illness, and discussions of controversial topics such as substance abuse and the use of antidepressants in children and adolescents. More than 8,000 physicians and researchers affiliated with the Harvard Medical School contribute articles to the newsletter. They cover common conditions such as attention deficit disorder and depression and discuss issues such as "How much therapy is enough?" and the risks and benefits of electroconvulsive therapy. This is a lively and informative publication of interest to both professional and lay readers.

JAMA: Journal of the American Medical Association. v. 1, American Medical Association, 1883.
http://jama.ama-assn.org
ISSN: 00987484
ISSN: 15383598 (Online)
See Also Chapter 1.9. Physician Assistants, Chapter 10: 10.10. Internal Medicine
Indexed in: MEDLINE, CINAHL
Recommended for: Hospital, Academic, Consumer Health Libraries
Brandon/Hill Selection

JAMA: Journal of the American Medical Association is the most widely circulated medical journal in the world. It publishes several international editions. It is also the source of many newspaper and television news reports about clinical advances and health policy. Consumers ask for it in the library so that they can see the original source. The journal has a "Patient Page" in each issue, available in English, Spanish, and French, with information about a disease or condition and its treatment options. This is a very useful resource. *JAMA* is available on the web and a number of its features are free to nonsubscribers. These include the Patient Pages, table of contents, abstracts, extracts, and excerpts from 1998 forward six months after publication. The archives are available from 1998 forward 12 months after publication.

Mayo Clinic Health Letter. v. 1, Mayo Clinic, 1998.
http://healthletter.mayoclinic.com
ISSN: 07416245
Indexed in: MEDLINE, CINAHL
Recommended for: Consumer Health Libraries

The *Mayo Clinic Health Letter* provides excellent information about health and preventive medicine, diseases and conditions, and nutrition and fitness. Among the topics covered are sinus inflammation, carotid artery disease, and kidney stones. The letter includes quizzes and healthy recipes. It also has coverage of topics such as service dogs, hand hygiene, and magnetic stimulation as therapy. There are advertisements, but they are for other Mayo Clinic books and newsletters. Articles are written by physicians on the staff of the Mayo Clinic. This is one of the oldest consumer health newsletters and it is very popular. A subscription to the print newsletter includes free online access.

New England Journal of Medicine. v. 198, Massachusetts Medical Society, 1928.
http://content.nejm.org
ISSN: 00284793
ISSN: 15334406 (Online)
See Also Chapter 1.9. Physician Assistants, Chapter 10: 10.10. Internal Medicine
Indexed in: MEDLINE, CINAHL
Recommended for: Hospital, Academic, Consumer Health Libraries
Brandon/Hill Selection

The *New England Journal of Medicine* (*NEJM*) is the oldest continuously published medical journal in the world. It is also one of the most prestigious. The research and policy issues discussed on its pages often turn up on the front page of the newspaper and on television newscasts. For this reason, consumers often ask for it. Although the language in this journal is technical, lay readers can understand it. They may need a medical dictionary, but, if they are motivated, they will make the effort. They often learn about new treatment options and clinical trials this way. *NEJM* is an important journal for consumer health collections because it is in demand. It is also available on the web, but, unless one subscribes, not all of the content is available.

NIH MedlinePlus. v. 1, National Library of Medicine, 2006.
http://medlineplus.gov
ISSN: 19374712
Recommended for: Consumer Health Libraries

NIH MedlinePlus the magazine is an extension of the MedlinePlus website. It features interviews with NIH researchers, current news about health and medical research, articles on diseases and conditions, and practical information about topics such as avoiding the flu. It is also available on the MedlinePlus website. A Spanish-language version, *NIH MedlinePlus Salud* has information about health topics of interest to the Hispanic community. The articles appear in both Spanish and English. Subscriptions to both versions of the magazine are free.

University of California, Berkeley Wellness Letter. v. 1, University of California School of Public Health, 1984.
http://www.wellnessletter.com
ISSN: 07489234
Indexed in: CINAHL
Recommended for: Consumer Health Libraries

This newsletter from the University of California, Berkeley School of Public Health focuses on prevention and maintaining a healthy lifestyle. It has outstanding coverage of nutrition and fitness, with excellent information about diet, exercise, and supplements that are worth taking. The contributors are faculty members and researchers at University of California Berkeley. They put current health news topics into perspective and evaluate and clarify them so that readers will understand them. This analysis should help readers make better decisions about their health. The newsletter has no advertisements and covers many subjects that readers will not find in other newsletters: drinking water quality and safety, equipment for an inexpensive home gym and exercises to go with it, and objective information about coffee. It is less expensive than some of the other health newsletters and well worth the price.

Databases and Other Electronic Resources

Genetics Home Reference. National Library of Medicine, 2009.
http://ghr.nlm.nih.gov/
Recommended for: Consumer Health Libraries

Genetics is a complex science that is difficult to understand. The National Library of Medicine's Genetics Home Reference website provides "consumer-friendly information about the effects of genetic variations on human health." The site has a "Help Me Understand Genetics Handbook" that explains basic concepts such as how genes and chromosomes work, mutations, and inherited conditions. It also has information on more than 450 genetic diseases and conditions, information on individual genes and chromosomes, a glossary, learning activities, information about newborn screening, and resources for patients and families, health professionals, and educators. This free site is excellent for answering questions from patients, students, and the general public.

MedlinePlus. National Library of Medicine, 1998.
http://medlineplus.gov
See Also Chapter 10.10. Internal Medicine
Recommended for: Consumer Health Libraries

The National Library of Medicine's MedlinePlus website is an outstanding resource for consumer health information. It contains current health news, a medical dictionary, a medical encyclopedia, information about more than 800 diseases and conditions, health issues in various demographic groups, and drug information. It also has health information in over 40 languages. The site has tutorials about diseases, diagnostic procedures, and surgeries as well as real time videos of surgical procedures. There are directories of hospitals, physicians, dentists, other health practitioners, and other facilities and services such as camps for children with chronic diseases and nursing home comparisons. There is a directory of consumer health libraries, too. This wonderful free resource is a foundation for consumer health and public libraries.

33.2. Health Communication

Role of communication theory, research and practice in health promotion and health care.

Contributors: Sharon Black, Marcia E. Zorn

Monographs

Applied Health Communication. Editors: Kevin B. Wright, Scott D. Moore. Hampton Press, 2008.
ISBN: 9781572737327
ISBN: 9781572737334
Recommended for: Hospital, Academic Libraries

This book promotes understanding of health communication processes and outcomes using practical application—or applied health communication—examples of theory and method. Contributors are respected scholars and educators of established and emerging areas of health communication research in a variety of health-related settings. This book supplements health communication textbooks focused on theory and method by providing "real world" examples of health communication in practice. It begins with a chapter aptly titled "Health Communication: Where Have We Been and Where Can We Go?" about the history of health communication research in the United States and the influential works that shaped the discipline. Of particular interest is the combined content analysis and discussion of the research scope of the two journals devoted to the study of health communication: *Health Communication* and *The Journal of Health Communication: International Perspectives*. Subsequent chapters focus on new technologies; social marketing and health campaigns; cultural competence and barriers to the delivery of health care; health beliefs; explaining illness to children; communication with the aging/geriatric patient; cross-cultural differences in choices of health information; end-of-life communication; communication and cancer; Alzheimer's care giving issues; interpersonal communication issues; and health narratives. Kevin Wright, who also serves as the editor of the *Journal of Computer-Mediated Communication*, and the book's contributors condense salient work into single chapters. The book ends with a nine-page list of references, which provide an excellent guide to more information sources for students, researchers, and/or practitioners.

Communicating About Health: Current Issues and Perspectives. 3rd ed. Author: Athena du Pré. Oxford University Press, 2010.
ISBN: 9780195380330
Recommended for: Academic Libraries

In its third edition, *Communicating About Health* updates coverage of the latest research topics and stories of people who embody health communication issues. Chapters explore the role of communication in actual health care delivery and health behavior change programs. As in the previous editions, this scholarly but practical book integrates evidence-based research with real-life examples. The book examines the context of communication theories and research with chapters on the roles of patients and caregivers; social and cultural issues; cultural conceptions of health and illness; culture and diversity in health organizations; public health (media, crisis communication, policy reform, and health promotion); health promotion campaigns; e-health; multicultural audiences; and risk communication. The third edition has some of the same educational features of the previous edition, including theoretical foundations boxes, perspectives boxes, resource boxes, communication skill builders, and communication technology features. Individual purchasers of this edition can now access new supplemental resources, such as the Instructor's Manual (in print or online format), an online test bank, and PowerPoint presentations at http://www.oup.com/us/dupre. More than 1,370 references can be used to discover and locate earlier, notable health communication works. This popular textbook for undergraduate and graduate students, as well as lay and professional caregivers, is among those listed in the article, "Health Communication Instruction: Toward Common Learning Goals, Course Content, and Pedagogical Strategies to Guide Curricular Development" (Query et al., *Health Communication*, 2007). It may also be useful to anyone seeking references to foundational health communication literature.

Cultural Sutures: Medicine and Media. Editor: Lester D. Friedman. Duke University Press, 2004.
http://www.ebrary.com/
ISBN: 9780822332947
ISBN: 9780822332565
ISBN: 9780822385530 (Online)
Recommended for: Hospital, Academic Libraries

This diverse collection of 21 original essays on the relationship between medicine and the media provocatively illustrates how communication in the medical world is culturally situated. Essays are arranged by genre: print media, advertisements, fiction films, television, documentaries, and computers. Lester Friedman explains that these essays offer "an expansive, interdisciplinary series of vantage points from which to contemplate, explore, understand, and (perhaps) challenge the ways different types of media present and affect the American health care system" (Introduction, p. 7). Chapters, written by scholars from health communication, social science, and the humanities, demonstrate how the world of medicine engages and permeates the media surrounding us. The collection covers such topics as psychotropic medication advertising from 1964–1985; news/television coverage of the Kervorkian-euthanasia controversy; managed-care billboard advertising; medical monsters in horror films; medical bureaucracies in film; content analysis of two popular television series, *ER* and *Chicago Hope*; disease and hygiene in World War II training films; and the Internet and patient-doctor relations. For further reading, the volume includes a bibliography of works cited in excess of 20 pages. This book is useful to stimulate class discussions of health communication in popular culture for residents in training, other health communication and/or media students, educators, and researchers. A longer review of *Cultural Sutures* can be located in *JAMA* 2004; 292(20):2524–5.

Emerging Perspectives in Health Communication: Meaning, Culture and Power. Editors: Heather M. Zoller, Mohan J. Dutta. Routledge, 2008.
http://extranet.netlibrary.com/TitleSelect/
http://www.ebrary.com/
ISBN: 9780805861952
ISBN: 9780805861969
ISBN: 9781410615503
ISBN: 9780203891223 (Online)
Recommended for: Academic Libraries

This book addresses the need for health messages, whether mass mediated or interpersonal, to engage recipients via their basic needs, motivations, and priorities. The book emphasizes an in-depth understanding of health constructions, assumptions about what it means to be healthy and what constitutes health, and how these affect health communication intervention objectives and evaluative criteria. A growing pluralism is presented as a strength of the health communication discipline. The editors want to draw attention to communication as a process beyond emphasis on messages, the need to understand meanings, and the ways meanings of health are constituted. The first part of the book is an overview of interpretive, critical, and cultural approaches to health communication. The second part is about culture in health communication (narratives and narration; influence—or not—of medical and social discourses; communicating healing holistically; and stigmatization). The third part focuses on culturally based health promotion using stories and culturally appropriate community-based research. The last part is devoted to medical communication, with an emphasis on health care delivery and health policy topics, including globalization, social justice movements, and the human genome diversity debates. The authors provide an initial discussion of the theoretical and practical contributions of interpretive, critical, and cultural research, and they conclude with emerging theoretical, methodological, and practical agendas and the challenge of multiple perspectives. An integrated index with both names and subjects is especially useful for researchers.

Handbook of Health Communication. Editors: Teresa L. Thompson, Alicia Dorsey, Katherine I. Miller, Roxanne Parrott. Lawrence Erlbaum Associates, 2003.
http://www.ebrary.com/
ISBN: 9780805838589
ISBN: 9780805838572
ISBN: 9781410607683 (Online)
Recommended for: Academic Libraries

This book is among the most frequently cited sources on syllabi for health communication courses. *Doody's Review Service* gives it a four-star rating for capturing the expanding body of health communication scholarship. The first edition, with 30 chapters, covers the field at its time of publication. A second edition is anticipated in May 2011, with at least 146 authors and 40 chapters. This work introduces and summarizes knowledge about communicative processes in health care contexts. Contributions are from top scholars in health communication, public health, and related areas. The editors include Professor Teresa Thompson, who was the 2009 recipient of the Outstanding Health Communication Scholar award from the National Communication Association *and* International Communication Association, Health Communication Division; she has also served as the senior editor of the journal *Health Communication* for over 20 years. Academic knowledge is combined with policy, practice, and research communication perspectives. Topics include illness narratives and the social construction of health; theory and meta-theory; the medical encounter and provider-patient issues; social and community health issues; organizational issues; media issues, including health campaigns and communication design strategies, narrowcast health messages, telemedicine, and health literacy; and lessons and challenges. This book belongs in all health communication collections, including even the smallest groupings. It is an important resource for anyone new to the study of health communication; health communication graduate students, educators, and researchers; and professionals in public health, psychology, and related areas.

Health Communication in Practice: A Case Study Approach. Editor: Eileen Berlin Ray. Lawrence Erlbaum Associates, 2005.
http://extranet.netlibrary.com/TitleSelect/
http://www.ebrary.com/
ISBN: 9780805847574
ISBN: 9780805847581
ISBN: 9781410612779 (Online)
Recommended for: Academic Libraries

In 2002, Eileen Berlin Ray won the National Communication Association's Gerald Phillips Applied Communication Scholar Award for her work in the application of health communication. This is her sixth book, and health communication course readings continue to be drawn from her case studies. Chapters are written by medical practitioners as well as communication scholars. The cases include provider-recipient communication and decision making; social identity; family and health care provider communication dynamics in health-related situations; delivery of health care; and health campaigns to change behaviors. Health communication with the elderly, delivering bad news, genetic testing, grieving families, and international campaigns are presented. This book includes a list of relevant concepts and definitions at the end of each case, along with references to scholarly health communication works and tables (such as "Key Variables of the Extended Parallel Process Model" by Kim Witte). The author and subject indexes are particularly impressive. This book is an instructional aid for educators, students, and researchers.

Health Communication in the 21st Century. Authors: Kevin B. Wright, Lisa Sparks, H. Dan O'Hair. Blackwell, 2008.
ISBN: 9781405155939
ISBN: 9781405155946
Recommended for: Hospital, Academic Libraries

This book examines key issues and theories related to health communication in provider-patient interaction; issues and theories related to care giving such as hospice and palliative care or end-of-life decision-making; social support theories and processes; cultural differences in beliefs about health and health care; and communication in the health organizations context. The authors draw on local, national, and international experience to highlight different aspects of health and a variety of intertwined communication processes. Twelve chapters examine growth and application of new communication technologies, mass media messages, and lifestyle choices. A risk communication theory and research chapter includes current approaches to terrorism and natural disaster responses. A final chapter focuses on growing areas of research: health literacy, breaking bad news to patients, and older adult health care issues. The book covers the current landscape of health communication research without being overwhelming. Useful and friendly features are chapter references to notable and still highly relevant research—book chapters, journal articles, reports, and websites—released since the 1970s; a glossary and discussion questions to reinforce learning; and an index with "see also" references to find particular, current and past theories and issues. A companion website is offered to instructors who purchase the print book and adopt this textbook. Links to PowerPoint slides, sample exams, classroom assignments, a syllabus to supplement and support lectures, and an Instructor's Manual are offered at http://www.blackwellpublishing.com/wright/. This book is clearly meant for educators and students; but, it is also useful for health communication researchers and health communication practitioners looking for research-based overviews of issues and developments.

Health Communication in the New Media Landscape. Editors: Jerry C. Parker, Esther Thorson. Springer, 2008.
http://extranet.netlibrary.com/TitleSelect/

http://www.ebrary.com/
ISBN: 9780826101228
ISBN: 9780826101235 (Online)
Recommended for: Academic Libraries

The author biographies, table of contents, and first chapter (available as an online sample at http://www.springerpub.com/samples/01224_chapter.pdf) introduce the broad, interdisciplinary scope and convergence of interests demonstrated in this book. The authors provide expertise about emerging health communication tools for specific populations and communities, such as the aged, those with poor health literacy, and recent immigrants or racial/ethnic groups. This book is a valuable addition to health communication scholarship in general. Contributors contextualize health communication theory and method in the emergent, "new media" environment. The first part of the book provides overviews of current trends and the status of useful, new media to enhance the availability of health information in forms appropriate to the needs of particular individuals and communities. Issues of patient activation and engagement, e-health for self-care, computer-mediated social support, and health literacy in the digital world form the second part. The third part discusses future directions, identification of evidence-based communication messages, knowledge translation, other challenges, and future directions. Various tables, charts, and figures capture and organize a great deal of cutting edge, "new media landscape" research for any audience. Examples of such entries include the "Summary of E-Health Interventions for Self-Management of Chronic Diseases" by Glueckauf and Lustria; "Overview of Case Studies and the Best Practices They Represent" by Haider, Ratzan, and Meltzer; and "Overlapping Research Foci and Variables" by Hensel, Boren, and Cameron.

Healthy People 2010 [Chapter 11: Health Communication]. U.S. Department of Health and Human Services, 2000.
http://www.healthypeople.gov/2010
See Also Chapter 10.15. Preventive Medicine
Recommended for: Hospital, Academic Libraries

The eleventh chapter, which introduces the concept of health communication and defines the basic terms in the field, is part of the two-volume work, *Healthy People 2010*. The set encompasses 28 chapters and 608 pages. The "Health Communication" chapter's overview section, glossary, and list of references alone are very useful for definitions and identification of foundational and influential health communication scholarship. Another feature is a chart of attributes of health communication. This chapter is frequently included on syllabi for health communication courses. *Healthy People 2020* launched on December 2, 2010, and is available at http://www.healthypeople.gov/.

Interactive Case Studies in Health Communication. Author: Michael P. Pagano. Jones & Bartlett, 2009.
ISBN: 9780763760182
Recommended for: Hospital, Academic Libraries

This book uses an interactive approach designed for classroom discussions of health communication situations. Readings and exercises encourage students' awareness, analysis, and understanding of "real life" situations to develop communication strategies that enhance information sharing, trust, and goal attainment. Michael Pagano's method for exploring health communication actions is based on his 30 years of experience as a health care provider and his 20 years as a health communication educator in medical schools, universities, and hospitals. He paraphrases and reconstructs communication he observed in clinical settings or from his experiences as a patient, family member, and friend. Chapters have key topics, such as learning to talk like a health care provider, included in the contents and then again before each chapter. The book includes narratives, questions for discussion, and other interactive features, including worksheets and scripts for communication role playing in a clinical setting. The workbook emphasizes the need to recognize and develop interpersonal and health communication behaviors in order to exchange information, empower patients, and enhance outcomes. A *Doody's* reviewer supplied a five-star rating or 100 points out of a possible 100.

Making Health Communication Programs Work: A Planner's Guide. National Cancer Institute, National Institutes of Health, 2002.
http://www.cancer.gov/pinkbook
http://www.nci.nih.gov/
ISBN: none
Recommended for: Academic Libraries

This "Pink Book," named for the color of the original print cover, is a classic "what works" guide for health communication based on evidence-based best practices of communication in general. Many well-known and respected health communication experts contributed to this book. This work is often included on syllabi of graduate courses in health communication. Hard copy and compact discs of *Making Health Communication Programs Work* are no longer produced; however, PDF and HTML versions of this revised edition, which was first printed in 1989, are freely available at the sites listed in this entry.

Patient-Centered Communication in Cancer Care: Promoting Healing and Reducing Suffering. Authors: Ronald M. Epstein, Richard L. Street Jr. National Cancer Institute, 2007.
http://outcomes.cancer.gov/areas/pcc/communication/monograph.html
ISBN: None/ NIH Publication No. 07-6225
Recommended for: Hospital, Academic Libraries

The National Cancer Institute commissioned this work to lay a foundation for future research in the area of patient-centered health communication. Richard Street is a research professor of medicine and the recipient of two outstanding health communication scholar awards from peers: the National Communication Association *and* the International Communication Association, Health Communication Divisions' Outstanding Health Communication Scholar, 2008. Ronald Epstein is director of research in family medicine and professor of family medicine at the University of Rochester School of Medicine & Dentistry. In 2008, they authored *Patient-Centered Care for the 21st Century: Physicians' Roles, Health Systems and Patients' Preferences* for the American Board of Internal Medicine Foundation. *Patient-Centered Communication in Cancer Care* is available in multiple electronic formats at the site listed, in print format by calling 1-800-4-CANCER, or by ordering online from NCI Publications Locator. Similarly, other NCI publications—such as *The Role of the Media in Promoting and Reducing Tobacco Use*, NCI Tobacco Control Monograph 19, Bethesda, MD: U.S. Department of Health and Human Services, National Institutes of Health, National Cancer Institute. NIH Publication No. 07-6242, June 2008—are available. These reports are in the public domain and may be reproduced or copied without permission.

Public Health Communication: Evidence for Behavior Change. Editor: Robert C. Hornik. Lawrence Erlbaum Associates, 2002.
http://extranet.netlibrary.com/TitleSelect/
http://www.ebrary.com/
ISBN: 9780805831764
ISBN: 9780805831771
ISBN: 9780585395227 (Online)
ISBN: 9781410603029 (Online)
Recommended for: Academic Libraries

This frequently cited book gathers 16 large-scale studies to support the editor's hypothesis that public health communication can affect health behavior. The studies—based on communication programs in the United States and other areas such as Europe, Asia, Africa, and Latin America—showcase a variety of global and national health issues: smoking, marijuana use, AIDS, family planning, heart disease, seat belt use, skin cancer, vasectomy promotion, vaccination, and childhood diseases. This is a "go-to" book for students and practitioners studying health communication campaigns. It tackles a variety of issues and populations, employs a range of methodological approaches from simple field experiments to complex, time-series designs using archival or newly collected data, and provides evidence of behavioral change in targeted populations. The studies are divided into three groups. In the book's introduction (pg. xii), Robert Hornik explains: "The first group presents the results of deliberate trials. The second group is evaluations done on 'real' interventions, which were not designed to accommodate the evaluations. The third set includes studies of the effects of normal media coverage on health behavior." The book is especially useful for addressing challenges associated with the effectiveness evaluation of campaigns. This book is required reading for students, practitioners, and policymakers in public health, health communication, social marketing, health psychology, and mass communication effects.

Speaking of Health: Assessing Health Communication Strategies for Diverse Populations. Author: Committee on Communication for Behavior Change in the 21st Century: Improving the Health of Diverse Populations, Board on Neuroscience and Behavioral Health. National Academies Press, 2002.
http://www.nap.edu/
http://www.ebrary.com/
ISBN: 9780309072717
ISBN: 9780309110617
Recommended for: Hospital, Academic Libraries

This important Institute of Medicine report continues, even seven years after release, to address the challenges of improving health communication in a diverse population. The challenge of categorizing audiences, the need for research that improves understanding of how information is received, and the evaluation of communication campaigns to determine effectiveness and design of future campaigns are discussed. The full online report is especially valuable for the contributions from members of the interdisciplinary committee comprised of experts in health behavior change, communication and the media, social marketing, and public health communication. The committee—which included Albert Bandura, Martin Fishbein, Robert C. Hornik, Barbara K. Rimer, and Everett Rogers, among others—addressed the following: (a) reviewed existing theory and research applications in health communication and health behavior change, especially related to culturally diverse populations, and defined research areas that would benefit from more research efforts; (b) evaluated specific examples of health communication interventions for whether and how those strategies affect culturally diverse groups; and (c) recommended how health communication strategies may be designed and implemented to help achieve sustained gains in public health across cultural groups. This is a core resource for health communication and public health communication researchers, educators, and students who are interested in using health communication to effect behavior change in diverse communities.

Journals

Health Communication. v. 1, Routledge, 1989.
http://www.tandf.co.uk/journals/hhth
ISSN: 10410236
ISSN: 15327027 (Online)
Indexed in: MEDLINE, CINAHL
Recommended for: Hospital, Academic Libraries

Since 1989, this journal has dedicated itself to improving practical communication between caregivers and patients *and* between institutions and the public. It is the older of the two journals devoted to the subject of health communication. All articles undergo anonymous, double-blind peer review by an editorial board from the communication, medical, and social science disciplines. The journal publishes pedagogical, methodological, theoretical, and applied health communication articles that use quantitative or qualitative evidence-based methods. Topics include provider-patient or family interaction, health campaigns, consumer health information, health promotion, interviewing, risk communication, mass media, Internet, direct-to-consumer, e-health, health public relations, organ donation, and gerontological concerns. *Health Communication* has a diverse readership of researchers, educators, and practitioners of communication, psychology, sociology, public health, medicine, nursing, dentistry, physical therapy, dietetics, pharmacy, and other allied health professions. A regular feature is a "Health Communication Bibliography" citing recent publications that feature original research or theory related to health communication. According to the 2009 *Journal Citation Reports*, this journal has an impact factor of 1.277 and is ranked fourteenth of 55 journals in the communication subject category and thirtieth of 49 journals in the health policy and services category. The journal is fully abstracted/indexed in numerous sources such as MEDLINE, PsycINFO, Communication Abstracts, Social Sciences Citation Index, CINAHL, and Scopus. Full online coverage back to volume 1, 1996 is available through the Informaworld platform.

JHC Link. Routledge, 2005.
http://www.gwu.edu/~cih/journal/JHClink/index.htm
Recommended for: Hospital, Academic Libraries

JHC Link is a quarterly email newsletter that alerts readers to newly published health communication research in the *Journal of Health Communication* (*JHC*). Anyone can register for this free e-newsletter and view all previous issues on a George Washington University Center for Global Health website. The newsletter provides links for free, full-text access to published editorials and abstracts archived from ten years of the *Journal of Health Communication*, book reviews, announcements, upcoming conferences, and meetings. The Johnson & Johnson Centre for Advancing Health Information contributes to improving health communication and patient information as a sponsor of this newsletter.

Journal of Health Communication: International Perspectives. v. 1, Taylor and Francis, 1996.
http://www.tandf.co.uk/journals/titles/10810730.html
http://www.informaworld.com/smpp/title~content=t713666566
http://www.gwu.edu/~cih/journal/
ISSN: 10810730
ISSN: 10870415 (Online)
Indexed in: MEDLINE
Recommended for: Hospital, Academic Libraries

The *Journal of Health Communication* features a timely, scholarly appraisal of the latest developments in the field of health communication. The editorial review board includes well-known health communication educators, researchers, and practitioners; articles are rigorously screened by editorial and double-blind peer review. The research includes the application of health communication principles to decision making, global health diplomacy, health literacy, e-health, computer mediated or web mediated communication, Internet and health communication, technology and public health, ethics, politics/policy, and health care in general. Evidence-based qualitative and quantitative studies, ethical essays, case studies, and book reviews are included. According to the 2009 *Journal Citation Reports*, this journal has the ninth highest impact factor in the communication category. It is fully abstracted/indexed in multiple sources such as MEDLINE, PsycINFO, Communication Abstracts,

Social Sciences Citation Index, and Health Education Abstracts. Full online coverage back to volume 1, 1996 is available through the Informaworld platform.

Journal of Medical Internet Research. v. 1, Gunther Eysenbach, JMIR, 1999.
http://www.jmir.org/
http://www.ncbi.nlm.nih.gov/pmc/journals/224/
ISSN: 14394456
ISSN: 14388871 (Online)
See Also Chapter 6.3. Informatics, Chapter 9.13. Telemedicine
Indexed in: MEDLINE
Recommended for: Hospital, Academic Libraries

Journal of Medical Internet Research (*JMIR*) is billed as "the leading Open Access peer-reviewed transdisciplinary journal on health and health care in the Internet age." It is a source of cutting-edge research and themed issues for evidence-based research on web-assisted interventions and other computer-mediated ("e-health") health communication research. According to the 2009 *Journal Citation Reports*, the *JMIR* impact factor is 3.924, up from the previous year's 3.6. Back issues are permanently archived in the National Library of Medicine's free digital archive, PubMed Central. In addition to MEDLINE, *JMIR* is indexed in Communication Abstracts, Information Science Abstracts, CINAHL Plus, INSPEC, LISA (Library and Information Science Abstracts), LISTA (Library, Information Science & Technology Abstracts) Embase, Scopus, Current Contents/Clinical Medicine, Science Citation Index Expanded (SCIE), Google Scholar, and PsycINFO. Founded in 1999 by scientists for scientists and the public, the clear writing and layout make this journal an accessible reference source for health communication research. The articles are appropriate for a wide audience, including but not limited to researchers and students. This should be an addition to any health communication collection.

Patient Education and Counseling. v. 5, Elsevier, 1983.
http://journals.elsevierhealth.com/periodicals/pec/home
http://www.sciencedirect.com/science/journal/07383991
ISSN: 07383991 (Print and online)
Indexed in: MEDLINE, CINAHL
Recommended for: Hospital, Academic Libraries

Patient Education and Counseling, formerly known as *Patient Counseling and Health Education*, is the official journal of the American Academy on Communication in Healthcare (AACH) and the European Association for Communication in Healthcare (EACH). This interdisciplinary, international journal explores health communication, health education, and counseling models in applied research. Many individual articles and special issues about health communication are authored or edited by well-known communication researchers and scholars. The journal seeks to elucidate educational, counseling, and communication models in health care for clinicians, patient and health education researchers, counselors, and others concerned with the communication of information, education, and counseling of patients. An aim is also to provide a forum for fundamental and applied research and to promote the study of patient education delivery, counseling, and health promotion services—including training models and organizational issues—for improved communication between providers and patients. According to the 2009 *Journal Citation Reports*, the journal's impact factor is 1.975. The journal is indexed in many abstracting and indexing sources, such as MEDLINE, PsycINFO, CINAHL, Embase, Scopus, Current Contents/Clinical Medicine and Current Contents/Social & Behavioral Sciences, and Health Promotion and Education Database.

34. General Reference

34.1. Bibliographic Sources for Monographs and Journals

Contributor: Jayson Felty

Databases and Other Electronic Resources

Amazon.com. Amazon.com, Inc., 1994.
http://www.amazon.com
Recommended for: Hospital, Academic, Consumer Health Libraries

Amazon is now one of the Internet's largest stores for books, DVDs, hardware, electronics, and various other items. The website provides a number of features to help librarians locate and purchase items of interest from the major science and medical book publishers and to verify book citation information quickly. While a general search will look for words in the author's name or title, Amazon also searches the full text of books in their "Search Inside the Book" program and returns the page number where the search terms appear. Advanced searching allows one to select specific fields to search, such as author or ISBN number, refine by format type, and limit by publication date. Subject browsing is also available. The details page for each book gives basic bibliographic information, along with editorial reviews by other sources (such as *Publisher's Weekly*), and reviews by other Amazon customers. The details page also provides information to purchase new and used copies from third parties. This is particularly useful when locating older or out-of-print materials. For many recently published books, the "Look Inside" feature shows searchable scans of a book's front and back covers, copyright page, table of contents, index, and a few pages from the text. One can also search the full text of the book and view the pages where the words appear. The site is recommended for librarians seeking basic book information as a supplement to their regular book vendors.

Journal Citation Reports. Thomson Reuters, 1997.
http://thomsonreuters.com/
Recommended for: Hospital, Academic Libraries

Those seeking to publish articles are frequently in need of guidance about potential journals. One measurement of a journal's research influence is its impact factor: "a measure of the frequency with which the 'average article' in a journal has been cited in a particular year." While there are many algorithms used to calculate a journal's impact, the most frequently touted is Thomson-Reuters' *Journal Citation Reports* (*JCR*). Based on the ISI Web of Science cited reference data from over 8,000 scholarly journals, coverage begins in 1997 with yearly updates for both the Science and Social Science editions. Individual journals can be searched by title or ISSN; journals can also be retrieved by subject category, publisher, and country. The original *JCR* Impact Factor compares citation data covering a two-year period: i.e., the 2009 impact factor score is calculated with the 2007 and 2008 citation data. *JCR* data also includes a five-year impact factor, immediacy index, Eigenfactor score (also available at http://eigenfactor.org/), article influence score, total cites, number of articles, and cited half-life. Search results can be sorted by any of the data points. The journal detail page illustrates how the impact factors are calculated and provides links to the cited and citing journal data behind the calculations. When properly used, the *JCR* is an effective tool to compare journals within the same subject for collection development and potential research influence and impact.

LocatorPlus. U.S. National Library of Medicine, 1998.
http://locatorplus.gov/
Recommended for: Hospital, Academic, Consumer Health Libraries

The U.S. National Library of Medicine (NLM) is the world's largest biomedical library and is committed to "acquiring, organizing, and preserving the world's scholarly biomedical literature." LocatorPlus is the NLM's online public catalog of over 1.2 million monographs, journals, and audiovisual titles available in the NLM collection or other regional libraries. Records contain links to online journals and other biomedical resources. The catalog can be searched and browsed by keyword, title, author, Medical Subject Heading, or PubMed journal title abbreviation. Search results can be refined using limits such as English-language materials, format type, or currently published journals. Advanced searching allows Boolean searching of any item record information: for example, publisher name or date. The catalog identifies NLM's item holdings and the circulation status of specific items. Additionally, MARC 21-formatted records can be searched and downloaded for both bibliographic records and title and name authority records. NLM's special collections, the History of Medicine Collections and History of Medicine images, are also indexed in LocatorPlus.

NLM Catalog (Entrez). U.S. National Library of Medicine, 2004.
http://www.ncbi.nlm.nih.gov/nlmcatalog
Recommended for: Hospital, Academic, Consumer Health Libraries

The National Library of Medicine Catalog is another interface for the NLM collections of monographs, journals, audiovisuals, and electronic resources. The catalog uses the familiar, PubMed-type interface of the other National Center for Biotechnology Information (NCBI) Entrez system databases. The catalog can be searched by subject, author, or title. To facilitate advanced searching of the catalog, expert searchers of PubMed can use PubMed field qualifier tags, such as [au] for author, [pd] for publication date, and [ti] for words in the title. Medical Subject Heading (MeSH) searching is supported and can be exploded or limited to major topic. Each record includes a link to LocatorPlus to determine item availability and holdings information. Records can be viewed and exported in XML format.

SCImago Journal & Country Rank. SCImago Research Group, 2007.
http://www.scimagojr.com/
Recommended for: Hospital, Academic Libraries

SCImago is a group of university researchers from Spain studying information analysis, representation, and analysis. The SCImago Journal & Country Rank is an open-access, freely available citation metric database, which is used to determine a journal's or country's research influence. The SCImago journal rank indicator (SJR), based on Elsevier's Scopus database of cited references from over 13,000 journals, uses an algorithm based on Google PageRank to calculate how often the average article in a journal has been cited for the previous three years. Higher SJRs indicate journals that are more influential. Unlike the *Journal Citation Reports* impact factor, self-citations are not included, and a citation from a citing journal with more citations or "prestige" is weighted more highly. Options include: search for journals by title, ISSN, or publisher; browse by Scopus subject areas and categories or country; or download as a Microsoft Excel spreadsheet. Other comparative information included in the rankings are h-index, total cites per journal, cites per document, and total published documents per journal. The journal detail page provides several graphs visualizing various comparisons of a journal's dataset: SJR vs. cites per document, cites per document for the past four years, etc. Historical charts display the data from the past 10 years. SCImago Journal & Country rank offers a good, complementary alternative to the traditionally used *Journal Citation Reports*.

Ulrichsweb. ProQuest, 200?
http://www.ulrichsweb.com/
Recommended for: Hospital, Academic, Consumer Health Libraries

In print, *Ulrich's Periodicals Directory* has long been an authoritative source for bibliographic information about serials and publishers, but the directory only offered a subset of the available serial titles. The subscription-based Ulrichsweb gives users full access to the information contained in the Ulrich's database of over 300,000 publications. Serials covered include academic and scholarly journals, business and trade magazines, open access journals, newspapers, and irregularly published titles. Each title's record contains detailed bibliographic information, purchase information, description, links to the online journal, title history, and a proprietary subject classification. With its vendor-neutral policy, Ulrichsweb comprehensively lists the coverage years of a title's full-text availability from publisher websites and aggregators, databases where journal content is indexed, reviews from Ulrich's *Magazines for Libraries*, and vendors supplying document delivery. Record information is completely searchable, and limits can be applied to locate refereed or open access journals, among others. The database is updated weekly.

WorldCat and ***xISSN History Visualization Tool (OCLC)***. OCLC Online Computer Library Center, Inc., 1971 (WorldCat).
http://www.worldcat.org
http://www.worldcat.org/xissn/titlehistory
Recommended for: Hospital, Academic, Consumer Health Libraries

From Dublin, Ohio, OCLC manages the shared cataloging records network used by thousands of libraries worldwide. Participating libraries update OCLC records to indicate their own individual item holdings, which facilitates resource sharing and interlibrary loan. WorldCat is the public, web-based interface that can be used to search over one billion items in OCLC's system. Because OCLC member libraries are so diverse, the books, journals, audiovisual titles, and indexed articles in WorldCat encompass more than just biomedical subject matter. Basic and advanced searching returns basic bibliographic information. When entering a ZIP Code or city name, WorldCat returns a list of nearby libraries that own the item, with links to search their online catalogs to verify availability. OCLC developed a separate application, the xISSN tool, which takes advantage of WorldCat's data. WorldCat records contain the unique ISSNs assigned to different editions of a serial (print or online) and the historical relationships based on title changes, splits, or mergers. Enter one ISSN, and the xISSN tool returns all the associated ISSNs found in the WorldCat database displayed in a flowchart highlighting formats and chronological name changes. This feature is particularly useful when publishers provide online access to older content under a serial's current title.

34.2. Indexing and Database Resources

Contributor: Jayson Felty

Databases and Other Electronic Resources

CINAHL. EBSCO, 1981.
http://www.ebscohost.com/
See Also Chapter 1. Allied Health, Chapter 12.1. Nursing Research
Recommended for: Hospital, Academic Libraries
Brandon/Hill Selection

CINAHL, the Cumulative Index to Nursing and Allied Health Literature, is a comprehensive bibliographic database of the nursing and allied health literature dating back to 1981. Covering almost 3,000 journals in nursing, biomedicine, health sciences librarianship, alternative and complementary medicine, and consumer health and allied health disciplines, CINAHL also contains complete coverage of English-language nursing journals and publications from the National League for Nursing and the American Nurses Association. The database indexes health care books, nursing dissertations, selected conference proceedings, standards of practice, educational software, audiovisuals, and book chapters. CINAHL subject headings were developed to reflect the terminology used by nursing and allied health professionals. An article's content may be described more fully with topical subheadings. Document types assigned to each record indicate the type of publication being indexed and the document type of the individual item. Starting with journals published after 2000, CINAHL includes searchable cited references for over 40 percent of their journals. CINAHL contains over 71 full-text journals. EBSCOhost offers other variations of the CINAHL database with citations going back to 1937 and additional full-text coverage. CINAHL is recommended for hospitals and academic institutions with nursing or allied health programs.

MEDLINE (via PubMed). National Center for Biotechnology Information, U.S. National Library of Medicine, 1996.
http://pubmed.gov
Brandon/Hill Selection
Recommended for: Hospital, Academic, Consumer Health Libraries

The U.S National Library of Medicine's MEDLINE is the world's premier database of biomedical and health literature, containing over 18 million citations to journal articles dating back to 1947. Journals, written in English or other languages, are selected for indexing based on scope and coverage, quality of content and editorial work, production quality, audience, and types of content. Thus, not every published journal is indexed in MEDLINE, and journals are dropped or added to the database every year. The power of the database lies with its use of the Medical Subject Headings (MeSH) controlled vocabulary to describe an article's topic. Through consistent assignment of MeSH terms by subject-expert indexers, searchers are able to retrieve relevant articles on their research subjects. MeSH terms can also contain qualifiers or subheadings to describe articles more specifically. In addition to MeSH terms, other article information includes the complete citation, article abstract (if available), author affiliation, chemical substances, and grant numbers acknowledged in the paper. Caveats to using MEDLINE are the lack of author disambiguation and the inclusion of only the first author's institutional affiliation. PubMed is NLM's freely available web interface to search MEDLINE. PubMed also includes new references not yet indexed and PubMed Central articles from journals not indexed in MEDLINE. Other vendors—such as Ovid, EBSCOhost, and Thomson Reuters/Web of Science—offer MEDLINE data on other platforms, which may contain additional functionality and features. MEDLINE is recommended for anyone searching the biomedical scholarly literature.

MICROMEDEX Healthcare Series. Thomson Reuters, 199?
http://www.micromedex.com
See Also Chapter 17.6. Clinical Pharmacology
Recommended for: Hospital, Academic Libraries

Thomson Reuters' MICROMEDEX platform is a collection of individual databases covering a broad range of drug information and toxicology. While some well-known books are included, such as the *Physician's Desk Reference* (FDA-approved product labels), *Martindale* (international drug products), and *Index Nominum* (international drug directory), MICROMEDEX has created their own proprietary databases prepared by the MICROMEDEX editorial board of physicians, pharmacists, nurses, and medical librarians. The main page has one search box that can search most of the databases simultaneously. Search results are organized in sections by type of information (drug information, disease information, toxicology, complementary and alternative medicine, and reproductive risk), with the links to the appropriate text in the individual databases. DRUGDEX provides unbiased, referenced information on FDA-approved and investigational drugs, over-the-counter and foreign preparations, and labeled and off-label indications. POISINDEX identifies ingredients for commercial, biological, and pharmaceutical products with links to information on clinical effects, toxicity, and treatment protocols. IDENTIDEX identifies prescription and over-the-counter drugs by imprint code, color, shape or logo. REPRORISK provides information on the reproductive risks of drugs, chemicals, and other environmental agents. Other tools include dosing calculators, drug interactions, alternative medicine, and patient information. MICROMEDEX is customizable with a combination of their available databases. This drug information resource is appropriate for academic health science libraries, hospitals, and clinics.

PsycINFO. American Psychological Association, 199?
http://www.apa.org/pubs/databases/psycinfo/index.aspx
See Also Chapter 17.7. Psychopharmacology
Recommended for: Hospital, Academic Libraries

Based on the original *Psychological Abstracts* index, PsycINFO contains bibliographic citations, abstracts, cited references, and descriptive information from a broad range of item types: international journals, books, book chapters, dissertations, technical reports, and other scholarly publications in the behavioral and social sciences. With entries going back to the 1800s, over 1,500 journals are indexed cover-to-cover; other journals' articles are selected for psychological relevance, such as the behavioral causes and effects of medical disorders and behavioral aspects of care. Books and book chapters make up 11 percent of the database, and selections from *Dissertation Abstracts International* make up another 12 percent. From 1967, each citation is extensively indexed with up to 15 terms from the controlled vocabulary in the American Psychological Association's *Thesaurus of Psychological Index Terms*. Items can also be retrieved by document type, population, age group, tests and measures, and methodology (interviews, clinical study, etc.). Because of its broader coverage of item types, PsycINFO complements a more general biomedical database like MEDLINE and is appropriate for academic and hospital libraries.

UpToDate. UpToDate, Inc., 2001?
http://www.uptodate.com
Recommended for: Hospital, Academic Libraries

UpToDate is a peer-reviewed subscription resource designed to give physicians current clinical information. Over 4,000 physicians, peer reviewers, and editors write topic reviews providing a synthesis of the literature, the latest evidence, and specific patient care recommendations for over 8,300 specific clinical conditions in 16 medical specialties. Authors combine their own clinical experience with a literature review, rather than performing a systematic review of the literature. Topic reviews can be searched by keyword or browsed by specialty. Each peer-reviewed topic review includes the major aspects of a particular condition, including symptoms, tests and diagnosis, and treatment options. Links to MEDLINE records of reviewed articles are included in the text, as well as links to drug information, information for patients, and other supporting materials. Some patient-level information is freely accessible through the "For Patients" link at the top of the UpToDate homepage. New versions of the database are released every four months as content is reviewed and updated by the authors. UpToDate is available in online, desktop, or mobile versions. UpToDate is recommended for libraries supporting physicians in clinical settings.

Web of Science. Thomson Reuters, 198?
http://thomsonreuters.com/
Recommended for: Academic Libraries

Web of Science from Thomson Reuters is based on the well-known Institute for Scientific Information citation indexes (Social Science, Science, and Arts & Humanities, along with a new Conference Proceedings index), which track cited references of articles in scholarly journals and conference proceedings as far back as 1900. The over

12,000 covered journals available in the three separate indexes are selected for timeliness of publication, English-language bibliographic information, editorial content, international diversity of authorship, and peer review process. The indexes are interdisciplinary, meaning articles may appear in multiple indexes when warranted by the subject. Each "source record" contains searchable bibliographic information, abstract, affiliations of all authors, author keywords, and funding acknowledgement (for the most recent articles). Most importantly, the records include the complete list of cited references from the paper, with a link to the Web of Science record if available, and a list of articles citing the paper with links to their records. When used with an author search or the author disambiguation tools, the "Create Citation Report" option calculates a number of bibliometric statistics based on Web of Science data. The "Cited Reference Search" is a special search option used to find citations of one specific paper based on author, publication name, and year even when cited incorrectly and not automatically matched in the database. While good as a discovery tool, the additional "Keywords Plus," based on article title words from cited references, can return irrelevant results if searching for papers on a specific topic. Web of Science is recommended for academic universities and other research-intensive institutions.

34.3. Terminology

Contributor: Katherine A. Prentice

Monographs

Dictionary of Epidemiology. 5th ed. Editor: Miquel S. Porta. Oxford University Press, 2008.
ISBN: 9780195314496
See Chapter 9.7. Epidemiology

A Dictionary of Medical Derivations: The Real Meaning of Medical Terms. Author: William Casselman. Informa Healthcare, 1998.
ISBN: 9781850707714
Recommended for: Hospital, Academic Libraries

A Dictionary of Medical Derivations covers the use of the 500 Greek and Latin words, along with word parts that make up most medical terms in use today. The book aims to help students effectively develop a medical vocabulary by learning how medical words are formed from Latin and Greek roots. The contents are listed in alphabetic order, and each listing includes word derivation and a brief description of meaning. This book is useful for libraries serving medical students and other health care trainees.

Dictionary of Medical Syndromes. 4th ed. Authors: Sergio I. Magalini, Sabina C. Magalini. Lippincott Williams & Wilkins, 1997.
ISBN: 9780397584185
Recommended for: Hospital, Academic, Consumer Health Libraries
Brandon/Hill Selection

The *Dictionary of Medical Syndromes* presents brief details on known syndromes from every branch of medicine. Each syndrome entry begins with the patient's concern and then follows a common format: synonyms, symptoms and signs, etiology, pathology, diagnostic procedures, therapy, prognosis, and related references. The entries are drawn from many medical periodicals and textbooks. The book contains newly reported, specialized, and common syndromes. The dictionary includes a cross-referenced index of synonyms for each syndrome. While this book has not been updated recently, it is still a useful and easy-to-use resource for consumer health libraries as well as academic and hospital libraries serving students.

Dorland's Illustrated Medical Dictionary. 31st ed. Author: W.A. Newman Dorland. Saunders, 2007.
ISBN: 9781416023647 (Print + CD-ROM)
Recommended for: Hospital, Academic, Consumer Health Libraries
Brandon/Hill Selection

Considered a standard medical dictionary, *Dorland's Illustrated Medical Dictionary* includes more than 120,000 entries. In addition to medical terms, it includes information about drugs and complementary and alternative medicine concepts and treatments. More than 1,500 terms include illustrations that contribute to understanding. The accompanying CD-ROM includes a medical spell check that integrates into most word processing software and an audio pronunciation guide for 35,000 terms. All libraries supporting patients and families, students, and health care professionals will find *Dorland's* to be an important, easy-to-use tool.

Medical Meanings: A Glossary of Word Origins. 2nd ed. Author: William S. Haubrich. American College of Physicians, 2003.
ISBN: 9781930513495
Recommended for: Hospital, Academic Libraries

Medical Meanings is a revision of Haubrich's 1984 *Medical Meanings*, which was an update of Henry Alan Skinner's *Origin of Medical Terms*, first published in 1949. Each entry includes a brief description, usually tracing the term to the old English, Latin, or Greek root. *Medical Meanings* stands out from other terminology books because of its focus on history and etymology rather than clinical usage only. This is a valuable tool for academic and hospital libraries.

Medical Phrase Index: A Comprehensive Reference to the Terminology of Medicine. 5th ed. Authors: Jean A. Lorenzini, Laura L. Ley. Practice Management Information Corporation (PMIC), 2006.
ISBN: 9781570663994
Recommended for: Hospital, Academic Libraries

Medical Phrase Index is a reference tool designed for health care professionals, students, medical transcriptionists, court reporters, and management personnel. It includes more than 50,000 entries of medical phrases. The entries are cross indexed under each word in the phrase and include sound alike words and common abbreviations. The *Medical Phrase Index* is a valuable tool for hospital and academic libraries serving a variety of students and professionals who may need a reference with an emphasis on phrases.

Medical Terminology: A Short Course. 5th ed. Author: Davi-Ellen Chabner. Saunders Elsevier, 2009.
See Chapter 1. Allied Health

Miller-Keane Encyclopedia & Dictionary of Medicine, Nursing, & Allied Health. 7th ed. Editor: Marie T. O'Toole. Saunders, 2005.
ISBN: 9781416026044
Recommended for: Hospital, Academic Libraries

The portable *Miller-Keane Encyclopedia & Dictionary of Medicine, Nursing, & Allied Health* features comprehensive entries and printed thumb tabs. Organized by major terms with related terms as subentries, entries are included on diseases, disorders, or conditions. The entries provide a definition and an overview of the most important information related to symptoms, treatment, patient care, and prevention. The seventh edition includes a 32-page color atlas of human anatomy and an expanded eight-page color atlas of common disorders. With extensive coverage of nursing, medicine, and allied health, hospital and academic libraries will find this book to be useful for a wide variety of students and faculty.

Slee's Health Care Terms. 5th ed. Authors: Debora A. Slee, Vergil N. Slee, H. Joachim Schmidt. Jones & Bartlett, 2008.
See Chapter 6. Health Services Administration

Stedman's Medical Abbreviations, Acronyms & Symbols. 4th ed. Author: Thomas L. Stedman. Lippincott Williams & Wilkins, 2008.
ISBN: 9780781772617
Recommended for: Hospital, Academic Libraries

Stedman's Medical Abbreviations, Acronyms & Symbols provides access to over 75,000 abbreviations, acronyms, and symbols primarily for medical, health, and nursing professionals. The critical "Do Not Use" abbreviations indicated by the Institute for Safe Medication Practices (ISMP) are also included and highlighted for readers. The book provides specialty abbreviations from anatomy, physiology, internal medicine, pathology, laboratory medicine, organisms, infectious diseases, plastic surgery, ENT, dentistry, alternative medicine, and endocrinology. The appendix includes content organized by professional titles and degrees, professional associations and organizations, chemotherapy and other drug regimens, and clinical trials. This book is an important work for hospital and academic collections; it is relevant for students and professionals.

Stedman's Medical Dictionary. 28th ed. Author: Thomas L. Stedman. Lippincott Williams & Wilkins, 2006.
http://online.statref.com/
ISBN: 9780781733908
Recommended for: Hospital, Academic, Consumer Health Libraries
Brandon/Hill Selection

Stedman's Medical Dictionary currently includes 107,000 terms and definitions, including more than 5,000 new terms added in the latest edition. *Stedman's* also includes around 1,500 images. Additionally, the dictionary includes notes to alert readers about common errors, including confusion between words of similar form and meaning. The print purchase is accompanied by a CD-ROM with *Stedman's Plus Medical/Pharmaceutical Spellchecker 2005*, which has nearly a half million medical, pharmaceutical, and bio-science terms. The CD-ROM also includes medical clip-art images that can add educational content to print, slide, and digital products. *Stedman's* is an important resource for all health science libraries because of the wide scope and usefulness of its content.

Taber's Cyclopedic Medical Dictionary. 21st ed. Editor: Donald Venes. F.A. Davis, 2009.
See Chapter 1. Allied Health

34.4. Statistics

Contributor: Jonquil D. Feldman

Monographs

AAMC Data Book: Medical Schools and Teaching Hospitals by the Numbers. 2010 ed. (Published annually) Editors: Peter Vassev, Wendy Geraci. Association of American Medical Colleges (AAMC), 2010.
ISBN: 9781577540892
Recommended for: Hospital, Academic Libraries

This publication reports data from U.S. medical schools and teaching hospitals. The book provides data about students, graduates, faculty, teaching hospitals, tuition, hospital financing, and physician compensation. Student information includes tables on application and enrollment, race and ethnicity, and states of residence. The section on graduate medical education provides data from the National Resident Matching Program on matches for PGY1 (Post Graduate Year One), PGY2, fellowship programs, and foreign medical graduates. The book includes data on resident and fellow stipends and benefits, along with a table reflecting trends in stipends for one to six years post graduation, from academic year 1968–1969 to 2009–2010. Faculty statistics includes counts by degree, department, race, and ethnicity. Also included is data on compensation for faculty with MDs, by specialty. The hospitals section includes bed and utilization data plus financial data addressing expenses and revenues, which include third-party revenues. Trend tables provide a historic perspective of changes since 1966, which was the first year the AAMC began recording the information. This is an essential resource for medical school applicants and those researching residency and fellowship programs. This publication is a valuable addition to collections in medical school and hospital libraries.

AHA Hospital Statistics. 2011 ed. (Published annually) Editor: Health Forum/American Hospital Association. American Hospital Association, 2010.
ISBN: 9780872588707 (print only)
ISBN: 9780872588714 (print & CD-ROM)
See Also Chapter 7: Hospital Administration
Recommended for: Hospital, Academic Libraries
Brandon/Hill Selection

Based on the results of the American Hospital Association's Annual Survey of Hospitals, this comprehensive resource analyzes and compares health care industry trends in U.S. hospitals. The publication provides data on five-year trends in utilization, personnel, revenues, expenses, and community health indicators. It is divided into eight sections or "Tables," which provide data on utilization, personnel, and finances. Utilization comprises inpatient data, such as admissions and length of stay, and outpatient data, such as number of outpatient emergency visits or surgeries. Personnel data includes types of health care providers, such as physicians, residents, registered nurses, licensed practical nurses, and other salaried personnel. Financial data include gross revenues, net patient revenue, other operating revenue, and total expenses. A table on U.S. Census geographical divisions provides five-year trends on bed size, location, control such as state or non-profit, personnel, revenue and expenses, and expense per capita. These same categories of data are arranged by individual state in another table. Other tables include data on facilities such as adult or pediatric care, cardiac, obstetrics, or burn units and long-term care facilities. The data in this resource can be used to bench mark hospitals of similar size and location for analysis and comparison, or to pinpoint emerging trends. This publication is an important resource for academic health sciences, hospital, or public health libraries.

Physician Characteristics and Distribution in the U.S., 2011. 2011 ed. (Published annually) American Medical Association, 2010.
ISBN: 9781603592253
Recommended for: Hospital, Academic, Consumer Health Libraries

This is a compilation of statistical data about more than 972,000 U.S. physicians. The preface makes a case that the current and future supply of physicians has become a significant component in planning for the nation's health care needs. The detailed tables on professional characteristics of physicians can be used in health work force planning, policy development, and research studies. The book is divided into six chapters: "Physician Preface," "Physician Distribution," "Analysis of Professional Activity by Self-Designated Specialty and Geography Region," "Primary Care Specialties," "Osteopathic Physicians," and "Physician Trends." Cross-tabulations include data on age, sex, major professional activity, specialty, geographic distribution, and race and ethnicity. Information on primary care physicians includes variables of board certification, school, and year of graduation. The chapter on trends includes national trend data for Metropolitan Statistical Areas, female physicians, and internal medicine graduates. This publication is suitable for hospital and medical libraries and others that support researchers of health care issues, trends in physician supply, and the availability of physician services.

State Medical Licensure Requirements and Statistics. 2010 ed. (Published annually) American Medical Association, 2010.
ISBN: 9781603591089
Recommended for: Hospital, Academic Libraries
Brandon/Hill Selection

This annual publication from the American Medical Association presents up-to-date information on medical licensure requirements and statistics in the United States. The data is compiled from information received from primary sources including state boards of medical and osteopathic examiners. Tables include state-by-state licensing requirements, including examination and endorsement fees; licensure re-registration; continuing medical education requirements; examination pass/fail percentages; and details about available licenses (including inactive, retired, and camp licenses) and fees. Information is also included on medical licensing examinations, such as the United States Medical Licensing Examination (USMLE) and descriptions of organizations such as the National Board of Medical Examiners. The publication contains a section for international medical graduates provided by the Educational Commission for Foreign Medical Graduates. Licensure requirements in the Air Force, Army, and Navy are provided. The QuickConsult section includes information on medical licensure and medical education organizations; a glossary that defines key medical licensure terminology; and contact information for United States medical and osteopathic boards, including phone, fax, e-mail, and website. This is a valuable reference tool for physicians who are relocating and for medical school graduates conducting research on credentialing and the licensure process.

Statistical Abstract of the United States. 129th ed. U.S. Census Bureau, 2010.
http://www.census.gov/compendia/statab/2010edition.html
ISBN: 9780160838859
Recommended for: Hospital, Academic, Consumer Health Libraries

This 985-page publication is the authoritative source for United States statistical information. Published by the U.S. Census Bureau, this tool includes federal statistics as well as data compiled from private sources. The *Statistical Abstract* provides a summary of both primary and secondary statistical information on a vast variety of subjects: vital statistics; health insurance coverage and expenditures; the land area of each state; school enrollment and degrees earned; law enforcement measures; summary tables for federal, state, and local government elections; business and banking data; travel trends; gross domestic product and the consumer price index; and Internet access and use. Footnotes for each table provide information on sources of the data and a URL for online information. The Statistical Abstract is also available online at the U.S. Census Bureau as an interactive website. This important reference and research tool is an essential addition for all types of libraries.

Survey of Dental Education. 2008–09 ed. American Dental Education Association, 2010.
http://www.ada.org/1621.aspx
ISBN: 9781601220905 (5 volume set)
Recommended for: Academic Libraries

This is a comprehensive survey of dental schools and educational programs accredited by the Commission on Dental Accreditation. A series of five volumes summarizes general information, student and graduate data, curriculum, and financial management of dental schools in the United States. The first volume provides tables on academic programs and focuses on first-year enrollment, attrition rates, tuition, and fees. The second volume summarizes the costs of attending dental school for state residents and non-residents, admissions requirements, and attrition rates. Trends in dental and clinical science faculty and support personnel, including tenure status, race, ethnicity, age, and gender, are provided in the third volume. The fourth volume, which is published biennially, summarizes clock hours of instruction in biomedical sciences, dental/clinical sciences, and behavioral, information, social, and research sciences by curriculum type and major teaching area. The last volume provides financial information from accredited U.S. dental schools. Revenues and expenditures are provided by categories and in total, and for private and public schools. Ratios and expenditures per student are included. The set is available in print format, and PDF versions of each volume are available online. This is an important resource for students seeking admission to dental schools, for dental school administrators, and for others researching dental education.

World Health Statistics 2010. World Health Organization (WHO), 2010.
http://www.who.int/whosis/whostat/EN_WHS10_Full.pdf
ISBN: 9789241563987
Recommended for: Academic Libraries

The World Health Organization's annual *World Health Statistics* presents health-related data statistics reported by 193 member countries. According to the introduction, the data has been compiled using publications and databases produced and maintained by the technical programs and regional offices of WHO. The indicators provide a comprehensive summary of the current status of national health and health systems in the following nine areas: mortality and burden of disease; cause-specific mortality and morbidity; selected infectious diseases; health service coverage; risk factors; health workforce, infrastructure, and essential medicines; health expenditures; health inequities; and demographic and socioeconomic statistics. The first part summarizes the progress made toward achieving the health-related Millennium Development Goals and associated targets such as a reduction in child mortality rates and increase in health interventions (e.g., immunizations, with charts that illustrate the trends). The second part covers life expectancy and mortality rates, which provide measures of overall population health. Tables present data on morbidity and mortality, prevalence of selected infectious diseases, availability of health service coverage such as antenatal care, immunization coverage, contraceptive prevalence, and antiretroviral therapy coverage for HIV patients. Other tables include data related to population risk factors such as sources of drinking water, obesity rates, tobacco and alcohol use, and condom use. Data is also included on numbers per population for health workers, hospital beds, availability of essential medicines, and health expenditures related to Gross Domestic Product or per capita. Demographic and socioeconomic statistics help to complete the overall picture of inequities in health service coverage among populations with contrasting conditions such as rural versus urban groups or low-versus high-income countries. This is an important tool for public health students, researchers, and health care workers in community service programs.

Databases and Other Electronic Resources

Health, United States, 2009: With Special Feature on Medical Technology. U.S. Department of Health and Human Services, Centers for Disease Control and Prevention, National Center for Health Statistics, 2010.
http://www.cdc.gov/nchs/hus.htm
Recommended for: Hospital, Academic, Consumer Health Libraries

This annual publication presents national trends in health statistics, providing an overall picture of the health of the population of the United States. As explained in the Executive Summary, monitoring the health of the American people is an essential step in making sound health policy and setting research and program priorities. Through the Chartbook and tables, the publication presents trends in health status, including risk factors, and health care utilization by age, race and ethnicity, gender, education and income level, disability measurements, and geographic location. *Health, United States* includes data on health spending per capita and as a portion of the Gross Domestic Product; utilization of insurance such as Medicaid; and health insurance coverage. A section on medical technology provides data on utilization of laboratory tests, imaging and invasive technologies, trends in the use of pharmaceuticals, and costs associated with hospitalizations for technologically complex procedures. The online version of this publication presents interactive links from summaries to relevant tables, and, where possible, additional data years provide comparative information in the form of Excel spreadsheet files. This is an essential tool for public health researchers and others seeking background information to support medical research projects.

U.S. Census Bureau. U.S. Census Bureau, 1994.
http://www.census.gov
Recommended for: Hospital, Academic, Consumer Health Libraries

The U.S. Census Bureau collects and publishes population, housing, and economic data, as well as economic indicators. The data is used to determine political seats and funding allocation for public health, education, social, and infrastructure development programs. The Bureau provides an "age search" service to provide genealogy data that can be used for verification of Social Security and retirement benefits, passport applications, estate settlements, and genealogical research. The Publications tab on the Census.gov website provides a subject guide to censuses, surveys, and other programs. Links are provided to actual tables of census data. The website also offers free PDFs of publications that are typically held by most libraries, such as the *Statistical Abstract of the United States*, *County and City Data Book*, and the *State and Metropolitan Area Data Book*. This is an essential resource for all types of libraries.

34.5. Directories and Biographical Sources

Contributor: Jonquil D. Feldman

Monographs

ADEA Official Guide to Dental Schools. 2010 ed. (Published annually) American Dental Education Association, 2010.
ISBN: 9780982095157
Recommended for: Academic Libraries

This is an authoritative directory of dental schools in the United States and Canada. The book's first section, "Becoming a Dentist," describes the range of careers in dentistry, provides pointers on the academic preparation and requirements for admission, defines important factors in selecting the right dental school, explores financing options, and lists additional resources. The second section contains a list of dental schools, first arranged by state and then alphabetically by institution. Each entry includes general contact information, admissions requirements, deadlines, degrees granted, estimated costs, financial aid information, special programs and services, and websites for additional information. This is an important reference tool for students applying to dental school, advisors, and parents.

AHA Guide to the Health Care Field. 2011 ed. (Published annually) Editors: Health Forum/American Hospital Association. American Hospital Association, 2010.
ISBN: 9780872588677 (Print only)
ISBN: 9780872588684 (CD-ROM only)
ISBN: 9780872588691 (Print + CD-ROM)
See Also Chapter 7: Hospital Administration
Recommended for: Hospital, Academic, Consumer Health Libraries
Brandon/Hill Selection

This annual publication lists hospitals in the United States alphabetically by state. The directory includes AHA member and non-member hospitals. The book is divided into three sections. Section A lists hospitals by state and city, followed alphabetically by hospital name. The section includes an index of hospital names and an index of health care professionals and administrators. Section B provides a geographical list of health care systems, networks, and alliances. Section C lists national, international, and regional health organizations; United States government, state, and provincial agencies; and other health care providers. Entries include hospital address, telephone number, and chief administrator. Listings in sections A and B include coded information on the hospital's facilities, services, governing structure, staff size, accreditation status by the Joint Commission on Accreditation of Healthcare Organizations (JCAHO), and utilization data (number of admissions, beds, outpatient visits, and births). This publication is useful for hospital administrators and for those doing research on hospital administration. This is an essential resource in hospital and academic health libraries.

Directory of American Medical Education. 2010 ed. (Published annually) Association of American Medical Colleges (AAMC), 2010.
ISBN: 9781577540908
Recommended for: Academic Libraries

This publication contains alphabetical and geographical listings of medical schools that are members of the AAMC. Each school entry includes address, telephone number for the dean's office, website, enrollment data, type of school (private or public), a brief historical statement, total enrollment, and affiliated clinical facilities. Also included are names of university administrators such as the president, chancellor, and provost; names of deans and assistant deans at the medical schools; and names of chairs or section heads of divisions or research units. The index provides an alphabetical listing of the faculty. This work assists college students preparing to apply to medical schools and serves as a useful directory of medical school administrators and division chairs. This book is an essential reference for a medical school library.

Directory of Physicians in the United States. 41st ed. American Medical Association (AMA), 2009.
http://extapps.ama-assn.org/doctorfinder/home.jsp
ISBN: 9781603590099
Recommended for: Hospital, Academic, Consumer Health Libraries
Brandon/Hill Selection

This four-volume resource includes demographic and professional information on practicing physicians, residents, administrators, researchers, and retired physicians located in the United States and U.S. territories, including Puerto Rico, U.S. Virgin Islands, Guam, and Palau. The first volume contains an alphabetical index, and the remaining volumes provide geographical listings arranged alphabetically by state and city. Each physician entry contains information on specialties, type of practice, medical school attended, and certification. Listings include AMA members and non-members. The web-based directory, DoctorFinder, includes basic address, specialization, and certification information about member and non-member physicians in the United States and territories. This is an essential reference tool for all types of libraries that serve patients, health care personnel, hospital administrators, and others who are researching a physician's background.

Graduate Medical Education Directory. 2010–2011 ed. American Medical Association, 2010.
http://www.ama-assn.org/
ISBN: 9781603592215
Recommended for: Hospital, Academic Libraries
Brandon/Hill, *Doody's Core Titles* Selection

The directory lists U.S. and Canadian medical schools and graduate medical education programs with descriptions of over 8,700 programs accredited by the Accreditation Council for Graduate Medical Education (ACGME), as well as over 200 combined specialty programs. The first section provides descriptions of organizations involved in graduated medical education, including the ACGME, the National Resident Matching Program (NRMP), Electronic Residency Application Service (ERAS), and Educational Commission for Foreign Medical Graduates (ECFMG). The second section contains a list of specialty and sub-specialty programs for residents and fellows. Each specialty includes a professional description and details of sub-specialties, prerequisites, and data tables that include the number of programs, number of residents or fellows, average number of faculty, work schedules, educational setting, and benefits. Programs are then listed by state and alphabetically by institution. Each program entry includes the title of the program, institution name, program director, address and contact information, length of the program, number of positions available, and the 10-digit program ID. The third section identifies new and withdrawn programs, and the fourth section provides a list of hospitals and organizations that sponsor or participate in residency or fellowship training. The online version of this resource, FREIDA Online (Fellowship and Residency Electronic Interactive Databases), includes expanded listings for those programs that provide data. FREIDA is searchable by specialty, location, and optional criteria such as program size or setting. This is a valuable resource for medical students and residents who are researching postgraduate options. Additionally, state licensing boards, specialty societies, and hospitals use this directory to verify the authenticity of programs presented by physicians seeking to qualify for licensure, certification, or hospital privileges.

The Official ABMS Directory of Board Certified Medical Specialists. 43rd ed. Editor: American Board of Medical Specialties. Saunders/Elsevier, 2010.
http://www.boardcertifieddocs.com/
ISBN: 9781437767490
Recommended for: Hospital, Academic, Consumer Health Libraries
Brandon/Hill Selection

This directory, authorized by the medical specialty boards of the American Board of Medical Specialists, is published annually in multiple volumes. It provides specialty and education information for more than 729,000 physicians, including specialists in foreign countries who are certified by American boards. The listings are arranged by specialty, then by state and city, making it easy to identify specialists in a geographic region. Biographies include medical school and year of degree, place and date of internship and residency, fellowship, academic and hospital appointments, professional associations, type of medical practice, and specialty and board certification. The master index is arranged alphabetically by last name. The directory also provides current names and addresses for U.S. and Canadian medical schools, state licensing boards, and major national and international medical associations. This publication is an essential reference tool that should be in every health sciences library collection and all hospital and consumer health libraries. Purchasers of the print publication receive access to a companion website; however the website and the print publication do not contain the same information.

Databases and Other Electronic Resources

Find a Dentist. American Dental Association (ADA), 199?
http://www.ada.org/
Recommended for: Hospital, Academic, Consumer Health Libraries

This free online directory locates ADA members who are actively practicing dentistry. The print version ceased publication in 2001. Information seekers can search the directory for specific dentists by name or street address. Search variables can be combined; for example, one can retrieve all dentists in a specific specialty practicing in a particular city or within a ZIP Code area. The database also includes ADA member dentists practicing in other countries. Search results include full name, type of practice, street address, telephone number, and a link to an interactive map. This web-based directory is recommended for all libraries that serve the public, especially hospital and health sciences libraries supporting patient populations.

34.6. Grant Sources

Contributor: Katherine A. Prentice

Monographs

Annual Register of Grant Support 2011: A Directory of Funding Sources. 44th ed. Editor: Beverley McDonough. Information Today, 2010.
ISBN: 9781573873871
Recommended for: Hospital, Academic, Consumer Health Libraries

The *Annual Register of Grant Support* is a guide to more than 3,000 granting organizations. Organized by 11 subject areas and 61 specific subcategories, *Grant Support* is a complete resource for researching and locating grants. It includes traditional corporate, private, and public funding programs, as well as educational, association, and union sources. Details include eligibility requirements, procedures, deadlines, and contact information. Intended for a broad audience, this book is recommended for all health sciences libraries that support programs and research involving grants.

Directory of Biomedical and Health Care Grants 2010. 21st ed. Editor: Louis S. Schafer. Schoolhouse Partners, 2010.
ISBN: 9780984172542
Recommended for: Hospital, Academic Libraries

The most recent update of the *Directory of Biomedical and Health Care Grants* covers over 3,500 funding sources from all levels of government, corporations, and foundations. It includes grant titles, descriptions, requirements, deadlines, contact information, URL, sponsor details, and awarded grant samples. It also includes four index selections: subject, organization, program type, and geographic. The book is especially useful for first-time grant writers due to the inclusion of awarded grant samples. It is recommended for academic and hospital libraries that support education and research.

The Foundation Directory 2010. 32nd ed. Editor: David G. Jacobs. Foundation Center, 2010.
http://fconline.foundationcenter.org/
ISBN: 9781595423030
Recommended for: Hospital, Academic, Consumer Health Libraries

The Foundation Directory 2010 subscription-based site contains detailed information on the 10,000 largest foundations in the United States. Foundation details include fields of interest, contact information, financial information, names of decision makers, and 60,000 sample grants. Complete indexing of content is available to assist the search process. The online edition includes weekly updates of new and updated company data. The online edition also includes content from IRS Forms 990 and 990-PF as the IRS makes it available. This resource is relevant for most health science libraries because of the variety of funding resources included, which are applicable to wide audiences.

The Grants Register 2011: The Complete Guide to Postgraduate Funding Worldwide. 29th ed. Palgrave Macmillan, 2010.
ISBN: 9780230206014
Recommended for: Hospital, Academic Libraries

The Grants Register is a comprehensive guide to postgraduate grants and professional funding opportunities. Each entry is updated annually and verified by the organization providing the award. It includes information from over 1,100 awarding bodies on more than 4,200 awards. Relevant details include subject areas, level of study, eligibility, and value of awards. In addition, details of application procedures and closing dates are shown for each listing. The guide includes complete indexing by award and awarding organizations. This book is recommended for hospital and academic libraries that support postgraduate and professional students.

Databases and Other Electronic Resources

Canadian Institutes of Health Research (CIHR) / Instituts de recherche en santé du Canada (IRSC). Canadian Institutes of Health Research, 19??
http://www.cihr-irsc.gc.ca/
Recommended for: Academic Libraries

Available in both French and English languages, the Canadian Institutes of Health Research website provides information about a variety of funding opportunities for health research, such as activities focusing on biomedical, clinical, and health systems services or social, cultural, environmental, and population health. Persons and organizations affiliated with an eligible Canadian institution or organization are eligible for support. CIHR funding is relevant to libraries in Canada and those libraries collaborating with Canadian organizations.

Community of Science Funding Opportunities. ProQuest, 199?
http://fundingopps.cos.com/
Recommended for: Hospital, Academic Libraries

The Community of Science Funding Opportunities subscription-based database is a comprehensive source of funding information, including more than 400,000 funding opportunities. Content includes information from private foundations, public agencies, national and local governments, and corporations. Grants are included for life sciences as well as health and medicine. Available funding options support research, travel, curriculum development, fellowships, and postdoctoral positions. All records include title and description, deadlines, and requirements. Records also include a COS Keyword drawn from a controlled vocabulary that is applied consistently to all funding opportunities. Academic and hospital libraries that support research and educational programs will find this resource to be particularly relevant.

Grants.gov. U.S. Department of Health and Human Services, 2002.
http://www.grants.gov/
Recommended for: Hospital, Academic, Consumer Health Libraries

Grants.gov was created as part of the President's Management Agenda, which charged federal grant-making agencies with the development of a single online system to locate and apply for federal grants. Grants.gov includes information on over 1,000 grant programs and provides access to approximately 500 billion dollars annually in federal funding. Grants are offered from 26 federal agencies in 21 support categories. This resource is a highly recommended resource for all libraries because of the interest in federal grant support.

GrantsNet. American Association for the Advancement of Science, 2000.
http://sciencecareers.sciencemag.org/funding
Recommended for: Academic Libraries

GrantsNet is a free online resource collaboration from the journal *Science* and the American Association for the Advancement of Science (AAAS). It is intended to help students and researchers find funding for research and training. The site also includes the "Funding News Index" of announcements and deadlines, "International Grants and Fellowship Index," and GrantsNet Express e-mail alert. Advanced search capabilities include the ability to search by experience level, research field, and deadline. GrantsNet is a relevant tool for academic libraries because of its advanced search features and wide scope of content.

NIH Guide for Grants and Contracts. National Institutes of Health (NIH), 19??
http://grants.nih.gov/grants/guide/index.html
Recommended for: Academic Libraries

The NIH Guide, produced at the National Institutes of Health, Office of Extramural Research, provides information on funding opportunities through Funding Opportunity Announcements, Program Announcements, Request for Applications, and Request for Proposals. Also available are notices related to grant support of basic or clinical biomedical, behavioral, and bioengineering research. In addition to NIH funding, NIH contracting offices and other Department of Health and Human Services agencies announce opportunities in the NIH Guide. The NIH Guide serves as an announcement tool in lieu of *Federal Register* announcements. NIH Guide updates are published online daily and updated weekly on a listserv. The NIH Guide is recommended for libraries that support biomedical research, health education, and public health programs.

Index of Monographs

C

D

E

F

G

H

I

J

K

L

M

N

O

Q

R

S

T

U

V

W

Y

Z

Index of Journals

A

B

C

D

E

F

G

H

I

J

K

L

M

N

O

P

Index of Databases and Electronic Resources

N

O

P

R

S

T

U

V

W

About the Editors

Laurie L. Thompson, MLS, AHIP, has over 30 years experience in health sciences libraries, including 6 years at the National Library of Medicine; 11 years in administrative positions at the Himmelfarb Health Sciences Library, George Washington University (including a year as interim director); and 5 years as Director of Libraries at SUNY Upstate Medical University in Syracuse, New York. She was appointed Director of Libraries at UT Southwestern in April 2003 and was named Assistant Vice President for Library Services soon thereafter. Ms. Thompson is active in the Medical Library Association and served on its Board of Directors 2006–2010. She is also active in the South Central Chapter of the MLA and the Association of Academic Health Sciences Libraries, and serves on several boards of directors. She is Chair of the University of Texas System Advisory Committee on Library Affairs and was appointed to the advisory board of the state resource sharing consortium, TexShare. She is an evaluator for the Commission on Higher Education's Southern Association of Colleges and Schools (SACS). Ms. Thompson's publications include "Journal Collection Development: Challenges, Issues and Strategies," co-authored with Mori Lou Higa (Wood, *Introduction to Health Sciences Librarianship*, 2008), which won the 2008 Dan Richards Prize for outstanding writing in collection development, and *Bibliographic Management of Resources in Health Sciences Libraries* (*Current Practices in Health Sciences Librarianship,* v. 6, 2001). She has written several articles on the licensing of electronic resources and has developed and teaches a day-long seminar in negotiating licenses for electronic resources. She received her MLS from the University of Hawaii.

Mori Lou Higa, MLS, AHIP, is Manager, Collection Development, Library, University of Texas Southwestern Medical Center, Dallas, TX. She holds a MLS from San Jose State University. Mori Lou joined UT Southwestern Medical Center in 1993 as an Information Services Librarian. Since then, she has managed the new North Campus branch library, led the library's strategic planning activities, and established the library's first digital infrastructure department, leading implementation efforts for the library's first link resolver and federated search engine. Mori Lou presently manages the library's collection development activities and a staff of three. She has authored articles on various collection topics, the use of focus groups in the strategic planning process, and the redesign of a library's organizational structure. She has also served as a column editor for the *Journal of Electronic Resources in Medical Libraries* and peer reviewer for *Health Information and Libraries Journal.*

Esther Carrigan, MLS, AHIP, is Associate Dean and Director at the Texas A&M University Medical Sciences Library. She earned her MLS in Library and Information Science from the State University of New York at Buffalo. Ms. Carrigan has been on the faculty of the Medical Sciences Library at Texas A&M University, College Station, Texas, since 1983, holds the rank of professor and is a distinguished member of the Academy of Health Information Professionals. She has served on a number of committees and has had leadership roles within the Medical Library Association, its Veterinary Medical Libraries Section and South Central Chapter. Her research interests include veterinary grey literature, collection development, organizational culture, and the assessment of library services and collections. She has presented her research in these areas at many national and international meetings and has published on these subjects in numerous journal articles.

Rajia Tobia, AMLS, AHIP, is Executive Director of Libraries at The University of Texas Health Science Center at San Antonio, where she has held a number of positions in public and technical services, including Associate Library Director for Collection Development. She began her career as Serials Librarian and Medical Center Librarian at the University of South Alabama Biomedical Library in Mobile, Alabama. She is a Distinguished Member of the Academy of Health Information Professionals and has served on a number of committees within the Medical Library Association and its regional chapter. She is a member of the Editorial Board of the *Journal of Electronic Resources in Medical Libraries* and has contributed articles to a number of journals during her career in health sciences librarianship. Ms. Tobia has participated in developing and implementing several National Library of Medicine grants and contracts aimed at outreach to health professionals and public librarians in the south Texas region. She received a MLS from the University of Michigan.